Anxiety Disorders

Anxiety Disorders

Edited by

D.J. Nutt

DM FRCP FRCPsych F.Med.Sci
Psychopharmacology Unit
School of Medical Sciences
University of Bristol
Bristol, UK

J.C. Ballenger

MD
Department of Psychiatry and Behavioral Sciences
Medical University of South Carolina
Charleston SC, USA

Blackwell
Science

© 2003 by Blackwell Science Ltd
a Blackwell Publishing company
Blackwell Science, Inc., 350 Main Street, Malden, Massachusetts 02148–5018, USA
Blackwell Science Ltd, Osney Mead, Oxford OX2 0EL, UK
Blackwell Science Asia Pty Ltd, 550 Swanston Street, Carlton South, Victoria 3053, Australia
Blackwell Wissenschafts Verlag, Kurfürstendamm 57, 10707 Berlin, Germany

First published 2003

Library of Congress Cataloging-in-Publication Data
Anxiety disorders / edited by D.J. Nutt, J.C. Ballenger.
    p. ; cm.
Includes index.
  ISBN 0–632–05938–9
  1. Anxiety.
  [DNLM: 1. Anxiety Disorders. 2. Anxiety Disorders—drug therapy. WM 172 A63719 2002] I. Nutt, David J., 1951– II. Ballenger, James C.
RC531 .A6118 2002
616.85′223061—dc21
2002009821

A catalogue record for this title is available from the British Library

Set in 9/11½pt Sabon by Graphicraft Limited, Hong Kong
Printed and bound in Great Britain, at the Bath Press, Bath, UK

Commissioning Editor: Stuart Taylor
Editorial Assistant: Rupal Malde
Production Editor: Rebecca Huxley
Production Controller: Chris Downs

For further information on Blackwell Science, visit our website:
http://www.blackwellpublishing.com

Contents

Contributors

R. Amiaz
Department of Psychiatry
Sheba Medical Center
Israel

S.V. Argyropoulos
Psychopharmacology Unit
School of Medical science
University Walk
University of Bristol
Bristol, UK

J.C. Ballenger
Department of Psychiatry and Behavioral Sciences
Medical University of South Carolina
Charleston SC, USA

K. Beesdo
Institute of Clinical Psychology and Psychotherapy
Technical University of Dresden
München, Germany

M. Bourin
EA 3256 Neurobiologie de l'anxiété et de la
    dépression
Faculté de Médecine, BP 5350, 44035 Nantes
Cedex 1, France

J. Bradwejn
Department of Psychiatry
University of Ottawa
Ottawa, Ontario, Canada

O. Brawman-Mintzer
Department of Psychiatry and Behavioral Sciences
Medical University of South Carolina
Charleston SC, USA

S.P. Cahill
Department of Psychiatry
University of Pennsylvania
Philadelphia PA, USA

M. Chopra
Department of Psychiatry
Sheba Medical Center
Israel

A. Combs-Lane
Department of Behavioral Medicine and Psychiatry
West Virginia School of Medicine
West Virginia, USA

J.R.T. Davidson
Department of Psychiatry and Behavioral Sciences
Duke University Medical Center
Durham NC , USA

J.L. Davis
Department of Psychology
University of Tulsa,
Tulsa OK, USA

R.A. Emsley
Department of Psychiatry
University of Stellenbosch
Cape Town, South Africa

S.A. Falsetti
National Crime Victims Research and Treatment
    Center
Department of Psychiatry and Behavioral Sciences
Medical University of South Carolina
Charleston SC, USA

C. Faravelli
Department of Neurology and Psychiatry
University of Florence
Florence, Italy

E.B. Foa
Department of Psychiatry
Center for the Treatment and Study of Anxiety
University of Pennsylvania
Philadelphia PA, USA

S.J. Fredman
University of North Carolina at Chapel Hill
Chapel Hill NC, USA

J. Gorman
Department of Psychiatry
University of Columbia
New York NY, USA

B.D. Greenberg
Department of Psychiatry and Human Behavior
Brown University
Providence RI, USA

E. Griez
University of Maastricht
Department of Psychiatry and Neuropsychology
6200 MD Maastricht, The Netherlands

R. Gross-Isseroff
Outpatient Department and Department of Research
Geha Psychiatric Hospital
Petah Tiqva and Sackler Faculty of Medicine
Tel Aviv University
Tel Aviv, Israel

S. Gur
Outpatient Department
Geha Psychiatric Hospital
Petah Tiqva and Sackler Faculty of Medicine
Tel Aviv University
Tel Aviv, Israel

R.B. Hidalgo
Department of Psychiatry and Behavioral Sciences
Duke University
Durham NC, USA

D.R. Hirshfeld-Becker
Pediatric Psychopharmacology Unit
Massachusetts General Hospital
Department of Psychiatry
Harvard Medical School
Boston MA, USA

W. Katon
Department of Psychiatry and Behavioral Sciences
University of Washington School of Medicine
Seattle WA, USA

S. Khalid-Khan
Mood and Anxiety Disorders Section
Department of Psychiatry
University of Pennsylvania
Philadelphia PA, USA

D.F. Klein
Columbia University College of Physicians and
    Surgeons
New York NY, USA

D. Koszycki
Department of Psychiatry
University of Ottawa
Ottawa, Ontario, Canada

N. Laufer
Outpatient Department and Department of Research
Geha Psychiatric Hospital
Petah Tiqva and Sackler Faculty of Medicine
Tel Aviv University
Tel Aviv, Israel

Y. Lecrubier
Hôpital de la Salpétrière, INSERM Unité 302
Paris, France

K.P. Lesch
Department of Psychiatry and Psychotherapy
University of Würzburg
Füchsleinstr. 15
97080 Würzburg, Germany

A.L. Malizia
Psychopharmacology Unit
University of Bristol
University Walk
Bristol, UK

R.D. Marshall
Trauma Studies, Anxiety Disorders Clinic
Columbia University College of Physicians and
    Surgeons
New York NY, USA

T.A. Mellman
Dartmouth Medical School
Department of Psychiatry
Lebanon, New Hampshire, USA

J. Monnier
Department of Psychiatry and Behavioral Sciences
Medical University of South Carolina
Charleston SC, USA

N. Nakash
Department of Psychiatry
Sheba Medical Center
Israel

A. Nocon
Institute of Clinical Psychology and Psychotherapy
Technical University of Dresden and Max Planck
  Institute of Psychiatry
München, Germany

D.J. Nutt
Psychopharmacology Unit
University of Bristol
Bristol, UK

G. Perna
Anxiety Disorders Clinical and Research Unit
Vita-Salute University, San Raffaele Hospital
Milan, Italy

S.A.M. Rauch
Center for the Treatment and Study of Anxiety
Department of Psychiatry
University of Pennsylvania,
Philadelphia PA, USA

K. Rickels
Mood and Anxiety Disorders Section
Department of Psychiatry
University of Pennsylvania
Philadelphia PA, USA

J.F. Rosenbaum
Chief of Psychiatry
Massachusetts General Hospital
Department of Psychiatry
Harvard Medical School
Boston MA, USA

R. Rosenberg
Department of Biological Psychiatry
Institute for Basic Psychiatric Research

Psychiatric University Hospital in Aarhus
DK-8240 Risskov
Denmark

S. Rosi
Department of Neurology and Psychiatry
University of Florence
Florence, Italy

M. Rynn
Mood and Anxiety Disorders Section
Department of Psychiatry
University of Pennsylvania
Philadelphia PA, USA

Y. Sasson
Department of Psychiatry
Sheba Medical Center
Israel

T.E. Schlaepfer
Psychiatric Neuroimaging Group
University Hospital Bern
Switzerland
and
Division of Psychiatric Neuroimaging
Department of Psychiatry
The Johns Hopkins Hospital
Baltimore MD, USA

J. Shlik
Department of Psychiatry
University of Tartu
Tartu, Estonia

S.S. Sinha
Department of Psychiatry
Columbia University
New York NY, USA

J.W. Smoller
Psychiatric Genetics Program in Mood and Anxiety
  Disorders
Outpatient Psychiatry Division
Massachusetts General Hospital
Department of Psychiatry
Harvard Medical School
Boston MA, USA

D.J. Stein
Medical Research Council Unit for Anxiety and Stress
  Related Disorders
University of Stellenbosch, Cape Town and
University of Florida
Gainesville FL, USA

J. Swain
Department of Psychiatry
University of Ottawa
Ottawa, Ontario, Canada

P.L. du Toit
MRC Cognition and Brain Sciences Unit
15 Chaucer Road
Cambridge, UK

E. Truglia
Department of Neurology and Psychiatry
University of Florence
Florence, Italy

M.M.M.P. Van Moffaert
Department of Psychiatry, Psychosomatic Medicine
  and Psychodermatology
Ghent University
Gent, Belgium

A. Weizman
Department of Research
Geha Psychiatric Hospital
Petah Tiqva and Sackler Faculty of Medicine
Tel Aviv University
Tel Aviv, Israel

H.-U. Wittchen
Institute of Clinical Psychology and Psychotherapy
Technical University of Dresden and Max Planck
  Institute of Psychiatry
München, Germany

T.S. Zaubler
Department of Psychiatry
Morristown Memorial Hospital
Morristown
New Jersey Medical School
Newark, NJ, USA

J. Zohar
Department of Psychiatry
Sheba Medical Center
Israel

Preface

The 1990s are sometimes called the 'decade of anxiety', and it may be that we will consider the 21st century the 'century of stress and anxiety'. There are many reasons for the increasing importance of anxiety disorders in society and they reflect a growing understanding of the neurobiology of the different types of anxiety disorder, and evidence of effective treatment by drugs and psychotherapies. Moreover, the pace of modern life, and the pressures that many of us are under, act as major stressors, which in an unfortunate number of people result in subsequent anxiety disorders.

As the genome is being unravelled, genetic mechanisms which predispose to anxiety are beginning to be understood and, in the long term, may lead to new diagnostics and targeted treatment interventions. A great hope is that appropriate early diagnosis and intervention will minimize the burden of disability, which is found as an inevitable corollary of the anxiety disorders and secondary psychiatric illnesses, especially depression.

This book pulls together state-of-the-art knowledge of the various anxiety disorders, and most appropriate and effective interventions, both pharmacological and psychotherapeutic. Each chapter is written by an expert or experts in the field, and thus is a stand alone up-to-date assessment of the area. However, taken together, the 28 chapters that make up this book synthesize into something much greater than the sum of its parts. We hope that it will be a landmark publication and will be of use to all practising and research psychiatrists and psychologists. Our ambition is for it to stand as the keystone of a much larger building of subsequent publications that will promote the better understanding and treatment of the anxiety disorders.

D.J. Nutt & J.C. Ballenger
2002

PART ONE

Introduction

1

Conceptual Antecedents of the Anxiety Disorders

R.D. Marshall & D.F. Klein

Introduction

The history of the "anxiety disorders" as currently recognized in the Diagnostic Statistical Manual, fourth edition (DSM-IV: American Psychiatric Association [APA] 1994) and International Classification of Diseases, 10th edition (ICD-10: World Health Organization [WHO] 1993) can neither be told as the history of terminology, nor the history of official nomenclatures. It must be the history of the *phenomena*—as best we can ascertain them from historical documents. This is particularly important in anxiety disorders because the phenomena are nothing new, and have been described over many centuries. There is, however, marked variation in their context of description (e.g. medical, psychological, religious, anthropologic, or philosophical); their relative emphasis; the etiologic assumptions which often determined their classification; and the assumed implications for obtaining relief, whether medical, psychological, or metaphysical (Berrios 1999).

Before the 1860s "such symptoms could be found in clinical realms as disparate as cardiovascular, inner ear, gastrointestinal, or neurological medicine" (Berrios 1999, p. 263). In general, the literature often appears divided between descriptions of psychological experiences such as anxiety, anguish, worry, depersonalization, rumination, etc.; and somatic experiences such as pain, vertigo, palpitations, suffocating sensations, hot flashes, and so forth (Berrios 1996).

As in all medicine, early formulations of anxiety, fear, and anguish mixed unsystematic observations with etiologic speculation in ways that now appear fanciful. The limitations which doctrine can impose on observation was recognized by Thomas Sydenham (1624–89), who complained of the disease descriptions of his day:

> It generally happens that even where we find a *specific* distribution [of symptoms], it has been done in subservience to some favourite hypothesis which lies at the bottom of the true phenomena; so that the distinction has been adapted not to the nature of the complaint, but to the views of the author and the character of his philosophy (Sydenham 1848).

A reliable and at least partially valid nomenclature facilitates collaborative progress in any scientific community. This chapter discusses some of the major ideas and figures in the history of mental health particularly relevant to contemporary scientific practice. As a comprehensive historical review is not possible, this chapter first discusses major conceptual issues from early nosologic models of illness and disease. We then emphasize highlights of the last century.

It has been observed by many historians of medicine and psychology that a few fundamental conceptual principles have been operative over many centuries, and appear to alternate between prominence and marginalization based on the dominant conceptual models of the time and culture. An appreciation of the historical context from which contemporary views on anxiety states have emerged can enhance the contemporary scientific practice of questioning and testing assumptions, as well as perhaps help to avoid the "rediscovery" of approaches already tested and discarded by previous generations of thinkers in psychiatry and psychology.

Conceptual issues in medical and psychiatric nosology

Concepts of illness and disease

The history of anxiety nosology is inextricable from the longstanding debate over the philosophical and sociological meanings of illness and disease. Within psychiatry, the three related concepts of *disease*, *illness*, and *disorder* are especially relevant to developing neurobiological models. The term disease is clearly a heterogeneous concept in current usage. This is not necessarily a limitation, because the ultimate value of a diagnostic system lies in its clinical utility, not its conceptual consistency or parsimony. Medical diagnoses also do not follow consistent principles: conditions may be defined by structural pathology (e.g. ulcerative colitis), symptom presentation (e.g. migraine), deviance from a physiological norm (e.g. hypertension), and etiology (e.g. pneumococcal pneumonia) (APA 1994, p. xxi).

The concept of disease is notoriously difficult to define satisfactorily. Klein (1978) proposed that, in general, disease implies a dysfunction of one or more evolved (naturally selected) functions within an organism. Optimum functioning of the organism, which is the comparison for defining diseased or defective states, is arguably determinable by empirical and rational analysis. It should be noted that a condition in which evolved functions are impaired in the absence of physiologic defect can be theoretically envisioned. In some cases, significant maladaptive mental functioning might be induced by trauma through negative conditioning, while physiology remains normally intact. Biological investigation, however, is driven by the hypothesis that physiologic dysfunction is likely to exist in serious psychiatric disorders.

The related concept of *illness* implies the dysfunction has significant potential implications for health and well-being. Thus, deviations from a normative standard (e.g. unusual height) do not imply disease in the absence of dysfunction.

The involuntary nature of *illness* may be inferred from features such as marked inflexibility, resistance to self-instruction, and persistence of the condition in the face of obvious negative consequences (Klein 1978). The definition of illness is subject to value-laden considerations, since the allocation of the sick role is grounded in its special significance for human suffering, and in social circumstances. If something has gone wrong within the organism (as in *disease*), it permits the individual to claim the sick role, which distinguishes illness from simple deviance from the norm and ordinary human unhappiness. The fact that disease is involuntary leads to the exemptions from normal obligations that the sick role provides. When disease is hypothesized without objective, obvious pathology, the suspicion of exploitative malingering arises, which may incite much social friction.

The distinction between disease and illness is further clarified by examples. An individual can be diseased without having an illness (e.g. asymptomatic carcinoma); or feel unwell without having a disease (as in severe fatigue). The notion of disease, but not illness, can apply to plants, and illness is often anthropomorphically inferred in animals.

These concepts accrue additional complexity in the realm of mental health, as is reflected by the use of the ambiguous term *disorder* for psychiatric syndromes. In particular, the term avoids commitment to an etiologic model (given the present paucity of knowledge), and allows syndromes to be derived from clinical manifestations.

The concept of mental disorder

Syndromes are defined from frequently coexisting manifestations of illness in many individuals. The widely cited monograph of Robins and Guze (1970) identified five phases of investigation toward validation of a syndrome: clinical description, laboratory study, exclusion of other disorders, follow-up study, and family study. The DSM and ICD have been guided by the premise that the identification of well-defined syndromal patterns would best advance reliable communication and facilitate valid investigations of treatment and etiology. Thus, at present the working taxonomy of mental disorder relies on manifestations of illness, emphasizing the importance of a systematic conceptual approach to diagnosis.

Mental illness has often been construed as the subset of illnesses which present evidence primarily in the cognitive, behavioral, affective, or motivational aspects of organismal functioning. However, certain problematic counterexamples (e.g. trigeminal neuralgia which presents with only the psychological symptom of pain) led Wakefield (1992) to critique the logic of the DSM-III (APA 1987) definition of disorder. He proposed that the definition of mental disorder be strictly derived as the failure of specific mental functions, as proposed, among others, by Lewis (1953) and Klein (1978).

Since many symptomatic states do overlap with normal emotions, the definition of disorder should serve to distinguish between normative and pathological forms of anxiety. The presence of distress or impairment is necessary but not sufficient to the definition of disorder, since normal emotional processes (such as intense fear or grief) may result in both. To this end, DSM-IV states that disorder must not be merely an "expectable" response, and must represent "dysfunction", without precisely defining the latter term. The stipulation that a mental condition be an unexpected response to the environment, however, introduces an essentially statistical requirement, which Wakefield (1992) argues is logically problematic. For example, skull fracture is an expectable result of serious head injury, and yet is clearly considered an organismic dysfunction.

The requirement that disorder involve "harmful dysfunction" arguably solves this dilemma (Wakefield 1992) by dividing the concept into a component requiring an evaluative judgement ("harm"), and a component which can be empirically established ("dysfunction"). This definition of dysfunction includes the concept of "part-dysfunction", defined as a physiologic defect which may not necessarily manifest itself as illness (Klein 1978). The problem of defining natural psychological and behavioral functions remains; however, Wakefield (1992) argues it is best informed by considerations of evolutionary design. Lilienfeld and Marino (1995) have contested Wakefield's model with a number of counterexamples, proposing, among other ideas, that evolutionary design is of limited relevance to many recognized disorders since disorders may also represent failures of functions not subject to the process of natural selection. They conclude that "mental disorder is a Roschian concept characterized by intrinsically fuzzy boundaries" (Lilienfeld & Marino 1995, p. 411), such that evaluative judgements are unavoidable in defining disorder criteria. Further debate and clarification on fundamental nosologic issues is critical; an historical perspective on the anxiety disorders suggests that such models heavily influence clinical and research practice.

Since the point of origin of a clinical syndrome is involuntary individual distress and impairment, it does not necessarily follow that the existence of a syndrome implies an underlying pathophysiologic disease process.

There is growing scientific attention, for example, to the influence of environmental and cultural context on the manifestation of mental illness. Some instances of behavioral dysfunction may be viewed as a response to an abnormally stressful environment, or as the maintenance of a learned response (e.g. fear and avoidance) which is maladaptive in a new environment. In keeping with these concepts, Spitzer and Endicott (1978), while developing the DSM-III revisions, proposed that the concept of medical disorder implied "negative consequences of the condition, an inferred or identified organismic dysfunction, and an implicit call for action. There is no assumption that the organismic dysfunction or its negative consequences are of a physical nature" (Spitzer & Endicott 1978, p. 17). Hence disorder is more inclusive than disease (which implies dysfunction usually due to pathophysiologic process in our view) and illness (which implies the clinical manifestations of a disease) as commonly used.

Categorical and dimensional models of anxiety symptoms

The ages-old debate between the utility of categorical models versus that of dimensional models in the anxiety disorders, as well as throughout psychiatry, continues until the present day. In many instances, the argument can be shown to be a false dichotomy, and can be rejected in favor of a synthetic model that appreciates the strengths and limitations of each approach, as well as the methodologic procedures that bias such studies (Klein & Davis 1969). For example, mathematical models that seek to identify clusters within a data matrix have underlying assumptions that bias the results toward finding such patterns (Torgerson 1967). Similarly, procedures that seek to identify dimensional variables within a data set are intrinsically biased toward such findings, and are notably dependent on the particular procedure for construction of the dimension. Most importantly, uncritical acceptance of such findings without entertaining alternative explanations or placing the observations in clinical context can lead to premature closure of an important question and thereby obscure rather than elucidate conceptual debate.

For example, advances in biotechnology have greatly increased the capacity to study the influence of genetic factors in the anxiety disorders, and a flurry of new studies will likely become available in the next decade.

Family studies to date have generally supported the view that most of the current anxiety disorders breed true. However genetic influences may also be discovered that function as nonspecific vulnerability factors across some or all of the anxiety disorders. It has been argued that such a finding reduces the usefulness of separate categories and supports a return to the more nonspecific general neuroticism model of anxiety and perhaps depression (Andrews *et al.* 1990). This argument, however, is flawed in that it does not follow from either historical or clinical principles of disease classification. Clinical syndromes are based primarily on phenomenological presentation. These, in turn, engage a body of knowledge concerning etiology and, more importantly, treatment. By analogy, multiple disease syndromes may be observed in an individual who is immunocompromised through an inborn genetic defect. However, treatment will be based on the specific syndrome diagnosed (pneumonia, encephalitis, carcinoma, and so forth), as well as, perhaps, knowledge of the underlying genetic defect. Since it is known that treatment differs dramatically between the various anxiety disorders, knowledge of shared genetic vulnerabilities would have limited practical utility until therapeutic models can make use of such data.

The syndromal model in anxiety disorders has also been challenged as an error of reification, i.e. a fallacy of misattributed concreteness to an amorphous flux or dynamic process. Although it is true that the existence of a discrete syndrome does not necessarily imply a single discrete pathology, the categorical model has been remarkably fruitful and supported by differential treatment findings. Nonetheless, future research will surely benefit from avoiding the two extremes of reification and classificatory nihilism that have at times dominated psychiatry in the last century.

Historical review of classification systems

Postmodern perspectives on history and culture have heightened our awareness of assumptions and context when approaching historical material. This brief historical review explicitly proceeds on the premise that the current empirical approach in medicine has produced tremendous gains in our knowledge of therapeutics and will play an essential role in future pathophysiologic studies. We therefore emphasize events and concepts especially relevant to contemporary priorities.

Early models of disease and illness

Medicine originated in the attempt to cure illness (rather than understand disease), at a time when systems of philosophy, medicine and religion had common sources (Cohen 1961). Cohen has broadly grouped theories of disease into two categories: (i) disease as a distinct entity (an ontological definition); (ii) disease as significant deviation from the normal (a statistical definition). These categories remain relevant for contemporary neurobiological research, as it may be that models of anxiety disorders will require elements from both models.

The earliest models of disease were demonologic-based views in which all illness, both mental and physical, was attributed to supernatural influences. Given the absence of any knowledge of physiology, this represented an attempt to account for involuntary afflictions with no apparent cause. Cure was determined by identifying and then eradicating the cause, through exorcism, offerings, amulets, trephining, or other methods consistent with the disease model of the culture. Philosophers of science have noted the similarities between this view of invisible external agents that invade the body, and modern knowledge of viruses and bacteria.

Views of disease as deviation from the norm, however, have been more influential in Western medicine. The humoral theory of disease dominated medicine for more than 2000 years. It can be traced to the writings of Hippocrates (460–377 BC), who argued that mental illness was caused by the interaction of the brain's physical condition (degree of moistness) with bodily humors (Spring *et al.* 1991). The system was reinterpreted with a de-emphasis on biology by Aristotle (384–322 BC), and was developed into an ordered, rationalist system of thought by Plato (428–348 BC) (Cohen 1961). Health was defined as harmony between the four humors (blood, phlegm, yellow bile, black bile), and illness resulted from defects, excesses, or imbalances of the humors. A corollary of this view was that illnesses were as varied as individuals—a biographical approach which did not encourage a search for general patterns. Galen (143–200 AD.) later revived Hippocrates' interest in the brain as the source of mental illness, and refined the diagnostic system which attributed causality to specific humoral imbalances (e.g. mania due to an excess of yellow bile) (Spring *et al.* 1991).

In the dominant Platonic, rationalist view of the time, the physician proceeded from a dogma, which explained disease and determined the treatment. Aristotle's teachings, by contrast, emphasized observation of the natural world and critical examination of axioms upon which reasoning is based, and influenced a school of medicine called the Empiricists (Cohen 1961). With the skeptic's belief in suspending judgement (since the true nature of things was unknowable) they did not aim to reason out causes, but instead applied their efforts to observation, primarily of treatment outcomes. The syndrome concept has been traced to this school, which defined disease as "a union of symptoms which are observed always in the same way in the human body" (Cohen 1961, p. 214), although the syndrome model did not appear in general medical thinking until centuries later.

Emergence of empirical principles

Histories of medical classification over the last three centuries emphasize the gradual shift toward attentive observation among scientist physicians. Thomas Sydenham (1624–89) best typifies the principles of the 17th century, or the "Age of Reason," in medicine. He was the first to stress the importance of combining careful observation with a deliberate effort to avoid "every philosophical hypothesis whatsoever that has previously occupied the mind of the author" (Sydenham 1848). Moreover, his observation that the course of illness is particularly important to validating syndromes is a fundamental principle in modern psychiatric nosology.

Perhaps because medicine was dominated by dogma rooted in *a priori* theories of disease, the recognition of the relevance of physiology to medicine came relatively late in history. The movement most relevant to the eventual development of neurobiological research was the study of pathological anatomy. Although the practice of occasional autopsies to determine cause of death dates to the middle ages, a work by Morgagni (derived from work by Bonet) in 1761 spurred a new era by gathering hundreds of case histories with postmortem findings, from which he attempted to make systematic generalizations.

Over several decades, the lessons of pathological anatomy were slowly integrated into existing clinical traditions. This constituted a paradigm shift in clinical science, during which traditional, fundamental concepts about disease and treatment were critically re-examined. Foucault (1963) observed that the new emphasis on description as the starting point of medical investigation created a need for a new common language of descriptive rigor, precision, and regularity in its correspondence to what is observed. It should not be forgotten, however, that during this same period in Europe supernatural explanations for unusual behavior and inexplicable events were widely accepted. The last documented European execution of a witch dates to 1782 (Spring *et al.* 1991).

Nineteenth and early 20th century

Until the mid-19th century the signs and symptoms of the anxiety disorders were found scattered throughout the medical literature. Morel (1866) was the first to suggest that pathology in the autonomic nervous system might give rise to the disparate psychological and somatic symptoms of pathological anxiety (Berrios 1999). This observation was based on his theory that classification should be based on etiologic reasoning from theorized pathology in known physiologic systems (Morel 1860).

Emil Kraepelin (1856–1926), following Sydenham, emphasized the crucial role of both cross-sectional and longitudinal clinical observation (Klein 1978; Kraepelin 1902). Working within the German neurological tradition which viewed mental illness as brain disease, he advocated intensive behavioral analysis, and also incorporated available methods from experimental psychology (e.g. studies of reaction-time, fatigue, and cognitive functions) in pursuit of classificatory hypotheses (Blashfield 1984). His ideas were summarized in a series of psychiatric textbooks, the sixth edition of which (Kraepelin 1899) contained the famous distinction between dementia praecox (schizophrenia) and manic-depressive insanity. The diagnosis of manic-depressive insanity linked the two previously independent syndromes of depression and mania (Blashfield 1984).

Kraepelin clearly described and classified together aspects of most contemporary anxiety disorders in his sixth edition textbook (Kraepelin 1899, pp. 138–9). He described symptoms of generalized anxiety (pervasive apprehensiveness and worry), obsessions (intrusive fears of contamination), compulsions (hoarding), the link between anxiety-provoking obsessions and anxiety-reducing compulsive behaviors, phobias (fear of insects), agoraphobia (fear of being alone, crowds, and crossing open spaces alone), specific social phobia (inability to urinate or write a letter while being observed), and generalized social phobia (avoidance of most interpersonal interactions).

Bergonzoli (1915) comprehensively reviewed the many manifestations of the anxiety disorders. He noted that the phenomena were quite complex, involved both psychological and somatic manifestations, appeared in a number of different mental disorders, and therefore should not be clustered as a single entity. He believed they did not represent extremes of normal emotions, but rather derived from constitutional factors that could be discovered in the autonomic nervous system and brain stem (Berrios 1999).

Psychoanalytic models of anxiety

Freud extensively developed the view that manifold phenomena could be explained through unitary etiologic constructs. Freud's classic paper of 1894 (Freud 1953) outlined the view of the psychoneuroses that would persist for many decades afterward. Concepts of anxiety were central to early psychoanalytic formulations, and took different forms through Freud's developing models. His earliest theory construed severe anxiety states and panic as the consequence of thwarted biological sexual drives. Hysteria (which included conversion, anxiety, and phobic symptoms) was viewed as a defense against becoming conscious of traumatic sexual memories. In Freud's later theories, anxiety became the signal of repressed unconscious sexual and aggressive infantile impulses whose threatened expression reinvoked infantile terrors within the adult. Infantile dangers derived from fears which were central to each developmental phase, such as loss of a necessary caretaker, castration, or punishment (Glick 1995). The detection of internal and external threats released anxiety, which in turn might promote an effective response (in normal anxiety), or a repressive response.

Much debate has surrounded the therapeutic mechanisms of psychodynamic therapy. Freud's later view was that psychoanalytic treatment heightened patients' awareness of these internal processes and thereby freed them from residual developmental influences. Clinical symptoms signified the failure of universal mechanisms; thus the symptom presentation was relatively unimportant, as the treatment recommendation was always the same.

In the later pluralistic environment, which began to emerge as Freud's followers developed alternative theoretical perspectives, the meaning of anxiety was given many interpretations. Anxiety may signify a real or a fantasized threat to the security and integrity of the self, the world view, or important interpersonal connections (Glick 1995). Most recently, efforts have been made to account for the distinction between normal human anxiety and pathological anxiety due to biological dysregulation. In this view, intrapsychic problems reflected in object relations, conflict, and distorted views of self and others are heavily influenced by attempts to cope with the disorganizing effects of a biologically driven disorder (Cooper 1985). In general, however, psychoanalytic theory presumes universal mechanisms for generating anxiety, and thus contributes minimally to nosology.

Adolf Meyer (1866–1950), one of the most influential psychiatrists in the early 20th century, began his career as a pathologist, and initially was an outspoken advocate of Kraepelin's ideas. Over the course of his celebrated chairmanship at Johns Hopkins University (1910–41) where he developed the psychobiological perspective, he became increasingly skeptical of classification and came to view it as reductionist. Integrating psychoanalytic, social, familial, and biologic theories, his view of psychiatric disorders as "reaction sets" influenced early DSM terminology (Blashfield 1984).

Laboratory studies of stress physiology

Early 19th century physiologists studied the relationship between fear and anxiety states and somatic functions. This represented a development of Renaissance interactionist ideas most widely associated with the deductive rationalist philosophies of Descartes and Hobbes. Relying primarily on syllogistic reasoning, Descartes (1596–1650), despite his absolute theoretical separation of soul from body, proposed a mechanistic model of the body which directly linked physiology and consciousness. Hobbes (1588–1679) emphasized the role of external stimuli and bodily sensations in generating the content of consciousness. In the 18th century, James Mill proposed an interactive relationship between emotions and physiologic states, in which sensations within the body (such as gastrointestinal contractions) could both give rise to anxiety, and be caused by it (Moehle & Levitt 1991).

A more unidirectional model rose to prominence in the 19th century, however, called the James–Lange theory of emotion. William James and Carl Lange independently proposed the view that emotions resulted from conscious awareness of somatic events, as opposed to being independent, meaningful responses to the environment. The implication was that anxiety responses were innate rather than learned, being the result of nonconscious, reflexive physiologic processes. The theory was later refuted by Walter B. Cannon (1871–1945) in a series of empirical tests of the James–Lange hypothesis, and replaced by Cannon's new emphasis on the thalamus as the originator of both emotion and its physiologic concomitants (Moehle & Levitt 1991).

Cannon devoted his career to the study of physiologic changes in animals under stress, which he elaborated into the "emergency theory" explaining the emotions of rage and fear. In 1929, he proposed a comprehensive model with several components: (i) epinephrine (adrenaline) was released as an adaptive component of the stress response, which also included the release of glucose, slowing of the gastrointestinal system, heightened energy and muscular tension, increased rapidity of coagulation, and orienting, vigilant behavior; (ii) the emotions of fear and rage were intimately associated with these physiologic events; (iii) this response was best understood as evolved to prepare for flight or attack (Cannon 1929). Darwin's emphasis on evolutionary explanations, rooted in mechanisms that promote adaptability and survival, figures prominently in Cannon's work. The idea that the functional significance of physiologic processes can be viewed in evolutionary terms is usually considered Cannon's major contribution. Furthermore, he compiled evidence from experimental, clinical, and pharmacologic observations to propose that the thalamus was the primary source of both emotion and visceral response. In his model, when a stimulus is registered, impulses travel either to the cortex, which then interprets and relays the signal, or directly to the thalamus. The net effect is the release of thalamic activity along pathways which innervate muscles and viscera as well as the cortex, resulting in experienced emotion (Cannon 1929, p. 369).

Learning theory

Pavlov believed conditioning could provide a physiologic explanation for the development of psychiatric symptoms. For example, he drew parallels between the "stereotypy, iteration, and perseveration" in his conditioned animals and compulsive neurosis (Pitman 1994, p. 8). In addition to conditioning mechanisms, Pavlov also posited an interaction between inherited temperament and learning based on the wide range of responses he observed in the same species of animals when exposed to identical stressors. Many authors since Pavlov have elaborated the conditioning model to explain both normal and pathological anxiety states, as well as to develop therapies. John B. Watson (1879–1952), considered the father of American behaviorism, believed human anxiety and fear were largely explainable as conditioned responses, but neglected Pavlov's earlier ideas on the influence of constitutional factors.

By the 1950s, common features between clinical anxiety symptoms and experimentally induced "neuroses" in chronically stressed animals had been widely appreciated, including (i) the induction of anxiety states by environmental experience; (ii) the tenacity of such responses in a variable reinforcement condition; (iii) the global responses of an organism to chronic inescapable stress (Liddell 1952).

Experimentally induced symptomatology in humans

A third body of research contributing to a neurobiological model of anxiety involved the study of experimentally induced psychiatric symptoms in human volunteers. During World War II the US government sponsored the Minnesota Experiment, a research program of controlled starvation of 36 male volunteer conscientious objectors over several months, followed by controlled nutritional rehabilitation. During the starvation phase, significant behavioral and psychological symptoms were observed in subjects, including depression, irritability, apathy, and erratic behavior. Most importantly, researchers found marked elevation of MMPI scores in the "neurosis triad" of hysteria, depression, and hypochondriasis. The scores and psychiatric symptoms normalized after nutritional balance was restored (Keys 1952). This finding was interpreted as evidence of the influence of physiology on producing psychological symptoms, although it seems likely in retrospect that environmental factors might also have been influential.

The discovery of lysergic acid diethylamide (LSD) also influenced etiologic concepts of mental illness, since for the first time symptoms similar to psychosis could be induced with a pharmacologic substance. It seemed more plausible therefore that neurotransmitter dysregulation might be implicated in psychological phenomena.

Integrating laboratory findings with clinical models

Laboratory models of anxiety had a minimal impact on clinical reasoning until Mowrer's classic paper (1939), credited as the first sophisticated attempt to introduce findings from experimental psychology into the predominantly Freudian clinical model of anxiety (from Moehle & Levitt 1991). Mowrer's major contribution was the use of learning theory to explain the development and maintenance of anxiety and avoidance behavior. Mowrer proposed that anxiety was learned, functioned as motivation, and operated to reinforce habits and associations by its reduction. These are now widely accepted concepts. Eysenck (1955) incorporated constitutional factors into a learning theory model of anxiety. His view was that the intrinsic lability and reactivity of the autonomic nervous system determined the range and intensity of anxiety responses, which in turn formed the basis of conditioning. During this same period, effective pharmacologic treatments created renewed clinical interest in the study of pathophysiology (see below).

Standardized classification systems of the 20th century (ICD and DSM)

DSM-I

> In writing the history of a disease, every philosophical hypothesis whatsoever, that has previously occupied the mind of the author, should lie in abeyance. This being done, the clear and natural phenomena of the disease should be noted—these, and these only. They should be noted accurately, and in all their minuteness; in imitation of the exquisite industry of those painters who represent in their portraits the smallest moles and the faintest spots (Sydenham 1848, preface).

The existence of a number of competing classification systems in the 19th and early 20th centuries impeded communication among clinicians and scientists, prevented the accumulation of a consistent body of reference literature, and greatly limited generalizability of pathophysiologic studies. Furthermore, empirical methods could not be applied to questions of nosology without a standardized classification from which to work. A plan for diagnostic uniformity in psychiatry was formulated as early as 1917, and the first official nomenclature, largely based on Kraepelin's work, was

published in 1934. The system was primarily for purposes of statistical classification in hospitals, however, and was never widely popularized (Blashfield 1984). In the late 1940s, growing international recognition of the need for scientific consensus on the terminology of mental illness—spurred by the creation of the National Institute of Mental Health in 1946—culminated in a project to develop an improved diagnostic system. The WHO published ICD-6 (WHO 1948) in the same time period, adding for the first time a section for mental disorders.

In DSM-I (APA 1952), the neurobiological consequences of overt brain disease were recognized as "disorders caused by or associated with impairment of brain tissue function" such as intoxication, infection, neurological trauma, and congenital disease. The anxiety disorders fell under the rubric of "disorders of psychogenic origin or without clearly defined physical cause or structural change in the brain" (APA 1952, p. 5). The following syndromes were designated as "psychoneurotic disorders": anxiety reaction, dissociative reaction, conversion reaction, phobic reaction, obsessive compulsive reaction, and depressive reaction. The syndromes were essentially prototypal narrative descriptions without clear boundaries or criteria.

Consistent with prevailing psychodynamic and Darwinian ideas, anxiety disorders were viewed as a "danger signal felt and perceived by the conscious portion of the personality" (APA 1952, p. 31). Emotional conflict generated by personality structure was the presumed primary etiology for all disorders. Overt symptoms were seen as shaped by defense mechanisms—hence the term "reaction" throughout DSM-I. Thus, anxiety disorders were located within a normative, dimensional model of anxiety, with an implied clinical emphasis on personality dynamics and the psychological meaning of anxiety over physiologic processes.

DSM-II

The second revision of DSM (DSM-II) published in 1968 (APA 1968) was similarly based more on committee consensus than scientific review, and was coordinated with the development of ICD-9 (WHO 1978). Lacking knowledge of etiology, DSM-II attempted "to provide a middle ground to satisfy the needs of psychiatrists of different schools of theoretical orientation" (APA 1968, p. XV). After a series of consultations with clinicians and experts, an APA committee reviewed and approved the new version. The process of development of DSM-II therefore emphasized the communicative function of a classification system, while relatively neglecting issues of reliability and validity.

In DSM-II, the relative emphasis on clinical description continued, but definitions still presented theoretical assumptions about etiology as factual. For example, phobias were "generally attributed to fears displaced to the phobic object or situation from some other object of which the patient is unaware" (APA 1968, p. 40). Panic attacks were recognized but remained within the category "anxiety neurosis." The other anxiety syndromes presented in DSM-II were obsessive-compulsive, depressive, dissociative, hysterical, phobic, neurasthenic, depersonalization, and hypochondriacal disorders.

Panic disorder and the discovery of effective pharmacotherapy

Perhaps the most important factor in stimulating nosologic progress in modern psychiatry was the serendipitous discovery of effective medications for severe mental illness such as lithium for manic-depressive illness (1949), followed by chlorpromazine for schizophrenia (1952), and later imipramine for depression and benzodiazepines for anxiety (chlordiazepoxide in 1960). The specific patterns of effectiveness of these drugs further validated the basic Kraepelinian approach to nosology, and allowed the creation of the first powerful biologically based method for refining nosology—pharmacologic dissection (Klein 1987).

In the 1950s, emotional conflict, and therefore anxiety, was assumed to be etiologic in not only the anxiety disorders, but in all mental illness. The result was a prevailing nosologic nihilism and relative dismissal of descriptive diagnosis. Not surprisingly, a number of studies found poor diagnostic agreement among clinicians due to inconsistencies in how observed phenomena were categorized. Hospitalized patients in the US with severe anxiety and agoraphobia were often diagnosed as schizophrenic, and clinical formulations emphasized prominent personality features and unconscious motivations. When preliminary clinical trials were conducted with the new medications, however, patients with psychotic symptoms improved on chlorpromazine, whereas patients with agoraphobia did not. Patients with agoraphobia did improve on imipramine, however, primarily due to the ablation of spontaneous

and situationally predisposed panic attacks (Klein & Fink 1962; Klein 1964).

Thus, the new drugs allowed pharmacologic dissection of distinct clinical syndromes within a heterogeneous population. The discovery of imipramine's effectiveness for the spontaneous panic attack itself, separate from generalized and anticipatory anxiety, was also important evidence that heterogeneous mechanisms for clinical anxiety might exist, further supporting a syndromal taxonomic approach to mental illness (Klein 1989).

The discovery of benzodiazepines also led to methodologic progress in neurobiological research by stimulating the development of animal models of anxiety. With respect to nosology, however, their *trans*diagnostic benefits appeared consonant with a continuum model of anxiety, or perhaps with the existence of a final common pathway. This also highlights the limitations of drawing taxonomic conclusions based solely on pharmacologic response. In other words, more valid conclusions can be drawn from pharmacologic dissection than pharmacologic amalgamation (Klein 1989).

DSM-III and the dissolution of the pyschoneuroses

> Our belief in any particular natural law cannot have a safer basis than our unsuccessful critical attempts to refute it (Popper 1963).

In their textbook *Diagnosis & Drug Treatment of Psychiatric Disorders* (Klein & Davis 1969), Klein and Davis reaffirmed the utility of descriptive diagnosis as a guide to proper treatment, while developing several new diagnostic categories. For DSM-III (APA 1980), there was better appreciation of the fundamental properties of classificatory systems, such as the constraints which reliability impose upon validity. Empirical evidence was available for the first time that could explicitly address nosologic issues such as syndromal coherence and discriminability (Spitzer & Fliess 1974). The existing nosology was in fact found to possess poor interrater reliability (Spitzer & Fleiss 1974). Two especially influential publications were Feighner *et al.*'s (1972) proposal of explicit criteria for 14 syndromes based on existing evidence (rather than committee consensus), and Spitzer *et al.*'s *Research Diagnostic Criteria* (1975) which served as a template for the DSM-III. The priorities of improving reliability and internal consistency are observable throughout DSM-III.

By this time well-developed, competing theoretical models of anxiety were in existence, and there was heightened appreciation of the paucity of available data which might inform diagnostic development. An attempt was made therefore to formulate disorders in neutral language with respect to etiology, in the tradition of Sydenham. When it was decided that both inclusion and exclusion criteria would be required for a syndrome definition, it became apparent the "psychoneuroses" as a group had no inclusion criteria. Their only commonality was an unsubstantiated etiological theory. Thus, the dissolution of the overall rubric of neurosis in DSM-III was the natural outcome of demanding descriptive inclusion/exclusion criteria that were not dependent upon theories of causation or inferred processes.

In addition, the multiaxial system was introduced in DSM-III, following the Meyerian tradition of comprehensive evaluation. It is worth noting that the DSM-III did not attempt, as has sometimes been claimed by critics, to be "atheoretical" in the broadest sense. It was explicitly based on the beliefs that empirical principles should take priority, and that achieving reliability and discriminant validity was important to progress (APA 1980, pp. 6–7).

Major features of the anxiety disorders section of DSM-III derived from newly available evidence from pharmacologic studies. In particular, the association between agoraphobia and panic attacks was recognized, and the symptom presentation redefined as a fear of "being alone or in public places from which escape might be difficult or help not available in case of sudden incapacitation, e.g. crowds, tunnels, bridges, public transportation" (APA 1974, p. 227). Panic disorder, generalized anxiety disorder, social phobia, and post-traumatic stress disorder were proposed as new diagnoses. New phenomenologic groups for somatoform, dissociative, psychosexual, and impulse control disorders were also created out of symptom clusters previously included in the single group of anxiety neuroses.

Increased awareness of the importance of the above issues seemed to accelerate the process of refinement and revision, culminating in the issue of DSM-III-R in 1987 (APA 1987), and DSM-IV in 1994 (APA 1994).

DSM-IV

For DSM-IV, persuasive empirical evidence was explicitly required to make further changes in diagnostic criteria. The availability of nosologically relevant data had increased dramatically during this period. DSM-IV diagnostic criteria are discussed at length elsewhere in this volume.

Individual DSM-IV disorders

Panic disorder

A number of medical scholars in the 18th and 19th centuries described paroxysmal attacks of overwhelming anxiety with dyspnea, vertigo, sweating, and palpitations, and often accompanied by dramatic avoidance and incapacitation (Berrios 1999). Often the term *anguish* (or its French or German equivalents) was used to differentiate these phenomena from general anxiety. Because of prominent dizziness and vertigo-like symptoms, frequently the cause was attributed to dysfunction of the inner ear. Following earlier Continental European writers, Freud made the observation in 1895: "In the case of agoraphobia, etc., we often find the recollection of a state of *panic*; and what the patient actually fears is a repetition of such an attack under those special conditions in which he believes he cannot escape it" (Freud 1895, p. 136). Freud (1926) eventually, however, proposed that the agoraphobic patient's avoidance served to prevent "the danger of giving way to his erotic desires". One of Kraepelin's lectures entitled "Irrepressible ideas and irresistible fears" contains a clear description of spontaneous panic attacks accompanied by fears of dying, morbid somatic preoccupations, and classic agoraphobia (Kraepelin 1904, pp. 262–4). Kraepelin essentially advocated exposure therapy (although with pessimistic expections) and cautioned against lengthy hospitalization in such cases.

The observation that imipramine was effective for panic attacks led Klein and Fink to take detailed histories and similarly observe that spontaneous panic attacks regularly anteceded agoraphobia. The history of panic disorder research is illustrative as a model integration of neurobiology and nosology (Klein & Klein 1989). Pharmacologic findings (imipramine response) led to creation of a new category (panic disorder), a redefinition of the concept of agoraphobia (from fear of open spaces, to fear of being away from home or otherwise in circumstances in which escape or getting help is limited), and ultimately new courses of rational neurobiological investigation into etiology (see Chapter 3).

A number of clinical and laboratory findings converge upon the conclusion that spontaneous panic attacks do not represent a sudden surge of normal anxiety, including the initial observation that imipramine was effective for panic attacks but relatively ineffective for anticipatory anxiety. Surprisingly, there is no sudden surge of hypothalamic–pituitary–adrenal (HPA) axis activation during a panic attack. Instead, there appears to be a moderate prepanic increase in cortisol, and subtle alterations in HPA axis activity which may correlate with severity of anticipatory anxiety, avoidance, and general illness severity (Abelson & Curtis 1996). Finally, the prominent symptom of dyspnea distinguishes the panic attack from normal fear. Instead, the panic attack may represent a suffocation false alarm related to dysregulation of a functional, respiratory-linked, behavioral regulatory system (Klein 1994). Alternatively, there may be a respiratory-dysfunction subtype of panic disorder characterized by prominent dyspnea, which might eventually prove relevant to future diagnostic revisions. Cognitive-behavioral views of the nature of panic disorder involve the anxiogenic effects of catastrophic misinterpretation of physiologic sensations, and have been discussed and reviewed elsewhere (Panzarella 1995; Antony & Barlow 1996). Conceptual efforts at integrating biological and cognitive behavioral models are consistent with Klein and Davis' early observations (1969) that spontaneous panic attacks appear distinct from accompanying generalized anxiety.

Social phobia

Kraepelin (1899) described the symptoms of both circumscribed and generalized social phobia. He noted that some patients experienced "overpowering feelings of aversion when they have to establish relations of any kind with other persons," whereas other individuals, who appeared otherwise healthy, were "unable to urinate or write a letter in the presence of other people" (Kraepelin 1904, p. 139).

Berrios notes that two books on social phobias (using the term "timidity") appeared at the turn of the century. The more important was by Hartenberg (1901) and presented a complete description with etiologic hypotheses. He theorized that it resulted from excessive fear, shame, and embarrassment in social situations; that it could cause serious social impairment; that it had multiple causes including environmental, dispositional, and hereditary factors; that it varied in a dimension from normal shyness to severe generalized fears; and that the best treatment was support with behavioral therapies (Berrios 1999).

Social phobia was also well-described by Isaac Marks (1969). Its recognition in DSM-III reflected early impressions that (i) most patients had only one social fear limited to a specific social situation, and (ii) social phobia should be meaningfully distinguished from avoidant personality disorder. The observation that pharmacotherapy might be effective for social phobia (Liebowitz et al. 1985) stimulated a proliferation of descriptive and treatment studies. As a result, the diagnosis was further refined in DSM-III-R to allow for a continuum of social fears and create the generalized subtype designation. Evidence that pharmacologic response was not influenced by the presence of comorbid avoidant personality disorder influenced the decision to allow making both diagnoses concurrently in DSM-III-R. The arbitrary distinction between severe generalized social phobia and avoidant personality disorder may represent a false dichotomy that is more reflective of historical precedent in the field than actual phenomenology.

As noted in DSM-IV, individuals with both panic attacks and social avoidance can sometimes pose a diagnostic problem. Individuals with social phobia may panic in their feared situations, although they generally do not develop dyspnea or fear they are going to die, nor do they experience nocturnal or spontaneous panic attacks. Many individuals with panic disorder fear being judged and humiliated if they panic in public, but will also report a history of unexpected panic attacks. Pathophysiologic studies support the current view that panic disorder and social phobia are distinct syndromes. Compared to individuals with social phobia, panic patients are significantly more likely to panic with lactate infusion. Panic patients also may respond better to tricyclic antidepressants (Klein 1996) than those with social phobia, although both respond to monoamine oxidase inhibitors (MAOIs).

In addition to studies of the clinical condition, a functional analysis of the social phobic syndrome suggests that future study of the neurophysiology of traits related to interpersonal sensitivity and attachment might be fruitful. In particular, functional systems that regulate social dominance and submission in a social hierarchy have been implicated in primate studies, and corroborative evidence in human studies of the D2 receptor has recently been discovered (Grant et al. 1998; Schneier et al. 2000).

Although individuals with a single circumscribed phobia are grouped within the same diagnosis as those with longstanding, pervasive social avoidance and impairment, it is possible these will emerge as pathophysiologically distinct conditions.

Obsessive-compulsive disorder

Descriptions of the phenomena of obsessions and compulsions can be found in historical documents over the past several centuries. Pitman (1994) provides several instances, which also illustrate the conceptual framework with which the symptoms were understood. A passage from the *Malleus Maleficarum* (the 15th century compendium of witchcraft and psychopathology) describes a priest brought to Rome for exorcism:

> When he passed any church, and genuflected in honour of the Glorious virgin, the devil made him thrust his tongue far out of this mouth when [he] tried to engage in prayer, [the devil] attacked him more violently (Pitman 1994, p. 3).

Although psychological symptoms have often been given metaphysical explanations, Pitman points out that common obsessional themes of guilt, doubt, doing harm, and determining right from wrong, made the phenomena even more convincing as a moral problem. Those with obsessional thoughts seemed "besieged" by the Devil, in contrast to psychotic individuals who appeared fully possessed.

The neurologist Carl Westphal in 1878 distinguished obsessions from depressive symptoms:

> Against the will of the person concerned, [the thoughts] come into the foreground of the consciousness. They cannot be dispelled, they hinder and frustrate the normal course of ideas, although the afflicted always recognizes them as abnormal and alien. Most of the time, [they are] absurd, and have no demonstrable connection with previous ideas, but rather [seem] even to the patient himself incomprehensible and appearing out of thin air (Pitman 1994, p. 6).

However, obsessions and compulsions were viewed as separate phenomena until the last few decades. Westphal's early observation of an association between obsessions, tic disorders and epilepsy presaged recent neuroanatomical and neurobiological findings in obsessive-compulsive disorder (OCD) (Insel 1992; Pitman 1994; see Chapter 6).

Although neurobiological hypotheses regarding obsessions and compulsions had been proposed, the discovery (1967) and confirmation of clomipramine's effectiveness initiated a new era of study, and, in particular, a focus on serotonergic mechanisms (Montgomery 1994). The pharmacologic finding that serotonergic agents are more effective for obsessions and compulsions than nonserotonergic antidepressants, and that their antiobsessive benefit is independent of antidepressant benefit, contributed to the separation of OCD from affective disorder (Dolberg *et al.* 1996).

There is perhaps more evidence in support of neurobiological origins for OCD than any other anxiety disorder, and is reviewed elsewhere in this volume. Since heterogeneity across individuals in these studies is common, future classification systems may be able to include subtypes of the disorder based on the pathophysiology involved.

Post-traumatic stress disorder

Descriptions of the consequences of severe trauma have existed since ancient times (Shay 1994). Several 18th century psychiatrists linked trauma and psychiatric disorder (van der Kolk & van der Hart 1989). John Ericksen described symptoms of increased arousal, nighmares, somatization, and increased startle following railroad accidents, and attributed them to spinal injury (railroad spine syndrome; Kinzie & Goetz 1996). The view that trauma was etiologic in anxiety symptoms was entertained at the turn of this century by a number of prominent authors, including Janet, Charcot, Briquet, and Freud (the seduction theory) before being replaced in the field by psychoanalytic theories emphasizing fantasy over actual experience as etiologic. As in all of psychiatry, the premature attempt to identify primary etiology (whether biological or psychological) before clear syndromes were established contributed to controversy and confusion (Kinzie & Goetz 1996).

War-related syndromes are especially prominent in the 19th and 20th century literature, and include "exhausted heart," "irritable heart syndrome" (American Civil War) and "neurocirculatory aesthenia" (World War I) (Jones 1995). The contemporary definition of post-traumatic stress disorder (PTSD) is usually traced to the World War I diagnosis of "shell shock," which was initially thought due to the actual concussive effects of the newly invented heavy artillery. Soldiers with the newly termed "war neuroses" were shown in 1918 to exhibit exaggerated stress responses when exposed to reminders of war (Southwick *et al.* 1994).

Studies of World War I veterans by Kardiner, Spiegel and Grinker (Grinker & Spiegel 1945; Kardiner & Spiegel 1947; Spiegel & Classen 1995) led to the theoretical integration of conditioning and psychoanalytic models. These authors also recognized the interaction of stressor severity with vulnerability in producing post-traumatic symptoms. Kardiner described traumatic neurosis as a "physioneurosis" based on the prominence of physiologic symptoms and somatic complaints. He emphasized its nosologic distinction from hysteria and compulsion neurosis since the operative fear in war neurosis was damage to the physical integrity of the self (Kardiner & Spiegel 1947, p. 336). Psychotherapy, support, and physical rehabilitation were the primary treatments. Hypnosis and narcosynthesis were used in some cases to facilitate an unproductive therapy or to accelerate the course of treatment. Abreaction involving reliving traumatic experiences was often advocated as a means of accessing memories to be later integrated in psychotherapy.

Between the World Wars, a clinical literature emerged dealing with the clinical consequences of industrial and occupational accidents, and the politics of compensation entered the literature as well (Kinzie & Goetz 1996). More clinical reports appeared in the 1940s and 1950s concerning not only war veterans, but also survivors of fire and Nazi concentration camps (Kinzie & Goetz 1996).

In spite of this early work, and perhaps in part because the prevailing psychoanalytic model minimized the importance of adult experience in explaining symptoms, a post-traumatic syndrome was not officially proposed until DSM-III (APA 1980). The DSM-I (APA 1952) diagnosis of "gross stress reaction" presented no criteria, and described a reaction to severe trauma in a "normal personality" which supposedly cleared rapidly in most cases. If it did not, a "definitive" diagnosis was to be made from other categories. This diagnosis was removed in DSM-II, and only the adjustment reactions were available to categorize post-traumatic symptoms.

Kolb proposed an influential model of PTSD in which traumatic exposure was hypothesized to produce cortical and synaptic changes through the mechanisms of conditioning, sensitization, and failure of normal habituation (Kolb 1987). The physiologic disturbance was regarded as primary, and the psychological symp-toms were viewed as the consequence of recurring, severe, uncontrollable symptoms of hyperarousal and intrusive memories.

The neurobiology of chronic PTSD has been an area of increasing investigation since its identification in DSM-III (see Chapter 5). However, most research to date has been conducted with war veterans, and it remains to be determined whether the generalizability of this research is limited by high comorbidity, unique aspects of war trauma, and the treatment-refractory status of many subjects in this population. Recent large multicenter clinical trials finding a significantly better response to medication than that seen in trials with war veterans supports this view, and emphasizes the likelihood that the diagnosis encompasses a high degree of heterogeneity (Brady *et al.* 2000; Marshall *et al.* 2001a).

The diagnosis of PTSD may prove to have several subtypes, depending upon such factors as the developmental phase during which the trauma occurred, presence or absence of impulsive dyscontrol, specific symptom profile (including dissociative symptoms), comorbidity, or pre-existing psychiatric disorder. In addition, several studies have found that individuals with subthreshold PTSD symptoms also experience significant impairment and have higher rates of comorbidity and suicidal ideation compared to controls (Weiss *et al.* 1992; Blanchard *et al.* 1996; Stein *et al.* 1997; Marshall *et al.* 2001c). This opens an important and relatively unexplored question in trauma research. By analogy, subthreshold major depressive disorder also has been found to be a legitimate focus of clinical attention.

The role of trauma as an etiologic factor in other psychiatric disorders and symptom domains remains to be clarified. For example, recent longitudinal studies confirm earlier retrospective studies in finding that childhood trauma is associated with adult personality disorders (Herman *et al.* 1989; Luntz & Widom 1994; Johnson *et al.* 1999; Shea *et al.* 1999). Epidemiologic studies have consistently found that childhood trauma increases risk for a range of adult disorders (Kessler *et al.* 1997). Trauma may function as a non-specific stressor within a stress-diathesis model, play a more specific causal role in some disorders, be irrelevant to the etiology of the disorder in question, or be an epiphenomenon of pre-existing disorder (such as impulse or substance abuse disorders). Such questions are especially relevant to understanding the pathophysiology of how different types of environmental experience are registered and subsequently influence synaptic networks, gene expression, and behavior. A high rate of comorbidity between PTSD and the affective, anxiety, and substance abuse disorders may indicate the existence of common etiologic mechanisms (Charney & Bremner 1999). However, important distinctions between PTSD and commonly comorbid disorders such as major depressive disorder (Yehuda *et al.* 1996) and panic disorder have been observed. For example, a recent study found that PTSD patients had significantly lower baseline cortisol, baseline MHPG, and lower volatility in response to clonidine challenge compared to those with panic disorder (Marshall *et al.* 2001b). The evolutionary utility of a functional neurophysiologic system for responding to danger and trauma and encoding the experience for purposes of survival has been appreciated for decades. This model figures importantly in distinctions between normal and pathological responses to trauma. It also raises the same controversial issues as the debate between normal and pathological anxiety. For example, vivid remembering of the trauma in the presence of stimuli resembling the traumatic event is so common that it might be considered a part of normal physiology. In fact, evidence to date suggests that each of the core clusters overlaps with the prospectively demonstrated normative response to severe trauma (Rothbaum *et al.* 1992; North *et al.* 1994).

Given the extensive comorbidity observed in PTSD using the current diagnostic system (Kessler *et al.* 1995), further nosologic research may suggest a more parsimonious nosology which recognizes a broader range of responses to severe trauma within a single syndrome. For example, Herman has proposed a diagnosis called disorders of extreme stress not otherwise specified (DESNOS), or complex PTSD, which would identify affective, dissociative, and somatic symptom clusters, disruptions of relationships, identity, and repeated experiences of self-harm in individuals with histories of severe childhood abuse (Herman 1993). Minimal empirical evidence is available at present in support of DESNOS. The essential issue is whether these symptoms cluster homogeneously and are not already captured by existing disorders of better established validity. Zlotnick *et al.* (1996) studied 108 women consecutively admitted to a psychiatric inpatient unit, 74 of whom reported serious childhood sexual abuse (90% had been raped). Diagnostic findings in the two groups were not reported. Childhood abuse victims had significantly higher scores on 8/9 scales, which were used to operationally define the DESNOS criteria. However, both groups were highly symptomatic, suggesting an alternative interpretation that childhood trauma was nonspecifically associated with increased severity of a range of symptom measures. Furthermore, the two groups were not matched on other variables that might account for the findings. Much more study is needed with diverse populations and methodologies.

Acute stress disorder

Acute stress disorder was added to the anxiety disorders in DSM-IV, and describes acute post-traumatic stress symptoms (re-experiencing, avoidance, and increased autonomic arousal) with prominent dissociative symptoms (Cardena *et al.* 1996) occurring in the immediate period after a traumatic event. The new diagnosis was proposed largely based on replicated findings that dissociative symptoms in the peritraumatic period increase risk for subsequently developing PTSD (Spiegel & Classen 1995).

Acute stress disorder identifies individuals who would meet criteria for post-traumatic stress disorder (except for the time restriction of being 1 month post-trauma) and also have prominent dissociative symptoms. Peritraumatic dissociation, however, is likely only one of several factors contributing to the development of PTSD, and thus it appears premature to narrow the focus of study to only those individuals with dissociative symptoms in addition to intrusive, avoidant, and arousal symptoms. Approximately 40% of subjects with PTSD symptoms in the 1st month post-trauma do not have prominent dissociative symptoms but still present with significant disability and distress and can develop chronic disorder (Marshall *et al.* 1999).

In contrast, ICD-10 is organized on different principles, and captures both relatively nonspecific acute responses to trauma (acute stress reaction, and adjustment disorder), and the specific, well-validated constellation of symptoms included in PTSD. It may be argued that this approach better serves the primary purpose of a clinical diagnosis, which is to identify the range of individual responses to trauma associated with significant impairment and/or distress. Instead, dissociative symptoms might be recognized as an associated feature of both acute and chronic PTSD in order to facilitate research and treatment studies.

Clarification of the relationship between the different dissociative symptoms, trauma, and psychiatric disorder is needed. For example, dissociation is not always associated with trauma, and is equally associated with general psychopathology (Waller *et al.* 1996; Mulder *et al.* 1998; Marshall *et al.* 2000).

Generalized anxiety disorder

Generalized anxiety disorder (GAD) remains perhaps the most provisional anxiety syndrome. GAD emerged as a residual category in DSM-III when the anxiety neurosis category was divided into multiple syndromes, and panic disorder was recognized separately. DSM-III allowed the diagnosis to be made after only 1 month of anxiety symptoms with motoric, autonomic, and cognitive manifestations. Since this potentially confounded the category with transient adjustment reactions, the time criteria was lengthened to 6 months in DSM-III-R to focus attention on a chronic, perhaps more endogenous form (Spitzer & Williams 1984). Excessive and/or unrealistic worry was made the key feature. The DSM-IV definition simplified the inclusion criteria and now emphasizes the uncontrollability of the worry. A core set of increased arousal and motor tension symptoms was also identified, based on validity studies (Brown *et al.* 1994). As currently defined, situational factors and the cognitive content of the worry must be carefully examined to exclude other disorders (Brown *et al.* 1994).

The clinical problem of defining excessive and unreasonable worry, given the influence of class, culture, personality, and values on what constitutes appropriate worry, remains a difficult diagnostic issue. Alternatively, GAD may be better conceptualized as a general trait/vulnerability factor (Brown *et al.* 1994), or a final common pathway for numerous disturbances.

To date, minimal differences have been found to distinguish qualitatively the physiology of GAD from normal physiology. The majority of studies of skin conductance, heart rate, respiration, epinephrine and norepinephrine (noradrenaline) levels, as well as urinary and plasma cortisol under rest and stress conditions, have shown no differences (Hoehn-Saric & McLeod 1993). However, heightened muscle tension and a narrowed range of autonomic responsiveness does appear to differentiate GAD patients from normal subjects (Hoehn-Saric & McLeod 1993).

Whether syndromal unity will emerge from further research is unclear. The issue of whether such symptoms might still be best understood as a general vulnerability to other disorders, a response to chronic and/or significant psychosocial stressors, or as the penumbra of subsyndromal disorders remains unresolved. Subgroups within GAD may show distinct resting or stress responses. Given the high rate of comorbidity in this disorder as in PTSD, heterogeneity is an important and increasingly debated issue. Research which excludes all other disorders possesses limited generalizability.

Neurobiological comparisons in patients with GAD and other anxiety disorders might be particularly pertinent to questions of nosologic validity. If replicated, the finding that major depression and GAD share the same genetic liability also suggests that further nosologic refinement of this syndrome may be necessary (Kendler *et al.* 1992).

Specific phobia

Clinical descriptions of phobic behavior can be found in the writings of Hippocrates, Shakespeare, Descartes, and Burton's *Anatomy of Melancholy*, in which he distinguishes between fear and depression (Marks 1969). The term phobia, derived from the Greek *phobos* meaning fear, acquired its modern definition (as an unreasonable, involuntary fear of an objectively nonthreatening situation or object) during the 19th century (Marks 1969).

Specific phobias are a clinically heterogeneous group of syndromes with the common feature of circumscribed fear and avoidance. Since phobias develop around a limited number of situations, objects, and animals, and usually are not the result of a conditioned reaction, this has been seen as evidence of a constitutional preparedness to develop fears of phylogenetically prepotent stimuli. It is also clear from primate studies that a fear reaction is evident on first exposure (e.g. to snakes) even in laboratory animals that have never been exposed in a natural environment. Evidence of pathophysiologic heterogeneity across the specific phobias are differences in age of onset, clinical course, familial aggregation, and autonomic response to the phobic stimulus (Fyer 1987). Blood- injury- needles-phobic individuals show a biphasic response on exposure characterized by an initial rise in blood pressure, followed by an overcompensatory vasovagal response of hypotension, bradycardia, and sometimes fainting

(Hoehn-Saric & McLeod 1993, p. 187). In contrast, all other phobic responses produce only inconstant autonomic arousal. Animal phobias have a consistently earlier onset than other phobias.

In contrast to earlier views that phobias were discrete entities which can be successfully and permanently treated in behavior therapy, one recent follow-up study indicated a more chronic, intermittent course for many individuals (Lipsitz *et al.* 1999).

Common mechanisms across diverse disorders

There is considerable evidence that the anxiety disorders share important common features, including high rates of symptom overlap and comorbidity across disorders, and the breadth of pharmacologic and psychosocial treatment efficacy. This suggests common underlying pathophysiologies. How to balance the differences and similarities is a critical issue that should be carefully considered in the field.

This historical review reveals an important pattern in the conceptual dialectic of psychiatry. *There is a clear oscillation between wholistic, integrative models* (e.g. the psychoneuroses, a general neurotic syndrome, an all encompassing model implicating final common pathways in brain circuitry) *and narrowly defined, carefully-observed syndrome or disease models* (e.g. in the writings of Kraepelin, and Bergonzoli, and the DSM-IV). Taking note of this pattern in the process of debate may allow real progress in this area.

Furthermore, common factors across psychosocial treatments must also be considered in future models. The utility of exposure-based treatments for a wide range of anxiety disorders is inarguable and may offer clues as to which neural circuits are common, or common final paths, across some disorders. Antidemoralization effects are also a common feature across psychosocial treatments, and may be the primary mechanism of the placebo effect. The fact that nonspecific interventions can produce true treatment response is as relevant to future research as findings of specific treatment interventions. For example, the fact that placebo response is quite low in OCD, moderate in social phobia, and high in panic disorder in recent clinical trials may offer important information. The fact that placebo response in PTSD has varied from 0% to 60% in clinical trials strongly supports the view that this diagnosis alone is insufficient to capture a homogeneous group.

It is unclear how the finding of common etiologic mechanisms in anxiety disorders would influence a diagnostic system. As discussed above, separate clinical syndromes might need to be preserved for diagnostic and treatment purposes regardless of common etiology, or conversely, in the presence of numerous phenocopies.

As scientific progress often consists of a series of successive approximations, future psychiatric classification will likely emerge from an ongoing dialectic between the fields of psychopharmacology, neurobiology, nosology, and various behavioral and psychological approaches.

Acknowlegements

This chapter is supported in part by National Institute of Mental Health (NIMH) grants MH01412 (Dr Marshall) and PHS grant MH-30906, MHCRC, New York State Psychiatric Institute (Dr Klein).

Portions of this chapter have been adapted from Marshall and Klein (1999) with permission from the publisher (Oxford University Press, New York.)

References

Abelson, J.L. & Curtis, G.C. (1996) Hypothalamic–pituitary–adrenal axis activity in panic disorder. *Arch Gen Psychiatry* 53, 323–38.

American Psychiatric Association (APA) (1952) *Diagnostic Statistical Manual of Mental Disorders*, 1st edn. American Psychiatric Association, Washington, D.C.

American Psychiatric Association (APA) (1968) *Diagnostic Statistical Manual of Mental Disorders*, 2nd edn. American Psychiatric Association, Washington, D.C.

American Psychiatric Association (APA) (1980) *Diagnostic Statistical Manual of Mental Disorders*, 3rd edn. American Psychiatric Association, Washington, D.C.

American Psychiatric Association (APA) (1987) *Diagnostic Statistical Manual of Mental Disorders*, 3rd edn revised. American Psychiatric Association, Washington, D.C.

American Psychiatric Association (APA) (1994) *Diagnostic Statistical Manual of Mental Disorders*, 4th edn. American Psychiatric Association, Washington, D.C.

Andrews, G., Stewart, G., Morris-Yates, A., Holt, P. & Henderson, H. (1990) Evidence for a general neurotic syndrome. *Br J Psychiatry* 157, 60–72.

Antony, M.M. & Barlow, D.H. (1996) Emotion theory as a framework for explaining panic attacks and panic disorder. In: *Current Controversies in the Anxiety Disorders* (R.M. Rapee (ed.)). Guilford Press, New York.

Bergonzoli, G. (1915) *Stati Ansiosi Nelle Malattie Mentali*, Borrioti, Vogera.

Berrios, G.E. (1996) *The History of Mental Symptoms: Descriptive Psychopathology Since the Nineteenth Century*. Cambridge University Press.

Berrios, G.E. (1999) Anxiety disorders: a conceptual history. *J Affect Disord* **56**, 83–94.

Blanchard, E.B., Hickling, E.J., Barton, K.A., Taylor, A.E., Loos, W.R. & Jones-Alexander, J. (1996) One year prospective follow-up of motor vehicle accident victims. *Behav Res Ther* **34**, 775–86.

Blashfield, R. (1984) *The Classification of Psychopathology: NeoKraepelinian and Quantitative Approaches*. Plenum Press, New York.

Brady, K., Pearlstein, T., Asnis, G.M. *et al.* (2000) Efficacy and safety of sertraline treatment of post-traumatic stress disorder. *JAMA* **283**, 1837–44.

Brown, T.A., Barlow, D.H. & Liebowitz, M.R. (1994) The empirical basis of generalized anxiety disorder. *Am J Psychiatry* **151**, 1272–80.

Cannon, W.B. (1929) *Bodily Changes in Pain, Hunger, Fear and Rage: An Account of Recent Researches into the Function of Emotional Excitement*, 2nd edn. D. Appleton, New York.

Cardena, E., Lewis-Fernandez, R., Bear, D., Pakianathan, I. & Spiegel, D. (1996) *Dissociative Disorders in the DSM-IV Sourcebook*, Vol. 2, American Psychiatric Association Press, Washington, D.C.

Charney, D.S. & Bremner, J.D. (1999) The neurobiology of anxiety disorders. In: *Neurobiology of Mental Illness* (D.S. Charney, E.J. Nestler & B.S. Bunney (eds), pp. 494–517). Oxford University Press, New York, Oxford.

Cohen, H. (1961) The evolution of the concept of disease. In: *Concepts of Medicine* (B. Lush (ed.), pp. 159–69). Pergamon Press, Oxford. Quoted from Caplan, A.L., Engelhardt, Jr, H.T. & McCartney, J.J. (eds) (1981) *Concepts of Health and Disease: Interdisciplinary Perspectives*. Addison-Wesley, London.

Cooper, A.M. (1985) Will neurobiology influence psychoanalysis? *Am J Psychiatry* **142**, 1395–402.

Dolberg, O.T., Iancu, I., Sasson, Y. & Zohar, J. (1996) The pathogenesis and treatment of obsessive-compulsive disorder. *Clin Neuropharmacol* **19**, 129–47.

Eysenck, H. (1955) A dynamic theory of anxiety and hysteria. *Journal of Medical Science* **101**, 28–51.

Feighner, J.P., Robins, E., Guze, S.B., Woodruff, R.A., Winokur, G. & Munoz, R. (1972) Diagnostic criteria for use in psychiatric research. *Arch Gen Psychiatry* **26**, 57–63.

Foucault, M. (1963) (translation by A.M. Sheridan. Published 1973) *The Birth of the Clinic: An Archaeology of Medical Perception*. Tavistock Publications, London. (Originally published as *Naissance de la Clinique* by Presses Universitaires de France, 1963, Paris.)

Freud, S. (1895) Obsessions and phobias; their psychical mechanisms and their aetiology. In: *Collected Papers*, Vol. 1 (translated by Jan Riviere). Hogarth Press, London, 1924.

Freud, S. (1953) The justification for detaching from neurasthenia a particular syndrome: the anxiety neurosis. In: *Collected Papers*, Vol 1. The Hogarth Press, London, pp. 76–106, 1894.

Fyer, A.J. (1987) Simple phobia. In: *Anxiety* (D.F. Klein (ed.), pp. 174–92). Karger, Basel.

Glick, R.A. (1995) Freudian and post-Freudian theories of anxiety. In: *Anxiety as Symptom and Signal* (S.P. Roose & R.A. Glick (eds), pp. 1–16). The Analytic Press, Hillsdale, NJ, London.

Grant, K.A., Sively, C.A., Nader, M.A. *et al.* (1998) Effect of social status on striatal DA D2 receptor binding characteristics in cynomolgus monkeys assessed with positron emission tomography. *Synapse* **29**, 80–3.

Grinker, R.R. & Spiegel, J.P. (1945) *Men Under Stress*. McGraw-Hill Book Co, Inc. New York.

Hartenberg, P. (1901) *Les Timides et la Timidité*. Alcan, Paris.

Herman, J.L. (1993) Sequelae of prolonged and repeated trauma: evidence for a complex post-traumatic syndrome (DESNOS). In: *Post-traumatic Stress Disorder: DSM-IV and Beyond* (J.R.T. Davidson & E.D. Foa (eds) pp. 213–28). American Psychiatric Press, Washington, D.C.

Herman, J.L., Perry, C. & van der Kolk, B.A. (1989) Childhood trauma in borderline personality disorder. *Am J Psychiatry* **146**, 490–5.

Hoehn-Saric, R. & McLeod, D.R. (1993) Somatic manifestations of normal and pathological anxiety. In: *Biology of Anxiety Disorders* (R. Hoehn-Saric & D.R. McLeod (eds), pp. 177–222). American Psychiatric Press, Washington, D.C.

Insel, T.R. (1992) Toward a neuroanatomy of obsessive-compulsive disorder. *Arch Gen Psychiatry* **49**, 739–44.

Johnson, J.G., Cohen, P., Brown, J., Smailes, E.M. & Bernstein, D.P. (1999) Childhood maltreatment increases risk for personality disorders during early adulthood. *Arch Gen Psychiatry* **56**, 600–6.

Jones, F.D. (1995) Psychiatry lessons of war. In: *War Psychiatry*. Office of the Surgeon General, US.

Kardiner, A. & Spiegel, H. (1947) *War Stress and Neurotic Illness*, 2nd edn. Paul B. Hoeber, Inc., Harper and Brothers, New York, London.

Kendler, K.S., Neale, M.C., Kessler, R.C., Heath, A.C. & Eaves, L.J. (1992) Major depression and generalized anxiety disorder: same genes, (partly) different environments? *Arch Gen Psychiatry* **49**, 716–22.

Kessler, R.C., Davis, C.G. & Kendler, K.S. (1997) Childhood adversity and adult psychiatric disorder in the US National Comorbidity Survey. *Psychol Med* **27**, 1101–19.

Keys, A. (1952) Experimental induction of psychoneuroses by starvation. In: *The Biology of Mental Health and Disease: The Twenty-seventh Annual Conference of the Milbank Memorial Fun* (symposium held at the New York Academy of Medicine, 1950). Paul B. Hoeber, Inc., Harper and Brothers, New York.

Kinzie, J.D. & Goetz, R.R. (1996) A century of controversy surrounding post-traumatic stress-spectrum syndromes: the impact on DSM-III and DSM-IV. *J Trauma Stress* **9**, 159–79.

Klein, D.F. (1964) Delineation of two drug responsive anxiety syndromes. *Psychopharmacologia* **5**, 397–408.

Klein, D.F. (1967) Diagnosis and pattern of reaction to drug treatment: clinically-derived formulations. In: *The Role and Methodology of Classification in Psychiatry and Psychopathology* (M.M. Katz, J.O. Cole & W.E. Barton (eds), pp. 466–83) US Department of Health, Education, and Welfare.

Klein, D.F. (1978) A proposed definition of mental illness. In: *Critical Issues in Psychiatric Diagnosis* (R.L. Spitzer & D.F. Klein (eds), pp. 41–71). Raven Press, New York.

Klein, D.F. (1987) Anxiety reconceptualized: gleaning from pharmacological dissection—early experience with imipramine and anxiety. In: *Anxiety*, Vol. 22 (D.F. Klein (ed.), pp. 1–35). Karger, New York.

Klein, D.F. (1989) The pharmacological validation of psychiatric diagnosis. In: *The Validity of Psychiatric Diagnosis* (L.N. Robins & J.E. Barrett (eds), pp. 203–16). Raven Press, New York.

Klein, D.F. (1994) Testing the suffocation false alarm theory of panic disorder. *Anxiety* **1**, 1–7.

Klein, D.F. (1996) The development of nosological concepts in anxiety disorders. In: *Implications of Psychopharmacology to Psychiatry: Biological, Nosological, and Therapeutical Concepts* (M. Ackenheil, B. Bond, R. Engel, M. Ermann & N. Nedopil (eds), pp. 89–100). Springer Verlag, Berlin Heidelberg.

Klein, D.F. & Davis, J.M. (1969) *Diagnosis and Drug Treatment of Psychiatric Disorders*. Williams & Wilkins Co., Baltimore, MD.

Klein, D.F. & Fink, M. (1962) Psychiatric reaction patterns to imipramine. *Am J Psychiatry* **119**, 432–8.

Klein, D.F. & Klein, H.M. (1989) The nosology, genetics, and theory of spontaneous panic and phobia: A critical review II. In: *Psychopharmacology of Anxiety* (P.J. Tyrer (ed.), pp. 135–62). Oxford University Press, New York.

Kolb, L.C. (1987) A neuropsychological hypothesis explaining post-traumatic stress disorders. *Am J Psychiatry* **144**, 989–95.

Kraepelin, E. (1899) Clinical psychiatry: a textbook for students and physicians, Vol. 1 In: *General Psychiatry* (J.M. Quen (ed.)). Science History Publications, Translated by Helga Metoui.

Kraepelin, E. (1902) *Clinical Psychiatry: A Textbook for Students and Physicians*, Macmillan, London. Translated by A.R. Diefendorf from the sixth edn of Kraepelin's textbook (1899).

Kraepelin, E. (1904) *Lectures on Clinical Psychiatry* (T. Johnstone (ed.)). Reprinted 1968 by Hafner Publishing Co., New York.

Lewis, A. (1953) Health as a social concept. *Br J Sociol* **4**, 109–24.

Liddell, H.S. (1952) Experimental induction of psychoneuroses by conditioned reflex with stress. In: *The Biology of Mental Health and Disease: The Twenty-seventh Annual Conference of the Milbank Memorial Fun* Symposium held at the New York Academy of Medicine, 1950.

Liebowitz, M.R., Gorman, J.M., Fyer, A.J. & Klein, D.F. (1985) Social phobia: review of a neglected anxiety disorder. *Arch Gen Psychiatry* **42**, 729–36.

Lilienfeld, S.O. & Marino, L. (1995) Mental disorder as a Roschian concept: a critique of Wakefield's "Harmful Dysfunction" analysis. *J Abnorm Psychol* **104**, 411–20.

Lipsitz, J.D., Mannuzza, S., Klein, D.F., Ross, D.C. & Fyer, A.J. (1999) Specific phobia 10–16 years after treatment. *Depress Anxiety* **10**, 105–11.

Luntz, B.K. & Widom, C.S. (1994) Antisocial personality disorder in abused and neglected children grown up. *Am J Psychiatry* **151**, 670–4.

Marks, I.M. (1969) *Fears and Phobias*. Academic Press, New York.

Marshall, R.D., Beebe, K.L., Oldham, M. & Zaninelli, R. (2001a) Efficacy and safety of paroxetine treatment of chronic PTSD: a fixed-dosage, multicenter, placebo-controlled study. *Am J Psychiatry* **158**, 1982–8.

Marshall, R.D., Blanco, C., Printz, D., Liebowitz, M.R., Klein, D.F. & Coplan, J. (2001b) Noradrenergic and HPA axis functioning in PTSD versus panic disorder. *Psych Res* **110**, 219–30.

Marshall, R.D. & Klein, D.F. (1999) Diagnostic classification of anxiety disorders: historical context and implications for neurobiology. In: *Neurobiology of Mental Illness* (D.S. Charney, E.J. Nestler & B.S. Bunney (eds), pp. 437–50). Oxford University Press, New York.

Marshall, R.D., Olfson, M., Hellman, F., Blanco, C., Guardino, M. & Struening, E. (2001c) Comorbidity, impairment, and suicidality in subthreshold PTSD. *Am J Psychiatry* **158**, 1467–73.

Marshall, R.D., Schneier, F.R., Lin, S.-H., Simpson, H.B., Vermes, D. & Liebowitz, M.R. (2000) Childhood trauma and dissociative symptoms in panic disorder. *Am J Psychiatry* **157**, 451–3.

Marshall, R.D., Spitzer, R. & Liebowitz, M.R. (1999) A review and critique of the new DSM-IV diagnosis of acute stress disorder. *Am J Psychiatry* **156**, 1677–85.

Moehle, K.A. & Levitt, E.E. (1991) The history of the concepts of fear and anxiety. In: *Clinical Psychology: Historical and Research Foundations* (C.E. Walker (ed.)). Plenum Press, New York.

Montgomery, S.A. (1994) Pharmacological treatment of obsessive-compulsive disorder. In: *Current Insights in Obsessive Compulsive Disorder* (E. Hollander, J. Zohar, D. Marazziti & B. Olivier (eds)). John Wiley and Sons, Chichester.

Morel, B.A. (1860) *Traité Des Maladies Mentales*. Masson, Paris.

Morel, B.A. (1866) Du délire émotif. Névrose du système nerveux ganglionnaire viscéral. *Archives Générales de Médecine* 7, 385–402, 530–51, 700–7.

Mulder, R.T., Beautrais, A.L., Joyce, P.R. & Fergusson, D.M. (1998) Relationship between dissociation childhood sexual abuse, childhood physical abuse, and mental illness in a general population sample. *Am J Psychiatry* **155**, 806–11.

North, C.S., Smith, E.M. & Spitznagel, E.L. (1994) Post-traumatic stress disorder in survivors of a mass shooting. *Am J Psychiatry* **151**, 82–8.

Panzarella, C. (1995) Klein's suffocation false alarm theory: another perspective. *Anxiety* 1, 144–9.

Pitman, R.K. (1994) Obsessive-compulsive disorder in Western history. In: *Current Insights in Obsessive Compulsive Disorder* (E. Hollander, J. Zohar, D. Marazziti & B. Olivier (eds), pp. 3–11). John Wiley and Sons, Chichester.

Popper (1963) Science: conjectures and refutations. In: *Conjectures and Refutations: The Growth of Scientific Knowledge*, p. 57. Routledge, New York.

Robins, E. & Guze, S.B. (1970) Establishment of diagnostic validity in psychiatric illness: its application to schizophrenia. *Am J Psychiatry* **126**, 107–11.

Rothbaum, B.O., Foa, E.B., Riggs, D.S., Murdock, T. & Walsh, W. (1992) A prospective examination of post-traumatic stress disorder in rape victims. *J Trauma Stress* 5, 455–75.

Schneier, F.R., Liebowitz, M.R., Abi-Dargham, A., Zea-Ponce, Y., Lin, S. & Laruelle, M. (2000) Low dopamine D2 receptor binding potential in social phobia. *Am J Psychiatry* 157, 457–9.

Shay, J. (1994) *Achilles in Vietnam: Combat Trauma and the Undoing of Character*. Simon and Schuster, New York.

Shea, M.T., Zlothick, C. & Weisberg, R.B. (1999) Comorbidty and specificity of personality disorder profiles in subjects with trauma histories. *J Personal Disord* 13, 199–210.

Southwick, S.M., Bremner, D., Krystal, J.H. & Charney, D.S. (1994) Psychobiologic research in post-traumatic stress disorder. *Psychiatr Clin North Am* 17, 251–65.

Spiegel, D. & Classen, C. (1995) Acute stress disorder. In: *Treatment of Psychiatric Disorders: The DSM-IV Edition* (G.O. Gabbard (ed.), pp. 1521–36). American Psychiatric Association Press, Washington, D.C.

Spitzer, R.L. & Endicott, J. (1978) Medical and mental disorder: proposed definition and criteria. In: *Critical Issues in Psychiatric Diagnosis* (R.L. Spitzer & D.F. Klein (eds), pp. 15–39). Raven Press, New York.

Spitzer, R.L., Endicott, J. & Robins, E. (1975) *Research Diagnostic Criteria (RDC) for a Selected Group of Functional Disorders*. New York State Psychiatric Institute, New York.

Spitzer, R.L. & Fliess, J.L. (1974) An analysis of the reliability of psychiatric diagnosis. *Br J Psychiatry* **125**, 341–7.

Spitzer, R.L. & Williams, J.B.W. (1984) Diagnostic issues in the DSM-IV classification of the anxiety disorders. In: *Psychiatry Update. American Psychiatric Association Annual Review*, Vol. 3 (L. Grinspoon (ed.), pp. 392–402). American Psychiatric Press, Washington D.C.

Spring, B.J., Weinstein, L., Lemon, M. & Haskell, A. (1991) Schizophrenia from Hippocrates to Kraepelin: intellectual foundations of contemporary research. In: *Clinical Psychology: Historical and Research Foundations* (C.E. Walker (ed.), pp. 259–77). Plenum Press, New York, London.

Stein, M.B., Walker, J.R., Hazen, A.L. & Forde, D.R. (1997) Full and partial post-traumatic stress disorder: findings from a community survey. *Am J Psychiatry* 154, 1114–19.

Sydenham, T. (1848) Preface to the third edn. *Observationes Medicae* from RG Latham, Transl, the Works of Thomas Sydenham, Vol. 1.

Torgerson, W.S. (1967) Multidimensional representation of similarity structures. In: *The Role and Methodology of Classification in Psychiatry and Psychopathology* (M.M. Katz, J.O. Cole & W.E. Barton (eds), pp. 212–20) US Department of Health, Education, and Welfare Washington, D.C.

Van der Kolk, B.A. & van der Hart, O. (1989) Pierre Janet and the breakdown of adaptation in psychological trauma. *Am J Psychiatry* **146**, 1530–40.

Wakefield, J.C. (1992) Disorder as harmful dysfunction: a conceptual critique of DSM-III-R's definition of mental disorder. *Psychol Rev* 99, 232–47.

Waller, N.G., Putnam, F.W. & Carlson, E.B. (1996) Types of dissociation and dissociative types: a taxometric analysis of dissociative experiences. *Psychol Methods* 1, 300–21.

Weiss, D.S., Marmar, C.R., Schlenger, W.E. *et al.* (1992) The prevalence of lifetime and partial post-traumatic stress disorder in Vietnam theater veterans. *Journal of Traumatic Stress*, 365–76.

World Health Organization (WHO) (1948) *Sixth Revision of the International Classification of Diseases Diagnostic*

Criteria for Research. World Health Organization, Geneva.

World Health Organization (WHO) (1978) *Ninth Revision of the International Classification of Diseases Diagnostic Criteria for Research.* World Health Organization, Geneva.

World Health Organization (WHO) (1993) *Tenth Revision of the International Classification of Diseases Diagnostic Criteria for Research.* World Health Organization, Geneva.

Yehuda, R., Teicher, M.H., Levengood, R., Trestman, R. & Siever, L.J. (1996) Cortisol regulation in post-traumatic stress disorder and major depression: a chronobiological analysis. *Biol Psychiatry* **40**, 79–88.

Zlotnick, C., Zakriski, A.L., Shea, M.T. *et al.* (1996) The long-term sequelae of sexual abuse: support for a complex post-traumatic stress disorder. *J Trauma Stress* **9**, 195–205.

PART TWO

Symptoms and Syndromes

2 Relationships Among Anxiety Disorders: Patterns and Implications

H.-U. Wittchen, Y. Lecrubier, K. Beesdo & A. Nocon

Introduction

The mandatory core element of all anxiety disorders as maladaptive human behavioral patterns is the occurrence of an anxiety reaction that may vary widely in terms of intensity, frequency, persistence, trigger situations, severity and consequences and other qualifying features. Given that such anxiety reactions, even in the context of clinically significant disorders, are universal primate experiences and behavioral patterns, with important evolutionary adaptive functions, one would expect a considerable degree of overlap between different forms of anxiety disorders, simply because of sharing this core element. This expectation is supported by the fact that our current diagnostic classification systems are almost exclusively based on descriptive phenomenology, using a patient's subjective verbal descriptions to classify his or her problem into one or more specific classes of anxiety disorders. Additionally, the introduction of descriptive explicit diagnostic criteria in modern classification systems (Diagnostic Statistical Manual, third edition [DSM-III: American Psychiatric Association, APA, 1980], third revised edition [DSM-III-R: APA 1987], fourth edition [DSM-IV: APA 1994], and the International Classification of Diseases, 10th edition [ICD-10: World Health Organization, WHO, 1993]), which replaced the former traditional broader distinction of anxiety neurosis and phobic neurosis by a large number of specific anxiety disorders, has considerably enhanced the probability that patients will receive more than one diagnosis ("comorbidity") from these various forms of anxiety disorders.

Although some of these "within-anxiety comorbidities" have certain nosological underpinnings, for example in the case of panic disorder and agoraphobia, the nature, the meaning and the implications of these associations remain poorly studied and understood. Whereas current clinical and treatment research is strongly focused on specific anxiety disorders, recent —yet controversial (Wittchen *et al.* 1999)—epidemiological modeling exercises came to the suggestion that there might actually be only very few indications for sufficiently different patterns of associations (Krueger 1999).

This chapter starts by summarizing the available evidence for overlap within the anxiety disorders from available epidemiological and clinical studies, but also voices some critical methodological concerns. In the second part of the chapter, various perspectives and conceptual frameworks for a better understanding of the relationship among different forms of anxiety disorders are discussed, focusing on the structure of phobic disorders, the panic-agoraphobia disorders, as well as generalized anxiety disorder (GAD).

Methodological considerations

The study of associations between disorders, usually termed "comorbidity" (Wittchen 1996), is a tricky process that requires a considerable degree of sophistication in order to avoid confusion and artefactual interpretations. Ideally, the study of associations amongst anxiety disorders should be based on epidemiological studies in representative population samples in order to avoid the risk of potentially biased estimates; such biases may result from sampling strategies typically used in clinical studies, and may be influenced, for example, by the patient's help seeking behavior, severity of symptoms, and stage of illness.

A fairly large number of such community studies have become available that have used modern operationalized diagnostic classification systems and standardized diagnostic instruments to document the considerable prevalence of specific anxiety disorders as well as some patterns of their comorbidity over lifetime and cross-sectionally. In studying comorbidity, particularly of highly prevalent disorders, one should be aware of the need to use appropriate statistical measures for associations that correct for chance agreement, such as the odds ratio (OR) statistic. The odds ratio is defined as the ratio of the odds of the two groups compared, whereby the odds is defined as the probability, p, that the event of interest occurred divided by the probability, l-p, that the event does not occur. This is essential, because one would expect increased rates of comorbid presentations simply by chance among highly prevalent conditions.

A second important consideration is the question of coverage of disorders. It is an important limitation of most of the available comorbidity studies that only a few have covered the full spectrum of anxiety disorders with the same degree of diagnostic sophistication, as the types and the frequencies of associations depend heavily on the number and the scope of anxiety disorders studied. For example, studies that examine only panic disorder, GAD, and phobias will result necessarily in lower numbers of comorbid conditions and consequently a higher number of "pure" disorders than studies that cover the full range of all types of phobic disorders (agoraphobia, social, specific phobia—animal type, situational type, etc.).

Other important considerations in evaluating the relationship between anxiety disorders are, for example, whether the respective study: (a) focuses on lifetime vs. 12-month or current diagnoses; (b) looks at patterns among children and adolescents who have not gone through the entire time period of risk for onset of each disorder as compared to adults; (c) uses diagnostic hierarchy rules, for example, not diagnosing agoraphobia as a separate disorder if criteria for panic disorder are met. All these aspects have tremendous effects on findings and, thus, it is not surprising that there is considerable variability between studies when it comes to the indication of estimates for pure and comorbid anxiety disorders as well as their patterns of associations.

One also needs to consider that comorbidity, defined as the "presence of specified disorders in a defined period of time" (Wittchen 1996) frequently disregards the dimensional nature of mental disorders and the problem of appropriate thresholds. Highlighting this problem, which is particularly relevant for cross-sectional studies, is the fact that a person with one threshold disorder might actually have one or more subthreshold diagnoses, just falling short of the mandatory criteria for these disorders (for example, having four instead of the five symptoms for major depression). Thus, it is possible that comorbidity estimates based on categorical diagnoses might considerably underestimate the "true" overlap of psychopathological syndromes (Goldberg 1996). The problem of a sometimes arbitrary diagnostic threshold has been highlighted by Weiller et al. (1998) and Angst and Dobler-Mikola (1985), who demonstrated that clinical severity and disability associated with subthreshold disorders are not that different from threshold disorders. Even when selecting patients after suicide attempts, more than 10% present with subthreshold diagnoses (Balazs et al. 2000).

Types and frequency of comorbid patterns in the spectrum of anxiety disorders

With these methodological limitations in mind, Table 2.1 reports patterns of associations between anxiety disorders from a community study of 14–24 year olds, covering all types of anxiety disorders, assessed with the DSM-IV version of the composite international diag-nostic interview, without using diagnostic hierarchies.

Table 2.1 documents that there is indeed a considerable degree of overlap of anxiety disorders. This generally supports Boyd et al.'s (1984) and Kessler et al.'s (1994) notion for comorbidity within anxiety disorders as well, that having one disorder enhances considerably the probability of having more disorders. The data come from a community survey of 3021 subjects aged 14–24 (Wittchen et al. 1998a) and reveal that the vast majority of anxiety disorders, including subtypes of specific phobias are significantly associated (only significant ORs are given) with each other, with only a few exceptions. To highlight as an example one interesting pattern of associations we want to focus on GAD, believed to rank among the most comorbid conditions. Unexpectedly, in this sample GAD does not seem to be more frequently comorbid than most of the other

Table 2.1 EDSP-community sample: lifetime associations (%, odds ratio) of anxiety disorders among 14–24-year olds (N = 3021).

Conditional probability of DSM-IV anxiety disorders for having other anxiety disorders and odds ratio (OR)

DSM-IV disorders	Prev. %	PD % (OR)	AG % (OR)	GAD % (OR)	SOC % (OR)	SP % (OR)	SP-a % (OR)	SP-e % (OR)	SP-s % (OR)	SP-b % (OR)	SP-o % (OR)	PNOS % (OR)	PTSD % (OR)	OCD % (OR)
							Specific phobia and subtypes						Other phobias	
Panic disorder	1.6	—	—	12.7 (7.5)	6.2 (4.1)	3.7 (2.7)	1.5 (NS)	6.8 (4.8)	1.5 (NS)	11.2 (7.7)	19.1 (9+)	0	20.4 (9+)	9.1 (5.7)
Agoraphobia	2.3	—	—	13.2 (6.1)	8.8 (4.6)	6.2 (3.6)	6.8 (2.7)	4.1 (NS)	8.2 (4.2)	8.1 (3.2)	8.2 (NS)	0	24.6 (9+)	20.7 (9+)
GAD	2.1	16.5 (7.5)	12.1 (6.2)	—	8.0 (4.0)	3.5 (NS)	5.8 (2.7)	2.7 (NS)	2.7 (NS)	3.5 (NS)	6.7 (NS)	4.5 (NS)	11.0 (4.5)	19.0 (9+)
Social phobia	7.3	27.6 (4.1)	27.6 (4.6)	27.3 (4.0)	—	18.3 (3.9)	19.3 (3.0)	18.6 (3.0)	18.9 (3.2)	22.9 (3.5)	28.3 (4.3)	10.1 (NS)	32.5 (5.1)	23.4 (3.7)
Specific phobia	16.2	36.6 (2.7)	43.4 (3.6)	26.4 (NS)	40.9 (3.9)	—	—	—	—	—	—	42.0 (3.9)	33.0 (NS)	29.2 (NS)
Animal type	5.8	5.2 (NS)	16.8 (2.7)	15.7 (2.7)	15.3 (3.0)	—	—	16.2 (3.5)	12.4 (2.4)	12.7 (NS)	20.4 (NS)	11.7 (2.0)	12.2 (NS)	11.3 (NS)
Environmental type	4.7	19.7 (4.8)	8.2 (NS)	5.9 (NS)	12.0 (3.0)	—	13.2 (3.5)	—	8.5 (2.0)	18.1 (4.8)	44.2 (9+)	15.3 (4.3)	9.0 (NS)	9.5 (NS)
Situational type	5.4	5.0 (NS)	19.3 (4.2)	6.9 (NS)	14.1 (3.2)	—	11.7 (2.4)	9.9 (2.0)	—	16.5 (3.5)	8.3 (NS)	13.1 (2.7)	14.2 (2.7)	14.5 (NS)
Blood-injury type	3.1	21.3 (7.6)	10.8 (3.2)	5.1 (NS)	9.7 (3.5)	—	6.8 (NS)	12.0 (4.8)	9.4 (3.5)	—	37.8 (9+)	13.1 (5.1)	14.1 (4.1)	3.7 (NS)
Other	0.8	9.9 (9+)	3.0 (NS)	2.7 (NS)	3.3 (4.4)	—	3.0 (NS)	8.0 (9+)	1.3 (NS)	10.3 (9+)	—	1.1 (NS)	6.4 (NS)	0
Phobia NOS	5.2	0	0	11.1 (NS)	7.2 (NS)	13.5 (3.9)	10.5 (2.0)	17.0 (4.3)	12.5 (2.7)	22.0 (5.1)	6.5 (NS)	—	14.0 (NS)	15.9 (NS)
PTSD	1.3	16.7 (9+)	14.1 (9+)	6.9 (4.3)	5.9 (5.1)	2.7 (NS)	2.8 (NS)	2.5 (NS)	3.5 (2.7)	6.1 (4.1)	10.1 (NS)	3.6 (NS)	—	9.6 (7.2)
OCD	0.7	4.0 (5.4)	6.4 (9+)	6.5 (9+)	2.3 (3.6)	1.3 (NS)	1.4 (NS)	1.5 (NS)	1.9 (NS)	0.9 (NS)	0	2.2 (3.2)	5.2 (7.0)	—

AG, agoraphobia; EDSP, Early Developmental Stages of Psychopathology Study; GAD, generalized anxiety disorder; NS, no significant odds ratio; OCD, obsessive compulsive disorder; OR, odds ratio; PD, panic disorder; PNOS, phobia not otherwise specified; Prev., prevalence; PTSD, post-traumatic stress disorder; SOC, social phobia; SP, specific phobia; SP-a, specific phobia-animal type; SP-b, specific phobia-blood injury type; SP-e, specific phobia-environmental type; SP-s, specific phobia-situational type.

Odds ratio adjusted for age and gender.
Odds ratios above 9.9 are indicated by 9+.

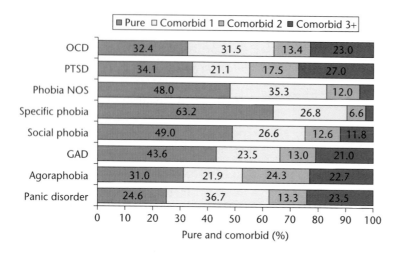

Fig. 2.1 Proportions of anxiety disorders, that are pure, comorbid with one, two, and three or more other anxiety disorders.

anxiety disorders, and actually reveals the highest proportion of non-significant associations. This finding is even more remarkable, because we deliberately chose to present findings from a younger age group that should give us considerably higher chances of pure disorders than samples based on older subjects.

Figure 2.1 demonstrates that the situation is even more complex, because of the fact that the vast majority of comorbid cases have not just *one* other anxiety disorder, but even two, or three or more out of the total of 13 specific forms of anxiety disorders included in the analyses. The three disorders with the highest number of additional diagnoses in this young sample are post-traumatic stress disorder (PTSD), panic disorder and agoraphobia. Further analyses of these data also reveal indication for a systematic increase with regard to a number of comorbid conditions over time and age. For example, the proportion of pure anxiety disorders in all disorders considered is high among 14–16 year olds, and then decreases fairly steadily with increasing age. By age 25 and above—in contradistinction to 14–16 year olds—only a minority of subjects presents with a pure anxiety disorder. This suggests that cross-sectional and lifetime comorbidity even within the anxiety disorders increases considerably with age. The consistently elevated significant ORs in Table 2.1 clearly demonstrate that the associations between anxiety disorders are not artefactual and cannot be explained by chance agreement. Instead, we have come to the conclusion that the comorbid presentations bear some meaningful implications from a patho-genetic, clinical and public health perspective.

The meaning of comorbidity patterns in anxiety disorders

Such patterns of comorbidities can be addressed from various perspectives (Merikangas *et al.* 1996). First, we would like to address the structure of specific fears and phobias and review the evidence for delineating different types of specific phobias as suggested by DSM-IV. Among this group a rare search for communalities amongst the phobic disorders has been conducted. Contingent upon Isaac Marks' phenomenological distinctions (1970), studies have examined more recently the interrelations and common latent structure of phobias. This group of studies is mostly descriptive and phenomenological. Secondly, we will examine more closely the association of panic disorder with agoraphobia and other disorders, before turning to GAD as a third example.

The common structure of specific fears and phobias

Curtis *et al.* (1998), using data from the National Comorbidity Survey (NCS; Kessler *et al.* 1994) demonstrated that specific fears are widespread in the community, whereas only one out of four subjects with fears meets criteria for specific phobias according to DSM-III-R criteria. The most robust finding of this study was that most simple phobias involve multiple fears.

This contrasts with the widespread notion that these specific phobias are isolated and circumscribed. Without reporting actual data, for example, Marks (1970) commented that people with phobias tended to report several lesser phobias in addition to the one for which they sought treatment. This impression has persisted among clinicians, though without much documentation. Yet, in a small community sample of women, Costello (1982) did observe a small but statistically significant tendency of one fear to be accompanied by others. Therefore a closer inspection of Curtis *et al.*'s (1998) work is informative.

In the NCS study 49.5% of respondents reported the lifetime occurrence of an unreasonably strong fear of one or more phobic stimuli. Fear of animals (22.2%) and of heights (20.4%) were reported significantly more often than other specific fears. Fear of being alone (7.3%), of storms (8.7%) and of water (9.4%) were the least prevalent. Only 22.7% of respondents with one or more lifetime fears met full NCS or DSM-III-R criteria for lifetime simple phobia. It is also noteworthy that the most common fears are least likely to be associated with a diagnosis of simple phobia (rank–order correlation = −0.94). Although most specific fears are accompanied by others, the prevalence in the population declines with the number of specific fears, from 22.23% with one fear to 2.1% for persons with 6–8 fears. The probability of meeting criteria for simple phobia increases consistently with the number of specific fears, from 12.1% for persons with a single fear to 56.9% for persons with 6–8 fears.

Interestingly, the examination of co-occurrence among specific fears and phobias revealed that only 24.2% of the people with lifetime simple phobias reported only a single specific fear. The vast majority had a lifetime history of two (26.4%), three (23.5%), four (10.4%) and more than four (17.3%) specific fears, respectively. In fact, high tetrachoric correlations (removing artificial reasons for differential bivariate correlations due to variation in prevalence of fears) were found among all pairs of the eight specific fears (range: 0.67–0.88). Factor analysis of this matrix documented a strong first principal factor. Attempted solutions with more dimensions failed to uncover evidence of interpretable dimensions.

One possible reason for this failure is that factor analysis uses only two-way relationships. To determine whether a meaningful subtyping could be obtained with higher-order information, the authors examined the full cross-classification among the specific fear/phobia types, with an unexpected finding: Among all ($N = 915$) NCS subjects with lifetime simple phobias, 141(!) multivariate profiles of specific fears were found out of a logically possible maximum of 255 (8^2). None contained enough cases to constitute a meaningful type.

Despite the relative rarity of pure simple phobias, the four most common profiles were all pure: namely animal, blood/illness, heights and closed spaces, in descending order of frequency. An additional latent class analysis (Lazarsfeld & Henry 1968; McCutcheon 1987) was used to determine whether a small set of underlying subtypes could account for the distribution of cases across the 141 reported profiles. Taking data from the total NCS population, the best-fitting model was a four-class solution characterized primarily by: (a) non-cases; (b) profiles with blood/illness and animal (two of the more prevalent) fears; (c) profiles with height fears (one of the more prevalent) and, to a lesser degree, flying, closed spaces, and animal fears; and (d) profiles with many specific fears.

It is remarkable that on factor analysis and other tests of association, the subtypes of specific fears and phobias studied in the NCS do not cluster in any predominant patterns. At first glance this appears to differ from research that shows separate animal and blood-injury factors (Arrindell *et al.* 1991) and that predispositions to these factors show evidence of heritability (Phillips *et al.* 1987). Actually, these analyses show that persons who fear one animal or one blood-injury situation also tend to fear others. In the present study, all such items were collapsed into one, so that there was no opportunity for multiple animal fears and multiple blood-injury fears to load on common factors.

To summarize, this pattern of findings from cross-setional epidemiological data does not support strongly the current DSM-IV subtyping of specific subtypes of specific phobias.

Implications of multiple phobias

The main differentiating feature of the latent class solution in the Curtis *et al.* (1998) study was the number of fears. Although this could be seen as a discouraging finding, it is noteworthy that subsequent analyses showed that it was an important distinction with many implications: Increasing numbers of specific fears, independent of content, are associated with more likelihood of full criteria simple/specific phobia diagnoses, more disability, and more comorbidity with other anxiety disorders. This suggests that the number of fears may mark some general predisposition to anxiety disorders (Table 2.2).

Table 2.2 demonstrates that the number of fears seems to be associated with various outcome measures, such as impairment, comorbidity with other anxiety dis-

Table 2.2 Impairment, comorbidity with anxiety disorders, and family psychopathology in simple phobia as a function of the number of specific fears.

	Only 1 fear			2–3 fears			4–5 fears			6–8 fears		
	%	OR	(95%CI)	%	OR	(95%CI)	%	OR	(95%CI)	%	OR	(95%CI)
Impairment												
Interfere a lot	17	1.0	—	36.3	2.7	(1.4–5.2)	40.9	3.3	(1.7–6.5)	54.5	5.8	(3.0–11.1)
See professional	25	1.0	—	32.4	1.4	(0.7–2.7)	28.3	1.2	(0.6–2.3)	35.5	1.6	(0.8–3.3)
Take medicine	9	1.0	—	5.8	0.6	(0.2–1.7)	8.2	0.9	(0.3–3.2)	16.0	1.9	(0.7–5.2)
Any of them	40	1.0	—	53.5	1.7	(1.0–3.1)	55.1	1.8	(1.1–3.1)	73.5	4.2	(2.3–7.8)
Comorbidity with other anxiety disorders												
Agoraphobia	12	3.5	(2.3–5.3)	21.5	6.3	(4.9–8.2)	42.7	22.6	(16.2–31.7)	48.1	23.6	(15.6–35.8)
Generalized anxiety disorder	9	3.2	(2.1–4.9)	16.2	4.7	(3.6–6.3)	18.4	4.8	(3.1–7.5)	32.1	10.8	(6.8–16.9)
Panic disorder	6	3.7	(2.2–6.3)	14.2	9.4	(6.9–12.6)	18.4	8.5	(5.3–13.5)	24.1	11.1	(8.5–18.7)
Social phobia	29	3.6	(2.7–4.9)	42.4	7.3	(5.9–8.9)	53.5	11.3	(8.2–15.7)	74.7	32.5	(20.1–52.4)
Any	42	3.8	(2.9–6.1)	62.6	9.1	(7.3–11.1)	76.1	22.2	(14.9–33.3)	84.1	45.8	(24.1–87.3)
Father's history												
Major depression	16	1.2	(0.9–1.7)	25.9	2.3*	(1.7–3.1)	21.4	1.8*	(1.1–2.9)	18.3	1.5	(0.6–3.6)
Generalized anxiety disorder	15	1.4	(1.0–2.1)	20.4	2.0*	(1.6–2.6)	21.1	2.1*	(1.3–3.5)	15.8	1.5	(0.7–3.8)
Substance dependence	24	1.5*	(1.0–2.2)	25.4	1.6*	(1.2–2.1)	29.5	2.0*	(1.3–3.0)	26.5	1.9	(0.9–3.2)
Mother's history												
Major depression	28	1.5	(1.0–2.2)	39.7	2.5*	(1.9–3.3)	44.6	3.1*	(2.0–4.7)	47.1	3.4*	(1.8–6.2)
Generalized anxiety disorder	24	1.7*	(1.1–2.7)	33.8	2.8*	(2.2–3.6)	36.5	3.2*	(2.1–4.8)	35.1	3.0*	(1.6–6.4)
Substance dependence	7	1.1	(0.7–1.8)	10.6	1.9*	(1.3–2.8)	11.9	2.2*	(1.3–3.6)	9.9	1.8	(0.7–4.7)

*Significant at the 0.05 level, two-sided test. Contrast group for odds ratios was the no phobia group.
OR, odds ratio; CI, confidence interval.

orders and several aspects of family psychopathology, most of which increase significantly with increasing numbers of specific fears. The most dramatic indicator of the trend in impairment is in reports that fears interfered "a lot" with life and activities. There are more modest elevations in the number of fears in people who sought help from a professional or took medication more than once because of their fears. As is also shown in Table 2.2, simple phobia is highly comorbid with other lifetime anxiety disorders. While 42% of the people with lifetime simple phobias with only one fear meet criteria for at least one other anxiety disorder, this percentage increases to 84.1% among those with 6–8 specific fears. The table also presents the associations between the number of specific fears in respondents with simple phobia and histories of major depression, GAD, substance dependence and antisocial personality disorder in their mothers and fathers. Almost all ORs were greater than 1.0, indicating a positive association between simple phobia and a family history of these mental disorders. In all cases the odds ratios were smaller for respondents with pure simple phobias than for those with multiple fears. It was also remarkable that age of onset curves were found to be virtually identical for respondents with a pure simple phobia and those with multiple specific fears. The median age of onset is about 12 years, and acquisition was about 90% complete by age 25. The finding that more fears predict more parental depression, substance dependence and antisocial personality disorders along with similar age of onset characteristics suggests that the number of fears may mark something broader, perhaps a general predisposition to psychopathology.

It is also noteworthy that the probability of recovery is inversely and significantly related to number of specific fears. While 60% of people with pure simple phobias eventually recover, this is true of only 30% of people with simple phobias plus 2–3 specific fears and only 20% of those with 5–8 fears.

Specific phobias: implications and future directions
These results provide slight support for heterogeneity of the specific phobia category, but strongly suggest underlying common factors. This is consistent with the ICD-10 classification system and with the dominant trend of the DSM system. However, the results do not rule out heterogeneity nor negate other evidence supporting it. It would not be surprising if there proved to be both a disposition to particular phobias and also a

more general disposition to all phobias. In a large-scale twin study, Kendler found exactly this: "strong evidence of the existence both of genetic and environmental risk factors unique to each kind of phobia and for genetic and environmental risk factors that influenced all phobia subtypes" (Kendler *et al.* 1992, p. 279).

In order to resolve the issue of combining or splitting the specific phobia category using the approaches currently in vogue, it will be necessary for future research to collect detailed and separate information about every irrational fear reported, including age of onset; whether it reaches full phobia criteria; its course, including age of remission, if any; detailed comorbidity history and information from family members, at least about fears and phobias, but ideally about a range or other mental disorders. The labor and cost of this undertaking can be minimized by making detailed inquiries in subsets of respondents from larger surveys. The purpose of the exercise would be, of course, to arrive at a classification which is etiologically and therapeutically meaningful. Among the questions hinging on the outcome are whether all simple/specific phobias should continue to be treated in the same way and whether treatment of all or some of them early in their course might reduce the later onset of more serious disorders for which they appear to signal an increased risk.

Separation anxiety/panic attacks/expectation anxiety/agoraphobia/depression

Probably the most stimulating approach to explain a considerable part of within anxiety comorbidity has been Donald Klein's "symptom progression model," which ultimately has lead to the distinction of panic disorder from GAD in DSM-III-R. Klein (1981) hypothesized that spontaneous panic attacks are responsible for triggering agoraphobic avoidance behavior, leading in the majority of subjects to the development of secondary agoraphobia and possibly other complications (depression and substance abuse). Within this framework, Gittelman and Klein (1984) also linked separation anxiety disorders in early childhood as a potentially additional "tracer" condition for subsequent panic-agoraphobia (Klein *et al.* 1992). From this etiologically exciting and clinically fruitful perspective that has led to the DSM-III-R decision to put panic disorder higher in the diagnostic hierarchy than agoraphobia, one would expect that subjects experiencing panic attacks and panic disorder are at an increased risk of

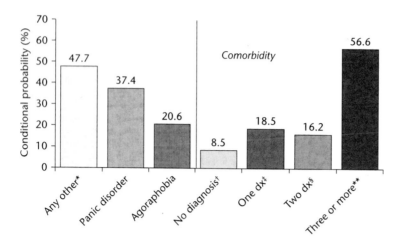

Fig. 2.2 Conditional probability of subjects with primary panic attacks to develop other mental disorders and to stay well (modified from Reed & Wittchen 1998, p. 341, with permission). *Any other mental disorder (except panic disorder and agoraphobia). †No diagnosis = no threshold DSM-IV diagnosis. ‡One dx = one additional diagnosis. §Two dx = two additional diagnoses. **Three or more = three or more additional diagnoses.

developing secondary agoraphobia and other comorbid conditions, such as depression and substance abuse. Another implication of this hypothesis is that one might expect that agoraphobia rarely or never occurs without panic or panic-like experiences.

Although a number of clinical studies focusing on clinical cases with panic disorder and agoraphobia provide, retrospectively, some considerable evidence for this model, prospective-longitudinal studies have failed so far to fully confirm the model. In a large prospective-longitudinal community sample of over 3000 adolescents and young adults, Reed and Wittchen (1998) examined whether primary panic attacks are associated with significantly increased risk of developing first panic disorder and then later on agoraphobia and other conditions. Their study showed first, consistent with Klein's model, that panic attacks are indeed associated significantly with both (a) the subsequent onset of panic disorder and agoraphobia, and (b) an increased subsequent risk of developing secondary depression and substance abuse. However, they further demonstrated that panic attacks are also strongly associated with numerous other conditions in the absence of panic disorder and agoraphobia, for example: PTSD (OR 17.8), dysthymia (OR 17.7), alcohol dependence (OR 11.5), social phobia (OR 5.0), and specific phobia (OR 6.1). Further, the association with separation anxiety disorder was significant not only for panic disorder and agoraphobia, but also for most other disorders. Another core finding of this study, which is inconsistent with the model, is the fact that even after the most careful and elaborate psychopathological distinctions among cases, the majority of cases

with agoraphobia did not reveal any signs of panic disorder, nor even of panic-like experiences (Wittchen *et al.* 1998b).

In fact these study findings, summarized in Fig. 2.2, suggest that panic attacks are overall fairly unspecific for the development of either panic disorder or agoraphobia. Rather, they seem to be unspecific yet sensitive markers for any type of secondary clinically significant psychopathology. They significantly predict the secondary onset of a wide variety of mental disorders and particularly of being multimorbid. Yet, the conditional probability of those who have experienced at least one DSM-IV panic attack to develop subsequently other mental disorders is, consistent with Klein's model, high for panic disorder (37.4%) and agoraphobia (20.6%), but also high for almost all other disorders (47.7%), whether they be social or specific phobias, GAD, affective, substance or stress-related disorders. Particularly noteworthy is the finding that subjects with primary panic attacks rarely continue with no specific mental disorder (8.5%), but go on frequently to develop three or more mental disorders in their further course (56.6%). Similar evidence has also been presented in the WHO primary care study (Lecrubier & Üstün 1998) conducted in 26 916 consecutive primary care patients. In this study 45.6% of those with lifetime panic attacks fulfilled diagnostic criteria for major depression, while only 42.6% reached criteria for panic disorder. In the same sample, out of 227 patients with lifetime signs of panic, all but two had an Axis I mental disorder. Whether this finding can be generalized is unclear; however, in samples with a high severity of mental disorders, such as suicide attempters,

Isometsä *et al.* (1996) and Johnson *et al.* (1999) also found that all patients with panic also had other Axis I mental disorders.

This finding is in line with previous longitudinal studies in adults (Wittchen & Perkonigg 1993; Goodwin & Hamilton 2001) concerning the relationship of comorbidity and extends to Barlow *et al.* (1985) work as well as DSM-IV claims that panic attacks may occur in all other (anxiety) disorders. Unlike Barlow *et al.*, however, we did not find that the frequency and number of symptoms differed between those panickers who developed panic disorder and those who did not. In our sample we found more evidence that the frequency and severity of associated avoidance behavior as well as cognitive correlates of panic are different in those panickers with and without panic disorder. The conditional probability after first onset of a panic attack of developing panic disorder (37.4%) or agoraphobia (20.6%) was similar for both sexes, but early onset males—unlike late onset panickers—seemed to have a lower probability than females of developing panic disorder and agoraphobia. Instead, such males were significantly more likely to develop other forms of mental disorders, particularly affective disorders. This suggests that the existence of various pathogenic pathways in early and late onset panic disorders are in need of further exploration. Similar indications were recently reported by Roy-Byrne *et al.* (2000) with regard to the association of panic disorder, panic attacks and depressive disorders. This analysis of NCS data also revealed that panic attacks and panic disorder are associated in a much more complex way to each other in terms of temporal ordering as well as impact on disability, course, severity and risk factors. However, does this entirely invalidate the panic symptom progression model? We suggest that this is not the case. Rather, we suggest that among young subjects up to the age 29, different pathways are possible, of which the symptom progression model is just one important model; however, we cannot exclude from such data the possibility that, for example, among older subjects a different picture emerges.

Comorbidity of GAD: do multiple phobias lead to GAD?

In light of the fact that comorbidity has been suggested to be a fundamental characteristic of the nature and course of GAD (Judd *et al.* 1998), it is surprising that, so far, most studies have been focused on comorbidity patterns with affective disorders and its nosological status in the anxiety–depressive spectrum disorders. Leaving aside the issue that it can be disputed whether the proportion of pure and comorbid presentations of GAD is really different from comorbidity rates observed in other disorders (see Kessler 2000), it is remarkable that few studies have up to now examined the hypothesis that GAD might be a consequence of preexisting multiple phobias in the patient's illness course. This hypothesis is consistent with a number of traditional writings by Freud (1962) and Isaac Marks (1987) that all suggested that multiple phobias and free-floating anxiety form a core basis of GAD.

An examinination of the temporal patterns of onset of comorbid disorders among sufferers with GAD in the NCS (retrospective data) indeed supports this hypotheses at first sight. Among all comorbid conditions examined in the NCS, social and specific phobias are the only two conditions that do precede the onset of GAD by at least 1 year in about two-thirds of all affected.

These retrospective figures were recently reexamined using a prospective-longitudinal design (Nocon, unpublished thesis). This study examined the baseline diagnostic status of a community sample yet unaffected by GAD and then observed for different baseline diagnostic groups the development of GAD as an outcome over a period of 5 years. Table 2.3 summarizes the outcome of this exercise. The upper portion of the table shows the conditional probabilities of subjects with no, one, two or three or more phobic disorders to develop GAD. Table 2.3 also gives information about the risk of subjects with other primary disorders (as compared to subjects with no mental disorders).

It is first noteworthy that the risk among baseline subjects with no disorder (cumulative incidence: 4.3%) to develop GAD is about the same as among cases with no phobic disorder (3.5%). (Note, other disorders might be present!) Having one or two phobic disorders, including specific phobia subtypes in the count, increases the risk moderately to 6.8% and 6.7%, respectively, whereas three or more phobias result in a significant increase to 13.6%, resulting in an OR of 2.7. Only one other primary mental disorder was found to be more strongly related to subsequent GAD development in this sample, namely PTSD (23.5%; OR: 5.9).

These findings suggest that there is some moderate support for the hypothesis that multiple phobias

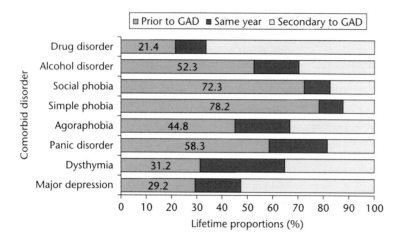

Fig. 2.3 Comorbidity: what comes first?

Status prior onset GAD at baseline	Conditional 5-years risk for secondary onset of GAD	
	Cond. prob. (% weighted)	OR (95%CI)
No phobic disorder at baseline (ref)	3.5	1.0 (ref. category)
One phobic disorder	6.8	1.48 (0.79–2.75)
Two phobic disorders	6.7	1.50 (0.65–4.42)
Three or more phobic disorders	**13.6**	**2.65 (1.11–6.33)**
No mental disorder (ref)	4.3	1.0 (ref. category)
Panic disorder	13.8	2.60 (0.84–8.10)
OCD	15.4	3.33 (0.64–17.40)
PTSD	**23.5**	**5.89 (2.13–16.27)**
Depressive disorders	5.2	1.06 (0.54–2.07)
Substance use disorder	3.1	0.78 (0.41–1.46)
Somatoform disorders	5.4	1.26 (0.69–2.32)
Eating disorder	8.8	1.40 (0.56–3.53)

Table 2.3 EDSP-longitudinal sample (N = 2548) subjects followed over 5 years after baseline: conditional probability of baseline cases to develop GAD in the follow-up period.

CI, confidence interval; EDSP, Early Developmental Stages of Psychopathology Study; GAD, generalized anxiety disorder; OCD, obsessive-compulsive disorder; OR, odds ratio; PTSD, post-traumatic stress disorder.

lead to GAD. At the same time, one needs to acknowledge that the association of primary PTSD with GAD is more impressive, suggesting at least one other pathway.

The lack of associations with other depressive, somatoform, substance and eating disorders lends further support to the general finding that among the vast majority of all people affected by major mental disorders with comorbid anxiety, the anxiety disorder starts first (Kessler *et al.* 1996; Regier *et al.* 1998). This seems to be true also for patterns of GAD, a disorder that might not necessarily occur with the same frequency as phobic disorders as the very first diagnosis in a patient's life, however, for which we also see in the majority other anxiety manifestations as temporally primary manifestations (Fig. 2.3).

Summary and outlook: comorbidity of anxiety disorders

The data discussed above demonstrate that we are still just beginning to understand comorbidity in general and within anxiety disorders, in particular.

In the past decade a vast number of studies have clarified the role of primary anxiety disorders in the development of secondary depressive and substance disorders as well as their effects on depression recurrence risk, length of depressive episodes, and type of onset in the community (e.g. Wittchen *et al.* 2000), primary care (e.g. Lecrubier 1998b) and clinical settings (Lecrubier 1998a). Yet, patterns within the anxiety disorders have been so far largely neglected. Therefore, we have focused and restricted our contribution to some associations of specific anxiety disorders, assuming that they are, in themselves valuable targets and valid diagnostic classes. However other perspectives to study comorbidity both within anxiety disorders and with other mental disorders, particularly from the affective spectrum, should not be neglected.

For example, although depression has been found to be the most common longitudinal outcome of most anxiety disorders, we cannot entirely rule out at this point the possibility that early and first manifestations of anxiety are simply "expressions" of the same type of underlying vulnerability for all types of anxiety disorders and maybe also for example prodromal stages of depressive disorders. The type of subsequent anxiety disorder expressed, the age when it is expressed, and the environmental events and other social factors available during the same period may organize the psychopathology and its further evolution in a yet unknown manner. Thus, we might be well advised to consider these issues within a broader framework, highlighting especially the partially "artificial" nature of our current classification systems.

Recent advances in the development of the classification of anxiety disorders through the adoption of a basically "atheoretical," empirically based, descriptive approach have enhanced the reliability, coverage across diverse settings, and clinical and research utility of explicit diagnostic criteria and specified diagnostic algorithms (APA 1994; WHO 1993). However, the diagnoses of anxiety and affective disorders are still heavily dependent on the outcome of diagnostic interviews rather than pathognomonic markers, and convincing clinical and nosological validation is still largely lacking in terms of prognostic value and stability, family and genetic findings, and laboratory findings (Robins & Guze 1970). Further, it is fair to state, that the goal of broader coverage of current psychopathological classification systems has naturally induced more, sometimes artificial, comorbidity than previous diagnostic systems based on questionable nosological and hierarchical assumptions (Wittchen 1996).

However, it should be stressed again, that the magnitude of comorbidity between disorders has been consistently highlighted by both epidemiological and clinical studies, irrespective of the type of diagnostic assessment interview used. For example, in the Epidemiological Catchment Area Study (Boyd *et al.* 1984) and the National Comorbidity Survey (Kessler *et al.* 1994), the odds of a single disorder increased the odds of a second, and the presence of three or more disorders was far more common than expected by chance. Further analyses in adults and adolescents (Brady & Kendall 1992; Wittchen 1996) demonstrated that patterns of comorbidity were caused by neither a methodological artifact nor help-seeking bias, but might have diagnosis-specific implications for improved etiological models and treatments as well as understanding severity, impairment (Kessler *et al.* 1996), course, and outcome (Wittchen & Essau 1989), at least for the majority of disorders studied so far.

Another alternative and controversial approach to study comorbidity was recently explored by Krueger (1999). He addressed the issue of diagnostic overlap by investigating the factor structure underlying some of the more common DSM-III-R mental disorders in an effort to elucidate the broad "higher-order structure of phenotypic psychopathology". By focusing on comorbidity as a potentially important "signal" indicating that current diagnostic systems lack parsimony, he conceptualizes comorbidity as meaningful covariance among putatively separate mental disorders. He argues that mental disorders or "core psychopathological processes" that might be more meaningful than specific disorders for research on treatment, prevention, and etiology. His chief finding—that a 3-factor mode labeled as anxious-misery and fear (representing facets of a higher-order internalizing factor)—as the two that basically represent the anxiety and depressive spectrum —and a broader externalizing factor (i.e. antisocial and substance use disorders) provides the best fit to the correlations among the 10 disorders—is remarkable. At first sight his finding matches data from child and genetic psychiatry and psychopharmacological intervention research showing considerable overlap in phenomenology, underlying genetic risks, and treatment response among the internalizing disorders. On this basis, Krueger suggests that his model might be not only phenotypically relevant, but may actually organize common psychopathological variance in terms of common genetic factors, a scheme that is particularly relevant for anxiety disorders.

There are several significant limitations to this study and approach dealing with the comorbidity phenomenon that suggest it would be unwise and premature to draw strong and dogmatic conclusions on the basis of Krueger's current analyses, which were recently discussed in greater detail by Wittchen *et al.* (1999). The findings are far too speculative to warrant the author's conclusion that the proposed model suggests key directions for diagnostic nomenclature and future research in psychiatric epidemiology, genetics, pharmacology, and intervention research. Yet despite limitations, Krueger's work on what might be labeled "common core diagnostic features" is a fruitful initial step complementing the type of "mainstream" comorbidity analyses. Both approaches should stimulate further research to enhance our understanding of the core processes underlying psychopathology of both anxiety and affective disorders.

References

American Psychiatric Association (APA) (1980) *Diagnostic Statistical Manual of Mental Disorders*, 3rd edn. American Psychiatric Association, Washington, D.C.

American Psychiatric Association (APA) (1987) *Diagnostic Statistical Manual of Mental Disorders*, 3rd edn, revised. American Psychiatric Association, Washington, D.C.

American Psychiatric Association (APA) (1994) *Diagnostic Statistical Manual of Mental Disorders*, 4th edn. American Psychiatric Association, Washington, D.C.

Angst, J. & Dobler-Mikola, A. (1985) The Zurich Study, V: anxiety and phobia in young adults. *European Archives of Psychiatric Neurological Science* **234**, 408–18.

Arrindell, W.A., Oei, T.P.S., Evans, L. *et al.* (1991) Agoraphobic, animal, death-injury-illness and social stimuli clusters as major elements in a four-dimensional taxonomy of self-rated fears: first order level confirmatory evidence from an Australian sample of anxiety disorder patients. *Advances in Behavioral Research Therapy* **13**, 227–49.

Balazs, J., Bitter, I., Lecrubier, Y., Csiszér, N. & Ostorharics, G. (2000) Prevalence of subthreshold forms of psychiatric disorders in persons making suicide attempts in Hungary. *Eur Psychiatry* **15**, 354–61.

Barlow, D.H., Vermilyea, J., Blanchard, E.B., Vermilyea, B.B., DiNerdo, P.A. & Cerny, J.A. (1985) The phenomenon of panic. *J Abnorm Psychol* **94**, 320–8.

Boyd, J.H., Burke, J.D., Gruenberg, E. *et al.* (1984) Exclusion criteria of DSM-III: a study of co-occurrence of hierarchy-free syndromes. *Arch Gen Psychiatry* **41**, 983–9.

Brady, E. & Kendall, P. (1992) Comorbidity of anxiety and depression in children and adolescents. *Psychological Bulletin* **111**(2), 244–255.

Costello, C.G. (1982) Fears and phobias in women: a community study. *J Abnorm Psychol* **91**, 280–6.

Curtis, G.C., Magee, W.J., Eaton, W.W., Wittchen, H.-U. & Kessler, R.C. (1998) Specific fears and phobias. epidemiology and classification. *Br J Psychiatry* **173**, 212–17.

Freud, S. (1962) On the grounds for detaching a particular syndrome from neurasthenia under the description 'anxiety neurosis.' In: *Standard Edition of the Complete Psychological Work of Sigmund Freud*, Vol. 3. Hogarth Press, London.

Gittelman, R. & Klein, D.F. (1984) Relationship between separation anxiety and agoraphobic disorders. *Psychopathology* **17** (Suppl. 1), 56–65.

Goldberg, D. (1996) A dimensional model for common mental disorders. *British Journal of Psychiatry* **168** (Suppl. 30), 44–9.

Goodwin, R.D. & Hamilton, S.P. (2001) Panic attack as a marker of core psychopathological processes. *Psychopathology* **34**(6), 278–8.

Isometsä, E., Henriksson, M., Heikkinen, M. *et al.* (1996) Suicide among subjects with personality disorders. *Am J Psychiatry* **153**, 667–73.

Johnson, J., Weissman, M. & Klerman, G. (1990) Panic disorder, comorbidity and suicide attempts. *Arch Gen Psychiatry* **47**, 805–8.

Judd, L.L., Kessler, R.C., Paulus, M.P., Zeller, P.V., Wittchen, H.-U. & Kunovac, J.L. (1998) Comorbidity as a fundamental feature of generalized anxiety disorders: results from the National Comorbidity Study (NCS). *Acta Psychiatr Scand* **98** (Suppl. 393), 6–11.

Kendler, R., Neale, M.C., Kessler, R.C. *et al.* (1992) The genetic epidemiology of phobias in women. The interrelationship of agoraphobia, social phobia, situational phobia and simple phobia. *Arch Gen Psychiatry* **49**, 273–81.

Kessler, R.C. (2000) The epidemiology of pure and comorbid generalized anxiety disorder: a review and evaluation of recent research. *Acta Psychiatrica Scandinavica* **102** (Suppl. 406), 7–13.

Kessler, R.C., McGonagle, K.A., Zhao, S. *et al.* (1994) Lifetime and 12-month prevalence of DSM-III-R psychiatric disorders in the United States: results from the National Comorbidity Survey. *Arch Gen Psychiatry* **51**, 8–19.

Kessler, R.C., Nelson, C.B., McGonagle, K.A., Swartz, M. & Blazer, D.G. (1996) Comorbidity of DSM-III-R major depressive disorder in the general population: results from the US National Comorbidity Survey. *Br J Psychiatry* **168** (Suppl. 30), 7–30.

Klein, D.F. (1981) Anxiety reconceptualized. In: *Anxiety: New Research and Changing Concepts* (D.F. Klein & J.G. Rabkin (eds), pp. 235–63). Raven, New York.

Klein, D.F., Mannuzza, S., Chapman, T. & Fyer, A.J. (1992) Child panic revisited. *J Am Acad Child Adolesc Psychiatry* **31**, 112–16.

Krueger, R.F. (1999) The structure of common mental disorders. *Arch Gen Psychiatry* **56**, 921–6.

Lazarsfeld, P.R. & Henry, N.W. (1968) *Latent Structure Analysis.* Houghton-Miffin, Boston, MA.

Lecrubier, Y. (1998a) Comorbidity in social anxiety disorder: impact on disease burden and management. *J Clin Psychiatry* **59** (Suppl. 17), 33–9.

Lecrubier, Y. (1998b) The impact of comorbidity on the treatment of panic disorder. *J Clin Psychiatry Supplement* (Suppl. 8), 11–14.

Lecrubier, Y. & Üstün, T.B. (1998) Panic and depression: a worldwide primary care perspective. *Int Clin Psychopharmacol* **13** (Suppl. 4), 7–11.

Marks, I.M. (1970) The classification of phobic disorders. *Br J Psychiatry* **116**, 377–86.

Marks, I.M. (1987) *Fears, Phobias, and Rituals. Panic, Anxiety, and their Disorders.* Oxford University Press, Oxford.

McCutcheon, A.L. (1987) *Latent Class Analysis.* Sage Publications, Newbury Park, CA.

Merikangas, K.R., Angst, J., Eaton, W. *et al.* (1996) Comorbidity and boundaries of affective disorders with anxiety disorders and substance misuse: results of an international task force. *Br J Psychiatry* **168** (Suppl. 30), 58–67.

Phillips, K., Fulker, D.W. & Rose, R.J. (1987) Path analysis of seven fear factors in adult twin and sibling pairs and their parents. *Genet Epidemiol* **4**, 345–55.

Reed, V. & Wittchen, H.-U. (1998) DSM-IV panic attacks and panic disorder in a community sample of adolescents and young adults: how specific are panic attacks? *J Psychiatr Res* **32**, 335–45.

Regier, D.A., Rae, D.S., Narrow, W.E., Kaelber, C.T. & Schatzberg, A.F. (1998) Prevalence of anxiety disorders and their comorbidity with mood and addictive disorders. *British Journal of Psychiatry* **173** (Suppl. 34), 24–8.

Robins, E. & Guze, S.B. (1970) Establishment of diagnostic validity in psychiatric illness: its application to schizophrenia. *Am J Psychiatry* **126**, 983–7.

Roy-Byrne, P.P., Stang, P., Wittchen, H.-U., Üstün, B., Walters, E.E. & Kessler, R.C. (2000) Lifetime panic depression comorbidity in the National Comorbidity Survey. *Br J Psychiatry* **176**, 229–35.

Weiller, E., Bisserbe, J.C., Maier, W. & Lecrubier, Y. (1998) Prevalence and recognition of anxiety syndromes in five European primary care settings from the WHO study on psychological problems in general health care settings. *Br J Psychiatry* **173**(34), 18–23.

Wittchen, H.-U. (1996) Critical issues in the evaluation of comorbidity of psychiatric disorders. *Br J Psychiatry* **168**, 9–16.

Wittchen, H.-U. & Essau, C.A. (1989) Comorbidity of anxiety disorders and depression. Does it affect course and outcome? *Journal of Psychiatry Psychobiology* **4**, 315–23.

Wittchen, H.-U., Höfler, M. & Merikangas, K. (1999) Toward the identification of core psychopathological processes? *Arch Gen Psychiatry* **56**, 929–31.

Wittchen, H.-U., Kessler, R.C., Pfister, H. & Lieb, R. (2000) Why do people with anxiety disorders become depressed? A prospective-longitudinal community study. *Acta Psychiatr Scand* **102**(406), 14–23.

Wittchen, H.-U. & Perkonigg, A. (1993) Panikattacken mit frühem und spätem Beginn: unterschiedliche pathogenetische mechanismen? *Verhaltenstherapie—Praxis, Forschung, Perspektiven* **3**(4), 296–303.

Wittchen, H.-U., Perkonigg, A., Lachner, G. & Nelson, C.B. (1998a) Early Developmental Stages of Psychopathology Study (EDSP). Objectives and design. *European Addiction Research* **4**, 18–27.

Wittchen, H.-U., Reed, V. & Kessler, R.C. (1998b) The relationship of agoraphobia and panic in a community sample of adolescents and young adults. *Arch Gen Psychiatry* **55**, 1017–24.

World Health Organization (WHO) (1993) Mental and behavioral disorders. In: *Tenth Revision of the International Classification of Diseases Diagnostic Criteria for Research.* World Health Organization, Geneva.

3

Panic Disorder: Symptoms and Syndromes

S.S. Sinha & J. Gorman

Introduction

Panic disorder (PD) was officially introduced into the psychiatric nomenclature as a distinct illness in 1980 with the publication of the Diagnostic Statistical Manual, third edition (DSM-III: American Psychiatric Association [APA] 1980). Its recognition was prompted by the qualitative distinction Donald Klein made between panic attacks and more generalized anxiety following his seminal discovery of the specifically antipanic effects of imipramine (Klein 1964). Prior to the publication of DSM-III panic attacks had been subsumed under the broad category of "anxiety neurosis." Klein's reconceptualization of anxiety differed from the prevailing continuum model of anxiety, which traditionally viewed panic as simply the most severe manifestation of general anxiety.

Klein's "pharmacological dissection" of panic from general anxiety allowed him to conceptualize three key aspects of the PD syndrome that figure in the current DSM-IV (APA 1994) formulation. These involve spontaneous panic attacks, anticipatory anxiety, and agoraphobic avoidance (Klein 1981).

The central clinical feature of PD is the spontaneous panic attack, a rapid crescendo of intense anxiety or fear that develops abruptly and peaks within 2–10 min, and involves numerous cognitive and physical symptoms in multiple body systems. According to the DSM-IV criteria, it involves at least four of the following: palpitations, sweating, trembling, shortness of breath, choking feelings, chest pain or discomfort, nausea, dizziness, derealization, fear of losing control or going crazy, fear of dying, numbness or tingling, and chills or hot flushes (APA 1994).

Spontaneous panic attacks, by definition, occur "out of the blue," without any obvious environmental or situational triggers. The DSM-IV also identifies situationally bound panic attacks (those that occur only in a certain situation) and situationally predisposed panic attacks (those that are more likely to occur with certain situations). Panic attacks occur in a wide range of psychiatric disorders, including other anxiety disorders, particularly social phobia and PTSD, as well as schizophrenia and depression. However, for the diagnosis of PD to be made the patient must have recurrent unexpected or spontaneous attacks.

The development of PD has its beginnings in the experience of an initial, spontaneous panic attack. As attacks recur and become more frequent, the patient develops intense worry about the occurrence and consequences of future attacks. This fear is known as anticipatory anxiety. The unfortunate consequence of such pervasive worry is a tendency for the patient to avoid situations in which a panic attack has occurred in the past or seems likely to occur in the future. A prime factor driving this avoidance behavior is the patient's belief that escape from such situations may prove difficult or embarrassing. Consequently, attempts to venture into these situations are avoided. Avoidance behavior can become so marked that it generalizes to several situations and may eventually render the patient housebound, unwilling to travel outside the house unless with a trusted companion. This severe form of avoidance behavior is agoraphobia.

According to the DSM-IV criteria, agoraphobia entails anxiety about being in places where help might be difficult or embarrassing, or in which help may not be available in the event of a panic attack. Typical situations involve being outside the home, being in a crowd or a line, being on a bridge, or in a bus, subway or car (APA 1994). The diagnosis of PD can be made with or without agoraphobia.

Agoraphobia

The "American" perspective that agoraphobia is a conditioned avoidance behavior secondary to the experience of spontaneous panic attacks has received considerable support from the available research. According to this model, agoraphobia is viewed exclusively as a consequence of panic. Indeed, that agoraphobia may be a distinct illness itself has not been supported by empirical evidence. In fact, the initially high estimations of agoraphobia without panic in epidemiological studies of the community may have largely been due to diagnostic error.

Most studies confirm that panic attacks antecede avoidance behavior. Garvey & Tuason (1984) showed that panic attacks were not preceded by agoraphobia in 12 patients. Thyer and Himle (1985) showed that approximately 80% of panic patients stated that agoraphobia developed after PD. Uhde *et al.* (1985) found that, of 32 panic patients, 31 developed phobic avoidance after panic attacks started. Aronson and Logue (1987), in a longitudinal assessment of 46 panic patients, showed that pathological anxiety and agoraphobic avoidance occurred after the onset of panic.

To address whether agoraphobia can stand on its own as a nosological entity, Goisman *et al.* (1995) identified the clinical characteristics of 26 subjects initially diagnosed with agoraphobia without a history of PD. Upon re-examination, the majority of subjects (73%) reported experiences resembling situational or limited symptom attacks. Eighty-one percent of subjects reported a high number of catastrophic cognitions, most prominent of which was fear of doing something embarrassing, followed by fears of fainting or losing control. Twenty-five percent reported a precipitating factor 1 month prior to the onset of the agoraphobia, and 30% reported a precipitating factor 6 months prior to onset, the most common of these being recent surgery or having medical symptoms in public, such as vomiting. Recent life stress, particularly onset of illness or changes in health, preceded the agoraphobia in 36% of cases. The situational or limited symptom attacks reported preceded the onset of the agoraphobia by at least 2 months in 29%, and appeared simultaneously in 67%. Most of the patients would have been diagnosed as PD with agoraphobia if they experienced a few more symptoms allowing them to meet criteria for full panic attacks. Thus, this study suggests that agoraphobia without panic may be an uncomplicated or less severe form of true PD, rather than a qualitatively distinct illness.

Horwath *et al.* (1993) blindly reinterviewed after 7–8 years 22 patients from the Epidemiologic Catchment Area (ECA) study who had been diagnosed with agoraphobia without panic. The instrument used was the SADS-LA, and the data were blindly reviewed by a research psychiatrist. Nineteen of the 22 originally classified agoraphobics actually had simple phobias or fears; one patient had agoraphobia with limited symptom attacks; and the other had PD that was missed in the ECA. This study provides strong evidence that the high prevalence of agoraphobia without panic in the ECA study may have been significantly overestimated due to imprecise interviewing.

Yet, a persisting question in panic research is why some patients develop agoraphobia and others do not. One possibility is the specific contextual features of the first panic attack. Some research suggests that agoraphobia is more likely to develop when the first panic attack occurs in a place that is classically agoraphobic, such as an open place with several people. Interestingly, this is consonant with the notion that agoraphobia is maintained through predominantly cognitive mechanisms, notably fear of being trapped and fear of doing something embarrassing.

Lelliot *et al.* (1989) studied 57 patients with panic and agoraphobia and found that 81% of all first panics occurred in public places. Similarly, Shulman *et al.* (1994) compared minimal versus extensive avoiders and found that extensive avoiders were more likely to have experienced the initial panic attack in classic agoraphobic situations.

Amering *et al.* (1997) interviewed 60 patients with agoraphobia and 30 patients without agoraphobia about their first panic attack. Agoraphobia prior to the first panic attack was relatively uncommon in the sample (10%) and did not predict the presence or absence of agoraphobia at the time of assessment. Feelings of embarrassment about experiencing the panic attack, and whether the panic attack occurred in a public place, were significantly associated with the later development of agoraphobia.

Langs *et al.* (2000) examined specific characteristics of PD with agoraphobia versus those without to determine if specific factors could predict the development of agoraphobia. They studied 84 outpatients, 24 without agoraphobia and 58 with agoraphobia. The authors found that age of onset of PD, the experience of fear of going crazy, and the experience of chills or hot flushes predicted whether agoraphobia would develop. Interestingly, the experience of chest pain or discomfort reduced the risk of agoraphobia.

Other literature indicates that a propensity towards agoraphobic avoidance may already exist prior to the first panic attack, suggesting that agoraphobia is not wholly a conditioned phenomenon. Roth (1984) suggests that patients with agoraphobia already have a complex repertoire of avoidance behaviors and tendencies to be dependent on others long before they experience the first panic attack.

Fava et al. (1988) studied 20 PD patients and found that 18 of these experienced significant agoraphobic avoidance, generalized anxiety and hypochondriacal concerns before the occurrence of the first panic attack. Lelliot et al. (1989) found that of 57 patients with PD and agoraphobia, 23% had agoraphobic avoidance evident before the first panic attack. Seventy percent of this sample had prodromal anxiety and depressive symptoms. Argyle and Roth (1989) studied 56 PD patients with agoraphobia and found that 20% of patients had agoraphobia that preceded the panic.

Subtypes of panic: respiratory and nonrespiratory

Although the hallmark of PD is the spontaneous panic attack, manifestations of panic attacks are largely nonuniform. The heterogeneous presentation of the spontaneous panic attack has stimulated interest in defining subtypes of the illness characterized by particular symptom patterns.

One potential subtype of PD is that defined by the presence of salient respiratory symptoms, notably shortness of breath, choking and smothering sensations, and hyperventilation. Briggs et al. (1993) analysed data from Phase Two of the Cross National Panic Study. Descriptions of the last severe panic attack for 1168 panic patients were collected. The major finding of this study was that PD patients could be phenomenologically dissected into two main groups: those with prominent respiratory symptoms and those without. The group with prominent respiratory symptoms experienced more choking and smothering sensations, chest pain, numbness/tingling and fear of dying. The group without prominent respiratory symptoms experienced more palpitations, dizziness, flushes, trembling, sweating, fear of going crazy or losing control, nausea and depersonalization. Interestingly, the group with prominent respiratory symptoms responded to imipramine, and suffered more spontaneous attacks. In contrast, the group without prominent respiratory symptoms had more situationally bound panic attacks and responded better to alprazolam.

Biological studies of panic also point to the likelihood of a respiratory subtype of panic. Challenge studies with agents such as lactate and CO_2 produce intense panic attacks characterized by intense respiratory distress, particularly shortness of breath, and physiological changes such as increased respiratory rate and tidal volume (Papp et al. 1997). These attacks are also blocked by imipramine as well as the newer selective serotonin reuptake inhibitors (SSRIs; Sinha et al. 2000). It is beyond the scope of this chapter to review the literature regarding challenge studies in PD.

Biber and Alkin (1999) demonstrated that challenge with a mixture of 35% CO_2 and 65% oxygen (O_2) provoked more robust behavioral and physiological responses in patients who routinely reported a greater number of respiratory symptoms in their panic attacks than in patients who did not. The patients in the respiratory group had more severe panic and phobic symptoms and longer duration of illness. Seventy-eight percent (22/28) patients in the respiratory group panicked to CO_2, whereas 48% (11/23) of the nonrespiratory group panicked. Patients in the respiratory group had significantly higher scores on the Panic and Agoraphobia Scale and had a longer duration of illness.

Beck et al. (2000) examined how respiratory and nonrespiratory panickers respond to a hypoxic challenge of 12% O_2. Although both groups showed equivalent increases in anxiety and panic symptoms, the respiratory subgroup showed greater fluctuation in tidal volume during and after the challenge. In addition, the respiratory subgroup showed overall lower levels of endtidal CO_2, a long established finding in the respiratory panic literature (Sinha et al. 2000).

Cox et al. (1994) examined panic attack symptomatology in 212 PD patients using the Panic Attack Questionnaire. They found strong evidence for three clusters of panic symptoms that could differentiate patients: cardiorespiratory distress (particularly tachycardia and palpitations), dizziness-related symptoms (items with highest loading were dizziness, vertigo, unsteady feelings and faintness), and cognitive/psychological symptoms (items with highest loading were fear of going crazy and fear of losing control). The three clusters had good internal consistency and were only modestly intercorrelated (0.5 or less).

Limited symptom attacks

Limited symptom attacks (LSA) are "near-panic" attacks that do not meet the four-symptom requirement as specified in the DSM-IV. Early studies suggest that LSA are less severe, less frequent and shorter in duration (Krystal *et al.* 1991). LSA are actually common and occur in 40% of PD patients with agoraphobia. They also appear with relatively high frequency in people without PD. Kanterndahl and Realini (1993) found the prevalence of LSA in the community to be between 2.2 and 8.5%. PD in its early stages may present exclusively with LSA.

Katerndahl (1990) addressed the validity of the symptom requirement criteria (at least four) of the DSM-III and suggested that this quantity of symptoms is largely arbitrary and does not meaningfully distinguish such patients from those experiencing fewer symptoms. Of 68 patients studied, 27 (40%) had LSA. He found no demographic distinctions between those with LSA and those with full-blown attacks. Interestingly, frequencies of symptoms were greater in full blown attacks, with the exception of the cognitive symptoms such as fear of dying, going crazy or losing control. The number of symptoms experienced did not affect the likelihood of agoraphobia development. Interestingly, cognitive symptoms may particularly contribute to the maintenance of agoraphobic fears. This study underscores the importance of recognizing LSA as a harbinger or variant of typical PD.

Katerndahl and Realini (1998) compared patients with LSA to patients with PD. LSA subjects reported lower mean symptom severity but longer duration of the disorder than PD patients. Also, LSA had lower overall health care utilization.

Katerndahl (1999) followed 21 patients with LSA. After 1 year, four (19%) of the patients stated their attacks had progressed to full-blown panic attacks. Three of these four met criteria for PD.

Rosenbaum (1987) found that out of 35 patients, 94% had experienced some LSA. Fifty percent of all panic attacks were LSA. Since the early stages of PD may present exclusively as LSA, these attacks can themselves be extremely disabling and lead to comorbidity. After treatment, 19% had only LSA. LSA may be present in the residual phase of PD.

Nocturnal panic

A substantial proportion of PD patients experience, in addition to recurring daytime panic attacks, the phenomenon of nocturnal panic. These attacks are characterized by sudden awakening, terror and marked physiological activation (Craske & Barlow 1989).

Nocturnal panic attacks occur during nonREM sleep, primarily in stages 2 and 3, usually between 24 and 225 min after sleep onset (Mellman & Uhde 1990; McNally 1994) They can be distinguished from night terrors and panic attacks that occur while dreaming. Approximately 70% of panic patients have experienced nocturnal panics; however, very few panic patients report nocturnal panic exclusively (Mellman & Uhde 1989). Sleep panic has been of interest to researchers since the phenomenon occurs during a time when intermediary cognitive factors are quiescent.

Whether nocturnal panic represents a more severe form of PD is as yet unclear. Krystal *et al.* (1991) compared sleep panic attacks with daytime spontaneous and situational attacks and found no differences with respect to severity and length of the attacks. Frequency of sleep panic was lower than daytime panic. However, this study did not report the particular symptoms endorsed by patients during sleep panic attacks.

Norton *et al.* (1999) compared the frequency and symptomatology of panic attacks in PD patients with (22) and without (21) a history of nocturnal panic attacks. Although no differences were found in the actual number of attacks, the nocturnal panic group experienced more panic symptoms during expected diurnal panic attacks, but not during unexpected or spontaneous diurnal panic attacks. The nocturnal panic group experienced more chest pain and endorsed more fears of dying.

Labatte *et al.* (1994) examined the characteristics of patients with sleep panic attacks. Of 95 panic patients, 38 (40%) reported at least one sleep panic attack. Patients with sleep panic had a higher prevalence and a longer duration of illness, and greater severity of illness as mea-sured by the CGI. They also showed higher rates of comorbidity with other anxiety disorders and major de-pression. In addition, they were more likely to have a history of childhood anxiety. The authors conclude from these results that sleep panic suggests a greater severity of illness.

Late onset PD

Initial presentation of panic in late life, though not uncommon, usually suggests a general medical condition as the prime etiologic factor. If panic attacks do begin at a later age, the ensuing anticipatory anxiety and agoraphobic avoidance follow a course similar to typical PD.

Segui *et al.* (2000) studied the sociodemographic and clinical characteristics of PD patients with onset after 60 years. Sixty-four PD patients were assessed; 27 of these were late onset panic, and the remainder earlier onset panic. Late onset PD had less family history of PD (compared to earlier onset), had less disability, and reported fewer and milder panic symptoms. There was also more comorbidity with dysthymia than with depression in late onset panickers.

Raj *et al.* (1993) examined 51 PD patients whose onset was after 60 years. Though the phenomenology of the panic was similar to patients in the earlier onset group, the late onset group experienced more shortness of breath. This group was also more likely to have medical disorders such as chronic obstructive pulmonary disease (COPD), vertigo and Parkinson's disease. Shortness of breath in this group clearly relates to the presence of chronic illnesses that make the experience of respiratory symptoms more likely. Beitman *et al.* (1991) showed that PD can begin after age 65 and present with chest pain with no actual cardiac pathology.

Childhood antecedents of adult PD

The initial childhood link to adult PD was thought to be separation anxiety (Gittelman & Klein 1984). One of the few prospective studies in this area found that children with separation anxiety were specifically prone to the development of adult PD (Klein *et al.* 1992). However, other studies have since challenged this specificity. Indeed, it is now clear that childhood separation anxiety can predispose an individual to the breadth of anxiety disorders, including obsessive-compulsive disorder (Raskin *et al.* 1982). It is also likely that other childhood anxiety disorders, such as overanxious disorder, as well as inborn patterns of temperament, such as behavioral inhibition, can lead to PD.

Lipsitz *et al.* (1994) examined the relation between retrospectively reported childhood separation anxiety disorder and adult anxiety disorders in 252 outpatients. Patients with one or more adult anxiety disorders were significantly more likely than those with only one anxiety disorder to have separation anxiety in childhood. This study did not support a specific association between childhood separation anxiety and adult PD, suggesting a more complex relationship between childhood anxiety and adult psychopathology

Pollack *et al.* (1996) investigated the relationship between childhood anxiety and adult PD. PD patients were more likely to have an anxiety disorder in childhood, particularly social anxiety and overanxious disorder. Patients with childhood anxiety were more likely to have a comorbid anxiety disorder in adulthood (74%) compared to those who did not (25%). Childhood anxiety also significantly increased the risk for comorbid depression in adulthood (68%) compared to those without childhood anxiety (27%). Severity of PD as measured by age of onset, duration of illness in adult PD was not significantly influenced by the presence of childhood anxiety, although the relationship to comorbid depression does suggest that childhood anxiety predicts a more severe course of illness.

Otto *et al.* (1994) studied 100 PD patients, 26 of whom had no agoraphobia, while the remainder had varying degrees of agoraphobia. Fifty-five percent of the patients had at least one childhood anxiety disorder. The most frequent childhood anxiety disorders were social phobia (35%) and overanxious disorder (31%), followed by avoidant disorder (20%), separation anxiety disorder (19%), and agoraphobia (16%). Patients with childhood anxiety also had greater agoraphobic avoidance in adulthood.

Behavioral inhibition to the unfamiliar is an extensively studied temperamental construct initially described by Kagan *et al.* (1984). It is quite common and occurs in an estimated 10–15% of all children. This trait can be recognized in toddlers and involves a tendency to be cautious, quiet and behaviorally restrained and fearful. As infants, they are generally irritable and emotionally reactive. Generally, this group will withdraw when exposed to novelty. By school age they are readily considered shy and introverted. Behavioral inhibition is now recognized as a risk factor for the development of adult anxiety disorders.

Rosenbaaum *et al.* (1988) found that offspring of patients with PD have higher rates of behavioral inhibition (85%) compared to controls (15%). Reznick *et al.* (1992), in a retrospective study, found that PD patients had a higher rate of behavioral inhibition than controls. A prospective study by Caspi *et al.* (1996), however, did not find elevated risk for anxiety disorders in a sample of behaviorally inhibited children followed to age 21, but did find a higher risk for the development of major depression. In addition, Biederman *et al.* (1993) found a higher rate of social phobia than PD in a prospective follow up of inhibited children. More recently, Rosenbaum *et al.* (2000)

suggested that much of the observed link between parental PD and behavioral inhibition can be accounted for by comorbid panic and depression.

Craske *et al.* (2001) attempted to identify childhood temperamental traits and early experiences with medical illness as factors in the etiology of adult PD. An analysis of 992 children aged from 3 to 18 from the Dunedin New Zealand Longitudinal Follow-up of Children Study was carried out. Assessments of these children were made every 2 years from ages 3 to 18. Forty-four were diagnosed with PD at 18 years and 42 at 21 years. Seventy of these cases were agoraphobia with panic, 10 were panic without agoraphobia, and 4 were panic with agoraphobia. All subjects had endorsed at least one panic attack symptom. Anxious temperament was measured on a 5-point scale of emotional reactivity during a set of cognitive and motor tasks at age 3. Medical health measurements at ages 3, 15 and 18 were used.

Of particular relevance to the phenomenology of panic was the finding that presence of respiratory disturbance (asthma, colds, ear infections) at a young age predicted the development of PD and differentiated PD patients from other anxiety disorders as well as controls. Interestingly, respiratory disturbance was predictive of later panic only in those patients found to be emotionally hyper-reactive. Males diagnosed as high on emotional reactivity at age 3 and were identified as behaviorally inhibited were more likely to develop PD. Separation anxiety was not assessed. History of asthma may confer particular vulnerability to the development of PD in those individuals with high emotional reactivity.

Panic and depression

An emerging diagnostic consideration within the PD syndrome is the significant overlap of major depression with panic. Extensive research has demonstrated a close association between panic and depressive symptoms. The co-occurrence of panic and depression has important implications for clinical course, response to treatment, and overall prognosis.

The comorbidity of panic with depression has been documented in numerous studies. The World Health Organization (WHO) collaborative study found a strong association between depression and anxiety disorders, including PD (Lecrubier & Ustun 1998). Studies have shown approximately 30–60% of depressed patients had secondary PD (Coryell *et al.* 1988; Keller & Hanks 1995). Kessler *et al.* (1997) showed that 21.6% of patients with major depression experience panic at least once in their lifetime. Similarly, Stein *et al.* (1990) showed that 63% of patients with PD had at least one major depressive episode. The National Comorbidity Survey (NCS) Study showed that 55.6% of subjects with PD had a history of major depression (Kessler 1997). That panic and depression frequently cluster together suggests their co-occurrence is not due to chance, and may actually represent a specific syndrome having a unique symptomatological and potentially pathophysiological profile.

Panic with depression has been shown to have greater symptom severity (Brown *et al.* 1996), and involves a greater number of symptoms. In addition, comorbid panic and depression leads to poorer outcome, poorer response to treatment and greater disability and functional impairment. The overall disability of panic patients is markedly increased once depressive symptoms become prominent in the clinical picture. In addition, there is a greater likelihood of professional-help seeking (Kessler *et al.* 1994). PD patients who present with depression required more immediate treatment or hospitalization (Grunhaus *et al.* 1994).

Roy-Byrne *et al.* (2000) examined the NCS data that surveyed the general population for mental disorders and looked at the association of lifetime and recent (12 month) panic depression comorbidity with symptom severity, impairment, course and help seeking. Results showed a lifetime and current comorbidity between panic and depression was stronger than that for any other anxiety disorder. Comorbid panic and depression was associated with a significantly greater number of physiological symptoms experienced during spontaneous panic attacks than those without depression. When other comorbid diagnoses were controlled for, this relationship was even stronger. Major depression with comorbid panic was associated with widespread increase in medical and mental health service utilization. In addition, current or recent (12 month) depression was associated with greater role impairment and disability. Comorbid panic and depression also had a more persistent course than either disorder alone.

Brown *et al.* (1996) found that depressed patients with lifetime PD had greater depressive severity, greater impairment in physical and psychosocial functioning, and were more likely to have a history of alcohol dependence, somatization disorder, and avoidant personality disorder. Depressed patients with panic are more likely to prematurely terminate both pharmacotherapy and psychotherapy.

The association of panic with depression has implications for suicide risk. However, the relationship of suicide to PD is complex. Several studies have shown that panic patients that attempt suicide have more comorbid depression that those who do not (Cox *et al.* 1994; Warshaw *et al.* 1995). Similarly, mood disorder patients with a history of panic attacks also have been shown to have a higher incidence of suicide (King *et al.* 1995; Keller 1996). However, this relationship has been recently questioned by Placidi *et al.* (2000), who found that the presence of comorbid PD in depressed melancholic inpatients did not increase the risk for lifetime suicide attempt, and was more related to the presence of aggression and impulsivity. Roy-Byrne *et al.* (2000) found a higher incidence of suicide in panic patients with depression compared to panickers without depression. Yet, they also found a higher incidence of suicide in depressed patients with panic attacks that, similar to Placidi *et al.*'s (2000) study, was accounted for by additional comorbidities such as personality disorders and substance abuse.

Comorbid panic and depression generally has a detrimental effect on treatment outcome. Van Valkenburg *et al.* (1984) found a poor treatment response in 55% of depressed patients with panic compared to a poor response in 28% of panic alone patients. Scheibe and Albus (1994) followed 52 PD patients prospectively over a 2-year period. They found that after 2 years of treatment, panic patients with depression had more severe symptoms and were more impaired in work and family life than patients with PD alone.

Panic and bipolar disease

A longstanding clinical observation is that panic attacks are a frequent concomitant of bipolar disease. One of first to document this phenomenon was Campbell in *Manic Depressive Disease: Clinical and Psychiatric Significance* (1953). Campbell succinctly describes panic and notes its appearance in both the depressive and, counterintuitively, manic phases of the illness.

Systematic evaluation of the overlap between panic and bipolar disease began with the ECA Study (Chen & Dilsaver 1995). Among the landmark findings reported was that 20% of bipolar patients had comorbid PD, a rate surpassing even that for major depression. Other studies have largely reinforced these findings. Grunhaus *et al.* (1994) found that 20% of patients with panic and depression had bipolar disorder. Pini *et al.* (1997) found that the most prevalent comorbid disorder in bipolar depressives was panic.

Genetic studies provide evidence for a subtype of panic that co-occurs with bipolar illness. Mackinnon *et al.* (1997) found that, in a group of bipolar probands, 88% of panic patients had comorbid bipolar disorder. Further, panic was diagnosed in 18% of family members with bipolar disorder. The same group reported chromosome 18 linkage data showing that linkage scores were highest in the families of probands with comorbid PD (Mackinnon *et al.* 1998).

PD with concomitant bipolar disorder has substantial implications for morbidity and mortality. Fawcett *et al.* (1987), in a controlled prospective study, reported that panic significantly increased the risk of suicidal behavior in bipolar patients. Young *et al.* (1993) found that anxious bipolar patients had a higher incidence of alcohol use than nonanxious bipolars.

Panic with bipolar illness may respond to mood stabilizers, and may be preferentially responsive to valproate as compared to lithium. Young *et al.* (1993) demonstrated a trend towards lithium nonresponsiveness in panicking bipolar patients. Baetz and Bowen (1998) found that panic patients with an underlying mood instability who were nonresponsive to typical antipanic agents, responded to valproate with amelioration of panic attacks.

PD and asthma

There is a strong relationship between panic and asthma. Asthma is a reversible airway obstructive disease characterized by airway inflammation and hyperreactive airways. An asthmatic attack involves wheezing, shortness of breath, cough and congestion, and hyperventilation. The panic–asthma association has implications for the suffocation false alarm hypothesis of panic neurobiology postulated by Klein (1993). Chronic hyperventilation may ultimately sensitize CO_2 centers in the brain stem, leading to exaggerated physiological and behavioral responses to changes in CO_2.

Though there is a degree of phenomenological overlap, the panic attack and the asthma attack are not identical. Schmaling and Bell (1997) compared 71 patients with PD without medical illness and 71 patients with asthma. They found that clusters of symptoms reflecting panic fear, hyperventilation and hypocapnia were more strongly endorsed by subjects with PD, whereas airway obstruction symptom clusters were more prominent in asthma attacks. Experientially, there are important differences between panic and asthma. Asthma is often felt as a difficulty with getting air out of the lungs, while panic is felt as a difficulty getting air into the lungs.

Asthma is a highly anxiety provoking illness. Carr (1999) found that 22.6% of asthmatics report having experienced panic attacks and 9.7% report PD. Yellowlees *et al.* (1987) and Shavitte *et al.* (1992) reported a lifetime prevalence of PD in asthmatics ranging from 6.5% to 24%, which is significantly higher than that for the general population. The prevalence of PD among asthmatics is approximately 8–10 times that of the general population.

Perna *et al.* (1997) investigated the comorbidity of panic and asthma. They evaluated 51 patients with allergic asthma and assessed the prevalence of PD and sporadic panic attacks, the temporal relationship between the two disorders, and the familial risk for PD in families of asthmatics. The psychiatric disorder with the highest prevalence in their sample was PD (20%). Social phobia was next highest at 9.8%. In addition, 13 asthmatics (25.5%) had positive histories for unexpected sporadic panic attacks but did not meet criteria for PD. 45% of asthmatics experienced at least one panic attack, and 96% of these described these panic attacks as qualitatively distinct from their typical asthmatic attacks. Women also had more comorbidity than men for PD (29.6% vs. 8.3%) and panic attacks (37% vs. 12.5%). Also, the morbidity risk for PD was higher for first degree relatives of asthmatics who never had experienced panic attacks. Interestingly, 9 of 10 of asthmatics with PD had the asthmatic symptoms precede the PD, suggesting that the presence of asthma confers specific vulnerability to the development of PD.

The presence of panic and panic-fear negatively affects the course of asthma. It is associated with longer and more frequent hospitalizations. In addition, it increases the use of steroids as well as more prn medications. These effects have been shown to be due to the panic symptoms themselves and not the degree of respiratory compromise (Dirks *et al.* 1977).

Panic and irritable bowel syndrome

IBS is the most common functional GI disorder. The diagnosis of IBS involves recurrent (at least 3-month duration) of abdominal pain that often is relieved with defecation, as well as disturbed defecation at least 25% of the time, manifested by three or more of change in stool frequency, form, passage, or bloating and abdominal distension. The symptoms must occur in the absence of organic pathology, such as positive findings on laboratory evaluation or sigmoidoscopy. IBS is a chronic, debilitating condition that affects twice as many females as males and is responsible for substantial health care expenditure.

There is clear overlap between PD and IBS. Lydiard *et al.* (1993) found that of 35 patients with IBS, 94% had psychiatric illness. Of these, 66% had a current anxiety disorder and 34% had a current mood disorder. Walker *et al.* (1995) compared 71 patients with IBS and 40 patients with inflammatory bowel disease (IBD) and found that IBS patients had a much higher prevalence of current (28%) and lifetime PD (41%). A previous study by the same group (Walker *et al.* 1990) found that 29% of IBS patients had PD. Analysis of the ECA data showed that persons with PD had the highest rates of unexplained GI symptoms.

Kaplan *et al.* (1996) studied the prevalence of IBS in a sample of 41 PD outpatients seeking treatment in a general medical office. Of these, 46.3% met criteria for full IBS and 8% met criteria for partial IBS. Patients with panic and IBS reported more personal history of back pain compared to panickers without IBS. Panic preceded the IBS in 10 patients and followed it in 8 patients.

Lydiard *et al.* (1994) assessed the prevalence of GI symptoms from the somatization section of the Diagnostic Interview Schedule (DIS) used in the ECA study. A total of 194 persons were identified as having PD. GI symptoms were reported more frequently by subjects with PD than by those without PD. Individuals with PD had the highest rate of endorsing GI symptoms compared with any other psychiatric disorder. There was a 4.6-fold greater risk for persons with PD to have IBS-like symptoms than those without PD. The results remained significant when 10 patients meeting criteria for somatization disorder were removed from the analysis. The results were also similar in patients who did not meet criteria for PD, but were experiencing panic attacks. The IBS symptoms were more likely to be present in patients with current or recent PD, rather than occurring as an antecedent or consequence of PD. This study did not include GI symptoms that were already part of the diagnostic criteria for panic attacks, thus suggesting true diagnostic overlap between the two disorders.

Panic and noncardiac chest pain

A striking number of chest pain patients who present

to emergency departments or who are referred for angiography and have normal angiograms have a diagnosis of PD. Panic attacks can mimic the symptoms of acute coronary insufficiency, leading to costly and unnecessary medical evaluations and prolonged mismanagement of underlying panic.

Katon *et al.* (1988) studied 74 patients with chest pain and no previous history of coronary artery disease (CAD). He found that 12 of 28 patients with normal angiograms (43%) met PD criteria; in contrast 6.5% of patients with positive angiograms had PD. Beitman *et al.* (1989) studied 94 chest pain patients with normal cardiac angiographies. He found 32 of 94 (34%) met the diagnosis for PD. Beitman *et al.* (1987) also studied 103 patients with atypical or nonanginal chest pain patients from a cardiology clinic and found that 59 (57%) met PD criteria.

Panic and cardiac illness

PD overlaps considerably with true cardiac illness. It is especially prominent in patients with documented CAD. Morris *et al.* (1997) evaluated the comorbidity of PD with heart disease and prevalence of PD in 128 outpatients presenting to cardiologists. They found that 16 patients (12%) met the criteria for PD, and 73 patients (57%) were determined to have actual cardiac illness; of these, 10 patients (14%) had PD. Basha *et al.* (1989) examined 49 CAD patients and found 13 (27%) with a diagnosis of PD.

Chernen *et al.* (1995) found that of 18 patients with CAD determined by exercise electrocardiogram (ECG) thallium studies, two (11%) had PD. Goldberg *et al.* (1990) estimated the prevalence of PD in 414 cardiology outpatients. Of the 310 patients that participated, 104 (34%) of the patients had definite or probable PD. Of these patients, 34% had evidence of CAD.

Carter *et al.* (1992) studied chest pain patients admitted to the coronary care unit (CCU). They found that one-third met the criteria for PD. Seventy-nine percent of these had no evidence of CAD, and 21% of these patients had actual CAD.

Fleet *et al.* (1998) examined PD prevalence in 250 patients presenting to an emergency department with noncardiac chest pain. All patients underwent a structured psychiatric interview and completed psychological scales. Seventy-four of these patients had actual CAD, and of these 74 a total of 25 (34%) met the criteria for current PD. Self report measures of psychological distress or disability were not different between CAD

patients with PD and those without PD. Thus, the presence of PD may actually mask underlying CAD.

PD and cigarette smoking

A growing body of evidence suggests that cigarette smoking is closely connected to the phenomenon of panic. The available research suggests that smoking may antecede panic, and subsequently affect the clinical course, particularly age of onset, and the symptom profile.

Amering *et al.* (1999) surveyed 102 PD patients, 31 of whom had PD with agoraphobia. Eighty-two percent of the patients were current or ex-smokers. Seventy-three percent of these patients smoked in excess of 20 cigarettes per day. At the time of onset of PD, 72% of the patients had been smokers. Patients who were smokers at the onset of the illness, when compared to patients who were nonsmokers at the onset, did not differ in terms of duration of illness of presence of agoraphobia. Interestingly, smoking was associated with a significantly earlier onset of the illness compared to the nonsmoking group.

Breslau and Klein (1999) estimated the risk for onset of panic attacks associated with prior smoking, as well as the risk of smoking onset with prior panic. The authors analysed data from two epidemiologic studies, the Epidemiologic Study of Young Adults in South-east Michigan ($N = 1007$) and the NCS Tobacco Supplement ($N = 4411$). Daily smoking was associated with increased risk for first time occurrence of panic attack; the risk for first panic attack was higher in active than in past smokers. There was no evidence that prior panic attacks increased the risk for daily smoking. The authors suggest that lung disease may be a potential mechanism whereby smoking induces panic.

Johnson *et al.* (2000) examined a sample of 688 youths at the mean age of 16 years and again at the mean age of 22 years. Heavy cigarette smoking (>20 cigarettes per day) was associated with a higher risk of PD, agoraphobia, and generalized anxiety disorder after controlling for several potentially confounding factors, such as temperament, substance abuse, adolescent anxiety and depression, and parental smoking, education, and psychopathology. Evidence was not found for an effect in the reverse direction; that is, anxiety disorders in adolescence were not associated with cigarette smoking in adulthood.

Biber and Alkin (1999) found that out of 51 PD patients, 37 (73%) of patients had a history of smoking, and 14 (27%) had never smoked. The lifetime smoking habits revealed that for 21 (75%) of patients in the respiratory symptom subgroup and 16 (70%) in the nonrespiratory symptom subgroup, smoking preceded the onset of PD. Cigarette consumption in the respiratory subgroup was greater (12.5 package years) than that in the nonrespiratory symptom subgroup (mean = 4.83 package years). In addition, the mean duration of smoking was longer in the respiratory symptom subgroup (150.21 months) versus the nonrespiratory symptom subgroup (120.39).

Conclusion

PD has evolved considerably from its original formulation as a relatively unitary disorder into a more heterogeneous "syndrome," encompassing a range of symptom profiles and unique associations with specific psychiatric and medical conditions. The complexity of this syndrome highlights the severity of panic and suggests that its diagnosis can only be enabled by careful, comprehensive evaluation. Recognition and study of varying aspects of the panic spectrum will shed important light on its underlying neurobiology and ultimately inform the development of novel treatments.

References

American Psychiatric Association (APA) (1980) *Diagnostic Statistical Manual of Mental Disorders*, 3rd edn. American Psychiatric Association, Washington, D.C.

American Psychiatric Association (APA) (1994) *Diagnostic Statistical Manual of Mental Disorders*, 4th edn. American Psychiatric Association, Washington, D.C.

Amering, M., Bankier, B., Berger, P., Griengl, H., Windhaber, J. & Katschnig, H. (1999) Panic disorder and cigarette smoking behavior. *Compr Psychiatry* 40, 35–8.

Amering, M., Katschnig, H., Berger, P. et al. (1997) Embarassment about the first panic attack predicts agoraphobia in panic disorder patients. *Behav Res Ther* 35, 517–21.

Argyle, N. & Roth, M. (1989) The phenomenological study of 90 patients with panic disorder: part 2. *Psychiatric Developments* 3, 187–209.

Aronson, T. & Logue, C. (1987) On the longitudinal course of panic disorder. *Compr Psychiatry* 28, 344–55.

Baetz, M. & Bowen, R. (1998) Efficacy of divalproex sodium in patients with panic disorder and mood instability who have not responded to conventional therapy. *Can J Psychiatry* 43, 73–7.

Basha, I., Mukerji, P. & Langevin, V. (1989) Atypical angina in patients with coronary artery disease suggests panic disorder. *Int J Psych Med* 19, 341–6.

Beck, J., Shipherd, J. & Ohtake, P. (2000) Do panic symptom profiles influence response to a hypoxic challenge in patients with panic disorder? A preliminary report. *Psychosomatic Medicine* 62(5), 678–83.

Beitman, B., Basha, I. & Flaker, G. (1987) Atypical or nonanginal chest pain. Panic disorder or coronary artery disease? *Arch Intern Med* 147, 1548–52.

Beitman, B., Kusher, M. & Grossberg, G. (1991) Late onset panic disorder: evidence from a study of patients with chest pain and normal cardiac evaluations. *Int J Psychiatry Med* 21(2), 29–35.

Beitman, B., Mukerji, V. & Lamberti, J. (1989) Panic disorder in patients with chest pain and angiographically normal coronary arteries. *Am J Cardiol* 63, 1399–403.

Biber, B. & Alkin, T. (1999) Panic disorder subtypes: differential response to CO_2 challenge. *Am J Psychiatry* 156, 739–44.

Biederman, J., Rosenbaum, J., Bolduc-Murphy, E. et al. (1993) A 3-year follow up of children with and without behavioral inhibition. *J Am Acad Child Adolesc Psychiatry* 32(4), 814–21.

Breslau, N. & Klein, D. (1999) Smoking and panic attacks. *Arch Gen Psychiatry* 56, 1141–7.

Briggs, A., Stretch, D. & Brandon, S. (1993) Subtyping of panic disorder by symptom profile. *Br J Psychiatry* 163, 201–9.

Brown, C., Schulberg, H., Madonia, M., Shear, M. & Houck, M. (1996) Treatment outcomes for primary care patients with major depression and lifetime anxiety disorders. *Am J Psychiatry* 153, 1293–300.

Campbell, J.D. (1953) *Manic Depressive Disease: Clinical and Psychiatric Significance.* J.B. Lippincott, Philadelphia.

Carr, R. (1999) Panic disorder and asthma. *J Asthma* 36(2), 143–52.

Carter, C., Maddock, R., Amsterdam, E. et al. (1992) Panic disorder and chest pain in the coronary care unit. *Psychosomatics* 33(3), 302–9.

Caspi, A., Moffit, T. & Newman, D. (1996) Behavioral observations at age 3 years predict adult psychiatric disorders: longitudinal evidence from a birth cohort. *Arch Gen Psychiatry* 53(11), 1033–9.

Chen, Y. & Dilsaver, S. (1995) Comorbidity of panic disorder in bipolar illness: evidence from the Epidemiological Catchment Area Survey. *Am J Psychiatry* 13, 633–49.

Chernen, L., Friedman, S. & Goldberg, N. (1995) Cardiac disease and non cardiac chest pain: factors leading to disability. *Cardiology* 86, 15–21.

Coryell, W., Endicott, J., Andreason, N., Keller, M., Clayton, P. & Hirschfield, R. (1988) Depression and panic attacks. *Am J Psychiatry* 145, 293–300.

Cox, B., Swinson, R., Endler, N. & Norton, G. (1994) The symptom structure of panic attacks. *Compr Psychiatry* 35, 349–53.

Craske, M. & Barlow, D. (1989) Nocturnal panic. *J Nerv Ment Dis* 177, 160–7.

Craske, M., Poulton, R., Tsao, J. *et al.* (2001) Paths to panic disorder/agoraphobia: an exploratory analysis from age 3 to 21 in an unselected birth cohort. *J Am Acad Child Adolec Psychiatry* **40**, 556–63.

Dirks, J., Jones, N. & Kinsman, R. (1977) Panic fear: a personality dimension related to intractability in asthma. *Psychosom Med* **39**(2), 120–6.

Fava, G., Grandi, S. & Canestrari, R. (1988) Prodromal symptoms in panic disorder with agoraphobia. *Am J Psychiatry* **145**, 1564–7.

Fawcett, J., Scheftner, W., Fogg, L. *et al.* (1987) Clinical predictors of suicide in patients with major affective disorders: a controlled prospective study. *Am J Psychiatry* **144**, 35–40.

Fleet, R., Dupuis, G. & Marchand, A. (1998) Panic disorder in coronary artery disease patients with noncardiac chest pain. *J Psychosom Res* **44**, 15–21.

Garvey, M. & Tuason, V. (1984) The relationship of panic disorder to agoraphobia. *Compr Psychiatry* **25**, 529–31.

Gittelman, R. & Klein, D. (1984) Relationship between separation anxiety and panic and agoraphobic disorders. *Psychopathology* **17**, 56–65.

Goisman, R., Warshaw, M., Stekete, G. *et al.* (1995) DSM-IV and the disappearance of agoraphobia without a history of panic disorder. New data on a controversial diagnosis. *Am J Psychiatry* **152**, 1438–43.

Goldberg, R., Morris, F. & Christian, P. (1990) Panic disorder in cardiac outpatients. *Psychosomatics* **31**, 168–73.

Grunhaus, L., Pande, A., Brown, M. & Greden, J. (1994) Clinical characteristics of patients with concurrent major depressive disorder and panic disorder. *Am J Psychiatry* **151**, 541–6.

Horwath, E., Lish, J., Johnson, J., Hornig, C. & Weissman, M. (1993) Agoraphobia without panic: clinical reappraisal of an epidemiologic finding. *Am J Psychiatry* **150**, 1496–501.

Johnson, J., Cohen, P., Pine, D. *et al.* (2000) Association between cigarette smoking and anxiety disorders during adolescence and early adulthood. *JAMA* **284**, 2348–51.

Kagan, J., Reznick, J., Snidman, N. & Garcia-Coll, C. (1984) Behavioral inhibition to the unfamiliar. *Child Dev* **55**, 2212–25.

Kaplan, D., Masand, P. & Gupta, S. (1996) The relationship between irritable bowel syndrome and panic disorder. *Ann Clin Psychiatry* **8**, 81–8.

Katerndahl, D. (1990) Infrequent and limited symptom panic attacks. *J Nerv Ment Dis* **178**, 313–17.

Katerndahl, D. (1999) Progression of limited symptom attacks. *Depress Anxiety* **9**, 138–40.

Katerndahl, D. & Realini, J. (1993) Lifetime prevalence of panic states. *Am J Psychiatry* **150**, 246–9.

Katerndahl, D. & Realini, J. (1998) Associations with subsyndromal panic and the validity of DSM-IV criteria. *Depress Anxiety* **8**(1), 33–8.

Katon, W., Hall, M. & Russo, J. (1988) Chest pain: relationship of psychiatric illness to coronary arteriographic results. *Am J Med* **84**, 1–9.

Keller, F. (1996) Suicidal ideation in depressed patients with concomitant anxiety symptoms. *J Psychiatric Prac* **23**, 135–8.

Keller, M. & Hanks, D. (1995) Anxiety symptom relief in depression treatment outcomes. *J Clin Psychiatry* **56** (Suppl. 6), 22–9.

Kessler, R., McGonagle, K., Zhao, S., Nelson, C., Hughes, M. & Eshelman, S. (1997) Lifetime and 12 month prevalence of DSM-III-R psychiatric disorders in the National Comorbidity Survey. *Arch Gen Psychiatry* **54**, 313–21.

King, M., Schmaling, K., Cowley, D. & Dunner, D. (1995) Suicide attempt history in depressed patients with and without a history of panic attacks. *Compr Psychiatry* **36**, 25–30.

Klein, D. (1964) Delineation of two drug responsive anxiety syndromes. *Psychopharmacologia* **5**, 397–408.

Klein, D. (1981) Anxiety reconceptualized. In: *Anxiety New Research and Changing Concepts* (D. Klein & J. Rabkin (eds), pp. 235–63). Raven Press, New York.

Klein, D. (1993) False suffocation alarms, spontaneous panics and related conditions: an integrative hypothesis. *Arch Gen Psychiatry* **50**, 306–17.

Klein, D., Mannuzza, S., Chapman, T. *et al.* (1992) Child panic revisited. *J Am Acad Child Adolesc Psychiatry* **31**(1), 112–14.

Krystal, J., Woods, S., Hill, C. & Charney, D. (1991) Characteristics of panic attack subtypes: assessment of spontaneous panic, situational panic, sleep panic, and limited symptom attacks. *Compr Psychiatry* **32**, 474–80.

Labatte, L., Pollack, M., Otto, M., Langenhauer, S. & Rosenbaum, J. (1994) Sleep panic attacks: an association with childhood anxiety and adult psychopathology. *Biol Psychiatry* **36**, 57–60.

Langs, G., Quehenberger, F., Fabisch, K. *et al.* (2000) The development of agoraphobia in panic disorder: a predictable process? *J Affect Disord* **58**(1), 43–50.

Lecrubier, Y. & Ustun, T. (1998) Panic and depression: a worldwide primary care perspective. *Int Clin Psychopharmacol* **13** (Suppl. 4), 7–11.

Lelliot, P., Marks, I., McNamee, G. & Tobena, A. (1989) Onset of panic disorder with agoraphobia: towards an integrated model. *Arch Gen Psychiatry* **46**, 1000–4.

Lipsitz, J., Martin, L., Mannuzza, S. *et al.* (1994) Childhood separation anxiety disorder in patients with adult anxiety disorder. *Am J Psychiatry* **151**, 927–9.

Lydiard, B., Fossey, M., Marsh, W. & Ballenger, J. (1993) Prevalence of psychiatric disorders in patients with the irritable bowel syndrome. *Psychosomatics* **34**, 229–34.

Lydiard, B., Greenwald, S., Weissman, M. *et al.* (1994) Panic disorder and gastrointestinal symptoms: findings from the NIMH epidemiologic catchment area project. *Am J Psychiatry* **151**, 64–70.

Mackinnon, D., Xu, J., McMahon, F. *et al.* (1998) Bipolar disorder and panic disorder in families: an analysis of chromosome 18 data. *Am J Psychiatry* **155**(6), 829–31.

Mackinnon, D., Xu, J., McMahon, F. *et al.* (1997) Panic disorder with familial bipolar disorder. *Biol Psychiatry* **42**, 90–5.

McNally, R. (1994) *Panic Disorder*. The Guilford Press, New York.

Mellman, T. & Uhde, T. (1989) Sleep panic attacks: new clinical findings and theoretical implications. *Am J Psychiatry* **146**, 1204–7.

Mellman, T. & Uhde, T. (1990) Sleep in panic and generalized anxiety disorders. In: *Neurobiology of Panic Disorder* (J.C. Ballenger (ed.), 365–76). Wiley Liss, New York.

Morris, A., Baker, B. & Devins, G. (1997) Prevalence of panic disorder in cardiac outpatients. *Can J Psychiatry* **42**, 185–90.

Norton, G., Norton, P., Walker, J., Cox, B. & Stein, M. (1999) A comparison of people with and without nocturnal panic attacks. *J Behav Ther Exp Psychiatry* **30**, 37–44.

Otto, M., Pollack, M., Rosenbaum, J. *et al.* (1994) Childhood history of anxiety in adults with panic disorder: association with anxiety sensitivity and comorbidity. *Harv Rev Psychiatry* **15**, 288–93.

Papp, L., Martinez, J., Klein, D. *et al.* (1997) Respiratory psychophysiology of panic disorder: three respiratory challenges in 98 subjects. *Am J Psychiatry* **154**(11), 1557–65.

Perna, G., Bertani, A., Politi, E. *et al.* (1997) Asthma and panic attacks. *Biol Psychiatry* **42**(7), 625–30.

Pini, S., Cassano, G., Simonini, E., Savini, M., Russo, A. & Montgomery, S. (1997) Prevalence of anxiety disorders comorbidity in bipolar depression, unipolar depression and dysthymia. *J Affect Disord* **42**, 145–53.

Placidi, G., Oquendo, M., Malone, K. *et al.* (2000) Anxiety in major depression: relationship to suicide attempts. *Am J Psychiatry* **157**, 1614–18.

Pollack, M., Otto, M., Sabatino, S. *et al.* (1996) Relationship of childhood anxiety to adult PD. Correlates and influence on course. *Am J Psychiatry* **153**, 376–81.

Raj, B., Corvea, M. & Dagon, E. (1993) The clinical characteristics of panic disorder in the elderly: a retrospective study. *J Clin Psychiatry* **54**(4), 150–5.

Raskin, M., Peeke, H., Dickman, W. & Pinsker, H. (1982) Panic and generalized anxiety disorders. Developmental antecedents and precipitants. *Arch Gen Psychiatry* **39**, 687–9.

Rosenbaum, J. (1987) Limited symptom panic attacks: mixed and masked diagnosis. *Psychosomatics* **28**, 407–12.

Rosenbaum, J., Biederman, J., Gersten, M. *et al.* (1988) Behavioral inhibition in children of parents with panic disorder and agoraphobia: a controlled study. *Arch Gen Psychiatry* **45**, 463–70.

Rosenbaum, J., Biederman, J., Hirschfeld-Becker, D. *et al.* (2000) A controlled study of behavioral inhibition in children of parents with panic disorder and depression. *Am J Psychiatry* **157**, 2002–10.

Roth, M. (1984) Agoraphobia, panic disorder and generalized anxiety disorder: some implications of recent advances. *Psychiatric Developments* **2**, 31–52.

Roy-Byrne, P., Stang, P., Wittchen, H., Ustun, B. & Walters, E. (2000) Lifetime panic-depression comorbidity in the National Comorbidity Survey. *Br J Psychiatry* **176**, 229–35.

Scheibe, G. & Albus, M. (1994) Prospective follow up study lasting 2 years in patients with panic disorder with and without depressive disorders. *Eur Arch Psychiatry Clin Neurosci* **244**, 39–44.

Schmaling, K. & Bell, J. (1997) Asthma and panic disorder. *Arch Fam Med* **6**(1), 20–3.

Segui, J., Salvador-Carulla, L., Marquez, M. *et al.* (2000) Differential clinical features of late-onset panic disorder. *J Affect Disord* **57**, 115–24.

Shulman, I., Cox, B., Swinson, R. *et al.* (1994) Precipitating events, locations and reactions associated with initial unexpected panic attacks. *Behav Res Ther* **32**, 17–20.

Sinha, S., Papp, L., Gorman, J. (2000) How study of respiratory physiology aided our understanding of abnormal brain function in panic disorder. *J Affect Disord* **61**(3), 191–200.

Stein, M., Tancer, M. & Uhde, T. (1990) Major depression in patients with panic disorder: factors associated with course and recurrence. *J Affect Disord* **19**, 287–96.

Thyer, B. & Himle, J. (1985) Temporal relationship between panic attack onset and phobic avoidance in agoraphobia. *Behav Res Ther* **23**, 607–8.

Uhde, T., Boulenger, J., Geraci, H., Vittone, B. & Post, R. (1985) Longitudinal course of panic disorder. *Prog Neuropsychopharmacol Biol Psychiatry* **9**, 39–51.

Van Valkenburg, C., Akiskal, H., Puzantian, V. & Rosenthal, T. (1984) Anxious depressions. *J Affect Disord* **6**, 67–82.

Walker, E., Gelfand, A., Gelfand, M. *et al.* (1995) Psychiatric diagnoses, sexual and physical victimization and disability in patients with irritable bowel syndrome or inflammatory bowel disease. *Psychol Med* **25**(6), 1259–67.

Walker, E., Roy-Byrne, P., Katon, W., Li, L., Amos, D. & Jiranek, G. (1990) Psychiatric illness and irritable bowel syndrome: a comparison with inflammatory bowel disease. *Am J Psychiatry* **147**, 1656–61.

Warshaw, M., Massion, A., Peterson, L. *et al.* (1995) Suicidal behavior in patients with panic disorder: retrospective and prospective data. *J Affect Disord* **34**, 235–47.

Yellowlees, P., Alpers, J., Bowden, J., Bryant, G. & Ruffin, R. (1987) Psychiatric morbidity in patients with chronic airflow obstruction. *Med J Aust* **146**, 305–7.

Young, L., Cooke, R., Robb, J., Levitt, A. & Joffe, R. (1993) Anxious and nonanxious bipolar disorder. *J Affect Disord* **29**, 49–52.

4 Generalized Anxiety Disorder

J. Monnier & O. Brawman-Mintzer

Introduction

Anxiety disorders, in general, are the most common form of mental illness in the US (DuPont *et al.* 1996). Generalized anxiety disorder (GAD) is one of the most common anxiety disorders, with a lifetime prevalence of 5.1% in the adult US population (Kessler *et al.* 1994). GAD typically occurs before the age of 40, runs a chronic, fluctuating course, and affects women twice as often as men (American Psychiatric Association, APA, 1994; Walley *et al.* 1994). Despite historic controversy to the contrary, numerous studies have demonstrated that GAD is a distinct illness, which occurs at a significant rate with serious consequences (Noyes *et al.* 1987; Rickels & Schweizer 1990; Kendler *et al.* 1992; Noyes *et al.* 1992; Brown *et al.* 1994; Wittchen *et al.* 1994). Additionally, GAD has been found to confer disability at approximately the same level as depression and other chronic medical illnesses (Kessler *et al.* 1999).

With such a high prevalence rate and serious consequences, GAD should be an important concern for health care providers. Unfortunately, anxiety symptoms often go unnoticed, especially in primary care settings (Kessler *et al.* 1994). In this chapter, we present information on diagnosis, epidemiology, comorbidity, differential diagnosis, course, social impact, and pathogenesis of GAD, with the intention that this information will promote efforts to detect and treat GAD in individuals seeking mental health and medical treatment alike.

Diagnosis

It is probably safe to say that, of all anxiety disorders,

the diagnostic criteria for GAD have been revised most frequently. As defined in the recent version of the Diagnostic Statistical Manual (DSM-IV: APA 1994), GAD diagnosis differs considerably from the preceding definitions.

The entity of general anxiety was originally conceptualized by Freud, who coined the term "anxiety neurosis." This term, as originally defined, included four major clinical syndromes: general irritability, chronic apprehension/anxious expectation, anxiety attacks, and secondary phobic avoidance (Freud 1957). Over time, this definition has evolved into numerous, separate anxiety disorders, one of them being GAD.

Both the first edition of DSM (DSM-I: APA 1952) and the second edition of DSM (DSM-II: APA 1968) used the term neurosis in referring to anxiety disorders and presented conceptualizations for all psychopathology as stemming from such neuroses. Following the publication of the DSM-II, Feighner *et al.* (1972) published diagnostic criteria for use in psychiatric research, in an effort to improve the reliability and validity of these diagnoses. Unlike the previous DSM criteria, the role of neurosis in psychopathology was not viewed as primary. With the revision of DSM-II into DSM-III (APA 1980), these research criteria were incorporated in the diagnostic criteria for anxiety. By the time DSM-IV was published, reference to neurosis was eliminated altogether (APA 1994).

The term GAD was introduced in the DSM-III, which evolved from the anxiety neurosis category in DSM-II that included two core components: panic symptoms and generalized symptoms of anxiety (APA 1968). In the DSM-III, a diagnosis of GAD required uncontrollable and diffuse anxiety or worry that was excessive or unrealistic in relation to objective life circumstance that persisted for 1 month or more. In addition, several psychophysiological symptoms were required to occur with the anxiety or worry. These symptoms needed to be present for the duration of 1 month for a diagnosis of GAD to be met. Finally, the diagnosis of GAD could not be assigned if subjects met criteria for another mental disorder. Early clinical studies evaluating GAD according to the DSM-III definition found that the disorder seldom occurred in the absence of some other anxiety or mood disorder. The comorbidity between GAD and major depression was especially strong (Breslau 1985; Breslau & Davis 1985a). Due to this high comorbidity, it was suggested that GAD would be better conceptualized as a prodrome, residual, or severity maker than as an independent disorder (Breslau & Davis 1985b; Clayton *et al.* 1991; Noyes *et al.* 1992). However, the comorbidity of GAD with other disorders was found to decrease as the duration of GAD increased (Breslau & Davis 1985a). Based on this finding, the DSM-III-R (APA 1987) committee on GAD recommended that the duration requirement for the disorder be increased to six months. This change was implemented in the DSM-III-R (APA 1987). In addition, the hierarchical exclusion rules were dropped in DSM-III-R, and a narrower diagnostic hierarchy rule, which required that GAD could not be assigned if occurring only during the course of a mood or psychotic disorder, was adopted.

Current DSM (DSM-IV) criteria for GAD include excessive anxiety and worry about a number of events or activities, occurring for at least 6 months (APA 1994). The worry must be difficult to control. The anxiety and worry needs to be associated with three or more of the following six symptoms: (i) restlessness or feeling keyed up or on edge; (ii) being easily fatigued; (iii) difficulty concentrating or mind going blank; (iv) irritability; (v) muscle tension; and (vi) sleep disturbance. The anxiety, worry, or physical symptoms need to cause clinically significant distress or impairment in social, occupational, or other important areas of functioning, and cannot be confined to features of other DSM IV Axis I disorders (e.g. panic disorder [PD]).

The International Classification of Disease, 10th edition (ICD-10: World Health Organization [WHO] 1993) defines GAD similarly in their Clinical Descriptions and Diagnostic Guidelines, with anxiety being generalized and persistent, and free floating. A variety of worries and a sense of foreboding also need to be present. Several months of feelings of anxiety and worry need to be present. An unspecified number of the following symptoms also need to be present: motor tension (restless, fidgeting, tension headaches, trembling, inability to relax); apprehension (worry about future, feeling "on edge", difficulty concentrating); autonomic over-activity (light-headedness, sweating, tachycardia, epigastric discomfort, dizziness, dry mouth, etc.). Additionally, in order to receive an ICD-10 diagnosis of GAD individuals must not meet full criteria for depressive episode, phobic disorder, PD, or obsessive-compulsive disorder (OCD).

More specific research diagnostic criteria (The Diagnostic Criteria for Research) were developed for the ICD-10 (WHO 1993). These research criteria increased the duration criterion from "several months" to "at least 6 months," and required the presence of at least four of 22 specific symptoms. These symptoms are divided into five groups: (i) autonomic symptoms ($N = 4$); (ii) symptoms of chest/abdomen ($N = 4$); (iii) symptoms involving mental state ($N = 4$); (iv) general symptoms ($N = 6$); and (v) nonspecific symptoms ($N = 4$).

Some believe that the ICD-10's diagnostic criteria is more accurate than the DSM-IV, lacking the DSM's excessive focus on worry while still listing "apprehension" as one of anxiety's key symptoms (Rickels & Rynn 2001). Evidence suggests that worry may not be the most important discriminator of GAD. For example, Bienvenue *et al.* (1998) examined the Diagnostic Interview Schedule data from the 1993 follow-up study of the Epidemiologic Catchment Area (ECA) Study (Baltimore cohort) and found that the most important differentiating factor between the ill and not ill groups was the presence of at least six associated symptoms, not worry or duration.

Epidemiology

The prevalence of anxiety disorders, as assessed prior to the introduction of GAD as a separate diagnostic entity in the DSM-III, was evaluated in several epidemiological surveys in general populations. For example, the Stirling County Study (Blazer *et al.* 1991) sampled approximately 1000 subjects from Eastern Canada who were evaluated by psychiatrists on the basis of the Health Opinion Survey (HOS) and also collected information from physicians and other health-care providers. Psychiatric diagnoses were assigned according to DSM-I criteria. The overall prevalence of anxiety, with no distinction between generalized anxiety and PD, was 2.9%.

Following the introduction of DSM-III, several community-based surveys estimated the current prevalence rates for GAD at 1.2% to 6.4% with a lifetime prevalence of 4% to 6.6%. Using the Schedule for Affective Disorders and Schizophrenia (SADS), 720 individuals were evaluated for specific psychiatric disorders in New Haven, Connecticut, between 1975 and 1976 (Weissman *et al.* 1978). Psychiatric diagnoses were assigned based on Research Diagnostic Criteria (RDC). Results from this survey of a US urban community found that 2.4% of the population had a current diagnosis of GAD. It is important to note that over 80% of the subjects who met positive criteria for GAD in this study would have been excluded had DSM-III criteria been used, because they also met criteria for phobic disorder, PD, or OCD.

In the first study to estimate the prevalence rates of DSM-III disorders on a national scale, 1-year prevalence rates of major depression, agoraphobia-panic, GAD, and other phobias in a large sample (3161 household interviews) were evaluated in a 1979 National Survey of psychotherapeutic drug use (Uhlenhuth *et al.* 1983). The authors developed a method for classifying survey respondents by DSM-III-compatible syndromes using the modified Hopkins Symptom Checklist. GAD was found to be the most common psychiatric disorder, with a 1-year prevalence of 6.4%.

In the first DSM-III-based longitudinal epidemiological study, a cohort of 292 males and 299 females aged 19–20 years were evaluated from the Canton of Zurich in Switzerland in 1979, 1981, and 1986 (Angst & Vollrath 1991) using the 90-item Hopkins Symptom Checklist and a semistructured interview. One-year prevalence for GAD appeared stable, with a 2.0% prevalence in 1979, 1.3% in 1981, and 1.9% in 1986.

The ECA Study was a five-center epidemiological study of the prevalence of DSM-III psychiatric disorders in the US (Blazer *et al.* 1991). Interviews were conducted using the Diagnostic Interview Schedule on more than 20 000 community and institutionalized adults. GAD was assessed in only three of the five ECA sites (Durham, NC, St. Louis, MO, and Los Angeles, CA). The data indicated that GAD was a common disorder with reported lifetime prevalence of 4.1% to 6.6%.

Two small regional epidemiological studies reported the prevalence of DSM-III-R GAD. Faravelli *et al.* (1989) evaluated prevalence of GAD in a population survey (1100 interviews) of Florence, Italy. Prevalence rates of 2% and 3.9% were found for current and lifetime GAD, respectively. In the second study, Wacker *et al.* (1992) reported a 1.9% lifetime prevalence of GAD in a population in Basel, Switzerland. Prevalence rates of GAD as diagnosed with the DSM-III-R and the ICD-10 were also compared in this study. Using the ICD-10 criteria, lifetime prevalence of GAD (9.2%) was found to be over four times higher than that found using the DSM-III-R. The authors argued that this may be due to the ICD-10's broader definition of worrying and the ICD-10 requirement of only four associated somatic symptoms versus six symptoms in DSM-III-R.

The most recent epidemiological survey of DSM-III-R GAD was conducted as a part of the National Comorbidity Survey of psychiatric disorders in the US by Kessler and colleagues (Kessler *et al.* 1994; Wittchen *et al.* 1994). The Composite International Diagnostic Interview, a structured psychiatric interview, was administered to a representative national sample and evaluated lifetime and 12-month prevalence of 14 DSM-III-R psychiatric disorders. Prevalence rates in the total sample (*N* = 8098) were 1.6% for current GAD (defined as the most recent 6-month period of anxiety), 3.1% for 12-month GAD, and 5.1% for lifetime GAD. These rates were higher than those for PD, and again, when ICD-10 criteria were used, the lifetime prevalence of GAD was considerably higher (8.9%).

The prevalence of GAD appears to be even higher in clinical settings, particularly in primary care settings. For example, Shear *et al.* (1994, Meeting of the Association for Primary Care) found prevalence rates of GAD, reported by patients at four primary care centers, to be twice as high as those reported in community samples (i.e. 10% vs. 5.1%). Another study found a prevalence rate of 2.9% for GAD, indicating that GAD was the most common anxiety disorder observed in the primary care setting (Barrett *et al.* 1988). Similarly, a collaborative study by WHO in primary care settings across 15 international sites reported prevalence rates of GAD at approximately 8% (Sartorius *et al.* 1996).

In addition to high rates of treatment seeking in the primary care setting, those with GAD also seek treatment specifically for GAD at high rates. For example, those meeting criteria for GAD in the ECA study reported receiving more outpatient mental services during the previous year than those diagnosed with other psychiatric disorders (Blazer *et al.* 1991). The

National Comorbidity Survey demonstrated that a large portion of individuals with GAD sought professional help for GAD (66% of participants), and used medications to reduce their symptoms of GAD (44% of participants; Wittchen *et al.* 1994). Similarly, the Harvard/Brown Anxiety disorders Research Program (HARP) data indicated over 80% of the GAD group received psychotherapy and/or pharmacotherapy (Yonkers *et al.* 1996).

Rates of GAD appear similar in special populations such as children and the elderly. For example, Anderson and colleagues (Anderson *et al.* 1987) reported a 1-year prevalence rate of 2.9% for overanxious anxiety disorder. In a community sample of 150 adolescents, Kashani and Orvaschel (1988) found a 6-month prevalence of 7.3% for overanxious disorder. The prevalence of childhood overanxious anxiety disorder appears to be even higher in a clinical setting, with up to 52% of the sampled children seen meeting criteria for the disorder (Last *et al.* 1987). It should be mentioned that in DSM-IV the diagnosis of childhood overanxious anxiety disorder was subsumed within the diagnosis of GAD. Epidemiological data on prevalence of GAD in childhood using DSM-IV criteria are lacking. In the elderly, GAD appears to account for the majority of anxiety disorders, with prevalence rates ranging from 0.7% to 7.3% (Flint 1994; Beekman *et al.* 1998).

Clinical features

Symptoms

The presence of *anxiety and worry* has been an essential part of GAD diagnosis. Worry was been further defined as *apprehensive expectation* in DSM-III-R. Without the presence of *apprehensive expectation* or *worry*, regardless of how many anxiety symptoms are present, the diagnosis of GAD cannot be made. A substantial revision between DSM-III-R and DSM-IV is the greater emphasis on the uncontrollability of worry (Brown *et al.* 1994). DSM-IV further departed from the focus on somatic symptoms. The ancillary symptoms associated with anxiety and worry have been reduced in DSM-IV to three of six symptoms reflecting motor tension and vigilance. Symptoms reflecting autonomic hyperactivity, which were present in DSM-III-R, were deleted.

The shift away from autonomic symptoms as the primary criteria has been based on studies examining symptom endorsement patterns among GAD patients.

For example, Marten *et al.* (1993) evaluated the 18 ratings that comprise the symptom criterion of DSM-III-R GAD. Endorsement rates and inter-rater reliability were calculated using interview-based ratings of patients with GAD at four study sites ($N = 204$) for each symptom. For most of the 18 symptoms, the interrater reliability analyses demonstrated high agreement. Spearman correlation in symptom endorsement revealed marked consistency across the four study sites (range 0.69–0.94). Seven "satisfactory" symptoms were identified from those meeting specific reliability and endorsement criteria: irritability, restlessness, muscle tension, difficulty concentrating, sleep difficulties, feeling keyed up, and easy fatigability. All these symptoms belong to either the motor tension or vigilance and scanning clusters of the DSM-III-R. Symptoms that belong to the autonomic hyperactivity cluster were infrequently endorsed. Thus, the authors concluded that these findings suggest that the associated symptom criterion of GAD should be revised.

In recent research, Starcevic and Bogojevic (1999) examined rates of GAD symptoms using the Structured Clinical Interview for DSM-III-R modified for DSM-IV and ICD-10 Diagnostic Criteria for Research. Because they were endorsed by large proportions of GAD patients, seven symptoms emerged in the first rank and five symptoms emerged in the second rank (see Table 4.1;

Table 4.1 First- and second-rank symptoms using the Structured Clinical Interview for the DSM-III-R modified for DSM-IV and ICD-10. (From Starcevic & Bogojevic 1999, pp. 5–11.)

First rank

An inability to relax, restlessness, or a mentally tense or "keyed-up" state
Fatigability
Exaggerated startle response
Muscle tension
Sleep disturbance
Difficulty in concentrating
Irritability

Second rank

Nausea or abdominal complaints
Perspiring
Dry mouth
Tachycardia/palpitations
Tremor

Starcevic & Bogojevic 1999). The presence of at least four of seven "first rank" symptoms and one of five "second-rank" symptoms assisted in better differentiating GAD from other anxiety disorders or depression. (Starcevic & Bogojevic 1999).

Finally, Brawman-Mintzer *et al.* (1994) compared the distribution of somatic symptoms associated with DSM-III-R GAD in 28 patients with GAD-only and 77 patients with GAD plus comorbid current or lifetime psychiatric diagnoses. No significant differences were noted in individual GAD symptom endorsement between the two groups. Thus, the authors concluded that the basic symptoms of GAD are disorder specific.

Patterns of cognitions also appear to be disorder specific. Breitholtz *et al.* (1999) used self-report of the frequency of anxiety, worry, or panic attacks among patients with GAD (*N* = 38) and PD (*N* = 36), as well as the severity of anxiety associated with each. Thirty-four percent of GAD patients' cognitions centred on interpersonal conflict or the issue of acceptance by others, while only 1.4% of PD patients reported such concerns. Patients with GAD also had exaggerated worries over relatively minor matters. PD patients, however, reported a significantly greater frequency of cognitions concerning physical dangers or catastrophes (e.g. accident, injury, death).

Onset

Epidemiology studies (Burke *et al.* 1991; Kendler *et al.* 1992) and clinical studies (Barlow *et al.* 1986; Rogers *et al.* 1999) suggest that onset of GAD typically begins between the late teens and late twenties.

Course

Retrospective and prospective reports indicate that course of GAD is chronic, persisting for a decade or longer (Angst & Vollrath 1991; Blazer *et al.* 1991; Mancuso *et al.* 1993; Noyes *et al.* 1996). HARP, a prospective, naturalistic study of 711 adults with DSM-III-R anxiety disorders, recruited initially from psychiatric clinics and hospitals in the Boston Metropolitan area, indicated that only 15% of those with GAD at baseline experienced a full remission for 2 months or longer at any time during the first year after baseline, and only 25% had a full remission in the 2 years after baseline (Yonkers *et al.* 1996). The disability associated with GAD was found to be similar to that found in individuals with PD or major depression (Kessler *et al.* 1999).

Comorbidity

As diagnostic criteria for GAD changed with the DSM-III-R, comorbid diagnoses were permitted and the high rate of comorbid psychiatric disorders with GAD was evident. Research studies conducted in relatively small treatment samples revealed that psychiatric comorbidity in GAD is very common. For example, in some studies more than 90% of GAD patients fulfilled criteria for at least one or more concurrent disorders (range of 45%–91%; Sanderson & Barlow 1990; Brawman-Mintzer *et al.* 1993). Similarly, Angst (1993) evaluated psychiatric comorbidity in a longitudinal epidemiological study in Zurich, Switzerland. Strong associations (expressed as odds ratio [OR]) between GAD and major depression (OR of an individual with GAD also having major depression of 4.2), and dysthymia (OR of 3.8) were found, but a relatively low association with PD (OR of 1.8) was found. Interestingly, the authors found high comorbidity of GAD with hypomania (OR of 3.7). The presence of comorbidity was also associated with a high suicide attempt risk (OR of 3.6). In addition, individuals with comorbid disorders were treated more frequently and endorsed more work impairment than GAD patients without comorbid disorders.

Similar findings have been reported from large epidemiological studies. For example, the National Comorbidity Survey showed 90% of respondents with lifetime GAD has at least one other lifetime disorder and of those with current GAD, 66% had at least one other current disorder (Wittchen *et al.* 1994). When DSM-III-R diagnostic hierarchy rules were applied, insignificant changes were noted (lifetime comorbidity of 89.8%, and current comorbidity of 65%). The most common comorbidities were found for mood disorders (major depression and dysthymia), PD, and (for current comorbidity only) agoraphobia.

The ECA Study found that 58% to 65% (depending on the site) of subjects who have ever suffered from GAD also have at least one other DSM-III disorder (Blazer *et al.* 1991). The highest comorbidities were with depressive disorders, and PDs (Angst 1993; Brawman-Mintzer *et al.* 1993; Fifer *et al.* 1994; Wittchen *et al.* 1994; Sartorius *et al.* 1996; Yonkers *et al.* 1996). In addition to high rates of comorbidity in those with GAD, studies suggest that GAD is often present in those diagnosed with other disorders. Rates of GAD are particularly high in those with PD and depressive disorders (Sanderson *et al.* 1990; Brown & Barlow 1992; Starcevic *et al.* 1992; Pini *et al.* 1997).

Studies examining order of onset of GAD and other comorbid disorders suggest that GAD usually has an earlier onset than other anxiety and depressive disorders (Brown & Barlow 1992). Brawman-Mintzer *et al.* (1993) found that GAD had an onset before dysthymia and PD and after simple and social phobia. Further, onset of major depression seemed to follow the onset of anxiety. Similar findings have been reported by other investigators (Fava *et al.* 1992; Massion *et al.* 1993; Kessler *et al.* 2000).

High rates of comorbidity have also been found in children and adolescents with GAD. For example, children with overanxious anxiety disorder also exhibit an unusual degree (over 50%) of comorbidity (Kashani *et al.* 1988). Among the most prevalent current comorbid diagnoses are social phobia (16% to 59%), simple (or specific) phobia (21% to 55%), PD (3% to 27%) and major depression (8%–39%). Furthermore, Masi *et al.* (1999) found, in those children and adolescents they sampled, 87% had a comorbid disorder. In particular, high rates of separation anxiety, social anxiety, and depressive disorders were found. Community samples have demonstrated similar findings (Kashani & Overschel 1990; McGee *et al.* 1990). Along these same lines, Lindesay *et al.* (1989) found a comorbidity rate of 91% in a sample of older adults with GAD.

In addition to high rates of comorbidity with other Axis I disorders, GAD also appears to co-occur with personality disorders. For example, rates of GAD and personality disorders in clinical populations have ranged from 31%–46% (Gasperini *et al.* 1990; Sanderson & Wetzler 1991; Mauri *et al.* 1992; Mavissakalian *et al.* 1993; Starcevic *et al.* 1995). These rates are similar to rates observed with other anxiety disorders (Mauri *et al.* 1992; Mavissakalian *et al.* 1993). Not surprisingly those with GAD were most likely to have Cluster C personality disorders, such as avoidant personality disorder, dependent personality disorder, and obsessive-compulsive personality disorder (Mauri *et al.* 1992; Mavissakalian *et al.* 1993).

Comorbid GAD appears to have a significant relationship to negative outcome. For example, comorbid GAD is associated with increased severity of secondary disorders (Kessler *et al.* 2000). The presence of comorbid disorders in GAD patients is related to increased rates of negative outcomes such as disability, impairment, and cost of care (Noyes *et al.* 1980; Murphy *et al.* 1986; Angst 1993; Massion *et al.* 1993; Souetre *et al.* 1994; Yonkers *et al.* 1996). For example, rates of

relapse for GAD patients with comorbid depression appear higher than in noncomorbid GAD patients (Yonkers *et al.* 1996). Further, comorbidity is also associated with greater treatment seeking (Bland *et al.* 1997). Data indicate that patients with comorbid GAD and depression may have poorer response to treatment than patients with an uncomplicated disorder (Joffe *et al.* 1993; Brown *et al.* 1996). Moreover, comorbidity in general in those with GAD impacts treatment outcome (Brown & Barlow 1992).

The frequent coexistence of more than one psychiatric disorder in an individual has important clinical and scientific implications. Specifically, the presence of more than one disorder may influence the diagnostic process, treatment response, course, and the prognosis of a disorder. Due to the high rates of comorbidity, some have suggested comorbid disorders should be taken into account to further our understanding of GAD (Maser 1998).

Differential diagnosis

Anxiety can be present as prominent feature of many psychiatric and medical conditions. In addition, the overlap of several common symptoms between GAD and other psychiatric disorders, such as major depression, as well as the substantial comorbidity with these disorders, often leads to difficulty distinguishing GAD from other disorders. This may complicate the task of differential diagnosis and treatment planning, particularly in a nonpsychiatric setting. Disorders that require consideration in the differential diagnosis of GAD are briefly discussed below.

Major depression

As mentioned, some researchers raised concerns that GAD may represent a prodromal phase of major depression. However, investigators have shown specificity at a symptom level for GAD compared with depression. Brown *et al.* (1994) found in their analysis separate latent factors of positive affectivity, negative affectivity, and autonomic suppression (related to GAD). They concluded that their findings support the notion that GAD and major depression can be distinguished despite overlap in some symptoms. Further, in contrast to major depression, which is characterized by variable presentation (such as increased vs. decreased appetite, insomnia vs.

hypersomnia, retardation vs. restlessness), GAD represents a relatively homogenous diagnostic group.

Anxiety disorders

Other anxiety disorders also require consideration in the differential diagnosis of GAD. Some researchers suggested that GAD is attributable to other anxiety disorders, such as social phobia (Mennin *et al.* 1998, 18th National Conference of Anxiety Disorders Association of America, Boston), or PD (Uhde *et al.* 1985). However, longitudinal follow-up studies, show significant stability of GAD over the years. Further research of gen-etic influences, such as candidate genes and abnormalities in specific neurotransmitter systems, together with re-search focusing on fear circuitry, will hopefully help elucidate factors influencing the different anxiety disorders.

General medical conditions

Many general medical conditions and medications may present with prominent anxiety symptoms. If not identified and properly addressed, these conditions may adversely affect the treatment outcome of the anxious patient. Such medical conditions include cardiovascular syndromes with endocrine causes, such as hyperthyroidism, hyperparathyroidism, hypoparathyroidism, pheochromocytoma, hypoglycemia, and Cushing's syndrome. These syndromes, although not very common, are possible causes of anxiety symptoms. Some neurologic conditions, such as complex partial seizures, intracranial tumors, strokes, and cerebral ischemia, may be associated with symptoms observed in GAD, and require appropriate evaluation.

Many drugs and substances commonly cause anxiety symptoms. Excessive caffeine use or withdrawal may cause significant anxiety symptoms (Bruce *et al.* 1992). The use of various commonly prescribed medications may cause side-effects manifesting as anxiety. Such medications include adrenergic agonists, bronchodilators, corticosteroids, thyroid supplements, antihypertensives, and cardiovascular medications, such as digitalis. Psychotropic medications, such as neuroleptics, and, less frequently, the selective serotonin reuptake inhibitors (SSRIs) may cause akathisia, which may be indistinguishable from anxiety.

Although alcohol withdrawal is a well-recognized cause of anxiety and agitation, sedative-hypnotic withdrawal symptoms are often underestimated as a potential cause of anxiety. The clinical phenomenology observed in alcohol and sedative-hypnotic drug withdrawal and in anxiety disorders, may be highly similar. In both conditions, nervousness, tachycardia, tremulousness, sweating, or nausea occur prominently. Further, the same drugs (e.g. benzodiazepines) may be used to treat anxiety symptoms, and alcohol may be used to alleviate anxiety. Thus, the symptoms of an underlying anxiety disorder may be difficult to differentiate from withdrawal symptoms associated with the use of these substances.

Social impact of GAD

For many years GAD was conceptualized as a "mild disorder," which received clinical attention only if a comorbid condition such as depression developed (APA 1987). However, increasingly data are indicating that GAD is a serious illness that frequently causes moderate impairment (Wittchen *et al.* 1994). The ECA study was the first to investigate risk factors and associated impairments occurring in individuals with GAD (Blazer *et al.* 1991). The ECA investigators found that DSM-III GAD (defined without the hierarchy rules) is more prevalent in women, African-Americans, and in young persons (i.e. under the age of 30). Additionally, lifetime GAD was more prevalent in urban areas, individuals in lower income brackets, but no clear association with education level was found.

Massion *et al.* (1993) examined the effects of GAD on role functioning, social life, overall functioning and emotional health ratings in a clinical population of individuals with GAD who participated in HARP. Only one-half of these individuals reported full-time employment and almost 40% reported receiving public assistance. In addition to poor occupational functioning, GAD patients reported poor social relationships, limited engagement in recreational activities, and low satisfaction with their lives. GAD, which almost universally co-occurred with other disorders, was found to be associated with a reduction in overall emotional health.

Consistent with data from the HARP study, 49% of participants diagnosed with GAD in the National Comorbidity Survey reported substantial interference with their lives due to GAD symptoms (Wittchen *et al.* 1994). Further analysis revealed that women had a higher prevalence of GAD than men, individuals who were older than 24, were previously married, unemployed, were a homemaker, and were living in the North-East of the US were significantly more likely to have a current diagnosis of GAD. The majority of individuals with GAD reported substantial interference with their lives (49% of subjects), had a high probability for seeking professional help for GAD (66% of subjects), and used medications for GAD (44% of subjects). While the presence of a comorbid disorder in subjects with GAD was associated with greater impairment in daily activities, the investigators noted that 59% of subjects with pure GAD reported similar impairment. Additionally, Kessler *et al.* (2000) found similar levels of disability between those with GAD and those with major depression.

Pathogenesis

Studies have indicated that one's vulnerability to develop GAD may be, at least in part, genetic. For example, Noyes *et al.* (1987) found that 19.5% of first-degree relatives of GAD probands developed GAD compared to only 3.5% of control subjects' families. Skre *et al.* (1994) reported similar findings with GAD being diagnosed in 22% of first-degree relatives of 33 probands with anxiety disorders. Twin studies have suggested a higher rate of concordance in monozygotic twins than dizygotic twins (Andrews *et al.* 1990; Skre *et al.* 1993). However, other studies have suggested that while genetic factors may predispose a person to GAD, unique and familial environmental factors play an important role in the development of GAD (Kendler *et al.* 1995; Scherrer *et al.* 2000), while others have found no support for the role of inheritance in GAD (Mendlewicz *et al.* 1993). Research in the area of molecular genetic studies of anxiety disorders have not yet added clarity to this debate (Jetty *et al.* 2001).

GABA$_A$ receptors and benzodiazepine receptors are thought to play an important role in GAD. Studies examining response following exposure to stressful stimuli in animal models (e.g. cold swim) have shown a decrease in benzodiazepine receptor binding in the frontal cortex, hippocampus, and hypothalamus, which are areas related to fear and anxiety (Drugan *et al.* 1989). Models using γ_2 knockout mice have shown a reduction in GABA$_A$ receptor clustering in the hippocampus and cerebral cortex, along with behavioral inhibition to aversive stimuli and increased responsiveness in

trace fear conditioning (see Chapter 13). Research with humans also supports the role of benzodiapine receptor problems in anxiety reactions (Dorow *et al.* 1987; Rickels *et al.* 1988; Ferrarese *et al.* 1990; Rocca *et al.* 1998). For example, researchers have shown low levels of peripheral lymphocyte benzodiazepine receptors, which are reversed with effective treatment (Ferrarese *et al.* 1990; Rocca *et al.* 1998). Interestingly, benzodiazepine-induced chemotaxis is also impaired in GAD patients, but is not restored with diazepam treatment (Sacerdote *et al.* 1999).

Abnormalities in the noradrenergic system (NE system) long have been implicated in the pathophysiology of anxiety disorders. However, data in GAD have been mixed and inconclusive. For example, some researchers found increased NE and free 3-methoxy-4-hydroxyphenylethylene glycol (MHPG) levels in GAD patients, and decreased presynaptic α_2-adrenoreceptors, while others did not confirm these findings (TiiMathew *et al.* 1982; Munjack *et al.* 1990; Honen *et al.* 1997). Abelson (1991) found a blunted growth hormone response to the α_2 partial agonist clonidine in GAD patients, possibly indicating presynaptic autoreceptor hypersensitivity or postsynaptic hyposensitivity in GAD. Charney *et al.* (1989) failed to find differences between GAD patients and controls in cardiovascular responses, self-rated anxiety, and plasma MHPG following challenge with the α_2-adrenergic antagonist yohimbine.

Serotonin (5-HT) system has also been shown to play a role in fear and anxiety responses in animal models (Taylor *et al.* 1985; Ramboz *et al.* 1998) and in humans (Kahn *et al.* 1991; Garvey *et al.* 1993; Iny *et al.* 1994; Garvey *et al.* 1995). Researchers demonstrated that agents that selectively impact serotonergic activity, such as the 5-HT1A agonists buspirone and gepirone decrease the firing rate of serotonergic neurones in the dorsal raphe nucleus in animal models and exert antianxiety effects in GAD patients (Tye *et al.* 1979; Engel *et al.* 1984). Further, serotonin receptor 1A (5-HT1A) knockout mice show behaviors consistent with heightened anxiety (Ramboz *et al.* 1998). In GAD subjects, Iny *et al.* (1994) have shown a decreased platelet paroxetine binding, and Garvey *et al.* (1995) found elevated urinary levels of 5-hydroxyindoleacetic acid, which predicted higher anxiety levels in GAD patients. Germine *et al.* (1992) found that the administration of *m*-chlorophenylpiperazine (mCPP) a mixed postsnaptic 5-HT agonist-antagonist, causes greater anxiety and "anger" responses in patients with GAD than in normals. Examining the role of 5-HT2 receptors, da Roza Davis *et al.* (1992) evaluated the effects of ritanserin treatment on slow wave sleep in a small number of GAD patients and normals, and found no differences between the two groups. Thus, given the available data, the question of whether overactivity or underact-ivity of the 5-HT system is the mechanism for GAD development still remains unclear (Jetty *et al.* 2001; Nutt 2001).

In recent years additional neurotransmitter systems have been examined as potentially involved in the pathogenesis of GAD. The cholecystokinin (CCK) system is one of the neuropeptides implicated in anxiety in animal models (Woodruff & Hughes 1991; Harro *et al.* 1993; Lydiard 1994). The CCK system has also been implicated in humans (Bradwejn & Koszycki 1992; Adams *et al.* 1995; Brawman-Mintzer *et al.* 1997; Goddard *et al.* 1999; Kennedy *et al.* 1999). Corticotropin-releasing factor (CRF) has been shown to contribute to behavioral responses to stress (Koob 1999). Administration on CRF to various parts of animal brains has elicited anxiety and fear responses (e.g. suppression of exploratory behavior, shock-induced freezing; Butler *et al.* 1990; Koob & Gold 1997; Griebel 1999). Koob (1999) proposed a model in which episodic or chronic stress results in increased CRF and norepinephrine (noradrenaline) interactions, resulting in an increase in overall CRF release. Evidence also suggests that neuropeptide Y (Widerlov *et al.* 1988; Boulenger *et al.* 1996; Stein *et al.* 1996; Britton *et al.* 1997) and tachykinins (Beresford *et al.* 1995) play a role in anxiety. Research has also suggested that glutamate may play a role in anxiety in both animal models and human studies (Trullas *et al.* 1989; Miserendino *et al.* 1990; Moghaddam *et al.* 1994).

Unfortunately, there have been few functional imaging studies in GAD. Data from two clinical imaging studies suggest the involvement of the occipital cortex in GAD (Buchsbaum *et al.* 1987; Wu *et al.* 1991). Wu *et al.* (1991) also found higher relative metabolic rates for GAD patients in parts of the occipital, temporal, frontal lobe, and cerebellum relative to normal controls, and a decrease in basal ganglia metabolism. The authors did not find right–left hippocampal asymmetry in GAD patients. After benzodiazepine treatment in these same patients, there was a reduction in glucose metabolism in the cortex, limbic system, and basal ganglia compared to controls. Using magnetic resonance imaging (MRI) and single photon emission computerized tomography (SPECT), Tiihonen *et al.* (1997) found that those with GAD had decreased benzodiazepine receptor binding in the left temporal pole. In the most recent study using functional MRI in GAD patients, Lorberbaum *et al.* (2001, 21st National Conference of Anxiety Disorders Association of America, Atlanta) found greater activity in the right cingulate, right medial prefrontal and orbitofrontal cortex, right temporal poles, and right dorsomedial thalamus, during periods of anticipatory anxiety, compared with rest periods, than matched control subjects. Further, only matched control subjects displayed increased activity in the medial prefronatal cortex. Overall, more data is needed to determine the central circuits of pathogenesis of GAD in humans.

Conclusions

In summary, despite the considerable heterogeneity of the diagnostic criteria among the various surveys, available data indicate that GAD is one of the most common of the anxiety disorders. Further, epidemiological surveys of community and clinical population indicate that GAD is a chronic illness, which can lead to significant morbidity. Additional work in the area of pathogenesis of GAD is needed.

Individuals suffering from GAD often experience significant distress and impairment. Additionally, those with GAD frequently seek treatment for their symptoms, whether in a mental health setting or a primary care setting. Thus, in view of the prevalence of GAD, the significant impact of the disorder, and the help-seeking behavior in primary care settings, greater attention should be devoted to educating both primary care and mental health professionals about GAD. It appears that education and specific psychiatric training for general practitioners is needed if they are to provide appropriately improved care for this patient population.

References

Abelson, J.L. (1991) Blunted growth hormone response to clonidine in patients with generalized anxiety disorder. *Arch Gen Psychiatry* 48, 157–62.

Adams, J.B., Pyke, R.E., Costa, J. *et al.* (1995) A double-blind, placebo-controlled study of a CCK-B receptor antagonist, CI-988, in patients with generalized anxiety disorder. *J Clin Psychopharmacol* **15** (6), 428–34.

American Psychiatric Association (APA) (1952) *Diagnostic Statistical Manual of Mental Disorders*, 1st edn. American Psychiatric Association, Washington, D.C.

American Psychiatric Association (APA) (1968) *Diagnostic Statistical Manual of Mental Disorders*, 2nd edn. American Psychiatric Association, Washington, D.C.

American Psychiatric Association (APA) (1980) *Diagnostic Statistical Manual of Mental Disorders*, 3rd edn. American Psychiatric Association, Washington, D.C.

American Psychiatric Association (APA) (1987) *Diagnostic Statistical Manual of Mental Disorders*, 3rd edn, revised. American Psychiatric Association, Washington, D.C.

American Psychiatric Association (APA) (1994) Adjustment disorders. In: *Diagnostic and Statistical Manual of Mental Disorders*, 4th edn (American Psychiatric Association, 623–7). American Psychiatric Association, Washington, D.C.

American Psychiatric Association (APA) (1994) *Diagnostic Statistical Manual of Mental Disorders*, 4th edn. American Psychiatric Association, Washington, D.C.

Anderson, J.C., Williams, S. & McGee, R. (1987) DSM-III disorders in preadolescent children: prevalence in a large sample from the general population. *Arch Gen Psychiatry* **44**, 69–76.

Andrews, G., Stewart, G., Allen, R. & Henderson, A.S. (1990) The genetics of six neurotic disorders: a twin study. *J Affect Disord* **19** (1), 23–9.

Angst, J. (1993) Comorbidity of anxiety, phobia, compulsion and depression. *International J Clin Psychopharmacol* **8** (Suppl. 1), 21–5.

Angst, J. & Vollrath, M. (1991) The natural history of anxiety disorder and generalized anxiety disorder. *Acta Psychiatr Scand* **141**, 572–5.

Barlow, D.H., Blanchard, R.B., Vermilyea, J.B., Vermilyea, B.B. & DiNardo, P.A. (1986) Generalized anxiety and generalized anxiety disorder: description and reconceptualization. *Am J Psychiatry* **143**, 40–4.

Barrett, J.E., Barrett, J.A., Oxman, T.E. & Gerber, P.D. (1988) The prevalence of psychiatric disorders in a primary care practice. *Arch Gen Psychiatry* **45**, 1100–6.

Beekman, A.T., Bremmer, M.A., Deeg, D.J *et al.* (1998) Anxiety disorder later in life: a report from the Longitudinal Aging Study Amsterdam. *Int J Geriatr Psychiatry* **13**(10), 717–26.

Beresford, I.J., Sheldrick, R.L., Ball, D.I. *et al.* (1995) GR159897, a potent nonpeptide antagonist at tachykinin NK2 receptors. *European Journal of Psychopharmacology* **272**(2–3), 241–8.

Bienvenue, O.J., Nestadt, G. & Eaton, W.W. (1998) Characterizing generalized anxiety: temporal and symptomatic thresholds. *J Nerv Ment Dis* **186**, 51–6.

Bland, R.C., Newman, S.C. & Orn, H. (1997) Help-seeking for psychiatric disorders. *Can J Psychiatry* **42**, 935–42.

Blazer, D.G., Hughes, D., George, L.K., Swartz, M. & Boyer, R. (1991) Generalized anxiety disorder. In: *Psychiatric Disorders in America: the Epidemiologic Catchment Area Study* (L.N. Robins & D.A. Regier (eds), pp. 180–203). The Free Press, New York.

Boulenger, J.P., Jerabek, I., Jolicoeur, F.B., Lavallee, Y.J., Leduc, R. & Cadieux, A. (1996) Elevated plasma levels of neuropeptide Y in patients with panic disorders. *Am J Psychiatry* **153**(1), 114–16.

Bradwejn, J. & Koszycki, D. (1992) The cholecystokinin hypothesis of panic and anxiety disorders: a review. *Annals of the New York Academy of Sciences* **713**, 273–82.

Brawman-Mintzer, O., Lydiard, R.B., Bradwejn, J. *et al.* (1997) Effects of the cholecystokinin agonist pentagastrin in patients with generalized anxiety disorder. *Am J Psychiatry* **154**(5), 700–2.

Brawman-Mintzer, O., Lydiard, R.B., Crawford, M.M *et al.* (1994) Somatic symptoms in generalized anxiety disorder with and without comorbid psychiatric disorders. *Am J Psychiatry* **151**, 930–2.

Brawman-Mintzer, O., Lydiard, R.B., Emmanuel, N. *et al.* (1993) Psychiatric comorbidity in patients with generalized anxiety disorder. *Am J Psychiatry* **150**, 1216–18.

Breitholtz, E., Johansson, B. & Öst, L.G. (1999) Cognitions in generalized anxiety disorder and panic disorder patients: a prospective approach. *Behav Res Ther* **37**, 533–44.

Breslau, N. (1985) Depressive symptoms, major depression and generalized anxiety: a comparison of self-reports on CES-D and results from diagnostic interviews. *Psychiatric Research* **15**, 219–29.

Breslau, N. & Davis, G.C. (1985a) DSM-III generalized anxiety disorder: an empirical investigation of more stringent criteria. *Psychiatric Research* **15**, 213–38.

Breslau, N. & Davis, G.C. (1985b) Further evidence on the doubtful validity of generalized anxiety disorder [letter]. *Psychiatric Research* **16**, 177–9.

Britton, K.T., Southerland, S., Van Uden, E., Kirby, D., Rivier, J. & Koob, G. (1997) Anxiolytic activity of NPY receptor agonists in the conflict test. *Psychopharmacology* **132**(1), 6–13.

Brown, T.A. & Barlow, D.H. (1992) Comorbidity among anxiety disorders: implications for treatment and DSM-IV. *J Consult Clin Psychol* **60**, 835–55.

Brown, T.A., Barlow, D.H. & Liebowitz, M.R. (1994) The empirical basis of generalized anxiety disorder. *Am J Psychiatry* **151**(9), 1272–80.

Brown, C., Schulberg, H.C., Madonia, M.J., Shear, M.K. & Houck, P.R. (1996) Treatment outcomes for primary care patients with major depression and lifetime anxiety disorders. *Am J Psychiatry* **153**, 1293–300.

Bruce, M., Scott, N., Shine, P. & Lader, M. (1992) Anxiogenic effects of caffeine in patients with anxiety disorders. *Arch Gen Psychiatry* **49**(11), 867–9.

Buchsbaum, M.S., Wu, J., Haier, R. et al. (1987) Positron emission tomography assessment of effects of benzodiazepines on regional glucose metabolic rate in patients with anxiety disorder. Life Sci 40(25), 2393–400.

Burke, K.C., Burke, J.D. Jr, Rae, D.S. & Reigier, D.A. (1991) Comparing age at onset of major depression and other psychiatric disorders by birth cohorts in five US community populations. Arch Gen Psychiatry 48(9), 789–95.

Butler, P.D., Weiss, J.M., Stout, J.C. & Nemeroff, C.B. (1990) Corticotropin-releasing factor produces fear-enhancing and behavioral activating effects following infusion into the locus coeruleus. J Neurosci 10(1), 176–83.

Charney, D.S., Woods, S.W. & Heninger, G.R. (1989) Noradrenergic function in generalized anxiety disorder: effects of yohimbine in healthy subjects and patients with generalized disorders. Critical Review of Neurobiology 10, 419–46.

Clayton, P.J., Grove, W.M., Coryell, W., Keller, M., Hirschfeld, R. & Fawcett, J. (1991) Follow-up and family study of anxious depression. Am J Psychiatry 148, 1512–17.

Dorow, R., Duka, T., Holler, L. & Sauerbrey, N. (1987) Clinical perspectives of β-carbolines from first studies in humans. Brain Res Bull 19(3), 319–26.

Drugan, R.C., Skolnick, P., Paul, S.M. & Crawley, J.N. (1989) A pretest procedure reliably predicts performance in two animal models of inescapable stress. Pharmacol Biochem Behav 33(3), 649–54.

DuPont, R.L., Rice, D.P., Miller, L.S., Shiraki, S.S., Rowland, C.R. & Harwood, H.J. (1996) Economic costs of anxiety disorders. Anxiety 2, 167–72.

Engel, J.A., Hjorth, S., Svensson, K., Carlsson, A. & Liljequist, S. (1984) Anticonflict effect of the putative serotonin receptor agonist 8-hydroxy-2 (di-n-propylamino) tetraline (8-OH-DPAT). Eur J of Pharmacol 105, 365–8.

Faravelli, C., Degl'Innocenti, G. & Giardinelli, L. (1989) Epidemiology of anxiety in Florence. Acta Psychiatr Scand 79, 308–12.

Fava, G.A., Grandi, S., Rafanelli, C. & Canestrati, R. (1992) Prodromal symptoms in panic disorder with agoraphobia: a replication study. J Affect Disord 26, 85–8.

Feighner, J.P., Robins, E., Guze, S.B., Woodruff, R.A., Winokur, G. & Munoz, R. (1972) Diagnostic criteria for use in psychiatric research. Arch Gen Psychiatry 124, 57–63.

Ferrarese, C., Appollonio, I., Frigo, M. et al. (1990) Decreased density of benzodiazepine receptors in lymphocytes of anxious patients: Reversal after chronic diazepam treatment. Acta Psychiatr Scand 82(2), 169–73.

Fifer, S.K., Mathias, S.D., Patrick, D.L., Mazonson, P.D., Lubeck, D.P. & Buesching, D.P. (1994) Untreated anxiety among primary care patients in a health maintenance organization. Arch Gen Psychiatry 51, 740–50.

Flint, A.J. (1994) Epidemiology and comorbidity of anxiety disorders in the elderly. Am J Psychiatry 151, 640–9.

Freud, S. (1957) Collected Papers, Vol. 1. Hogarth Press, London.

Garvey, M.J., Noyes, R. Jr, Woodman, C. & Laukes, C. (1993) A biological difference between panic disorder and generalized anxiety disorder. Biol Psychiatry 34(8), 572–5.

Garvey, M.J., Noyes, R. Jr, Woodman, C. & Laukes, C. (1995) Relationship of generalized anxiety symptoms to urinary 5-hydroxyindoleacetic acid and vanillymandelic acid. Psychiatry Res 57(1), 1–5.

Gasperini, M., Battaglia, M., Daiferia, G. & Bellodi, L. (1990) Personality features related to generalized anxiety disorder. Comprehensive Psychiatry 31, 363–8.

Germine, M., Goddard, A.W., Woods, S.W., Charney, D.S. & Henninger, G.R. (1992) Anger and anxiety responses to m-chlorophenylpiperazine in generalized anxiety disorder. Biol Psychiatry 32(5), 457–61.

Goddard, A.W., Woods, S.W., Money, R. et al. (1999) Effects of the CCK antagonist CI-988 on responses to mCPP in generalized anxiety disorder. Psychiatry Res 85, 225–40.

Griebel, G. (1999) Is there a future for neuropeptide receptor ligands in the treatment of anxiety disorders? Pharmacology Therapy 82(1), 1–61.

Harro, J., Vasar, E. & Bradwejn, J. (1993) CCK in animal and human research on anxiety. TIPS 14, 244–9.

Iny, L.J., Pecknold, J., Suranyi-Cadotte, B.E. et al. (1994) Studies of a neurochemical link between depression, anxiety, and stress from [3H]imipramine and [3H]paroxetine binding on human platelets. Biol Psychiatry 36(5), 281–91.

Jetty, P.V., Charney, D.S. & Goodard, A.W. (2001) Neurobiology of generalized anxiety disorder. The Psychiatr Clin North Am 24(1), 75–98.

Joffe, R.T., Bagby, R.M. & Levitt, A. (1993) Anxious and nonanxious depression. Am J Psychiatry 150(8), 1257–8.

Kahn, R.S., Wetzler, S., Asnis, G.M., Kling, M.A., Suckrow, R.F. & van Praag, H.M. (1991) Pituitary hormone response to meta-chlorophenylpiperazine in panic disorder and healthy control subjects. Psychiatry Res 37(1), 25–34.

Kashani, J.H. & Orvaschel, H. (1988) Anxiety disorders in mid-adolescence: a community sample. Am J Psychiatry 145, 960–4.

Kashani, J.H. & Overschel, H. (1990) A community study of anxiety in children and adolescents. Am J Psychiatry 147, 313–18.

Kendler, K.S., Neale, M.C., Kessler, R.C., Heath, A.C. & Eaves, L.J. (1992) Generalized anxiety disorder in women: a population based twin study. Arch Gen Psychiatry 49, 267–72.

Kendler, K.S., Walters, E.E., Neale, M.C., Kessler, R.C., Heath, A.C. & Eaves, L.J. (1995) The structure of the genetic and environmental risk factors for six major psychiatric disorders in women: phobia, generalized anxiety disorder, panic disorder, bulimia, major depression, and alcoholism. *Arch Gen Psychiatry* **52**(5), 374–83.

Kennedy, J.L., Bradwejn, J., Koszycki, D. *et al.* (1999) Investigation of cholestokinin system genes in panic disorder. *Mol Psychiatry* **4**(3), 284–5.

Kessler, R.C., DuPont, R.L., Berglund, P. & Wittchen, H.U. (1999) Impairment in pure and comorbid generalized anxiety disorder and major depression at 12 months in two national surveys. *Am J Psychiatry* **15**(6), 1915–23.

Kessler, R.C., Keller, M.B. & Wittchen, H.U. (2000) The epidemiology of generalized anxiety disorder. *Psychiatr Clin North Am* **24**(1), 19–40.

Kessler, R.C., McGonagle, K.A., Zhao. S. *et al.* (1994) Lifetime and 12-month prevalence of DSM-III-R psychiatric disorders in the United States: results from the National Comorbidity Survey. *Arch Gen Psychiatry* **51**, 8–19.

Koob, G.F. (1999) Cortiocotropin-releasing factor, norepinephrine, and stress. *Biol Psychiatry* **46**(9), 1167–80.

Koob, G.F. & Gold, L.H. (1997) Molecular biological approaches in the behavioural pharmacology of anxiety and depression. *Behav Pharmacol* **8**, 652.

Last, C.G., Hersen, M. & Kazdin, A.E. (1987) Comparison of DSM-III separation anxiety and overanxious disorders: demographic characteristics and pattern of comorbidity. *J Am Acad Child Adolesc Psychiatry* **4**, 527–31.

Lindesay, J., Briggs, K. & Murphy, E. (1989) The Guy's/Age Concern Survey: prevalence rates of cognitive impairment, depression, and anxiety in an urban elderly community. *Br J Psychiatry* **155**, 317–29.

Lydiard, R.B. (1994) Neuropeptides and anxiety: focus on cholecystokinin. *Clin Chem* **40**, 315–18.

Mancuso, D.M., Townsend, M.H. & Mercante, D.E. (1993) Long-term follow-up of generalized anxiety disorder. *Comprehensive Psychiatry* **34**, 441–6.

Marten, P.A., Brown, T.A., Barlow, D.H., Borkovec, T.D., Shear, M.K. & Lydiard, R.B. (1993) Evaluation of the ratings comprising the associated symptom criterion of DSM-III-R generalized anxiety disorder. *J Nerv Ment Dis* **181**, 676–82.

Maser, J.D. (1998) Generalized anxiety disorder and its comorbidities: disputes at the boundaries. *Acta Psychiatr Scand* **98** (Suppl. 393), 12–22.

Masi, G., Mucci, M., Favilla, L., Romano, R. & Poli, P. (1999) Symptomatology and comorbidity of generalized anxiety disorder in children and adolescents. *Comprehensive Psychiatry* **40**, 210–15.

Massion, A.O., Warshaw, M.G. & Keller, M.B. (1993) Quality of life and psychiatric morbidity in panic disorder and generalized anxiety disorder. *Am J Psychiatry* **150**, 600–7.

Mathew, R.J., Ho, B.T., Franics, D.J., Taylor, D.L. & Weinman, M.L. (1982) Catecholamines and anxiety. *Acta Psychiatr Scand* **63**, 142–7.

Mauri, M., Sarno, N., Rossi, V.M. *et al.* (1992) Personality disorders associated with generalized anxiety, panic, and recurrent depressive disorders. *J Personal Disord* **6**, 162–7.

Mavissakalian, M.R., Hamann, M.S., Abou Haidar, S. & de Groot, C.M. (1993) DSM-III personality disorders in generalized anxiety, panic/agoraphobia, and obsessive-compulsive disorders. *Comprehensive Psychiatry* **34**(4), 243–8.

McGee, R., Feehan, M., Williams, S., Patridge, F., Silva, P.A. & Kelly, J. (1990) DSM-III disorders in a large sample of adolescents. *J Am Acad Child Adolesc Psychiatry* **29**, 611–19.

Mendlewicz, J., Papadimitriou, G. & Wimotte, J. (1993) Family study of panic disorder: comparison to generalized anxiety disorder, major depression, and normal subjects. *Psychiatry Genetics* **3**, 73–8.

Miserendino, M.J., Sananes, C.B., Melia, K.R. & Davis, M. (1990) Blocking of acquisition but not expression of conditioned fear-potentiated startle by NMDA antagonists in the amygdala. *Nature* **345**(6277), 716–18.

Moghaddam, B., Bolinao, M.L., Stein-Behrens, B. & Sapolsky, R. (1994) Glucocorticoids mediate the stress-induced extracellular accumulation of glutamate. *Brain Res* **655** (1–2), 251–4.

Munjack, D.J., Baltazar, P.L., DeQuattro, V. *et al.* (1990) Generalized anxiety disorder: some biochemical aspects. *Psychiatry Res* **32**, 35–43.

Murphy, J.M., Olivier, D.C., Sobol, A.M., Monson, R.R. & Leighton, A.H. (1986) Diagnosis and outcome: depression and anxiety in a general population. *Psychol Med* **16**(1), 117–26.

Noyes, R. Jr, Clancy, J., Hoenk, P.R. & Slymen, D.J. (1980) The prognosis of anxiety neurosis. *Arch Gen Psychiatry* **37**(2), 173–8.

Noyes, R. Jr, Clarkson, C., Crowe, R.R., Yates, W.R. & McChesney, C.M. (1987) A family study of generalized anxiety disorder. *Am J Psychiatry* **144**(8), 1019–24.

Noyes, R. Jr, Holt, C.S. & Woodman, C.L. (1996) Natural course of anxiety disorders. In: *Long-Term Treatments of Anxiety Disorders* (M.R. Mavissakalian & R.F. Prien (eds)). American Psychiatric Press, Washington, D.C.

Noyes, R. Jr, Woodman, C., Garvey, M.J. *et al.* (1992) Generalized anxiety disorder versus panic disorder: distinguishing characteristics and patterns of comorbidity. *J Nerv Ment Dis* **180**, 369–79.

Nutt, D.J. (2001) Neurobiological mechanisms in generalized anxiety disorder. *J Clin Psychiatry* **62** (Suppl. 11), 22–7.

Pini, S., Cassano, G.B., Simonini, E., Sarino, M., Russo, A. & Montgomery, S.A. (1997) Prevalence of anxiety disorders comorbidity in bipolar depression unipolar depression and dysthymia. *J Affect Disord* **42**, 145–53.

Ramboz, S., Oosting, R., Amara, D.A. *et al.* (1998) Serotonin receptor 1A knockout: an animal model of anxiety-related disorder. *Proc Natl Acad Sci USA* **95**(24), 14 476–81.

Rickels, K., Case, W.G. & Schweizer, E. (1988) The drug treatment of anxiety and panic disorder. *Stress Medicine* **4**(4), 231–9.

Rickels, K. & Rynn, M. (2001) Overview and clinical presentation of generalized anxiety disorder. *Psychiatr Clin North Am* **24**(1), 1–18.

Rickels, K. & Schweizer, E. (1990) The spectrum of generalized anxiety in clinical practice: The role of short-term, intermittent treatment. *Br J Psychiatry* **173** (Suppl. 34), 49–54.

Rocca, P., Beoni, A.M., Eva, C., Ferrero, P., Zanalda, E. & Ravizza, L. (1998) Peripheral benzodiazepine receptor messenger RNA is decreased in lymphocytes of generalized anxiety disorder patients. *Biol Psychiatry* **43**(10), 767–73.

Rogers, M.P., Warshaw, M.G., Goisman, R.M. *et al.* (1999) Comparing primary and secondary generalized anxiety disorder in a long-term naturalistic study of anxiety disorder. *Depress Anxiety* **10**, 1–7.

da Roza Davis, J.M., Sharpley, A.L. & Cowen, P.J. (1992) Slow wave sleep and 5-HT2 receptor sensitivity in generalized anxiety disorder: a pilot study with ritanserin. *Psychopharmacology* **108**, 387–9.

Sacerdote, P., Panerai, A.E., Frattola, L. & Ferrarese, C. (1999) Benzodiazepine-induced chemotaxis is impaired in monocytes from patients with generalized anxiety disorder. *Psychoneuroendocrinology* **24**(2), 243–9.

Sanderson, W.C. & Barlow, D.H. (1990) A description of patients diagnosed with DSM-III-R generalized anxiety disorder. *J Nerv Ment Dis* **178**, 588–91.

Sanderson, W.C., Beck, A.T. & Beck, J. (1990) Syndrome comorbidity in patients with major depression or dysthymia: prevalence and temporal relationships. *Am J Psychiatry* **147**, 1025–8.

Sanderson, W.C. & Wetzler, S. (1991) Chronic anxiety and generalized anxiety disorder: issues in comorbidity. In: *Chronic Anxiety: Generalized Anxiety Disorder and Mixed Anxiety-Depression* (R. M. Rapee & D. H. Barlow (eds), pp. 119–35). Guilford Press, New York.

Sartorius, N., Ustun, T.B., Lecrubier, Y. & Wittchen, H.U. (1996) Depression comorbid with anxiety: Results from the WHO study on psychological disorders in primary health care. *Br J Psychiatry* **June** (30), 38–43.

Scherrer, J.F., True, W.R., Xian, H. *et al.* (2000) Evidence for genetic influences common and specific to symptoms of generalized anxiety disorder and panic. *J Affect Disord* **57**(1–3), 25–35.

Skre, I., Onstad, S., Evardsen, J., Torgersen, S. & Kringlen, E. (1994) A family study of generalized anxiety disorders: familial transmission and relationship to mood disorder and psychoactive substance use disorder. *Acta Psychiatr Scand* **90**(5), 366–74.

Skre, I., Onstad, S., Torgersen, S., Lygren, S. & Kringlen, E. (1993) A twin study of DSM-III-R anxiety disorders. *Acta Psychiatr Scand* **88**(2), 85–92.

Souetre, E., Lozet, H., Cimarosti, I. *et al.* (1994) Cost of anxiety disorders: impact of comorbidity. *J Psychosom Res* **38** (Suppl. 1), 151–60.

Starcevic, V. & Bogojevic, G. (1999) The concept of generalized anxiety disorder: between the too narrow and too wide diagnostic criteria. *Psychopathology* **32**, 5–11.

Starcevic, V., Uhlenhuth, E.H. & Fallon, S. (1995) The tridimensional personality questionnaire as an instrument for screening personality disorders: use in patients with generalized anxiety disorder. *J Personal Disord* **9**, 247–53.

Starcevic, V., Uhlenhuth, E.H., Kellner, R. & Pathak, D. (1992) Matters of comorbidity and panic disorder and agoraphobia. *Psychiatric Research* **42**, 171–83.

Stein, M.B., Hauger, R.L., Dhalla, K.S., Chartier, M.J. & Asmundson, G.J. (1996) Plasma neuropeptide Y in anxiety disorders: findings in panic disorder and social phobia. *Psychiatry Res* **59**(3), 183–8.

Taylor, D.P., Eison, M.S., Riblet, L.A. & Vandermaelen, C.P. (1985) Pharmacological and clinical effects of buspirone. *Pharmacol Biochem Behav* **23**(4), 687–94.

Tiihonen, J., Kuikka, J., Rasanen, P. *et al.* (1997) Cerebral benzodiazepine receptor binding and distribution in generalized anxiety disorder: a fractal analysis. *Mol Psychiatry* **2**(6), 463–71.

Trullas, R.B., Jackson, B. & Skolnick, P. (1989) Anxiolytic properties of 1-aminocyclopropanecarboxylic acid, a ligand at strychnine-insensitive glycine receptors. *Pharmacol Biochem Behav* **34**(2), 313–16.

Tye, N.C., Iversen, S.D. & Green, A.R. (1979) The effects of benzodiazepines and serotonergic manipulations on punished responding. *Neuropharmacology* **18**, 689–95.

Uhde, T.W., Boulenger, J.P., Roy-Byrne, P.P., Geraci, M.F., Vittone, B.J. & Post, R.M. (1985) Longitudinal course of panic disorder. Clinical and biological considerations. *Program of Neuropsychopharmacology and Biol Psychiatry* **9**, 39–51.

Uhlenhuth, E.H., Mitchell, B.B., Mellinger, G.D., Cisin, I.H. & Clinthorne, J. (1983) Symptom checklist syndromes in the general population. *Arch Gen Psychiatry* **40**, 1167–73.

Wacker, H.R., Mullejans, R., Klein, K.H. & Battegay, R. (1992) Identification of cases of anxiety disorders and affective disorders in the community according to ICD-10 and DSM-III-R using the Composite International Diagnostic Interview (CIDI). *International Journal of Methods in Psychiatry Res* **2**, 91–100.

Walley, E.J., Beebe, D.K. & Clark, J.L. (1994) Management of common anxiety disorders. *Am Fam Physician* **50**, 1745–53.

Weissman, M.M., Myers, J.K. & Harding, P.S. (1978) Psychiatric disorders in a US urban community. *Am J Psychiatry* **135**(4), 459–61.

Widerlov, E., Lindstrom, L.H., Wahlestedt, C. & Ekman, R. (1988) Neuropeptide Y and peptide YY as possible cerebrospinal fluid makers for major depression and schizophrenia, respectively. *J Psychiatr Res* **22**(1), 69–79.

Wittchen, H.U., Zhao, S., Kessler, R.C. & Eaton, W.W. (1994) DSM-III-R generalized anxiety disorder in the National Comorbidity Survey. *Arch Gen Psychiatry* **51**, 355–64.

Woodruff, G.N. & Hughes, J. (1991) Cholecystokinin antagonists. Annual review of. *Pharmacol Toxicol* **31**, 469–501.

World Health Organization (WHO) (1993) *ICD-10 Classification of Mental and Behavioural Disorders: Diagnostic Criteria for Research*. World Health Organization, Geneva, Switzerland.

Wu, J.C., Buchsbaum, M.S., Hershey, T.G., Hazlett, E., Sicotte, N. & Johnson, J.C. (1991) PET in generalized anxiety disorder. *Biol Psychiatry* **29**(12), 1181–9.

Yonkers, K.A., Massion, A., Warshaw, M. & Keller, M.B. (1996) Phenomenology and course of generalized anxiety disorder. *Br J Psychiatry* **168**, 308–13.

Post-traumatic Stress Disorder

S.A.M. Rauch & E.B. Foa

Introduction and diagnosis

Post-traumatic stress disorder (PTSD) is an anxiety disorder precipitated by exposure to an event which involves actual or threatened death or serious injury, or threat to the personal integrity of self or others that causes intense fear, helplessness, or horror. Typical post-trauma symptoms are re-experiencing some aspects of the trauma, avoidance of trauma-related stimuli, numbing, and increased arousal. The Diagnostic Statistical Manual, fourth edition (DSM-IV: American Psychiatric Association [APA] 1994) criteria for PTSD are presented in Table 5.1. PTSD can be acute (1–3 months duration of symptoms), chronic (more than 3 months in duration), or delayed (symptoms appear at least 6 months after the trauma). The diagnosis requires that the onset of the symptoms of re-experiencing, avoidance, numbing, and arousal be related to exposure to the traumatic event.

A related diagnosis, acute stress disorder (ASD), is given to traumatized individuals who exhibit symptoms of dissociation and numbing, re-experiencing, avoidance, and arousal within 1 month of exposure to a traumatic event. The DSM-IV criteria for ASD are presented in Table 5.2. Thus, if an individual is highly symptomatic within the first 4 weeks after the trauma, the diagnosis of ASD should be considered. If the symptoms persist, a PTSD diagnosis may be appropriate.

What is a traumatic event?

Previous versions of the DSM defined a traumatic event according to its prevalence in the population (i.e. an event outside the range of normal human experience).

In the DSM-IV, the definition emphasizes the characteristics of the event and the person's response to the event. Specifically, DSM-IV requires: (i) "the person experienced, witnessed or was confronted with an event or events that involved actual or threatened death or serious injury, or a threat to the physical integrity of self or others," and (ii) "the person's response involved intense fear, helplessness, or horror" (APA 1994, pp. 427–8). The abandoning of the normative definition was prompted by the realization that traumatic events are not rare but rather are experienced by a large percentage of the general population during their lifetimes (e.g. Kessler *et al.* 1995).

The inclusion of the subjective aspect of the trauma (e.g. feelings of fear, helpless or horror) has been supported by March's (1993) review of the literature and was corroborated by later research suggesting that the interpretation of the event impacts the probability of development of PTSD (Blanchard *et al.* 1995; Solomon & Davidson 1997; Bernat *et al.* 1998; Ehlers *et al.* 1998).

In a prospective study, following crime survivors from 1 month to 6 months postcrime, Brewin *et al.* (2000) examined whether experiencing intense emotions at the time of the trauma predicted the presence of DSM-III-R criteria of PTSD at 6 months postcrime. Consistent with the DSM-IV criterion (i), participants who reported having intense experiences of horror, helplessness, and fear during the crime were more likely to have PTSD 6 months later than participants who did not report these experiences. Further, all participants who developed PTSD in the absence of horror, helplessness, or fear reported intense anger or shame during the trauma.

Table 5.1 DSM-IV diagnostic criteria for PTSD. (From APA 1994, pp. 427–9, with permission. Copyright 1994 American Psychiatric Association.)

A. The person has been exposed to a traumatic event in which both of the following were present:
  1 The person experienced, witnessed, or was confronted with an event or events that involved actual or threatened death or serious injury, or a threat to the physical integrity of self or others
  2 The person's response involved intense fear, helplessness, or horror. Note: in children, this may be expressed instead by disorganized or agitated behavior

B. The traumatic event is persistently re-experienced in one (or more) of the following ways:
  1 Recurrent and intrusive distressing recollections of the event, including images, thoughts, or perceptions. Note: In young children, repetitive play may occur in which themes or aspects of the trauma are expressed
  2 Recurrent distressing dreams of the event. Note: In children, there may be frightening dreams without recognizable content
  3 Acting or feeling as if the traumatic event were recurring (includes a sense of reliving the experience, illusions, hallucinations, and dissociative flashback episodes, including those that occur on awakening or when intoxicated). Note: In young children, trauma-specific re-enactment may occur
  4 Intense psychological distress at exposure to internal or external cues that symbolize or resemble an aspect of the traumatic event
  5 Physiological reactivity on exposure to internal or external cues that symbolize or resemble an aspect of the traumatic event

C. Persistent avoidance of stimuli associated with the trauma and numbing of general responsiveness (not present before the trauma), as indicated by three (or more) of the following:
  1 Efforts to avoid thoughts, feelings, or conversations associated with the trauma
  2 Efforts to avoid activities, places, individuals that arouse recollections of the trauma
  3 Inability to recall an important aspect of the trauma
  4 Markedly diminished interest or participation in significant activities
  5 Feeling of detachment or estrangement from others
  6 Restricted range of affect (e.g. unable to have loving feelings)
  7 Sense of foreshortened future (e.g. does not expect to have a career, marriage, children, or a normal life span)

D. Persistent symptoms of increased arousal (not present before the trauma), as indicated by two (or more) of the following:
  1 Difficulty falling or staying asleep
  2 Irritability or outbursts of anger
  3 Difficulty concentrating
  4 Hypervigilance
  5 Exaggerated startle response

E. Duration of the disturbance (symptoms in criteria B, C, and D) is more than 1 month

F. The disturbance causes clinically significant distress or impairment in social, occupational, or other important areas of functioning

Specify if:
Acute: if duration of symptoms is less than 3 months
Chronic: if duration of symptoms 3 months or more

Specify if:
With delayed onset: if onset of symptoms is at least 6 months after stressor

Table 5.2 DSM-IV Diagnostic Criteria for ASD. (From APA 1994, pp. 427–9, with permission. Copyright 1994 American Psychiatric Association.)

A. The person has been exposed to a traumatic event in which both of the following were present:
  1 The person experienced, witnessed, or was confronted with an event or events that involved actual or threatened death or serious injury, or a threat to the physical integrity of self or others
  2 The person's response involved intense fear, helplessness, or horror. Note: In children, this may be expressed instead by disorganized or agitated behavior

B. Either while experiencing or after experiencing the distressing event, the individual has three (or more) of the following dissociative symptoms:
  1 A subjective sense of numbing, detachment, or absence of emotional responsiveness
  2 A reduction in awareness of his or her surroundings (e.g. "being in a daze")
  3 Derealization
  4 Depersonalization
  5 Dissociative amnesia (i.e. inability to recall an important aspect of the trauma)

C. The traumatic event is persistently re-experienced in at least one of the following ways:
Recurrent images, thoughts, dreams, illusions, flashback episodes, or a sense of reliving the experience: or distress on exposure to reminders of the traumatic event

D. Marked avoidance of stimuli that arouse recollections of the trauma (e.g. thoughts, feelings, conversations, activities, places, and individuals)

E. Marked symptoms of anxiety or increased arousal (e.g. difficulty sleeping, irritability, poor concentration, hypervigilance, exaggerated startle response, motor restlessness)

F. The disturbance causes clinically significant distress or impairment in social occupational, or other important areas of functioning or impairs the individual's ability to pursue some necessary task, such as obtaining necessary assistance or mobilizing personal resources by telling family members about the traumatic experience

G. The disturbance lasts for a minimum of 2 days and a maximum of 4 weeks and occurs within 4 weeks of the traumatic event

H. The disturbance is not due to the direct psychological effects of a substance (e.g. a drug of abuse, a medication) or a general medical condition, is not better accounted for by brief psychotic disorder, and is not merely an exacerbation of a pre-existing Axis I or Axis II disorder

Assessment

As with most psychiatric disturbances, assessment is a critical part of the diagnosis and treatment of PTSD. As noted by Foa and Rothbaum (1998), assessment serves several goals: it helps establish the diagnosis of PTSD and related psychopathology and assists in determining which diagnosis is primary; it provides a baseline for symptom severity in order to evaluate progress or deterioration associated with treatment; it enables the clinician to evaluate the response to treatment; it offers an opportunity for validation, normalization, and education about PTSD.

Nonstandardized assessment
Self-monitoring of target difficulties or symptoms is a common and often useful form of nonstandardized assessment. With this technique, the client keeps a record of the occurrence of target behaviors (e.g. nightmares, angry outbursts, etc.). Such recording often includes the date and time of the occurrence, the situation during which the symptom is apparent, thoughts at the time of the symptom, and the client's emotional reactions during the occurrence of the symptom. These reactions are often measured using the Subjective Units of Distress scale (SUDs) where 100 indicates the maximum distress possible and 0 indicates no distress.

The information obtained by self-monitoring (e.g. symptoms, triggers, avoidance, dysfunctional thoughts, and reaction patterns) can be used in the description and treatment of PTSD. For a more detailed account of self-monitoring along with examples of self-monitoring forms see Foa and Rothbaum (1998). Despite the rich information obtained from self-monitoring, it is underutilized because it requires a lot of effort during both recording and reviewing.

A second more commonly used nonstandardized assessment technique is the clinical interview. Such interviews usually include a general psychosocial assessment including history of the psychosocial problems, previous treatment and outcome, familial difficulties, educational and employment functioning, etc. (see Cormier & Cormier 1991 for discussion). Following such a general assessment, specific information related to the client's history of traumatic experiences and current difficulties should follow. This includes details about the precipitating trauma, such as what type of trauma, when it happened, who was involved, duration, etc. This inquiry also includes previous traumatic experiences and how they impacted on the patient. Foa and Rothbaum (1998) offer an example of such an interview format with survivors of sexual assault. This format addresses the main areas of concern of many trauma survivors and can be altered to address other specific traumatic events. While nonstandardized clinical interviews offer flexibility to the clinician, important information may be missed and the assessment may take longer than standardized techniques. These drawbacks may be especially pertinent with clinicians inexperienced with PTSD.

Standardized assessment

Standardized assessments offer several advantages over nonstandardized measures including efficiency, validity, and reliability in measurement of symptom severity and change. Standardized measures include both clinician interview and self-report instruments. Several such measures have been developed for PTSD diagnosis and severity. Only the most commonly used will be reviewed here.

Clinician interview The 30-item Clinician-administered PTSD Scale (CAPS; Blake *et al.* 1990) assesses frequency and intensity of individual PTSD symptoms as well as associated features. In addition to the 17 DSM-IV symptoms of PTSD, the CAPS assesses guilt, depression, and functional impairment in job and social performance.

The CAPS contains three subscales which coincide with the three symptom clusters of the DSM: re-experiencing, avoidance and numbing, and arousal. With combat veterans, the CAPS has yielded excellent inter-rater reliability for all three subscales ($r = 0.92–0.99$). It also has good concurrent validity as indicated by its high correlations with other measures of PTSD symptoms: Keane PTSD subscale (PK) of the Minnesota Multiphasic Personality Inventory (MMPI) ($r = 0.77$: Keane *et al.* 1984) and Mississippi Scale for Combat-related PTSD ($r = 0.91$: Keane *et al.* 1988). The CAPS has been found to be sensitive to treatment outcome (van der Kolk *et al.* 1994). Studies on psychometric properties of the CAPS with trauma populations other than combat veterans are scarce. While a psychometrically sound instrument, the CAPS has been criticized for the length of administration (between 40 and 60 min: Newman *et al.* 1996; Foa & Tolin 2000).

The PTSD Symptom Scale-Interview The PTSD Symptom Scale-Interview (PSS-I; Foa *et al.* 1993) is a 7-item scale that assesses the presence of DSM-IV PTSD diagnosis and the severity of the PTSD symptoms. Each item is rated on a scale of 0 ("not at all") to 3 ("very much"). Symptoms are clustered into the DSM-IV symptom clusters of re-experiencing, avoidance, numbing, and arousal. This interview has excellent test–retest reliability over 1 month ($r = 0.80$). Inter-rater reliability was excellent with a κ of 0.91 for PTSD diagnosis. Foa *et al.* (1993) demonstrated that the PSS-I has good concurrent validity as determined by high correlation with other measures of PTSD symptoms: Impact of Event Scale (IES)-Intrusion ($r = 0.69$: Horowitz *et al.* 1979) and IES-Avoidance ($r = 0.56$: Horowitz *et al.* 1979). The PSS-I also correlates highly with other measures of psychological distress: Beck Depression Inventory (BDI; $r = 0.72$: Beck *et al.* 1961) and State-Trait Anxiety Inventory-State (STAI-S; $r = 0.48$: Spielberger *et al.* 1970). Finally, the PSS-I has been found to be sensitive to treatment outcome (Foa *et al.* 1999). The interview takes approximately 20 min to administer. In a psychometric study comparing the CAPS and the PSS-I, Foa and Tolin (2000) found that the PSS-I and CAPS performed equally well with regard to diagnosis and psychometrics properties, with the PSS-I taking an average of 22 min and the CAPS 32 min.

The Structured Clinical Interview for DSM-IV The Structured Clinical Interview for DSM-IV (SCID-IV;

First *et al.* 1997) assesses lifetime and current diagnosis of various DSM-IV diagnoses (e.g. depression, mania, PTSD, etc.). The PTSD module is often used to ascertain the presence of PTSD. Inter-rater reliability of a previous version of this measure (Structured Clinical Interview for DSM-III-R [SCID]) based upon DSM-III-R (APA 1987) was moderate ($\kappa = 0.68$; diagnostic agreement 78%: Keane *et al.* 1998). However, the complete SCID-IV requires 1–2 hours to complete and an administrator with appropriate clinical background and training.

The Anxiety Disorders Interview Schedule-IV The Anxiety Disorders Interview Schedule-IV (ADIS-IV; DiNardo *et al.* 1994) is a semistructured clinical interview which focuses on anxiety and affective disorders. The ADIS-IV provides assessment of lifetime and current disorders and onset, duration, and severity of symptoms. Inter-rater reliability as assessed by κ ($\kappa = 0.59$) and lifetime diagnosis of PTSD ($\alpha = 0.61$) are moderate. The ADIS-IV takes about 2 hours to complete and requires a general knowledge of diagnostic categories and experience with the measure.

Self-report measures The PTSD Diagnostic Scale (PDS; Foa *et al.* 1997) is a 49-item, self-report measure that assesses presence and severity of the DSM-IV 17 PTSD symptoms as well as trauma history, reactions to the most salient trauma, and general functioning. The PDS has three subscales: re-experiencing, avoidance and numbing, and arousal. It has demonstrated excellent test–retest reliability ($r = 0.83$) and internal consistency ($\alpha = 0.92$) with mixed trauma populations. The diagnosis derived from the PDS corresponds highly with that derived by the SCID with excellent sensitivity (0.89) and specificity (0.75). The PDS demonstrated very good concurrent validity as reflected in high correlation with other measures of PTSD symptoms, depression, and anxiety (Foa *et al.* 1997). The excellent psychometric properties of the PDS, the ease of administration (about 10 min), and the complete mapping on DSM-IV criteria for PTSD render the scale a useful tool for diagnostic screening and assessment of PTSD severity in clinical and research settings.

The Impact of Event Scale The Impact of Event Scale is a 15-item scale developed by Horowitz *et al.* (1979) to assess intrusion and avoidance symptoms. More

recently it was revised by Weiss and Marmar (IES-R; 1997) to include seven additional items that assess hyperarousal and the event criterion. Thus, the IES-R consists of 22 items assessing intrusion, avoidance, and hyperarousal. Internal consistency of the items of the IES-R is good: intrusion, $\alpha = 0.87$; avoidance, $\alpha = 0.85$; and hyperarousal, $\alpha = 0.79$. Test–retest reliability was less satisfactory: intrusion, $r = 0.57$; avoidance, $r = 0.51$; and hyperarousal, $r = 0.59$. The scale requires about 15 min to complete.

The Mississippi Scale The Mississippi Scale (Keane *et al.* 1988) includes 35-items designed to measure PTSD in combat veterans. The items were selected from a pool of 200 items generated by experts to closely resemble DSM-III (APA 1980) criteria for PTSD. The scale has excellent test–retest reliability over a 1 week interval ($r = 0.97$) and excellent internal consistency ($\alpha = 0.94$). The scale also has excellent diagnostic sensitivity (0.93) and specificity (0.89) with a cut-off score of 107 (Keane *et al.* 1988; McFall *et al.* 1990). The measure takes roughly 15 min to complete. The disadvantage of this measure is a lack of mapping with DSM-IV diagnosis.

Clinical features

As is apparent in Table 5.1, the DSM-IV divides the 17 symptoms of PTSD into three clusters: re-experiencing of the trauma (e.g. intrusive thoughts, nightmares, flashbacks, and emotional or physiological reactivity with reminders), avoidance/numbing of trauma reminders (e.g. avoidance of thoughts, feeling, conversations, activities, individuals or places that are reminders, inability to recall portions of the trauma, decreased interest in pleasurable activities, detachment or estrangement from others, restricted affect, and foreshortened future) and arousal (e.g. sleep problems, irritability and anger, difficulty concentrating, hypervigilance, and exaggerated startle).

Studies examining the validity of the three symptom clusters yielded mixed results. Using a factor analytical method in a sample of sexual and nonsexual assault survivors 3 months postassault, Foa *et al.* (1995) found a three-factor solution. However, the breakdown of symptoms was somewhat different from that of the DSM-IV. The first factor included primarily arousal and avoidance symptoms. The second factor included primarily numbing symptoms along with irritability and anger (which can be conceptualized as avoidance of fear and anxiety). The third factor was composed of intrusive symptoms along with difficulty sleeping. Thus, this study tends to support a separation of the numbing and avoidance symptoms which are combined into one cluster in the DSM-IV. Further, severe avoidance and arousal symptoms independently increased the likelihood of numbing symptoms. Consistent with the above results, Litz *et al.* (1997) and Flack *et al.* (2000) found that emotional numbing was more robustly predicted by arousal cluster symptoms than avoidance symptoms.

Comorbidity

PTSD often co-occurs with other psychosocial difficulties. In an adult sample of individuals diagnosed with PTSD, 62% met criteria for another diagnosis (Davidson *et al.* 1991). The most common comorbid diagnosis was generalized anxiety disorder (53%) followed by simple phobia (50%). In the Epidemiological Catchment Area Study (Helzer *et al.* 1987) individuals with PTSD were twice as likely to have another disorder than individuals without PTSD, with the greatest increase in risk for obsessive-compulsive disorder, dysthymia, and bipolar disorder. The two most prevalent comorbid diagnoses in a sample of young adults with PTSD were major depressive disorder (MDD) (37%) and alcohol abuse/dependence (31%; Breslau *et al.* 1991). Similar results were obtained in the National Comorbidity Survey where alcohol abuse or dependence, major depressive episode, and simple phobia were the most common comorbid diagnoses (Kessler *et al.* 1995). These studies did not provide information about which diagnosis occurred first. Therefore, comorbid psychiatric disorders may have either preceded or succeeded PTSD. To address this problem, Kessler *et al.* (1995) provided estimates of the percentage of cases in which PTSD began at an earlier or later age than the comorbid disorders. These estimates suggest that while PTSD often precedes other comorbid diagnoses, it usually succeeds at least one diagnosis (Kessler *et al.* 1995). Closer examination of which disorder preceded the others is necessary to determine: (i) whether individuals with PTSD are more vulnerable to developing other problems or vice versa, and (ii) which disorders are more likely to precede PTSD and which are more likely to succeed PTSD.

Differential diagnosis

Several other psychiatric disorders may resemble PTSD. For instance, if a person experiences symptoms of PTSD in response to a stressor that does not qualify as a traumatic event, as previously defined, the diagnosis of adjustment disorder would be warranted. This diagnosis can also be appropriate when a person has symptoms following a qualifying traumatic event but does not meet full PTSD diagnostic criteria.

Embedded in the diagnosis of PTSD is the notion that avoidance and fear associated with the trauma generalize to many areas of life. If the avoidance and fear is limited to a specific aspect of the trauma or to a specific object or situation, a diagnosis of specific phobia may be more appropriate. For example, if a person who survived drowning simply avoids swimming and is unaffected in other areas of life, specific phobia would be the appropriate diagnosis. If, however, the person avoids swimming, cannot be near a lake, or drive near water, cannot sleep, alternates between numbing and high arousal, and is constantly irritable, a diagnosis of PTSD should be considered.

Distinguishing panic disorder from PTSD can be a difficult task. Both diagnoses involve a significant amount of avoidance in response to feared stimuli. Also, PTSD patients may experience panic attacks in response to reminders of the trauma. However, one distinguishing characteristic which appears to separate panic disorder from PTSD involves the cognitions associated with the avoidance. The panic disordered individual typically avoids situations in order to prevent the occurrence of a panic attack and the feared consequences of these attacks (e.g. dying of a heart attack). In PTSD the person avoids trauma-related situations in order to prevent the distress associated with the traumatic memory. Further, the diagnosis of panic disorder requires the presence of uncued panic attacks which appear to "come out of the blue." In patients with PTSD, the panic attacks are likely to be triggered by specific cues (i.e. by trauma reminders). Finally, the possibility of comorbidity between panic disorder and PTSD should not be discounted.

While there is significant overlap between the symptoms of a major depressive episode (MDE) and numbing symptoms of PTSD, the re-experiencing and avoidance symptoms of PTSD can be an effective way to distinguish these diagnoses. If the patient reports nightmares, repeated thoughts or flashbacks of a traumatic event, PTSD should be considered. Also, if the patient is reporting significant avoidance related to the traumatic experience rather than avoidance of activities due to fatigue and disinterest, PTSD should be considered. Comorbid diagnosis of MDD and PTSD should also be considered (see previous comorbidity discussion).

Epidemiology

How common are traumatic events?

The prevalence of trauma varies greatly across community studies suggesting that between 39% and 90% of individuals have had at least one traumatic experience in their lifetime (e.g. Breslau *et al.* 1991; BresNorris 1992; Resnick *et al.* 1993; Kessler *et al.* 1995; Solomon & Davidson 1997; Lau *et al.* 1998). The large differences across studies are often attributed to differences in the screening methods and instruments used. Among a sample from a health maintenance organization (HMO), who were of moderate socioeconomic status (SES) and relatively young (Breslau *et al.* 1991) lifetime prevalence of trauma exposure was about 39%. This rate may underestimate the pre-valence of trauma in the general population of the US because of the insensitivity of the Diagnostic Interview Schedule (DIS; Robins *et al.* 1981) version to several trauma types (e.g. rape; Solomon & Davidson 1997). Further, the DIS recorded only three traumatic events, which may also result in underestimation of trauma rates.

A higher prevalence of trauma exposure was reported by Norris (1992) who used a more sensitive screening instrument to examine the rates of 10 traumatic events involving violent encounters with natural or technical disasters or human violence in a large urban sample from the South-Eastern US. Sixty-nine percent reported experiencing at least one traumatic event in their lifetime. Similar rates were reported by Resnick *et al.* (1993) in a representative sample of women in the US. Again, 69% of women reported exposure to a traumatic event during their lifetime. These higher prevalence rates may be due to both studies using a trauma screen that included multiple behaviorally specific questions in order to increase detection of traumatic experiences.

A considerably higher rate of trauma exposure, 89.6%, was reported more recently, in a representative sample of adults in the Detroit, Michigan area (Breslau

et al. 1998). The authors suggested that both the recording of all traumatic experiences and the inclusion of the new category of sudden unexpected death of a loved one may account for the higher prevalence, since 60% of the sample reported unexpected death of a loved one.

In the Breslau *et al.* (1991) study, the most common traumatic events were sudden injury or serious accident (9.4%), physical assault (8.3%), seeing someone seriously injured or killed (7.1%), and news of the sudden death or injury of a relative or close friend (5.7%). Only 2% of this sample reported having been raped. Using the more sensitive assessment procedure described earlier, Norris (1992) found that the most frequent lifetime event was tragic death of a loved one (30%), an event not included in the previous study. As noted above, the high prevalence of this traumatic event, 60%, was also noted by Breslau *et al.* (1998). Seven percent of women and 1% of men in Norris's sample reported having been raped, and 15% of the sample reported having been physically assaulted. Within a sample of women, Resnick *et al.* (1993) found a higher prevalence of rape and sexual assault (12.7% rape; 14.3% other sexual assault), but lower prevalence of physical assault (10.3%). These higher overall rates may be attributed to the sensitive screening procedure with multiple behaviorally specific anchors and the consistent finding that reported rape rates are higher in samples of women than men (e.g. Kessler *et al.* 1995; Breslau *et al.* 1998).

When considering gender differences in trauma exposure, two questions must be addressed: Are observed differences in rates between genders clinically significant? and, what gender-related factors contribute to the observed differences? In the Breslau *et al.* (1991) study, men reported more overall traumatic events than women (43% vs. 37%, respectively). Later, in assessing all traumas in a representative sample from Detroit, Breslau *et al.* (1999) found that 92% of men and 88% of women reported exposure to traumatic events. Although the two studies differed in the overall rates of trauma exposure (due to methodological differences discussed above), gender differences were quite small. Among young adults, no gender differences were found (Breslau *et al.* 1997). Somewhat larger gender differences were reported by Norris (1992): 74% for men and 65% for women. Importantly, Norris reported that sexual assault was significantly higher for women (7.3%) than men (1.3%) while men were more likely to have been in a motor vehicle accident (MVA) (27.9% and 20.1%, respectively) or physically assaulted (18.7% and 11.7%, respectively) than women. Similarly, Breslau *et al.* (1998) found that although women were less exposed to assaultive violence (a composite of specific traumas involving personal attack) than men (32.4% and 43.3%, respectively), they had higher levels of exposure to rape (9.4% and 1.1%, respectively) and other sexual assault (9.4% and 2.8%, respectively).

In summary, differences in prevalence estimates vary with the assessment utilized (cf. Solomon & Davidson 1997). When behaviorally specific questions are used to assess for traumatic events, especially for sexual assault and rape, prevalence estimates are typically higher and probably more accurate. Irrespective of the method of data collection, several patterns emerged from all studies: (a) rates of trauma exposure are high enough to suggest that traumatic events and their impact on the survivor represent an important societal issue worthy of closer examination; (b) adult men are more likely to be exposed to traumatic experiences than adult women; and (c) the rates of different trauma vary across genders with men more likely to be exposed to physical assault and traffic accidents and women more likely to experience sexual assault.

How common is PTSD?

Prospective and retrospective studies suggest that the majority of individuals naturally recover from trauma (e.g. Rothbaum *et al.* 1992; Riggs *et al.* 1995; Brewin *et al.* 1999). Riggs *et al.* (1995) followed survivors of nonsexual assault for 12 weeks with weekly assessments. Seventy-one percent of women and 50% of men met symptom criteria for PTSD at the initial assessment (an average of 19 days postassault). At 4 weeks postassault, the rates decreased to 42% of women and 32% of men with PTSD. At 12 weeks postassault, 21% of women and none of the men met criteria for PTSD. While this chronic group of women did not show decline in symptoms over the 12 weeks, there were no survivors who showed increased symptoms over time. While most survivors showed recovery and did not meet criteria for PTSD at 12 weeks, many still experienced some symptoms.

In a longitudinal study examining reactions of sexual assault survivors, 94% met criteria for PTSD (except for duration) at their initial assessment (Rothbaum *et al.* 1992). Sixty-five percent had PTSD at 4 weeks

postassault, and 47% at 12 weeks postassault. As in the previous study, women who did not have PTSD at 12 weeks showed steady decreases in symptoms over the 12 weeks while those who did have PTSD at 12 weeks showed no decrease in symptoms after 4 weeks.

When examining prevalence of PTSD, two conditional probabilities are important: the probability of PTSD in the general population and the probability of PTSD within specific trauma populations. General population prevalence estimates range from 1% to 9%. The differences in estimates can be attributed to: (i) the sensitivity of the assessment techniques to detect traumatic events and PTSD symptoms (e.g. Solomon & Davidson 1997), and (ii) the traumatic event under study (e.g. Rothbaum *et al.* 1992; Foa & Riggs 1995; Kessler 1995).

Helzer *et al.* (1987) found a PTSD prevalence rate of 1% in an adult sample using the DIS which is based on the DSM-III criteria. Utilizing the same version of the DIS with a North Carolina community sample, Davidson *et al.* (1991) found a similar lifetime prevalence of 1.3%. As noted by Solomon and Davidson (1997), the insensitivity of the DIS may have resulted in a underestimation of PTSD prevalence. Using the DSM-III-R criteria and a more sensitive assessment procedure (previously described), Breslau *et al.* (1991) found a 9.2% lifetime prevalence of PTSD in their HMO sample. Also using more sensitive trauma assessment, Norris (1992) reported a rate of 5.1% and Kessler *et al.* (1995) reported a rate of 7.8%. A somewhat higher rate was reported for a national sample of women (12.3%: Resnick *et al.* 1993).

Among individuals who had traumatic events and were assessed with an insensitive trauma screen, higher rates of PTSD were found (24%: Breslau *et al.* 1991). However, with the more sensitive assessment, Norris (1992) found that only 7% of individuals with a positive trauma history currently met criteria for PTSD. Correspondingly, Breslau *et al.* (1998) reported that 9.2% of individuals with a positive trauma history currently had PTSD*.

*Lower rates were reported by Helzer *et al.* (1987) who found that 3.3% of men who reported combat as their most distressing trauma developed PTSD and 1.7% of men who reported their most distressing trauma as seeing someone hurt or killed. Among women, who reported physical assault as their most distressing trauma, 4.6% developed PTSD. These low rates may be due to the relatively insensitivity of the original DIS discussed earlier.

Pathogenesis

Several studies have examined predictors of PTSD following a traumatic event (see Brewin *et al.* 2000 for a meta-analytic review). On the basis of their meta-analysis, Brewin *et al.* (2000) concluded that there were three categories of predictors. First, factors that predict PTSD in some but not in all populations; these include gender, age at trauma, and race. Second, factors that predict PTSD in many populations but show some variation across populations and methods; these include education, previous trauma, and general childhood adversity. Finally, factors that predict PTSD across studies and populations; these include psychiatric history, reported childhood abuse, and family psychiatric history. Brewin *et al.* (2000) further concluded that while all of the effect sizes associated with predictors of PTSD are modest, factors that operate during or after the trauma, such as trauma severity, lack of social support, and additional life stress, have somewhat larger effects than pretrauma factors.

Trauma type

One potential predictor of PTSD is type of trauma. Rates of PTSD have been found to reliably differ from one type of trauma to another with some events, such as rape, leading to extremely high rates of PTSD and other events, such as natural disasters, leading to lower rates of PTSD (e.g. Kilpatrick *et al.* 1989; Rothbaum *et al.* 1992; Foa & Riggs 1995). For example, in a national sample of women, Resnick *et al.* (1993) found a higher prevalence rate among survivors of crime than noncrime traumas. Among crime survivors somewhat lower rates of PTSD were associated with rape (32%) than physical assault (38.5%: Resnick *et al.* 1993).

Using a more precise methodology assessing all traumatic events, Breslau *et al.* (1998) examined the conditional probability of developing PTSD following 19 specific types of traumatic events. The highest conditional risk of PTSD diagnosis was associated with assaultive violence (including rape) after which 20.9% of survivors met PTSD diagnosis. Among the assaultive events, the highest risk was associated with being captured, kidnapped, and tortured with 53.8% developing PTSD. Forty-nine percent of rape survivors and 31.9% of those who were badly beaten

up developed PTSD. Higher rates of PTSD among women following rape (80%) were reported by Breslau *et al.* (1991). However, these higher rates may have been attributable to a lower sensitivity of the measure used to assess for rape and sexual assault leading to detecting only the most severe rapes and thus inflating the probability of PTSD in the reported rapes. Notably, high rates of PTSD (60%) were also reported by Rothbaum *et al.* (1992), in a prospective study of a convenient sample that did not suffer from the above methodological problems.

Breslau *et al.*'s (1998) rates of PTSD are similar to those reported by Kessler (1995) in the National Comorbidity Survey, where 65% of men and 46% of women who reported rape as their most upsetting trauma had a lifetime diagnosis of PTSD. Lower rates were reported by men with combat as their most upsetting traumatic experience (39% develop PTSD: Kessler *et al.* 1995). In the Kessler *et al.* sample, 3.7% of men and 5.4% of women who reported natural disaster as their most upsetting trauma developed PTSD; these rates were similar to those reported by Breslau *et al.* (3.8%).

Despite the high conditional risk associated with assaultive violence, studies suggest that other, less potent but more common, traumatic experiences may actually account for more cases of PTSD. Thirty-one percent of participants diagnosed with PTSD in the Breslau *et al.* (1998) sample reported the unexpected death of a loved one as the precipitating event. Sixty percent of the sample experienced such a trauma with a moderate risk of PTSD development (14.3%: Breslau *et al.* 1998). Other studies have also found that the unexpected loss of a loved one accounts for a large percentage of cases of PTSD (e.g. 26.6% of women with PTSD and 38.5% of men with PTSD: Breslau *et al.* 1999).

Trauma severity

Another predictor of PTSD is the severity of the trauma exposure, as measured by the proximity to the traumatic event and physical injury resulting from the event. Traumatic events which were directly experienced resulted in a longer average duration of PTSD symptoms than traumatic events which were indirectly experienced, such as learning about the unexpected loss or trauma of a loved one (48 months vs. 12 months: Breslau *et al.* 1998). Similarly, Resnick *et al.* (1993)

found that direct threat to life or personal injury was a predictor of PTSD in a national sample of women. Epstein *et al.* (1998) also reported that health care workers who directly worked with the most severe burn victims following an air disaster were more likely to develop PTSD at 6, 12 or 18 months post-trauma than those not exposed to the most severe victims. Two direct measures of severity of physical injury (i.e. unconsciousness at the time of the accident and persistent medical problems at 3 months post-accident) were related to PTSD severity at 3 months post-trauma in a sample of MVA survivors assessed in the emergency room immediately following the accident and again at 3 months postaccident (Ehlers *et al.* 1998). Comparable results were found when medical personnel completed an objective measure of injury severity following MVA. Severity of injury as assessed by medical personnel predicted PTSD symptom severity and diagnosis between 1 and 4 months post-trauma (Blanchard *et al.* 1995). Also, perceived life threat assessed immediately after the MVA predicted PTSD symptoms at 1 and 4 months postMVA (Blanchard *et al.* 1995). Similar results were found in a sample of women who survived physical assault; individuals who perceived their lives to be in danger during the assault were more likely to develop persistent PTSD (Riggs *et al.* 1995). Earlier studies also support the conclusion that individuals who have experienced more severe traumatic events have a higher risk of developing PTSD (e.g. McFarlane 1988; Kilpatrick *et al.* 1989).

Developmental factors

Several personal vulnerability factors have also been implicated in the development of PTSD. In their earlier retrospective study, Breslau *et al.* (1991) found that early separation from parents, neuroticism, pretrauma anxiety or depression, and family history of anxiety, all predicted PTSD development following trauma exposure. Again using a retrospective design, Davidson *et al.* (1991) found that individuals with PTSD had more family history of psychiatric illness, more job instability, parental poverty, child abuse, and lower subjective social support. As another indication of early environmental stress, the parents of individuals with PTSD were more likely to have separated or divorced in their childhood (prior to the age of 10:

Davidson *et al.* 1991). Behavioral problems before the age of 15 have also been found to be associated with increased rates of PTSD (Helzer *et al.* 1987). Taken together, these findings suggest that growing up in a less advantaged home environment renders the person vulnerable to develop PTSD. When such an environment is combined with early psychological difficulties, the probability of developing PTSD is greater. The retrospective nature of these studies weakens the conclusions about the causal relationships between these variables and later PTSD.

Other psychopathology

Another factor that was found to be associated with PTSD is the presence of other psychopathology. Accordingly, PTSD was associated with greater psychiatric comorbidity and a history of attempted suicide in adult samples (Helzer *et al.* 1987; Davidson *et al.* 1991). While these studies and others (e.g. Breslau *et al.* 1991; Kessler *et al.* 1995) suggest that PTSD is associated with general psychopathology, the retrospective design does not allow for causal inferences.

History of traumatic events

Many individuals have experienced more than one trauma (Kessler *et al.* 1995). The mean number of lifetime traumatic events among adults is 4.8 (Breslau *et al.* 1998). A history of prior victimization has been found to increase the likelihood of developing PTSD following an index trauma (e.g. Ellis *et al.* 1981; Resnick *et al.* 1993; Bernat *et al.* 1998). Also, increased frequency of traumatic events was predictive of greater PTSD severity among young adults (Bernat *et al.* 1998). In a meta-analysis, Brewin *et al.* (2000) found that child abuse history was a relatively consistent predictor of PTSD across studies. In an attempt to explain the relationship between early environmental factors, multiple traumatic events, and PTSD, Bolstad and Zinbarg (1997) examined retrospectively in young, adult women factors related to PTSD symptom severity following adult victimization. Multiple experiences of childhood sexual abuse was associated with a decreased perception of control and this, in turn, was associated with greater PTSD symptom severity.

Dissociation and numbing during or shortly after the trauma

Dissociation and numbing during and immediately after the traumatic event has been implicated in the development of chronic PTSD. In retrospective studies, dissociative symptoms during or immediately after other types of traumatic events (i.e. natural disasters, combat, and MVA) have been found to predict later PTSD (Koopman *et al.* 1994; Marmar *et al.* 1994; Tichenor *et al.* 1996; Ehlers *et al.* 1998). In a sample of health care workers who cared for victims of an air disaster, those individuals who experienced emotional numbness immediately following the disaster were more likely to develop PTSD (Epstein *et al.* 1998). In a prospective study, Gilboa-Schechtman & Foa 2001) found that participants with delayed peak reactions as measured by severity of PTSD symptoms, depression, and trait anxiety exhibited more psychopathology 12 weeks post-trauma than those with early peaks. While numbing and dissociation were not directly assessed in this study, the authors suggested that lower levels of expressed distress shortly after the trauma may be indicative of low emotional engagement, or dissociation. In another prospective study, dissociation within 2 weeks of physical assault was predictive of PTSD symptoms at 3 months postassault† (Dancu *et al.* 1996).

Severe negative emotional reactions during the trauma

Focusing more broadly on severe emotional reactions, Bernat *et al.* (1998) found that in addition to dissociation, retrospective report of intense negative emotional reactions and panic symptoms during the trauma were associated with greater PTSD symptoms severity at the time of assessment. Notably, this effect remained significant after controlling for vulnerability factors (gender and number of traumas) and objective characteristics of the trauma (personal injury, life threat, and other killed or injured). Consistent results have been found in MVA survivor populations. MVA survivors' ratings of perceived fright and dissociation during the accident predicted PTSD symptom severity at 3 and 12 months postaccident (Ehlers *et al.* 1998).

†This was not true for sexual assault survivors who generally reported more dissociation (Dancu *et al.* 1996).

Coping

Coping following the trauma may also increase the risk for PTSD. For example, diagnosis of ASD and high levels of re-experiencing and arousal symptoms within the 1st month after crime exposure, independently contributed to the prediction of PTSD at 6 months postcrime (Brewin *et al.* 1999). One coping factor which was found to be related to PTSD severity is anger. High anger was predictive of more severe PTSD symptoms in a veteran population with chronic PTSD (Frueh *et al.* 1997). However, since this sample was composed of chronic PTSD patients, the results do not provide information regarding anger's contribution to the development of PTSD. In two prospective studies of female assault survivors, initial anger was related to PTSD (Riggs *et al.* 1992; Feeny *et al.* 2000). Using a more extended follow-up in a sample of MVA survivors, Ehlers *et al.* (1998) found that individuals who report anger immediately following MVA were more likely to be diagnosed with PTSD at 3 and 12-months postaccident.

The effects of other coping strategies on PTSD have also been examined. Wishful thinking was related to higher PTSD symptoms at 3 months postassault in female sexual and nonsexual assault survivors (Valentiner *et al.* 1996). Shame has also been implicated in the development of PTSD. For instance, after controlling for shame and anger at others as assessed 1-month post-trauma, shame at 6 months post-trauma predicted PTSD symptom severity at 6 months post-trauma in violent crime survivors (Andrews *et al.* 2000).

Reactions of others

Along with the survivors' reactions to the trauma, reactions of significant others may also increase the risk of PTSD. The degree of reported interpersonal friction shortly after assault was predictive of PTSD severity at 3 months postassault while degree of positive social support was not related to later PTSD severity (Zoellner *et al.* 1999). Indeed, individuals who experienced more stressful life events (including interpersonal strain) in the 6 months following caring for survivors of an air disaster were more likely to develop PTSD (Epstein *et al.* 1998).

Gender

Gender has been related to PTSD as women are twice as likely to develop the disorder than men (e.g. Kessler *et al.* 1995; Breslau *et al.* 1997; Breslau *et al.* 1999). However, researchers have suggested that observed gender differences are at least partially due to higher prevalence of traumas with high likelihood of PTSD among women. Also, women are thought to have greater likelihood of perception of life threat during physical attack than men (Kessler *et al.* 1995; Solomon & Davidson 1997; Tolin & Foa, unpublished manuscript, 2002). Support for this hypothesis came from Kessler *et al.* (1995) who reported higher lifetime prevalence rates of PTSD in women (10.4%) than in men (5.0%). Among those exposed to trauma, more women (20%) than men (8%) developed PTSD in this adult sample. However, while men were more likely than women to experience trauma, women were more likely than men to experience a trauma associated with a high probability of PTSD, such as rape (Kessler *et al.* 1995).

While some studies suggest that gender difference remains even after the type of trauma is controlled, these studies have often not separated rape from other personal violence. For example, Breslau *et al.* (1999) found that 13% of women and 6.2% of men who reported trauma exposure developed PTSD and suggested that the higher risk of PTSD for women was primarily due to differences in likelihood of developing PTSD following exposure to assaultive violence. Among those exposed to assaultive violence, 36% of women and only 6% of men developed PTSD. However, the gender difference revealed in this category is primarily due to the high conditional probability of developing PTSD after rape (49%), an experience reported primarily by women. The higher rates of PTSD after rape than after other assaultive violence and the higher rates of rape among women may account for some portion of the observed gender difference in PTSD rates. However, rape was not the only type of assaultive violence in which gender differences were apparent. Women also had a higher conditional risk of developing PTSD following being kidnapped, tortured, or captured than men (78% vs. 0%). Due to the low rates of reported exposure to being kidnapped, tortured, or captured in the overall sample of women and men (2.0% and 1.7%, respectively), the conditional probabilities associated with the small number of exposed cases can be imprecise. Also, the assumption that abduction experiences are a homogeneous category does not consider the variation in treatment of the victim during the abduction. Sexual assault, physical assault, and other experiences that can occur during abduction may result in higher conditional probabilities of PTSD and may be unevenly distributed between genders. Therefore, while differences in exposure to high risk traumatic events between men and women contribute to the overall gender difference in PTSD observed in this study, it does not entirely explain the results.

Women were twice as likely as men to develop PTSD following trauma exposure in a young adult sample gathered at an HMO in Detroit, MI, (Breslau *et al.* 1997). The magnitude of this difference decreased after controlling for history of pre-existing anxiety disorders or depression, but was still significant. When the trauma occurred in childhood, the gender difference was larger than when the trauma occurred in adolescence or later. Interestingly, women reporting first trauma exposure prior to age 15 were more likely to report their first traumatic event as rape or ongoing physical and sexual abuse than men victimized prior to this age. Men victimized prior to age 15 were more likely to report serious accident or injury. These results suggest that differences between men and women in the likelihood of traumatic events with a high risk of PTSD contributed to the observed gender difference in PTSD prevalence in this study. Again, this may not entirely explain the observed gender differences.

An alternate explanation for the observed gender differences in PTSD prevalence is suggested by the finding that PTSD symptoms may persist longer in women than men (48 vs. 12 months) in a representative adult sample (Breslau *et al.* 1998). If women experience symptoms longer than men, they would be more likely to meet diagnostic criteria for PTSD at any given time than men. Inconsistent with this hypothesis is the findings by Ehlers *et al.* (1998) that gender predicted PTSD symptom severity at 3 months, but not at 12 months. For a more complete discussion of gender differences in PTSD rates see Tolin and Foa (unpublished manuscript 2002).

Social impact of PTSD

As noted earlier, PTSD often exists with other problems, including depression, substance abuse or dependence, poor physical health, and poor social or occupational functioning. For an extensive review of the social impact of PTSD see Kessler (2000). While little research has focused specifically on the financial costs of PTSD, in the year 1990, the direct and indirect costs of anxiety disorders in general were estimated to be US$46.6 billion. This constitutes 32% of the mental health costs for that year in the US and represents an increase of 38% over estimates from 1985 (Dupont et al. 1996). Direct costs include increased doctor visits, emergency rooms visits, psychiatric hospitalization, and outpatient psychotherapy. Indirect costs include missed work, decreased productivity, and job loss.

PTSD and physical health

While several studies have examined increased somatic symptoms and medical utilization among victims of different traumatic experiences, few studies examined these factors in PTSD and nonPTSD populations. One study examining sexual assault survivors (Waigandt et al. 1990) found that in the 2 years following an assault, women survivors reported more negative health perceptions, more physical symptoms, more negative health behaviors (e.g. smoking, lack of exercise), more doctor visits per year, and more reproductive physiology illnesses than women who had not been assaulted. Women survivors of criminal assault incurred 2.5 times the outpatient costs of nonvictims in the 2 years following the crime, including making twice as many doctor visits. This rate of utilization significantly increased relative to the 2 years prior to the crime. Also, the degree of violence of the crime predicted more doctor visits (Koss et al. 1991). Increased somatic complaints, poorer health perceptions, and increased medical utilization have been reported up to 1 year following victimization in sexual assault victims versus nonvictims (Kimerling & Calhoun 1994). Accordingly, the medical costs of victimization appear to be extremely high.

Studies that focus on PTSD compared to nonPTSD populations, found the expected increased use of medical services when the traumatic experience involved physical injury. However, several studies have found that PTSD was associated with increased use of medical services irrespective of injury (for a full review see Jaycox & Foa 1999). The majority of the available studies comparing people with and without PTSD have been conducted in veteran populations. Veterans

with PTSD had increased incidence of hypertension, bronchial asthma, and peptic ulcers (Davidson et al. 1991) and used more inpatient medical services following discharge (Kulka et al. 1990) than veterans without PTSD. Veterans with PTSD also had more unfavorable lipid profiles compared to veterans without PTSD (Kagan et al. 1999). Following a review of research examining the medical impact of PTSD, Friedman and Schnurr (1995) concluded on the basis of available studies, that PTSD is associated with higher rates of cardiovascular morbidity.

In a sample of female veterans, PTSD was associated with an increased likelihood of cardiovascular, gastrointestinal, gynecological, dermatological, opthalmological, and pain problems even after controlling for war-zone exposure (Wolfe et al. 1994). In a follow-up study, PTSD symptoms in women veterans predicted both physical symptoms and reported health perceptions (Kimerling et al. 2000). Also, the hyperarousal cluster predicted health complaints beyond the other two symptom clusters. To address the hypothesis that the health problems preceded PTSD, a prospective design was used in a sample of male and female Gulf War veterans. PTSD symptoms assessed immediately upon returning from the war predicted self-reported health problems 18–24 months later (Wagner et al. 2000). In a study comparing individuals with and without PTSD in nonveteran, female survivors of crime, PTSD severity predicted self-reported physical symptoms beyond negative life events, anger, and depression (Zoellner et al. 2000). Taken together, the studies described above suggest that PTSD uniquely contributes, either directly or indirectly, to negative health and to increased health costs beyond what is attributable to the traumatic experience *per se*.

PTSD and mental health

As mentioned earlier, comorbidity rates between PTSD and depression are high with 26–68% of individuals with PTSD having met criteria for major depression and 34% having met criteria for dysthymic disorders (Kilpatrick et al. 1987; Keane & Wolfe 1990; Kulka et al. 1990). Individuals with comorbid disorders are likely to experience even greater difficulties in social and occupational functioning than those with PTSD alone. Indeed, more severely impaired functioning can be apparent in an inability to care for children, marital discord, and job loss resulting in high social costs.

Individuals with PTSD have higher rates and risk of suicide than individuals without PTSD (e.g. Davidson *et al.* 1991; Kessler 2000; Kotler *et al.* 2001). Among a sample of political refugees diagnosed with PTSD, 57% reported suicidal behavior (including thoughts, plan, and attempt) with similar rates in those individuals with a comorbid diagnosis of depression (56%) and those without such a comorbid diagnosis (58%: Ferrada-Noli *et al.* 1998). The social cost of the impact of suicide and attempted suicide on the victim and those close to the victim is understandably high. As discussed previously, the unexpected loss of a loved one is one of the most frequent precipitating events for PTSD (e.g. Norris 1992; Breslau *et al.* 1998). Indeed, it is possible that suicide may create a cycle of PTSD in which the suicide of one individual precipitates PTSD in another individual.

The negative impact of PTSD on social relationships results in high social costs. Feelings of emotional detachment and estrangement from others are defining features of PTSD. While many of the symptoms of PTSD can result in interpersonal difficulties (e.g. angry outbursts, avoidance of social contact, avoidance of sexual contact), estrangement and detachment can be especially detrimental. Individuals with PTSD often report feeling unable to emotionally care for their children or unresponsive to the needs of those closest to them. For instance, sexual dysfunction and dissatisfaction are common among sexual assault survivors (e.g. Letourneau *et al.* 1996; Jaycox & Foa 1999). These problems affect not only the quality of life for the survivor, but also the quality of significant relationships which can potentially increase interpersonal stress and impede recovery from trauma as previously discussed. Such problems can result in separation or divorce from significant others and social isolation from friends.

As previously mentioned, alcohol abuse and PTSD commonly co-occur (e.g. Kilpatrick & Resnick 1993). Research has also demonstrated that the prevalence and severity of alcohol dependence are related to the severity of PTSD (Breslau & Davis 1992; McFall *et al.* 1992). The comorbidity of these disorders is also related to more dissociative symptoms and more borderline personality characteristics and elevated avoidance and arousal symptoms (Behar 1987; Saladin *et al.* 1995; Ouimette *et al.* 1996). The high rate of this comorbidity also increases the social cost of PTSD in both loss of social and occupational functioning and increases in societal problems which coincide with substance abuse and dependence (e.g. crimes to pay for the substance, loss of ability to care for children and self, etc.).

Conclusions

PTSD is an anxiety disorder precipitated by exposure to an event which involves actual or threatened death or serious injury or threat to the personal integrity of self or others that causes intense fear, helplessness, or horror. The defining symptoms include re-experiencing aspects of the trauma, avoidance of trauma-related stimuli, numbing, and arousal. PTSD often co-occurs with other psychiatric diagnoses, most commonly MDD and alcohol and substance abuse or dependence.

Several factors may be useful in identifying individuals most at risk for PTSD. First, individuals who have experienced assaultive violence, especially rape and physical assault, are more likely to develop PTSD than other trauma populations. However, this does not mean that other traumatic experiences cannot lead to PTSD. Indeed, unexpected loss of a loved one is one of the most commonly reported precipitating events for PTSD (Breslau *et al.* 1998, 1999). Second, individuals who have experienced multiple traumatic experiences are more likely to be diagnosed with PTSD. Third, high levels of emotional reactions (such as fear and anger), dissociation, and numbing are all predictive of PTSD severity and development. Also, more interpersonal stress following traumatic events is predictive of PTSD severity. Finally, women are more likely to be diagnosed with PTSD than men. Research is necessary to clarify the specific nature of and reasons for this observed difference.

Due to the extreme negative impact of PTSD on the social and occupational functioning of individuals with this disorder, PTSD extracts an extremely high negative social impact. As such, continued research into the factors which predict those most vulnerable to the development of PTSD, along with continued examination of effective treatment strategies for PTSD are imperative.

References

American Psychiatric Association (APA) (1980) *Diagnostic Statistical Manual of Mental Disorders*, 3rd edn. American Psychiatric Association, Washington, D.C.

American Psychiatric Association (APA) (1987) *Diagnostic Statistical Manual of Mental Disorders*, 3rd edn, revised. American Psychiatric Association, Washington, D.C.

American Psychiatric Association (APA) (1994) *Diagnostic Statistical Manual of Mental Disorders*, 4th edn. American Psychiatric Association, Washington, D.C.

Andrews, B., Brewin, C.R., Rose, S. *et al.* (2000) Predicting symptoms in survivors of violent crime: the role of shame, anger, and childhood abuse. *J Abnorm Psychol* **109**(1), 69–73.

Beck, A.T., Ward, C.H., Mendelsohn, M., Mock, J. & Erbaugh, J. (1961) An inventory for measuring depression. *Arch Gen Psychiatry* **4**, 561–71.

Behar, D. (1987) Flashbacks and post-traumatic stress in combat veterans. *Comprehensive Psychiatry* **28**(6), 459–66.

Bernat, J.A., Ronfeldt, H.M., Calhoun, K.S. *et al.* (1998) Prevalence of traumatic events and peritraumatic predictors of post-traumatic stress symptoms in a nonclinical sample of college students. *J Trauma Stress* **11**(4), 645–64.

Blake, D.D., Weathers, F.W., Nagy, L.M. *et al.* (1990) A clinician rating scale for assessing current and lifetime PTSD: the CAPS-1. *Behavior Therapist* **18**, 187–8.

Blanchard, E.B., Hickling, E.J., Mitnick, N. *et al.* (1995) The impact of severity of physical injury and perception of life threat in the development of post-traumatic stress disorder in motor vehicle accident survivors. *Behav Res Ther* **33**(5), 529–34.

Bolstad, B.R. & Zinbarg, R.E. (1997) Sexual victimization, generalized perception of control, and post-traumatic stress disorder symptom severity. *J Anxiety Disord* **11**(5), 523–40.

Breslau, N., Chilcoat, H.D., Kessler, R.C. *et al.* (1999) Vulnerability to assaultive violence: Further specification of the sex difference in post-traumatic stress disorder. *Psychol Med* **29**, 813–21.

Breslau, N. & Davis, G.C. (1992) Post-traumatic stress disorder in an urban population of young adults: risk factors for chronicity. *Am J Psychiatry* **149**, 671–5.

Breslau, N., Davis, G.C., Andreski, P. *et al.* (1991) Traumatic events and post-traumatic stress disorder in an urban population of young adults. *Arch Gen Psychiatry* **48**, 216–22.

Breslau, N., Davis, G.N., Andreski, P. *et al.* (1997) Sex differences in post-traumatic stress disorder. *Arch Gen Psychiatry* **54**(11), 1044–8.

Breslau, N., Kessler, R.C., Chilcoat, H.D. *et al.* (1998) Trauma and post-traumatic stress disorder in the community: the 1996 Detroit area survey of trauma. *Arch Gen Psychiatry* **55**(7), 626–32.

Brewin, C.R., Andrews, B. & Rose, S. (2000) Fear, helplessness, and horror in post-traumatic stress disorder: investigating DSM-IV criterion A2 in survivors of violent crime. *J Trauma Stress* **13**(3), 499–509.

Brewin, C.R., Andrews, B., Rose, S. *et al.* (1999) Acute stress disorder and post-traumatic stress disorder in survivors of violent crime. *Am J Psychiatry* **156**(3), 360–6.

Brewin, C.R., Andrews, B. & Valentine, J.D. (2000) Meta-analysis of risk factors for post-traumatic stress disorder in trauma-exposed adults. *J Consult Clin Psychol* **68**(5), 748–66.

Cormier, W.H. & Cormier, L.S. (1991) Defining client problems with an interview assessment. In: *Interviewing Strategies for Helpers* (W.H. Cormier & L.S. Cormier (eds), pp. 171–215). Brooks/Cole Publishing Co., Pacific Grove, CA.

Dancu, C.V., Riggs, D.S., Hearst-Ikeda, D. *et al.* (1996) Dissociative experiences and post-traumatic stress disorder among female survivors of criminal assault and rape. *J Trauma Stress* **9**(2), 253–67.

Davidson, J.T., Hughes, D., Blazer, D.G. *et al.* (1991) Post-traumatic stress disorder in the community: an epidemiological study. *Psychological Medicine* **21**, 713–21.

DiNardo, P.A., Brown, T.A. & Barlow, D.H. (1994) *Anxiety Disorders Interview Schedule for DSM-IV: Lifetime Version (ADIS-IV-L)*. Psychological Corporation, San Antonio, TX.

DuPont, R.L., Rise, D.P., Miller, L.S., Shiraki, S.S., Rowland, C.R., Harwood, H.J. (1996) Economic costs of anxiety disorders. *Anxiety* **2**, 167–72.

Ehlers, A., Mayou, R.A. & Bryant, B. (1998) Psychological predictors of chronic post-traumatic stress disorder after motor vehicle accidents. *J Abnorm Psychol* **107**(3), 508–19.

Ellis, E.M., Atkeson, B.M. & Calhoun, K.S. (1981) An assessment of long-term reactions to rape. *J Abnorm Psychol* **90**(3), 263–6.

Epstein, R.S., Fullerton, C.S. & Ursano, R.J. (1998) Post-traumatic stress disorder following an air disaster: a prospective study. *Am J Psychiatry* **155**(7), 934–8.

Feeny, N.C., Zoellner, L.A. & Foa, E.B. (2000) Anger, dissociation, and post-traumatic stress disorder among female assault survivors. *J Trauma Stress* **13**(1), 89–100.

Ferrada-Noli, M., Asberg, M., Ormstad, K. *et al.* (1998) Suicidal behavior after severe trauma. Part 1: PTSD diagnosis, psychiatric comorbidity, and assessments of suicidal behavior. *J Trauma Stress* **11**(1), 103–24.

First, M.B., Spitzer, R.L., Gibbon, M. *et al.* (1997) *Structured Clinical Interview for DSM-IV Axis I Disorders: Clinician Version (SCID-IV)*. American Psychiatric Press, Washington, D.C.

Flack, W.F., Litz, B.T., Hsieh, F.Y. *et al.* (2000) Predictors of emotional numbing, revisited: a replication and extension. *J Trauma Stress* **13**(4), 611–18.

Foa, E.B., Cashman, L., Jaycox, L. *et al.* (1997) The validation of a self-report measure of post-traumatic stress disorder: the Post-traumatic Diagnostic Scale. *Psychol Assess* **9**, 445–51.

Foa, E.B., Dancu, C.V., Hembree, E.A. *et al.* (1999) A comparison of exposure therapy, stress inoculation training, and their combination for reducing post-traumatic stress disorder in female assault victims. *J Consult Clin Psychol* **67**, 194–200.

Foa, E.B. & Riggs, D.S. (1995) Post-traumatic stress disorder following assault: theoretical considerations and empirical findings. *Current Directions in Psychological Science* **2**, 61–5.

Foa, E.B., Riggs, D.S., Dancu, C.V. *et al.* (1993) Reliability and validity of a brief instrument for assessing post-traumatic stress disorder. *J Trauma Stress* **6**, 459–73.

Foa, E.B., Riggs, D.S. & Gershuny, B.S. (1995) Arousal, numbing, and intrusion: symptom structure of PTSD following assault. *Am J Psychiatry* **152**(1), 116–20.

Foa, E.B. & Rothbaum, B.O. (1998) *Treating the Trauma of Rape: Cognitive-Behavioral Therapy for PTSD.* Guilford Press, New York.

Foa, E.B. & Tolin, D.F. (2000) Comparison of the PTSD Symptom Scale-Interview version and the Clinician-Administered PTSD Scale. *J Trauma Stress* **13**(2), 181–91.

Friedman, M.J. & Schnurr, P.P. (1995) The relationship between trauma, post-traumatic stress disorder, and physical health. In: *Neurobiological and Clinical Consequences* (M.J. Friedman, D.S. Charney & A.Y. Deutch (eds), pp. 507–24). Lippincott–Raven Publishers, Philadelphia, PA.

Frueh, B.C., Henning, K.R., Pellegrin, K.L. *et al.* (1997) Relationship between scores on anger measures and PTSD symptomatology, employment, and compensation seeking status in combat veterans. *Journal of Clin Psychol* **53**(8), 871–8.

Gilboa-Schechtman, E. & Foa, E.B. (2001) Patterns of recovery from trauma: the use of intraindividual analysis. *Journal of Abnormal Psychology* **110**(3), 392–400.

Helzer, J.E., Robins, L.N. & McEvoy, L. (1987) Post-traumatic stress disorder in the general population: findings of the Epidemiological Catchment Area survey. *N Engl J Med* **317**(26), 1630–4.

Horowitz, M.J., Wilner, N. & Alvarez, W. (1979) Impact of Event Scale: a measure of subjective distress. *Psychosomatic Medicine* **41**, 209–18.

Jaycox, L.H. & Foa, E.B. (1999) Cost-effectiveness issues in the treatment of post-traumatic stress disorder. In: *Cost-Effectiveness of Psychotherapy* (N.E. Miller & K.M. Magruder (eds), pp. 259–69). Oxford University Press, Inc., New York, NY.

Kagan, B.L., Leskin, G., Haas, B., Wilkins, J., Foy, D. (1999) Elevated lipid levels in Vietnam veterans with chronic post-traumatic stress disorder. *Biological Psychiatry* **45**(3), 374–7.

Keane, T.M., Caddell, J.M. & Taylor, K.L. (1988) Mississippi scale for combat-related PTSD: three studies in reliability and validity. *J Consult Clin Psychol* **56**, 85–90.

Keane, T.M., Kolb, L.C., Kaloupek, D.G. *et al.* (1998) Utility of psychophysiological measurement in the diagnosis of post-traumatic stress disorder: results from a Department of Veterans Affairs Cooperative Study. *J Consult Clin Psychol* **66**, 914–23.

Keane, T.M., Malloy, P.F. & Fairbank, J.A. (1984) Empirical development of an MMPI subscale for the assessment of combat-related post-traumatic stress disorder. *J Consult Clin Psychol* **52**, 888–91.

Keane, T.M. & Wolfe, J. (1990) Comorbidity in post-traumatic stress disorder: an analysis of clinical and community studies. *J Appl Soc Psychol* **20**, 1176–88.

Kessler, R.C. (2000) Post-traumatic stress disorder: the burden to the individual and society. *J Clin Psychiatry* **61** (Suppl. 5), 4–14.

Kessler, R.C., Sonnega, A., Bromet, E. *et al.* (1995) Post-traumatic stress disorder in the National Comorbidity Survey. *Arch Gen Psychiatry* **52**, 1048–60.

Kilpatrick, D.G. & Resnick, H.S. (1993) Post-traumatic stress disorder associated with exposure to criminal victimization in clinical and community populations. In: *Post-traumatic Stress Disorder: DSM-IV and Beyond* (R.T. Davidson & E.B. Foa (eds), pp. 113–43). American Psychiatric Press, Washington, D.C.

Kilpatrick, D.G., Saunders, B.E., Amick-McMullan, A. *et al.* (1989) Survivor and crime factors associated with the development of crime-related post-traumatic stress disorder. *Behavior Therapy* **20**, 199–214.

Kilpatrick, D.G., Saunders, B.E., Veronen, L.J. *et al.* (1987) Criminal victimization: lifetime prevalence, reporting to police, and psychological impact. *Crime and Delinquency* **33**, 479–89.

Kimerling, R. & Calhoun, K.S. (1994) Somatic symptoms, social support, and treatment seeking among sexual assault victims. *J Consult Clin Psychol* **62**(2), 333–40.

Kimerling, R., Clum, G.A. & Wolfe, J. (2000) Relationships among trauma exposure, chronic post-traumatic stress disorder symptoms, and self-reported health in women: replication and extension. *J Trauma Stress* **13**(1), 115–28.

van der Kolk, B.A., Dreyfuss, D., Michaels, M. *et al.* (1994) Fluoxetine in post-traumatic stress disorder. *J Clin Psychiatry* **55**(12), 517–22.

Koopman, C., Classen, C. & Spiegel, D. (1994) Predictors of post-traumatic stress symptoms among Oakland/Berkeley firestorm survivors. *Am J Psychiatry* **151**, 888–94.

Koss, M.P., Koss, P.G. & Woodruff, W.J. (1991) Deleterious effects of criminal victimization on women's health and medical utilization. *Arch Intern Med* **151**, 342–7.

Kotler, M., Iancu, I., Efroni, R. *et al.* (2001) Anger, impulsivity, social support, and suicide risk in patients with post-traumatic stress disorder. *J Nerv Ment Dis* **189**(3), 162–7.

Kulka, R.A., Schlenger, W.E., Fairbank, J.A. *et al.* (1990) *Trauma and the Vietnam War Generation. Report of findings from the National Vietnam Veterans Readjustment Study.* Brunner/Mazel, New York.

Letourneau, E.J., Resnick, H.S., Kilpatrick, D.G. *et al.* (1996) Comorbidity of sexual problems and post-traumatic stress disorder in female crime victims. *Behavior Therapy* **27**, 321–36.

Litz, B.T., Schlenger, W.E., Weathers, F.W. *et al.* (1997) Predictors of emotional numbing in post-traumatic stress disorder. *J Trauma Stress* **10**(4), 607–18.

March, J.S. (1993) What constitutes a stressor? The "criterion A" issue. In: *Post-traumatic Stress Disorder: DSM-IV and Beyond* (J.T. Davidson & E.B. Foa (eds), pp. 37–54). American Psychiatric Press, Washington, D.C.

Marmar, C.R., Weiss, D.S., Schlenger, D.S. *et al.* (1994) Peritraumatic dissociation and post-traumatic stress in male Vietnam theater veterans. *Am J Psychiatry* **151**, 902–7.

McFall, M.E., Mackay, P.W. & Donovan, D.M. (1992) Combat-related post-traumatic stress disorder and severity of substance abuse in Vietnam veterans. *J Stud Alcohol* **53**(4), 357–63.

McFall, M.E., Smith, D.E., Mackay, P.W. *et al.* (1990) Reliability and validity of the Mississippi Scale for combat-related post-traumatic stress disorder. *Psychol Assess* **2**, 114–21.

McFarlane, A.C. (1988) The aetiology of post-traumatic stress disorders following natural disaster. *Br J Psychiatry* **152**, 116–21.

Newman, E., Kaloupek, D.G. & Keane, T.M. (1996) Assessment of post-traumatic stress disorder in clinical and research settings. In: *Traumatic Stress: The Effects of Overwhelming Experience on Mind, Body Society* (B.A. van der Kolk, A.C. McFarlane & L. Weisaeth (eds), pp. 242–73). Guilford Press, New York.

Norris, F.H. (1992) Epidemiology of trauma: frequency and impact of different potentially traumatic events on different demographic groups. *J Consult Clin Psychol* **60**(3), 409–18.

Ouimette, P.C., Wolfe, J. & Chrestman, K.R. (1996) Characteristics of post-traumatic stress disorder-alcohol abuse comorbidity in women. *J Subst Abuse* **8**(3), 335–46.

Resnick, H.S., Kilpatrick, D.G., Dansky, B.S. *et al.* (1993) Prevalence of civilian trauma and post-traumatic stress disorder in a representative national sample of women. *J Consult Clin Psychol* **61**(6), 984–91.

Riggs, D.S., Dancu, C.V., Gershuny, B.S. *et al.* (1992) Anger and post-traumatic stress disorder in female crime survivors. *J Trauma Stress* **5**(4), 613–25.

Riggs, D.S., Rothbaum, B.O. & Foa, E.B. (1995) A prospective examination of post-traumatic stress disorder in survivors of nonsexual assault. *Journal of Interpersonal Violence* **10**(2), 201–14.

Robins, L.N., Helzer, J.E., Croughland, J.L., Williams, J.B.W. & Spitzer, R.L. (1981) *NIMH Diagnostic Interview Schedule—Version III. Public Health Services (PHS)*, publication ADM-T-42-3 (5-8-81). NIMH, Rockville, MD.

Rothbaum, B.O., Foa, E.B., Riggs, D.S. *et al.* (1992) A prospective examination of post-traumatic stress disorder in rape survivors. *J Trauma Stress* **5**(3), 455–75.

Saladin, M.E., Brady, K.T., Dansky, B.S. *et al.* (1995) Understanding comorbidity between PTSD and substance use disorders: two preliminary investigations. *Addict Behav* **20**(5), 643–55.

Solomon, S.D. & Davidson, J.T. (1997) Trauma: prevalence, impairment, service use, and cost. *J Clin Psychiatry* **58** (Suppl. 9), 5–11.

Spielberger, C.D., Gorsuch, R.L. & Lushene, R.E. (1970) *Manual for the State-Trait Anxiety Inventory (Self-Evaluation Questionnaire)*. Consulting Psychological Press, Palo Alto, CA.

Tichenor, V., Marmar, C.R., Weiss, D.S. *et al.* (1996) The relationship of peritrauamtic dissociation and post-traumatic stress: findings in female Vietnam theater veterans. *J Consult Clin Psychol* **64**(5), 1054–9.

Valentiner, D.P., Riggs, D.S., Foa, E.B. *et al.* (1996) Coping strategies and post-traumatic stress disorder in female survivors of sexual and nonsexual assault. *J Abnorm Psychol* **105**(3), 455–8.

Wagner, A.W., Wolfe, J., Rotnitsky, A. *et al.* (2000) An investigation of the impact of post-traumatic stress disorder on physical health. *J Trauma Stress* **13**(1), 41–55.

Waigandt, Wallace, Phelps & Miller (1990) The impact of sexual assault on physical health status. *J Trauma Stress* **3**(1), 93–102.

Weiss, D.S. & Marmar, C.R. (1997) The impact of Event Scale-Revised. In: *Assessing Psychological Trauma and PTSD* (J.P. Wilson & T.M. Keane (eds), pp. 399–428). Guilford Press, New York.

Wolfe, J., Schnurr, P.P., Brown, P.J. *et al.* (1994) PTSD and war-zone exposure as correlates of perceived health in female Vietnam veterans. *J Consult Clin Psychol* **62**, 1235–40.

Zoellner, L.A., Foa, E.B. & Brigidi, B.D. (1999) Interpersonal friction and PTSD in female survivors of sexual and nonsexual assault. *J Trauma Stress* **12**(4), 689–99.

Zoellner, L.A., Goodwin, M.L. & Foa, E.B. (2000) PTSD severity and health perceptions in female victims of sexual assault. *J Trauma Stress* **13**(4), 635–49.

Obsessive-compulsive Disorder

J. Zohar, Y. Sasson, M. Chopra, R. Amiaz & N. Nakash

Introduction

Obsessive-compulsive disorder (OCD) is a common, chronic, and disabling disorder characterized by obsessions and/or compulsions. These symptoms are egodystonic and cause significant distress to patients and their families. Up to the early 1980s, OCD was considered a rare, treatment-refractory, chronic condition, of psychological origin. Since then, however, several researchers have reported that the prevalence of OCD is around 2% in the general population (Robins *et al.* 1984; Weissman *et al.* 1994) and it is almost equally distributed between males and females.

Clinical features

The diagnosis of OCD according to the Diagnostic Statistical Manual, fourth edition (DSM-IV: American Psychiatric Association 1994) is based on the presence of either obsessions or compulsions. Obsessions are recurrent, intrusive and distressing thoughts, images or impulses, while compulsions are repetitive, seemingly purposeful behaviors that a person feels driven to perform. Obsessions are usually unpleasant and increase a person's anxiety, whereas carrying out compulsions reduces it. Resisting carrying out a compulsion, however, results in increased anxiety. The patient usually realizes that the obsessions are irrational and experiences both the obsession and the compulsion as egodystonic.

The obsessions and compulsions cause marked distress, are time-consuming (more than 1 h per day) and interfere significantly with the person's normal routine and social and occupational activities. At some point during the course of the disorder, but not necessarily during the current episode, the diagnosis requires for the person to have recognized that the obsessions or compulsions are excessive or unreasonable. However, if during most of the current episode the patient does not have this recognition, the diagnosis of OCD with poor insight might be most appropriate.

If another Axis I disorder is present, it is mandatory that the content of the obsessions or compulsions not be restricted to it (e.g., preoccupation with food or weight in eating disorders, or guilt ruminations in the presence of major depressive episode). The disturbance should not be due to the direct effects of a substance (e.g., a drug of abuse or a medication), or a general medical condition.

The DSM-IV diagnostic criteria for OCD are presented in Table 6.1.

Symptom clusters

The number and types of obsessions and compulsions are remarkably limited and stereotypical, and can generally be classified into several major symptom clusters.

The most prevalent obsession is concerned with contamination by dirt and/or germs; its accompanying compulsion is *washing*. Such patients may spend several hours daily washing their hands, showering or cleaning. Typically, they attempt to avoid sources of "contamination" such as door knobs, electric switches and newspapers. Paradoxically, some of these patients are actually quite slovenly. While they recognize that nothing will happen if they resist washing, they may refuse to touch even their own bodies, knowing that if

Table 6.1 Diagnostic criteria for OCD (DSM-IV).

A. Either obsessions or compulsions
Obsessions as defined by 1, 2, 3 and 4:
  1 Recurrent and persistent thoughts, impulses, or images
  2 The thoughts, impulses, or images are not simply excessive worries about real-life problems
  3 The person attempts to ignore or suppress such thoughts, impulses, or images, or to neutralize them
  4 The person recognizes that the obsessional thoughts, impulses, or images are a product of his or her own mind (not imposed from without as in thought insertion)
Compulsions are defined by 1 and 2:
  1 Repetitive behaviors (e.g., hand washing, ordering, checking) or mental acts (e.g., praying, counting, repeating words silently) that the person feels driven to perform
  2 The behaviors or mental acts are aimed at preventing or reducing distress or preventing some dreaded event or situation

B. At some point during the course of the disorder, the person has recognized that the obsessions or compulsions are excessive or unreasonable. Note: this does not apply to children

C. The obsessions or compulsions cause marked distress, are time consuming (take more than 1 h a day), or significantly interfere with the person's normal routine

D. If another Axis 1 disorder is present, the content of the obsessions or compulsions is not restricted to it (e.g., preoccupation with food in the presence of an eating disorder; ruminations in the presence of major depressive disorder)

E. The disturbance is not due to the direct physiological effects of a substance (e.g., a drug of abuse, a medication) or a general medical condition

Specify **with poor insight** if, for most of the time during the current episode, the person does not recognize that the obsessions and compulsions are excessive or unreasonable.

they do, they will not be at ease unless they carry out extensive washing rituals.

Another symptom cluster is that of *checking*. These patients are obsessed with doubt, usually tinged with guilt, and are frequently concerned that if they do not check carefully enough they will harm others. Yet instead of resolving uncertainty, their checking often only contributes to even greater doubt, which leads to further checking. Often these patients will enlist the help of family and friends to ensure they have checked enough or correctly. By some inscrutable means, the checker ultimately resolves a particular doubt, only to have it replaced by a new one. Resistance, which in this case involves the attempt to refrain from checking, leads to difficulty in concentrating and to exhaustion from the endless intrusion of nagging uncertainties.

Common examples of such doubts are the fear of causing a fire, that leads to checking the stove (even to the extent that the patient cannot leave home), or the fear of hurting someone while driving, leading to repetitive driving back over the same spot after hitting a bump in the road. Some checkers may not even be sure why they are checking, merely led by the inexplicable "urge" to do so. Checkers may also engage in related compulsive behaviors. Sometimes, uncertain whether the checking is sufficient, patients may develop "undoing" rituals such as counting to a certain number in their head, repeating actions a specific number of times, or avoiding particular numbers.

Another symptom cluster is that of *pure obsessions*. The pure obsessional patient experiences repetitive, intrusive thoughts which are usually somatic, aggressive, or sexual, and are always reprehensible to the thinker. In the absence of what appears to be discrete compulsion, these obsessions may be associated with impulses or fearful images. When the obsession is an aggressive impulse, it is usually directed at the one person most valuable to the patient. The obsession may also be a fear of acting on other impulses (e.g., killing someone, robbing a bank, stealing), or a fear of being held responsible for something terrible (e.g., fire, plague). Often, there may be subtle rituals surrounding these obsessive thoughts. For example, a mother who is afraid she will stab her daughter may struggle with this impulse by avoiding sharp objects, then by avoiding touching her daughter and ultimately by leaving the house altogether.

Although such avoidant behavior may not appear as an actual repetitive behavior or compulsion, it does share other properties of compulsion in that it is an intentional attempt to neutralize the obsession. Patients may seek treatment claiming they have a phobia, when in fact their avoidance is motivated by obsessions. Often, close examination of the patient history will reveal the presence of other obsessions or compulsions as well.

Sexual obsessions include forbidden or perverse sexual thoughts, images, or impulses that may involve children, animals, incest, homosexuality, etc. Obsessional thoughts may also be of a religious rather than sexual or violent nature. Such thoughts can lead to repetitive silent prayer or confession or result in more apparent rituals such as repeated bowing or trips to temple, church or synagogue. Such behavior presents a particular problem to both clinicians and clergy as they attempt to draw the line between disorder and devotion.

Obsessional slowness involves the obsession to have objects or events in a certain order or position, to do and undo certain motor actions in an exact way, or to have things perfectly symmetrical or "just right." Such patients require an inordinate amount of time to complete even the simplest of tasks; thus, merely getting dressed may take a couple of hours. Unlike most obsessive-compulsive patients, these patients usually do not resist their symptoms. Instead, they seem to be consumed with completing their routine precisely. Although this subtype of OCD is rare, aspects of slowness often appear along with other obsessions and compulsions, and may be the major source of interference in daily functioning.

Another noncommon OCD subtype, where patients also make little attempt to resist their symptoms is hoarding behavior. These patients may refuse to throw out junk mail, old newspapers or used tissues, for example, because they fear throwing away something important in the process.

Many OCD patients have a combination of symptoms, although one symptom type, be it washing, checking, pure obsessions or obsessional slowness, may predominate. In addition to the lack of pure subtypes is the phenomenon of symptom shifting. At different points in the course of their illness, patients

Table 6.2 Commonly occurring obsessions and compulsions (from Rasmussen 1986).

Obsessions	%	Compulsions	%
Contamination	45	Checking	60
Pathological doubt	42	Washing	50
Somatic	36	Counting	36
Need for symmetry	31	Need to ask or confess	31
Aggressive impulse	28	Symmetry/precision	28
Sexual impulse	26	Hoarding	18
Other	13	Multiple compulsions	48
Multiple obsessions	60		

report that different OCD symptoms are predominant. Thus, a patient who in childhood may have had predominantly washing rituals may have checking rituals as an adult. The principal reason for noting this symptom shift is not in terms of treatment but in order to increase the level of confidence in making the OCD diagnosis.

Recent dimensional approaches have been utilized in order to analyse these characteristic subtypes, and present the different symptoms in an innovative way. Leckman *et al.* (1997) have examined the symptom dimensions of OCD in two groups of OCD patients ($N = 300$) using factor analysis. Four factors emerged: obsessions and checking, symmetry and ordering, cleanliness and washing, and hoarding, in total accounting for more than 60% of the variance.

Table 6.2 presents commonly occurring obsessions and compulsions.

Pathogenesis of OCD

Serotonin reuptake inhibitors are effective in the treatment of OCD while nonserotonergic reuptake inhibitors do not display antiobsessional effects (Zohar *et al.* 1992). This drug-specific response renders OCD unique among affective and anxiety disorders, which respond to both serotonergic and nonserotonergic reuptake inhibitors, and lends support to the serotonergic hypothesis for this disorder (Zohar & Insel 1987).

Abnormality of the serotonin system and particularly hypersensitivity of postsynaptic 5-HT receptors remains the leading hypothesis for the underlying pathophysiology of OCD. A number of lines of evidence support this serotonergic hypothesis, not least treatment studies which demonstrated clearly and consistently that anti-obsessional efficacy was a function of serotonin reuptake inhibition (Zohar & Kindler 1992a). Studies of markers and biological probes provided further evidence: platelet studies, for example, linked reductions in 5-HT activity with clinical response (Flament *et al.* 1988), and treatment response was correlated with decreased 5-hydroxyindoleacetic acid (5-HIAA) levels within the cerebrospinal fluid of OCD patients (Thoren *et al.* 1980). Added to this was the evidence from the behavioral or physiological responses observed following serotonergic challenge with the serotonin agonists *m*-chlorophenylpiperazine (mCPP), a compound with high affinity for 5-HT1A, 5-HT1D and 5-HT2C receptors (Zohar *et al.* 1987).

As an array of 5-HT receptors subtypes have been identified, researchers have endeavored to determine which subtype might be primarily implicated in OCD (Zohar & Kindler 1992b). Lesch *et al.* (1991) administered the 5-HT1A receptor ligand ipsapirone to drug-free patients and found that it induced hypothermia and release of corticotrophin and cortisol but had no effect on OCD symptoms. The study concluded that 5-HT1A did not seem to be the likely candidate. Furthermore, a double blind buspirone augmentation study by McDougle *et al.* (1993) found no added beneficial effect of augmentation and hence supported the general consensus regarding the limited therapeutic value of 5-HT1A agonists in OCD.

Administration of MK-212, a serotonin agonist with a high affinity for 5-HT1A and 5-HT2C receptors, similarly had no effect on behavior in OCD patients or controls (Bastani *et al.* 1990). Taken together, these challenge studies suggest that 5-HT2C and 5-HT1D receptors may be possible candidates. A pilot study with the specific 5-HT1D agonist sumatriptan in patients with OCD supports a potential role for the 5-HT1D receptor in some OCD patients (Stern *et al.* 1998). Further support for the role of 5-HT1D in OCD has emerged from the genetic study by Mundo *et al.* (2000).

Although attention has been focused on the postsynaptic serotonin receptor, presynaptic mechanisms may also be implicated. Marazziti *et al.* (1993) reported a decreased number of platelet 3H-imipramine and 3H-paroxetine binding sites, peripheral markers of the presynaptic 5-HT transporter in drug-free OCD patients compared with healthy controls and patients with

other anxiety disorders. Reassessment after 8 weeks of treatment with either clomipramine or fluvoxamine showed that 3H-imipramine density had significantly increased over baseline towards normal values. This suggests that the 5-HT transporter has a role in OCD and may be linked to recovery and positive response to serotonergic drugs.

The serotonergic hypothesis remains a necessary but not sufficient explanation for the pathogenesis of OCD. Most evidence remains focused on the basal ganglia and on a 5-HT/dopamine inter-relationship. Given that the basal ganglia receive such rich enervation from both 5-HT and dopamine neurones it has been postulated that OCD is subserved by a neuronal dysfunction in the basal ganglia and orbitofrontal cortex circuit. However, other systems, such as the neuropeptides arginine, vasopressin, oxytocin and somatostatin have also been suggested. Clinical association between obsessive-compulsive symptoms, autoimmune diseases and D8/17 positive response in OCD patients with childhood onset of OCD suggests the presence of an autoimmune mechanism. An initial attempt to utilize these findings in a clinical intervention via plasmaphoresis in these cases was encouraging (Perlmutter *et al.* 1999). Further studies are required to understand the relevance of the serotonergic and nonserotonergic systems in different subtypes of OCD.

Epidemiology

In the last decade, the prevalence of OCD symptoms in the general population has been found to be remarkably high. Until 1984, the most quoted figure was 0.05% (Woodruff & Pitts 1969). However, since 1984, at least three studies carried out in North America found the prevalence of OCD in the general population to be greater than 2%, which is 40 times higher than the earlier estimation from the 1950s. Robins *et al.* (1984) found a prevalence figure of 2.5%, Bland *et al.* (1988) found a prevalence figure of 3.0% and Karno *et al.* (1988) found a prevalence figure of 2.5% of OCD in the general population.

The prevalence of OCD in countries other than North America has also been examined. A major study carried out by Weissmann *et al.* (1994) in over four different continents examined the prevalence of OCD across the globe. This study found OCD prevalence to be approximately 2% in the US, Canada, Latin

Table 6.3 OCD prevalence worldwide.

Study	Location	Prevalence (%)
Robins et al. (1984)	US	2.5
Bland et al. (1988)	Canada	3.0
Karno et al. (1988)	US	2.5
Sasson et al. (1997)	Israel	3.6*
Reinherz et al. (1993)	US	2.1*
Chen et al. (1993)	Hong Kong	2.1
Lindal and Stefannson (1993)	Iceland	2.0
	US	2.3
	Canada	2.3
Weissman et al. (1994)	Puerto Rico	2.5
	Germany	2.1
	Taiwan	0.7
	Korea	1.9
	New Zealand	2.2
Valleni-Basile et al. (1994)	US	3.0

*Adolescent population.

America and Puerto Rico. The findings were the same in Europe and New Zealand, while in Asia and Korea, OCD prevalence was found to be 1.9%, and in Taiwan 0.7%. Therefore, with the exception of Taiwan, where the prevalence of all psychiatric disorders is relatively low, OCD prevalence worldwide is approximately 2%. With these findings, OCD has been placed prevalence-wise between major depressive disorder and schizophrenia. They also define OCD as a global problem, as the estimated total number of patients who suffer from the disorder worldwide appears to be at least 50 million. Table 6.3 presents data regarding the worldwide prevalence of OCD.

However, it should be noted that not all the authors agree with these figures. For example, Nelson and Rice (1997) and Stein et al. (1997) have suggested that diagnosis of OCD by the Diagnostic Interview Schedule and by laypersons may lead to over-diagnosis, and proposed lower prevalence rates of 1–2%.

Cultural aspects

The universality of obsessive-compulsive symptoms poses the question of what role culture plays in the content of obsessions. Thomsen (1995) found only a few cross-cultural differences in obsessive-compulsive symptoms between Denmark and the US. Various studies carried out among OCD sufferers in the US, India, England, Japan, Denmark and Israel found the content of obsessions to be relatively similar across locations (Greenberg & Wtzum 1994; Okasha et al. 1994; Foa & Kozak et al. 1995; Sasson et al. 1997). The most common obsession across these six countries, regardless of cultural background, appears to be the obsession about dirt or contamination. The second most common obsession is harm or aggression, the third is somatic, the fourth is religious, and the last is sexual obsessions. It appears therefore that the content of obsessions is remarkably similar regardless of cultural or geographic location. The commonly occurring obsessions, according to country, are presented in Table 6.4.

Additional demographic findings from the Cross-National Collaborative Study (Weissmann et al. 1994) show the mean age of onset of OCD to be roughly in the twenties; female : male ratio to be roughly 1 : 2; and the course of OCD to be usually chronic. The prevalence of OCD among children and adolescents appears to be as high as among adults (Flament et al. 1988).

Table 6.4 Content of obsessions in different countries (%).

Country	Dirt/ contamination	Harm/ aggression	Somatic	Religious	Sexual
US (N = 425)	38	24	7	6	6
India (N = 410)	32	20	14	5	6
UK (N = 86)	47	27	—	5	10
Japan (N = 61)	39	12	13	—	5
Denmark (N = 61)	34	23	18	8	6
Israel (N = 34)	50	20	3	9	6

Diagnostic issues

The DSM-IV classifies OCD as part of the anxiety disorders which include phobias (specific and social), panic disorder (with and without agoraphobia), post-traumatic stress disorder, generalized anxiety disorder, anxiety disorder due to medical condition or substance abuse, and acute stress disorders.

However, there are some important differences between OCD and other anxiety disorders. They include: age of onset (younger in OCD patients than in those with panic disorder), sex distribution (equal distribution of males and females among OCD patients compared to greater prevalence among females for other anxiety disorders), responses to anxiogenic and anxiolytic compounds, and selective responsivity of serotonergic medications (cf. Zohar & Pato 1991).

Although both obsessions and compulsions are found in a variety of psychiatric disorders, as well as in normal mental life, OCD is distinguished by two principal features. First, the symptoms are egodystonic —the individual attempts to ignore or suppress them and recognizes these preoccupations to be excessive or unreasonable. Second, the obsessions and the compulsions cause marked distress, are time consuming (should occupy more than 1 h per day, according to the DSM-IV), and lead to significant interference in functioning.

Although OCD is an anxiety disorder in the DSM-IV classification, according to the International Classification of Diseases, 10th edition (ICD-10: World Health Organization 1993) it belongs to the "Neurotic, stress-related and somatoform disorders" group as a stand-alone disorder (and not to the "Anxiety disorders" group). According to this classification, the obsessions or compulsions (or both) should be present for a period of at least 2 weeks. Otherwise, the diagnostic criteria and clinical features are quite similar to those in the DSM-IV.

Reasons for underestimation of OCD

If OCD is indeed the second most prevalent psychiatric disorder, why we do not diagnose OCD more often? The answer to this question lies in the egodystonic nature of the disorder. Patients will often attempt to disguise their symptoms due to the shame or embarrassment associated with the disorder. Thus, they will not reveal their obsessive-compulsive symptoms unless asked about them directly.

Therefore, in order to identify an OCD sufferer, every mental status examination should include five specific questions about OCD. These questions are as follows:

1 Do you wash or clean a lot?
2 Do you check things a lot?
3 Is there any thought that keeps bothering you that you would like ot get rid of but can't?
4 Do your daily activities take a lot of time to complete?
5. Are you concerned about orderliness or symmetry?

If these five questions are not asked, it is likely the diagnosis of OCD patients will elude the clinician, since, unless they are questioned directly, these patients will probably not reveal their symptoms. The crucial importance of diagnosing OCD lies in the fact that with appropriate treatment many patients will show substantial improvement, not only in their obsessive compulsive symptoms but also in their quality of life (Koran et al. 1996) and will experience a significant decrease in suffering as well.

Differential diagnosis

Certain patients with OCD may appear to resemble simple or social phobic individuals. Patients with obsessions about contamination may even describe their problem as "germ phobia." Although in individual cases it may be difficult to distinguish between OCD and phobia, unlike the phobic patient, the OCD patient's fear often involves harming others rather than the self. Furthermore, the "phobic" OCD patient is usually concerned with avoiding a stimulus that is unavoidable, such as germs, dirt, or a virus, rather than "classic" phobic objects such as crowds, bridges or tunnels.

According to the DSM-IV, another Axis I disorder may be present. However, the content of the obsession should be unrelated to it (e.g., guilty thoughts in the presence of major depressive disorder, or thoughts about food in the presence of a eating disorder should not be considered symptoms of OCD).

OCD behaviors which are engaged in excessively, with a sense of compulsion, such as pathological gambling, overeating, alcohol or drug abuse and sexuality, can also be distinguished from true compulsions, as to some degree they are exerienced as pleasurable, while compulsions are not.

There may be some similarities in the diagnosis of OCD, an Axis I disorder in DSM-IV, and of obsessive-compulsive personality disorder (OCPD), an Axis II disorder in DSM-IV. Compulsive personality disorder refers to individuals afflicted with perfectionism, orderliness, and rigidity, for whom these traits are egosyntonic. Both disorders reveal a preoccupation with aggression and control, both use the defenses of reaction formation, undoing, intellectualization, denial and isolation of affect. The psychoanalytic formulation suggests that OCD develops when these defenses fail to contain the obsessional character's anxiety. In this view, OCD is often considered to be on a continuum with OCPD pathology.

However, epidemiological evidence reveals that a concurrent diagnosis of OCPD is neither necessary nor sufficient for the development of OCD on Axis I, in most OCD patients. Moreover epidemiological evidence reveals that a substantial number of patients with OCD do not exhibit premorbid compulsive traits (Rasmussen & Tsuang 1986; Black et al. 1993; Mavissakalian et al. 1993; Thomsen & Mikkelsen 1993). These two disorders are not on a continuum, and thus, if an individual meets the criteria for both disorders, both diagnoses should be recorded.

Another source of diagnostic difficulty may arise in very severe OCD patients who may briefly relinquish the struggle against their symptoms. At such times the obsessions or compulsions may appear to shift from an egodystonic intrusion to a psychotic delusion. Since follow-up data reveal that such psychotic-like decompensations may occur in patients with OCD who never go on to develop schizophrenia, Insel and Akiskal (1986) suggested that these patients should be considered as having "obsessive-compulsive psychosis," analogous to the association between psychotic depression and depression. Indeed, the DSM-IV includes the subtype "with poor insight" which specifically refers to this status.

Prognosis and life course

OCD is characterized by a slow onset of symptoms and it may take years for symptoms to become full-blown. However, a rapid onset of symptoms may occur, sometimes associated with a traumatic event, such as pregnancy or loss. Due to the secretive nature of the disorder, there is often a delay of more than 10 years before patients come to psychiatric attention (Hollander et al. 1996). However, this delay may be shortened by the increasing public awareness regarding the disorder, through a proliferation of articles, books and movies on the subject. The course is usually long, with most patients experiencing a chronic course, while others experience a fluctuating one (Sasson et al. 1997).

A poor prognosis is indicated by yielding to (rather than resisting) compulsions. Further indications include childhood onset, bizarre compulsions, the need for hospitalization, coexisting major depressive episode, delusional beliefs, the presence of overvalued ideas (that is, some acceptance of the obsessions and compulsions), and the presence of a personality disorder (especially schizotypal personality disorder). A good prognosis is indicated by good social and occupational adjustment, the presence of a precipitating event, and an episodic nature to the symptoms. Obsessional content does not appear to be related to prognosis. However, further research is needed in order to examine the nature and determinants of prognosis in OCD.

Comorbidity

Coexisting Axis I diagnoses in primary OCD are major depressive disorder (67%), simple phobia (22%), social phobia (18%), and eating disorder (17%) (Rasmussen & Eisen 1990). Major depressive disorder, which as we have noted is the most prevalent coexisting Axis I diagnosis with primary OCD, may develop as a secondary disorder among individuals who find themselves wasting long hours each day washing or checking, or obsessing on a persistently recurring thought, which prevents them from leading fully productive lives.

OCD and tic disorder

The comorbidity with tic disorders suggests interesting pathophysiological and therapeutic implications. In juvenile OCD the rate of tic disorders reaches up to 40% of cases and there is a substantial increase in the prevalence of Tourette's syndrome among relatives of OCD patients (Pauls 1992). Tic-related OCD may constitute a separate OCD phenotype, on the basis of symptom profiles, sex ratio, age of onset, family and genetic data, neurochemical and neuroendocrine findings, and patterns of response to treatment.

OCD and depression

Depression is the most common complication of OCD and, by recognizing this relationship, DSM-IV no longer excludes a diagnosis of OCD if depression is present. Instead, it stipulates that the obsession may not be related in content to the guilt-ridden rumination of major depression. However, a precise definition of the relationship between OCD and depression remains elusive. At the clinical level, the illnesses often seem inseparable—one worsening or improving in synchrony with the other. However, in some clinical cases, OCD symptoms may remain in remission while depression recurs. Although researchers have reported some similarities in the biological markers for depression and OCD, the differences between the two outweigh their similarities (see Zohar & Insel 1987 for review).

The most striking difference is that antidepressants with excellent efficacy, such as the norardenergic reuptake inhibitor desipramine, appear to be totally ineffective in the treatment of OCD (Goodman *et al.* 1990). Only medications possessing serotonergic properties, such as clomipramine, fluoxetine, fluvoxamine, paroxetine, sertraline and citalopram, have consistent efficacy in decreasing OCD symptoms. Other differences relate again to the lack of therapeutic effect of electroconvulsive therapy or lithium augmentation in OCD, as compared to their proven efficacy in depression (McDougle *et al.* 1991; Jenicke & Rauch 1994).

OCD and other anxiety disorders

Despite the DSM-IV classification of OCD as an anxiety disorder, there are some important differences between OCD and other anxiety disorders. These include: age of onset (younger in OCD patients as compared to those with panic disorder), sex distribution (equal distribution of males and females among OCD patients as compared to greater prevalence among females of other anxiety disorders), lack of response to nonserotonergic, anxiogenic and anxiolytic compounds

(Zohar & Insel 1987b; Gross *et al.* 1998), and selective responsivity of serotonergic medications (cf. Zohar & Pato 1991).

OCD and phobia

Phobias are distinguished from OCD by the absence of a relation between the phobic objects and the obsessive thoughts or compulsive behaviors. The fears in OCD often involve harm to others rather than harm to oneself. In addition, the OCD patient when "phobic," is usually afraid of a stimulus that is unavoidable (i.e., virus, germs or dirt) as opposed to the classic phobic objects, like tunnels, bridges or crowds.

OCD and OCPD

The relationship between OCD and OCPD has been a focus of debate. This is due to the presence of certain similarities in the diagnosis of OCD, an Axis I disorder in DSM-IV, and of OCPD, an Axis II disorder in DSM-IV. Both disorders reveal a preoccupation with aggression and control, both use the defences of reaction formation, undoing, intellectualization, denial and isolation of affect. The psychoanalytic formulation suggests that OCD develops when these defences fail to contain the obsessional character's anxiety. In this view, OCD is often considered to be on a continuum with OCPD pathology.

Diagnostic confusion can be lessened if one remembers that OCD symptoms are usually egodystonic, while compulsive character traits are egosyntonic and rarely provoke resistance. Moreover, OCPD does not have the degree of functional impairment characteristic of OCD.

OCD and schizophrenia

About 10–25% of chronic schizophrenia patients may also present with OCD symptoms (range 5–45%) (Berman *et al.* 1995), and 15% may qualify for the diagnosis of OCD. As in OCD, the OCD symptoms in these patients will not necessarily surface unless specific questions are asked. Many patients with schizophrenia can distinguish the egodystonic OC symptoms, perceived as coming from within, from the egosyntonic delusions perceived as intruding from the outside. Follow-up studies demonstrate diagnostic stability over time and it seems that the presence of OCD in schizophrenia predicts a poor prognosis (Fenton & McGlashan 1986; Berman *et al.* 1995). Several studies among patients with schizophrenia and OCD reported an improvement in OCD symptomatology after the addition of a specific antiobsessive medication (Zohar 1997).

Due to the different (poorer) prognosis of patients with schizo-obsessive symptoms, as well as preliminary data regarding their response to specific therapeutic intervention (i.e., the combination of antipsychotic and antiobsessive medications), and taking into account the high prevalence of this presentation, several researchers have suggested that a "schizo-obsessive" category may be considered (Zohar 1997).

Social and economic costs

While the introduction of effective pharmacological treatments for OCD has considerably improved course and outcome for the disorder, recent studies have shown OCD to have an acute effect on psychosocial functioning and on quality of life (Stein *et al.* 1996, 1997). Frequently reported consequences of obsessive-compulsive symptoms include decreased self esteem, lowered career aspirations, a troubled relationship with one's spouse, having fewer friends and decreased academic achievement (Hollander *et al.* 1997). OCD has also been shown to have a negative impact on other family members, who often become involved in the patient's symptoms. OCD may also interfere with family members' social and work function.

With regard to quality of life, obsessive-compulsive symptoms can lead to substantial distress and to critical interference in numerous areas of functioning, including family relations, socialization and work and study (Hollander *et al.* 1997; Stein *et al.* 1997). Thus, OCD can have a widespread effect on patients, families, friends and employers.

Pharmacoeconomic studies have indicated that OCD can cost billions of US dollars to the world's economy (DuPont *et al.* 1995; Stein *et al.* 1997). The majority of costs associated with OCD result either from underdiagnosis or misdiagnosis and the receipt of ineffective treatment, or, indirectly, as a result of work loss and absenteeism (Hollander *et al.* 1997).

The estimated direct cost of OCD in the US, according to cost studies, is approximately US$2 billion per year, including medications, professional service fees, health care use (inpatient and outpatient), housing/nursing home costs, social welfare, and support. Hollander *et al.* (1997) reported in their study that 41% of patients were unable to work due to obsessive-compulsive symptoms, with a mean work time loss of 2.5 years. In addition, suicide attempts were reported in 12% of patients.

In summary, it is clear from these findings that OCD can have staggering emotional, social and financial costs, accenting the great need for appropriate diagnostic, treatment, and educational interventions.

References

American Psychiatric Association (1994) *Diagnostic Statistical Manual of Mental Disorders*, 4th edn. American Psychiatric Association, Washington, D.C.

Bastani, B., Nash, J.F. & Meltzer, H.Y. (1990) Prolactin and cortisol responses to MK-212, a serotonin agonist, in obsessive-compulsive disorder. *Arch Gen Psychiat* **47**, 833–9.

Berman, I., Kalinowski, A., Berman, S.M., Lengua, J. & Green, A.I. (1995) Obsessive and compulsive symptoms in chronic schizophrenia. *Compr Psychiatry* **36**, 6–10.

Black, D.W., Noyes, R., Pfohl, B. *et al.* (1993) Personality disorder in obsessive-compulsive volunteers, well comparison subjects and their first-degree relatives. *Americal J Psychiatry* **150**, 1226–32.

Bland, R.C., Newman, S.C. & Orn, H. (1988) Age of onset of psychiatric disorders. *Acta Psychiatr Scand* **77** (Suppl. 338), 43–9.

Chen, C.N., Wong, J., Lee, N., Chan-Ho, M.W., Lau, J.T., Fung, M. (1993) The Shatin community mental health survey in Hong Kong. II. Major Findings. *Arch Gen Psychiatry* **50**, 125–33.

Dupont, R.L., Rice, D.P., Shiraki, S. *et al.* (1995) Economic costs of obsessive-compulsive disorder. *Med Interface* **8**, 102–9.

Fenton, W.S. & McGlashan, S. (1986) The prognostic significance of obsessive-compulsive symptoms in chronic schizophrenia. *Am J Psychiatry* **143**, 437–41.

Flament, M.F., Whitaker, A., Rapoport, J.L. *et al.* (1988) Obsessive-compulsive disorder in adolescence: an epidemiological study. *J Am Acad Child Adolesc Psychiatry* **27**, 764–71.

Foa, E.B. & Kozak, M.J. (1995) DSM-IV field trial: obsessive compulsive disorder. *Am J Psychiatry* **152**, 90–6.

Goodman, W.K., Price, L.H., Delgado, P.L. *et al.* (1990) Specificity of serotonin reuptake inhibitors in the treatment of obsessive-compulsive disorder. Comparison of fluvoxamine and desipramine. *Arch Gen Psychiatry* **47**, 577–85.

Greenberg, D. & Wtzum, E. (1994) Cultural aspect of OCD. In: *Current Insights in Obsessive Compulsive Disorder* (E. Hollander, J. Zohar, D. Marazziti *et al.* (eds), p. 17). John Wiley & Sons, Chichester, England.

Gross, R., Sasson, Y., Chopra M. & Zohar, J. (1998) Biological models of obsessive-compulsive disorder: the serotonin hypothesis. In: *Obsessive-compulsive Disorder: Theory, Research and Treatment* (R.P. Swinson, M.M. Antony, S. Rachman & M.A. Richter (eds), pp. 141–53). Guilford Publications, New York.

Hollander, E., Greenwald, S., Neville, D. *et al.* (1996) Uncomplicated and comorbid obsessive-compulsive disorder in epidemiological sample. *Depress Anxiety* **4**, 111–19.

Insel, T. & Akiskal, H. (1986) Obsessive-compulsive disorder with psychotic features: a phenomenological analysis. *Am J Psychiatry* **143**, 1527–33.

Jenike, M.A. & Rauch, S.L. (1994) Managing the patient with treatment-resistant obsessive-compulsive disorder. *J Clin Psychiatry* **55** (Suppl. 3), 11–17.

Karno, M., Golding, J.M., Sorenson, S.B. & Burnam, M.A. (1988) The epidemiology of obsessive-compulsive disorder in five US communities. *Arch Gen Psychiatry* **45**, 1094–9.

Koran, L.M., McElroy, S.L., Davidson, J.R. *et al.* (1996) Fluvoxamine versus clomipramine for obsessive-compulsive disorder: a double-blind comparison. *J Clin Psychopharmacol* **16**(2) 121–9.

Leckman, J.F., Grice, D.E., Boardman, J. *et al.* (1997) Symptoms of OCD. *Am J Psychiatry* **154**, 911–17.

Lesch, K.P., Hoh, A., Dissellcamp-Tieze, J. *et al.* (1991) Hydroxytyptamine-1A receptor receptivity in obsessive-compulsive disorder: comparison of patients and controls. *Arch Gen Psychiatry* **48**, 540–7.

Lindal, E. & Stefannson, J.G. (1993) The lifetime prevalence of anxiety disorders in Iceland as estimated by the US National Institute of Mental Health Diagnostic Interview Schedule. *Acta Psychiatr Scand* **88**, 29–34.

Marazziti, D., Lensi, P., Ravagli, S. *et al.* (1993) Peripheral CNS markers in OCD. Proceedings of the First International OCD Conference, p. 51.

Mavissakalian, M.R., Hamann, M.S., Haidar, S.A. & deGroot, C.M. (1993) DSM-III personality disorders in generalized anxiety, panic/agoraphobia, and obsessive-compulsive disorders. *Compr Psychiatry* **34**, 243–8.

McDougle, C.J., Goodman, W.K., Leckman, J.F. *et al.* (1993) Limited therapeutic effect of addition of buspirone in fluvoxamine refractory obsessive-compulsive disorder. *Am J Psychiatry* **150**, 647–9.

McDougle, C.J., Price, L.H., Goodman, W.K. *et al.* (1991) A controlled trial of lithium augmentation in fluvoxamine-refractory obsessive-compulsive disorder: lack of efficacy. *J Clin Psychopharmacol* **11**, 175–84.

Mundo, E., Richter, M.A., Sam, F., Macciardi, F. & Kennedy, J.L. (2000) Is the 5-HT1Db receptor gene implicated in the pathogenesis of obsessive-compulsive disorder? *Am J Psychiatry* **157**, 1160–1.

Nelson, E. & Rice, J. (1997) Stability of diagnosis of obsessive-compulsive disorder in the epidemiologic catchment area study. *Am J Psychiatry* **154**, 826–31.

Okasha, A., Saad, A., Khalil, A.H. *et al.* Phenomenology of obsessive compulsive disorder: a transcultural study. *Compr Psychiatry* **35**, 191–7.

Pauls, D. (1992) The genetics of OCD and Gilles de la Tourette's syndrome. *Psychiatr Clin North Am* **15**, 759–66.

Perlmutter, S.J., Leitman, S.F., Garvey, M.A. *et al.* (1999) Therapeutic plasma exchange and intravenous immunoglobulin for obsessive-compulsive disorder and tic disorders in childhood. *Lancet* **354**, 1153–8.

Rasmussen, S.A. & Tsuang, M.T. (1986) The epidemiology of obsessive-compulsive disorder. *J Clin Psychiatry* **45**, 450–7.

Rasmussen, S.A. & Eisen, J.L. (1990) Epidemiology of obsessive-compulsive disorder. *J Clin Psychiatry* **51** (Suppl.), 10–13.

Rasmussen, S.A. & Tsuang, M.T. (1986) Clinical characteristics and family history in DSM-III obsessive-compulsive disorder. *Am J Psychiat* **143**, 317–22.

Reinherz, H.Z., Giaconia, R.M., Lefkowitz, E.S. *et al.* (1993) Prevalence of psychiatric disorders in a community population of older adolescents. *J Am Acad Child Adolesc Psychiatry* **32**, 369–77.

Robins, L.N., Helzer, J.E., Weissman, M.M. *et al.* (1984) Lifetime prevalence of specific psychiatric disorders in three sites. *Arch Gen Psychiatry* **138**, 949–58.

Sasson, Y., Zohar, J., Chopra, M., Lustig, M., Iancu, I. & Hendler, T. (1997) Epidemiology of obsessive-compulsive disorder: a world view. *J Clin Psychiatry* **58** (Suppl. 12), 7–10.

Stein, D.J., Roberts, M., Hollander, E. *et al.* (1996) Quality of life and pharmaco-economic aspects of obsessive-compulsive disorder. A South African survey. *S Afr Med J*, **8** (Suppl. 12), 1579–85.

Stein, M.B., Forde, D.R., Anderson, G. & Walker, J.R. (1997) Obsessive-compulsive disorder in the community: an epidemiologic survey with clinical reappraisal. *Am J Psychiatry* **154**, 1120–6.

Stern, L., Zohar, J., Cohen, R. & Zohar, J. (1998) Treatment of severe, drug resistant obsessive-compulsive disorder with the 5-HT1D agonist sumatriptan. *Eur Neuropsychopharmacol* **8**(4), 325–8.

Thomsen, P.H. (1995) Obsessive-compulsive disorder in children and adolescents: predictors in childhood for long-term phenomenological course. *Acta Psychiatr Scand*, **92**, 255–9.

Thomsen, P.H. & Mikkelsen, H.U. (1993) Development of personality disorders in children and adolescents with obsessive-compulsive disorder: a 6- to 22-year follow-up study. *Acta Psychiatr Scand* **87**, 456–62.

Thoren, P., Crohnholm, B., Jornestedt, L. *et al.* (1980) Clomipramine treatment of OCD. I. A controlled clinical trial. *Br J Psychiatry* **161**, 665–70.

Valleni-Basile, L.A., Garrison, C.Z., Jackson, K.L. *et al.* (1994) Frequency of obsessive-compulsive disorder in a community sample of young adolescents. *J Am Acad Child Adolesc Psychiatry* **33**, 782–91.

Weissman, M.M., Bland, R.C., Canino, G.J. *et al.* (1994) The cross-national epidemiology of obsessive-compulsive disorder. *J Clin Psychiat* **55** (Suppl. 3), 5–10.

Woodruff, R. & Pitts, F. (1969) Monozygotic twins with obsessional illness. *Am J Psychiatry* **120**, 1075–80.

World Health Organization (WHO) (1993) *Tenth Revision of the International Classification of Diseases Diagnostic Criteria for Research*. World Health Organization, Geneva.

Zohar, J. (1997) Is there room for a new diagnostic subtype—the schizo-obsessive subtype? *CNS Spectrums* **2**(3), 49–50.

Zohar, J. & Insel, T.R. (1987) Obsessive-compulsive disorder. psychobiological approaches to diagnosis, treatment and pathophysiology. *Biol Psychiatry* **22**(6), 667–87.

Zohar, J. & Kindler, S. (1992b) Serotonergic probes in obsessive-compulsive disorder. *Int. Clin. Psychopharmacol* **7** (Suppl. 1), 39–40.

Zohar, J. & Kindler, S. (1992a) Update of the serotonergic hypothesis of obsessive-compulsive disorder. *Clin. Neuropharmacol* **15** (Suppl. 1), 257A–8A.

Zohar, J., Mueller, E.A., Insel, T.R., Zohar-Kadouch, R.C. & Murphy, D.L. (1987) Serotonergic responsivity in obsessive-compulsive disorder: comparison of patients and healthy controls. *Arch Gen Psychiatry* **446**, 946–51.

Zohar, J. & Pato, M.T. (1991) Diagnostic considerations. In: *Current Treatments of Obsessive-compulsive Disorder* (Pato, M.T. & Zohar, J. (eds), pp. 1–9). American Psychiatric Press, Washington, D.C.

Zohar, J, Zohar-Kadouch, R.C., Kindler, S. (1992) Current concepts in the pharmacological treatment of obsessive-compulsive disorder. *Drugs* **43**(2), 210–18.

7

Social Anxiety Disorder

P.L. du Toit & D.J. Stein

Introduction

Social anxiety disorder (also known as social phobia), once a "neglected anxiety disorder" (Liebowitz *et al.* 1985), has been gaining recognition as a chronic psychiatric problem associated with considerable functional impairment. Although the Diagnostic Statistical Manual, fourth edition (DSM-IV; American Psychiatric Association [APA] 1994) recognizes both social phobia and social anxiety disorder as descriptors for the condition, many patients and advocacy groups feel that the term social phobia trivializes the disorder and that social anxiety disorder better describes the condition (Liebowitz *et al.* 2000). The patients with this condition can have social anxiety and either have no avoidance, endure social situations with considerable distress but do not avoid them, or have varying levels of phobic avoidance (Ballenger 1998). For these reasons, the term social anxiety disorder will be preferred over social phobia in the present chapter.

With a lifetime prevalence of about 13% and a 1 month prevalence rate of 4.5%, social anxiety disorder is the most prevalent of the anxiety disorders (Magee *et al.* 1996) and the third most frequently occurring disorder after depression and generalized anxiety disorder (GAD) (Goldberg & Lecrubier 1995; Kessler *et al.* 1994). However, epidemiological studies indicate that less than 5% of people with social anxiety disorder seek treatment for their disorder (Schneier *et al.* 1992; Magee *et al.* 1996). Despite the under-recognition and under-reporting of social anxiety disorder, recent years have seen major advances in the development of a number of effective pharmacotherapeutic as well as

psychotherapeutic approaches for treating social anxiety disorder. The present chapter aims to review the clinical features, diagnosis, pathogenesis and social impact of social anxiety disorder.

Clinical features

Social anxiety disorder is characterized by the fear of humiliation or embarrassment in social or performance situations as well as the avoidance of such social and performance situations. The diagnostic criteria for DSM-IV social anxiety disorder and for International Classification of Diseases, 10th edition (ICD-10; WHO 1993) social anxiety disorder are presented in Table 7.1.

Feared situations

The extent of situations feared by people with social anxiety disorder ranges from fear of a single, discrete setting, such as performing on stage, to a fear of virtually all forms of interpersonal contact. Generally, most people with social anxiety disorder fear a number of social situations (Holt *et al.* 1992). Public speaking tends to be the most commonly feared social situation (Rapee *et al.* 1988; Holt *et al.* 1992; Schneier *et al.* 1992; Turner *et al.* 1992) followed by situations such as meetings, social events (e.g. parties) and interacting with authority figures (Rapee *et al.* 1988). Women report experiencing greater fear across a range of social situations when compared to men (Turk *et al.* 1998).

In a recent study, Faravelli *et al.* (2000) found that 86.9% of patients with social anxiety disorder had more than one fear, with the most common fear being

Table 7.1 ICD-10 and DSM-IV criteria for social anxiety disorder.

SP ICD-10

(A) SP is centred around a fear of scrutiny by other people in comparatively small groups (as opposed to crowds), usually leading to avoidance of social situations*

(B) SP is usually associated with low self-esteem and fear of criticism*

(C) May present as complaint of blushing, tremor, nausea, or urgency of micturition. These symptoms may progress to panic attacks*

(D) The feared situation is avoided whenever possible or endured with dread. Avoidance is often marked and in extreme cases may result in almost complete social isolation*

(E) Anxiety must be restricted to or predominate in particular social situations*

(F) If the distinction between SP and agoraphobia is difficult, precedence should be given to agoraphobia. Panic disorder should only be diagnosed in the absence of phobia*

(G) Psychological, behavioral or autonomic symptoms must be primary manifestations of anxiety and not secondary to other symptoms such as delusions or obsessional thoughts*

(H) May be discrete (restricted to eating in public, public speaking, encounters with the opposite sex) or diffuse (involving almost all social situations)*

DSM-IV

(A) Marked and persistent fear of one or more social or performance situations in which the person is exposed to unfamiliar people or possible scrutiny by others, and fearing he/she will act or show anxiety symptoms that will be humiliating or embarrassing

(B) Exposure to the feared situation provokes anxiety, which may take the form of a situationally bound/predisposed panic attack

(C) The person recognizes that the fear is excessive and unreasonable

(D) The feared situations are either avoided or endured with intense anxiety or distress

(E) The person has marked distress about having the phobia or the avoidance, anticipatory anxiety, or distress in the feared situation(s) interferes significantly with the person's normal routine, occupational or academic functioning, or social relationships

(F) For individuals younger than 18 years, the duration is at least 6 months

(G) The fear or avoidance behavior is not better accounted for by another mental disorder, e.g. panic disorder with or without agoraphobia or body dysmorphic disorder

(H) If medical or other psychiatric condition coexists, the fear is unrelated to that condition

SP, social phobia.

*Generalized social anxiety disorder is specified as a fear of most social situations.

speaking in public (89.4%), followed by entering a room occupied by others (63.1%) and meeting with strangers (47.3%). Although researchers have investigated whether distinct clusters of feared situations can be distinguished (e.g. the distinction between performance-related concerns and concerns relating to social interaction) (Liebowitz 1987; Turner *et al.* 1992), such distinctions have arguably not received conclusive empirical support (Rapee 1995). It has been noted that the degree of fear experienced in social anxiety disorder is moderated by a number of variables (e.g. the degree of formality of the situation and the size and gender of an audience) (Rapee 1995).

Fear response

Somatic symptoms

Most people with social anxiety disorder experience some somatic symptoms, although a number experience only self-consciousness and fear. Patients with social anxiety disorder are more likely than patients with panic disorder to report blushing, twitching and stammering (Amies *et al.* 1983; Solyom *et al.* 1986). Panic disorder symptoms such as dizziness and dyspnea are less common in social anxiety disorder. Some somatic symptoms such as palpitations, sweating, trembling, muscle-tension and gastrointestinal discomfort are common to both social anxiety disorder and other anxiety disorders. In social anxiety disorder, these somatic symptoms are usually clearly related to an actual social or performance situation or to the recollection or anticipation of such situations.

Behavioral symptoms

Avoidance behaviors are often the greatest source of impairment in social anxiety disorder and range from relatively subtle in-situation safety behaviors (e.g. avoiding eye contact) to the avoidance of all interpersonal contact outside the patient's immediate family. In-situation safety behaviors and avoidance of social situations prevent exposure to feared situations and their consequences, and may, paradoxically, make feared outcomes more likely (Clark & Wells 1995).

Actual performance and social skills

Although it has been hypothesized that social anxiety disorder is associated with certain deficits in social and performance-related skills, the evidence for such deficits is mixed (Rapee 1995). Various studies have not found differences in social or performance-related skills between normal controls and patients with social anxiety disorder (Clark & Arkowitz 1975; Pilkonis 1977b; Rapee & Lim 1992). Other studies have found differences between socially anxious and nonanxious people on global measures of performance, but not on specific social skills (e.g. eye contact) (Beidel et al. 1985). These differences may reflect the inhibition of social skills within feared situations rather than being indicative of actual skills deficits (Rapee 1995).

Clinical subtypes

Two subtypes of social anxiety disorder have been distinguished on the basis of the number of situations feared by patients with social anxiety disorder, namely generalized or diffuse social anxiety disorder (fear of most social and performance situations) and non-generalized social anxiety disorder (fear of only two or three social or performance situations). Also, it has been suggested that public-speaking social anxiety disorder (in which only public speaking situations are feared) represents a distinct subtype of social anxiety disorder (Kessler et al. 1998; Stein et al. 1998a). Both DSM-IV and ICD-10 recognize the distinction between generalized and nongeneralized social anxiety disorder

and a number of studies have offered support for the distinction between the two subtypes of social anxiety disorder (Heimberg et al. 1990; Turner et al. 1992; Stein et al. 1998a).

People with generalized social anxiety disorder are less well educated, are more likely to be unemployed and are more likely never to have married than people with nongeneralized social anxiety disorder (Heimberg et al. 1990; Mannuzza et al. 1995). The age at onset of generalized social anxiety disorder is generally also younger than in nongeneralized social anxiety disorder (Mannuzza et al. 1995; Wittchen et al. 1999), although not all data are consistent (Weinshenker et al. 1996). A number of studies have found that people with generalized social anxiety disorder reported more severe anxiety symptoms, higher general levels of distress, greater functional impairment, and greater lifetime comorbidity with other disorders than people with the nongeneralized subtype (Heimberg et al. 1990; Turner et al. 1992; Mannuzza et al. 1995; Wittchen et al. 1999).

Mannuzza et al. (1995) reported that the rate of social anxiety disorder was significantly greater in first-degree relatives of patients with generalized versus nongeneralized social phobia; however, the prevalence rates of social anxiety disorder were identical for relatives of patients with nongeneralized social anxiety disorder and healthy controls. Stein et al. (1998a) performed a direct-interview family study to investigate differences in the rates of generalized, nongeneralized, and discrete social anxiety disorder in the first-degree relatives of patients with generalized social anxiety disorder and healthy controls. It was found that first-degree relatives of probands with generalized social anxiety disorder had an approximately 10-fold greater risk for generalized social anxiety disorder and for avoidant personality disorder when compared to first-degree relatives of healthy controls and of patients with discrete or nongeneralized social anxiety disorder.

The existing data therefore seems to confirm that there may be some validity in distinguishing between generalized and nongeneralized subtypes of social anxiety disorder.

Social anxiety disorder in children

In DSM-IV, social anxiety disorder in childhood/adolescence replaced avoidant and overanxious disorder. Children and adults show similarities in the types of social situations feared as well as in the somatic symptoms associated with social anxiety disorder (Beidel *et al*. 1999). The behavioral manifestations of social anxiety disorder in children and adolescents may differ according to the developmental level of the child and include behaviors such as clinging and crying in younger children (Albano *et al*. 1995) as well as school refusal, vague somatic complaints, stuttering, fidgeting, and test-anxiety in addition to manifestations typical in adults with social anxiety disorder (Beidel 1991; Albano *et al*. 1995; Schneier & Welkowitz 1996).

There exists a strong association between selective mutism, i.e. the consistent failure to speak in specific social situations but not in others, and social anxiety disorder in children (Black & Uhde 1992). In a study of 50 children with selective mutism, Dummit *et al*. (1997) found that all of the children included in their sample had comorbid DSM-III-R (APA 1987) social phobia or avoidant disorder.

In diagnosing social anxiety disorder in children, attention has to be paid to developmental processes (Kaminer & Stein 1999). Furthermore, there must be evidence that the child is capable of establishing age-appropriate social relationships with familiar people. The clinician also needs to establish that social anxiety is not limited to interactions with adults (since many children fear such interactions) but also occurs in social interactions with peers. Children may lack the cognitive sophistication to recognize the unreasonable and excessive nature of their social anxiety. Since children and adolescents may experience transient shyness and social evaluative fears during particular developmental periods, DSM-IV requires that social anxiety disorder-symptoms have a duration of at least 6 months in people younger than 18 years.

As in adults, social anxiety disorder is associated with considerable comorbidity in children (Last *et al*. 1992; Strauss & Last 1993; Beidel *et al*. 1999). Social anxiety disorder in children and adolescents is also associated with considerable distress and impairment (Beidel 1998; Beidel *et al*. 1999; Kaminer & Stein 1999). Social anxiety disorder during childhood and adolescence may interfere with the normal development of the child thus contributing to the functional impairment associated with social anxiety disorder in adults. For instance the avoidance of social situations during childhood and adolescence may decrease the child's opportunities to develop the social skills necessary for later academic, social and work-related functioning. In addition, adult sufferers of social anxiety disorder report a significantly higher incidence of problem behaviors (e.g. fighting, running away from home, and stealing) during adolescence than do healthy controls (Davidson *et al*. 1993a). Social anxiety disorder during adolescence also commonly leads to truancy (Beidel 1998). These problem behaviors may not be recognized as secondary problems resulting from social anxiety disorder and may themselves have deleterious developmental outcomes.

Cultural variations in the presentation of social anxiety disorder

Clinicians need to be sensitive to differences in the presentation of social anxiety disorder. The well-documented psychiatric syndrome "taijin kyofusho" (TKS)—meaning "fear of facing other people"—shares a number of characteristics with social anxiety disorder and occurs commonly in certain East Asian societies (Chang 1984; Prince 1993; Ono *et al*. 1996). Individuals suffering from TKS experience intense shame about, and persistent irrational fears of, causing others offense, embarrassment or even harm, through some perceived personal inadequacy or shortcoming. Common specific manifestations of TKS include fear of blushing (erythrophobia), fear of emitting body odor (dysosmophobia), and fear of displaying unsightly body parts (dysmorphophobia) (Chang 1984). Whereas DSM-IV criteria for social anxiety disorder tend to focus on patients' concern with the negative evaluation of their behavior, patients with TKS are more concerned about the offense that they may cause to others. One of the interesting things about TKS is that insight can be poor, this raises the question of whether poor insight can be found in Western social anxiety disorder patients.

Diagnostic thresholds

Shyness and social anxiety disorder

It has been suggested that social anxiety disorder may be an extreme on a putative continuum of shyness (Heckelman & Schneier 1995; Hirshfeld-Becker *et al*. 1999). If shyness is defined as the fear of social or performance situations involving exposure to strangers or scrutiny by others, then per definition, all people with social anxiety disorder suffer from excessive shyness in some contexts. However, shyness is a heterogeneous concept often poorly defined and operationalized in research (Heckelman & Schneier 1995; Hirshfeld-Becker et al. 1999). Certain similarities exist between shy individuals and patients with social anxiety disorder: Similar physical symptoms are experienced by people with self-defined shyness as well as people with social anxiety disorder (Ludwig & Lazarus 1983; Kagan et al. 1988), both groups experience fear of negative evaluation and may show certain social skills deficits (see Turner et al. 1990 for a review). Whereas the prevalence rates of self-described shyness are 20–40% (Turner et al. 1990), prevalence rates of social anxiety disorder range from 3% to 13% (Kessler et al. 1994). Further research into the relationship between shyness and social anxiety disorder is necessary in order to determine whether qualitative differences exist between shy individuals and people with social anxiety disorder, and whether social anxiety disorder and avoidant personality disorder form part of a putative shyness continuum.

Test-anxiety and social anxiety disorder secondary to another psychiatric or medical illness

A number of studies have reported a positive relationship between test-anxiety (i.e. the intense anxiety in anticipation of and response to tests or evaluations of knowledge or skills) and social anxiety or social anxiety disorder (Pilkonis 1977a; Turner et al. 1986; Beidel 1988). The DSM-IV workgroup on social phobia (Schneier et al. 1996) recommended that test-anxiety should be diagnosed as a form of discrete social anxiety disorder providing it meets DSM-IV criteria for social anxiety disorder.

In addition, the DSM-IV workgroup on social phobia recommended that the diagnosis of social anxiety disorder excludes social fears secondary to medical conditions such as stuttering and benign tremor and psychiatric conditions such as Parkinson's disease, and classifies them under "Anxiety disorder not otherwise specified" (APA 1994). However, patients with such medical and psychiatric conditions often report significant social anxiety symptoms. For instance, it has been found that people with stuttering suffer significant impairment due to their social fears and that—if the DSM-IV exclusion criteria is waived—a large proportion of such patients qualify for a DSM-IV diagnosis of social anxiety disorder (Stein et al. 1996; Schneier et al. 1997). In addition, it has been shown that patients with

social anxiety disorder secondary to disfiguring or disabling medical conditions, may respond to the monoamine oxidase inhibitor (MAOI) phenelzine (Oberlander et al. 1994). Since DSM-IV exclusion criteria may hinder the identification and treatment of these disorders, a number of researchers have suggested that social anxiety disorder secondary to medical conditions and certain psychiatric conditions should be conceptualized as social anxiety disorder and treated accordingly (Stein et al. 1996; Schneier et al. 1997).

Clinical course of the disorder

Age at onset

The mean age at onset of social anxiety disorder is around the mid to late teen years (Mannuzza et al. 1990). This is later than is found for many specific phobias, but considerably earlier than age at onset of panic disorder (Marks & Gelder 1966; Öst 1987). In the subgroup of subjects with uncomplicated social anxiety disorder included in the US Epidemiologic Catchment Area (ECA) study, the overall age of onset occurred in a bimodal distribution with mean reported age of 15.5 years and peaks at the interval between 0 and 5 years and at 13 years. As many as 47% of patients with social anxiety disorder report that the disorder had been present for their whole lives or, at least, had an onset before the age of 10 (Schneier et al. 1992). In the early developmental stages of psychopathology (EDSP) study conducted among young German subjects, the generalized subtype of social anxiety disorder appeared to have a significantly lower median age at onset (males: 11.5 years; females: 12.5 years) than non-generalized social anxiety disorder (males: 14 years; females: 15 years) (Wittchen et al. 1999).

Since there may exist inaccuracies in retrospective self-reported age at onset (Rapee 1995), it may well be that social anxiety disorder has an earlier age at onset than is generally reported. Certainly, social anxiety disorder is commonly diagnosed in children below the age of 10 (Beidel 1991). Furthermore, unlike other childhood fears, social fears often appear to be non-transitory (Beidel 1999).

Age at presentation

The mean age at presentation for treatment of social anxiety disorder appears to be about 30 years (Rapee et al. 1988; Heimberg et al. 1990). This is perhaps earlier than that of patients with other anxiety disorders

(Amies *et al.* 1983; Solyom *et al.* 1986; Rapee *et al.* 1988). However, most people with social anxiety disorder present for treatment between 15 and 25 years after the onset of their disorder; this is a considerably longer duration of illness than is found in people with, say, panic disorder (Solyom *et al.* 1986). This delay could be ascribed to less public awareness of the disorder and treatment options. In addition, people with social anxiety disorder may be more likely to ascribe symptoms to intractable personality traits than are people with other anxiety disorders (Rapee 1995).

Clinical course

Concern over social threat appears to be relatively stable across the lifespan (Lovibond & Rapee 1993; Campbell & Rapee 1994). Davidson *et al.* (1993a) reported a 1-year recovery rate of 27% in social anxiety disorder at the Duke site of the ECA study. Good prognostic predictors that emerged were: onset of social anxiety disorder after age 11, absence of psychiatric comorbidity, and higher levels of education. As part of the longitudinal study by the Harvard/Brown Anxiety disorders Research Project (HARP) (Reich *et al.* 1994a), a sample of 140 patients with a DSM-III-R diagnosis of social anxiety disorder was monitored on the Psychiatric Status Rating, a standardized measure of the severity of the disorder, for a period of 65 weeks. The mean duration of illness was about 18 years, and only 39% of patients had uncomplicated social anxiety disorder. The probability of good outcome during the 65-week follow-up period was only 11% for complete remission, 25% for partial remission and 43% for minimal remission. The probability for remission was the same for the generalized and specific subtypes of social anxiety disorder (Reich *et al.* 1994b).

In summary, social anxiety disorder is unlikely to remit spontaneously; it is a chronic condition with a relatively stable course that typically has its onset by the mid-teens and that has an average duration of 20 years at the time of presentation (Davidson *et al.* 1993a; Wittchen & Beloch 1996).

Epidemiology

In the past two decades, numerous studies have investigated the prevalence of social anxiety disorder. A number of definitional as well as methodological differences exist between the various surveys (Lépine &

Pelissolo 1999). For instance, differences between ICD and DSM criteria sets as well as changes in the criteria sets of these two classification systems may contribute to differences found in the estimates of the prevalence of social anxiety disorder.

Studies determining the lifetime prevalence of DSM-III social anxiety disorder in community samples using the Diagnostic Interview Schedule (DIS) (Robins *et al.* 1981), have found lifetime prevalence rates of DSM-III (APA 1980) social anxiety disorder to range from 0.5% to 3.5% (Hwu *et al.* 1989; Wells *et al.* 1989; Lee *et al.* 1990; Schneier *et al.* 1992; Weissman *et al.* 1996). The DIS may have had a higher diagnostic threshold than the DSM, since it requires that social anxiety disorder-symptoms must interfere with life and activities, whereas DSM-III, DSM-III-R and DSM-IV require that the anxiety symptoms cause significant distress *or* are associated with significant interference in activities (Walker & Stein 1995). In addition, the version of the DIS used in these surveys covered only a limited range of social fear situations (Davidson *et al.* 1993a; Walker & Stein 1995; Magee *et al.* 1996).

More recently, studies determining the prevalence of DSM-III-R social anxiety disorder as assessed by the CIDI have found considerably higher lifetime prevalence rates. In the National Comorbidity Survey (NCS) (Kessler *et al.* 1994) DSM-III-R social anxiety disorder had a lifetime prevalence rate of 13.3%. Using the CIDI, Wacker *et al.* (1992) found lifetime prevalence rates of 16.0% for social anxiety disorder as defined by the DSM-III-R, and 9.6% for social anxiety disorder as defined by the ICD-10 in a community study in Switzerland.

As part of the EDSP study, Wittchen *et al.* (1999) investigated the prevalence rate of DSM-IV social anxiety disorder and social fears in a community sample of 3021 14–24 year-old Germans by means of a computerized version of the CIDI. The total lifetime prevalence of DSM-IV social anxiety disorder was 7.3% and the 12-month prevalence of social anxiety disorder for the total sample was 5.2%, indicating a significant degree of persistence in symptoms. Social anxiety disorder had a lifetime prevalence of 9.5% in females and 4.9% in males and about one-third of the total sample met the criteria for generalized social anxiety disorder (Wittchen *et al.* 1999).

A number of studies have shown that social anxiety disorder has high prevalence rates in patients attending general medical clinics (Fifer *et al.* 1994; Sherbourne *et al.* 1996; Schonfeld *et al.* 1997). Weiller *et al.* (1996) reported a lifetime prevalence rate of 14.4% and a 1-month prevalence rate of 4.9% for DSM-III-R social anxiety disorder in a study of 2096 consecutive primary care patients, whereas a slightly higher prevalence rate in DSM-IV social anxiety disorder (7%) was reported by Stein *et al.* (1999) in their study of 511 primary care patients.

Cross-cultural differences in epidemiology

A number of studies assessing DSM-III social anxiety disorder with the DIS in East Asian countries have reported significantly lower lifetime prevalence rates than studies conducted in Western countries. In a Korean study, Lee *et al.* (1990) found a lifetime prevalence of 0.53% of DIS/DSM-III social anxiety disorder and Hwu *et al.* (1989) reported a lifetime prevalence of 0.6% for DSM-III social anxiety disorder in a Taiwanese study. The lower rates of social anxiety disorder in Taiwan may, however, reflect the lower rates of psychiatric disorders in general in Taiwan. In a cross-national study conducted in the US, Canada, Puerto Rico and Korea, Weissman *et al.* (1996) found that the prevalence rates of social anxiety disorder differed by country: from 2.6% in the US to as low as 0.5% in Korea, although there were similar rates in most countries. In addition, there were cross-national differences in the expression of social anxiety disorder symptoms (Weissman *et al.* 1996).

Differences in the cross-cultural prevalence of social anxiety disorder may derive from cultural differences with regard to the willingness to divulge information assessed in structured clinical interviews. In addition, assessment instruments such as the DIS may not be adequately sensitized to nonWestern expressions of psychiatric disorders such as social anxiety disorder (Chapman *et al.* 1995). For instance, as noted earlier, TKS is a psychiatric syndrome that may be quite common in East Asia (Ono *et al.* 1996).

Gender ratio

In epidemiological studies of social anxiety disorder in the general population, social anxiety disorder is generally found to be more prevalent in women than in men. In the ECA study, the female : male ratio was about 1.5 : 1, with DSM-III social anxiety disorder having a lifetime prevalence of 3.1% of females and

2.0% of males (Schneier *et al.* 1992). The female : male ratio found in the NCS was about 1.4 : 1; DSM-III-R social anxiety disorder had a lifetime prevalence of 15.5% among females and 11.1% among males (Kessler *et al.* 1994). In general, the female : male ratio for the lifetime prevalence of social anxiety disorder varies between 1.5 and 2 females for 1 male. In clinical settings, though, social anxiety disorder is more or less equally common in males and females (Solyom *et al.* 1986; Rapee *et al.* 1988; Weiller *et al.* 1996). It therefore seems that, as is the case with other anxiety disorders, females are more likely than males to suffer from social anxiety disorder, but males may be more likely to seek treatment.

Pathogenesis

Biological factors

Evolutionary perspective
Seligman proposed that human and nonhuman primates may have an evolutionary predisposition to acquire fears and phobias that once facilitated the survival of their evolutionary ancestors (Seligman 1971). Support for the preparedness theory has been provided by (a) studies that indicate a higher than expected prevalence of certain phobias (snakes, heights, places of restricted escape) (McNally 1987) that may be related to common environmental threats to human and nonhuman primates, and (b) the ease of conditioning fears in humans and primates to certain specific phobic stimuli (e.g. snakes) and not to others (e.g. flowers) (Mineka & Zinbarg 1995). Research suggests that humans are biologically prepared to fear angry, threatening or rejecting faces (Öhman 1986; Öhman *et al.* 1989) and scrutiny or evaluation by others (Rosenbaum *et al.* 1994). These social fears may have facilitated survival of human and nonhuman primates in a dominance hierarchy (Öhman 1986; Mattick & Lampe 1995). In dominance hierarchies, less dominant members display fear and submissive behaviors in the presence of more dominant members, thereby remaining affiliated with the group and the benefits associated with this affiliation. Human blushing speculatively serves as an analogue of appeasement displays in other species, so that social anxiety disorder can be conceptualized in terms of a false appeasement display (Stein & Bouwer 1997). The existence of a specific social alarm would be supported if pathological absence could be found. Indeed,

patients with Williams syndrome (a nonhereditary genetic disorder caused by a microdeletion of the elastin gene on chromosome 7) are characterized by a range of physical, behavioral, psychological and developmental features including hypersociability and impaired social judgement (Gosch & Pankau 1997; Davies *et al.* 1998).

Biological perspective

A number of different methodologies have been used in the investigation of the role of neurobiological factors in social anxiety disorder. These methodologies include: pharmacological challenge studies, naturalistic challenges, and neuroimaging studies. Psychoneuroendocrine assessment studies of the hypothalamic–pituitary–adrenal and hypothalamic–pituitary–thyroid axes have been largely unrevealing (Potts *et al.* 1996; see Mendlowicz & Stein 1999 for a review).

Pharmacological challenge studies
Various pharmacological compounds have been administered to patients with social anxiety disorder in order to investigate provocation of anxiety symptoms. These paradigms have also been used to investigate possible differences between neurochemical factors in social anxiety disorder and other anxiety disorders such as panic disorder. Although there is still a relative paucity of challenge studies in social anxiety disorder when compared to other anxiety disorders, the existing literature indicates that carbon dioxide (CO_2), caffeine, pentagastrin, and nicotinic acid are anxiogenic in social anxiety disorder and that epinephrine (adrenaline) and lactate are not.

Patients with panic disorder have been shown to be hypersensitive to CO_2 challenge (Gorman *et al.* 1984; Griez *et al.* 1987). In contrast, patients with social anxiety disorder have fewer panic attacks and less intense anxiety symptoms than patients with panic disorder in response to low concentrations of CO_2 (Holt & Andrews 1989). However, higher concentrations of CO_2 (35%) may induce panic attacks in comparable proportions in both patient groups (Gorman *et al.* 1990; Caldirola *et al.* 1997). The common hypersensitivity of social anxiety disorder and panic disorder to CO_2 might indicate that these disorders form part of a putative panic-social anxiety disorder spectrum distinct from anxiety disorders with normal sensitivity to 35% CO_2 (Caldirola *et al.* 1997).

A similar proportion of social anxiety disorder and panic disorder patients, greater than that of controls, experience panic attacks in response to the administration of caffeine (480 mg) (Tancer *et al.* 1991).

Challenge studies have suggested the involvement of cholecystokinin (CCK) in social anxiety disorder. McCann *et al.* (1997) found that pentagastrin, a CCK agonist, produces anxiety and panic in 64% of patients with panic disorder, 47% of patients with social anxiety disorder, and 11% of healthy controls. van Vliet *et al.* (1997) found that pentagastrin was anxiogenic in 71% of social anxiety disorder patients and 29% of healthy controls. Although further research is needed to determine the mechanisms involved, these findings suggest that the CCK system is involved in the genesis of anxiety in both panic disorder and social anxiety disorder. Bouwer and Stein (1998) reported that administration of nicotinic acid (100 mg), a substance which induces vasodilation by increasing the synthesis of prostaglandins, was associated with increased flushing, anxiety, autonomic activity and temperature in patients with social anxiety disorder compared with normal controls.

Studies examining the anxiogenic effects of epinephrine, have shown that epinephrine challenges do not induce anxiety in most patients with social anxiety disorder (Papp *et al.* 1988) and that the rate of epinephrine induced panic attacks is the same in patients with panic disorder and social anxiety disorder (Veltman *et al.* 1996). Similarly, although it has been shown that sodium lactate is panicogenic in panic disorder (Liebowitz *et al.* 1984), significantly fewer patients with social anxiety disorder experience panic attacks in response to sodium lactate when compared to patients with panic disorder and patients with agoraphobia with panic attacks (Liebowitz *et al.* 1985a).

In summary, the existing literature suggests that patients with social anxiety disorder show hypersensitivity to CO_2, caffeine, pentagastrin, and nicotinic acid, but not to epinephrine and lactate.

Neurochemistry

Dopaminergic function The increased prevalence of social anxiety disorder in patients who later developed Parkinson's disease as well as the exacerbation of social anxiety disorder in response to dopamine blockers and the clinical observation of increased anxiety in patients on neuroleptics, offer indirect evidence for an association between dopaminergic dysfunction and social anxiety disorder (Liebowitz *et al.* 1987; Mendlowicz & Stein 1999). Using a levodopa-challenge, Tancer (1993) failed to demonstrate differences in dopaminergic dysfunction in people with social anxiety disorder versus healthy controls. However, Tiihonen *et al.* (1997) found lower striatal dopamine reuptake site densities in people with social anxiety disorder. Furthermore, Schneier *et al.* (2000) found that people with social anxiety disorder showed significantly lower mean D2 receptor binding than controls. Notably, Rowe *et al.* (1998) found evidence for an association between a particular polymorphism of the dopamine transporter gene (DAT1) and social anxiety disorder. Taken together with trials showing the efficacy of MAOIs in social anxiety disorder, these studies suggest that the dopamine system may well play a role in mediating the symptoms of social anxiety disorder.

Serotonergic function The effectiveness of various serotonin reuptake inhibitors (SSRIs) in the treatment of social anxiety disorder (e.g. van der Linden *et al.* 2000), seems to suggest that the serotonin system may play a role in mediating some of the symptoms of social anxiety disorder.

Studies examining differences between patients with social anxiety disorder and normal controls have failed to demonstrate differences in 5-HT2 binding to platelets. Stein *et al.* (1995) reported no significant differences between patients with social anxiety disorder, patients with panic disorder and healthy controls in the density and affinity of ^{3}H-paroxetine binding sites. Similarly, Chatterjee *et al.* (1997) did not find differences between 20 patients with social anxiety disorder and a normal comparison group in platelet 5-HT2 receptor density.

On the other hand, challenge studies have provided some evidence for serotonergic dysfunction in social anxiety disorder. When compared to controls, patients with social anxiety disorder show a significantly greater cortisol response to fenfluramine (a nonspecific serotonin-releasing agent) (Tancer *et al.* 1994). Hollander *et al.* (1998) reported that, compared to healthy controls, patients with social anxiety disorder showed increased cortisol responses to orally administered m-chlorophenylpiperazine (m-CPP), a partial serotonin agonist.

With regard to molecular genetics, Stein *et al.* (1998b) reported no genetic link between generalized social anxiety disorder and either the serotonin transporter protein [5-HTT] gene or the 5-HT2 receptor gene. However, other 5-HT receptor subtypes or indirect modulatory effects of 5-HT on other neurotransmitters remain to be studied (Stein *et al.* 1998).

Adrenergic function The presence of autonomic symptoms (e.g. blushing, sweating and tremor) associated with increased activation of peripheral β-receptors as well as the efficacy of β-blockers in treating these symptoms in patients with social anxiety disorder, suggest that the adrenergic system is involved in social anxiety disorder. A number of studies involving public speaking challenges have indicated that patients with non-generalized social anxiety disorder (but not patients with generalized social anxiety disorder) exhibit increased cardiovascular reactivity in response to public speaking challenges (Heimberg *et al.* 1990; Hofmann *et al.* 1995). Patients with social anxiety disorder also show increased blood pressure responsivity to the Valsalva maneuver, exaggerated vagal withdrawal in response to isometric exercise, and a smaller immediate fall in blood pressure upon standing (Stein *et al.* 1994; Coupland *et al.* 1995). Abnormalities in plasma levels of epinephrine and norepinephrine (noradrenaline) in people with social anxiety disorder have not been conclusively demonstrated.

GABA function Nutt *et al.* (1999) have suggested that gamma-aminobutyric acid (GABA) dysfunction may be associated with social anxiety disorder. Benzodiazepines, which have proven efficacy in the amelioration of symptoms associated with social anxiety disorder, enhance GABA neurotransmission. However, a recent study that investigated the effects of flumazenil, a benzodiazepine antagonist on people with social anxiety disorder, failed to show differences between social anxiety disorder and control subjects in the rate of panic attacks and the severity of panic symptoms following the flumazenil challenge (Coupland *et al.* 2000). This contrasts with the situation in panic disorder where flumazenil is highly anxiogenic (Nutt *et al.* 1990).

Neuroanatomy

A number of neuroimaging studies have been conducted on patients with social anxiety disorder, providing more information on structural and functional abnormalities in social anxiety disorder.

Proton-localized magnetic resonance spectroscopy (MRS) has revealed significant differences in signal-to-noise ratios (SNRs) between patients with social anxiety disorder and healthy controls with regard to cortical gray matter as well as—to a lesser degree—subcortical gray matter (caudate, thalamus and putamen) (Davidson *et al.* 1993b; Tupler *et al.* 1997). In a magnetic resonance imaging (MRI) study, Potts *et al.* (1994) found no significant difference between patients with social anxiety disorder and normal controls with respect to total cerebral, caudate, putamen and thalamic volumes, although patients with social anxiety disorder showed a greater age-related reduction in putamen volume.

Stein and Leslie (1996) found no significant difference between patients and healthy subjects in regional cerebral blood flow using single photon emission computerized tomography (SPECT). More recently, Van der Linden *et al.* (2000) studied patients with social anxiety disorder with SPECT before and after an 8-week trial of pharmacotherapy with the SSRI citalopram. Post-treatment SPECT indicated significantly reduced activity in the anterior and lateral part of the left temporal cortex; the anterior, lateral and posterior part of the left mid frontal cortex; and the left cingulum. Furthermore, nonresponders showed higher activity at baseline in the anterior and lateral part of the left temporal cortex and the lateral part of the left mid frontal regions than responders.

Birbaumer *et al.* (1998) used fMRI to investigate differential activation of the amygdala in patients with social anxiety disorder and healthy controls in response to slides of neutral faces as well as aversive odor stimuli. Only patients with social anxiety disorder showed selective activation of the amygdala during the presentation of the face stimuli. Schneider *et al.* (1999) examined differences between patients with social anxiety disorder and healthy controls in brain activity in subcortical and cortical regions involved in the processing of negative affect during presentation of paired conditioned stimuli (neutral facial expressions) and unconditioned stimuli (negative odor vs. unmanipulated air). For patients with social anxiety disorder, the presentation of neutral facial stimuli associated with negative odor led to signal increases in both the amygdala and hippocampus, whereas healthy subjects showed decreases in activity in the amygdala and hippocampus.

Bell *et al.* (1999) investigated neural activation using ^{15}O-water blood flow positron emission tomography (PET) in patients with social anxiety disorder in a symptom provocation study. Using formal conjunction analysis, cerebral blood flow patterns in patients with social anxiety disorder were compared to patterns previously observed in conditioned anxiety. Increases in blood flow in the anterior cingulate and the insulae were found in both social anxiety and conditioned anxiety. However, increases in blood flow in the right dorsolateral prefrontal cortex and in the left parietal cortex were found only in social anxiety disorder— these areas involve functions associated with social anxiety disorder namely awareness of body position as well as planning of affective responses (Nutt *et al.* 1999).

Tillfors *et al.* (2001) conducted a symptom provocation study of 18 people with social anxiety disorder and a healthy comparison group using ^{15}O-water PET. The social anxiety disorder group reported a greater increase in subjective anxiety during public versus private speaking. It was found that increased anxiety was associated with enhanced regional cortical blood flow (rCBF) in the amygdaloid complex in socially anxious subjects relative to healthy subjects. Interestingly, subjects with social anxiety disorder showed a decrease in rCBF whereas comparison subjects showed an increase in rCBF during public speaking (as opposed to private speaking) in the orbitofrontal and insular cortices as well as in the temporal pole. The increase in rCBF was also less in subjects with social anxiety relative to the comparison group, in the parietal and secondary visual cortices. Increases of rCBF in the perirhinal and retrosplenial cortices occurred in the comparison group but not in subjects with social anxiety disorder. Tillfors *et al.* (2001) interpreted the relatively increased cortical rather than subcortical perfusion in the comparison group as indicating that cortical evaluation may be taxed by public performance situations. In contrast, people with social anxiety disorder respond to symptom challenge with increased subcortical activation.

In summary, functional neuroimaging studies suggest that patients with social anxiety disorder differ from normals with regard to the processing of social-threat related stimuli and conditioned aversive stimuli.

Genetic risk factors

Family studies (Reich & Yates 1988; Fyer *et al.* 1993, 1995; Chapman *et al.* 1995) and twin studies (Kendler *et al.* 1992) have provided evidence for a heritable component to social anxiety disorder. Reich and Yates

(1988) found that first-degree relatives of probands with uncomplicated social anxiety disorder had a higher incidence of social anxiety disorder (6.6%) than first-degree relatives of probands with panic disorder (0.4%) or healthy controls (2.2%). Fyer *et al.* (1993) found that a significantly greater proportion of the relatives of patients with social anxiety disorder had social anxiety disorder (16%; relative risk = 3.12), than did relatives of healthy controls (5%). Mannuzza *et al.* (1995) reanalysed their initial family study findings (Fyer *et al.* 1993) in order to determine whether differences exist between generalized and nongeneralized social anxiety disorder with regard to familial transmission. They found that prevalence rates of social anxiety disorder were significantly higher in first-degree relatives of patients with generalized social anxiety disorder than in nongeneralized social anxiety disorder and normal controls. Furthermore, relatives with either generalized or nongeneralized social anxiety disorder were more likely to have nongeneralized social anxiety disorder (Mannuzza *et al.* 1995).

Similarly, Stein *et al.* (1998a) found that generalized social anxiety disorder "bred true." They found that the rate of generalized social anxiety disorder, but not nongeneralized or discrete (performance situations only) social anxiety disorder was approximately 10 times higher (26.4% vs. 2.7%) among the first-degree relatives of probands with generalized social anxiety disorder than among the first-degree relatives of comparison subjects.

Furthermore, in a high risk study, Mancini *et al.* (1996) found that children of adults with social anxiety disorder have a higher incidence of social anxiety disorder as well as other anxiety disorders that reported community prevalences of these disorders (Mancini *et al.* 1995).

Although these studies have provided evidence for familial transmission of social anxiety disorder, they do not indicate whether such transmission is due to genetic factors or to family environmental factors (Hirshfeld-Becker *et al.* 1999). In contrast, twin studies provide data on the relative role of genetics versus family environment. In a study of 654 twins who met criteria for agoraphobia, social anxiety disorder, animal phobia and situational specific phobia, Kendler *et al.* (1992) found that the concordance rate for social anxiety disorder was 24.4% in monozygotic and 15.3% in dizygotic twins. They estimated that the heritability

of social anxiety disorder was 30% and that general familial environmental factors did not play a significant role in the transmission of social anxiety disorder. Kendler *et al.* (1992) postulated that, instead, more specific, individual life experiences may account for nongenetic factors in the etiology of social anxiety disorder. More recently, Kendler *et al.* (1999) obtained two assessments, 8 years apart, of lifetime history of agoraphobia, social anxiety disorder, situational and animal and blood-injury phobia in a community sample of 1708 female twins. Findings indicated that the estimated total genetic heritability of social anxiety disorder was 51%. It was also found that individual-specific environmental differences, and not familial-environmental factors, play an important role in the etiology of social anxiety disorder and other phobic conditions.

Transmission of general anxiety-proneness or anxiety diathesis may play a role in the etiology of social anxiety disorder (Barlow 1988; Rosenbaum *et al.* 1991; Turner *et al.* 1991; Rosenbaum *et al.* 1994; Hirshfeld-Becker *et al.* 1999). Thus, in the study by Kendler *et al.* (1992), it was found that both a general risk for anxiety proneness as well as disorder specific genetic risks account for the genetic transmission of social anxiety disorder. Further support for a general anxiety diathesis in social anxiety disorder derives from studies that found an increased risk for social anxiety disorder in the first-degree relatives of probands with panic disorder (Goldstein *et al.* 1994; Horwarth *et al.* 1995). Further research is necessary to clarify the contribution of a general anxiety diathesis and social anxiety disorder-specific genetic risk factors in the etiology of social anxiety disorder.

The role of temperament
Various researchers have suggested that the temperamental factor, behavioral inhibition (BI) to the unfamiliar, may predispose individuals to the development of social anxiety disorder (Rosenbaum *et al.* 1991; Hayward *et al.* 1998; Mick & Telch 1998; Hirshfeld-Becker *et al.* 1999; Schwartz *et al.* 1999). Children with BI towards the unfamiliar demonstrate retreat, avoidance and fear, or restraint when confronted with unfamiliar situations, objects, people or events (Kagan *et al.* 1988a). Kagan and Snidman (1999) estimate that about 20% of healthy children are behaviorally inhibited towards the unfamiliar and that about a third

of these children will develop serious social anxiety. Precursors to BI have been identified in children as young as 4 months, although BI is usually identified from about 2.5 years (Kagan 1997).

Longitudinal studies have provided evidence for the preservation of these temperamental characteristics: compared to less inhibited infants, behaviorally inhibited infants are more likely to be timid, reticent and socially avoidant throughout childhood (Kagan 1989; Kagan 1994). Twin studies have provided evidence for the heritability of BI (Emde et al. 1992; Robinson et al. 1992; DiLalla et al. 1994). Primate studies have confirmed the existence and persistence of BI similar to that found in humans in nonhuman primates (Mineka & Zinbarg 1995; Suomi 1997).

Mick and Telch (1998) investigated the association between a retrospective self-report measure of BI and anxiety symptomatology in 76 undergraduates with social anxiety, generalized anxiety, comorbid social and generalized anxiety, and minimal social and generalized anxiety. They found that BI was a specific risk-factor for social anxiety disorder, but not for GAD. Hayward et al. (1998) reported a four-fold higher risk for developing social anxiety disorder in high-school students with features of BI (as measured by retrospective self-report) compared to students without BI features.

Using the Diagnostic Interview Schedule for Children (DISC; Costello et al. 1985) as well as behavioral observation, Schwartz et al. (1999) assessed 79 13 year olds who were classified as inhibited or uninhibited at 21 and 31 months (Kagan et al. 1988). They found that adolescents who were classified as being behaviorally inhibited at 21 and 31 months, had a significantly higher prevalence rate of generalized social anxiety disorder (34%) than adolescents who were classified as uninhibited as infants (9%). However, the inhibited and uninhibited groups did not differ significantly with regard to the prevalence of specific fears, performance anxiety or separation anxiety.

It has been suggested that the increased physiological arousal present in some children with BI could make these children more prone to conditioning by adverse experiences (Nickel & Uhde 1995), thereby placing such children at greater risk for developing social anxiety disorder (Hirshfeld-Becker et al. 1999).

Behavioral influences

From a behavioral perspective, it has been proposed that three main processes may play a role in the development of social anxiety disorder, namely direct conditioning, vicarious (or observational) learning, and information transfer.

Some researchers have reported that about half of patients with social anxiety disorder are able to identify a specific negative social experience (e.g. negative performance situations or embarrassing social interactions) that initiated or exacerbated the onset of their social anxiety (Öst 1985; Stemberger et al. 1995). Direct conditioning may also play a role in erythrophobia (fear of blushing). In addition to single-trial direct conditioning, repetitive, less dramatic noxious experiences (e.g. teasing by peers) may also eventually lead to social anxiety and avoidance (Beidel & Turner 1998).

Indirect or vicarious learning may also be involved in the acquisition of social fears. Vicarious learning involves the acquisition of fears through the observation of the fearful reaction of another person in response to a specific stimulus or situation (Rachman 1991). Öst and Hugdahl (1981) reported that 13% of people with social anxiety disorder included in their study, reported the acquisition of social fears after seeing another person undergo traumatic social experiences. Information transfer, in which information regarding social situations is verbally or nonverbally transmitted, accounted for only 3% of the acquisition of social anxiety disorder in the study by Öst and Hughdal (1981).

These studies have relied on retrospective recall of traumatic events and may reflect memory biases associated with social anxiety disorder (Mattick & Lampe 1995; Hirshfeld-Becker et al. 1999). Additionally, numerous variables (including genetic vulnerability and experiential factors) influence the degree to which specific fears are conditioned and maintained (Mineka & Zinbarg 1995).

Cognitive and behavioral factors

Cognitive–behavioral theories of social anxiety disorder emphasize the role of certain cognitive processes (e.g. biases in processing social cues and performance-related deficits, anticipatory and postevent processing, self-focused attention), cognitive content (e.g. negative expectations, dysfunctional assumptions and self-schemas) and behaviors (e.g. avoidance and in-situation safety behaviors) in the maintenance of social anxiety (Heimberg & Barlow 1991; Clark & Wells 1995; Wells et al. 1995; Otto 1999).

The anticipatory anxiety often reported by people with social anxiety disorder, may be related to their tendency to overestimate the possibility of negative outcomes and to underestimate the possibility of positive outcomes for social events (Foa *et al.* 1996). When people with social anxiety disorder enter into social situations, these negative expectations lead to a hypervigilance for potential signs of threat. Such attentional biases involve a hypersensitivity to somatic reactions that are likely to be viewed as particularly conspicuous to others (Clark & Wells 1995). People with social anxiety disorder also show a negative bias towards detecting negative audience responses while disregarding positive audience responses (Veljaca & Rapee 1998) and tend to interpret ambiguous social scenarios as negative when compared to people with other anxiety disorders and normal controls (Amin *et al.* 1998). Studies using information-processing paradigms such as the modified Stroop task have shown hypervigilance to social-threat related words in people with social anxiety disorder compared to healthy controls, thus providing further evidence for threat-related information-processing biases in this condition (Cloitre *et al.* 1992; Mattia *et al.* 1993).

An increase in self-focused attention is also characteristic of people with social anxiety disorder (Ingram 1990). When compared to healthy controls, people with social anxiety disorder report making more negative self-evaluative comments in social or performance situations (Stopa & Clark 1993) and devote excessive attention to aspects of their self-representation (increased public self-consciousness) (Rapee & Heimberg 1997). This self-focused attention as well as the attentional focus on social threat cues seem to exacerbate social anxiety (Woody 1996) and to contribute to actual deficits in social performance (Stopa & Clark 1993). In addition, people with social anxiety disorder tend to have various unconditional dysfunctional beliefs about themselves and about social performance and evaluation (Clark & Wells 1995). These cognitive contents and processes result in a vicious cycle, which has various behavioral consequences beyond single social or performance situations.

People with social anxiety disorder tend to avoid social situations and also tend to engage in subtle in-situation safety behaviors (e.g. avoiding eye contact), thereby reducing the opportunities for testing dysfunctional cognitive contents, for lowering social anxiety through continued exposure, and for improving social skills (Clark & Wells 1995). Cognitive-behavioral interventions are aimed at modifying those cognitive processes and content as well as decreasing avoidance behaviors in order to break the vicious cycle involved in sustaining social anxiety disorder.

Diagnosis and differential diagnosis

History of social anxiety disorder diagnosis

Although there has long been an interest in studying fears relating to social interaction (e.g. erythrophobia —the fear of blushing in front of others), the term "social phobia" was first used by Janet (1903) to describe patients who feared being observed while speaking, playing the piano, or writing. In the first and second editions of the DSM (APA 1952, 1968), all phobias were grouped together on the basis of the psychoanalytic assumption that all phobias were related to unacceptable instinctual urges (Freud 1926, 1961). However, on the basis of findings by Marks and Gelder (1966) that provided evidence for considering the different phobias to be discrete diagnostic entities, social anxiety disorder emerged as a distinct disorder with the advent of DSM-III (APA 1980).

As defined in the DSM-III, social anxiety disorder was characterized by an excessive fear of observation or scrutiny in discrete, performance related situations accompanied by significant distress. Patients who met criteria for avoidant personality disorder (i.e. who feared multiple situations) did not receive a diagnosis of social anxiety disorder. The most deleterious effect of the arbitrary exclusion from social anxiety disorder of individuals with multiple social fears, was that such individuals were less likely to receive pharmacotherapy for their disorder than patients who met the criteria for DSM-III social anxiety disorder (Liebowitz *et al.* 1985). Consequently, criteria for DSM-III-R (APA 1987) social anxiety disorder were revised and broadened to include a generalized subtype of social anxiety disorder. In addition, DSM-III-R social anxiety disorder no longer excluded individuals with avoidant personality disorder. The subtype of social anxiety disorder characterized by more specific situational fears was referred to as "nongeneralized," "circumscribed," "discrete," or "specific" (Heimberg *et al.* 1993). Although the DSM-IV task force examined the reliability and validity of alternative subtyping systems, it was decided that more research was needed before implementing changes to the DSM-III-R classification of social anxiety disorder subtypes.

However, based on the recommendations of the DSM-IV task force, it was decided to recognize the continuity of social anxiety disorder from childhood into adulthood (Beidel 1991) by including features specific to the childhood presentation of social anxiety disorder. In addition, DSM-IV no longer included avoidant and overanxious disorders of childhood.

The major difference between ICD-10 and DSM-IV criteria sets (see Table 7.1) is that the DSM-IV diagnosis requires persistent fear of social situations, fear of humiliation and avoidance, whereas the ICD-10 requires only one of these criteria to be present. In addition, ICD-10 does not consider fear of public speaking in front of large audiences as a pathological phobic condition and specifies that the fear of scrutiny should be related to small groups of people (and not crowds). The DSM-IV specifies that social anxiety disorder should be associated with significant functional impairment, whereas ICD-10 does not. Furthermore, DSM-IV includes child specifiers and ICD-10 does not. Finally, DSM-IV does not specify somatic anxiety symptoms associated with social anxiety disorder, whereas ICD-10 does.

Panic disorder with agoraphobia

Avoidance of certain social situations is a common feature in panic disorder with agoraphobia, agoraphobia without a history of panic disorder, and social anxiety disorder. In addition, panic attacks related to interaction fears may occur in social anxiety disorder. Patients with panic disorder with agoraphobia and patients with social anxiety disorder can, however, be distinguished on the basis of their feared situations, their feared outcomes and the nature of the symptoms experienced during panic attacks (Page 1994). In social anxiety disorder, social situations are directly associated with a fear of embarrassment and negative evaluation by others, whereas the social fears of patients with panic disorder with agoraphobia are secondary to fears of panic attacks and the possible consequences of such attacks (losing control, dying, collapsing).

In addition, patients with panic disorder with agoraphobia are more likely to experience symptoms of paraesthesias, choking sensations, feelings of dizziness and feelings of faintness in addition to fears of dying,

losing control or going mad (Page 1994). Typically, blushing, muscle twitching and stammering are more commonly found in patients with social anxiety disorder (Amies et al. 1983; Solyom et al. 1986; Reich et al. 1988). Furthermore, uncued panic attacks or nocturnal panic attacks while sleeping occur only rarely in patients with social anxiety disorder (Heckelman & Schneier 1995; Stein et al. 1993). In patients with comorbid panic disorder and social anxiety disorder, social anxiety disorder usually precedes the onset of uncued panic attacks by several years (Yu Moutier & Stein 1999). Patients with social anxiety disorder generally report feeling less anxious when alone, whereas patients with panic disorder with agoraphobia and patients with agoraphobia generally report feeling safer in the company of others (Heckelman & Schneier 1995). Panic disorder with agoraphobia tends to have its onset in the mid-twenties, whereas social anxiety disorder has an onset in the mid-teen years (Mannuzza et al. 1990).

Avoidant personality disorder

The degree of comorbidity between avoidant personality disorder and social anxiety disorder is particularly high, with more than half the patients with either diagnosis qualifying for a diagnosis of the other comorbid condition (Reich et al. 1994a). The high degree of overlap may be ascribed to similarities between DSM-III-R and DSM-IV criteria sets for these conditions. Social anxiety disorder and avoidant personality disorder further share onset by mid-teens and chronic and stable course. In addition, although intensive psychotherapy has traditionally been recommended in patients with avoidant personality disorder, these patients have been shown to respond to briefer cognitive-behavior therapy (see Heimberg & Juster 1995 for a review) as well as to pharmacotherapy (Liebowitz et al. 1992).

Individuals with comorbid avoidant personality disorder and social anxiety disorder exhibit a greater degree of psychiatric comorbidity and social impairment than people with uncomplicated social anxiety disorder (Herbert et al. 1992). This has led to the proposal that social anxiety disorder and avoidant personality form part of a single continuum of psychopathology, with avoidant personality representing a severe form of social anxiety (Schneier et al. 1991; Herbert et al. 1992; Turner et al. 1992).

Depressive disorders

Patients with depressive disorders (perhaps particularly patients with atypical depressive disorder) may also show symptoms of social withdrawal and social isolation. It has been found that atypical depression has a higher prevalence rate (54.8%) in patients with comorbid avoidant personality disorder and social anxiety disorder compared to patients with neither social anxiety disorder nor avoidant personality disorder (31.1%) (Alpert *et al.* 1997).

Atypical depression is characterized by hypersensitivity to rejection and criticism and has been shown to have a preferential response to MAOIs over tricyclic antidepressants (Liebowitz *et al.* 1992). However, unlike social anxiety disorder, social avoidance in depressive disorders is usually not associated with intense fears of scrutiny and negative evaluation by others. Instead, depressed patients are usually socially withdrawn because of anhedonia or a lack of energy. In addition, although some people with depressive disorders experience true social fears, such fears usually co-occur with depressive episodes and remit between depressive episodes (Disalver *et al.* 1992). In cases where both a depressive disorder and social anxiety disorder are present, it is therefore advisable to ascertain whether a history of social anxiety disorder predates the onset of the depressive disorder (Heckelman & Schneier 1995).

Generalized anxiety disorder

Although patients with GAD may have worries about social situations in addition to nonsocial worries, social anxiety disorder can be distinguished from GAD by the presence of significant fear of scrutiny or negative evaluation. However, it may be necessary to conduct a thorough diagnostic interview in order to determine whether worries reflect underlying fears of social interaction, in which case a diagnosis of social anxiety disorder may be more appropriate. Certain symptoms may also help to distinguish GAD from social anxiety disorder; patients with GAD may experience insomnia, headaches and fears of dying more frequently than patients with social anxiety disorder (Reich *et al.* 1988).

Anxiety disorder not otherwise specified

DSM-IV excludes the diagnosis of social anxiety disorder in patients whose social fears and avoidance is secondary to other psychiatric illnesses (e.g. Parkinson's disease) or medical problems (e.g. benign tremor and stuttering). Such "secondary social phobia" (Liebowitz *et al.* 1985b) is currently classified under "anxiety disorder not otherwise specified" in DSM-IV. However, patients with social anxiety secondary to disfiguring or disabling medical conditions experience significant social anxiety and avoidance, and since such symptoms have been shown to respond to the MAOI phenelzine (Oberlander *et al.* 1994), clinicians should treat social anxiety and avoidance in such patient groups (Yu Moutier & Stein 1999).

Obsessive-compulsive disorder

Generally, it is not problematic to distinguish between obsessive-compulsive disorder (OCD) and social anxiety disorder. However, certain obsessions and compulsions of patients with OCD may be associated with considerable social fears and social avoidance. In such cases it is important to determine whether the manifested social fears and avoidance behaviors are secondary to the anxiety associated with the compulsions and obsessions or whether fears of scrutiny and negative evaluation by others are distinct from the symptoms of OCD.

Body dysmorphic disorder

Social anxiety disorder has relatively high comorbidity with body dysmorphic disorder (Wilhelm *et al.* 1997; Zimmerman & Mattia 1998). Clinicians must determine whether the social avoidance and fear is directly related to the patient's imagined defect in appearance.

Recently, it has been suggested that olfactory reference syndrome, a psychiatric condition characterized by persistent preoccupations with body odor accompanied by persistent shame and embarrassment (Pryse-Phillips 1971), shares various phenomenological features with body dysmorphic disorder (Stein *et al.* 1998). However, olfactory reference syndrome may also overlap significantly with social anxiety disorder, in particular with culture-bound expressions of social anxiety disorder such as TKS. Additional research is required to determine whether olfactory reference syndrome can be conceptualized as lying somewhere between social anxiety disorder and body dysmorphic disorder.

Other conditions

Although certain psychotic disorders such as schizophrena and a number of schizophrena spectrum disorders (such as schizotypal personality disorder) may be associated with social fears and avoidance behaviors, such fears and avoidance behaviors are mostly due to avolition or delusional fears. In contrast to people with social anxiety disorder, people with delusional disorders show an inability to recognize the excessive and unreasonable nature of their fears.

Schizoid personality disorder is characterized by a pervasive pattern of detachment from social relationships and a restricted range of expression of emotions in interpersonal contexts. In schizoid personality disorder, social situations are avoided because of a lack of interest in interpersonal interaction. In contrast, people with social anxiety disorder do not have a profound lack of interest in social contact (indeed, they may desperately yearn for such interaction). Rather, people with social anxiety disorder avoid social situations because of their intense social anxiety.

Differential diagnosis of social anxiety disorder in children

Clinicians need to consider additional differential diagnoses and developmental factors in diagnosing social anxiety disorder in children. In order to rule out misdiagnoses of social anxiety disorder in children with pervasive developmental disorders or mental retardation, it is necessary to establish that the child displays the capacity for age-appropriate social interaction and interpersonal relationships. For instance, Asperger's disorder is characterized by marked impairment in social interaction. However, in contrast to social anxiety disorder, children with Asperger's disorder do not display the capacity for age-appropriate social interactions. Furthermore, the social avoidance and social fears must not be transient shyness or fear of negative evaluation by others associated with a particular developmental stage (i.e. symptoms must have a duration of at least 6 months). It is also necessary to establish that the social fears and avoidance behaviors do not occur only in relation to interaction with adults, but also occur in peer settings.

In the light of the high prevalence of social anxiety

disorder in children with selective mutism (Dummit *et al.* 1997), i.e. the consistent failure to speak in specific social situations but not in others, it has been suggested that selective mutism may be a variant of social anxiety disorder in children (Black & Uhde 1992). In addition, some studies indicate that selective mutism responds to pharmacotherapy used in treating social anxiety disorder (Dummit *et al.* 1996; Golwyn & Sevlie 1999). In cases where children meet criteria for both social anxiety disorder and selective mutism, both diagnoses may be assigned (Albano *et al.* 1995). When differentiating between social anxiety disorder and specific phobia, it is necessary to determine whether the child's social fears and avoidance of social situations are associated with a fear of embarrassment and scrutiny or negative evaluation by others. Furthermore, children with social anxiety disorder may show more severe impairment and higher levels of comorbid depression than children with specific phobia (Last *et al.* 1992).

Assessment

A number of inventories and interview schedules are available for diagnosing social anxiety disorder and for determining the severity of the condition. Some of these measures are presented in Table 7.2 (see pp. 111 & 112).

Comorbidity

The majority of people with social anxiety disorder report the lifetime prevalence of at least one other psychiatric disorder (Schneier *et al.* 1992; Magee *et al.* 1996). Schneier *et al.* (1992) reported that 69% of people with DSM-III social anxiety disorder included in the ECA study had at least one additional lifetime disorder. In the NCS, 81% of people with social anxiety disorder reported a lifetime history of at least one additional DSM-III-R disorder (Magee *et al.* 1996). Interestingly, findings from the EDSP study revealed that the high degree of comorbidity between DSM-IV social anxiety disorder and other disorders was mainly attributable to generalized social anxiety disorder, whereas ORs for lifetime comorbidity were lower in nongeneralized DSM-IV social anxiety disorder (Wittchen *et al.* 1999).

Table 7.2 Selected inventories used in the assessment of social anxiety disorder.

Name of instrument	Description	Rationale of scale	Reliability and validity	Reference
Diagnostic interviews				
Structured Clinical Interview for DSM-IV (SCID-I/P)	Structured, DSM-IV-based criteria sets grouped into modules	Comprehensive structured clinical interview for most DSM-IV Axis I disorders	Inter-rater reliability for DSM-III-R social anxiety disorder ranged from poor to fair (Spitzer et al. 1992; Williams et al. 1992). Good clinical utility overall	First et al. 1996
Social phobia module of Anxiety Disorders Interview Schedule for DSM-IV (ADIS-IV-L)	Assesses current and lifetime anxiety disorders as well as other disorders (e.g. mood disorders). Also inquires about situational and cognitive cues for anxiety	Comprehensive interview schedule for diagnosis of DSM-IV anxiety disorders	Adequate reliability ($k = 0.64$) for social anxiety disorder (DiNardo et al. 1995). Good reliability and clinical utility overall	DiNardo et al. 1994
Clinician-administered social anxiety inventories				
Liebowitz Social Anxiety Scale (LSAS)	Evaluates fear and avoidance of 11 social- and 13 performance-related situations using a four point Likert-type scale. Yields four subscales (performance fear, performance avoidance, social fear, social avoidance) as well as total fear and avoidance scores	Evaluates severity of fear and avoidance symptoms for social and performance-related situations	Good internal consistency (Heimberg et al. 1999). Good reliability, validity and clinical utility overall	Liebowitz 1987
Brief Social Phobia Scale (BSPS)	Rates fear and avoidance of seven social situations and severity of four somatic symptoms on a 0–4 Likert-type scale	Measurement of severity of fear and avoidance as well as somatic symptoms	Satisfactory test-retest reliability (Davidson et al. 1997) and excellent inter-rater reliability (Davidson et al. 1991). Good internal consistency (Davidson et al. 1991)	Davidson et al. 1991, 1997

(Continued on p. 112)

Table 7.2 (*cont'd*)

Name of instrument	Description	Rationale of scale	Reliability and validity	Reference
Patient-rated social anxiety inventories				
Fear of Negative Evaluation Scale	Thirty-item true/false self-report inventory	Designed to measure the cognitive construct of fear of negative evaluation	Excellent inter-item reliability and test–retest reliability (Heimberg *et al.* 1988). May assess both nonspecific and disorder-specific features of social anxiety disorder (Elting & Hope 1995)	Watson & Friend 1969
Social phobia subscale of the Fear Questionnaire	Five-item measure on a nine-point Likert-type scale	Assesses fear motivated avoidance of situations involving being observed, performing, being criticized or interacting with authority figures	Adequate 1-week test–retest reliability (Marks & Mathews 1979) and adequate internal consistency (Oei *et al.* 1991). Measure of behavioral avoidance that does not measure the full range of social anxiety disorder symptomatology	Marks & Mathews 1979
Social Phobia and Anxiety Inventory (SPAI)	Forty-five-item scale of which 21 items require multiple responses, yielding 109 items in total rated on a seven-point Likert-type scale. Includes a social phobia and agoraphobia subscale	Assesses somatic, cognitive and behavioral responses to a variety of social and performance situations	Adequate internal consistency (Turner *et al.* 1989), good concurrent validity (Herbert *et al.* 1991; Turner *et al.* 1989)	Turner *et al.* 1989
Social Interaction Anxiety Scale (SIAS)	Twenty-item self-report inventory with five-point Likert-type scale	Designed to assess fear of interacting in dyads and groups and fear of scrutiny	Adequate test–retest reliability and excellent internal consistency (Mattrick & Clarke 1998)	Mattrick & Clarke 1998

Anxiety disorders

Other anxiety disorders are frequently comorbid with social anxiety disorder. In their analysis of the ECA data, Schneier et al. (1992) reported that the anxiety disorders with the highest increased rates of co-occurrence with social anxiety disorder were agoraphobia (OR = 11.81), simple phobia (OR = 9.44) and obsessive compulsive disorder (OR = 4.36). In patients with DSM-III social anxiety disorder, the most commonly occurring comorbid conditions were simple phobia (59%) and agoraphobia (44.9%) (Schneier et al. 1992).

Similarly, Magee et al. (1996) reported that people with DSM-III-R social anxiety disorder included in the NCS had a higher risk for having any other anxiety disorder in their lifetime than for developing any substance abuse, dependence, or mood disorder. In addition, the disorders with the highest increased rate of co-occurrence with social anxiety disorder were agoraphobia (23.3%; OR = 7.06) and simple phobia (37.6%; OR = 7.75). In 46.5% of those with agoraphobia and 44.5% of simple phobia had a lifetime prevalence of DSM-III-R social anxiety disorder. Social anxiety disorder generally precedes agoraphobia, whereas simple phobia and social anxiety disorder both seem to have relatively early ages at onset (Magee et al. 1996). The lifetime prevalence rate of GAD in DSM-III-R social anxiety disorder patients included in the NCS was 13.3% (OR = 3.77) (Magee et al. 1996). Although comorbidity rates as high as 32% have been found for GAD and social anxiety disorder (Yonkers et al. 1996), other clinical studies have not found significant associations between GAD and social anxiety disorder (Lecrubier & Weiller 1997).

Mood disorders

A number of community and clinical studies have found that social anxiety disorder is significantly comorbid with mood disorders (Schneier et al. 1992; Lecrubier & Weiller 1997; Kessler et al. 1999). Social anxiety disorder and avoidant personality disorder have high prevalence rates among patients with major depressive disorder (MDD) and dysthymia (Sanderson et al. 1990, 1992, 1994; Magee et al. 1996). As mentioned earlier, social anxiety disorder may well have a particularly strong relationship with atypical depression (Mannuzza et al. 1995; Alpert et al. 1997).

Schneier et al. (1992) found increased rates of co-occurrence between DSM-III social anxiety disorder and dysthymia (12.5%; OR = 4.3), bipolar disorder (4.7%; OR = 4.09) and major depressive disorder (16.6%; OR = 4.41). Of people with social anxiety disorder included in the NCS study, 41.4% (OR = 3.74) reported the lifetime prevalence of any other mood disorder. Major depressive disorder was found to occur in 37.2% (OR = 3.65) of people with social anxiety disorder and dysthymia was found to occur in 14.6% (OR = 3.15) (Magee et al. 1996). More recently, Kessler et al. (1999) reported that the ORs between social anxiety disorder and lifetime mood disorders are 2.9 for major depression, 2.7 for dysthymia, and 5.9 for bipolar disorder. In addition, pure public speaking social anxiety disorder was associated with lower ORs than other forms of social anxiety disorder, indicating that the type of social fear as well as the number of social fears influence comorbidity with other disorders.

In the majority of patients with social anxiety disorder and comorbid mood disorder, social anxiety disorder comes before the mood disorder (Schneier et al. 1992; Merikangas et al. 1996; Regier et al. 1998). Schneier et al. (1992) found that social anxiety disorder comes before the mood disorder in 70.9% of social anxiety disorder patients included in the ECA study. In an analysis of NCS data, Kessler et al. (1999) also found that social anxiety disorder preceded comorbid mood disorders in 68.5% of respondents, whereas 21.9% of respondents reported social anxiety disorder temporally secondary to mood disorders. In 9.6% of respondents, social anxiety disorder and mood disorders had an onset in the same year. Social anxiety disorder was temporally primary in 71.9% of patients with comorbid major depression and 76% of patients with comorbid dysthymia; however, onset of social anxiety disorder preceded the onset of bipolar disorder in only 47% of respondents with comorbid bipolar disorder (Kessler et al. 1999). In addition, Kessler et al. (1999) also found that temporally primary social anxiety disorder was associated with severity and persistence of comorbid mood disorders, a finding consistent with earlier studies (Alpert et al. 1997). The data indicate that social anxiety disorder is an extremely important risk factor for developing major depressive disorder.

Substance use disorders

Community studies have generally found high prevalence rates of substance abuse dependence, particularly alcohol abuse/dependence, in respondents with social anxiety disorder. In an analysis of the ECA data, Schneier *et al.* (1992) found a lifetime prevalence rate of 18.8% (OR = 2.20) for alcohol abuse and 13.0% (OR = 2.85) for drug abuse in people with social anxiety disorder. In the NCS study, 39.6% (OR = 2.01) of respondents with social anxiety disorder reported the presence of a lifetime substance use disorder with 23.9% (OR = 2.17) reporting lifetime alcohol dependence and 10.9% (OR = 1.20) reporting alcohol abuse (Magee *et al.* 1996). In addition, 14.8% (OR = 2.56) of respondents with social anxiety disorder reported drug dependence and 5.3% (OR = 1.24) reported drug abuse (Magee *et al.* 1996). In a study by Regier *et al.* (1998), it was found that 14.3% of respondents with social anxiety disorder reported having a comorbid substance use disorder and that 6.2% of respondents with substance use disorders reported having comorbid social anxiety disorder in a 1-year period.

In clinical settings, the rates of substance use disorders have been somewhat lower than in community surveys, varying between about 2% (Turner *et al.* 1991, 1992; Herbert *et al.* 1992) and 16% (Schneier *et al.* 1989).

Social anxiety disorder is usually temporally primary to substance use disorders (Schneier *et al.* 1992; Magee *et al.* 1996; Regier *et al.* 1998). Schneier *et al.* (1992) reported that social anxiety disorder preceded alcohol abuse in 85% and drug abuse in 76.7% of community-based respondents with these comorbid conditions. Conversely, Magee *et al.* (1996) found that alcohol dependence or abuse was temporally primary in only 6.4% of community-based respondents with comorbid social anxiety disorder, and drug dependence or abuse in only 3.8% of respondents.

A recent study investigating the effects of alcohol versus placebo utilizing a public-speaking challenge showed that alcohol does not directly reduce social anxiety in patients with social anxiety disorder, although the belief that one has received alcohol was associated with a reduction in social anxiety (Himle *et al.* 1999). Indeed, patients with social anxiety disorder may be more prone to develop substance use disorders, since they may attempt to self-medicate their social anxiety with such substances.

Social and economic impact

A number of factors contribute to the morbidity associated with social anxiety disorder. Social anxiety disorder has a relatively early onset and chronic course and patients with social anxiety disorder often develop comorbid conditions such as depression and substance abuse. Furthermore, the symptoms of social anxiety disorder intrinsically affect social interactions and relationships in a range of settings.

In an important paper, Schneier *et al.* (1994) used the Disability Profile and the Liebowitz Self-Rated Disability Scale, two disorder measures of current and lifetime functional impairment in social anxiety disorder to investigate functional impairment in 32 patients with social anxiety disorder and 14 controls. More than half of the patients with social anxiety disorder reported at least moderate impairment at some time in their lives of this was due to social anxiety and avoidance in a number of domains, including education, employment, family relationships, marriage/romantic relationships, friendships/social network, and other interests. Patients with social anxiety disorder were more impaired than normal controls on both the clinician-rated and well as the patient-rated scales.

People with social anxiety disorder are significantly more likely to report troubled relationships or dissatisfaction with interpersonal relationships (Schneier *et al.* 1994; Stein & Kean 2000). People with social anxiety disorder are also more likely to be unmarried (Schneier *et al.* 1992; Magee *et al.* 1996). Furthermore, elevated rates of social anxiety disorder have been reported in widowed, separated or divorced subjects (Lépine & Lellouch 1995).

Wittchen and Beloch (1996) compared 65 patients meeting DSM-III-R social anxiety disorder-criteria and 65 matched controls (patients with a history of herpes infection as a control for chronicity of illness) on the Social Function Survey (SF-36), a 36-item questionnaire developed for the Medical Outcomes Study (Ware *et al.* 1994). Patients with social anxiety disorder had significantly lower quality of life, particularly in the domains of mental health, general health, vitality, role limitations and social function. Differences between people with social anxiety disorder and matched control subjects on the subscales of the SF-36 are shown in Fig. 7.1.

On scores for mental health, 23.1% of patients with social anxiety disorder were severely impaired

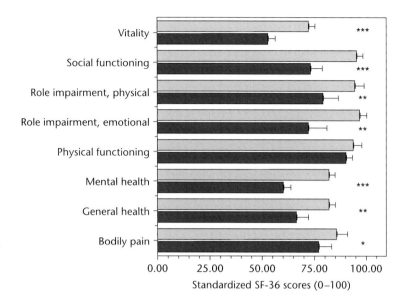

Fig. 7.1 Comparison of SF-36 dimensions of quality life in patients with social anxiety disorder and matched controls. ▨ Healthy controls, ■ Social anxiety disorder. (Adapted with permission from Wittchen & Beloch 1996, p. 19.)

and 24.6% were significantly impaired, whereas only 4.5% of controls were impaired. In addition, patients with social anxiety disorder showed a reduction in work productivity of around 12% compared with control subjects; 11% of patients with social anxiety disorder (vs. 3% of controls) were unemployed and 23% reported that social anxiety disorder symptoms were associated with substantially impaired work performance. Patients with social anxiety disorder indicated that the worst affected areas of functioning were partner and family relationships, education and career development, and household or work management as measured by the Liebowitz Self-Rated Disability Scale.

Bech and Angst (1996) reported on the quality of life of people with DSM-III social anxiety disorder drawn from a community study originally conducted in 1978 in Zurich (Angst *et al.* 1984). The quality of life of people with social anxiety disorder and people with subthreshold social anxiety disorder as measured by the Zurich Quality of Life Scale, was significantly poorer than people with mood disorders or other anxiety disorders such as panic disorder. The domains of quality of life that were most affected were work, relationships (partners and friends) and retrospective perceptions of childhood (Bech & Angst 1996). In the EDSP study (Wittchen *et al.* 1998) conducted in Munich among adolescents and young adults, it was found that

social anxiety disorder had a considerable impact on work, school and household management.

Despite the high level of impairment, patients with social anxiety disorder are less likely than people with other anxiety disorders (e.g. agoraphobia) to seek help for their psychiatric problems. In the Duke ECA study, it was found that although 32.6% of the respondents with social anxiety disorder reported having seen their physicians for psychological problems, only 3% reported seeking help for social anxiety (Davidson *et al.* 1993a). Similarly, in the NCS, when people with social anxiety disorder were compared to people with agoraphobia, it was found that significantly fewer people with social anxiety disorder had sought professional help (19% vs. 41%) or had ever used medication (6.2% vs. 21.6%) (Magee *et al.* 1996). Similar results have been obtained in clinical settings. As part of the WHO's study on psychiatric disorders in primary care, Weiller *et al.* (1996) assessed 2096 patients with the General Health Questionnaire (GHQ; Goldberg & Williams 1988) and conducted structured diagnostic interviews with 405 patients. Compared to patients without social anxiety disorder, patients with social anxiety disorder had higher scores on the GHQ, more alcohol-related problems, and a greater tendency to have suicidal ideation. Despite these problems, only 5% of patients with uncomplicated social anxiety disorder consulted their physicians for

115

psychological problems or mentioned their concerns to their physicians.

In a comparative study by Antony *et al.* (1998) differences between patients with panic disorder, OCD and social anxiety disorder in Quality of Life as measured by the Illness Intrusiveness Rating Scale (IIRS), a scale that assesses perception of interference in 13 domains of functioning, were investigated. Although the groups did not differ on total scores on the IIRS, group differences emerged for particular domains of functioning. Patients with social anxiety disorder reported more impairment in social relationships and self-expression/self-improvement than did the other two groups. In addition, all three groups experienced significantly more impairment as measured by the IIRS than populations with a variety of other chronic illnesses (e.g. multiple sclerosis and rheumatoid arthritis).

Social anxiety disorder is frequently comorbid with other psychiatric conditions, with around 80% of patients developing additional disorders such as depression or alcoholism (Schneier *et al.* 1992; Magee *et al.* 1996). Patients with comorbid conditions evidence even greater impairment than those with uncomplicated social anxiety disorder (Wittchen *et al.* 1999; Katzelnick *et al.* 2001). Individuals with social anxiety disorder with comorbid depression are also at greater risk for suicide attempts (Schneier *et al.* 1992; Lépine & Lellouch 1995). Katzelnick *et al.* (2001) reported that 21.9% of subjects with noncomorbid generalized social anxiety disorder in a community cohort of HMO members had attempted suicide. Wittchen *et al.* (2000) compared quality of life, work productivity, and social impairments in 65 patients with uncomplicated social anxiety disorder, 51 with comorbidity and 34 with subthreshold social anxiety disorder to controls. Current quality of life, particularly in vitality, general health, mental health, role limitations, and social functioning, was significantly reduced in all social anxiety disorder groups. However, patients with comorbidity revealed more severe reductions in quality of life than patients with uncomplicated and patients with subthreshold social anxiety disorder. Overall impairment for the group with subthreshold social anxiety disorder was slightly lower than for the group with uncomplicated social anxiety disorder.

Few studies have measured the economic costs associated with social anxiety disorder. DuPont *et al.* (1996) found that anxiety disorders contributed to a third of all costs of psychiatric disorders. However, less than a quarter of costs associated with anxiety disorders were for the treatment of these disorders, whereas three-quarters of costs were attributable to lost or reduced work productivity. Compared to controls, people with social anxiety disorder are more likely to be unemployed, show reduced work performance and are more absent from work due to social anxiety disorder (Wittchen *et al.* 2000; Katzelnick *et al.* 2001).

Conclusion

Social anxiety disorder had the third highest lifetime prevalence rate of all psychiatric disorders in the NCS (Kessler *et al.* 1994). This disorder has been shown to have high degrees of comorbidity with other psychiatric disorders and leads to considerable functional impairment. There is a growing body of data on the pathogenesis of social anxiety disorder, and an integrated account that incorporates neurobiological, temperamental, cognitive-behavioral, and cultural factors is gradually being consolidated. Fortunately, there is also growing evidence that certain pharmacological and psychotherapeutic interventions can be effective in the management of this disorder; it is therefore crucial that the current underrecognition and undertreatment of this disorder are tackled.

Acknowledgements

Mr du Toit is supported by an Association of Commonwealth Universities scholarship. Professor Stein is supported by the Medical Research Council of South Africa.

References

Albano, A.M., DiBartolo, P.M., Heimberg, R.G. & Barlow, D.H. (1995) Children and adolescents: assessment and treatment. In: *Social Phobia: Diagnosis, Assessment and Treatment* (R.G. Heimberg, M.R. Liebowitz, D.A. Hope & F.R. Schneier (eds), pp. 387–425). The Guilford Press, New York.

Alpert, J.E., Uebelacker, L.A., McLean, N.E. *et al.* (1997) Social phobia, avoidant personality disorder and atypical depression: co-occurrence and clinical implications. *Psychol Med* 27(3), 627–33.

American Psychiatric Association (APA) (1952) *Diagnostic Statistical Manual of Mental Disorders*, 1st edn. American Psychiatric Association, Washington, D.C.

American Psychiatric Association (APA) (1968) *Diagnostic Statistical Manual of Mental Disorders*, 2nd edn. American Psychiatric Association, Washington, D.C.

American Psychiatric Association (APA) (1980) *Diagnostic Statistical Manual of Mental Disorders*, 3rd edn. American Psychiatric Association, Washington, D.C.

American Psychiatric Association (APA) (1987) *Diagnostic Statistical Manual of Mental Disorders*, 3rd edn, revised. American Psychiatric Association, Washington, D.C.

American Psychiatric Association (APA) (1994) *Diagnostic Statistical Manual of Mental Disorders*, 4th edn. American Psychiatric Association, Washington, D.C.

Amies, P.L., Gelder, M.G. & Shaw, P.M. (1983) Social phobia: a comparative clinical study. *Br J Psychiatry* **142**, 174–9.

Amin, N., Foa, E.B. & Coles, M.E. (1998) Negative interpretation bias in social phobia. *Behav Res Ther* **36**, 945–57.

Angst, J., Dobler, M.A. & Binder, J. (1984) The Zurich study: a prospective epidemiological study of depressive, neurotic and psychosomatic syndromes. I. Problem, methodology. *Archiv Fuer Psychiatrie und Nervenkrankheiten* **234**(1), 13–20.

Antony, M.M., Roth, D., Swinson, R.P., Huta, V. & Devins, G.M. (1998) Illness intrusiveness in individuals with panic disorder, obsessive-compulsive disorder, or social phobia. *J Nerv Ment Dis* **186**(5), 311–15.

Ballenger, J.C. (1998) Introduction: focus on social anxiety disorder. *J Clin Psychiatry* **59** (Suppl. 17), 3.

Barlow, D. (1988) *Anxiety and its Disorders*. Guilford Press, New York.

Bech, P. & Angst, J. (1996) Quality of life in anxiety and social phobia. *Int Clin Psychopharmacol* **3**, 97–100.

Beidel, D.C. (1988) Psychophysiological assessment of anxious emotional states in children. *J Abnorm Psychol* **97**, 80–2.

Beidel, D.C. (1991) Social phobia and overanxious disorder in school-age children. *J Am Acad Child Adolesc Psychiatry* **30**, 545–52.

Beidel, D.C. (1998) Social anxiety disorder: etiology and early clinical presentation. *J Clin Psychiatry* **59** (Suppl. 17), 27–31.

Beidel, D.C. & Turner, S. (1998) *Shy Children, Phobic Adults*. American Psychiatric Association, Washington, D.C.

Beidel, D.C., Turner, S.M. & Dancu, C.V. (1985) Physiological, cognitive and behavioral aspects of social anxiety. *Behav Res Ther* **23**, 109–17.

Beidel, D.C., Turner, S.M. & Morris, T.L. (1999) Psychopathology of childhood social phobia. *J Am Acad Child Adolesc Psychiatry* **38**(6), 643–50.

Bell, C.J., Malizia, A.L. & Nutt, D.J. (1999) The neurobiology of social phobia. *Eur Arch Psychiatry Clin Neurosci* **249** (Suppl. 1), S11–S18.

Birbaumer, N., Grodd, W., Diedrich, O. *et al.* (1998) fMRI reveals amygdala activation to human faces in social phobics. *Neuroreport* **9**(6), 1223–6.

Black, B. & Uhde, T.W. (1992) Case study: elective mutism as a variant of social phobia. *J Am Acad Child Adolesc Psychiatry* **31**(6), 1090–4.

Bouwer, C. & Stein, D.J. (1998) Hyper-responsivity to nicotinic acid challenge in generalized social phobia: a pilot study. *Eur Neuropsychopharmacol* **8**, 311–13.

Caldirola, D., Perna, G., Arancio, C., Bertani, A. & Bellodi, L. (1997) The 35% CO_2 challenge test in patients with social phobia. *Psychiatry Res* **71**, 41–8.

Campbell, M.A. & Rapee, R.M. (1994) The nature of feared outcome representations in children. *J Abnorm Child Psychol* **22**, 99–111.

Chang, S.C. (1984) English-language review of Yamashita, I. *Taijin-Kyofu*. Kenehara, Tokyo. *Transcultural Psychiatry Review* **21**, 283–8.

Chapman, T.F., Manuzza, S. & Fyer, A.J. (1995) Epidemiology and family studies of social phobia. In: *Social Phobia: Diagnosis, Assessment and Treatment* (R.G. Heimberg, M.R. Liebowitz, D.A. Hope & F.R. Schneier (eds), pp. 21–40). The Guilford Press, New York.

Chatterjee, S., Sunitha, T.A., Velayudhan, A. & Khanna, S. (1997) An investigation into the psychobiology of social phobia: personality domains and serotonergic function. *Acta Psychiatr Scand* **95**(6), 544–50.

Clark, D.M. & Wells, A. (1995) A cognitive model of social phobia. In: *Social Phobia: Diagnosis, Assessment and Treatment* (R.G. Heimberg, M.R. Liebowitz, D.A. Hope & F.R. Schneier (eds), pp. 69–93). The Guilford Press, New York.

Clark, J.V. & Arkowitz, H. (1975) Social anxiety and self-evaluation of interpersonal performance. *Psychol Rep* **36**, 211–21.

Cloitre, M., Heimberg, R.G., Holt, C.S. & Liebowitz, M.R. (1992) Reaction time to threat stimuli in panic disorder and social phobia. *Behav Res Ther* **30**, 609–18.

Costello, E.J., Edelbrock, C.S. & Costello, A.J. (1985) Validity of the NIMH Diagnostic Interview Schedule for children: a comparison between psychiatric and pediatric referrals. *J Abnorm Child Psychol* **13**, 579–95.

Coupland, N.J., Bailey, J.E., Potakar, J.E. *et al.* (1995) Abnormal cardiovascular response to standing in panic disorder and social phobia [abstract]. *J Psychopharmacol* **9** (Suppl. 3), A73.

Coupland, N.J., Bell, C., Potokar, J.P., Dorkins, E. & Nutt, D.J. (2000) Flumazenil challenge in social phobia. *Depress Anxiety* **11**(1), 27–30.

Davidson, J.R.T., Hughes, D.L., George, L.K. *et al.* (1993a) The epidemiology of social phobia: findings from the Duke Epidemiological Catchment Area Study. *Psychol Med* **23**, 709–18.

Davidson, J.R.T., Krishnan, K.R., Charles, H.C. *et al.* (1993b) Magnetic resonance spectroscopy in social phobia: preliminary findings. *J Clin Psychiatry* **54**, 19–25.

Davidson, J.R., Miner, C.M., De Veaugh Geiss, J., Tupler, L.A., Colket, J.T. & Potts, N.L. (1997) The Brief Social Phobia Scale: a psychometric evaluation. *Psychol Med* **27**(1), 161–6.

Davidson, J.R., Potts, N.L., Richichi, E.A. *et al.* (1991) The Brief Social Phobia Scale. *J Clin Psychiatry* **52**, 48–51.

Davies, M., Udwin, O. & Howlin, P. (1998) Adults with Williams syndrome. Preliminary study of social, emotional and behavioral difficulties. *Br J Psychiatry* **172**, 273–6.

DiLalla, L.F., Kagan, J. & Reznick, J. (1994) Genetic etiology of behavioral inhibition among 2-year-old children. *Infant Behavior and Development* **17**(4), 405–12.

DiNardo, P.A., Brown, T.A. & Barlow, D.H. (1994) *Anxiety Disorders Interview Schedule for DSM-IV: Lifetime Version (ADIS-IV-L)*. Graywind Publications, Albany, NY.

Disalver, S.C., Qamar, A.B. & Del Medico, V.J. (1992) Secondary social phobia in patients with major depression. *Psychiatry Res* **44**, 33–40.

Dummit, E.S., 3rd, Klein, R.G., Tancer, N.K., Asche, B., Martin, J. & Fairbanks, J.A. (1997) Systematic assessment of 50 children with selective mutism. *J Am Acad Child Adolesc Psychiatry* **36**(5), 653–60.

Dummit, E.S., 3rd, Klein, R.G., Tancer, N.K., Asche, B. & Martin, J. (1996) Fluoxetine treatment of children with selective mutism: an open trial. *J Am Acad Child Adolesc Psychiatry* **35**(5), 615–21.

DuPont, R.L., Rice, D.P., Miller, L.S., Shiraki, S.S., Rowland, C.R. & Harwood, H.J. (1996) Economic costs of anxiety disorders. *Anxiety* **2**(4), 167–72.

Elting, D.T. & Hope, D.A. (1995) Cognitive assessment. In: *Social Phobia: Diagnosis, Assessment and Treatment* (R.G. Heimberg, M.R. Liebowitz, D.A. Hope & F.R. Schneier (eds), pp. 232–58). The Guilford Press, New York.

Emde, R.N., Plomin, R., Robinson, J. *et al.* (1992) Temperament, emotion and cognition at 14 months. The MacArthur Longitudinal Twin Study. *Child Dev* **63**, 1437–55.

Faravelli, C., Zucchi, T., Viviani, B. *et al.* (2000) Epidemiology of social phobia: a clinical approach. *Eur Psychiatry* **15**(1), 17–24.

Fifer, S.K., Mathias, S.D., Patrick, D.L., Mazonson, P.D., Lubeck, D.P. & Buesching, D.P. (1994) Untreated anxiety among adult primary care patients in a health maintenance organization. *Arch Gen Psychiatry* **51**, 740–50.

First, M.B., Spitzer, R.L., Gibbon, M. & Williams, J. (1996) *Structured Clinical Interview for DSM-IV Axis I Disorders. Patient Edition (SCID-I/P)*, Version 2.0. New York State Psychiatric Institute, New York.

Foa, E., Franklin, M., Perry, K. & Herbert, J. (1996) Cognitive biases in generalized social phobia. *J Abnorm Psychol* **105**, 433–9.

Freud, S. (1961) Inhibitions, symptoms and anxiety. In: *The Standard Edition of the Complete Works of Sigmund Freud*, Vol. 20 (J. Strachey (ed.), pp. 87–157). Hogarth Press, London.

Fyer, A.J., Mannuzza, S., Chapman, T., Liebowitz, M. & Klein, D. (1993) A direct interview family study of social phobia. *Arch Gen Psychiatry* **50**, 286–93.

Fyer, A.J., Mannuzza, S., Chapman, T.F., Martin, L.Y. & Klein, D.F. (1995) Specificity in familial aggregation of phobic disorders. *Arch Gen Psychiatry* **52**(7), 564–73.

Goldberg, D.P. & Lecrubier, Y. (1995) Form and frequency of mental disorders across centers. In: *Mental Illness in General Health Care: an International Study* (T.B.Üstun & N. Sartorius (eds), pp. 323–34). John Wiley & Sons, New York.

Goldberg, D.P. & Williams, P. (1988) *A User's Guide to the General Health Questionnaire: GHO*. Nfer–Nelson, Windsor, UK.

Goldstein, R.B., Weissman, M.M., Adamas, P.B. *et al.* (1994) Psychiatric disorders in relatives of probands with panic disorder and/or major depression. *Arch Gen Psychiatry* **51**, 383–94.

Golwyn, D.H. & Sevlie, C.P. (1999) Phenelzine treatment of selective mutism in four prepubertal children. *J Child Adolesc Psychopharmacol* **9**(2), 109–13.

Gorman, J.M., Askanazi, J., Liebowitz, M.R. *et al.* (1984) Response to hyperventilation in a group of patients with panic disorder. *Am J Psychiatry* **141**, 857–61.

Gorman, J.M., Papp, L.A., Martinez, J. *et al.* (1990) High dose CO_2 challenge test in anxiety disorder patients. *Biol Psychiatry* **28**, 743–57.

Gosch, A. & Pankau, R. (1997) Personality characteristics and behavior problems in individuals of different ages with Williams syndrome. *Dev Med Child Neurol* **39**(8), 527–33.

Griez, E.J., Lousberg, H., van den Hout, M.A. & van der Molen, G.M. (1987) CO_2 vulnerability in panic disorder. *Psychiatry Res* **20**, 87–95.

Hayward, C., Killen, J.D., Kraemer, K. & Taylor, C. (1998) Linking self-reported childhood behavioral inhibition to adolescent social phobia. *J Am Acad Child Adolesc Psychiatry* **37**(12), 1308–16.

Heckelman, L.R. & Schneier, F.R. (1995) Diagnostic issues. In: *Social Phobia: Diagnosis, Assessment and Treatment* (R.G. Heimberg, M.R. Liebowitz, D.A. Hope & F.R. Schneier (eds), pp. 3–20). The Guilford Press, New York.

Heimberg, R.G. & Barlow, D.H. (1991) New developments in cognitive-behavioral therapy for social phobia. *J Clin Psychiatry* **52** (Suppl. 11), 21–30.

Heimberg, R.G., Holt, C.S., Schneier, F.R., Spitzer, R.L. & Liebowitz, M.R. (1993) The issue of subtypes in the diagnosis of social phobia. *J Anx Disord* **7**, 249–69.

Heimberg, R.G., Hope, D.A., Dodge, C.S. & Becker, R.E. (1990) DSM-III-R subtypes of SP: comparison of generalized social phobics and public speaking phobics. *J Nerv Ment Dis* **178**, 172–9.

Heimberg, R.G., Hope, D.A., Rapee, R.M. & Bruch, M.A. (1988) The validity of the Social Avoidance and Distress Scale and the Fear of Negative Evaluation Scale with social phobic patients. *Behav Res Ther* **26**(5), 407–10.

Heimberg, R.G., Horner, K.J., Juster, H.R. *et al.* (1999) Psychometric properties of the Liebowitz Social Anxiety Scale. *Psychol Med* **29**(1), 199–212.

Heimberg, R.G. & Juster, H.R. (1995) Cognitive-behavioral treatments: literature review. In: *Social Phobia: Diagnosis, Assessment and Treatment* (R.G. Heimberg, M.R. Liebowitz, D.A. Hope & F.R. Schneier (eds), pp. 261–309). The Guilford Press, New York.

Herbert, J.D., Bellack, A.S. & Hope, D.A. (1991) Concurrent validity of the Social Phobia and Anxiety Inventory. *Journal of Psychopathology and Behavioral Assessment* **13**, 357–68.

Herbert, J.D., Hope, D.A. & Bellack, A.S. (1992) Validity of the distinction between generalized social phobia and avoidant personality disorder. *J Abnorm Psychol* **101**(2), 340–3.

Himle, J.A., Abelson, J.L., Haghightgou, H., Hill, E.M., Nesse, R.M. & Curtis, G.C. (1999) Effect of alcohol on social phobic anxiety. *Am J Psychiatry* **156**(8), 1237–43.

Hirshfeld-Becker, D.R., Fredman, S.J., Robin, J.A. & Rosenbaum, J.F. (1999) The etiology of social anxiety disorder. In: *Social Anxiety Disorder* (H.G.M. Westenberg & J.A. den Boer (eds), pp. 47–79). Synthesis, Amsterdam.

Hofmann, S.G., Newham, M.G., Ehlers, A. & Roth, W.T. (1995) Psychophysiological differences between subgroups of social phobia. *J Abnorm Psychol* **104**, 224–31.

Hollander, E., Kwon, J., Weiller, E. *et al.* (1998) Serotonergic function in social phobia: comparison to normal control and obsessive-compulsive disorder subjects. *Psychiatry Res* **79**, 213–17.

Holt, C.S., Heimberg, R.G. & Hope, D.A. (1992) Avoidant personality disorder and the generalized subtype of social phobia. *J Abnorm Psychol* **101**, 318–25.

Holt, P.E. & Andrews, G. (1989) Provocation of panic: three elements of the panic reaction in four anxiety disorders. *Behav Res Ther* **27**, 253–61.

Horwarth, E., Wolk, S.I., Goldstein, R.B. *et al.* (1995) Is the comorbidity between social phobia and panic disorder due to the familial cotransmission or other factors? *Arch Gen Psychiatry* **52**, 574–82.

Hwu, H.G., Yeh, E.K. & Chang, L.Y. (1989) Prevalence of psychiatric disorders in Taiwan defined by the Chinese Diagnostic Interview Schedule. *Acta Psychiatr Scand* **79**, 136–47.

Ingram, R.E. (1990) Self-focused attention in clinical disorders: review and conceptual model. *Psychol Bull* **107**, 156–76.

Janet, P. (1903) *Les Obsessions et la Psychasténie*. F. Alcan, Paris.

Kagan, J. (1989) Temperamental contributions to social behavior. *Am Psychol* **44**, 668–74.

Kagan, J. (1994) *Galen's Prophecy: Temperament and Human Nature*. Basic Books, New York.

Kagan, J. (1997) Temperament and the reactions to unfamiliarity. *Child Dev* **68**(1), 139–43.

Kagan, J., Reznick, J.S. & Snidman, N. (1988) Biological bases of childhood shyness. *Science* **240**, 167–71.

Kagan, J. & Snidman, N. (1999) Early childhood predictors of adult anxiety disorders. *Biol Psychiatry* **46**(11), 1536–41.

Kaminer, D.B. & Stein, D.J. (1999) Social anxiety disorder in children and adolescents. In: *Social Anxiety Disorder* (H.G.M. Westenberg & J.A. den Boer (eds), pp. 117–31). Synthesis, Amsterdam.

Katzelnick, D.J., Kobak, K.A., DeLeire, T. *et al.* (2001) Impact of generalized anxiety disorder in managed care. *Am J Psychiatry* **158**(12), 1999–2007.

Kendler, K.S., Karkowski, L.M. & Prescott, C.A. (1999) Fears and phobias: reliability and heritability. *Psychol Med* **29**(3), 539–53.

Kendler, K., Neale, M., Kessler, R., Heath, A. & Eaves, L. (1992) The Genet Epidemiol of phobias in women: the interrelationship of agoraphobia, social phobia, situational phobia and simple phobia. *Arch Gen Psychiatry* **49**, 273–81.

Kessler, R.C., McGonagle, K.A., Zhao, S. (1994) Lifetime and 12-month prevalence of DSM-III-R psychiatric disorders in the United States. Results from the National Comorbidity Survey. *Arch Gen Psychiatry* **51**(1), 8–19.

Kessler, R.C., Stang, P., Wittchen, H.U., Stein, M. & Walters, E.E. (1999) Lifetime co-morbidities between social phobia and mood disorders in the US National Comorbidity Survey. *Psychol Med* **29**(3), 555–67.

Kessler, R.C., Stein, M.B. & Berglund, P. (1998) Social phobia subtypes in the National Comorbidity Survey. *Am J Psychiatry* **155**, 613–19.

Last, C.G., Perrin, S., Hersen, M. & Kazdin, A.E. (1992) DSM-III-R anxiety disorders in children: sociodemographic and clinical characteristics. *J Am Acad Child Adolesc Psychiatry* **31**(6), 1070–6.

Lecrubier, Y. & Weiller, E. (1997) Comorbidities in social phobia. *Int Clin Psychopharmacol* **12** (Suppl. 6), 517–21.

Lee, C.K., Kwak, Y.S., Yamamoto, J. *et al.* (1990) Psychiatric epidemiology in Korea. Part I: gender and age differences in Seoul. *J Nerv Ment Dis* **178**, 242–6.

Lépine, J.P. & Lellouch, J. (1995) Diagnosis and epidemiology of agoraphobia and social phobia. *Clin Neuropharmacol* **18** (Suppl. 2), S15–S26.

Lépine, J.P. & Pelissolo, A. (1999) Epidemiology and co-morbidity of social anxiety disorder. In: *Social Anxiety Disorder* (H.G.M. Westenberg & J.A. den Boer (eds), pp. 29–45). Synthesis, Amsterdam.

Liebowitz, M.R. (1987) Social phobia. *Mod Prob Pharmacopsychiatry* **22**, 141–73.

Liebowitz, M.R., Campeas, R., Levin, A., Sandberg, D., Hollander, E. & Papp, I. (1987) Pharmacotherapy of social phobia: a condition distinct from panic attacks. *Psychosomatics* **28**, 305–8.

Liebowitz, M.R., Fyer, A., Gorman, J.M. *et al.* (1984) Lactate provocation of panic attacks. I. Clinical and behavioral findings. *Arch Gen Psychiatry* **41**, 764–70.

Liebowitz, M.R., Fyer, A.J., Gorman, J.M. *et al.* (1985a) Specificity of lactate infusions in social phobia versus panic disorders. *Am J Psychiatry* **42**, 947–50.

Liebowitz, M.R., Gorman, J.M., Fyer, A.J. & Klein, D.F. (1985b) Social phobia. Review of a neglected anxiety disorder. *Arch Gen Psychiatry* **42**, 729–36.

Liebowitz, M.R., Heimberg, R.G., Fresco, D.M., Travers, J. & Stein, M.B. (2000) Social phobia or social anxiety disorder: what's in a name? [letter]. *Arch Gen Psychiatry* **57**(2), 191–2.

Liebowitz, M.R., Schneier, F., Campeas, R. *et al.* (1992) Phenelzine versus atenolol in social phobia: a placebo-controlled comparison. *Arch Gen Psychiatry* **49**, 290–300.

van der Linden, G., Van Heerden, B., Warwick, J. *et al.* (2000) Functional brain imaging and pharmacotherapy in social phobia: Single photon emission computed tomography before and after treatment with the selective serotonin reuptake inhibitor citalopram. *Prog Neuropsychopharmacol Biol Psychiatry* **24**, 419–38.

Lovibond, P.F. & Rapee, R.M. (1993) The representation of feared outcomes. *Behav Res Ther* **31**, 595–608.

Ludwig, R.P. & Lazarus, P.J. (1983) Relationship between shyness in children and constricted cognitive control as measured by the Stroop color-word test. *J Consult Clin Psychol* **51**, 386–9.

Magee, W.J., Eaton, W.W., Wittchen, H.U., McGonagle, K.A. & Kessler, R.C. (1996) Agoraphobia, simple phobia, and social phobia in the National Comorbidity Survey. *Arch Gen Psychiatry* **53**, 159–68.

Mancini, A., van Ameringen, M., Szatmari, P., Fugere, C. & Boyle, M. (1996) A high-risk study of the children of adults with social phobia. *J Am Acad Child Adolesc Psychiatry* **35**, 1511–17.

Mannuzza, S., Fyer, A.J., Liebowitz, M.R. & Klein, D.F. (1990) Delineating the boundaries of social phobia: its relationship to panic disorder and agoraphobia. *J Anxiety Disord* **4**(1), 41–59.

Mannuzza, S., Schneier, F.R., Chapman, T.F., Liebowitz, M.R., Klein, D.F. & Fyer, A.J. (1995) Generalized social phobia. Reliability and validity. *Arch Gen Psychiatry* **52**(3), 230–7.

Marks, I.M. & Gelder, M.G. (1966) Different ages of onset in varieties of phobias. *Am J Psychiatry* **123**, 218–21.

Marks, I.M. & Mathews, A.M. (1979) Brief standard self-rating for phobic patients. *Behav Res Ther* **17**, 263–7.

Mattia, J.I., Heimberg, R.G. & Hope, D.A. (1993) The revised Stroop color-naming task in social phobics. *Behav Res Ther* **31**, 305–13.

Mattick, R.P. & Clarke, J.C. (1998) Development and validation of measures of social phobia scrutiny fear and social interaction anxiety. *Behav Res Ther* **36**(4), 455–70.

Mattick, R.A.P. & Lampe, L. (1995) Cognitive and behavioral aspects. In: *Social Phobia Clinical and Research Perspectives* (M.B. Stein (ed.), pp. 189–228). American Psychiatric Press, Washington, D.C.

McCann, U.D., Slate, S.O., Geraci, M., Roscow-Terrill, D. *et al.* (1997) A comparison of the effects of intravenous pentagastrin on patients with social phobia, panic disorder and healthy controls. *Neuropsychopharmacology* **16**(3), 229–37.

McNally, R. (1987) Preparedness and phobias: a review. *Psychol Bull* **101**, 283–303.

Mendlowicz, M.V. & Stein, M.B. (1999) The biological basis of social anxiety disorder. In: *Social Anxiety Disorder* (H.G.M. Westenberg & J.A. den Boer (eds), pp. 81–108). Synthesis, Amsterdam.

Merikangas, K.R., Angst, J., Eaton, W. *et al.* (1996) Comorbidity and boundaries of affective disorders with anxiety disorders and substance misuse: results of an international task force. *Br J Psychiatry* **30**, 58–67.

Mick, M. & Telch, M. (1998) Social anxiety disorder and history of behavioral inhibition in young adults. *J Anxiety Disord* **12**, 1–20.

Mineka, S. & Zinbarg, R. (1995) Conditioning and ethological models of social phobia. In: *Social Phobia: Diagnosis, Assessment and Treatment* (R.G. Heimberg, M.R. Liebowitz, D.A. Hope & F.R. Schneier (eds), pp. 134–62). The Guilford Press, New York.

Nickell, P. & Uhde, T. (1995) Neurobiology of social phobia. In: *Social Phobia: Diagnosis, Assessment and Treatment* (R.G. Heimberg, M.R. Liebowitz, D.A. Hope & F.R. Schneier (eds), pp. 113–33). The Guilford Press, New York.

Nutt, D.J., Bell, C.J. & Malizia, A.L. (1999) Brain mechanisms of social anxiety disorder. *J Clin Psychiatry* **59** (Suppl. 17), 4–9.

Nutt, D.J., Glue, P., Lawson, C. & Wilson, S. (1990) Flumazenil provocation of panic attacks. Evidence for altered benzodiazepine receptor sensitivity in panic disorder. *Arch Gen Psychiatry* **47**(10), 917–25.

Oberlander, E.L., Schneier, F.R. & Liebowitz, M.R. (1994) Physical disability and social phobia. *J Clin Psychopharmacol* **14**(2), 136–43.

Oei, T.P.S., Moylan, A. & Evans, L. (1991) Validity and clinical utility of the Fear Questionnaire for anxiety-disorder patients. *Psychol Assess* **3**, 391–7.

Öhman, A. (1986) Face the beast and fear the face: animal and social fears as prototypes for evolutionary analyses of emotion. *Psychophysiology* **23**, 123–45.

Öhman, A., Dimberg, U. & Esteves, F. (1989) Preattentive activation of aversive emotions. In: *Aversion, Avoidance and Anxiety: Perspectives on Aversively Motivated Behavior* (T. Archer & L.-G. Nilsson (eds), pp. 123–75). Erlbaum, Hillsdale, NJ.

Ono, Y., Yoshimura, K., Sueoka, R. *et al.* (1996) Avoidant personality disorder and taijin kyoufu: sociocultural implications of theWHO/ADAMHA International Study of Personality Disorders in Japan. *Acta Psychiatr Scand* **93**, 172–6.

Öst, L.G. (1985) Ways of acquiring phobias and outcome of behavioral treatments. *Behav Res Ther* **23**, 683–9.

Öst, L.G. (1987) Age of onset in different phobias. *J Abnorm Psychol* **96**, 223–9.

Öst, L.G. & Hugdahl, K. (1981) Acquisition of phobias and anxiety response patterns in clinic patients. *Behav Res Ther* **16**, 439–47.

Otto, M.W. (1999) Cognitive-behavioral therapy for social anxiety disorder: model, methods and outcome. *J Clin Psychiatry* **60** (Suppl. 9), 14–19.

Page, A.C. (1994) Distinguishing panic disorder and agoraphobia from social phobia. *J Nerv Ment Dis* **182**(11), 611–17.

Papp, L.A., Gorman, J.M., Liebowitz, M.R., Fyer, A.J., Cohen, B. & Klein, D.F. (1988) Epinephrine infusions in patients with social phobia. *Am J Psychiatry* **145**, 733–6.

Pilkonis, P.A. (1977a) Shyness, public and private and its relationship to other measures of social behavior. *J Pers* **45**, 585–97.

Pilkonis, P.A. (1977b) The behavioral consequences of shyness. *J Pers* **45**, 598–611.

Potts, N.L.S., Book, S. & Davidson, J.R.T. (1996) The neurobiology of social phobia. *Int Clin Psychopharmacol* **11** (Suppl. 3), 43–8.

Potts, N.L., Davidson, J.R., Krishnan, K.R. & Doraiswamy, P.M. (1994) Magnetic resonance imaging in social phobia. *Psychiatry Res* **52**, 35–42.

Prince, R.H. (1993) Culture bound syndromes. The example of social phobias. In: *Environment and Psychopathology* (A. Ghadirian & H.E. Lehman (eds), pp. 55–72). Springer, New York.

Pryse-Phillips, W. (1971) An olfactory reference syndrome. *Acta Psychiat Scan* **47**, 484–509.

Rachman, S. (1991) Neo-conditioning and the classical theory of fear acquisition. *Clin Psychol Rev* **11**, 155–73.

Rapee, R.M. (1995) Descriptive psychopathology of social phobia. In: *Social Phobia: Diagnosis, Assessment and Treatment* (R.G. Heimberg, M.R. Liebowitz, D.A. Hope & F.R. Schneier (eds), pp. 41–66). The Guilford Press, New York.

Rapee, R.M. & Lim, L. (1992) Discrepancy between self and observer ratings of performance in social phobics. *J Abnorm Psychol* **101**, 727–31.

Rapee, R.M. & Heimberg, R.G. (1997) A cognitive-behavioral model of anxiety in social phobia. *Behav Res Ther* **35**, 741–56.

Rapee, R.M., Sanderson, W.C. & Barlow, D.H. (1988) Social phobia features across the DSM-III-R anxiety disorders. *Journal of Psychopathology and Behavioral Assessment* **10**, 287–99.

Regier, D.A., Rae, D.S., Narrow, W.E., Kaelber, C.T. & Schatzberg, A.F. (1998) Prevalence of anxiety disorders and their comorbidity with mood and addictive disorders. *Br J Psychiatry* **34**, 24–8.

Reich, J., Goldenberg, I., Goisman, R., Vasile, R. & Keller, M. (1994b) A prospective follow-up study of the course of social phobia. II. Testing for basic predictors of course. *J Nerv Ment Dis* **182**, 297–301.

Reich, J., Goldenberg, I., Vasile, R., Goisman, R. & Keller, M. (1994a) A prospective, follow-along study of the course of social phobia. *Psychiatry Res* **54**, 249–58.

Reich, J.H., Noyes, R. & Yates, W. (1988) Anxiety symptoms distinguishing social phobia from panic and generalized anxiety disorders. *J Nerv Ment Dis* **176**, 510–13.

Reich, J. & Yates, W. (1988) Family history of psychiatric disorders in social phobia. *Compr Psychiatry* **29**, 72–5.

Robins, L.N., Helzer, J.E., Croughan, J. & Ratcliff, K.S. (1981) National Institute of Mental Health Diagnostic Interview Schedule: Its history, characteristics, and validity. *Arch Gen Psychiatry* **38**, 381–9.

Robinson, J.L., Kagan, J., Reznick, J.S. & Corley, R. (1992) The heritability of inhibited and uninhibited behavior: a twin study. *Dev Psychol* **28**(6), 1030–7.

Rosenbaum, J., Biederman, J., Hirshfeld, D., Bolduc, E. & Chaloff, J. (1991) Behavioral inhibition in children: a possible precursor to panic disorder or social phobia. *J Clin Psychiatry* **52** (Suppl. 11), 5–9.

Rosenbaum, J.F., Biederman, J., Pollock, R.A. & Hirshfeld, D.R. (1994) The etiology of social phobia. *J Clin Psychiatry* **55**, 10–16.

Rowe, D.C., Stever, C., Gard, J.M.C. *et al.* (1998) The relation of the dopamine transporter gene (DAT1) to symptoms of internalizing disorders in children. *Behav Genet* **28**(3), 215–25.

Sanderson, W.C., Beck, A.T. & Beck, J. (1990) Syndrome comorbidity in patients with major depression or dysthymia: prevalence and temporal relationships. *Am J Psychiatry* **147**(8), 1025–8.

Sanderson, W.C., Wetzler, S., Beck, A.T. & Betz, F. (1992) Prevalence of personality disorders in patients with major depression and dysthymia. *Psychiatry Res* **42**(1), 93–9.

Sanderson, W.C., Wetzler, S., Beck, A.T. & Betz, F. (1994) Prevalence of personality disorders among patients with anxiety disorders. *Psychiatry Res* **51**(2), 167–74.

Schneider, F., Weiss, U., Kessler, C. *et al.* (1999) Subcortical correlates of differential classical conditioning of aversive emotional reactions in social phobia. *Biol Psychiatry* **45**(7), 863–71.

Schneier, F.R., Heckelman, L.R., Garfinkel, R., Campeas, R. et al. (1994) Functional impairment in social phobia. *J Clin Psychiatry* **55**(8), 322–31.

Schneier, F.R., Liebowitz, M.R., Abi-Dargham, A., Zea-Ponce, Y., Lin, S.-H. & Laruelle, M. (2000) Low dopamine D2 receptor binding potential in social phobia. *Am J Psychiatry* **157**(3), 457–9.

Schneier, F.R., Liebowitz, M.R., Beidel, D.C. et al. (eds) (1995) *DSM-IV Sourcebook*, Vol. 2. American Psychiatric Association, Washington, D.C, pp. 507–48.

Schneier, F.R., Martin, L.Y., Liebowitz, M.R., Gorman, J.M. et al. (1989) Alcohol abuse in social phobia. *J Anxiety Disord* **3**(1), 15–23.

Schneier, F.R., Spitzer, R.L., Gibbon, D., Fyer, A. & Liebowitz, M.R. (1991) The relationship of social phobia subtypes and avoidant personality disorder. *Compr Psychiatry* **32**, 496–502.

Schneier, F.R., Spitzer, R.L., Gibbon, M., Fyer, A.J., Liebowitz, M.R. & Weissman, M.M. (1992) Social phobia. Comorbidity in an epidemiological sample. *Arch Gen Psychiatry* **49**, 282–8.

Schneier, F.R. & Welkowitz, L. (1996) *The Hidden Face of Shyness: Understanding and Overcoming Social Anxiety*. Avon Books, New York.

Schneier, F.R., Wexler, K.B. & Liebowitz, M.R. (1997) Social phobia and stuttering. *Am J Psychiatry* **154**(1), 131.

Schonfeld, W.H., Verboncoeur, C.J., Fifer, S.K., Lipschutz, R.C., Lubeck, D.P. & Buesching, D.P. (1997) The functioning and well-being of patients with unrecognized anxiety disorders and major depressive disorder. *J Affect Disord* **43**, 105–19.

Schwartz, C.E., Snidman, N. & Kagan, J. (1999) Adolescent social anxiety as an outcome of inhibited temperament in childhood. *J Am Acad Child Adolesc Psychiatry* **38**(8), 1008–15.

Seligman, M. (1971) Phobias and preparedness. *Behavior Therapy* **2**, 307–20.

Sherbourne, C.D., Jackson, C.A., Meredith, L.S., Camp, P. & Wells, K.B. (1996) Prevalence of comorbid anxiety disorders in primary care outpatients. *Arch Fam Med* **5**, 27–34.

Solyom, L., Ledwidge, B. & Solyom, C. (1986) Delineating social phobia. *Br J Psychiatry* **149**, 464–70.

Spitzer, R.L., Williams, J.B., Gibbon, M. & First, M.B. (1992) The Structured Clinical Interview for DSM-III-R (SCID). I: History, rationale, and description. *Arch Gen Psychiatry* **49**(8), 624–9.

Stein, M.B., Asmundson, G.J. & Chartier, M. (1994) Autonomic responsivity in generalized social phobia. *J Affect Disord* **31**, 211–21.

Stein, M.B., Baird, A. & Walker, J.R. (1996) Social phobia in adults with stuttering. *Am J Psychiatry* **153**, 278–80.

Stein, D.J. & Bouwer, C. (1997) Blushing and social phobia: a neuroethological speculation. *Med Hypotheses* **49**, 101–8.

Stein, M.B., Chartier, M.J., Hazen, A.L. et al. (1998a) A direct-interview family study of generalized social phobia. *Am J Psychiatry* **155**, 90–7.

Stein, M.B., Chartier, M.J., Kozak, M.V., King, N. & Kennedy, J.L. (1998b) Genetic linkage to the serotonin transporter protein and 5HT-$_{2A}$ receptor genes excluded in generalized social phobia. *Psychiatry Res* **81**(3), 283–91.

Stein, M.B., Chartier, M. & Walker, J.R. (1993) Sleep in nondepressed patients with panic disorder. I. Systematic assessment of subjective sleep quality and sleep disturbance. *Sleep* **16**(8), 724–6.

Stein, M.B., Delaney, S.M., Chartier, M.J., Kroft, C.D.L. et al. (1995) $_{-3H}$Paroxetine binding to platelets of patients with social phobia: comparison to patients with panic disorder and healthy volunteers. *Biol Psychiatry* **37**(4), 224–8.

Stein, M.B. & Kean, Y.M. (2000) Disability and quality of life in social phobia: epidemiological findings. *Am J Psychiatry* **157**, 1606–13.

Stein, D.J., Le Roux, L., Bouwer, C. & Van Heerden, B. (1998) Is olfactory reference syndrome an obsessive-compulsive spectrum disorder? Two cases and a discussion. *J Neuropsychiatry Clin Neurosci* **10**(1), 96–9.

Stein, M.B. & Leslie, W.D. (1996) A brain single photon-emission computed tomography (SPECT) study of generalized social phobia. *Biol Psychiatry* **39**, 825–8.

Stein, M.B., McQuaid, J.R., Laffaye, C. & McCahill, M.E. (1999) Social phobia in the primary care medical setting. *J Fam Pract* **49**(7), 514–19.

Stemberger, R., Turner, S., Beidel, D.C. & Calhoun, K. (1995) Social phobia: an analysis of possible developmental factors. *J Abnorm Psychol* **104**, 526–31.

Stopa, L. & Clark, D. (1993) Cognitive processes in social phobia. *Behav Res Ther* **31**, 255–67.

Strauss, C.C. & Last, C.G. (1993) Social and simple phobias in children. *J Anxiety Disord* **7**, 141–52.

Suomi, S.J. (1997) Early determinants of behavior: evidence from primate studies. *Br Med Bull* **53**(1), 170–84.

Tancer, M.E. (1993) Neurobiology of social phobia. *J Clin Psychiatry* **54** (Suppl. 12), 26–30.

Tancer, M.E., Mailman, R.B., Stein, M.B., Mason, G.A., Carson, S.W. & Golden, R.N. (1994) Neuroendocrine responsivity to monoaminergic system probes in generalized social phobia. *Anxiety* **1**(216–23).

Tancer, M.E., Stein, M.B. & Uhde, T.W. (1991) Lactate response to caffeine in panic disorder: a replication using an "anxious" control group. *Biol Psychiatry* **29**, 57.

Tiihonen, J., Kuikka, J., Bergstroem, K., Lepola, U. *et al.* (1997) Dopamine reuptake site densities in patients with social phobia. *Am J Psychiatry* **154**(2), 239–42.

Tillfors, M., Furmark, T., Marteinsdottir, I. *et al.* (2001) Cerebral blood flow in subjects with social phobia during stressful speaking tasks: a PET Study. *Am J Psychiatry* **158**(8), 1220–6.

Tupler, L.A., Davidson, J.R.T., Smith, R.D., Lazeyras, F., Charles, H.C. & Krishnan, K.R. (1997) A repeat proton magnetic resonance spectroscopy study in social phobia. *Biol Psychiatry* **42**, 419–24.

Turk, C.L., Heimberg, R.G., Orsillo, S.M. *et al.* (1998) An investigation of gender differences in social phobia. *J Anxiety Disord* **12**(3), 209–23.

Turner, S.M., Beidel, D.C., Dancu, C.V. & Stanley, M.A. (1989) An empirically derived inventory to measure social fears and anxiety: the Social Phobia and Anxiety Inventory. *Psychol Assess* **1**, 35–40.

Turner, S.M., Beidel, D.C. & Epstein, L.H. (1991) Vulnerability and risk for anxiety disorders. *J Anxiety Disord* **5**, 151–66.

Turner, S.M., Beidel, D.C. & Larkin, K.T. (1986) Situational determinants of social anxiety in clinic and nonclinic samples: physiological and cognitive correlates. *J Consult Clin Psychol* **1**, 35–40.

Turner, S.M., Beidel, D.C. & Townsley, R.M. (1992) Social phobia: a comparison of specific and generalized subtypes and avoidant personality disorder. *J Abnorm Psychol* **101**, 326–31.

Veljaca, K.A. & Rapee, R.M. (1998) Detection of negative and positive audience behaviors by socially anxious subjects. *Behav Res Ther* **36**(3), 311–21.

Veltman, D.J., van Zijderveld, G., Tilders, F.J.H. & van Dyck, R. (1996) Epinephrine and fear of bodily sensations in panic disorder and social phobia. *J Psychopharmacol* **10**(4), 259–65.

van Vliet, I.M., Westenberg, H.G.M., Slaap, B.R., den Boer, J.A. & Ho Pian, K.L. (1997) Anxiogenic effects of pentagastrin in patients with social phobia and healthy controls. *Biol Psychiatry* **42**(1), 76–8.

Wacker, H.R., Müllejans, R., Klein, K.H. & Battegay, R. (1992) Identification of cases of anxiety disorders and affective disorders in the community according to ICD-10 and DSM-III-R by using the Composite International Diagnostic Interview (CIDI). *Intl J Meth Psych Res* **2**, 91–100.

Walker, J.R. & Stein, M.B. (1995) Epidemiology. In: *Social Phobia Clinical and Research Perspectives* (M.B. Stein (ed.), pp. 43–75). American Psychiatric Press, Washington, D.C.

Ware, J.E., Gandek, B. & Group, I.P. (1994) The SF-36 Health Survey: development and use in mental health research and the IQOLA project. *International Journal of Mental Health* **23**(2), 49–73.

Watson, D. & Friend, R. (1969) Measurement of social-evaluative anxiety. *J Consult Clin Psychol* **33**, 448–57.

Weiller, E., Bisserbe, J.C., Boyer, P., Lepine, J.P. & Lecrubier, Y. (1996) Social phobia in general health care: an unrecognized, undertreated disabling condition. *Br J Psychiatry* **168**, 169–74.

Weinshenker, N.J., Goldenberg, I. & Rogers, M.P. (1996) Profile of a large sample of patients with social phobia: comparison between generalized and specific social phobia. *Depress Anxiety* **4**(5), 209–16.

Weissman, M.M., Bland, R.C., Canino, G.J. *et al.* (1996) The cross-national epidemiology of social phobia: a preliminary report. *Int Clin Psychopharmacol* **11** (Suppl. 3), 9–14.

Wells, J.E., Bushnell, J.A., Hornblow, A.R., Joyce, P.R. & Oakley-Browne, M.A. (1989) Christchurch psychiatric epidemiology study. I. Methodology and lifetime prevalence for specific psychiatric disorders. *Aust N Z J Psychiatry* **23**, 315–26.

Wells, A., Clark, D.M., Salkovskis, P. *et al.* (1995) Social phobia: the role of in-situation safety behaviors in maintaining anxiety and negative beliefs. *Behavioral Therapy* **26**, 153–61.

Wilhelm, S., Otto, M.W., Zucker, B.G. & Pollack, M.H. (1997) Prevalence of body dysmorphic disorder in patients with anxiety disorders. *J Anxiety Disord* **11**(5), 499–502.

Williams, J.B., Gibbon, M., First, M.B. *et al.* (1992) The Structured Clinical Interview for DSM-III-R (SCID). II. Multisite test–retest reliability. *Arch Gen Psychiatry* **49**(8), 630–36.

Wittchen, H.U. & Beloch, E. (1996) The impact of social phobia on quality of life. *Int Clin Psychopharmacol* **11** (Suppl. 3), 15–23.

Wittchen, M., Sonntag, H., Mueller, N. & Liebowitz, M. (2000) Disability and quality of life in pure and co-morbid social phobia: findings from a controlled study. *Eur Psychiatry* **15**(1), 46–58.

Wittchen, H.-U., Perkonigg, A., Lachner, G., Nelson, C.B. (1998) Early developmental stages of psychopathology study (EDSP): objectives and design. *Eur Addict Res* **4**(1–2), 18–27.

Wittchen, H.U., Stein, M.B. & Kessler, R.C. (1999) Social fears and social phobia in a community sample of adolescents and young adults: prevalence, risk factors and comorbidity. *Psychol Med* **29**, 309–323.

Woody, S. (1996) Effects of focus of attention on anxiety levels and social performance of individuals with social phobia. *J Abnorm Psychol* **105**, 61–9.

World Health Organization (WHO) (1990) *Composite International Diagnostic Interview (CIDI)*. World Health Organization, Geneva, Switzerland.

World Health Organization (WHO) (1993) *ICD-10 Classification of Mental and Behavioural Disorders: Diagnostic Criteria for Research*. World Health Organization, Geneva, Switzerland.

Yonkers, K.A., Warshaw, M.G., Massion, A.O., Keller, M.B. (1996) Phenomenology and course of generalized anxiety disorder. *Br J Psychiatry* **168**(3), 308–13.

Yu Moutier, C. & Stein, M.B. (1999) The history, epidemiology, and differential diagnosis of social anxiety disorder. *J Clin Psychiatry* **60** (Suppl. 9), 4–8.

Zimmerman, M. & Mattia, J.I. (1998) Body dysmorphic disorder in psychiatric outpatients: recognition, prevalence, comorbidity, demographic, and clinical correlates. *Compr Psychiatry* **39**(5), 265–70.

8 Sleep Aspects of Anxiety Disorders

T.A. Mellman

Introduction

Other chapters in this volume document the considerable recent advances in delineating phenomenology, probing pathophysiology, and the development of effective treatments for anxiety disorders. There has been parallel progress in advancing the nosology, basic understanding and treatment efficacy for sleep disorders. Disorders of sleep, most notably insomnia, and anxiety appear to have considerable overlap. Insomnia populations typically manifest anxiety. Sleep disturbances are included among the diagnostic features of two of the six categories for anxiety disorders in the Diagnostic Statistical Manual, fourth edition (DSM-IV; American Psychiatric Association [APA] 1994)—post-traumatic stress disorder and generalized anxiety disorder—and are commonly associated with others (e.g. panic disorder). Interventions designated as targeting insomnia and other sleep disorders and those targeting worry, tension and other manifestations of anxiety often employ similar approaches (e.g. relaxation, cognitive restructuring, benzodiazepine medications).

There are also theoretical links between anxiety and sleep disorders. Sleep is a necessary and restorative state of diminished cortical arousal. Anxiety and fear states manifest with heightened cortical and peripheral arousal. Increased arousal is also implicated when sleep initiation or maintenance are disturbed. Thus, insights on mechanisms of arousal regulation would be dually applicable to anxiety and sleep disorders (and their overlapping features).

Sleep has been a productive focus for biologically orientated research of psychiatric conditions. Sleep is less encumbered by direct environmental influence, relative to wake behaviors. Normal sleep features a well-characterized progression of discrete psychophysiologic states. Basic aspects of the neuroanatomical and neurochemical regulation of these states are known. Thus, investigations utilizing sleep as a "window" into psychopathologic conditions has been the most extensively applied in researching depression. Studies of sleep in depression have evaluated endocrine secretion, response to neurochemical challenges and, recently, functional brain activation, in addition to the most common method, polysomnography (PSG) (Gillin *et al.* 1984). In the anxiety disorders, with the exception of a limited number of challenge studies, the laboratory methodology has been limited to PSG.

PSG studies of anxiety disorders provide information regarding measurable objective disturbances in sleep initiation and maintenance, as well as the presence of primary sleep pathology. PSG studies also address the structure of sleep (e.g. sleep architecture which usually refers to the percentage of sleep comprised of specific sleep stages, and the timing and intensity of rapid eye movement [REM] sleep). These parameters can be informative as to the function of the neurobiological systems implicated in sleep regulation that are also important to the regulation of mood and arousal (i.e. locus coeruleus, pontine cholinergic nucleii; noradrenergic and cholinergic activity). A more unique focus in panic and post-traumatic stress disorders, relates to the core paroxysmal events that can manifest in relation to sleep (e.g. panic attacks, nightmares). The goal for the remainder of the chapter, is to review and summarize the current state of knowledge of subjective complaints, PSG evaluations of sleep disturbances and structure, and symptomatic events that occur in relation to sleep among the anxiety disorders.

Sleep in specific and social phobias

The key feature of phobic disorders is fear and avoidance of situations. As these situations are encountered in the environment when awake, sleep disturbances are not typically considered core or commonly associated features of these conditions. Agoraphobia when it occurs with panic disorder is an exception that will be considered later. It is possible that individuals with phobic disorders experience anticipatory anxiety that would impact on their sleep and dreams. In fact, the one report identified that specifically focused on subjective sleep in patients with social phobia found reports of poorer sleep quality, longer sleep latency, and more frequent sleep disturbance and daytime dysfunction compared to controls (Stein *et al.* 1993c). The one pilot study of social phobia identified utilizing PSG, however, reported normal findings (Brown *et al.* 1994).

Investigations relating sleep to specific phobias are also quite limited. Sleep architecture was not found to be different in depressed patients with and without simple phobias (the term that predated DSM-IV) (Clark *et al.* 1995). A study investigating parasomnias (sleep terrors and sleepwalking) in adolescents found increased comorbidity with simple phobias as well as other anxiety disorders (Gau & Soong 1999).

Sleep in obsessive-compulsive disorder

Similar to the nonpanic phobic disorders, neither the core syndromal manifestations nor prominent associated features of obsessive-compulsive disorder (OCD) include sleep disturbances. Reasons to consider sleep aspects of OCD include sleep disturbance as an index of general distress, and a means of evaluating biological relationships with major depression. An early study that employed PSG did find evidence for impaired sleep maintenance, as well as reduced latency to REM sleep in a group with OCD. These findings were presented as supporting a link between OCD and affective illness. A majority of these cases were reported to feature histories of abnormal sleep patterns (Insel *et al.* 1982). Two more recent PSG studies of OCD patients have not replicated these findings and have concluded sleep patterns of OCD patients are essentially normal (Hohagan *et al.* 1994; Robinson *et al.* 1998).

Sleep in generalized anxiety disorder

Sleep disturbance, further defined as difficulty initiating or maintaining sleep, or sleep that is restless and unsatisfying, is one of the six features that are associated with chronic worry in the DSM-IV criteria for generalized anxiety disorder (GAD) (three are needed to establish a diagnosis). Two of the other features, fatigue and irritability, can be consequences of sleep loss. The core cognitive feature of GAD, "excessive worry (apprehensive expectation)" is commonly implicated in the genesis and maintenance of insomnia problems. The several PSG studies of GAD support the occurrence of impaired initiation and maintenance of sleep relative to healthy controls. These studies also provide evidence that GAD can be differentiated from major depression in terms of not being associated with a reduction in the latency to REM sleep (Papdimitriou *et al.* 1988; Arriaga & Paiva 1990; Saletu-Zyhlarz *et al.* 1997). Thus, despite the frequent comorbidity of GAD and major depression, a well-established marker of endogenous major depression does not appear characteristic of GAD.

The overlap of issues that appear to underlie GAD and chronic insomnia appears to be relevant to intervention. There is documentation of utilizing the same benzodiazepine treatment to target comorbid GAD and insomnia, and evidence for differential combined efficacy related to the active duration of the agents (Saletu *et al.* 1994). The potential efficiency of integrating psychotherapeutic interventions that target excessive generalized worries, and worries about sleep, warrants exploration.

Sleep in panic disorder

Sleep complaints appear to be a salient feature of panic disorder. Clinical data document a high frequency of sleep complaints in panic disorder populations. Panic attacks, which are the core feature of the disorder, can emerge directly from sleep. Panic attacks in panic disorder generally feature sudden episodes of severe anxiety that at times occur unpredictably, including under circumstances where arousal is not increased or is diminished. This illness phenomenology is suggestive of disturbed mechanisms of arousal regulation. Thus, there is a conceptual link between panic disorder and sleep regulation, which involves a discrete progression of states of diminished arousal.

Survey studies document increased complaints of insomnia in panic disorder patients compared to control populations (Mellman & Uhde 1989a; Stein et al. 1993a). Most PSG studies (Lydiard et al. 1989; Mellman & Uhde 1989b; Arriaga et al. 1996; Sloan et al. 1999), but not all (Stein et al. 1993b; Uhde et al. 1984) have found decreased sleep efficiency and sleep duration with panic disorder. Greater motor activity during sleep as evidenced by increased epochs of movement time has also been reported with panic disorder (Uhde et al. 1984). The two studies not finding impaired sleep duration and maintenance are noteworthy for specifying exclusion of comorbid depression. Survey data noted a high correlation of sleep complaints and depression comorbid with panic disorder (Stein et al. 1993b). This suggested relationship and possible dependence of sleep disturbance on depression with panic disorder can be interpreted in several ways. The most straightforward is that much of the associated sleep disturbance is a function of depressive illness that is commonly comorbid with panic disorder. However, at least one of the "positive" studies excluded depressive illness and it is not clear that depression accounts for all of the sleep disturbance documented in the remaining positive studies. Another consideration is that depression may serve as a marker of a more severe variant of panic disorder. A third possibility is that depression is more likely to evolve as a comorbid condition when panic disorder features disturbed sleep.

Several surveys and studies of populations with panic disorder have documented the occurrence of panic attacks emerging from sleep as a not uncommon feature of the disorder. Eighteen percent of panic attacks were found to occur during sleep hours (Taylor et al. 1986) and 33–71% of panic disorder populations report sleep panic (Craske & Barlow 1989; Mellman & Uhde 1989a; Krystal et al. 1991; Shapiro & Sloan 1998). These episodes are often described as being awakened "like a jolt" out of sleep with the experience of apprehension and somatic symptoms that are also characteristic of panic attacks from wake states. Two studies have captured the occurrence of sleep panic attacks with PSG recording. The two studies were consistent in reporting that the sleep panic attack episodes were preceded by either stage 2 or stage 3 sleep (Hauri et al. 1986; Mellman & Uhde 1989b). This association can be further understood as suggesting a relationship between diminishing arousal during nonREM sleep (i.e. transition into early slow wave sleep) and the onset of sleep panic attacks. The paradoxical triggering of panic from states of diminished arousal has been suggested to have implications regarding the nature of panic disorder. It is more straightforward to conceptualize crescendo-like occurrences of severe anxiety evolving from states of already heightened arousal (e.g. when encountering a feared situation). Sleep panic attacks would therefore seem to implicate a more endogenous, physiological mechanism for triggering anxiety. Specific mechanisms that have been proposed include sensitivity to subtle increases in blood carbon dioxide levels (Klein 1993) and irregular breathing (Stein et al. 1995) during slow wave sleep, and a rebound increase of noradrenergic activity (Mellman & Uhde 1989b; Sloan et al. 1999). Data have also been elicited in support of a role for cognitive factors related to sensitivity to interoceptive stimuli (Craske & Barlow 1989).

Clinical implications of sleep panic include recognition of their status as a not uncommon component of the disorder and not necessarily indicative of an additional medical condition. (One should nonetheless be thorough and there have been cases reported where sleep panic occurred in association with sleep breathing disorders: Enns et al. 1995.) Reports of sleep panic being associated within panic disorder populations with early illness onset, higher symptom load, depression and suicidal ideation are collectively suggestive of their marking a more severe variant of the illness (Krystal et al. 1991; Labbate et al. 1994). Preliminary observations support that sleep panic attacks are responsive to antidepressant/antipanic medications (Mellman & Uhde 1990).

The link to salient clinical phenomenology in panic disorder to sleep appears to have influenced the development of research that utilizes sleep states as a means of reducing the influence of cognitive expectancy and environmental stimuli. Koenigsberg and colleagues have demonstrated elicitation of panic attacks from slow wave sleep by caffeine infusions. That the more fully elaborated attacks were preceded by a period of lighter sleep prior to awakening was suggested to support a mixture of physiological and cognitive influences on sleep panic (Koenigsberg et al. 1998). This group has also demonstrated greater cardiac and respiratory response to lactate infusion during sleep (Koenigsberg et al. 1994). Subgroups with sleep panic have also been shown to demonstrate greater heart rate variability during nonREM sleep consistent with sympathetic/noradrenergic activation (Sloan et al. 1999).

Sleep in post-traumatic stress disorder

Post-traumatic stress disorder (PTSD) features two distinct (albeit possibly inter-related) types of sleep complaints. These are denoted in the diagnostic criteria for the disorder by nightmares that replicate traumatic events, and impairment in initiating and maintaining sleep. Thus, there are two main domains of sleep disturbance in PTSD, one featuring insomnia categorized as an arousal symptom, and the other relating to patterns of memory activation and recall from sleep. Survey studies confirm that insomnia complaints are very common symptoms of PTSD; however, nightmares are more specific manifestations of the disorder (Green 1993; Neylan et al. 1998). Clinical and survey data further suggest that sleep manifestations of heightened arousal in PTSD also include excessive motor activity and awakenings with somatic anxiety symptoms (Inman et al. 1990; Mellman et al. 1995b).

Almost all of the initial PSG studies of PTSD subjects have featured male combat veterans during a chronic phase of the disorder. Findings are mixed with respect to the presence of impaired sleep initiation and maintenance. Several studies reported reduced sleep time or efficiency, or increased awakenings in the PTSD patients (Hefez et al. 1987; Glaubman et al. 1990; Mellman et al. 1995b; Dow et al. 1996). In other studies measures of sleep maintenance did not differ between PTSD patients and controls (Dagan et al. 1991; Ross et al. 1994a; Hurwitz et al. 1998). A "paradoxical" finding of increased thresholds to arouse from sleep to white noise have also been reported and replicated (Dagan et al. 1991; Lavie et al. 1998). There are two published studies that tend to corroborate the complaint of excessive motor activity by documenting frequent limb or gross body movement during sleep (Mellman et al. 1995b; Brown & Boudewyns 1996). Several of the aforementioned studies have found subgroups of PTSD patients to have evidence of sleep breathing disorders. In a recent study of civilian PTSD sleep breathing disorders were present in all but four of the 44 subjects (Krakow et al. 2001). Thus studies of chronic PTSD present a somewhat confusing and contradictory picture. Questions raised include why there are negative PSG findings in subgroups with prominent sleep complaints, what accounts for the deeper sleep suggested by the arousal threshold data, and the true base rates, and causal relationships

of sleep disordered breathing and sleep movement disorders.

It seems intuitive that sleep would be disrupted in the acute aftermath of trauma and that common sequellae of sleep loss would contribute to the symptom profile of PTSD. PSG studies from more acute stages of trauma response are very limited. However, PSG findings from three acute combat fatigue cases were described to include marked fragmentation of sleep (Schlosberg & Benjamin 1978). In a study conducted 6–8 months after a natural disaster, subjects with PTSD did demonstrate some tendencies toward impaired sleep continuity (Mellman et al. 1995a). In our recent, presently unpublished, study of severely injured patients recorded within a month of the traumatic incident, sleep duration and maintenance did not differ between injured subjects developing versus not developing PTSD.

The prominence and specificity of nightmare complaints in PTSD and the strong association of the REM state and dream mentation (Foulkes 1962) has focused interest on REM sleep variables. The variance between the "stereotypic, replicative" nightmare in PSTD (Ross et al. 1989) and the more typical REM-related dream report which features mixtures of past and present, and does not conform to actual memories (Dow et al. 1996; Hobson et al. 1998) is also an issue of interest.

Nightmares in PTSD subjects have been reported in association with both REM and nonREM sleep stages (van der Kolk et al. 1984; Kramer & Kinney 1988). The preponderance of reports, however, suggests that PTSD nightmares most typically arise from REM sleep (Hefez et al. 1987; Ross et al. 1994a; Mellman et al. 1995b; Woodward 2000). Overall studies have not revealed consistent abnormalities regarding the timing or amount of REM sleep in PTSD (Hefez et al. 1987; Glaubman et al. 1990; Ross et al. 1994a; Dow et al. 1996; Mellman et al. 1997). Two studies of combat veterans with chronic PTSD have reported increases in the frequency of eye movements within REM periods (REM density) (Ross et al. 1994a; Mellman et al. 1997). Increased phasic muscle activation during REM sleep with PTSD has also been reported (Ross et al. 1994b). Symptomatic awakenings with and without dream recall were found to more commonly have been preceded by REM than other sleep stages (Mellman et al. 1995b). These observations preliminarily suggest greater arousal during REM sleep and the possibility of REM sleep sometimes being disrupted with chronic PTSD.

With respect to the limited available information on REM sleep activity in the acute aftermath of trauma, the aforementioned case study of combat fatigue noted very brief periods of REM sleep. In our recent study of early trauma reactions, the group that manifested PTSD symptoms 2 months after the trauma (approximately 1 month after the PSG recording) had a greater number of discrete REM periods and shorter average duration of continuous (uninterrupted) REM sleep. Thus the development of PTSD was associated with a more fragmented REM sleep. Consistent with the diagnostic criteria, the group with PTSD was also more likely to report recall of disturbing dream content that was similar to the traumatic incident (Mellman *et al.* 2001). While preliminary, the data suggest that the development of PTSD may be contributed to by activation of relatively unaltered memories of the traumatic event and a more fragmented pattern of REM sleep. These findings are also suggestive of the possibility of adaptive functions for (less disrupted) REM sleep in emotional adaptation that has been supported by other research (Cartwright *et al.* 1991).

Summary and conclusions

In the preceding sections, associations of each anxiety disorder with sleep complaints, the evidence for sleep disturbances from PSG studies, conceptual links between anxiety, sleep and arousal regulation, and investigations of sleep in anxiety that are focused on mechanisms were reviewed. The main findings are also summarized in Table 8.1. Common themes are discussed and integrated in this closing section.

The introduction pointed out the overlap of phenomenology, conceptual frameworks, and treatment between anxiety disorders and insomnia. Clinical surveys of social phobia, GAD, panic, and PTSD document associations with subjective reports of difficulty with sleep initiation and maintenance, and/or nonrestorative sleep. These associations are incorporated into the DSM-IV diagnostic criteria for GAD and PTSD. Studies specifically relating specific phobias and OCD to insomnia were not identified in a Medline search. The not infrequent occurrences of panic attacks and re-experiencing trauma from sleep are also of clinical significance.

There are a number of implications of these relationships for clinical management. The first is recognition of the likelihood of many cases of anxiety disorders experiencing distress about sleep disturbance and that sleep loss and disruption may be exacerbating daytime symptoms. Interventions specifically targeting insomnia such as sleep hygiene education and/or use of hypnotic medications may be useful to include in the management of many patients with anxiety disorders. The overlap of interventions for anxiety and insomnia suggests potential therapeutic efficiencies. For example, the approach of addressing maladaptive cognitions that is widely utilized in anxiety disorder treatment, has also been demonstrated to be useful for treating insomnia (Edinger *et al.* 2001). Medications that are marketed for insomnia versus anxiety are typically from the same therapeutic class. In addition to benzodiazepines and related novel compounds, antidepressants that are increasingly considered first-line interventions for chronic anxiety disorders can directly benefit sleep. Direct sleep effects of antidepressant medication vary, however (Rush *et al.* 1998).

A challenge to a more straightforward interpretation of relationships of anxiety and insomnia has been the somewhat inconsistent documentation of shortened, or otherwise disrupted or altered sleep patterns by PSG studies. This discrepancy is not unique as insomnia literature also has long documented discrepancies between subjective sleep complaints and objective findings. A recent study that utilized modern techniques for analyzing EEG frequency spectra provides a novel perspective on subjective-objective discrepancies regarding sleep. The relative power for beta frequency (a relatively high frequency spectra reflecting greater cortical arousal) was increased in association with the degree of "sleep-state misperception" (Perlis *et al.* 2001). The one study identified that applied this technology to an anxiety disorder suggests complex relationships of cortical arousal during sleep and chronic PTSD. The patients did exhibit greater power for beta frequencies in REM relative to nonREM sleep, compared to the controls (Woodward *et al.* 2000).

Another issue that might relate to the variable presence of objective sleep disturbance on PSG studies is the potential effect of the laboratory environment. Conditioned apprehension related to environmental cues is a feature of insomnia and anxiety disorders. Thus, the absence of typical environmental stimuli and the safety of being observed might bring about a salutary effect of a laboratory environment in some cases. Finally, it may simply be that it is a subset of

Table 8.1 Sleep aspects of anxiety disorders.

Disorder	Subjective sleep disturbances	Sleep disturbance documented by PSG	Alterations of sleep architecture or REM	Paroxysmal events
Panic/agoraphobia	Insomnia complaints common Panic attacks can be triggered during sleep	Mixed evidence for increased sleep latency and reduced sleep efficiency Possible increased movement time	REM latency not reduced	Panic attacks arising from sleep are common feature of disorder Above associated with non-REM sleep
Social phobia	One study documents sleep complaints	No difference from controls	No difference from controls	
Specific phobias	Perhaps comorbid with parasomnias	No difference in depression with and without phobia	No difference in depression with and without phobia	
Generalized anxiety	Frequent insomnia complaints	Impaired sleep initiation and maintenance	Normal REM latency	
Obsessive-compulsive	Not well studied	One-third of studies only	One-third of studies only	
Post-traumatic stress	Insomnia complaints very common Nightmares related to trauma experience also common and specific to disorder	Data are mixed with four of seven studies reporting reduced sleep efficiency or sleep time Increases in motor activity during sleep also reported	No consistent abnormalities of sleep architecture, REM latency Increased REM density reported by two research groups	Trauma-related nightmares Above most often noted as arising from REM sleep but can also occur from other sleep stages Night terrors, sleep startle or panic also noted

PSG, polysomnography; REM, rapid eye movement.

patients, and a subset of those who perceive sleep disturbance, manifest measurable physiological indices of sleep disruption. These subgroups of people with anxiety disorders may manifest disturbances of arousal regulation that are more autonomous in nature than individuals whose symptoms are more dependent on an environmental context.

One of the main initial rationales for applying PSG technology to anxiety disorders was to evaluate biological relationships of anxiety and mood disorders. Anxiety and mood disorders often occur in the same individuals and have overlapping pharmacological treatments. The validity of their distinctiveness was viewed with greater skepticism during previous decades. Reduced latency to the onset of REM sleep is one of the best-established "markers" of major depression, particularly the melancholic subtype (Gillin *et al.* 1984). With a few exceptions that have been subsequently contradicted, the studies have demonstrated that reduced REM latency is not a feature of primary anxiety disorders. One might further postulate that mechanisms inferred to be related to reduced REM latency in major depression such as a phase advance mechanism and/or cholinergic hypersensitivity are not similarly applicable to anxiety disorders, individually, or as a group. Another parameter where mood and anxiety disorders appear to diverge is the response to sleep deprivation. In contrast to melancholic subtypes of depression where mood can paradoxically improve, anxiety disorders do not benefit, and can worsen from experimental sleep deprivation (Roy-Byrne *et al.* 1986; Labbate *et al.* 1997; Labbate *et al.* 1998).

The use of sleep as a "window" into basic mechanisms underlying psychopathological states has not been exploited in anxiety disorders to the same extent that it has been in affective illness. Nonetheless, investigations focused on sleep have revealed some important insights. That the core feature of panic disorder, panic attacks, can be triggered from a state of diminished arousal during which cognitive activity is at a relative low point has implications for conceptualizing the disorder. A limited number of challenge studies suggest that heightened sensitivities associated with panic disorder are demonstrable from sleep as well as wake states. It has been difficult to definitively pin down patterns of abnormality underlying the dream disturbance of PTSD. Some findings are suggestive of greater activation and/or disruption of the REM state. Putative adaptive functions of REM sleep may apply to responses to trauma and impaired functions contribute to the development of PTSD. Despite the limited number of definitively established findings, better understanding of anxiety disorders through the "window" of sleep remains a worthwhile goal. Advances in functional brain imaging, molecular biology and the cognitive neurosciences are being increasingly applied in sleep research. Application of these emerging perspectives and tools to sleep aspects of anxiety disorders could provide promising directions for future research.

References

American Psychiatric Association (APA) (1994) *Diagnostic Statistical Manual of Mental Disorders*, 4th edn. American Psychiatric Association, Washington, D.C.

Arriaga, F. & Paiva, T. (1990) Clinical and EEG sleep changes in primary dysthymia and generalized anxiety: a comparison with normal controls. *Neuropsychobiology* 24(3), 109–14.

Arriaga, F., Paiva, T., Matos-Pires, A., Cavaglia, F., Lara, E. & Bastos, L. (1996) The sleep of nondepressed patients with panic disorder: a comparison with normal controls. *Acta Psychiatr Scand* 93(3), 191–4.

Brown, T.M., Black, B. & Uhde, T.W. (1994) The sleep architecture of social phobia. *Biol Psychiatry* 35 (Suppl. 6), 420–1.

Brown, T.M. & Boudewyns, P.A. (1996) Periodic limb movements of sleep in combat veterans with post-traumatic stress disorder. *J Trauma Stress* 9, 129–36.

Cartwright, R.D., Kravitz, H., Eastman, C.I. & Wood, E. (1991) REM latency and the recovery from depression. Getting over divorce. *Am J Psychiatry* 148, 1530–5.

Clark, C.P., Gillin, J.C. & Golshan, S. (1995) Do differences in sleep architecture exist between depressives with co-morbid simple phobia as compared with pure depressives? *J Affect Disord* 33(4), 251–5.

Craske, M. & Barlow, D.H. (1989) Nocturnal panic. *Journal of Nerv Ment Disorder* 177, 160–7.

Dagan, Y., Lavie, P. & Bleich, A. (1991) Elevated awakening thresholds in sleep stage 3–4 in war-related post-traumatic stress disorder. *Biol Psychiatry* 30, 618–22.

Dow, B.M., Kelsoe, J.R. & Gillin, J.C. (1996) Sleep and dreams in Vietnam PTSD and depression. *Biol Psychiatry* 39, 42–50.

Edinger, J.D., Wohlgemuth, W.K., Radtke, R.A., Marsh, G.R. & Quillian, R.E. (2001) Does cognitive-behavioral insomnia therapy alter dysfunctional beliefs about sleep? *Sleep* 24(5), 591–9.

Enns, M.W., Stein, M. & Kryger, M. (1995) Successful treatment of comorbid panic disorder and sleep apnea with continuous positive airway pressure. *Psychosomatics* 36(6), 585–6.

Foulkes, W.D. (1962) Dream reports from different stages of sleep. *Journal of Abnormal Social Psychology* 65, 14–25.

Gau, S.F. & Soong, W.T. (1999) Psychiatric comorbidity of adolescents with sleep terrors or sleepwalking: a case-control study. *Aust N Z J Psychiatry* 33(5), 734–9.

Gillin, J.C., Sitaram, N., Wehr, T. *et al.* (1984) Sleep and affective illness. In: *Neurobiology of Mood Disorders* (R.M. Post & J.C. Ballenger (eds), pp. 157–89). Williams & Wilkins, Baltimore.

Glaubman, H., Mikulincer, M., Porat, A., Wasserman, O. & Birger, M. (1990) Sleep of chronic post-traumatic patients. *J Trauma Stress* 3, 255–63.

Green, B.L. (1993) Disasters and post-traumatic stress disorder. In: *Post-traumatic Stress Disorder DSM-IV and Beyond* (J.R.T. Davidson & E.B. Foa (eds)). American Psychiatric Press, Washington, D.C., pp. 75–97.

Hauri, P.J., Freidman, M., Ravaris, C.L. (1989) Sleep in patients with spontaneous panic attacks. *Sleep* 12, 323–37.

Hefez, A., Metz, L. & Lavie, P. (1987) Long-term effects of extreme situational stress on sleep and dreaming. *Am J Psychiatry* 144, 344–7.

Hobson, J.A., Stickgold, R. & Pace-Schott, E.F. (1998) The neuropsychology of REM sleep dreaming. *Neuroreport* 9, R1–R14.

Hohagan, F., Lis, S., Krieger, S. et al. (1994) Sleep EEG of patients with obsessive-compulsive disorder. *Eur Arch Psychiatry Clin Neurosci* **243**(5), 273–8.

Hurwitz, T.D., Mahawold, M.W., Kuzkowski, M., Engdahl, B.E. (1998) Polysomnographic sleep is not clinically impaired in Vietnam combat veterans with chronic post-traumatic stress disorder. *Biol Psychiatry* **44**, 1066–73.

Inman, D.J., Silver, S.M. & Doghramji, K. (1990) Sleep disturbance in post-traumatic stress disorder: a comparison with nonPTSD insomnia. *J Trauma Stress* **3**, 429–37.

Insel, T.R., Gillin, J.C., Moore, A., Mendelson, W.B., Loewenstein, R.J. & Murphy, D.L. (1982) The sleep of patients with obsessive-compulsive disorder. *Arch Gen Psychiatry* **39**(12), 1372–7.

Klein (1993) False suffocation alarms, spontaneous panics, and related conditions: an integrative hypothesis. *Arch Gen Psychiatry* **50**, 306–17.

Koenigsberg, H.W., Pollack, C.P. & Ferro, D. (1998) Can panic be induced in deep sleep? Examining the necessity of cognitive processing for panic. *Depress Anxiety* **8**(3), 126–30.

Koenigsberg, H.W., Pollack, C.P., Fine, J. & Kakuma, T. (1994) Cardiac and respiratory activity in panic disorder: effects of sleep and sleep lactate infusions. *Am J Psychiatry* **151**(8), 1148–52.

van der Kolk, B.A., Blitz, R., Burr, W.A., Sheery, S. & Hartmann, E. (1984) Nightmares and trauma: a comparison of nightmares after combat with lifelong nightmares in veterans. *Am J Psychiatry* **141**, 187–90.

Krakow, B., Melendrez, D., Pederson, B. et al. (2001) Complex insomnia: insomnia and sleep-disordered breathing in a consecutive series of crime victims with nightmares and PTSD. *Biol Psychiatry* **49**(11), 948–53.

Kramer, M. & Kinney, L. (1988) Sleep patterns in trauma victims with disturbed dreaming. *Psychiatric Journal of University of Ottawa* **13**, 12–16.

Krystal, J., Woods, S., Hill, C. & Charney, D. (1991) Characteristics of panic attack subtypes: assessment of spontaneous panic, situational panic, sleep panic, and limited symptom attacks. *Compr Psychiatry* **32**, 474–80.

Labbate, L.A., Johnson, M.R., Lydiard, R.B. et al. (1997) Sleep deprivation in panic disorder and obsessive-compulsive disorder. *Can J Psychiatry* **42**(9), 982–3.

Labbate, L.A., Johnson, M.R., Lydiard, R.B. et al. (1998) Sleep deprivation in social phobia and generalized anxiety disorder. *Biol Psychiatry* **43**(11), 840–2.

Labbate, L.A., Pollack, M.H., Otto, M.W., Langenauer, S. & Rosenbaum, J.F. (1994) Sleep panic attacks: an association with childhood anxiety and adult psychopathology. *Biol Psychiatry* **36**, 57–60.

Lavie, P., Katz, N., Pillar, G. & Zinger, Y. (1998) Elevated awaking thresholds during sleep: characteristics of chronic war-related post-traumatic stress disorder patients. *Biol Psychiatry* **44**(10), 1060–5.

Lydiard, R.B., Zealberg, J., Laraia, M.T. et al. (1989) Electroencephalography during sleep of patients with panic disorder. *J Neuropsychiatry Clin Neurosci* **1**(4), 372–6.

Mellman, T.A., David, D., Bustamante, V., Torres, J. & Fins, A. (2001) Dreams in the acute aftermath of trauma and their relationship to PTSD. *J Trauma Stress* **14**, 234–41.

Mellman, T.A., David, D., Kulick-Bell, R., Hebding, J. & Nolan, B. (1995a) Sleep disturbance and its relationship to psychiatric morbidity following Hurricane Andrew. *Am J Psychiatry* **152**, 1659–63.

Mellman, T.A., Kulick-Bell, R., Ashlock, L.E. & Nolan, B. (1995b) Sleep events in combat-related post-traumatic stress disorder. *Am J Psychiatry* **152**, 110–15.

Mellman, T.A., Nolan, B., Hebding, J., Kulick-Bell, R. & Dominguez, R. (1997) A polysomnographic comparison of veterans with combat-related PTSD, depressed men, and nonill controls. *Sleep* **20**, 46–51.

Mellman, T.A. & Uhde, T.W. (1989a) Sleep panic attacks: new clinical findings and theoretical implications. *Am J Psychiatry* **146**(9), 1204–7.

Mellman, T.A. & Uhde, T.W. (1989b) Electroencephalographic sleep in panic disorder. A focus on sleep-related panic attacks. *Arch Gen Psychiatry* **46**(2), 178–84.

Mellman, T.A. & Uhde, T.W. (1990) Patients with frequent sleep panic: clinical findings and response to medication treatment. *J Clin Psychiatry* **51**(12), 513–16.

Neylan, T.C., Marmar, C.R., Metzler, T.J. et al. (1998) Sleep disturbances from a nationally representative sample of male Vietnam veterans. *Am J Psychiatry* **155**(7), 929–33.

Papdimitriou, G.N., Kerkhofs, M., Kempenaers, C. & Mendlewicz, J. (1988) EEG sleep studies in patients with generalized anxiety disorder. *Psychiatry Res* **26**(2), 183–90.

Perlis, M.L., Smith, M.T., Andrews, P.J., Orff, H. & Giles, D.E. (2001) Beta/gamma EEG activity in patients with primary and secondary insomnia and good sleeper controls. *Sleep* **24**(1), 110–17.

Robinson, D., Walsleben, J., Pollack, S. & Lerner, G. (1998) Nocturnal polysomnography in obsessive-compulsive disorder. *Psychiatry Res* **80**(3), 257–63.

Ross, R.J., Ball, W.A., Dinges, D.F. et al. (1994a) Rapid eye movement sleep disturbance in post-traumatic stress disorder. *Biol Psychiatry* **35**, 195–202.

Ross, R.J., Ball, W.A., Dinges, D.F. et al. (1994b) Motor dysfunction during sleep in post-traumatic stress disorder. *Sleep* **17**, 723–32.

Ross, R.J., Ball, W.A., Sullivan, K.A. & Caroff, S.N. (1989) Sleep disturbance as the hallmark of post-traumatic stress disorder. *Am J Psychiatry* **146**, 697–707.

Roy-Byrne, P.P., Uhde, T.W. & Post, R.M. (1986) Effects of one night's sleep deprivation on mood and behavior in panic disorder. Patients with panic disorder compared with depressed patients and normal controls. *Arch Gen Psychiatry* **43**(9), 895–9.

Rush, A.J., Armitage, R., Gillin, J.C. *et al.* (1998) Comparative effects of nefazodone and fluoxetine on sleep in outpatients with major depressive disorder. *Biol Psychiatry* **44**(1), 3–14.

Saletu, B., Anderer, P., Brandstatter, N. *et al.* (1994) Insomnia in generalized anxiety disorder: polysomnographic, psychometric and clinical investigations before, during and after therapy with a long- versus a short-half-life benzodiazepine (quazepam versus triazolam). *Neuropsychobiology* **29**(2), 69–90.

Saletu-Zyhlarz, G., Saletu, B., Anderer, P. *et al.* (1997) Nonorganic insomnia in generalized anxiety disorder. Controlled studies on sleep, awakening and daytime vigilance utilizing polysomnography and EEG mapping. *Neuropsychobiology* **36**(3), 117–29.

Schlosberg, A. & Benjamin, M. (1978) Sleep patterns in three acute combat fatigue cases. *J Clin Psychiatry* **39**, 546–9.

Shapiro, C.M. & Sloan, E.P. (1998) Nocturnal panic: an under-recognized entity. *J Psychosom Res* **44**, 21–3.

Sloan, E.P., Natarajan, M., Baker, B. *et al.* (1999) Nocturnal and daytime panic attacks—comparison of sleep architecture, heart rate variability, and response to sodium lactate challenge. *Biol Psychiatry* **45**, 1313–20.

Stein, M.B., Chartier, M. & Walker, J.R. (1993a) Sleep in nondepressed patients with panic disorder. I. Systematic assessment of subjective sleep quality and sleep disturbance. *Sleep* **16**(8), 724–6.

Stein, M.B., Enns, M.W. & Kryger, M.H. (1993b) Sleep in nondepressed patients with panic disorder. II. Polysomnographic assessment of sleep architecture and sleep continuity. *J Affect Disord* **28**(1), 1–6.

Stein, M.B., Kroft, C.D. & Walker, J.R. (1993c) Sleep impairment in patients with social phobia. *Psychiatry Res* **49** (Suppl. 3), 251–6.

Stein, M.B., Millar, T.W., Larsen, D.K. & Kryger, M.H. (1995) Irregular breathing during sleep in patients with panic disorder. *Am J Psychiatry* **152**(8), 1168–73.

Taylor, C.B., Skeikh, J., Agras, S. *et al.* (1986) Ambulatory heart rate changes in patients with panic attacks. *Am J Psychiatry* **143**, 478–482.

Uhde, T.W., Roy-Byrne, P.P., Gillin, J.C. *et al.* (1984) The sleep of patients with panic disorder. *Psychiatry Res* **12**, 251–9.

Woodward, S.H. (2000) PTSD-related hyperarousal assessed during sleep. *Physiol Behav* **70**(1–2), 197–203.

Woodward, S.H., Arsenault, N.J., Santerre, C., Michel, G., Stewart, L.P., Stegman, W. (2000) Polysomnographic characteristics of trauma-related nightmares. *Sleep* **23**, 356.

Childhood Antecedents of Adult Anxiety Disorders

S.J. Fredman, D.R. Hirshfeld-Becker, J.W. Smoller &
J.F. Rosenbaum

Introduction

In many cases, adult anxiety disorders do not appear *de novo*. Instead, there is an earlier manifestation of anxiety that precedes them, most notably in childhood. In some cases, this may be the childhood expression of the same symptoms in adulthood (e.g. an adult with generalized anxiety disorder recalls excessive and uncontrollable worry as a child). In others, the marker may appear as a different anxiety disorder altogether (e.g. an adult with panic disorder recalls being anxious in response to separation as a child long before experiencing a panic attack). Alternatively, the early expression may not be in the form of an anxiety disorder *per se* but rather may manifest itself as anxious temperament or behavioral inhibition (e.g. an adult with social phobia recalls being shy and withdrawn in new situations as a child). In each of these cases, the anxious adults may be seen as possessing a pre-existing risk for the development of later anxiety, though the specific nature of the risk and the mechanism through which it develops into adult psychopathological states may vary.

The field of developmental psychopathology hypothesizes that there is a link between early and later functioning, suggesting that at-risk individuals develop along a trajectory that may result in either psychopathology or successful adaptation. During development, risk may be moderated by vulnerability or protective factors which interact with child characteristics, environmental variables, or their combination (Sroufe & Rutter 1984; Cicchetti & Cohen 1995). Consistent with this idea of dynamic and multidetermined development, developmental psychopathology recognizes that individuals may arrive at the same outcome through multiple pathways (equifinality). For example, equifinality is evident in the observation that genetic influences, temperament, parenting styles, or their combination may all contribute to later anxiety states. However, the field also recognizes the concept of multifinality, the idea that the same influences do not necessarily result in the same outcome. For example, not all children who are at increased genetic risk for anxiety disorders will suffer from adult anxiety disorders, suggesting opportunities for change and adaptation at multiple points in time. Consequently, the identification of risk factors that may serve as markers of later anxiety, as well as any moderating factors, offers tremendous potential for intervention.

We will use the framework of developmental psychopathology to review what is known about childhood precursors of adult anxiety disorders. Because the area of adult anxiety disorders is broad, we will focus mainly on antecedents of panic disorder and social phobia and will devote less attention to other disorders. We will review hypothesized precursors such as childhood anxiety disorders, temperamental features, genetic factors, cognitive biases, and influences of parents, life events, and peers. Our discussion will include findings from family studies, prospective studies of at-risk children, retrospective studies of anxious adults, and studies of environmental factors that may increase the risk of experiencing anxiety disorders in adulthood. The identification of potential risk factors and their associated vulnerability processes will serve as the basis for discussing potential opportunities for intervention that may shift an individual's trajectory from risk to resilience.

Childhood anxiety disorders

One potential precursor to adult anxiety disorders is the presence of anxiety disorders in childhood. Evidence for this association derives from retrospective studies of anxious adults, a few prospective studies of anxious children and adolescents, and studies of the offspring of adults with anxiety disorders.

The phenomenologic similarities between childhood and adult anxiety disorders have been acknowledged in the latest edition of the Diagnostic and Statistical Manual (DSM-IV; American Psychiatric Association [APA] 1994). Children may now be diagnosed with any of the adult anxiety disorders, including panic disorder, agoraphobia, generalized anxiety disorder (GAD), social phobia, specific phobia, obsessive-compulsive disorder (OCD), and post-traumatic stress disorder (PTSD). Whereas the DSM-III-R (APA 1987) had labeled socially anxious children with the diagnosis of avoidant disorder of childhood, the DSM-IV now subsumes childhood social anxiety under the category of social phobia. Similarly, overanxious disorder, previously a diagnosis that could be assigned only in childhood, is now eliminated and replaced by GAD. Separation anxiety disorder currently remains the only anxiety disorder diagnosed exclusively in childhood, although it has been suggested that some adults also meet these criteria (Manicavasagar *et al.* 2000). This nosological shift, as seen in the changes from the DSM-III-R to the DSM-IV, has been empirically validated (Kendall & Warman 1996; Spence 1997) and is consistent with the recognition by clinical researchers that childhood anxiety disorders are symptomatically more similar to adult anxiety disorders than they are different. Further research is needed to determine whether anxiety disorders diagnosed in children differ etiologically from the corresponding adult disorders, and in which cases these disorders are continuous with their adult counterparts.

Course and outcome of childhood anxiety disorders

For many children, anxiety disorders remit within several years (Last *et al.* 1996). However, in a number of cases, the disorders remain chronic or are followed by the emergence of new anxiety disorders in childhood or adolescence (Keller *et al.* 1992; Cohen *et al.* 1993; Orvaschel *et al.* 1995; Last *et al.* 1996). Prospective studies have also found that childhood and

adolescent anxiety disorders may predispose children to develop other disorders, such as depression (Orvaschel *et al.* 1995; Cole *et al.* 1998), and increase the risk for anxiety disorders and depression in adulthood (Klein & Last 1989; Pine *et al.* 1998).

A number of retrospective studies have found that childhood anxiety disorders precede adult anxiety disorders, panic disorder in particular. Based on the observation that separation-anxious children fear being apart from their parents and that agoraphobic individuals need the comfort of a familiar companion in order to feel safe, it has been hypothesized that separation anxiety disorder in childhood may be a specific risk factor for the development of adult panic disorder with agoraphobia (Klein 1964, 1981). However, more recent work suggests that although separation anxiety disorder may be a childhood precursor of adult agoraphobia, it does not appear to be uniquely associated with later panic disorder with agoraphobia (Silove & Manicavasagar 1993). Moreover, it has been observed that separation anxiety disorder, social phobia, and overanxious disorder are all common in the childhood histories of adults with panic disorder with agoraphobia (Aronson & Logue 1987; Otto *et al.* 1994). For example, Otto and colleagues (Otto *et al.* 1994) found that 55 of 100 panic disorder patients met the criteria for at least one childhood anxiety disorder based on structured retrospective interviews. Social phobia (36%) and overanxious disorder (28%) were the most frequently diagnosed disorders of childhood in this sample. Children with agoraphobia also tend to show a prior history of anxiety disorders. In a large sample of clinically referred children and adolescents ($N = 472$), Biederman and colleagues (Biederman *et al.* 1997) observed that agoraphobic children tended to show histories of simple phobia, avoidant disorder, and separation anxiety disorder prior to the onset of agoraphobia.

A prior history of childhood anxiety disorders is not unique to individuals with panic disorder and/or agoraphobia. For example, many adults with GAD recall being worriers for as long as they can remember (Rapee 1985), and a study found that rates of childhood separation anxiety disorder were comparable between adults with GAD and those with panic disorder (Silove & Manicavasagar 1993). Similarities have also been observed between adults with social phobia and those with panic disorder. Rapee and Melville conducted a retrospective study comparing the childhood histories of clinically referred socially phobic adults and adults with panic disorder (Rapee & Melville 1997). They found that both groups reported higher rates of introverted and anxious behaviors in childhood and fewer friends in childhood than nonclinical controls. This pattern was confirmed by reports from the mothers of the clinical subjects, although the pattern was more consistent for the socially phobic individuals. Phobic adults also commonly report that their specific phobias began in childhood (Öst 1987).

A history of childhood anxiety among anxious adults also appears to have implications for the severity of adult anxiety, particularly with respect to panic disorder. Otto and colleagues (Otto *et al*. 1994) compared adults with panic disorder who had childhood histories of anxiety disorders to adult panic patients without a history of anxiety in childhood. They found that those with a history of childhood anxiety developed panic attacks and phobic avoidance earlier, were more likely to develop agoraphobia, and were more likely to suffer from comorbid anxiety disorders as adults compared to those without a history of childhood anxiety disorders. The same investigators also found that anxiety disorders in childhood were associated with comorbid depression among adults with panic disorder (Pollack *et al*. 1996). In another retrospective study, Lipsitz and colleagues reported that childhood separation anxiety disorder conferred an increased risk for comorbidity of anxiety disorders in adulthood (Lipsitz *et al*. 1994). Prospective studies of anxious children are needed to further test the hypothesized connection between child and adulthood disorders.

It is important to note, in keeping with the principles of equifinality and multifinality, that not all anxious children develop adult disorders, nor do all anxious adults have childhood histories of anxiety disorders. For example, a prospective study of children with separation anxiety and school refusal found that only a small proportion (fewer than 10%) developed panic disorder by early adulthood (Klein & Last 1989). Nonetheless, there appears to be a subset of anxious children who are at increased risk for experiencing anxiety in adulthood. Additional prospective studies that follow anxious children into adulthood may help to clarify the extent to which childhood anxiety serves as a specific risk factor for the presence of anxiety disorders in adulthood.

Familiality of childhood anxiety disorders

Besides following anxious children to adulthood, or querying anxious adults about their childhood, another way to test the hypothesized connection between child and adulthood anxiety disorders is to examine the offspring of parents with anxiety disorders. Since these children are presumably at increased genetic risk for the adulthood disorders, the disorders they manifest may represent early prodromes of adulthood disorders. Moreover, if the sequence of disorders manifested by the offspring parallels those reported retrospectively by their parents, this lends further support to the hypothesis that the childhood disorders are the antecedents of the adulthood disorders.

Numerous studies have found that children of parents with anxiety disorders are at increased risk for a spectrum of anxiety disorders (Weissman *et al*. 1984; Sylvester *et al*. 1987; Turner *et al*. 1987; Biederman *et al*. 1991; Last *et al*. 1991; Capps *et al*. 1996; Mancini *et al*. 1996; Beidel & Turner 1997; Merikangas *et al*. 1998; Unnewehr *et al*. 1998; Biederman *et al*. 2001). Rates of any childhood anxiety disorder among young offspring of parents with anxiety disorders (in most studies either panic disorder or agoraphobia) range from 21% to 42%, compared with rates in the 2–10% range among children of comparison parents without anxiety disorders.

In some instances, there is concordance between specific parental and offspring anxiety disorders. For example, in a large prospective study of German adolescents aged 14–17, Lieb and colleagues found that the adolescents who were at the highest risk for social phobia were those whose parents had social phobia (Lieb *et al*. 2000). Another German study, conducted by Unnewehr and colleagues (Unnewehr *et al*. 1998), compared the rates of psychopathology in the offspring of parents with panic disorder, animal phobia, and no psychiatric disorder. The children of parents with panic disorder had higher rates of panic disorder or agoraphobia than did the other groups, and the children of parents with phobias had significantly higher rates of phobias than did the children of control parents. Interestingly, in 67% of the cases in which the children of phobic parents had phobias themselves, the phobic children and parents had identical phobias.

In other cases, offspring of parents with specific anxiety disorders such as panic disorder or social phobia are found to have increased rates of several different anxiety disorders (Weissman *et al.* 1984; Capps *et al.* 1996; Mancini *et al.* 1996). A recent study by Biederman and colleagues found evidence for both specific and nonspecific transmission of anxiety disorders (Biederman *et al.* 2001). The investigators compared the rates of psychopathology among the children of parents with comorbid panic disorder and depression, panic disorder only, depression only, and neither panic disorder nor depression. They found that parental panic disorder, with or without comorbid depression, was associated with increased risk for panic disorder and agoraphobia in offspring and that parental depression with or without comorbid panic disorder was associated with increased risk for depression, social phobia, and disruptive disorders in children. Panic disorder and major depression were each associated with increased risk for separation anxiety disorder and multiple anxiety disorders in the offspring.

We may conclude from these studies that children of parents with anxiety disorders, particularly panic disorder, agoraphobia, and social phobia, are at heightened risk for developing childhood anxiety disorders themselves. Children of parents with major depression may be similarly at risk. To the degree that these offspring are at risk for the parental disorders, the studies also add to the suggestion that childhood disorders may be precursors of adulthood anxiety disorders. However, studies that follow these children prospectively to adulthood are needed to clarify the course of psychopathology in these at-risk children and the extent to which parental psychopathology predicts specific forms of offspring adult psychopathology.

Temperament: focus on behavioral inhibition

Research suggests that certain temperamental markers may reflect the tendency to become anxious prior to the onset of clinically meaningful anxiety *per se*. One potential marker of an early predisposition to anxiety is "behavioral inhibition to the unfamiliar," which has been extensively investigated and described by Kagan and colleagues (Garcia-Coll *et al.* 1984; Reznick *et al.* 1986; Kagan *et al.* 1987, 1984, 1988a,b, 1989, 1998; Gersten 1989; Kagan 1989, 1994; Snidman 1989; Kagan & Snidman 1991a,b). Behavioral inhibition refers to the tendency to be cautious, quiet, and introverted in response to novel situations, events, or people.

Behavioral inhibition is estimated to occur in approximately 10–15% of middle-class Caucasian children (Kagan *et al.* 1988a), and it appears to be a moderately stable temperamental disposition (Asendorpf 1994; Kagan 1994; Caspi & Silva 1995; Scarpa *et al.* 1995; Gest 1997; Fordham & Stevenson-Hinde 1999; Goldsmith & Lemery 2000). Using laboratory measures, behavioral inhibition has been observed in children of preschool age and younger. The temperamental tendency manifests differently during different developmental stages. For instance, the tendency to be irritable and highly reactive during infancy, shy and fearful during toddlerhood, and cautious and introverted during school years are all believed to reflect the same temperamental trait. For example, children selected in toddlerhood as extremely fearful, distressed and clinging to mothers when presented in the laboratory with novel people, situations, and objects were more likely to be inhibited and avoidant with an unfamiliar adult or peer at age 4, and to be reticent with a group of peers at age 7 (Kagan *et al.* 1988a). When they examined children younger than toddlers, Kagan and colleagues found associations between high reactivity (high distress and motor activity in response to a battery of standard stimuli) at 4 months and anxiety symptoms (of all types) at age 7 (based on mother and teacher reports). The highly reactive children were also more subdued with an unfamiliar examiner at age 7 (Kagan *et al.* 1999). The highly reactive children who had shown more fears at age 21 months in laboratory observations with unfamiliar examiners were the ones most likely to have high anxiety symptoms at age 7.

Kagan and colleagues have hypothesized that behavioral inhibition reflects a lower threshold for arousal in the amygdala, hypothalamus and other brain regions that mediate arousal and fear responses, particularly when an individual is faced with unfamiliar situations (Kagan *et al.* 1987). Moderate support for this hypothesis comes from the observation that behavioral inhibition is associated with a number of biological correlates reflecting increased arousal, including increased sympathetic nervous system activation and increased noradrenergic function (see Hirshfeld *et al.* 1999 for a review).

Inhibited behavior in response to novel situations is not limited to humans. Suomi and colleagues describe similar behaviors in rhesus monkeys (Suomi *et al.* 1981; Suomi 1984, 1986, 1997, and unpublished papers [1986, 1996]), noting that 15% of rhesus monkeys are more likely than their peers to demonstrate behaviorally inhibited behaviors (e.g. diminished exploration and an increase in retreat behaviors) in the face of environmental stressors, such as repeated separation. This tendency is similar to that of behaviorally inhibited children who withdraw in the face of new people or situations and is consistent with the hypothesis that certain organisms may be biologically predisposed to experience extreme physiological reactivity and discomfort in the face of environmental change.

Behavioral inhibition as a marker for anxiety

Given the similarities among the descriptions of school-aged inhibited children and retrospective descriptions of adult agoraphobics' childhoods, Rosenbaum, Biederman, and colleagues hypothesized that behavioral inhibition may represent an early marker for a predisposition to develop later anxiety, particularly among offspring of adults with panic disorder. Several converging lines of evidence support this association, as we will discuss in this section. However, it should be noted that the association between behavioral inhibition in offspring and psychopathology in parents does not appear to be unique to panic and other anxiety disorders, since children of depressed parents are also characterized by high rates of behavioral inhibition (Kochanska 1991; Rosenbaum et al. 2000).

Several different research groups have found an association between behavioral inhibition and anxiety. In particular, studies have found elevated rates of behavioral inhibition in the offspring of adults with panic disorder (Rosenbaum et al. 1988; Manassis et al. 1995; Battaglia et al. 1997; Rosenbaum et al. 2000). These findings converge with those from "bottom-up" studies of inhibited or extremely shy children, which have revealed elevated rates of anxiety disorders in the parents, social phobia in particular (Rosenbaum et al. 1991; Cooper & Eke 1999). Cross-sectional studies reveal that inhibited children themselves are at an increased risk for anxiety. In a small, controlled study of children of parents with panic disorder, Biederman and colleagues (Biederman et al. 1990) observed that behaviorally inhibited children had higher rates of multiple anxiety disorders (two or more), overanxious, and phobic disorders, than did children who were not behaviorally inhibited. At 3-year follow-up, rates of anxiety disorders were significantly higher in children who were classified as inhibited at baseline

than among those who were not inhibited, and rates of anxiety disorders in inhibited children increased significantly from baseline to follow-up (Biederman et al. 1993). In a larger controlled study, the same investigators found that behavioral inhibition in children was exclusively associated with increased risk for social phobia and avoidant disorder and that this association was most pronounced for children of parents with panic disorder with or without comorbid depression (Biederman et al. 2001).

Inhibited children from a nonclinical, longitudinal study conducted by Kagan and colleagues were also at elevated risk for anxiety disorders compared to children who were not behaviorally inhibited (Biederman et al. 1990). Examination of the children from age 21 months through age 7 suggested that those children who were consistently inhibited over time were at the greatest risk for the development of anxiety (Hirshfeld et al. 1992). When these children (and others from a second cohort selected at age 31 months) were followed through age 13, the children who were classified as inhibited at age 2 were at significantly greater risk for generalized social anxiety than were the children who were classified as uninhibited. These findings were more robust for girls than for boys (Schwartz et al. 1999).

The assessments of behavioral inhibition discussed above used laboratory assessments on samples of young children. Recently, Muris and colleagues (Muris et al. 1999, 2001) have reported that behavioral inhibition, assessed in older children and adolescents using self-report measures, is also related to the presence of anxiety and depression. They observed that 12–14-year-old children who classified themselves as high in behavioral inhibition had higher self-reported levels of worry, depression, and anxiety. Their measure of self-reported behavioral inhibition was most highly correlated with the social phobia subscale of a self-report questionnaire of anxiety symptomatology, but significant associations were also found with the subscales for panic disorder, GAD, separation anxiety disorder, OCD, and blood-injection-injury phobia (Muris et al. 1999). The association among self-reported behavioral inhibition, anxiety, and depression was replicated in a second study of adolescents aged 12–18, and it appeared that the association between behavioral inhibition and depression was mediated by the presence of anxiety (Muris et al. 2001). A recent prospective study of more than 2000 ninth graders in the US found that self-reported behavioral inhibition as recalled from the elementary school years was significantly related to the subsequent development of social phobia by the end of high school (Hayward *et al.* 1998).

The association between behavioral inhibition in childhood and later psychopathology is also supported by retrospective studies in which adults report the extent to which they were behaviorally inhibited during the elementary school years (Reznick *et al.* 1992). Reznick and colleagues found that adult patients who had been successfully treated for either panic disorder or depression had significantly higher behavioral inhibition scores than did adults who had never been diagnosed with either disorder. In another study, retrospectively reported behavioral inhibition was significantly higher among college undergraduates with social anxiety than among those with generalized anxiety or controls with minimal social anxiety (Mick & Telch 1998).

Despite evidence that suggests an association between behavioral inhibition and anxiety disorders, it should be emphasized that behavioral inhibition is likely neither a necessary nor sufficient risk factor for anxiety. For example, not all inhibited children develop social phobia or other anxiety disorders and not all anxious adults were inhibited as children. As reviewed earlier, the link between behavioral inhibition in childhood and the development of anxiety disorders appears to be strongest among those children who remain consistently inhibited throughout early childhood. Longitudinal studies are needed to clarify the role that other child characteristics or environmental influences may play in determining how behavioral inhibition may or may not lead to later psychopathology.

Genetic influences on anxiety disorders and anxiety-related traits

The observation that anxiety disorders and behavioral inhibition are more common among children of parents affected with anxiety disorders leads naturally to the question of what role genes play in this familial transmission. The genetics of anxiety disorders are reviewed in detail in Chapter 13, but we summarize several pertinent findings here as well.

Family and twin studies have demonstrated that all of the major DSM-IV anxiety disorders are familial (with the exception of PTSD, for which data are limited)

and at least moderately heritable (Smoller & Tsuang 1998; Smoller *et al.* 2000). Estimates of the excess risk to first degree relatives of affected individuals ranges from about three-fold to seventeen-fold for panic disorder (Crowe *et al.* 1983; Noyes *et al.* 1986; Maier *et al.* 1993; Goldstein *et al.* 1997), three-fold to ten-fold for social phobia (Fyer *et al.* 1993, 1995; Stein *et al.* 1998), two-fold to three-fold for specific phobias, and five-fold for GAD (Noyes *et al.* 1987) and OCD (Pauls *et al.* 1995; Nestadt *et al.* 2000). The estimated heritability (or proportion of population phenotypic variance due to genetic factors) of these disorders has typically ranged from 30% to 50% (Kendler *et al.* 1992, 1993, 1999, 2001; True *et al.* 1993; Jonnal *et al.* 2000), suggesting that environmental factors are at least as influential. However, there is conflicting evidence about the relative importance of family and nonfamily environmental factors. For example, in a prospective longitudinal study by Lieb and colleagues (Lieb *et al.* 2000), parental anxiety and parenting style were associated with the development of social phobia in offspring. However, using model-fitting techniques in their large population-based twin sample, Kendler and colleagues (Kendler *et al.* 1999) found that individual-specific environment contributed to social phobia liability, but shared family environment appeared to have little impact.

Although the evidence that genes influence anxiety disorders is compelling, the specific identity of the genes involved remains unknown. Molecular genetic studies of the anxiety disorders have implicated several chromosomal regions and candidate genes, but none has been established (see Chapter 13, for review). Thus far, the most intriguing findings have been reported for panic disorder/agoraphobia and OCD. For example, genome scans of panic disorder/agoraphobia have provided evidence of possible linkage to regions of chromosomes 1 (Gelernter *et al.* 2001), 3 (for agoraphobia) (Gelernter *et al.* 2001), 7p (Knowles *et al.* 1998; Crowe *et al.* 2001), 11p (Gelernter *et al.* 2001), 12q (Smoller *et al.* 2001b), and 13q (Weissman *et al.* 2000). An interstitial duplication of chromosome 15q has recently been reported to be associated with panic and phobic anxiety disorders in combination with joint laxity (Gratacos *et al.* 2001). These findings and associations of candidate genes such as the MAO-A gene (Deckert *et al.* 1999) await replication. For OCD, several candidate genes have been associated with the disorder in independent samples, including the genes encoding catechol-O-methyltransferase (Karayiorgou *et al.* 1997, 1999), MAO-A (Karayiorgou *et al.* 1999; Camarena *et al.* 2001) and the serotonin transporter (McDougle *et al.* 1998; Bengel *et al.* 1999). Again, however, the precise role of these genes remains uncertain. Another area of uncertainty concerns the specificity of genetic influences on anxiety. Do genes influence risk for specific anxiety disorders, or do they impact a quantitative "anxiety proneness" that, in the extreme, may be expressed as a variety of clinical syndromes? Evidence for the specificity of gene effects comes from family studies that have suggested that panic and phobic disorders "breed true" (Fyer *et al.* 1995). That is, relatives of probands with panic disorder appear to be at greatest risk for panic disorder and relatives of probands with social phobia are at greatest risk for social phobia. On the other hand, the studies of high-risk children reviewed earlier are more consistent with the notion that a more general anxiety proneness is transmitted in families and can be expressed as several anxiety disorders and comorbid disorders. Other family and twin studies have indicated that there are shared genetic influences between panic and phobic disorders (Kendler *et al.* 1995), between panic and GAD (Scherrer *et al.* 2000), between OCD, GAD and agoraphobia (Nestadt *et al.* 2001), and among the different phobic disorders (social, specific, agoraphobia) (Kendler *et al.* 1999). Moreover, anxiety-related traits and temperaments appear to be more pronounced in relatives of probands with panic and phobic disorders (Perugi *et al.* 1998; Rosenbaum *et al.* 2000; Stein *et al.* 2001). Finally, molecular genetic studies have suggested that specific genetic loci may influence liability to multiple anxiety disorders (Gratacos *et al.* 2001; Smoller *et al.* 2001b). The most striking example of this is a recent report by Gratacos and colleagues (Gratacos *et al.* 2001) that a genomic duplication on chromosome 15q was strongly associated with a phenotype that included panic disorder, phobic disorders, and joint laxity. One interpretation of such findings is that there are latent, heritable anxiety traits underlying these disorders and that these traits cut across diagnostic categories. The boundaries among the phenotypes defined as anxiety disorders, then, may not be so distinct as implied by DSM-IV.

In addition to behavioral inhibition (Kagan *et al.* 1984), a number of anxiety-related traits and temperaments have been described including "neuroticism" (Eysenck 1967), "harm avoidance" (Cloninger 1986),

and "shyness/sociability" (Plomin & Daniels 1986). We review the genetic basis of these traits briefly here. The association between these traits and specific anxiety disorders has not been fully defined, and each may capture different elements of anxiety-proneness (Heath *et al.* 1994). The putative role of neuroticism, which refers to the predisposition to experience psychological distress and negative affect (Clark *et al.* 1994), is perhaps the broadest of these constructs. Neuroticism has been said to predispose to both anxiety disorders and depression (i.e. "neurotic disorders") (Andrews *et al.* 1990a,b; Clark *et al.* 1994; Bienvenu *et al.* 2001b) and to comorbidity among these disorders (Bienvenu *et al.* 2001a). It is also the most extensively studied of the anxiety-related traits, and numerous large twin studies have demonstrated that genes influence neuroticism with heritability estimates consistently in the range of 30–60% (Floderus-Myrhed *et al.* 1980; Rose *et al.* 1988; Mackinnon *et al.* 1990).

Harm avoidance was defined by Cloninger and colleagues as a heritable temperament encompassing "pessimistic worry in anticipation of future problems, passive avoidant behaviors such as fear of uncertainty and shyness of strangers, and rapid fatiguablity" (Cloninger *et al.* 1993). Elevated harm avoidance has been observed among patients with OCD (Richter *et al.* 1996), panic disorder and GAD (Starcevic *et al.* 1996), and among patients with social phobia (Kim & Hoover 1996) and their first-degree relatives (Stein *et al.* 2001). In an analysis of 2680 adult Australian twin pairs, Heath and colleagues (Heath *et al.* 1994) reported that the heritability of harm avoidance (44%) was comparable to that of neuroticism (35–45%), but they appeared to capture somewhat different dimensions of personality. As has been reported in twin studies of anxiety disorders, shared family environment did not appear to influence either trait. Interestingly, in the first study to associate an anxiety phenotype with a specific gene, Lesch and colleagues (Lesch *et al.* 1996) reported that a functional polymorphism in the serotonin transporter gene promoter (5-HTTLPR) was associated with both neuroticism and harm avoidance (see Chapter 13). Subsequently, a series of studies have attempted to replicate this finding with mixed results. Although some studies have found evidence of association (Katsuragi *et al.* 1999) or linkage (Mazzanti *et al.* 1998) between the 5-HTT promoter and neuroticism or harm avoidance, a larger number have not (Ball *et al.* 1997; Ebstein *et al.* 1997; Gelernter *et al.* 1998;

Jorm et al. 1998; Deary et al. 1999; Flory et al. 1999; Gustavsson et al. 1999; Herbst et al. 2000). Differences in populations, assessment methods, and statistical power may account for some of these discrepancies. Harm avoidance has also been linked to a locus on the short arm of chromosome 8 in a large genome scan of more than 750 sibling pairs (Cloninger et al. 1998). In that study, there was also evidence of gene–gene interaction (epistasis) between the chromosome 8p locus and loci on chromosomes 18p, 20p, and 21q, so that taken together, these loci explained nearly all of the genetic variance in the trait.

Twin and adoption studies have documented that genes contribute to shyness and behavioral inhibition, which are phenotypically related to social phobia, in children (Plomin & Daniels 1986; Matheny 1989; Robinson et al. 1992; Plomin et al. 1993; DiLalla et al. 1994). In the MacArthur Longitudinal Twin Study, estimated heritability was 18–60% for measures of shyness and 41% for behavioral inhibition in twins at ages 14 and 20 months (Plomin et al. 1993; Cherny et al. 1994). Furthermore, the stability of shyness and behavioral inhibition between these two ages appeared to be mediated by genetic factors. Additional analyses of subsamples of this cohort suggest that extreme behavioral inhibition is highly heritable (heritability >70% at 2 years of age), although the precision of these estimates is unclear because of the relatively small sample sizes involved (Robinson et al. 1992; DiLalla et al. 1994). In a linkage analysis of a large extended pedigree, Smoller and colleagues (Smoller et al. 2001a) observed suggestive evidence of linkage to a locus on chromosome 10 for a phenotype definition based on studies of the familial relationship between behavioral inhibition and panic disorder/agoraphobia. Candidate gene association studies of shyness and behavioral inhibition have begun to appear, but results to date have been largely negative (Jorm et al. 1998, 2000; Henderson et al. 2000; Smoller et al. 2001b).

To summarize, it is clear that genes influence the development of the major adult anxiety disorders. Childhood anxiety disorder symptoms and behavioral inhibition also appear to be heritable (Thapar & McGuffin 1995; Topolski et al. 1997; Warren et al. 1999). What is unclear, however, is the specificity of the genetic effects on anxiety disorders: are the heritable phenotypes discrete diagnostic categories or temperamental predispositions? Modeling of twin data has provided some evidence that genes affecting heritable temperament also affect childhood anxiety disorder symptoms (Goldsmith & Lemery 2000), and future genetic studies may benefit from incorporating assessments of both clinical diagnoses and temperamental traits.

Hypothesized cognitive risk factors

Cognitions indicating pathological fear or worry (e.g. "I'm going to lose control of myself if my heart races and I feel dizzy.") are common correlates of anxiety among adults, and emerging evidence suggests that anxious children may experience similar anxious thoughts. In the following section, we highlight some of these cognitive biases and also discuss what is known regarding the extent to which these cognitions may serve as potential risk factors for the development of later anxiety.

Anxiety sensitivity

It has been shown that adults with panic disorder tend to respond to physiological sensations of anxiety with alarm, believing that otherwise benign physical indicators of anxiety (e.g. a pounding heart) signify impending catastrophe (e.g. a heart attack) (Clark 1986). Consistent with this observation, adults with panic disorder tend to score approximately two standard deviations above the norm on the Anxiety Sensitivity Index (ASI) (Reiss et al. 2001), a 16-item questionnaire that measures fear of sensations of arousal in adults (Reiss et al. 1986). "Anxiety sensitivity," the tendency to fear arousal and anxiety-related sensations because of the belief that such symptoms are harbingers of physical catastrophe, public embarrassment, or mental incapacitation (Reiss 1991), is distinct from trait anxiety, a general proneness to respond anxiously across a wide range of situations (McNally 1996; Schmidt et al. 1997). Research on anxiety sensitivity as a correlate or predictor of anxiety has tended to focus on anxiety sensitivity's relation to panic disorder. Nonetheless, elevated anxiety sensitivity scores have also been observed among individuals with circumscribed social phobia (Norton et al. 1997), PTSD (McNally et al. 1987), and panic attacks (Donnell & McNally 1990; Asmundson & Norton 1993).

Anxiety sensitivity, as measured with the ASI, appears to represent both a higher order factor as well as three lower-order factors: physical concerns (a fear of somatic sensations of anxiety), mental incapacitation concerns (a fear of mental loss of control), and social concerns (a fear of public observation of anxiety sensations) (Zinbarg *et al.* 1997). However, due to the small number of items tapping social concerns, the social concerns factor may be less reliable than the physical or mental concerns factors, as measured with the existing version of the ASI (Zinbarg *et al.* 1999).

An early model suggested that fear of anxiety sensations in the context of panic disorder with agoraphobia is the classically conditioned response to the negative experience of a panic attack (Goldstein & Chambless 1978). More recently, though, researchers have suggested that anxiety sensitivity may actually serve as a cognitive risk factor for the development of anxiety rather than just a correlate or a consequence of anxiety or panic (Reiss 1991). Recent research has shown that anxiety sensitivity does, in fact, predict the development of spontaneous panic attacks and anxiety in non-clinical samples (Maller & Reiss 1992; Schmidt *et al.* 1997; Schmidt *et al.* 1999). Schmidt and colleagues (Schmidt *et al.* 1997) conducted a prospective study of more than 1400 US Air Force Academy cadets undergoing military basic training, a brief but intensely stressful 5-week period. The authors observed that anxiety sensitivity, but not trait anxiety, predicted the occurrence of spontaneous panic attacks, even after controlling for a prior history of panic attacks. The authors replicated these findings using another large sample of cadets undergoing basic training (Schmidt *et al.* 1999). They demonstrated that in addition to predicting the occurrence of spontaneous panic attacks, anxiety sensitivity predicted panic-related worry, somatic anxiety symptoms, and anxiety-related impairment, even after controlling for the effect of trait anxiety and a prior history of panic attacks. Anxiety sensitivity is also a reliable predictor of relapse and re-emergence in untreated panickers as well as a sensitive index of change when panic patients are treated with cognitive-behavioral therapy (Otto & Reilly-Harrington 1999).

Although less prevalent than in adulthood, panic attacks and panic disorder do occur in children and adolescents (Ollendick & King 1998), suggesting that similar cognitive correlates and precursors of panic may also be present in these youths. Researchers have investigated this hypothesis using the Child Anxiety Sensitivity Index (CASI), an 18-item version of the ASI

used to assess anxiety sensitivity in children and adolescents aged 6–17 (Silverman *et al.* 1991). Like its adult counterpart, the CASI is characterized by multiple dimensions, the most robust of which are fears of impending physical catastrophe (physical concerns) and loss of mental control (mental incapacitation) (Silverman *et al.* 1999a). In studies of young children, the CASI differentiated children with anxiety disorders from those without anxiety disorders (Rabian *et al.* 1993) and successfully differentiated children with panic disorder from those with anxiety disorders other than panic disorder (Kearney *et al.* 1997). Among adolescents, the CASI was significantly correlated with panic attack symptoms and was able to successfully differentiate between adolescents who experienced panic attacks and those who did not (Lau *et al.* 1996; Hayward *et al.* 1997). It also prospectively predicted the onset of panic attacks in a large sample of adolescents, even after controlling for negative affectivity and a prior history of major depression (Hayward *et al.* 2000).

There has been debate regarding the construct validity of anxiety sensitivity in preadolescent children. Chorpita *et al.* (1996) found that the CASI predicted trait anxiety in older children (age 12–17) but not in younger children (age 7–11). They suggested that preadolescent children lacked the cognitive abilities necessary to pair internal sensations of autonomic arousal or anxiety with the potential for future negative consequences of danger. However, recent studies have challenged these findings. Using a large sample of clinically referred children and adolescents, Weems and colleagues (Weems *et al.* 1998) found that the CASI did predict variance in fear beyond that accounted for by trait anxiety in both young children (age 6–11) and adolescents (age 12–17). In another study investigating the construct validity of anxiety sensitivity in preadolescent children, Mattis and Ollendick (1997) compared the cognitive responses of 8, 11, and 14-year-old children after they listened to a tape describing the physical symptoms of a panic attack and imagined that they were experiencing the same sensations. The authors did not observe age differences in the children's tendencies to make internal attributions regarding the origin of the panic attack. Furthermore, they found that the children's CASI scores predicted their tendency to make internal catastrophic attributions in response to the imagined panic attack. Additional support for the construct utility of anxiety sensitivity in preadolescent children comes from a behavioral validation of the CASI (Rabian *et al.* 1999). Using a sample of elementary school children (age 8–11), Rabian and colleagues found that the CASI predicted state anxiety and subjective fear in response to a physically challenging stair-stepping exercise, even after controlling for trait anxiety and pretest measures of state anxiety and fear.

Studies have demonstrated that anxiety sensitivity may be heritable and predictive of susceptibility to carbon dioxide (CO_2) induced panic attacks (McNally & Eke 1996). In one study of 337 adult twin pairs, the heritability of anxiety sensitivity was estimated to be 45% (Stein *et al.* 1999), although a subsequent analysis indicated that the trait is heritable only in women (Jang *et al.* 1999). Schmidt and colleagues (Schmidt *et al.* 2000) reported an interaction between anxiety sensitivity and a polymorphism in the serotonin transporter gene that may affect susceptibility to CO_2-induced panic. The polymorphism in the serotonin transporter promoter that increased expression of the gene (the "long" allele) was associated with increased fear response to CO_2 challenge. There also appeared to be an interaction between genotype and anxiety sensitivity such that subjects homozygous for the long allele who also scored highly on anxiety sensitivity had the lowest heart rate variability, a measure of autonomic arousal that has been associated with panic/anxiety.

Other studies have suggested that family environment factors may potentially play a role in the development of anxiety sensitivity as well. Several retrospective studies have found that individuals with high anxiety sensitivity reported greater childhood instrumental and vicarious learning experiences involving somatic symptoms that included both arousal and nonarousal sensations (Watt *et al.* 1998; Watt & Stewart 2000; Stewart *et al.* 2001). The role of arousal-related sensations may be particularly strong for the development of panic attacks. When individuals were compared on the basis of panic attacks versus no panic attacks, those with panic attacks report greater parental reinforcement of and vicarious learning for anxiety-related sensations (Ehlers 1993; Watt *et al.* 1998).

To date, no longitudinal studies have found that anxiety sensitivity in early childhood predicts the development of anxiety and panic disorder in adulthood, largely because prospective studies that follow children through different developmental stages have not yet extended into adulthood. It has been shown, however, that anxiety sensitivity does predict the development of anxiety and panic in adolescence and early adulthood. Thus, the identification of young children with high anxiety sensitivity may serve as an opportunity to identify those who are at significant risk for the later development of panic and other anxiety disorders. Furthermore, in light of the suggestion from retrospective studies that the development or reinforcement of anxiety sensitivity may be associated with parental modeling of maladaptive reactions to physical sensations, identification and modification of anxiogenic parental behaviors may also aid in the prevention and amelioration of later anxiety disorders.

Increased bias for threat and low perceived control

Adults with anxiety disorders tend to overestimate the likelihood of future negative events occurring and to underestimate their ability to cope under adverse circumstances (Beck *et al.* 1985). They tend to perceive threat in ambiguous situations (Butler & Matthews 1983), to regard negative events as unpredictable and uncontrollable, and to anticipate adverse outcomes (Barlow 1988; Alloy *et al.* 1990). These qualities appear to be common to a number of anxiety disorders. For instance, in the absence of legitimate cardiac or pulmonary pathology, individuals with panic disorder tend to misinterpret physical sensations of arousal as signs of impending physical catastrophe. Their coping style is generally characterized by avoidance of situations that are likely to precipitate uncomfortable physical sensations, often because they believe they will be unable to cope with having a panic attack. Socially phobic individuals often misperceive the extent to which others judge them harshly, overestimate the likelihood that they will be humiliated or embarrassed, and underestimate their ability to cope with such criticism; similarly, their preferred coping style tends to be characterized by avoidance. Individuals with OCD tend to perceive bizarre and extreme threat in situations that normals perceive as potentially hazardous but not overwhelming (e.g. contamination by germs or disease). They also respond catastrophically to fleeting unusual thoughts about dangers, violence, or sexual situations which normals might also have but dismiss without worry (Rachman & de Silva 1978). Individuals with OCD either avoid these situations or thoughts or use rituals to neutralize the distressing thoughts and accompanying anxiety. Failure to perform the compulsion is met with intense anxiety because the individual seems to believe that he or she could not cope with the feared outcome. Thus, empirically supported psychological treatments for each of these disorders generally involve principles of cognitive-behavioral therapy and/or exposure therapy (with response prevention added for OCD) (Chambless & Ollendick 2001) to decrease fear and to help the individual to more realistically appraise future threat as well as his or her perceived ability to cope.

Though we are aware of no prospective studies of cognitive biases in at-risk children, cross-sectional studies examining the cognitions of anxious children have tended to find cognitive biases similar to those found in anxious adults, particularly among children old enough to report on their cognitions (i.e. school-age and older). Barrett and colleagues found that clinically referred children seeking treatment for separation anxiety disorder, overanxious disorder, social anxiety, and simple phobia were more likely than nonclinic children to perceive hypothetical ambiguous situations as threatening and were also more likely to generate avoidant strategies to cope with these situations (Barrett et al. 1996a). Similar findings were observed by Bögels and Zigterman in a mixed group of anxious children (Bogels & Zigterman 2000). Other studies have found that anxious children tend to have lower self-perceived competence (Messer & Beidel 1994; Bogels & Zigterman 2000) and an external locus of control (the belief that events are controlled by factors external to oneself). In particular, it has been observed that children who have an external locus of control score higher in trait anxiety (Finch et al. 1975; Nunn 1988) and fearfulness (Ollendick & Francis 1988; Krohne 1992). Anxious children may also be characterized by a negative attributional style (for review see Bell-Dolan & Wessler 1994) or by the use of more negative self-statements when confronted with ambiguous or anxiety-provoking circumstances (Prins 1986; Treadwell & Kendall 1996; Bogels & Zigterman 2000; Muris et al. 2000).

Cross-sectional studies of both children and adults suggest that low perceived control and an increased bias for threat are common correlates of anxiety disorders. The extent to which these cognitive biases also serve as specific risk factors for the development of anxiety, however, is not clear. Chorpita and Barlow have proposed a model describing the mechanism through which low perceived control may itself serve as a cognitive risk factor for the later development of both anxiety and depression (for review see Chorpita & Barlow 1998). They suggest that individuals whose early lives are characterized by few experiences of perceived control are at risk of developing anxiety and depression because they learn to expect to be helpless when faced with stressful situations later in life. Over time they develop a bias toward interpreting later events as out of their control, which in turn reinforces a pattern of helpless passivity and continued anxiety. Longitudinal research is needed to test this hypothesis.

Parenting

We now highlight findings from studies that have examined the role parenting behaviors may play in increasing an individual's vulnerability to become anxious, or conversely, in decreasing that risk by serving as a protective influence.

A number of caveats are worth noting when discussing parenting behaviors in the context of offspring anxiety. First, there is no substantive evidence that specific parenting behaviors or attitudes cause anxiety disorders; on the other hand, certain parenting practices may be helpful to children who are predisposed to become anxious in the first place. As we have noted earlier, the relative helpfulness or unhelpfulness of given parental behaviors may depend, in part, on characteristics of the child (Hirshfeld et al. 1998). For instance, encouraging children to act cautiously may be helpful for an impulsive but not an inhibited child. On the other hand, if behavioral inhibition is in fact a predisposition factor for later anxiety, encouraging an inhibited child to take small risks may help to decrease anxiety. Second, children play an important role in shaping their interpersonal environments. Children may elicit particular responses from their parents and then react to these parental behaviors, the effect of which may be to reinforce a child's given temperamental style (Sameroff 1975a,b; Lerner & Lerner 1987; Caspi et al. 1989). Thus, in many cases parental behaviors may actually reflect reactions to anxiety in the child rather than serving as the cause of the child's anxiety (e.g. Rubin et al. 1999). For example, parents may be overprotective toward a child who appears to be distressed when faced with a feared situation; however, in the absence of the child's distress, the parents would not behave toward the child in this manner. As a result of these repeated interactions over time, the child may come to perceive himself as incapable of dealing with novel situations while not in the presence of the parent. Third, specific parenting practices are associated with only a small measure of explanatory power in elucidating the precise mechanism through which some individuals develop clinically meaningful anxiety (for review see Rapee 1997; Dadds & Roth 2001). Nonetheless, this small but significant amount of variance in offspring anxiety may prove informative, particularly for investigators and clinicians hoping to intervene with children at risk for developing adult anxiety disorders.

The specific mechanisms through which parental behaviors or attitudes may exacerbate a child's vulnerability are not known, but we suspect that parent–child interactions that amplify the cognitive distortions discussed earlier may play a role. Thus, parenting behaviors that may increase the likelihood that a child will become clinically anxious are those that influence a child to perceive negative events as uncontrollable or unpredictable, to anticipate adverse outcomes, to regard themselves as lacking a sense of personal efficacy, to overestimate the likelihood of threat, and to use avoidant coping strategies. Several theories have been proposed to explain how parents may interact with children to contribute to or exacerbate these vulnerabilities. Chorpita and Barlow have suggested that a controlling parenting style might undermine a child's sense of being able to control his or her own environment because the child has few opportunities to direct situations and bring about change by himself or herself (Chorpita & Barlow 1998). Spence has proposed other parental influences, which may be particularly common among anxious parents, such as modeling fearful behavior, encouraging avoidant coping strategies, encouraging children's perceptions of threat, and not promoting the child's development of active coping strategies (Spence 1994). Krohne has suggested that parental punitiveness, inconsistency, and restrictiveness contribute to a child's expectations of negative outcome and a diminished sense of being able to direct these outcomes (Krohne 1990, 1992).

Control and rejection

We are not aware of any prospective studies that demonstrate a link between specific parenting practices and the later development of adult anxiety, but a number of retrospective and cross-sectional studies suggest that high parental control and, to a lesser extent, criticism or low warmth, are associated with anxiety in offspring (for review see Rapee 1997; Waters & Barrett 2000; Dadds & Roth 2001). Retrospective studies of anxious adults (Parker 1979b; Arrindell et al. 1983; Arrindell et al. 1989; Gerlsma et al. 1990; Bruch & Heimberg 1994; Chambless et al. 1996; Rapee & Melville 1997) converge with cross-sectional studies of anxious children (Gruner et al. 1999; Lieb et al. 2000) to find reports of increased parental control and decreased warmth. These findings are supported by studies that examine the parents of anxious children. When parents are asked to speak about their children in an unstructured manner for 5 min, parental emotional overinvolvement (overprotective, self-sacrificing, or intrusive behavior) was associated with child anxiety in both an epidemiological sample (Stubbe et al. 1993) and a small at-risk sample (Hirshfeld et al. 1997b). Observational studies have confirmed that the interactions of anxious children and their parents tend to be characterized by high levels of parental control, overprotection, or criticism (Krohne & Hock 1991; Dumas et al. 1995; Siqueland et al. 1996; Hudson & Rapee 2001).

It has been suggested that the effect of controlling and rejecting parenting on anxious children may be to restrict opportunities to explore their environments. If children have been rejected, they may develop anxieties about dealing with others, particularly in social situations. This insecurity, in connection with overprotectiveness, may keep the children from engaging in unfamiliar situations, which in turn may undermine the children's autonomy and decrease opportunities for exposure to unfamiliar situations and the acquisition of new skills (Muris & Merckelbach 1998; Lieb et al. 2000). Nonetheless, the finding that this type of parenting is reported by anxious adults with different presentations of anxiety, such as fears, phobias, and compulsions (Parker 1979b; Arrindell et al. 1983, 1989; Gerlsma et al. 1990; Bruch & Heimberg 1994; Chambless et al. 1996; Rapee & Melville 1997), as well as depression (Parker 1979a), suggests that a controlling and/or rejecting parenting style is not linked to the development of specific forms of anxiety, nor to anxiety disorders exclusively. Instead, as suggested by Chambless and colleagues (Chambless et al. 1996), poor parental bonding likely constitutes a general risk factor for the development of psychopathology.

The quality of parental bonding is presumed to reflect the extent to which the child is securely versus insecurely attached to the caregiver. As described by Bowlby (1973), human infants are biologically programed to behave in ways that increase proximity to their caregivers and they engage in distress behaviors (e.g. crying) when separated in order to increase their safety. When caregivers respond in a sensitive and consistent manner, it is believed that infants develop an internal working model of parental responsiveness and stability. This, in turn, leads them to expect that their caregivers will be present when needed and will serve as a safe base to which they can return after exploring. These children are termed "securely attached" and are likely to behave in a self-confident and secure manner when older. In contrast, "insecurely attached" infants, who tend to perceive their caregivers as unresponsive or inconsistent, engage in less exploration and tend to be distressed and anxious while separated from their parents or primary caregiver. This model finds some empirical support in the findings of Warren and colleagues, who observed that children who were insecurely attached as infants were twice as likely to develop anxiety disorders by late adolescence (Warren *et al.* 1997).

Investigators have examined whether certain child characteristics may increase the likelihood of particular parental responses. However, because of the cross-sectional nature of many studies, the direction of causality regarding parental rearing practices and child anxiety has tended to be unclear. That is, are children anxious because the parents are controlling or critical towards them, or are the parents' behaviors a reaction to the presence of anxiety in children? In an attempt to answer this question, Rubin and colleagues examined parental perceptions of shyness in their children at age 2 and parental encouragement of exploration in unfamiliar situations at age 4 (Rubin *et al.* 1999). They found that parental perceptions of their children's shyness and social fears at age 2 predicted how encouraging the parents were 2 years later; in contrast, the parents' encouragement at age 2 did not predict how socially anxious the child was at age 4. Interestingly, this finding was evident only for parents' self-reported perceptions of children's social withdrawal and not with observational assessments made by objective raters, suggesting that it is the parents' subjective perception of children's behaviors which influences parental behaviors and attitudes towards

the child. Research that takes into account both the presence of parental psychopathology and child status would be helpful in determining whether these perceptions are more common among anxious parents.

Indeed, several studies have suggested that parental psychopathology contributes to the ways parents behave or respond toward their anxious or inhibited children. In their sample of adults with panic disorder and psychiatric controls, Hirshfeld and colleagues found that mothers with a lifetime history of anxiety disorder were more likely to express criticism when discussing their behaviorally inhibited child than were psychiatric control mothers without anxiety disorders (Hirshfeld *et al.* 1997a). A recent observational study yielded similar results. Whaley and colleagues compared the interactional patterns of anxious mothers, many of whom had panic disorder and agoraphobia, and their children to the patterns of anxiety- and depression-free controls mothers and their children (Whaley *et al.* 1999). The authors found that anxious mothers with anxious children were more controlling than were anxious mothers with nonanxious children or the control mothers with nonanxious children. Furthermore, compared to control mothers of non-anxious children, anxious mothers with anxious children were also more critical and catastrophizing toward their children than were control mothers. Anxious mothers, regardless of the child's anxiety status, were found to be less warm and positive, than were the control mothers. In addition, in an uncontrolled study, Manassis and colleagues found results suggesting that mothers with anxiety disorders had a high rate of forming insecure attachments with their young children (Manassis *et al.* 1994).

Reinforcement of avoidant coping strategies and modeling fearful behavior

Parents may also influence a child's anxiety directly by reinforcing the child's use of avoidant coping strategies or by fearful behavior. Barrett and colleagues reported that in families of clinically referred children with social anxiety, general anxiety, separation anxiety, or specific phobias, family discussions about suggestions for coping with hypothetical ambiguous situations served to increase the child's formulation of an avoidant coping response (Barrett *et al.* 1996a; Dadds *et al.* 1996). In the retrospective study of adults with social phobia, panic disorder, and their mothers by Rapee and Melville described earlier, the authors found that mothers of anxious adults were significantly less likely to engage in social activities than were mothers of nonanxious controls, suggesting a modeling mechanism (Rapee & Melville 1997). This hypothesis finds further support in the discovery that infant shyness is negatively related to sociability in adoptive as well as biological parents (Daniels & Plomin 1985).

Parental modeling and verbal transmission of threatening information have been identified as potential influences on the development of specific phobias in offspring, although it should be noted that there is also evidence for the role of nonassociative factors in the development of childhood fears (Menzies & Clarke 1993; for review see King *et al.* 1998; Menzies & Harris 2001; Muris & Merckelbach 2001). It has also been suggested that parental modeling of avoidant or compulsive behaviors may play a role in childhood OCD (Henin & Kendall 1997), and Silverman and colleagues have hypothesized that that anxious parents who avoid a wide range of situations may explicitly or implicitly encourage their children to avoid situations that they fear (Silverman *et al.* 1988). Consistent with the hypothesis of parental modeling, Capps and colleagues (Capps *et al.* 1996) observed that agoraphobic mothers' level of anxiety regarding separation from their children was negatively associated with the children's level of perceived control over environmental risks and stress. Therefore, parental facilitation of avoidant coping, modeling of anxious or avoidant responses, and transmission of threatening information may all play a role in fostering or maintaining a child's anxiety.

Life events

Retrospective studies of adults find that stressful life events are common in the histories of anxious individuals. In some studies, adults with anxiety disorders report the presence of early stressful life events that precede the onset of the disorder by a number of years. For example, adults with panic disorder and/or agoraphobia report a greater incidence of childhood parental separation (Faravelli *et al.* 1985; Laraia *et al.* 1994) and having household members with chronic physical illness or with substance use problems (Laraia *et al.* 1994) compared to nonpsychiatric controls. However,

comparisons of individuals with panic disorder to other anxious groups have yielded mixed results with respect to the specificity of negative events and the development of later panic disorder. For example, one study found that patients with panic disorder reported more adverse events over the total course of their lives compared to those with OCD (De Loof *et al.* 1989). In contrast, other investigations have found no differences in the rate of parental death among individuals with panic disorder, agoraphobia, or simple phobia (Thyer *et al.* 1988) and have observed that early traumatic events are common to many psychiatric groups (Jacobson 1989).

Investigations have also focused on the role of proximate triggering events in the onset of anxiety. In a naturalistic study of 223 panic disorder patients, Manfro and colleagues observed that 80% of the subjects reported having had at least one negative stressful event in the year prior to onset of the disorder (Manfro *et al.* 1996). Similarly, Faravelli found that panic patients reported a greater incidence of negative stressful events in the year prior to the onset of panic disorder compared to normal controls (Faravelli 1985). Faravelli and Pallanti (1989) found that patients with panic disorder had significantly higher life stress, particularly in the month prior to their first panic attack. Negative life events are also implicated in the development of other anxiety disorders, such as social phobia and PTSD, whose diagnosis specifically requires the occurrence of an identifiable traumatic event. Studies of socially phobic adults have found that individuals with social phobia often attribute the onset of their social anxiety to traumatic conditioning experiences, such as extreme embarrassment or humiliation (Öst 1987; Stemberger *et al.* 1995), particularly among individuals who fear specific social situations rather than social situations generally (Stemberger *et al.* 1995). However, the occurrence of negative experiences does not necessarily appear to be sufficient for the development of either social phobia or PTSD. For example, Stemberger and colleagues observed that 20% of nonsocially anxious controls reported traumatic social experiences (Stemberger *et al.* 1995), and individual differences appear to account more for the development of PTSD than do event characteristics (for review see Bowman 1999). As noted by Mineka and Zinbarg (1995), conditioning experiences or negative events may result in an acute anxiety disorder primarily among those who have a pre-existing vulnerability, such as an anxious temperament or low perceived control. Anxious individuals may be differentiated from nonanxious individuals less by the experience of more negative life events than by their perception that the events are more subjectively distressing (Rapee *et al.* 1990).

Two studies have found cross-sectional associations between specific types of adverse life events and anxiety in children and adolescents. However, in neither study was the temporal relation between the stressor and the onset of anxiety ascertained. In a large population sample of 13 years-old twins, Eley and Stevenson (2000) compared the occurrence of loss versus threat events in the previous year among children who scored high on measures of depression or trait anxiety. They observed that anxious children scored significantly higher than did nonanxious children for threat but not for loss events, and that the depressed children scored significantly higher on loss but not threat than did the nondepressed children. In addition, they found that anxious probands scored significantly higher on threat events than did their nonanxious cotwins, even when exclusively examining monozygotic twin pairs. The authors interpreted the latter finding to suggest that factors resulting in the association between threat events and anxiety are individual-specific and are not due to genetic influences (that is, they may be learned or acquired through unshared experiences). In another study, Tiet and colleagues (Tiet *et al.* 2001) assessed an epidemiological sample of 9–17 year-old children for rates of adverse life events in the past year that the children considered "negative experiences." Different patterns of life events emerged among children with different diagnoses. Overanxious disorder and separation anxiety disorder were associated with more negative life events than were agoraphobia and social phobia. Particularly strong associations were observed between child separation anxiety and the child starting a new school or a parent beginning a new job.

The precise mechanism through which adverse life events relate to anxiety is not known. As suggested by Eley and Stevenson (2000), a number of hypotheses exist: stressful events may precipitate anxiety, individuals who are predisposed to become anxious or already are anxious may bring about negative events, a third factor (e.g. chaotic living conditions) may account for both the occurrence of the event and the anxiety, or anxious individuals may over-report events or interpret them as more distressing because of cognitive biases. Given the observation that subjective distress related to a stressful life event differentiates anxious adults from nonanxious controls (Rapee *et al.* 1990), one may hypothesize that subjective distress and coping in response to negative life events may play a role in youth anxiety as well. Indeed, a recent study of normal adolescents found that rumination, self-blame, and catastrophizing as coping strategies in response to negative life events were associated with greater reported anxiety symptoms (Garnefski, Kraaj, & Spinhoven 2001). In contrast, self-reported use of positive reappraisal as a coping strategy was associated with lower self-reported anxiety. Thus, although adverse life events may be common in the histories of anxious individuals, subjective distress and coping styles may play an important role in determining the extent to which the stressor exerts a negative influence.

Peers

A number of studies have found that dysfunctional peer relationships are associated with anxiety disorders (for review see Masia & Morris 1998). For example, Strauss and colleagues found that 6–13 year-old anxious children were more likely to be neglected by their peers than were psychiatric and nonpsychiatric controls (Strauss *et al.* 1988). Similarly, LaGreca and colleagues observed that 7–11 year-old children who were neglected by their peers were more likely to report social anxiety and fear of negative evaluation than were children from other groups (LaGreca *et al.* 1988). In retrospective studies, shy adolescents or avoidant adults reported unpleasant experiences with peers (Ishiyama 1984), or bullying or harassment as children (Gilmartin 1987). However, based on these findings, it is not clear whether peer behavior influences child anxiety or whether anxious children elicit neglect or rejection from peers. A longitudinal study suggests that social withdrawal in children becomes increasingly unacceptable to peers as children become older and, in turn, contributes to later rejection. Rubin and colleagues followed 50 US second grade children over a 3-year period and found that the association between social withdrawal and peer rejection increased with age (Rubin & Mills 1988), as did a negative association between popularity and anxiety (Hymel *et al.* 1990). Thus, it may be that as withdrawn children become older and are rejected by their peers, their withdrawal and introversion are exacerbated by the development of low self-esteem and expectations of negative social events.

Summary of hypothesized risk factors and tentative etiological model

Although some individuals may experience the onset of clinically meaningful anxiety in adulthood, adult anxiety disorders are commonly characterized by childhood antecedents. As reviewed in this chapter and summarized in Table 9.1, children who may be at the greatest risk of experiencing anxiety in adulthood are those who: (i) demonstrate early signs of an anxious disposition (e.g. childhood anxiety disorders and/or inhibited temperament); (ii) have a family history of anxiety; (iii) fear physiological arousal (i.e. demonstrate anxiety sensitivity); and (iv) are biased toward interpretation of threat, overestimation of risk, and underestimation of perceived control, and the use of avoidance to cope with feared situations. Anxiety may be further influenced on the part of parents by modeling poor coping, facilitating anxious coping (e.g. through facilitating avoidance or overprotecting), or being overly restrictive, critical or rejecting. It may be influenced as well by stressful life events and dysfunctional peer relationships.

Although there is a growing body of literature on child antecedents, questions still remain regarding the specificity of these risk factors in relation to particular forms of adult anxiety disorders. Moreover, uncertainty also exists regarding the mechanism through which these risk factors may give rise to adult psychopathology. For example, one might speculate that as a result of genetics, certain children are biologically predisposed to have a low threshold for physiological arousal or to be easily conditioned to fear various objects, places, or situations. Behaviorally, this predisposition may manifest itself early in life as high reactivity, social withdrawal, and/or specific childhood anxiety syndromes such as separation anxiety, social phobia, agoraphobia, or specific phobias. Individual environmental moderators, such as parental modeling of anxiety, overprotectiveness, and criticism, stressful life events, and adverse peer relations, may interact with a child's pre-existing biological diathesis by psychologically reinforcing the child's belief that the world is a dangerous place and that he or she is incapable of coping (e.g. that signs of anxiety, obsessive thoughts, or peer interactions are harmful and uncontrollable).

Testing these hypothesized mechanisms would require a combination of longitudinal naturalistic studies, twin studies, adoption studies, and intervention studies. These might include the following examples of programatic research: (i) Research that identifies specific biological or behavioral markers of a vulnerability to become anxious prior to the acute onset of the anxiety and then longitudinally examines the environmental conditions and processes through which clinically meaningful anxiety ensues could be crucial to identifying at-risk children and informing preventive efforts. For instance, researchers could prospectively compare behaviorally inhibited children and noninhibited children of anxious parents to those of nonanxious parents to determine the relative influences of genes, child temperament, and parental anxiety on the development of child anxiety over time. Attention could also be devoted to identifying protective factors among children with one or more risk factor who do not develop psychopathology. The inclusion in longitudinal studies of observational measures of parent–child interactions at different developmental stages and the systematic assessment of life events and peer relations over the child's life would contribute to an enhanced understanding of how environmental variables may serve as moderators of outcome in at-risk children. (ii) Efforts to answer these questions would be greatly enhanced by twin studies of children (such as those conducted by Goldsmith & Lemery 2000), which would examine both child temperament and a full spectrum of child psychopathology. (iii) Ideally, the hypothesized mechanism could be tested through adoption studies, especially if, as may be increasingly the case with open adoptions in the US, the temperamental and psychiatric histories of biological as well as adoptive parents could be assessed. (iv) Finally, experimenters could randomize children from different (temperamental, familial, genetic, and environmental) risk groups to controlled interventions aimed to decrease child anxiety or inhibition and/or parental anxiety (or other environmental influences such as peer rejection) to help determine the extent to which these factors are malleable and the circumstances under which interventions may be most helpful. Looking toward the future, one would aim to be able to categorize a given child's profile of risk and to put together an individualized program of

Table 9.1 Potential indicators of risk for adult anxiety disorders. (Adapted from Hirshfeld *et al.* 1998.)

Constitutional factors	
Genetic factors	Family history of anxiety[a,b]
Childhood psychopathology	Childhood anxiety disorders[c,d]
Temperamental factors	Behavioral inhibition to the unfamiliar: a tendency to exhibit fear (toddlerhood) and quiet restraint (early childhood) in response to novel situations[c,d,e,j]
	Heightened limbic-sympathetic arousal in response to novel situations in some inhibited children[d]
	Anxiety sensitivity: a tendency to catastrophically misinterpret and fear physiological sensations associated with arousal[e,h,i,j]
	?Other cognitive biases: tendency to misperceive and magnify threat; tendency to underestimate competency for coping; expectations of unpredictability and uncontrollability of negative events; overestimation of risk of adverse outcome
Psychological vulnerability factors	
Cognitive predispositions	Anxiety sensitivity: a tendency to catastrophically misinterpret and fear physiological sensations associated with arousal[e,h,i,j]
	?Other cognitive biases: tendency to misperceive and magnify threat; tendency to underestimate competency for coping; expectations of unpredictability and uncontrollability of negative events; overestimation of risk of adverse outcome
Behavioral tendencies	[e]Tendency to cope via escape or avoidant strategies
	?Deficit of skills for coping with anxiety-inducing situations
Environmental factors	
Parental influences	Overprotection[c,e,f]
	Encouragement of avoidant behavior[c,g]
	Low warmth or high rejection[c,e]
	Parental restrictiveness and control[c,e,g]
	High criticism[g]
Life events	Negative life events associated with subjective distress serve as precipitants[c,?e]
	History of adverse or traumatic life events[c,?e]
Peers	Peer neglect[l]
	Peer rejection or humiliation[c,k]

Nature of supporting evidence: [a]Family studies. [b]Twin studies. [c]Retrospective accounts by anxious adults. [d]Studies of offspring of anxious patients. [e]Reports by children with anxiety disorders. [f]Reports by parents of patients with anxiety disorders. [g]Observations of parent–child interactions in families of anxiety-disordered or high-trait anxious children. [h]Prospective studies of adults who develop panic attacks. [i]Experiments with children. [j]Prospective studies of children and adolescents. [k]Prospective studies of anxious/withdrawn children. [l]Peer nomination studies.

Note: Question marks indicate hypothesized factors that are theoretically related but await empirical support.

intervention (drawing upon some of the strategies described below). This program would be geared to minimize both the child's anxiety, avoidance, physiologic arousal, and the environmental moderators of risk, as well as to teach adaptive coping and to maximize protective factors in the family, school, and community, in order to foster maximally adaptive and unconstrained functioning.

Clinical implications

Although anxiety disorders are among the most common psychiatric disorders in children (Anderson *et al.* 1987; Costello *et al.* 1988), anxious children are often not referred for treatment because they do not disrupt classrooms or family functioning to the same extent that children with disruptive behavior disorders do. Nonetheless, anxiety disorders and symptoms do impair social and academic functioning (Strauss *et al.* 1987; Ialongo *et al.* 1995), and if untreated can lead to worsening impairment as well as comorbidity. Therefore, identification of at-risk or clinically anxious children by clinicians, pediatricians, or teachers may facilitate early intervention efforts to improve coping and adaptation and, possibly, to reduce the likelihood of impairing anxiety or dysfunction continuing into adulthood. Children 4 years and older who are exhibiting maladaptive anxiety (e.g. worry, compulsions, panic) or phobic avoidance that interferes with their social, academic, or family functioning; or who are extremely behaviorally inhibited (shy to the degree of social impairment); or who are offspring or first-degree relatives of individuals with anxiety disorders and are already exhibiting inhibited temperament or anxious symptoms, ought to be referred for evaluation and for possible intervention.

Early psychological interventions with these children offer the possibility that later dysfunction may be prevented or, at least, ameliorated among children with mild to moderate anxiety (for review see Barrett 2001; Spence 2001). Successful outcomes have been reported using cognitive-behavioral treatments of anxiety disorders of childhood or adolescence (Kendall 1994; Barrett *et al.* 1996b; Kendall & Southam-Gerow 1996; Silverman *et al.* 1999b), cognitive-behavioral methods to teach young children and their parents to manage anxiety before it becomes debilitating (Hirshfeld-Becker, unpublished data), and concurrent management

of parent anxiety and child anxiety (Cobham *et al.* 1998). Other helpful interventions include those designed to reduce parental control and intrusiveness among anxious-withdrawn preschool children (LaFreniere & Capuano 1997), pairing peer-neglected children with popular children to increase social status and positive interactions with other children (Morris *et al.* 1995), and cognitive behavioral therapy, including exposure, skills training, and practice sessions for interacting with nonanxious peers, for social phobia (Beidel *et al.* 2000). For children with more severe or debilitating anxiety, pharmacological treatment may be indicated. Regardless of the cause, swift identification and treatment may offer the best possibility of minimizing future dysfunction and promoting maximally adaptive anxiety management and coping.

References

Alloy, L.B., Kelly, K.A., Mineka, S. & Clements, C.M. (1990) Comorbidity of anxiety and depressive disorders: a helplessness–hopelessness perspective. In: *Comorbidity of Mood and Anxiety Disorders* (J. Maser & C. Cloninger (eds), pp. 499–544). American Psychiatric Press, Washington, D.C.

American Psychiatric Association (APA) (1987) *Diagnostic Statistical Manual of Mental Disorders*, 3rd edn, revised. American Psychiatric Association, Washington, D.C.

American Psychiatric Association (APA) (1994) *Diagnostic Statistical Manual of Mental Disorders*, 4th edn. American Psychiatric Association, Washington, D.C.

Anderson, J., Williams, S., McGee, R. & Silva, P. (1987) DSM-III disorders in preadolescent children: prevalence in a large sample from the general population. *Arch Gen Psychiatry* **44**(1), 69–76.

Andrews, G., Stewart, G., Allen, R. & Henderson, A.S. (1990a) The genetics of six neurotic disorders: a twin study. *J Affect Disord* **19**, 23–9.

Andrews, G., Stewart, G., Morris-Yates, A., Holt, P. & Henderson, S. (1990b) Evidence for a general neurotic syndrome. *Br J Psychiatry* **157**, 6–12.

Aronson, T. & Logue, C. (1987) On the longitudinal course of panic disorder: developmental history and predictors of phobic complications. *Compr Psychiatry* **28**(4), 344–55.

Arrindell, W.A., Emmelkamp, P.M.G., Monsma, A. & Brilman, E. (1983) The role of perceived parental rearing practices in the etiology of phobic disorders: a controlled study. *Br J Psychiatry* **143**, 183–7.

Arrindell, W., Kwee, M., Methorst, G., Van der Ende, J., Pol, E. & Moritz, B. (1989) Perceived parental rearing styles of agoraphobic and socially phobic inpatients. *Br J Psychiatry* **155**, 526–35.

Asendorpf, J. (1994) The malleability of behavioral inhibition: a study of individual developmental functions. *Dev Psychol* **30**(6), 912–19.

Asmundson, G.J.G. & Norton, G.R. (1993) Anxiety sensitivity and its relationship to spontaneous and cued panic attacks in college students. *Behav Res Ther* **31**(2), 199–201.

Ball, D., Hill, L., Freeman, B. *et al.* (1997) The serotonin transporter gene and peer-rated neuroticism. *Neuroreport* **8**, 1301–4.

Barlow, D.H. (1988) *Anxiety and its Disorders: the Nature and Treatment of Anxiety and Panic.* Guilford Press, New York.

Barrett, P. (2001) Current issues in the treatment of childhood anxiety. In: *The Developmental Psychopathology of Anxiety* (M.W. Vasey & M.R. Dadds (eds), pp. 304–24). Oxford University Press, New York.

Barrett, P.M., Rapee, R.M. & Dadds, M.R. (1996b) Family treatment of childhood anxiety: a controlled trial. *J Consult Clin Psychol* **64**(2), 333–42.

Barrett, P.M., Rapee, R.M., Dadds, M.M. & Ryan, S.M. (1996a) Family enhancement of cognitive style in anxious and aggressive children. *J Abnorm Child Psychol* **24**(6), 187–203.

Battaglia, M., Bajo, S., Strambi, L.F. *et al.* (1997) Physiological and behavioral responses to minor stressors in offspring of patients with panic disorder. *J Psychiat Res* **31**(3), 365–76.

Beck, A.T., Emery, G. & Greenberg, R.L. (1985) *Anxiety Disorders and Phobias: a Cognitive Perspective.* Basic Books, New York.

Beidel, D. & Turner, S. (1997) At risk for anxiety. I. Psychopathology in the offspring of anxious parents. *J Am Acad Child Adolesc Psychiatry* **36**(7), 918–24.

Beidel, D.C., Turner, S.M. & Morris, T.L. (2000) Behavioral treatment of childhood social phobia. *J Consult Clin Psychol* **68**(6), 1072–80.

Bell-Dolan, D. & Wessler, A.E. (1994) Attributional style of anxious children: extensions from cognitive theory and research on adult anxiety. *J Anx Dis* **8**, 79–96.

Bengel, D., Greenberg, B., Cora-Locatelli, G. *et al.* (1999) Association of the serotonin transporter promoter regulatory polymorphism and obsessive-compulsive disorder. *Mol Psychiatry* **4**, 463–6.

Biederman, J., Faraone, S., Hirshfeld-Becker, D., Friedman, D., Robin, J. & Rosenbaum, J. (2001) Patterns of psychopathology and dysfunction in a large sample of high-risk children of parents with panic disorder and major depression: a controlled study. *Am J Psychiatry* **158**(1), 49–57.

Biederman, J., Faraone, S., Marrs, A. *et al.* (1997) Panic disorder and agoraphobia in consecutively referred children and adolescents. *J Am Acad Child Adolesc Psychiatry* **36**(2), 214–23.

Biederman, J., Hirshfeld-Becker, D.R., Rosenbaum, J. *et al.* (2001) Further evidence of association between behavioral inhibition and social anxiety in children. *Am J Psychiatry* **158**(10), 1673–9.

Biederman, J., Rosenbaum, J.F., Bolduc, E.A., Faraone, S.V. & Hirshfeld, D.R. (1991) A high-risk study of young children of parents with panic disorder and agoraphobia with and without major depression. *Psychiatry Res* **37**, 333–48.

Biederman, J., Rosenbaum, J.F., Bolduc-Murphy, E.A. *et al.* (1993) A 3-year follow-up of children with and without behavioral inhibition. *J Am Acad Child Adolesc Psychiatry* **32**(4), 814–21.

Biederman, J., Rosenbaum, J.F., Hirshfeld, D.R. *et al.* (1990) Psychiatric correlates of behavioral inhibition in young children of parents with and without psychiatric disorders. *Arch Gen Psychiatry* **47**, 21–6.

Bienvenu, O.J., Brown, C., Samuels, J.F. *et al.* (2001a) Normal personality traits and comorbidity among phobic, panic and major depressive disorders. *Psychiatry Res* **102**(1), 73–85.

Bienvenu, O.J., Nestadt, G., Samuels, J.F., Costa, P.T., Howard, W.T. & Eaton, W.W. (2001b) Phobic, panic, and major depressive disorders and the five-factor model of personality. *J Nerv Ment Dis* **189**(3), 154–61.

Bogels, S.M. & Zigterman, D. (2000) Dysfunctional cognitions in children with social phobia, separation anxiety disorder, and generalized anxiety disorder. *J Abnorm Child Psychol* **28**(2), 205–11.

Bowlby, J. (1973) *Separation: Anxiety and Anger*, Vol. 2. Basic Books, New York.

Bowman, M.L. (1999) Individual differences in post-traumatic distress: problems with the DSM-IV model. *Can J Psychiatry* **44**, 21–33.

Bruch, M. & Heimberg, R. (1994) Differences in perceptions of parental and personal characteristics between generalized and nongeneralized social phobics. *J Anxiety Disord* **8**(2), 155–68.

Butler, G. & Matthews, A. (1983) Cognitive processes in anxiety. *Adv Behav Res Ther* **5**, 51–62.

Camarena, B., Rinetti, G., Cruz, C., Gomez, A., de La Fuente, J.R. & Nicolini, H. (2001) Additional evidence that genetic variation of MAO-A gene supports a gender subtype in obsessive-compulsive disorder. *Am J Med Genet* **105**(3), 279–82.

Capps, L., Sigman, M., Sena, R. & Henker, B. (1996) Fear, anxiety, and perceived control in children of agoraphobic parents. *Journal of Clinical Psychology and Psychiatry* **37**(4), 445–54.

Caspi, A., Bem, D.J. & Elder, G.H. (1989) Continuities and consequences of interactional styles across the life course. *J Pers* **57**(2), 375–406.

Caspi, A. & Silva, P.A. (1995) Temperamental qualities at age 3 predict personality traits in young adulthood: longitudinal evidence from a birth cohort. *Child Dev* **66**, 486–98.

Chambless, D.L., Gillis, M.M., Tran, G.Q. & Steketee, G.S. (1996) Parental bonding reports of clients with obsessive-compulsive disorder and agoraphobia. *Clinical Psychology and Psychotherapy* 3(2), 77–85.

Chambless, D.L. & Ollendick, T.H. (2001) Empirically supported psychological interventions: controversies and evidence. *Annu Rev Psychol* 52, 685–716.

Cherny, S.S., Fulker, D.W., Corley, R.P., Plomin, R. & DeFries, J.C. (1994) Continuity and change in infant shyness from 14 to 20 months. *Behav Genet* 24(4), 365–79.

Chorpita, B.F., Albano, A.M. & Barlow, D.H. (1996) Child Anxiety Sensitivity Index: considerations for children with anxiety disorders. *J Clin Child Psychol* 25, 77–82.

Chorpita, B.F. & Barlow, D.H. (1998) The development of anxiety: the role of control in the early environment. *Psychol Bull* 124(1), 3–21.

Cicchetti, D. & Cohen, D.J. (1995) Perspectives on developmental psychopathology. In: *Developmental Psychopathology.*, Vol. 1. *Theory and Methods* (D. Cicchetti & D.J. Cohen (eds), pp. 3–20). Wiley, New York.

Clark, D. (1986) A cognitive approach to panic. *Behav Res Ther* 24, 461–70.

Clark, L., Watson, D. & Mineka, S. (1994) Temperament, personality and the mood and anxiety disorders. *J Abnorm Psychol* 103, 103–16.

Cloninger, C. (1986) A unified biosocial theory of personality and its role in the development of anxiety states. *Psychiatric Development* 3, 167–226.

Cloninger, C.R., Svrakic, D.M. & Przybeck, T.R. (1993) A psychobiological model of temperament and character. *Arch Gen Psychiatry* 50, 975–90.

Cloninger, C., Van Eerdewegh, P., Goate, A. *et al.* (1998) Anxiety proneness linked to epistatic loci in genome scan of human personality traits. *Am J Med Genet (Neuropsychiatric Genetics)* 81, 313–17.

Cobham, V., Dadds, M. & Spence, S. (1998) The role of parental anxiety in the treatment of childhood anxiety. *J Consult Clin Psychol* 66(6), 893–905.

Cohen, P., Cohen, J. & Brook, J. (1993) An epidemiological study of disorders in late childhood and adolescence. II. Persistence of disorders. *J Child Psychol Psychiatr* 34(6), 869–77.

Cole, D.A., Peeke, L.G., Martin, J.M., Truglio, R. & Seroczynski, A.D. (1998) A longitudinal look at the relation between Depress Anxiety in children and adolescents. *J Consult Clin Psychol* 66(3), 451–60.

Cooper, P.J. & Eke, M. (1999) Childhood shyness and maternal social phobia: a community study. *Br J Psychiatry* 174, 439–43.

Costello, E.J., Costello, A.J., Edelbrock, C. *et al.* (1988) Psychiatric disorders in pediatric primary care. *Arch Gen Psychiatry* 45, 1107–16.

Crowe, R.R., Goedken, R., Samuelson, S., Wilson, R., Nelson, J. & Noyes, R. Jr (2001) Genomewide survey of panic disorder. *Am J Med Genet* 105(1), 105–9.

Crowe, R.R., Noyes, R., Pauls, D.L. & Slymen, D. (1983) A family study of panic disorder. *Arch Gen Psychiatry* 40, 1065–69.

Dadds, M.R., Barrett, P.M., Rapee, R.M. & Ryan, S. (1996) Family process and child anxiety and aggression: an observational analysis. *J Abnorm Child Psychol* 24(6), 715–34.

Dadds, M.R. & Roth, J.H. (2001) Family processes in the development of anxiety problems. In: *The Developmental Psychopathology of Anxiety* (M.W. Vasey & M.R. Dadds (eds), pp. 278–303). Oxford University Press, New York.

Daniels, D. & Plomin, R. (1985) Origins of individual differences in infant shyness. *Dev Psychol* 21, 118–21.

De Loof, C., Zandbergen, J., Lousberg, H., Pols, H. & Griez, E. (1989) The role of life events in the onset of panic disorder. *Behav Res Ther* 27(4), 461–3.

Deary, I.J., Battersby, S., Whiteman, M.C., Connor, J.M., Fowkes, F.G. & Harmar, A. (1999) Neuroticism and polymorphisms in the serotonin transporter gene. *Psychol Med* 29(3), 735–9.

Deckert, J., Catalano, M., Syagailo, Y. *et al.* (1999) Excess of high activity monoamine oxidase A gene promoter alleles in female patients with panic disorder. *Hum Molecular Genetics* 8(4), 621–4.

DiLalla, L., Kagan, J. & Reznick, J. (1994) Genetic etiology of behavioral inhibition among 2-year-old children. *Infant Behavioral Development* 17, 405–12.

Donnell, C. & McNally, R. (1990) Anxiety sensitivity and panic attacks in a nonclinical population. *Behav Res Ther* 28, 83–5.

Dumas, J.E., LaFreniere, P. & Serketich, W.J. (1995) "Balance of power": a transactional analysis of control in mother-child dyads involving socially competent, aggressive, and anxious children. *J Abnorm Psychol* 104(1), 104–13.

Ebstein, R.P., Gritsenko, I., Nemanov, L., Frisch, A., Osher, Y. & Belmaker, R.H. (1997) No association between the serotonin transporter gene regulatory region polymorphism and the Tridimensional Personality Questionnaire (TPQ) temperament of harm avoidance. *Mol Psychiatry* 2(3), 224–6.

Ehlers, A. (1993) Somatic symptoms and panic attacks: a retrospective study of learning experiences. *Behav Res Ther* 31(3), 269–78.

Eley, T.C. & Stevenson, J. (2000) Specific life events and chronic experiences differentially associated with Depress Anxiety in young twins. *J Abnorm Child Psychol* 28(4), 383–94.

Eysenck, H. (1967) *Biological Bases of Personality*. Charles C. Thomas, Springfield, IL.

Faravelli, C. (1985) Life events preceding the onset of panic disorder. *J Affect Disord* 9, 103–5.

Faravelli, C. & Pallanti, S. (1989) Recent life events and panic disorder. *Am J Psychiatry* 146(5), 622–6.

Faravelli, C., Webb, T., Ambonetti, A., Fonnesu, F. & Sessarego, A. (1985) Prevalence of traumatic early life events in 31 agoraphobic patients with panic attacks. *Am J Psychiatry* **142**(12), 1493–4.

Finch, A.J., Kendall, P.C., Deardorff, P.A., Anderson, J. & Sitarz, A.M. (1975) Reflection-impulsivity, persistence behavior, and locus of control in emotionally disturbed children. *J Consult Clin Psychol* **43**(5), 748.

Floderus-Myrhed, B., Pedersen, N. & Rasmuson, I. (1980) Assessment of heritability for personality, based on a short-form of the Eysenck Personality Inventory: a study of 12 898 twin pairs. *Behav Genet* **10**, 153–62.

Flory, J.D., Manuck, S.B., Ferrell, R.E., Dent, K.M., Peters, D.G. & Muldoon, M.F. (1999) Neuroticism is not associated with the serotonin transporter (5-HTTLPR) polymorphism. *Mol Psychiatry* **4**(1), 93–6.

Fordham, K. & Stevenson-Hinde, J. (1999) Shyness, friendship quality, and adjustment during middle childhood. *J Child Psychol Psychiat* **40**(5), 757–68.

Fyer, A., Mannuzza, S., Chapman, T., Liebowitz, M. & Klein, D. (1993) A direct interview family study of social phobia. *Arch Gen Psychiatry* **50**, 286–93.

Fyer, A.J., Mannuzza, S., Chapman, T.F., Martin, L.Y. & Kelin, D.F. (1995) Specificity in familial aggregation of phobic disorders. *Arch Gen Psychiatry* **52**, 564–73.

Garcia-Coll, C., Kagan, J. & Reznick, J.S. (1984) Behavioral inhibition in young children. *Child Dev* **55**, 1005–19.

Garnefski, N., Kraaj, V. & Spinhoven, P. (2001) Negative life events, cognitive emotion regulation and emotional problems. *Pers Individ Dif* **30**, 1311–27.

Gelernter, J., Bonvicini, K., Page, G. *et al.* (2001) Linkage genome scan for loci predisposing to panic disorder or agoraphobia. *Am J Med Genet* **105**(6), 548–57.

Gelernter, J., Kranzler, H., Coccaro, E.F., Siever, L.J. & New, A.S. (1998) Serotonin transporter protein gene polymorphism and personality measures in African-American and European-American subjects. *Am J Psychiatry* **155**(10), 1332–8.

Gerlsma, C., Emmelkamp, P. & Arrindell, W. (1990) Anxiety, depression, and perception of early parenting: a meta-analysis. *Clin Psychol Rev* **10**, 251–77.

Gersten, M. (1989) Behavioral inhibition in the classroom. In: *Perspectives on Behavioral Inhibition* (J. Resnick (ed.), pp. 71–91). University of Chicago Press, Chicago.

Gest, S.D. (1997) Behavioral inhibition: stability and associations with adaptation from childhood to early adulthood. *J Pers Soc Psychol* **72**(2), 467–75.

Gilmartin, B.G. (1987) Peer group antecedents of severe love-shyness in males. *Journal of Personality* **55**, 467–89.

Goldsmith, H.H. & Lemery, K.S. (2000) Linking temperamental fearfulness and anxiety symptoms: a behavior-genetic perspective. *Biol Psychiatry* **48**(12), 1199–209.

Goldstein, A.J. & Chambless, D.L. (1978) A reanalysis of agoraphobia. *Behavior Therapy* **9**, 47–59.

Goldstein, R.B., Wickramaratne, P.J., Horwath, E. & Weissman, M.M. (1997) Familial aggregation and phenomenology of "early" onset (at or before age 20 years) panic disorder. *Arch Gen Psychiatry* **54**, 271–8.

Gratacos, M., Nadal, M., Martin-Santos, R. *et al.* (2001) A polymorphic genomic duplication on human chromosome 15 is a susceptibility factor for panic and phobic disorders. *Cell* **106**(3), 367–79.

Gruner, K., Muris, P. & Merckelbach, H. (1999) The relationship between anxious rearing behaviors and anxiety disorders symptomatology in normal children. *J Behav Ther Exp Psychiatry* **30**, 27–35.

Gustavsson, J.P., Nothen, M.M., Jonsson, E.G. *et al.* (1999) No association between serotonin transporter gene polymorphisms and personality traits. *Am J Med Genet* **88**(4), 430–6.

Hayward, C., Killen, J.D., Kraemer, H.C. *et al.* (1997) Assessment and phenomenology of nonclinical panic attacks in adolescent girls. *J Anxiety Disord* **11**, 17–32.

Hayward, C., Killen, J., Kraemer, K. & Taylor, C. (1998) Linking self-reported childhood behavioral inhibition to adolescent social phobia. *J Am Acad Child Adolesc Psychiatry* **37**(12), 1308–16.

Hayward, C., Killen, J.D., Kraemer, H.C. & Taylor, C.B. (2000) Predictors of panic attacks in adolescents. *J Am Acad Child Adolesc Psychiatry* **39**(2), 207–14.

Heath, A.C., Cloninger, C.R. & Martin, N.G. (1994) Testing a model for the genetic structure of personality: a comparison of the personality systems of Cloninger and Eysenck. *J Pers Soc Psychol* **66**(4), 762–75.

Henderson, A.S., Korten, A.E., Jorm, A.F. *et al.* (2000) COMT and DRD3 polymorphisms, environmental exposures, and personality traits related to common mental disorders. *Am J Med Genet* **96**(1), 102–7.

Henin, A. & Kendall, P.C. (1997) Obsessive-compulsive disorder in childhood and adolescence. *Advances in Clinical Child Psychology* **19**, 75–131.

Herbst, J.H., Zonderman, A.B., McCrae, R.R. & Costa, P.T., Jr (2000) Do the dimensions of the temperament and character inventory map a simple genetic architecture? Evidence from molecular genetics and factor analysis. *Am J Psychiatry* **157**(8), 1285–90.

Hirshfeld, D., Biederman, J., Brody, L., Faraone, S. & Rosenbaum, J. (1997a) Expressed emotion toward children with behavioral inhibition: associations with maternal anxiety disorders. *J Am Acad Child Adolesc Psychiatry* **36**, 910–17.

Hirshfeld, D.R., Biederman, J., Brody, L., Faraone, S.V. & Rosenbaum, J.R. (1997b) Associations between expressed emotion and child behavioral inhibition and psychopathology: a pilot study. *J Am Acad Child Adolesc Psychiatry* **36**, 205–13.

Hirshfeld, D.R., Rosenbaum, J.F., Biederman, J. *et al.* (1992) Stable behavioral inhibition and its association with anxiety disorder. *J Am Acad Child Adolesc Psychiatry* **31**(1), 103–11.

Hirshfeld, D.R., Rosenbaum, J.F., Fredman, S.J. & Kagan, J. (1999) Neurobiology of childhood anxiety disorders. In: *Neurobiological Foundations of Mental Illness* (D. Charney, E. Nestler & B. Bunney (eds), pp. 823–38). Oxford University Press, Oxford.

Hirshfeld, D., Smoller, J., Fredman, S., Bulzachelli, M. & Rosenbaum, J. (1998) Early antecedents of panic disorder. Genes, childhood, and the environment. In: *Panic Disorder and its Treatment* (J.F. Rosenbaum & M.H. Pollack (eds), pp. 93–151). Marcel Dekker, New York.

Hirshfeld-Becker, D.R., Fredman, S.J., Robin, J. & Rosenbaum, J.F. (1999). Etiology of social phobia. In: *Social Anxiety Disorder* (J.A. den Boer & H.M. Westenberg (eds), pp. 47–79). Synthesis, Amsterdam.

Hudson, J. & Rapee, R.M. (2001) Parent–child interactions and anxiety disorders: an observational study. *Behav Res Ther* **39**(12), 1411–27.

Hymel, S., Rubin, K., Rowden, L. & LeMare, L. (1990) Children's peer relationships: longitudinal prediction of internalizing and externalizing problems from middle to late childhood. *Child Dev* **61**, 2004–21.

Ialongo, N., Edelsohn, G., Werthamer-Larsson, L., Crockett, L. & Kellam, S. (1995) The significance of self-reported anxious symptoms in first-grade children: prediction to anxious symptoms and adaptive functioning in fifth grade. *J Child Psychol Psychiatry* **36**(3), 427–37.

Ishiyama, F. (1984) Shyness: anxious social sensitivity and self-isolating tendency. *Adolescence* **19**, 903–11.

Jacobson, A. (1989) Physical and sexual assault histories among psychiatric outpatients. *Am J Psychiatry* **146**(6), 755–8.

Jang, K.L., Stein, M.B., Taylor, S. & Livesley, W.J. (1999) Gender differences in the etiology of anxiety sensitivity: a twin study. *J Gend Specif Med* **2**(2), 39–44.

Jonnal, A.H., Gardner, C.O., Prescott, C.A. & Kendler, K.S. (2000) Obsessive and compulsive symptoms in a general population sample of female twins. *Am J Med Genet* **96**(6), 791–6.

Jorm, A.F., Henderson, A.S., Jacomb, P.A. *et al.* (1998) An association study of a functional polymorphism of the serotonin transporter gene with personality and psychiatric symptoms. *Mol Psychiatry* **3**(5), 449–51.

Jorm, A.F., Prior, M., Sanson, A., Smart, D., Zhang, Y. & Easteal, S. (2000) Association of a functional polymorphism of the serotonin transporter gene with anxiety-related temperament and behavior problems in children: a longitudinal study from infancy to the mid-teens. *Mol Psychiatry* **5**(5), 542–7.

Kagan, J. (1989) Temperamental contributions to social behavior. *Am Psychol* **44**(4), 668–74.

Kagan, J. (1994) *Galen's Prophecy: Temperament in Human Nature.* BasicBooks, New York.

Kagan, J., Reznick, J.S., Clarke, C., Snidman, N. & Garcia-Coll, C. (1984) Behavioral inhibition to the unfamiliar. *Child Dev* **55**, 2212–25.

Kagan, J., Reznick, J.S. & Gibbons, J. (1989) Inhibited and uninhibited types of children. *Child Dev* **60**, 838–45.

Kagan, J., Reznick, J.S. & Snidman, N. (1987) The physiology and psychology of behavioral inhibition in children. *Child Dev* **58**, 1459–73.

Kagan, J., Reznick, J.S. & Snidman, N. (1988a) Biological bases of childhood shyness. *Science* **240**, 167–71.

Kagan, J., Reznick, J.S., Snidman, N., Gibbons, J. & Johnson, M.O. (1988b) Childhood derivatives of inhibition and lack of inhibition to the unfamiliar. *Child Dev* **59**(6), 1580–9.

Kagan, J. & Snidman, N. (1991a) Infant predictors of inhibited and uninhibited profiles. *Psychol Sci* **2**(1), 40–4.

Kagan, J. & Snidman, N. (1991b) Temperamental factors in human development. *Am Psychol* **46**(8), 856–62.

Kagan, J., Snidman, S. & Arcus, D. (1998) Childhood derivatives of high and low reactivity in infancy. *Child Dev* **69**(6), 1483–93.

Kagan, J., Snidman, N., Zetner, M. & Peterson, E. (1999) Infant temperament and anxious symptoms in school age children. *Dev Psychopathol* **11**, 209–24.

Karayiorgou, M., Altemus, M., Galke, B.L. *et al.* (1997) Genotype determining low catechol-o-methyltransferase activity as a risk factor for obsessive-compulsive disorder. *Proc Natl Acad Sci U S A* **94**(9), 4572–5.

Karayiorgou, M., Sobin, C., Blundell, M.L. *et al.* (1999) Family-based association studies support a sexually dimorphic effect of COMT and MAOA on genetic susceptibility to obsessive-compulsive disorder [In Process Citation]. *Biol Psychiatry* **45**(9), 1178–89.

Katsuragi, S., Kunugi, H., Sano, A. *et al.* (1999) Association between serotonin transporter gene polymorphism and anxiety-related traits. *Biol Psychiatry* **45**(3), 368–70.

Kearney, C.A., Albano, A.M., Eisen, A.R., Allan, W.D. & Barlow, D.H. (1997) The phenomenology of panic disorder in youngsters: an empirical study of a clinical sample. *J Anx Dis* **11**, 49–62.

Keller, M., Lavori, P., Wunder, J., Beardslee, W., Schwartz, C. & Roth, J. (1992) Chronic course of anxiety disorders in children and adolescents. *J Am Acad Child Adolesc Psychiatry* **31**(4), 595–9.

Kendall, P.C. (1994) Treating anxiety disorders in children: results of a randomized clinical trial. *J Consult Clin Psychol* **62**(1), 100–10.

Kendall, P.C. & Southam-Gerow, M.A. (1996) Long-term follow-up of a cognitive-behavioral therapy for anxiety disordered youth. *J Consult Clin Psychol* **64**(4), 724–30.

Kendall, P.C. & Warman, M.J. (1996) Anxiety disorders in youth: diagnostic consistency across DSM-III-R and DSM-IV. *J Anxiety Disord* **10**, 453–63.

Kendler, K.S., Gardner, C.O. & Prescott, C.A. (2001) Panic syndromes in a population-based sample of male and female twins. *Psychol Med* **31**(6), 989–1000.

Kendler, K.S., Karkowski, L.M. & Prescott, C.A. (1999) Fears and phobias: reliability and heritability. *Psychol Med* **29**(3), 539–53.

Kendler, K.S., Neale, M.C., Kessler, R.C., Heath, A.C. & Eaves, L.J. (1992) Generalized anxiety disorder in women. *Arch Gen Psychiatry* **49**, 267–72.

Kendler, K.S., Neale, M.C., Kessler, R.C., Heath, A.C. & Eaves, L.J. (1993) Panic disorder in women: a population-based twin study. *Psychol Med* **23**, 397–406.

Kendler, K., Walters, E., Neale, M., Kessler, R., Heath, A. & Eaves, L. (1995) The structure of the genetic and environmental risk factors for six major psychiatric disorders in women. *Arch Gen Psychiatry* **52**, 374–83.

Kim, S.W. & Hoover, K.M. (1996) Tridimensional personality questionnaire: assessment in patients with social phobia and a control group. *Psychol Rep* **78**(1), 43–9.

King, N.J., Eleonora, G. & Ollendick, T.H. (1998) Etiology of childhood phobias: current status of Rachman's three pathways. *Behav Res Ther* **36**, 297–309.

Klein, D. (1964) Delineation of two-drug reponsive anxiety syndromes. *Psychopharmacologia* **5**, 397–408.

Klein, D.F. (1981) Anxiety reconceptualized. In: *Anxiety: New Research and Concepts* (D.F. Klein & J. Rabkin (eds), pp. 235–62). Raven Press, New York.

Klein, R.G. & Last, C.G. (1989) *Anxiety Disorders in Children*, Vol. 20. Sage Publications, Newbury Park.

Knowles, J.A., Fyer, A.J., Vieland, V.J. *et al.* (1998) Results of a genome-wide genetic screen for panic disorder. *Am J Med Genet* **81**(2), 139–47.

Kochanska, G. (1991) Patterns of inhibition to the unfamiliar in children of normal and affectively ill mothers. *Child Dev* **62**, 250–63.

Krohne, H. (1990) Parental child rearing and anxiety development. In: *Health Hazards in Adolescence: Prevention and Intervention in Childhood and Adolescence* (K. Hurrelmann & F. Losel (eds), pp. 115–30). DeGruyter, New York.

Krohne, H. (1992) Developmental conditions of anxiety and coping. A two-process model of child-rearing effects. In: *Advances in Test Anxiety Research*, Vol. 7. (K. Hagtvet & T. Johnsen (eds), pp. 143–55). Swets & Zeitlinger, Amsterdam.

Krohne, H. & Hock, M. (1991) Relationships between restrictive mother–child interactions and anxiety of the child. *Anxiety Research* **4**, 109–24.

LaFreniere, P.J. & Capuano, F. (1997) Preventive intervention as means of clarifying direction of effects in socialization: Anxious-withdrawn preschoolers case. *Dev Psychopathol* **9**, 551–64.

LaGreca, A., Dandes, S., Wick, P., Shaw, K. & Stone, W. (1988) Development of the social anxiety scale for children: reliability and concurrent validity. *J Clin Child Psychol* **17**(1), 84–91.

Laraia, M., Stuart, G., Grye, L., Lydiard, R. & Ballenger, J. (1994) Childhood environment of women having panic disorder and agoraphobia. *J Anx Dis* **8**(1), 1–17.

Last, C.G., Hersen, M., Kazdin, A.E., Orvaschel, H. & Perrin, S. (1991) Anxiety disorders in children and their families. *Arch Gen Psychiatry* **48**, 928–34.

Last, C., Perrin, S., Hersen, M. & Kazdin, A. (1996) A prospective study of childhood anxiety disorders. *J Am Acad Child Adolesc Psychiatry* **35**(11), 1502–10.

Lau, J.J., Calamari, J.E. & Waraczynski, M. (1996) Panic attack symptomatology and anxiety sensitivity in adolescents. *J Anxiety Disord* **10**, 355–64.

Lerner, R.M. & Lerner, J.V. (1987) Children in their contexts. A goodness-of-fit model. In: *Parenting Across the Lifespan* (J. Lancaster, J. Altman, A. Possi & L. Sheri (eds), pp. 377–403). Aldive de Gruyter, New York.

Lesch, K.-P., Bengel, D., Heils, A. *et al.* (1996) Association of anxiety-related traits with a polymorphism in the serotonin transporter gene regulatory region. *Science* **274**, 1527–31.

Lieb, R., Wittchen, H.U., Hofler, M., Fuetsch, M., Stein, M.B. & Merikangas, K.R. (2000) Parental psychopathology, parenting styles, and the risk of social phobia in offspring: a prospective-longitudinal community study. *Arch Gen Psychiatry* **57**(9), 859–66.

Lipsitz, J.D., Martin, L.Y., Mannuzza, S. *et al.* (1994) Childhood separation anxiety disorder in patients with adult anxiety disorders. *Am J Psychiatry* **151**(6), 927–9.

Mackinnon, A., Henderson, A. & Andrews, G. (1990) Genetic and environmental determinants of the lability of trait neuroticism and the symptoms of anxiety and depression. *Psychol Med* **20**, 581–90.

Maier, W., Lichtermann, D., Minges, J., Oehrlein, A. & Franke, P. (1993) A controlled family study in panic disorder. *J Psychiat Res* **27** (Suppl. 1), 79–87.

Maller, R.G. & Reiss, S. (1992) Anxiety sensitivity in 1984 and panic attacks in 1987. *J Anxiety Disord* **6**(3), 241–7.

Manassis, K., Bradley, S., Goldberg, S., Hood, J. & Swinson, R. (1994) Attachment in mothers with anxiety disorders and their children. *J Am Acad Child Adolesc Psychiatry* **33**(8), 1106–13.

Manassis, K., Bradley, S., Goldberg, S., Hood, J. & Swinson, R. (1995) Behavioral inhibition, attachment and anxiety in children of mothers with anxiety disorders. *Can J Psychiatry* **40**, 87–92.

Mancini, C., van Ameringen, M., Szatmari, P., Fugere, C. & Boyle, M. (1996) A high-risk pilot study of the children of adults with social phobia. *J Am Acad Child Adolesc Psychiatry* **35**(11), 1511–17.

Manfro, G.G., Otto, M.W., McArdle, E.T., Worthington, J.J., Rosenbaum, J.F. & Pollack, M.H. (1996) Relationship of antecedent stressful life events to childhood and family history of anxiety and the course of panic disorder. *J Affect Disord* **41**(12), 135–9.

Manicavasagar, V., Silove, D., Curtis, J. & Wagner, R. (2000) Continuities of separation anxiety from early life into adulthood. *J Anxiety Disord* **14**(1), 1–18.

Masia, C. & Morris, T. (1998) Parental factors associated with social anxiety: methodological limitations and suggestions for integrated behavioral research. *Clin Psychol Sci Prac* **5**, 211–28.

Matheny, A.P. (1989) Children's behavioral inhibition over age and across situations: genetic similarity for a trait during change. *J Pers* **57**(2), 215–35.

Mattis, S.G. & Ollendick, T.H. (1997) Children's cognitive responses to the somatic symptoms of panic. *J Abnorm Child Psychol* **25**, 47–57.

Mazzanti, C.M., Lappalainen, J., Long, J.C. *et al.* (1998) Role of the serotonin transporter promoter polymorphism in anxiety-related traits. *Arch Gen Psychiatry* **55**(10), 936–40.

McDougle, C., Epperson, C., Price, L. & Gelernter, J. (1998) Evidence for linkage disequilibrium between serotonin transporter protein gene (SLC6A4) and obsessive-compulsive disorder. *Mol Psychiatry* **3**, 270–3.

McNally, R.J. (1996) Anxiety sensitivity is distinguishable from trait anxiety. In: *Current Controversies in the Anxiety Disorders* (R.M. Rapee (ed.), pp. 214–27. Guilford Press, New York.

McNally, R.J. & Eke, M. (1996) Anxiety sensitivity, suffocation fear, and breath-holding duration as predictors of response to carbon dioxide challenge. *J Abnorm Psychol* **105**(1), 146–9.

McNally, R.J., Luedke, D.L., Besyner, J.K., Peterson, R.A., Bohm, K. & Lips, O.J. (1987) Sensitivity to stress-relevant stimuli in post-traumatic stress disorder. *J Anx Dis* **1**, 105–16.

Menzies, R.G. & Clarke, C.J. (1993) The etiology of childhood water phobia. *Behav Res Ther* **31**(5), 499–501.

Menzies, R.G. & Harris, L.M. (2001) Nonassociative factors in the development of phobias. In: *The Developmental Psychopathology of Anxiety* (M.W. Vasey & M.R. Dadds (eds), pp. 183–204. Oxford University Press, New York.

Merikangas, K.R., Dierker, L.C. & Szatmari, P. (1998) Psychopathology among offspring of parents with substance abuse and/or anxiety disorders: a high-risk study. *J Am Acad Child Adolesc Psychiatry* **39**(5), 711–20.

Messer, S.C. & Beidel, D.C. (1994) Psychosocial correlates of childhood anxiety disorders. *J Am Acad Child Adolesc Psychiatry* **33**(7), 975–83.

Mick, M. & Telch, M. (1998) Social anxiety and history of behavioral inhibition in young adults. *J Anx Disorders* **12**(1), 1–20.

Mineka, S. & Zinbarg, R. (1995) Conditioning and ethological models of social phobia. In: *Social Phobia: Diagnosis, Assessment, and Treatment* (R. Heimberg, M. Liebowitz, D. Hope & F. Schneier (eds), pp. 134–62). The Guilford Press, New York.

Morris, T.L., Messer, S.C. & Gross, A.M. (1995) Enhancement of the social interaction and status of neglected children: a peer-pairing approach. *J Clin Child Psychol* **24**(1), 11–20.

Muris, P. & Merckelbach, H. (1998) Perceived parental rearing behavior and anxiety disorders symptoms in normal children. *Pers Individ Dif* **25**, 1199–206.

Muris, P. & Merckelbach, H. (2001) The etiology of childhood specific phobia: a multifactorial model. In: *The Developmental Psychopathology of Anxiety* (M.W. Vasey & M.R. Dadds (eds), pp. 355–85. Oxford University Press, New York.

Muris, P., Merckelbach, H. & Damsma, E. (2000) Threat perception bias in nonreferred, socially anxious children. *J Clin Child Psychol* **29**(3), 348–59.

Muris, P., Merckelbach, H., Schmidt, H., Gadet, B. & Bogie, N. (2001) Anxiety and depression as correlates of self-reported behavioral inhibiton in normal adolescents. *Behavior Therapy and Research* **39**, 1051–61.

Muris, P., Merckelbach, H., Wessel, I. & van de Ven, M. (1999) Psychopathological correlates of self-reported behavioral inhibition in normal children. *Behav Res Ther* **37**(6), 575–84.

Nestadt, G., Samuels, J., Riddle, M. *et al.* (2000) A family study of obsessive-compulsive disorder. *Arch Gen Psychiatry* **57**(4), 358–63.

Nestadt, G., Samuels, J., Riddle, M.A. *et al.* (2001) The relationship between obsessive-compulsive disorder and anxiety and affective disorders: results from the Johns Hopkins OCD Family Study. *Psychol Med* **31**(3), 481–7.

Norton, G.R., Cox, B.J., Hewitt, P.L. & McLeod, L. (1997) Personality factors associated with generalized and nongeneralized social anxiety. *Pers Individ Dif* **22**(5), 655–60.

Noyes, R., Clarkson, C., Crowe, R.R., Yates, W.R. & McChesney, C.M. (1987) A family study of generalized anxiety disorder. *Am J Psychiatry* **144**, 1019–24.

Noyes, R., Crowe, R.R., Harris, E.L., Hamra, B.J., McChesney, C.M. & Chaudhry, D.R. (1986) Relationship between panic disorder and agoraphobia: a family study. *Arch Gen Psychiatry* **43**, 227–32.

Nunn, G. (1988) Concurrent validity between the Nowicki–Strickland Locus of Control Scale and the State–Trait Anxiety Inventory for Children. *Educational and Psychological Measurement* **48**, 435–8.

Ollendick, T. & Francis, G. (1988) Behavioral assessment and treatment of childhood phobias. *Beh Mod* **12**(2), 165–204.

Ollendick, T.H. & King, N.J. (1998) Empirically supported treatments for children with phobic and anxiety disorders: current status. *J Clin Child Psychol* **27**(2), 156–67.

Orvaschel, H., Lewinsohn, P. & Seeley, J.R. (1995) Continuity of psychopathology in a community sample of adolescents. *J Am Acad Child Adolesc Psychiatry* **34**(11), 1525–35.

Öst, L.-G. (1987) Age of onset of different phobias. *J Abnorm Psychol* **96**, 223–9.

Otto, M., Pollock, M., Rosenbaum, J.F., Sachs, G.S. & Asher, R.H. (1994) Childhood history of anxiety in adults with panic disorder: association with anxiety sensitivity and comorbidity. *Harv Rev Psychiatry* **1**, 288–93.

Otto, M.W. & Reilly-Harrington, N.A. (1999) Impact of treatment on anxiety sensitivity. In: *Anxiety Sensitivity: Theory, Research and Treatment of the Fear of Anxiety* (S.A. Taylor (ed.), pp. 321–38). Lawrence Erlbaum Associates, Mahwah, NJ.

Parker, G. (1979a) Parental characteristics in relation to depressive disorders. *Br J Psychiatry* **134**, 138–47.

Parker, G. (1979b) Reported parental characteristics of agoraphobics and social phobics. *Br J Psychiatry* **135**, 555–60.

Pauls, D., Alsobrook, J.I.I., Goodman, W., Rasmussen, S. & Leckman, J. (1995) A family study of obsessive-compulsive disorder. *Am J Psychiatry* **152**, 76–84.

Perugi, G., Toni, C., Benedetti, A. *et al.* (1998) Delineating a putative phobic-anxious temperament in 126 panic-agoraphobic patients: toward a rapprochement of European and US views. *J Affect Disord* **47**(1–3), 11–23.

Pine, D.S., Cohen, P., Gurley, D., Brook, J. & Ma, Y. (1998) The risk for early-adulthood anxiety and depressive disorders in adolescents with anxiety and depressive disorders. *Arch Gen Psychiatry* **55**(1), 56–64.

Plomin, R. & Daniels, D. (1986) Genetics and shyness. In: *Shyness: Perspectives on Research and Treatment* (W. Jones, J. Cheek & S. Briggs (eds)). Plenum, New York, pp. 63–80.

Plomin, R., Emde, R., Braungart, J. *et al.* (1993) Genetic change and continuity from 14 to 20 months: the MacArthur Longitudinal Twin Study. *Child Dev* **64**, 1354–76.

Pollack, M.H., Otto, M.W., Sabatino, S. *et al.* (1996) Relationship of childhood anxiety to adult panic disorder: correlates and influence on course. *Am J Psychiatry* **153**(3), 376–81.

Prins, P. (1986) Children's self-speech and self-regulation during a fear-provoking behavioral test. *Behav Res Ther* **24**(2), 181–91.

Rabian, B., Embry, L. & MacIntyre, D. (1999) Behavioral validation of the Childhood Anxiety Sensitivity Index in children. *J Clin Child Psychol* **28**, 105–12.

Rabian, B., Peterson, R.A., Richters, J. & Jensen, P.S. (1993) Anxiety sensitivity among anxious children. *J Clin Child Psychol* **22**, 441–6.

Rachman, S. & de Silva, P. (1978) Abnormal and normal obsessions. *Behav Res Ther* **16**, 233–48.

Rapee, R.M. (1985) Distinctions between panic disorder and generalised anxiety disorder. *Aust N Z J Psychiatry* **19**, 227–32.

Rapee, R. (1997) Potential role of child rearing practices in the development of anxiety and depression. *Clinical Psychological Review* **17**(1), 47–67.

Rapee, R.M., Litwin, E.M. & Barlow, D.H. (1990) Impact of life events on subjects with panic disorder and on comparison subjects. *Am J Psychiatry* **147**(5), 640–4.

Rapee, R.M. & Melville, L.F. (1997) Recall of family factors in social phobia and panic disorder: comparison of mother and offspring reports. *Depress Anxiety* **5**, 7–11.

Reiss, S. (1991) Expectancy model of fear, anxiety, and panic. *Clinical Psychology Review* **11**(2), 141–53.

Reiss, S., Peterson, R.A., Gursky, M. & McNally, R.J. (1986) Anxiety sensitivity, anxiety frequency, and the prediction of fearfulness. *Behav Res Ther* **24**, 1–8.

Reiss, S., Silverman, W.K. & Weems, C.F. (2001) Anxiety Sensitivity. In: *The Developmental Psychopathology of Anxiety* (M.W. Vasey & M.R. Dadds (eds), pp. 92–111). Oxford University Press, New York.

Reznick, J.S., Hegeman, I.M., Kaufman, E., Woods, S.W. & Jacobs, M. (1992) Retrospective and concurrent self-report of behavioral inhibition and their relation to adult mental health. *Dev Psychopathol* **4**, 301–21.

Reznick, J.S., Kagan, J., Snidman, N., Gersten, M., Baak, K. & Rosenberg, A. (1986) Inhibited and uninhibited behavior: a follow-up study. *Child Dev* **57**, 660–80.

Richter, M.A., Summerfeldt, L.J., Joffe, R.T. & Swinson, R.P. (1996) The Tridimensional Personality Questionnaire in obsessive-compulsive disorder. *Psychiatry Res* **65**(3), 185–8.

Robinson, J.L., Kagan, J., Reznick, J.S. & Corley, R. (1992) The heritability of inhibited and uninhibited behavior: a twin study. *Dev Psychol* **28**(6), 1030–7.

Rose, R., Koskenvuo, M., Kaprio, J., Sarna, S. & Langinvainio, H. (1988) Shared genes, shared experiences, and similarity of personality: data from 14 288 adult Finnish cotwins. *J Pers Soc Psychol* **54**, 161–71.

Rosenbaum, J.F., Biederman, J., Gersten, M. *et al.* (1988) Behavioral inhibition in children of parents with panic disorder and agoraphobia: a controlled study. *Arch Gen Psychiatry* **45**, 463–70.

Rosenbaum, J.F., Biederman, J., Hirshfeld, D.R. *et al.* (1991) Further evidence of an association between behavioral inhibition and anxiety disorders: results from a family study of children from a nonclinical sample. *J Psychiat Res* **25**(1–2), 49–65.

Rosenbaum, J.F., Biederman, J., Hirshfeld-Becker, D.R. *et al.* (2000) A controlled study of behavioral inhibition in children of parents with panic disorder and depression. *Am J Psychiatry* **157**(12), 2002–10.

Rubin, K. & Mills, R. (1988) The many faces of social isolation in childhood. *J Cons Clin Psychol* **56**(6), 916–24.

Rubin, K., Nelson, L., Hastings, P. & Asendorpf, J. (1999) The transaction between parents' perceptions of their children's shyness and their parenting styles. *International Journal of Behavioral Development* **23**(4), 937–57.

Sameroff, A. (1975a) Transactional models in early social relations. *Hum Dev* **18**, 65–79.

Sameroff, A.J. (1975b) Early influences on development: fact or fancy? *Merrility Palmer Quarterly* **21**(4), 267–94.

Scarpa, A., Raine, A., Venables, P. & Mednick, S. (1995) The stability of inhibited/uninhibited temperament from ages 3–11 years in Mauritian children. *J Abnorm Child Psychol* **23**(5), 607–18.

Scherrer, J.F., True, W.R., Xian, H. *et al.* (2000) Evidence for genetic influences common and specific to symptoms of generalized anxiety and panic. *J Affect Disord* **57**(1–3), 25–35.

Schmidt, N.B., Lerew, D.R. & Jackson, R.J. (1997) The role of anxiety sensitivity in the pathogenesis of panic: prospective evaluation of spontaneous panic attacks during acute stress. *J Abnorm Psychol* **106**(3), 355–64.

Schmidt, N.B., Lerew, D.R. & Jackson, R.J. (1999) Prospective evaluation of anxiety sensitivity in the pathogenesis of panic: replication and extension. *J Abnorm Psychol* **108**, 532–7.

Schmidt, N.B., Storey, J., Greenberg, B.D., Santiago, H.T., Li, Q. & Murphy, D.L. (2000) Evaluating gene X psychological risk factor effects in the pathogenesis of anxiety: a new model approach. *J Abnorm Psychol* **109**(2), 308–20.

Schwartz, C., Snidman, N. & Kagan, J. (1999) Adolescent social anxiety as an outcome of inhibited temperament in childhood. *J Am Acad Child Adolesc Psychiatry* **38**(8), 1008–15.

Silove, D. & Manicavasagar, V. (1993) Adults who feared school: is early separation anxiety specific to the pathogenesis of panic disorder? *Acta Psychiatr Scand* **88**, 385–90.

Silverman, W., Cerny, J., Nelles, W. & Burke, A. (1988) Behavior problems in children of parents with anxiety disorders. *J Am Acad Child Adolesc Psychiatry* **27**(6), 779–84.

Silverman, W.K., Fleisig, W., Rabian, B. & Peterson, R.A. (1991) Childhood Anxiety Sensitivity Index. *J Clin Child Psychol* **20**(2), 162–8.

Silverman, W.K., Ginsburg, G.S. & Goedhart, A.W. (1999a) Factor structure of the Child Anxiety Sensitivity Index. *Behav Res Ther* **37**, 903–17.

Silverman, W.K., Kurtines, W.M., Ginsburg, G.S., Weems, C.F., Lumpkin, P.W. & Carmichael, D.H. (1999b) Treating anxiety disorders in children with group cognitive-behavioral therapy: a randomized clinical trial. *J Consult Clin Psychol* **67**(6), 995–1003.

Siqueland, L., Kendall, P. & Steinberg, L. (1996) Anxiety in children: perceived family environments and observed family interaction. *J Clin Child Psychol* **25**(2), 225–37.

Smoller, J.W., Acierno, J.S. Jr, Rosenbaum, J.F. *et al.* (2001a) Targeted genome screen of panic disorder and anxiety disorder proneness using homology to murine QTL regions. *Am J Med Genet* **105**(2), 195–206.

Smoller, J., Finn, C. & White, C. (2000) The genetics of anxiety disorders: an overview. *Psychiatric Annals* **30**, 745–53.

Smoller, J.W., Rosenbaum, J.F., Biederman, J. *et al.* (2001b) Genetic association analysis of behavioral inhibition using candidate loci from mouse models. *Am J Med Genet* **105**(3), 226–35.

Smoller, J. & Tsuang, M. (1998) Panic and phobic anxiety: defining phenotypes for genetic studies. *Am J Psychiatry* **155**, 1152–62.

Snidman, N. (1989) Behavioral inhibition and sympathetic influence on the cardiovascular system. In: *Perspectives on Behavioral Inhibition* (J. Reznick (ed.), pp. 51–70). University of Chicago Press, Chicago.

Spence, S.H. (1994) Preventative strategies. In: *International Handbook of Phobic and Anxiety Disorders* (T.H. Ollendick, N.J. King & W. Yule (eds), pp. 453–74). Plenum, New York.

Spence, S.H. (1997) Structure of anxiety symptoms among children: a confirmatory factor-analytic study. *J Abnorm Psychol* **106**(2), 280–97.

Spence, S.H. (2001) Prevention strategies. In: *The Developmental Psychopathology of Anxiety* (M.W. Vasey & M.R. Dadds (eds), pp. 325–54). Oxford University Press, New York.

Sroufe, L.A. & Rutter, M. (1984) The domain of developmental psychopathology. *Child Dev* **55**, 17–29.

Starcevic, V., Uhlenhuth, E.H., Fallon, S. & Pathak, D. (1996) Personality dimensions in panic disorder and generalized anxiety disorder. *J Affect Disord* **37**(2–3), 75–9.

Stein, M., Chartier, M., Hazen, A. *et al.* (1998) A direct-interview family study of generalized social phobia. *Am J Psychiatry* **155**(1), 90–7.

Stein, M.B., Chartier, M.J., Lizak, M.V. & Jang, K.L. (2001) Familial aggregation of anxiety-related quantitative traits in generalized social phobia: clues to understanding "disorder" heritability? *Am J Med Genet* **105**(1), 79–83.

Stein, M., Jang, K. & Livesley, W. (1999) Heritability of anxiety sensitivity: a twin study. *Am J Psychiatry* **156**, 246–51.

Stemberger, R., Turner, S., Beidel, D. & Calhoun, K. (1995) Social phobia: an analysis of possible developmental factors. *J Abnorm Psychol* **104**(3), 526–31.

Stewart, S.H., Taylor, S., Jang, K.L. *et al.* (2001) Causal modeling of relations among learning history, anxiety sensitivity, and panic attacks. *Behav Res Ther* **39**, 443–56.

Strauss, C., Frame, C. & Forehand, R. (1987) Psychosocial impairment associated with anxiety in children. *J Clin Child Psychol* **16**(3), 235–9.

Strauss, C.C., Lahey, B.B., Frick, P., Frame, C.L. & Hynd, G.W. (1988) Peer social status of children with anxiety disorders. *J Consult Clin Psychol* **56**(1), 137–41.

Stubbe, D.E., Zahner, G., Goldstein, M.J. & Leckman, J.F. (1993) Diagnostic specificity of a brief measure of expressed emotion: a community study of children. *J Child Psychol Psychiat* **34**(2), 139–54.

Suomi, S.J. (1984) The development of affect in rhesus monkeys. In: *The Psychobiology of Affective Development*. (N. Fox & R. Davidson (eds)) Erlbaum, Hillsdale, NJ, 119–59.

Suomi, S.J. (1986) Anxiety-like disorders in young non-human primates. In: *Anxiety Disorders of Childhood*, (R. Gittleman (ed.), pp. 1–23). Guilford Press, New York.

Suomi, S.J. (1997) Early determinants of behavior: evidence from primate studies. *Br Med Bull* **53**, 170–84.

Suomi, S.J., Kraemer, G.W., Baysinger, C.M. & DeLizio, R.D. (1981) Inherited and experiential factors associated with individual differences in anxious behavior displayed by rhesus monkeys. In: *Anxiety: New Research and Changing Concepts* (D.F. Klein & J. Rabkin (eds), pp. 179–200). Raven Press, New York.

Sylvester, C.E., Hyde, T.S. & Reichler, R.J. (1987) The Diagnostic Interview for Children and the Personality Inventory for Children in studies of children at risk for anxiety disorders or depression. *J Am Acad Child Adolesc Psychiatry* **26**(5), 668–75.

Thapar, A. & McGuffin, P. (1995) Are anxiety symptoms in childhood heritable? *J Child Psychol Psychiat* **36**, 439–47.

Thyer, B.A., Himle, J. & Fischer, D. (1988) Is parental death a selective precursor to either panic disorder or agoraphobia? A test of the separation anxiety hypothesis. *J Anx Dis* **2**, 333–8.

Tiet, Q.Q., Bird, H.R., Hoven, C.W. *et al.* (2001) Relationship between specific adverse life events and psychiatric disorders. *J Abnorm Child Psychol* **29**(2), 153–64.

Topolski, T., Hewitt, J., Eaves, L. *et al.* (1997) Genetic and environmental influences on child reports of manifest anxiety and symptoms of separation anxiety and overanxious disorders: a community-based twin study. *Behav Genet* **27**, 15–28.

Treadwell, K.R. & Kendall, P.C. (1996) Self-talk in youth with anxiety disorders: states of mind, content specificity, and treatment outcome. *J Consult Clin Psychol* **64**(5), 941–50.

True, W.R., Rice, J., Eisen, S.A. *et al.* (1993) A twin study of genetic and environmental contributions to liability for post-traumatic stress symptoms [see comments]. *Arch Gen Psychiatry* **50**(4), 257–64.

Turner, S.M., Beidel, D.C. & Costello, A. (1987) Psychopathology in the offspring of anxiety disorders patients. *J Consult Clin Psychol* **55**(2), 229–35.

Unnewehr, S., Schneider, S., Florin, I. & Margraf, J. (1998) Psychopathology in children of patients with panic disorder or animal phobia. *Psychopathology* **31**, 69–84.

Warren, S., Huston, L., Egeland, B. & Sroufe, L. (1997) Child and adolescent anxiety disorders and early attachment. *J Am Acad Child Adolesc Psychiatry* **36**(5), 637–44.

Warren, S.L., Schmitz, S. & Emde, R.N. (1999) Behavioral genetic analysis of self-reported anxiety at 7 years of age. *J Am Acad Child Adolesc Psychiatry* **38**(11), 1403–8.

Waters, T.L. & Barrett, P.M. (2000) The role of the family in childhood obsessive-compulsive disorder. *Clin Child Fam Psychol Rev* **3**(3), 173–84.

Watt, M.C. & Stewart, S.H. (2000) Anxiety sensitivity mediates the relationships between childhood learning experiences and elevated hypochondriacal concerns in young adulthood. *J Psychosom Res* **49**(2), 107–18.

Watt, M., Stewart, S. & Cox, B. (1998) A retrospective study of the learning history origins of anxiety sensitivity. *Behav Res Ther* **36**, 505–25.

Weems, C.F., Hammond-Laurence, K., Silverman, W.K. & Ginsburg, G. (1998) Testing the utility of the anxiety sensitivity construct in children and adolescents referred for anxiety disorders. *J Clin Child Psychol* **24**, 69–77.

Weissman, M., Fyer, A., Haghighi, F. *et al.* (2000) Potential panic disorder syndrome: clinical and genetic linkage evidence. *Am J Med Genet (Neuropsychiatrics Genetics)* **96**, 24–35.

Weissman, M., Leckman, J., Merikangas, K., Gammon, G. & Prusoff, B. (1984) Depress Anxiety disorders in parents and children: results from the Yale Family Study. *Arch Gen Psychiatry* **41**, 845–52.

Whaley, S., Pinto, A. & Sigman, M. (1999) Characterizing interactions between anxious mothers and their children. *J Consult Clin Psychol* **67**(6), 826–36.

Zinbarg, R.E., Barlow, D.H. & Brown, T.A. (1997) The hierarchical structure and general factor saturation of the Anxiety Sensitivity Index: evidence and implications. *Psychol Assess* **9**, 277–84.

Zinbarg, R.E., Mohlman, J. & Hong, N.N. (1999) Dimensions of anxiety sensitivity. In: *Anxiety Sensitivity: Theory, Research, and Treatment of the Fear of Anxiety* (S.A. Taylor (ed.), pp. 83–114). Lawrence Erlbaum Associates, Mahwah, NJ.

10 Anxiety and Schizophrenia

R.A. Emsley & D.J. Stein

Introduction

Schizophrenia is a disease of the brain that expresses itself with a mixture of characteristic signs and symptoms involving perception, thought, language and communication, behavior, movement, affect, volition and attention. These signs and symptoms are usually associated with marked social and vocational impairment. Indeed, schizophrenia is *the* most severe and debilitating of all psychiatric disorders, and exacts enormous emotional and economic costs worldwide.

Symptoms of anxiety are frequently encountered during the course of schizophrenia. They may occur during any phase of the illness. There are many reasons why patients with schizophrenia may develop symptoms of anxiety, such as: response to adverse life-events (e.g. involuntary hospitalization, unemployment, broken relationships); reaction to terrifying psychotic experiences; substance intoxication or withdrawal (there is a very high incidence of substance abuse in patients with schizophrenia); neuroleptic-induced anxiety (either directly, e.g. akathisia, or indirectly, e.g. in reaction to the distressing experience of developing an acute dystonic reaction); comorbid anxiety disorders; comorbid major depression; or the possibility that affective symptoms are a core feature of the schizophrenic illness itself.

This chapter will deal with the following topics relevant to anxiety in schizophrenia:
- Epidemiological aspects of anxiety in schizophrenia.
- Anxiety symptoms as a core dimension of schizophrenia.
- Obsessive-compulsive disorder (OCD) and schizophrenia.
- Panic disorder and schizophrenia.
- Post-traumatic stress disorder (PTSD) and schizophrenia.
- Social phobia and schizophrenia.
- Anxiety and antipsychotic agents.

Epidemiology

Estimates of the frequency of anxiety symptoms and syndromes in schizophrenia vary widely, depending on which populations of subjects are investigated, and which instruments are used to assess anxiety. So, for example, studies estimating the prevalence of comorbid anxiety disorders in schizophrenia have reported different findings. In a study in which the patterns and clinical correlates of psychiatric comorbidity were explored in a sample of 96 hospitalized patients with psychotic symptoms (schizophrenia spectrum and mood spectrum psychoses), the total lifetime prevalence of comorbid psychiatric disorders in the entire cohort was 57.3% (Cassano *et al.* 1998). Of these, 32.3% had more than two comorbid diagnoses. Anxiety disorders featured prominently. The most frequently observed comorbid disorders among the schizophrenia spectrum disorders were OCD (29%), panic disorder (19.4%), major depressive disorder (19.4%), social phobia (16.1%), substance abuse/dependence (9.7%), alcohol abuse/dependence (6.5%) and simple phobia (3.2%). It was noted that generalized anxiety disorder was difficult to assess in psychotic patients. Comorbid social phobia, substance abuse disorder and panic disorder showed the greatest association with psychotic symptoms. No significant differences in gender, educational and employment status were found between those with, and those without comorbid psychiatric disorders. Somatic delusions were more frequent in subjects with comorbidity, while delusions of control were more frequent in subjects without comorbidity. Frequency of hallucinations and other behavioral symptoms did not differ between subjects with and without comorbidity.

These authors suggest that psychiatric comorbidity has been relatively less investigated in psychotic disorders for three main reasons. First, it has frequently been assumed that any concomitant psychiatric disorder that is hierarchically lower than the principal diagnosis may not require an adjunctive diagnosis. Second, concomitant psychiatric syndromes in psychosis may represent nonspecific by-products of psychosis rather than distinct co-occurring disorders and, third, the validity of multiple diagnoses in psychotic disorders may be confounded by factors such as symptom overlap, effects of treatments and information bias.

Considerably lower prevalence rates of comorbid disorders were found in a study investigating a sample of 102 first-hospitalized psychotic patients (schizophrenia spectrum, mood disorders and delusional disorder) (Strakowski *et al.* 1995). The overall psychiatric comorbidity was 40.2%. Substance abuse was the most commonly diagnosed disorder in this sample, with alcohol abuse/dependence being reported in 18.6% and other substance abuse/dependence in 13.7% of the subjects. Regarding the anxiety disorders, OCD was diagnosed in 7.8%, simple or social phobia in 6.9% and panic disorder in 5.9%. Patients with schizophrenia spectrum disorders had the highest rate of comorbid diagnoses. The presence of a comorbid diagnosis in these patients was associated with longer hospitalization.

On the other hand, in a cohort of subjects with nonaffective psychoses ascertained from the general population in the National Comorbidity Survey, prevalence rates of psychiatric comorbidity were considerably higher (Kendler *et al.* 1996). In this survey, only 7% of subjects did *not* receive at least one additional psychiatric diagnosis. The most common comorbid disorders were alcohol dependence (43.2%), other substance dependence (37.7%), social phobia (39.5%), simple phobia (30.8%), and panic disorder (25.5%). One reason for the high levels of comorbid diagnoses in this study is that a community-based sample is more likely to include patients with untreated forms of illness.

Cosoff and Hafner (1998) evaluated the prevalence of anxiety disorders in 100 inpatients with a Diagnostic Statistical Manual, fourth edition (DSM-IV; American Psychiatric Association [APA] 1994) diagnosis of schizophrenia, schizoaffective disorder or bipolar disorder. The proportion of subjects with an anxiety disorder was similar across the three diagnostic groups (43–45%). The most common disorders in the schizophrenia group were social phobia (17%), OCD (13%) and generalized anxiety disorder, while in the bipolar group the most common comorbid diagnoses were OCD (30%) and panic disorder (15%). Almost none of the subjects were receiving treatment for their comorbid anxiety disorders, and in fact these conditions were rarely recognized. The authors point out that, in view of the fact that anxiety disorders are relatively responsive to treatment, greater recognition of their coexistence with psychotic disorders should yield worthwhile clinical benefits.

Aspects of the epidemiology of specific anxiety disorders in schizophrenia will be discussed in the relevant sections below.

Anxiety symptoms as a core dimension of schizophrenia

It has become clear that affective symptoms are frequently encountered in patients with schizophrenia, in spite of the fact that diminished affective response, as initially described by both Kraepelin and Bleuler, is a key feature of the illness. These anxious and depressive symptoms do not appear to be ascribable to comorbid mood and anxiety disorders—they coexist with the acute psychotic symptoms, and usually resolve with successful antipsychotic treatment (Koreen *et al.* 1993).

Clinical features

For many years, when investigating the symptoms of schizophrenia, the focus of attention fell on the positive and the negative symptoms. Crow (1980) introduced the concept of two broad dimensions—positive and negative symptoms—that represented different subtypes of schizophrenia. However, subsequent studies preferentially yielded a three-dimensional model of negative, psychosis and disorganization factors. More recently, and particularly with the advent of the second-generation antipsychotics, attention has shifted to other symptoms that accompany the illness. The Positive and Negative Syndrome Scale (PANSS) (Kay 1991) identified an affective dimension, comprising anxiety and depressive symptoms. Using principal component and factor analytical techniques, Kay (1991) found that anxiety and depressive symptoms clustered together as a single factor. This finding has been replicated in subsequent work (Hansen *et al*. 1998; Lykouras *et al*. 2000).

In a study, for example, in which we investigated depressive and anxiety symptoms in a sample of 177 subjects with schizophrenia or schizophreniform disorder who were assessed by means of the PANSS (Emsley *et al*. 1999a), we were initially interested in looking at anxiety and depressive symptoms separately. To determine whether these were in fact separate entities, we selected the PANSS items that we considered to represent "pure" anxiety symptoms (G2 [anxiety] and G4 [tension]) and depressive (G3 [guilt feelings] and G6 [depression]) symptoms and correlated them. A highly significant correlation was found between these factors, indicating that depressive and anxiety symptoms largely occurred together in our sample of patients. We therefore examined depression and anxiety factors together, using the items identified by Kay for the affective factor (G1 [somatic concern], G2 [anxiety], G3 [guilt feelings] and G6 [depression]) (Kay 1991). Of particular interest was that depressive and anxiety symptoms were more common in patients with predominantly positive symptoms. Positive symptoms in turn are more common in younger patients, in first psychotic episode, and in women—findings that may account also for the association of affective symptoms with these clinical and demographic variables. Furthermore, depressive and anxiety symptoms predicted a positive response to pharmacotherapy.

The significant correlation that we found between affective symptoms and positive symptoms is consistent with other studies reporting a similar association (Norman & Malla 1994; Lysaker *et al*. 1995). Several possible explanations exist for this finding. First, according to the stress-diathesis model, these affective symptoms may constitute a stressor that triggers a psychotic episode (Siris 1993). Second, the affective symptoms could be secondary to the positive symptoms and, third, it could be that affective symptoms and positive symptoms are common manifestations of the same underlying pathologic process. The latter

explanation is consistent with a previous proposal that affective symptoms are a core part of schizophrenia that occur at the height of the psychosis and diminish over time with treatment (Koreen *et al*. 1993).

Course

Whatever the origins of these affective symptoms in schizophrenia, they are of considerable clinical importance. Their existence may compromise social and vocational functioning, they may detrimentally effect compliance, and they are associated with an increased risk of relapse (Birchwood *et al*. 1993) and suicide (Roy *et al*. 1983).

The presence of affective symptoms in the acute phases of schizophrenia appears to be associated with a favorable outcome (Kay & Lindenmayer 1987; Siris 1991; Emsley *et al*. 1999a). In fact, Kay (1991), in his factor analysis of PANSS scores, found that the affective dimension was the only clinical variable to emerge as a reliable predictor of good outcome. However, in the chronic course of the illness affective symptoms are associated with a poorer outcome (McGlashan & Carpenter 1976; Mandel *et al*. 1982).

Pathogenesis

Considerable progress has been made over the past decade or so in our understanding of the biological basis of many psychiatric disorders, including schizophrenia and the anxiety disorders. Accumulating evidence indicates that the symptoms of schizophrenia are related to neurochemical and/or morphological brain abnormalities. Particularly from a neurochemical and psychopharmacological point of view, there are interesting points of convergence between schizophrenia and the anxiety disorders. This raises the possibility that interplay between neurotransmitter systems could account for at least some of the circumstances where schizophrenia and anxiety disorders coexist. Of particular interest in this regard are the dopaminergic and serotonergic systems. Although a range of additional neurochemical systems (glutamate, benzodiazepine, peptide, hormonal) may also be pertinent, we will focus on these two systems.

Dopamine and schizophrenia

For decades, the "dopamine (DA) hypothesis" was regarded as the most likely model for explaining the pathophysiology of schizophrenia. This hypothesis proposes that the symptoms of the illness are related to increased central dopaminergic neurotransmission (Davis *et al.* 1991). Supportive evidence includes the following: DA receptor blockers are effective in treating the illness (Snyder 1976); DA agonists are known to exacerbate the symptoms of schizophrenia (Snyder 1972); increased numbers of D2 receptors have been found in postmortem schizophrenic brains (Clardy *et al.* 1993); positron-emission tomography (PET) studies show a relationship between striatal D2 receptor occupancy and clinical efficacy (Kapur & Remington 1996); and PET studies indicate an abnormal function of presynaptic dopaminergic neurones (Farde 1997). Although the DA hypothesis has proven untenable in its original form, research over the past decade or so gives compelling evidence for a role for DA.

One of the problems with the original hypothesis was that not all of the core symptoms of the illness are equally responsive to treatment with DA antagonists. The negative symptoms and cognitive deficits are particularly difficult to treat with conventional antipsychotic agents. Another problem was that the second generation antipsychotic clozapine, while being the most effective treatment for chronic schizophrenia, has the lowest levels of D2 occupancy of all the antipsychotic agents (Farde *et al.* 1994) indicating that other pathways are also likely to be involved.

Serotonin and schizophrenia

Serotonin (5-hydroxytryptamine [5-HT]) has frequently been implicated in the etiology of schizophrenia. Recently, interest in the relationship between 5-HT and schizophrenia has been rekindled due to the fact that the second-generation antipsychotic agents are potent 5-HT2A receptor antagonists and relatively weak D2 antagonists (Iqbal & van Praag 1995). These drugs have a reduced potential for inducing extrapyramidal side-effects, and as a group appear to have greater efficacy in treating negative and mood symptoms and in improving cognitive function in schizophrenia (Meltzer 1999).

However, studies report variable and inconsistent results, and the nature of 5-HT involvement in schizophrenia is still unclear. While postmortem brain tissue analysis, cerebrospinal fluid studies, and pharmacological challenges point to a deficit in 5-HT function in the cortex of patients with schizophrenia, 5-HT2

antagonism is claimed to have beneficial effects on both positive and negative symptoms of the illness (Abi *et al.* 1997). Although postmortem studies have been mostly inconclusive, the most promising findings involve a reduction in 5-HT2 receptors and 5-HT re-uptake sites in the prefrontal cortex of schizophrenic patients (Ohuoha *et al.* 1993). However, recently (Lewis *et al.* 1999) in a PET study of 13 drug-free schizophrenics and 26 matched controls, failed to find a decrease in 5-HT receptors. These authors concluded that a primary serotonergic abnormality in schizophrenia, if one exists, is either minor, or unlikely to involve the 5-HT2 receptors. They suggest that the therapeutic contribution for 5-HT2 antagonists is likely to be an indirect one. Bleich *et al.* (1988) proposed that 5-HT postsynaptic receptor hypersensitivity could be related to the negative symptoms of schizophrenia.

Dopamine–serotonin interaction

There are various complex anatomical and functional interactions between DA and 5-HT. Overall, reduced 5-HT activity is associated with enhancement of DA activity. This interaction may account for the beneficial effects of the second-generation antipsychotics. Meltzer (1989) formulated a serotonin-dopamine hypothesis, proposing that abnormalities in serotonergic modulation of dopaminergic activity played a role in schizophrenia. He also proposed that the enhanced antipsychotic effect of clozapine and other second-generation antipsychotics might be due to normalization of the interactions between 5-HT and DA systems, as all of these compounds have strong 5-HT antagonistic properties. On the basis of molecular biological studies suggesting that allelic variations of 5-HT receptor genes may affect both susceptibility to schizophrenia and clinical response to atypical antipsychotics, it has been suggested that 5-HT receptors are critical sites of second-generation antipsychotic action (Busatto & Kerwin 1997). While the association between striatal D2 receptor occupancy rates and antipsychotic efficacy is not entirely clear-cut, 5-HT2A occupancy rates are associated with favorable treatment outcome for depressive symptoms and cognitive function in schizophrenia (Kasper *et al.* 1999).

Taken together, strong evidence exists for the involvement—either directly or indirectly—of dopaminergic and serotonergic systems in both schizophrenia and the anxiety disorders. It seems likely that these two systems are particularly relevant in patients with comorbid schizophrenia and anxiety disorders. The underlying mechanisms involved appear to be complex, and different patterns of dysregulation of these neurotransmitter systems may explain the emergence of different anxiety syndromes in subjects with schizophrenia. Also, the effect of antipsychotic medication, particularly the new 5-HT2 D2 antagonists, seems to be considerable.

Treatment

Of further importance is the fact that these affective symptoms appear to be amenable to treatment. In the acute phase, most affective symptoms resolve with successful treatment of the psychosis with antipsychotics (Koreen et al. 1993). Perhaps because of their serotonergic effects (see above), the atypical antipsychotics may be particularly valuable in treating the affective dimension of schizophrenia symptoms. Recently, olanzapine was found to be more effective than haloperidol in reducing depressive signs and symptoms in patients with schizophrenia—an effect that was independent of improvement in psychotic symptoms (Tollefson et al. 1998). In two other trials, the efficacy of olanzapine in treating anxious and depressive symptoms accompanying schizophrenia was assessed. In the first study the sample comprised 335 subjects with chronic schizophrenia in acute exacerbation. Anxiety and depressive symptoms were assessed by means of the Brief Psychiatric Rating Scale (BPRS) cluster (items 1, 2, 5, 9). Three fixed doses of olanzapine (5, 10 or 15 mg ± 2.5 mg) were compared to haloperidol 10–20 mg or placebo over 6 weeks. Two dose ranges of olanzapine (10 and 15 mg) were superior to placebo, whereas haloperidol was not (Tollefson et al. 1998). The second study was a posthoc analysis of the BPRS anxiety-depression cluster in a sample of 1996 subjects with schizophrenia or a related diagnosis randomly assigned to olanzapine (5–20 mg/day) or haloperidol (5–20 mg/day) in a multinational, double-blind trial. Olanzapine therapy was associated with a significantly greater baseline to endpoint improvement in the affective cluster compared to haloperidol therapy (Tollefson & Sanger 1999). Also, decreased levels of depression and suicidality have been reported in treatment-refractory patients who were treated with clozapine (Meltzer & Okayli 1995).

OCD and schizophrenia

It has been long recognized that there are similarities between the symptoms of OCD and schizophrenia. The first description of obsessive-compulsive (OC) symptoms in patients with schizophrenia appeared in the literature in 1878 (Westphal 1878). In fact, early descriptions of OCD regarded the condition as having intrinsic connections to psychotic disorders, and patients with combined OC and psychotic symptoms were considered to be suffering from a variant of schizophrenia. However, the later development of a fundamental dichotomy between neurotic and psychotic disorders resulted in OCD coming to be regarded as a neurosis. Insel and Akiskal (1986) argue that the tradition of labeling OCD as a neurosis has resulted in clinicians overlooking aspects of the syndrome that resemble psychotic rather than neurotic psychopathology.

Recently, however, the association between OCD and schizophrenia has again become a topic of interest. Not only does this association raise important clinical considerations, but also investigation of subjects with comorbid OCD and schizophrenia may shed new light on the pathogenesis of the two disorders. Generally, researchers have investigated an association between the two disorders from two different perspectives: OC symptoms in patients with schizophrenia and other psychotic disorders; and psychotic symptoms in patients with diagnosed OCD.

Clinical features

Earlier studies, which suffered from various methodological shortcomings, reported a variable rate of comorbidity between these two disorders. More recent work, in which systematic diagnostic criteria have been used, suggest that the rate of coexistence of symptoms of the two disorders is higher than previously thought, and higher than could be expected by chance (Berman et al. 1998; Emsley et al. 1999b).

Obsessive-compulsive symptoms in schizophrenia
The frequency of occurrence of OC symptoms in patients with schizophrenia has been reported as between 3.5% and 25% (Rosen 1957; Fenton & McGlashan 1986; Poyurovsky et al. 1999; Kruger et al. 2000). The wide variation in frequency probably reflects different methods of assessment, different samples studied and

Table 10.1 Reported prevalence of OC symptoms and OCD in patients with schizophrenia

Study	Sample	Sample size	% OC symptoms	% OCD symptoms
Rosen (1957)	Schizophrenia	848	3.5	—
Fenton & McGlashan (1986)	Schizophrenia	163	12.9	—
Strakowski *et al.* (1993)	First-hospitalized psychosis	102	—	7.8
Berman *et al.* (1995a)	Chronic schizophrenia	102	25.0	—
Eisen *et al.* (1997)	Schizophrenia, schizoaffective	77	—	7.8
Cassano *et al.* (1998)	Schizophrenia spectrum	31	—	29.0
Cosoff & Haffner (1998)	Schizophrenia	—	—	13.0
Poyurovsky *et al.* (1999)	First-episode schizophrenia spectrum	50	—	14.0
Kruger *et al.* (2000)	Schizophrenia	76	—	15.8

OC, obsessive compulsive; OCD, obsessive-compulsive disorder.

different criteria used to diagnose OC symptoms as well as schizophrenia.

Early studies used retrospective or other problematic methodologies. Rosen (1957) retrospectively reviewed the charts of 848 patients with schizophrenia and found prominent OC features in 30 (3.5%). These patients had more prominent depressive and paranoid features and appeared to have a favorable prognosis. The OC symptoms either preceded or coincided with the onset of the psychotic symptoms in every case. However, in only 7 of these cases did the delusion represent a transition from an obsession. In another retrospective review of 163 patients with DSM-III (APA 1980) diagnosed schizophrenia, Fenton and McGlashan (1986) found that 21 (12.9%) of their subjects with schizophrenia had prominent OC symptoms. Berman *et al.* (1995a) interviewed the treating physicians in a sample of 102 patients with chronic schizophrenia. Prominent OC symptoms were reported in 27 (25%) (Table 10.1).

More recent studies have used prospective designs with structured interviews. Eisen *et al.* (1997) found that only 6 (7.8%) of 77 patients with schizophrenia or schizoaffective disorder also met DSM-III-R (APA 1987) criteria for OCD. This was a well-designed study that utilized the Structured Interview for DSM-III-R (SCID) and the Yale–Brown Obsessive Compulsive Scale (Y-BOCS), as well as a review of the patients' charts and an interview with the treating clinicians. In another methodologically sound study 50 hospitalized patients with first-episode psychosis

who met DSM-IV criteria for schizophrenia spectrum disorders were assessed for OCD (Poyurovsky *et al.* 1999). Patients were again assessed by means of the SCID and Y-BOCS, as well as the Schedule for the Assessment of Positive Symptoms (SAPS) and the Schedule for the Assessment of Negative Symptoms (SANS). Seven patients (14%) met DSM-IV criteria for OCD. The subjects with OCD had significantly lower scores than the subjects without OCD on the formal thought disorder subscale of the SAPS and the flattened affect subscale of the SANS. The authors proposed that the coexistence of OCD with schizophrenia might have a "protective" effect on some of the symptoms of schizophrenia. Finally, Kruger *et al.* (2000) found that 12 of 76 patients (15.8%) with schizophrenia met the criteria for OCD. Compared to the schizophrenic subjects without OCD, these subjects had more motor symptoms, including catatonia. This finding was regarded as supportive of a basal ganglia-frontal lobe connection linking OCD with schizophrenia.

While the latter three studies looked at the coexistence of OC *disorder* in patients with schizophrenia, the incidence of OC *symptoms* is likely to be considerably higher. In a sample of 13 patients with schizophrenia, Yaryura-Tobias *et al.* (1995) found higher than expected scores on the Y-BOCS and the Self Rated Symptom Scale for OCD. They also found great similarities in thought process impairment and perceptual deficits when these patients were compared with 22 OCD subjects.

Using neurocognitive testing, Berman *et al.* (1998) investigated whether the presence of obsessions and compulsions represented a distinct cluster of symptoms in schizophrenia. Patients with coexisting OC symptoms performed worse than those without such symptoms in several cognitive areas, and severity of OC scores correlated significantly with poor performance. These results were interpreted as supporting the hypothesis that OC symptoms may constitute a distinct cluster separate from psychosis, and raise the possibility of a distinct subtype of schizophrenia.

Psychotic symptoms in OCD

OCD patients represent a heterogeneous mix of clinical phenotypes (Sobin *et al.* 2000). Clinical observations indicate that not all OCD patients recognize their obsessions as being irrational or excessive. These ideas have usually been described as overvalued or delusional. From their review of the literature concerning insight amongst patients with OCD, Kozak and Foa (1994) concluded that OC ideas cannot be dichotomised according to patients' insight, and proposed that a continuum representing the strength of OC beliefs is more appropriate. They emphasized that the relationship between the strength of OC conviction and treatment outcome remains unclear.

As far back as 1875, du Saulle (Berrois 1989) reported psychotic symptoms in some of the 27 OCD patients he described. He noted that the patients with psychotic symptoms also had more severe pathology and poorer insight. Janet (Pittman 1987) reported psychotic symptoms in 7.7% of patients with OCD. Insel and Akiskal (1986) reviewed the literature of OCD with psychotic features. They list nine studies (Muller 1953; Rudin 1953; Pollit 1957; Ingram 1961; Kringlen 1965; Lo 1967; Rosenberg 1968; Bratfos 1970; Welner *et al.* 1976) in which patients who had been diagnosed as OCD were investigated for the presence of psychotic symptoms. The incidence of schizophrenia in these studies ranged from 0.7% to 12.3%. The authors caution that these were retrospective studies with the diagnoses being made by chart review, and that standardized diagnostic criteria were not used. Some patients were regarded as being psychotic in the sense of a transient loss of insight or the emergence of paranoid ideas.

There appears to be considerable heterogeneity in the clinical features of the OCD patients who also have psychotic symptoms. Eisen and Rasmussen (1993) attempted to identify and characterize the demographic and clinical features of subjects with OCD and psychotic symptoms. From a sample of 475 patients meeting DSM-III criteria for OCD they identified 67 (14%) as having psychotic symptoms, defined as hallucinations, delusions, or thought disorder. However, in 27 (6%), the only "psychotic" symptom was lack of insight and strong conviction about the reasonableness of the obsessions, and 14 (3%) met criteria for schizotypal personality disorder. The remainder of the subjects met criteria for specific psychotic disorders. Eighteen (4%) met criteria for schizophrenia and eight (2%) for delusional disorder. Compared to the OCD patients without psychosis, the subjects with OCD and psychotic features were more likely to be male, single, have a deteriorating course, and to have had their first treatment at a younger age. The data suggested that these features were largely explained by those patients with schizophrenia spectrum disorders.

A recent study (Sobin *et al.* 2000) investigated the possibility that schizotypal traits could distinguish a subtype of OCD. They obtained schizotypy scores from 119 subjects who met lifetime criteria for DSM-IV OCD. They found that 50% of the sample had mild to severe schizotypy scores. The variables that distinguished OCD patients with schizotypy were: earlier age of onset, greater number of comorbid diagnoses, increased rates of learning disability, counting compulsions, and a history of specific phobia. Indeed, OCD with schizotypal traits may be characterized by particular neurobiological factors (see below).

The coexistence of OCD and schizophrenia appears to be greater than could be expected on the basis of calculated comorbidity figures (Tibbo & Warneke 1999). Taken together, the evidence points to a small but significant subset of patients sharing OCD and schizophrenia symptoms. It is not clear whether this represents a distinct clinical entity, or the extremes of a continuum. Future studies need to focus on possible risk factors, clinical features, underlying mechanisms and whether these patients respond differentially to various treatment options.

Outcome

Some of the earlier studies reported a relatively favorable outcome in OCD patients with psychotic features. Insel and Akiskal (1986) noted that the deteriorating course that is often characteristic of schizophrenia is extremely rare in OCD patients with psychotic symptoms. Thus, the occurrence of psychotic features in patients with OCD may often be due to a delusional disorder or a mood disorder rather than a schizophrenic illness. However, in contrast to many of the other studies, Eisen and Rasmussen (1993) found that OCD patients with features of schizophrenia had a poorer outcome.

OCD and schizophrenia: pathogenesis

Evidence from various sources suggests that dopaminergic and serotonergic pathways are important in both schizophrenia and OCD. Dopamine-blocking agents have been the mainstay of the treatment of schizophrenia for many years, and striatal D2 receptor occupancy above about 70% consistently predicts antipsychotic efficacy (Nyberg et al. 1996; Remington & Kapur 1999). Preclinical and clinical studies have reported that dopamine plays a role in OCD and in related disorders such as Tourette's disorder (Goodman et al. 1990; Hollander et al. 1992; Szechtman et al. 1999).

Furthermore, OCD patients with comorbid tics are more likely to fail treatment with serotonin reuptake inhibitors, but in such patients augmentation with haloperidol has been found to be effective (McDougle et al. 1994). The second generation antipsychotics are of particular interest, because of their combined dopaminergic and serotonergic antagonistic properties. Indeed, several open-label studies suggest improved efficacy with atypical antipsychotic augmentation in treatment-refractory OCD (Jacobsen 1995; McDougle et al. 1995; Ravizza et al. 1996; Saxena et al. 1996; Stein et al. 1997), and there is now also a confirmatory controlled study (McDougle et al. 2000).

On the other hand, cases have been reported of patients with schizophrenia who have developed OC symptoms while being treated with the novel antipsychotics clozapine (Baker et al. 1992; Patil 1992; Patel & Tandon 1993; Allen & Tejera 1994; Eales & Layeni 1994) risperidone (Kopala & Honer 1994; Remington & Adams 1994; Dryden-Edwards & Reiss 1996) and olanzapine (Marazziti et al. 1996; Koran et al. 2000). The emergence of OC symptoms appears to be differentiated from the antipsychotic effect of risperidone. In a single case study psychotic symptoms ceased during treatment with risperidone, but the patient experienced an incapacitating exacerbation of pre-existing OC symptoms. These symptoms were only briefly and partially improved with the addition of a serotonin reuptake inhibitor (SSRI), but subsided after discontinuation of risperidone (Dryden-Edwards & Reiss 1996). The frequency of treatment-emergent OC symptoms with second-generation antipsychotics in patients with schizophrenia is not known. It may be very rare, as a retrospective review of 142 randomly selected hospital files of patients on clozapine treatment failed to identify a single case of OC symptoms worsening or emerging during treatment (Ghaemi et al. 1995). Also, in a subanalysis of a prospective study of olanzapine versus placebo in schizophrenia, OC symptoms were no more frequent in the olanzapine group than in the placebo group. To complicate matters further, the emergence of OC symptoms during clozapine withdrawal has been reported in two schizophrenic patients. Resumption of the clozapine led to complete resolution of the OC symptoms in both cases (Poyurovsky et al. 1998).

These apparently paradoxical findings with the second-generation antipsychotics—i.e. efficacy in treatment-refractory OCD on the one hand and treatment-emergent OC symptoms in patients with schizophrenia on the other—point to a complex interrelationship between serotonergic and dopaminergic systems in the pathogenesis of OC symptoms in schizophrenia. It would appear that there is significant overlap in neurotransmitter dysfunction in the putative circuits of OCD and schizophrenia, which may lead to the coexpression of symptoms of both disorders. It is possible that the emergence of OC symptoms during treatment with the second-generation antipsychotics is a coincidental occurrence, or it may represent a rare idiosyncratic reaction. However, it could also be argued that patients with coexisting OC symptoms and psychosis and those with treatment-resistant OCD represent two subgroups of patients with distinct underlying disorders of dopaminergic and serotonergic function (Emsley et al. 1999b). Thus, patients with coexisting OCD and psychosis may experience exacerbation of OC symptoms with combined dopamine and serotonin blockade, while patients with treatment-refractory OCD appear to respond favorably to this intervention. Evidence from other sources may partly explain the differential effect on OC symptoms in patients with psychosis and in patients with OCD—functional brain-imaging studies have reported an opposite pattern of frontal lobe activity in OCD and schizophrenia (Buchsbaum et al. 1997). Furthermore, a neuropsychological study has described a double dissociation of frontal lobe functioning in subjects with OCD and those with schizophrenia (Abbruzzese *et al.* 1997), arguably reflecting a dorsolateral prefrontal cortex deficit in schizophrenia and orbitofrontal cortex involvement in OCD.

The study mentioned above in which more motor symptoms in schizophrenia subjects with OCD were reported compared to those without (Kruger *et al.* 2000), supports the hypothesis of a basal ganglia-frontal lobe connection linking OCD with schizophrenia. The relationship between OCD and psychosis was also examined in a functional magnetic resonance imaging (fMRI) study on a group of schizophrenic patients with varying degrees of OC symptomatology (Levine *et al.* 1998). In this study, in a subset of patients a significant negative relationship was found between OC symptoms and activation of the left dorsolateral prefrontal cortex, suggesting that circuits other than the orbito-frontal-striatal connections known to be significant in OCD, may be important in patients with both schizophrenia and OCD.

Treatment

Several reports have suggested that treatment of OC symptoms in schizophrenia with a serotonin reuptake inhibitor (SRI) in conjunction with antipsychotic medication may be effective. In a more persuasive double-blind, crossover study, six subjects with DSM-III-R chronic schizophrenia with OC symptoms were treated with clomipramine or placebo, added to their maintenance antipsychotic medication. Patients were rated according to the PANSS and Y-BOCS scales. Patients on clomipramine showed significantly greater improvement of OC symptoms. No patients experienced an exacerbation of psychotic symptoms (Berman *et al.* 1995b). OCD subjects with delusions respond poorly to antipsychotic medication, but may improve on SSRIs and behavior therapy (O'Dwyer & Marks 2000).

Panic disorder and schizophrenia

Despite the fact that patients suffering from schizophrenia frequently report experiencing panic attacks, little research has been done in this area. Consequently little is known about the association between these two conditions.

Clinical features

Studies investigating the frequency of comorbid psychiatric disorders in schizophrenia report the frequency of panic attacks as between 5.9% and 25.5% (Argyle 1990; Strakowski *et al.* 1993; Kendler *et al.* 1996; Labbate *et al.* 1999). Labbate *et al.* (1999), for example, examined 49 subjects meeting DSM-IV criteria for chronic schizophrenia or schizoaffective disorder by administering appropriate sections of the SCID. The subjects who reported panic attacks were further questioned about treatment and about the onset of panic attacks relative to psychotic symptoms. Twenty-one (43%) experienced panic attacks, and 16 (33%) had a current or past panic disorder. Eight (50%) of the latter had received treatment for panic attacks. Patients with paranoid schizophrenia were more likely to have panic attacks or panic disorder. Substance dependence was not associated with panic attacks or panic disorder.

Approximately one-quarter of schizophrenic and schizoaffective patients with postpsychotic depression were found to experience panic attacks (Cutler & Siris 1991). This may be a particularly important group of patients to identify, as the risk of suicide appears to be increased in these patients. Siris *et al.* (1993) found significant associations between lifetime history of suicidal ideation and a lifetime history of panic attacks or panic disorder in a sample of 40 schizophrenic patients with postpsychotic depression (Table 10.2).

Pathogenesis

Although panic attacks and schizophrenia commonly coexist, little is known about the reason for this association. Hofmann (1999) proposes four possibilities. First, it could simply be due to a methodological artefact. Second, it may be that panic attacks cause schizophrenic symptoms. Third, schizophrenic symptoms may cause or precipitate panic attacks. Fourth, panic attacks and schizophrenic symptoms may share a common etiology. The latter is arguably the most likely reason. Another possibility, at least in some patients, is that the panic attacks are induced by antipsychotic medication. Higuchi *et al.* (1999) found that nine (20%) of 45 patients with chronic schizophrenia met DSM-III-R criteria for panic disorder, and all nine were taking antipsychotics in higher doses than the others. New onset panic attacks have also been reported

Table 10.2 Reported prevalence of panic attacks and PD in patients with schizophrenia.

Study	Sample	Sample size	% Panic attacks	% PD
Strakowski *et al.* (1993)	First-hospitalized psychosis	102	—	5.9
Cassano *et al.* (1998)	Schizophrenia spectrum	31	—	19.4
Kendler *et al.* (1996)	Nonaffective psychoses	74	—	25.5
Argyle (1990)	Schizophrenia	20	35	—
Labbate *et al.* (1999)	Schizophrenia schizoaffective	49	43	33.0
Higuchi *et al.* (1999)	Chronic schizophrenia	45	—	20.0
Cutler & Siris (1991)	Schizophrenia with postpsychotic depression	45	25	—

PD, panic disorder.

in a patient being treated with olanzapine (Mandalos & Szarek 1999).

Heun and Maier (1995) conducted a family study to investigate the relationship between schizophrenia and panic disorder. The sample comprised 59 patients with schizophrenia, 54 with panic disorder and 29 patients with comorbid diagnoses of panic disorder and schizophrenia. A significant difference was found in the familial loading for primary panic disorders in schizophrenics (4.3%) compared to controls (0.9%), while the risk for schizophrenia was not enhanced in relatives of patients with panic disorder (0%) compared to controls (0.3%). These results were interpreted as suggesting an etiological relationship between schizophrenia and panic disorder, or at least a relationship between subgroups of these disorders.

Treatment

Few studies have examined the treatment of panic attacks in schizophrenia. Arlow *et al.* (1997) conducted an open label 16-week clinical trial of cognitive behavioral therapy for the treatment of panic attacks in eight patients with DSM-III-R schizophrenia. There was a significant reduction in panic symptoms as well as in the number of attacks compared with baseline ratings, suggesting that this is a worthwhile treatment approach. In a single case report, alprazolam added to antipsychotic medication was effective in treating panic attacks in a patient with schizophrenia (Sandberg & Siris 1987). Similar findings were also reported in seven patients with schizophrenia (Kahn *et al.* 1988). Interestingly, these latter patients all showed marked improvement of positive and negative symptoms as

well as reduction of panic attacks with alprazolam. This finding was replicated in a sample of 12 schizophrenic patients without panic attacks—the addition of alprazolam was associated with significant, albeit modest, reductions in psychotic features (Wolkowitz *et al.* 1988). In a recent literature review of the SSRIs in schizophrenia with panic attacks no studies were found, in spite of the fact that these drugs have become first-line pharmacotherapy for panic disorder (Pollack & Marzol 2000).

PTSD and schizophrenia

Once again, there is a relative paucity of good research into the associations between these two disorders.

Clinical features

The association between PTSD and psychosis has been investigated from two angles: psychotic symptoms have been studied in PTSD patients, and PTSD symptoms have been explored in patients with schizophrenia.

Psychotic symptoms in PTSD

Psychotic symptoms occur frequently in PTSD, and they appear to correlate with severity of PTSD symptoms (Hamner *et al.* 2000) and comorbid depression (Hamner 1997; David *et al.* 1999). It has been suggested that these patients represent a distinct subtype of PTSD (Hamner *et al.* 2000). The psychotic features that have been reported include auditory and visual hallucinations, and delusions that are frequently paranoid in nature. For example, in a study assessing 53 combat

Table 10.3 Reported prevalence of PTSD in patients with schizophrenia.

Study	Sample	Sample size	% PTSD
Strakowski *et al.* (1993)	First-hospitalized psychosis	102	1.0
Kendler *et al.* (1996)	Nonaffective psychoses	74	28.9
Priebe *et al.* (1998)	Schizophrenia	105	51.0
Meyer *et al.* (1999)	Schizophrenia and delusional	46	11.0

PTSD, post-traumatic stress disorder.

veterans with PTSD it was found that 40% reported experiencing psychotic symptoms in the preceding 6 months. These symptoms featured auditory hallucinations in all but one case, and typically reflected combat scenes and guilt, were nonbizarre, and were not usually associated with other features of schizophrenia such as formal thought disorder or flat or inappropriate affect.

In comparing 40 subjects with chronic PTSD and well-defined psychotic features with 40 subjects with schizophrenia, it was found that the two groups of subjects were remarkably similar with regard not only to positive symptoms, but negative symptoms as well (Hamner *et al.* 2000). In fact, it has been proposed, rather speculatively, that negative symptoms are manifestations of a traumatic stress disorder that is fundamentally similar to chronic PTSD (Stampfer 1990). Compared to PTSD patients without psychosis on the one hand, and patients with psychosis without PTSD on the other, patients with PTSD and a comorbid psychotic disorder showed excessive cognitive, emotional and behavioral disturbances (Sautter *et al.* 1999).

The treatment of PTSD with psychotic symptoms has only recently received attention. Preliminary work suggests that the atypical antipsychotics may be useful in such patients (Hamner *et al.* 2000).

PTSD in schizophrenia

Psychosis has been regarded as one of the most severe stressors to which one can be subjected (Lundy 1992). It could therefore be expected that some patients who experience psychotic episodes would develop symptoms of PTSD. In fact, PTSD is a common comorbid disorder in schizophrenia that is frequently unrecognized in clinical settings. The prevalence of PTSD in psychotic disorders has been reported as between 11% and 51% (Shaw *et al.* 1997; Mueser *et al.* 1998; Priebe

et al. 1998; Meyer *et al.* 1999). Comorbid PTSD is rarely recognized in these patients—the rate of PTSD was found to be 43% in a sample of severe mental illnesses (e.g. schizophrenia and bipolar disorder)—but in only 2% of these subjects had this diagnosis been made clinically (Mueser *et al.* 1998) (Table 10.3).

Pathogenesis

It has been suggested that PTSD may be a useful paradigm for assessing the psychological response to the distressing experience of hospitalization and psychosis. Meyer *et al.* (1999) assessed 46 schizophrenic and delusional patients and found the prevalence of PTSD to be 11%. Traumatic symptoms were related to psychosis in 69%, and to hospitalization in 24%, suggesting that psychotic symptoms are more traumatic to patients than the coercive measures that are used to control them. Additional evidence also suggests that the consequences of hospitalization are less important in the genesis of PTSD symptoms in psychotic patients. In a sample of 105 community-care patients with schizophrenia it was found that 51% fulfilled criteria for PTSD (Priebe *et al.* 1998). In this sample the role of involuntary admissions was examined as a possible contributing factor, and found not to correlate with PTSD symptoms.

Social phobia and schizophrenia

Clinical features

Many patients with schizophrenia exhibit features of social phobia, namely social anxiety and avoidance of social situations. The prevalence of social phobia has been reported as 16.1% in hospitalized patients with schizophrenia spectrum disorders (Cassano *et al.*

Table 10.4 Reported prevalence of social phobia in patients with schizophrenia.

Study	Sample	Sample size	% Social phobia
Strakowski et al. (1993)	First-hospitalized psychosis	102	6.9
Cassano et al. (1998)	Schizophrenia spectrum	31	16.1
Kendler et al. (1996)	Nonaffective psychoses	74	39.5

1998), 17% in a sample of patients with schizophrenia, schizoaffective and bipolar disorder (Cosoff & Hafner 1998) and 39.5% in a community sample of subjects with nonaffective psychosis (Kendler et al. 1996). The prevalence of simple and social phobia was reported as 6.9% in a group of first-hospitalized psychotic patients (Strakowski et al. 1993). In the Cassano et al. study (1998) of all the comorbid disorders, social phobia together with panic disorder and substance abuse disorder, showed the greatest association with psychotic features (Table 10.4).

The relationship between social anxiety and the positive and negative symptoms of schizophrenia was investigated in a sample of 38 inpatients with schizophrenia who completed self-report measures of anxiety, a modified Stroop task, and an unstructured role play activity (Penn et al. 1994). Positive symptoms were significantly related to fear in a number of self-report domains (i.e. social and agoraphobic). Negative symptoms were related to a global observational rating of anxiety during the role-play activity, as well as to specific behaviors associated with self-reported social anxiety (i.e. speech rate and fluency). The authors concluded that specific behaviors related to social anxiety appear to be associated with negative symptoms of schizophrenia, while self-report social anxiety is associated with positive symptoms. However, Stern et al. (1999) did not find a significant correlation between severity of social phobia symptoms and positive and negative symptoms in schizophrenia.

The possibility of social phobia being a precursor to schizophrenia has been addressed in a prospective analysis of antecedent psychopathological features and socio-demographic risk factors in schizophrenia with data from community sites in the Epidemiologic Catchment Area Study (Tien & Eaton 1992). It was found that social phobia (and OCD) were associated with more than three and a half times increased odds of developing schizophrenia.

Pathogenesis and treatment

Speculation for an underlying neurochemical basis for an association between social phobia and schizophrenia is based on indications of serotonergic and dopaminergic dysfunction in both disorders. The atypical antipsychotic clozapine has been reported to induce anxiety symptoms, possibly due to its known effect on serotonergic pathways. Pallanti et al. (1999), for example, reported 12 patients with schizophrenia who developed social phobia during clozapine treatment. These patients represented 43% of a subgroup of patients who were treated with clozapine after being resistant to, or intolerant of, conventional antipsychotics. Fluoxetine was added to their treatment for a period of 12 weeks. In eight cases, symptoms improved according to a priori criteria (≥ 35% reduction in Liebowitz Social Phobia Scale score). Social phobia has also been reported as a treatment-emergent effect of haloperidol (Mikkelsen et al. 1981), suggesting a role for dopamine, which fits with the finding of increased social anxiety in patients with Parkinson's disease (see Chapter 7).

Antipsychotics and anxiety

Patients with schizophrenia require long-term treatment with antipsychotic agents, and there are various important associations between these drugs and anxiety. First, antipsychotics are effective in treating anxiety symptoms in nonpsychotic subjects. The conventional antipsychotics have been used in low dose for many years to treat anxiety states. Also, the second-generation antipsychotics in particular have been recommended as add-on treatment in refractory OCD (McDougle et al. 2000). Second, anxiety may be a direct manifestation of an untoward effect of antipsychotic agents. Akathisia is an extremely common side-effect of conventional antipsychotics, having been reported in up to 75% of schizophrenics on maintenance therapy (Van-Putten *et al.* 1984). Akathisia is less common, but still occurs with the second generation antipsychotics (Jauss *et al.* 1998). A subjective sense of intense anxiety accompanies the motor restlessness in these patients, who report akathisia as extremely distressing. Third, anxiety may be an indirect consequence of the development of side-effects such as acute dystonias, which may be terrifying to patients. Fourth, antipsychotic agents, via an as yet unknown mechanism, may precipitate anxiety symptoms or disorders. Risperidone was reported to cause acute separation anxiety in two adolescents with OCD (Hanna *et al.* 1999), which resolved when risperidone was discontinued. Clozapine has precipitated social phobia in patients with schizophrenia (Pallanti *et al.* 1999), and treatment-emergent OCD has been reported with clozapine (Baker *et al.* 1992; Patil 1992; Patel & Tandon 1993; Allen & Tejera 1994; Eales & Layeni 1994), risperidone (Kopala & Honer 1994; Remington & Adams 1994; Dryden-Edwards & Reiss 1996), and olanzapine (Marazziti *et al.* 1996; Koran *et al.* 2000) (see p. 170).

Finally, antipsychotics have been effectively used to treat anxiety symptoms and comorbid anxiety disorders in psychotic patients. In a posthoc analysis of two randomised clinical trials, risperidone was superior to haloperidol in reducing anxiety/depression symptoms in chronic schizophrenia (Marder *et al.* 1997). Anxiety symptoms were significantly more reduced in risperidone compared to haloperidol patients in 62 subjects with acute exacerbations of schizophrenia (Blin *et al.* 1996). The response of anxiety and depressive symptoms, as assessed by the anxiety-depression cluster of the Brief Psychiatric Rating Scale (BPRS), to olanzapine, haloperidol and placebo, was assessed in a randomised sample of 335 subjects with chronic schizophrenia (Tollefson *et al.* 1998). Two dose-ranges of olanzapine (10 mg and 15 mg/day) were superior to placebo, whereas haloperidol (10–20 mg/day) was not. The authors speculate that this differential benefit seen with olanzapine could be attributed to the drug's more selective mesolimbic dopaminergic profile, D1 or D4 activity, the release of dopamine/norepinephrine (noradrenaline) in the prefrontal cortex, or 5-HT2A antagonism. The beneficial effect in anxiety and depressive symptoms in schizophrenia may not be shared equally by all of the second-generation antipsychotics. In a

sample of 30 treatment-refractory chronic psychotic patients, the BPRS anxiety-depression factor was the factor least influenced by clozapine (Abraham *et al.* 1997).

Conclusion

Anxiety symptoms are common and varied in schizophrenia. Whether representing a reaction to adverse experiences, or due to medication side-effects, comorbid anxiety syndromes, or whether core features of schizophrenia itself, a heightened clinician awareness is clearly indicated. These anxiety symptoms are rarely recognized by treating physicians, in spite of the fact that they may be amenable to treatment intervention. Further research into comorbid anxiety and psychosis may shed light on the pathogenesis not only of this subset of patients, but of schizophrenia and the anxiety disorders as well.

References

Abbruzzese, M., Ferri, S. & Scarone, S. (1997) The selective breakdown of frontal functions in patients with obsessive-compulsive disorder and in patients with schizophrenia: a double dissociation experimental finding. *Neuropsychologia* 35(6), 907–12.

Abi, D.A., Laruelle, M., Aghajanian, G.K., Charney, D. & Krystal, J. (1997) The role of serotonin in the pathophysiology and treatment of schizophrenia. *J Neuropsychiatry Clin Neurosci* 9(1), 1–17.

Abraham, G., Nair, C., Tracy, J.I., Simpson, G.M. & Josiassen, R.C. (1997) The effects of clozapine on symptom clusters in treatment-refractory patients. *J Clin Psychopharmacol* 17(1), 49–53.

Allen, L. & Tejera, C. (1994) Treatment of clozapine-induced obsessive-compulsive symptoms with sertraline. *Am J Psychiatry* 151(7), 1096–7.

American Psychiatric Association (APA) (1980) *Diagnostic Statistical Manual of Mental Disorders*, 3rd edn. American Psychiatric Association, Washington, D.C.

American Psychiatric Association (APA) (1987) *Diagnostic Statistical Manual of Mental Disorders*, 3rd edn, revised. American Psychiatric Association, Washington, D.C.

American Psychiatric Association (APA) (1994) *Diagnostic Statistical Manual of Mental Disorders*, 4th edn. American Psychiatric Association, Washington, D.C.

Argyle, N. (1990) Panic attacks in chronic schizophrenia. *Br J Psychiatry* 157, 430–3.

Arlow, P.B., Moran, M.E., Bermanzohn, P.C., Stronger, R. & Siris, S.G. (1997) Cognitive-behavioral treatment of panic attacks in chronic schizophrenia. *J Psychother Pract Res* 6(2), 145–50.

Baker, R.W., Chengappa, K.N., Baird, J.W., Steingard, S., Christ, M.A. & Schooler, N.R. (1992) Emergence of obsessive-compulsive symptoms during treatment with clozapine [see comments]. *J Clin Psychiatry* 53(12), 439–42.

Berman, I., Kalinowski, A., Berman, S.M., Lengua, J. & Green, A.I. (1995a) Obsessive and compulsive symptoms in chronic schizophrenia. *Compr Psychiatry* 36(1), 6–10.

Berman, I., Merson, A., Viegner, B., Losonczy, M.F., Pappas, D. & Green, A.I. (1998) Obsessions and compulsions as a distinct cluster of symptoms in schizophrenia: a neuropsychological study. *J Nerv Ment Dis* 186(3), 150–6.

Berman, I., Sapers, B.L., Chang, H.H., Losonczy, M.F., Schmildler, J. & Green, A.I. (1995b) Treatment of obsessive-compulsive symptoms in schizophrenic patients with clomipramine. *J Clin Psychopharmacol* 15(3), 206–10.

Berrois, G.E. (1989) Obsessive-compulsive disorder: its conceptual history in France during the 19th century. *Compr Psychiatry* 44, 226–32.

Birchwood, M., Mason, R. & Macmillan, F. (1993) Depression, demoralization and control over psychotic illness: a comparison of depressed and nondepressed patients. *Psychol Med* 23, 387–95.

Bleich, A., Brown, S.L., Kahn, R. & van Praag, H.M. (1988) The role of serotonin in schizophrenia. *Schizophr Bull* 14(2), 297–315.

Blin, O., Azorin, J.M. & Boulhours, P. (1996) Antipsychotic and anxiolytic properties of risperidone, haloperidol, and methotrimeprazine in schizophrenic patients. *J Clin Psychopharmacol* 16, 38–44.

Bratfos, O. (1970) Transition of neuroses and other minor mental disorders into psychoses. *Acta Psychiatr Scand* 46, 35–49.

Buchsbaum, M.S., Spiegel-Cohen, J. & Wei, T. (1997) Three dimensional PET/MRI images in OCD and schizophrenia. *CNS Spectrums* 2, 26–31.

Busatto, G.F. & Kerwin, R.W. (1997) Perspectives on the role of serotonergic mechanisms in the pharmacology of schizophrenia. *J Psychopharmacol* 11(1), 3–12.

Cassano, G.B., Pini, S., Saettoni, M., Rucci, P. & Dell'Osso, L. (1998) Occurrence and clinical correlates of psychiatric comorbidity in patients with psychotic disorders. *J Clin Psychiatry* 59(2), 60–8.

Clardy, J.A., Hyde, T.M. & Kleinman, J.E. (1993) Postmortem neurochemical and neuropathological studies in schizophrenia. In: *Schizophrenia: from Mind to Molecule* (N.C. Andreasen (ed.)) American Psychiatric Press, Washington, D.C., pp. 123–45.

Cosoff, S.J. & Hafner, R.J. (1998) The prevalence of co-morbid anxiety in schizophrenia, schizoaffective disorder and bipolar disorder [see comments]. *Aust N Z J Psychiatry* 32(1), 67–72.

Crow, T. (1980) Molecular pathology of schizophrenia: more than one disease process?. *Br Medical J* 2280, 66–8.

Cutler, J.L. & Siris, S.G. (1991) "Panic-like" symptomatology in schizophrenic and schizoaffective patients with postpsychotic depression: observations and implications. *Compr Psychiatry* 32(6), 465–73.

David, D., Kutcher, G.S., Jackson, E.I. & Mellman, T.A. (1999) Psychotic symptoms in combat-related post-traumatic stress disorder [see comments]. *J Clin Psychiatry* 60(1), 29–32.

Davis, K.L., Kahn, R.S. & Ko, G. (1991) Dopamine in schizophrenia: a review and reconceptualization. *Am J Psychiatry* 148, 1474–86.

Dryden-Edwards, R.C. & Reiss, A.L. (1996) Differential response of psychotic and obsessive symptoms to risperidone in an adolescent. *J Child Adolesc Psychopharmacol* 6(2), 139–45.

Eales, M.J. & Layeni, A.O. (1994) Exacerbation of obsessive-compulsive symptoms associated with clozapine [see comments]. *Br J Psychiatry* 164(5) 687–8.

Eisen, J.L., Beer, D.A., Pato, M.T., Venditto, T.A. & Rasmussen, S.A. (1997) Obsessive-compulsive disorder in patients with schizophrenia or schizoaffective disorder [see comments]. *Am J Psychiatry* 154(2), 271–3.

Eisen, J.L. & Rasmussen, S.A. (1993) Obsessive-compulsive disorder with psychotic features. *J Clin Psychiatry* 54(10), 373–9.

Emsley, R.A., Oosthuizen, P.P., Joubert, A.F., Roberts, M.C. & Stein, D.J. (1999a) Depressive and anxiety symptoms in patients with schizophrenia and schizophreniform disorder. *J Clin Psychiatry* 60(11), 747–51.

Emsley, R.A., Stein, D.J. & Oosthuizen, P.P. (1999b) Co-occurrence of schizophrenia and obsessive-compulsive disorder—a literature review. *S Afr Med J* 9, 1000–2.

Farde, L. (1997) Brain imaging of schizophrenia—the dopamine hypothesis. *Schizophr Res* 28, 157–62.

Farde, L., Nordstrom, A.L., Nyberg, S., Halldin, C. & Sedvall, G. (1994) D1, D2, and 5-HT2 receptor occupancy in clozapine-treated patients. *J Clin Psychiatry* 55 (Suppl. B), 67–9.

Fenton, W.S. & McGlashan, T. (1986) The prognostic significance of obsessive-compulsive symptoms in schizophrenia. *Am J Psychiatry* 143, 437–41.

Ghaemi, S.N., Zarate, C.A. Jr, Popli, A.P., Pillay, S.S. & Cole, J.O. (1995) Is there a relationship between clozapine and obsessive-compulsive disorder? A retrospective chart review [see comments]. *Compr Psychiatry*, 36(4), 267–70.

Goodman, W.K., McDougle, C.J. & Price, L.H. (1990) Beyond the serotonin hypothesis: a role for dopamine in some forms of obsessive-compulsive disorder? *J Clin Psychiatry* **51** (Suppl. 8), 36–43.

Hamner, M.B. (1997) Psychotic features and combat-associated PTSD. *Depress Anxiety* **5**(1), 34–8.

Hamner, M.B., Frueh, B.C., Ulmer, H.G. *et al.* (2000) Psychotic features in chronic post-traumatic stress disorder and schizophrenia: comparative severity. *J Nerv Ment Dis* **188**(4), 217–21.

Hanna, G.L., Fluent, T.E. & Fischer, D.J. (1999) Separation anxiety in children and adolescents treated with risperidone. *J Child Adolesc Psychopharmacol* **9**, 277–83.

Hansen, C., Sanders, S.L., Massaro, S. & Last, C.G. (1998) Predictors of severity of absenteeism in children with anxiety-based school refusal. *J Clin Child Psychol* **27**(3), 246–54.

Heun, R. & Maier, W. (1995) Relation of schizophrenia and panic disorder: evidence from a controlled family study. *Am J Med Genet* **60**(2), 127–32.

Higuchi, H., Kamata, M., Yoshimoto, M., Shimisu, T. & Hishikawa, Y. (1999) Panic attacks in patients with chronic schizophrenia: a complication of long-term neuroleptic treatment. *Psychiatry Clin Neurosci* **53**(1), 91–4.

Hofmann, S.G. (1999) Relationship between panic and schizophrenia. *Depress Anxiety* **9**, 101–6.

Hollander, E., Stein, D.J. & Saoud, J.B. (1992) Effects of fenfluramine on plasma pHVA in OCD. *Psychiatry Res* **42**, 185–8.

Ingram, I.M. (1961) Obsessional illness in mental hospital patients. *J Ment Sci* **107**, 382–402.

Insel, T.R. & Akiskal, H.S. (1986) Obsessive-compulsive disorder with psychotic features: a phenomenologic analysis. *Am J Psychiatry* **143**, 1527–1533.

Iqbal, N. & van Praag, H.M. (1995) The role of serotonin in schizophrenia. *Eur Neuropsychopharmacol* **5** (Suppl.) 11–23.

Jacobsen, F.M. (1995) Risperidone in the treatment of affective illness and obsessive-compulsive disorder. *J Clin Psychiatry* **56**(9), 423–9.

Jauss, M., Schroder, J., Pantel, J., Bachmann, S., Gerdsen, I. & Mundt, C. (1998) Severe akathisia during olanzapine treatment of acute schizophrenia. *Pharmacopsychiatry* **31**, 146–8.

Kahn, J.P., Puertollano, M.A., Schane, M.D. & Klein, D.F. (1988) Adjunctive alprazolam for schizophrenia with panic anxiety: clinical observation and pathogenetic implications. *Am J Psychiatry* **145**(6), 742–4.

Kapur, S. & Remington, G. (1996) Serotonin–dopamine interaction and its relevance to schizophrenia. *Am J Psychiatry* **153**(4), 466–76.

Kasper, S., Tauscher, J., Kufferle, B., Barnas, C., Pezawas, L. & Quiner, S. (1999) Dopamine- and serotonin-receptors in schizophrenia: results of imaging-studies and implications for pharmacotherapy in schizophrenia. *Eur Arch Psychiatry Clin Neurosci* **249** (Suppl. 4), 83–9.

Kay, S. (1991) *Positive and Negative Syndromes in Schizophrenia: Assessment and Research. Clinical and Experimental Psychiatry Monograph No. 5* Brunner/Mazel, New York.

Kay, S.R. & Lindenmayer, J.P. (1987) Outcome predictors in acute schizophrenia: prospective significance of background and clinical dimensions. *J Nerv Ment Dis* **175**, 152–60.

Kendler, K.S., Gallagher, T.J., Abelson, J.M. & Kessler, R.C. (1996) Lifetime prevalence, demographic risk factors, and diagnostic validity of nonaffective psychosis as assessed in a US community sample. The National Comorbidity Survey. *Arch Gen Psychiatry* **53**(11), 1022–31.

Kopala, L. & Honer, W.G. (1994) Risperidone, serotonergic mechanisms, and obsessive-compulsive symptoms in schizophrenia [letter]. *Am J Psychiatry* **151**(11), 1714–15.

Koran, L.M., Ringold, A.L. & Elliott, M.A. (2000) Olanzapine augmentation for treatment-resistant obsessive-compulsive disorder [In process citation]. *J Clin Psychiatry* **61**(7), 514–17.

Koreen, A.R., Siris, S.G., Chakos, M., Alvir, J., Mayerhoff, D. & Lieberman, J. (1993) Depression in first-episode schizophrenia [see comments]. *Am J Psychiatry* **150**(11), 1643–8.

Kozak, M.J. & Foa, E.B. (1994) Obsessions, overvalued ideas, and delusions in obsessive-compulsive disorder. *Behav Res Ther* **32**(3), 343–53.

Kringlen, E. (1965) Obsessional neurotic: a long-term follow-up. *Br J Psychiatry* **111**, 709–22.

Kruger, S., Braunig, P., Hoffler, J., Shugar, G., Borner, I. & Langkrar, J. (2000) Prevalence of obsessive-compulsive disorder in schizophrenia and significance of motor symptoms. *J Neuropsychiatry Clin Neurosci*, **12**(1), 16–24.

Labbate, L.A., Young, P.C. & Arana, G.W. (1999) Panic disorder in schizophrenia. *Can J Psychiatry* **44**(5), 488–90.

Levine, J.B., Gruber, S.A., Baird, A.A. & Yurgelun-Todd, D. (1998) Obsessive-compulsive disorder among schizophrenic patients: an exploratory study using functional magnetic resonance imaging data. *Compr Psychiatry* **39**(5), 308–11.

Lewis, R., Kapur, S., Jones, C. *et al.* (1999) Serotonin 5-HT2 receptors in schizophrenia: a PET study using [18F]setoperone in neuroleptic-naive patients and normal subjects. *Am J Psychiatry* **156**(1), 72–8.

Lo, W.H. (1967) A follow-up study of obsessional neurotics in Hong Kong Chinese. *Br J Psychiatry* **113**(501), 823–32.

Lundy, M.S. (1992) Psychosis-induced post-traumatic stress disorder. *Am J Psychother* **46**(3), 485–91.

Lykouras, L., Oulis, P., Psarros, K. *et al.* (2000) Five-factor model of schizophrenic psychopathology: how valid is it? *Eur Arch Psychiatry Clin Neurosci* **250**, 93–100.

Lysaker, P.H., Bell, M.D., Bioty, S.M. & Zito, W.S. (1995) The frequency of associations between positive and negative symptoms and dysphoria in schizophrenia. *Compr Psychiatry* **36**(2), 113–17.

Mandalos, G.E. & Szarek, B.L. (1999) New-onset panic attacks in a patient treated with olanzapine [letter]. *J Clin Psychopharmacol* **19**(2), 191.

Mandel, M.R., Severe, J.B. & Schooler, N.R. (1982) Development and prediction of postpsychotic depression in neuroleptic-treated schizophrenics. *Arch Gen Psychiatry* **39**, 197–203.

Marazziti, D., Giannaccini, G., Martini, C. *et al.* (1996) Benzodiazepine binding inhibitory activity: new supportive findings on its presence in psychiatric patients and further biochemical analyses. *Neuropsychobiology* **34**(1), 9–13.

Marder, S.R., Davis, J.M. & Chouinard, G. (1997) The effects of risperidone on the five dimensions of schizophrenia derived by factor analysis: combined results of the North American trials [published erratum appears in *J Clin Psychiatry* (1998) **59**(4), 200]. *J Clin Psychiatry* **58**(12), 538–46.

McDougle, C.J., Epperson, C.N., Pelton, G.H., Waslyink, S. & Price, L.H. (2000) A double-blind, placebo-controlled study of risperidone addition in serotonin reuptake inhibitor-refractory obsessive-compulsive disorder. *Arch Gen Psychiatry* **57**, 794–801.

McDougle, C.J., Fleischman, R.L., Epperson, C.N., Wasylink, S.L.J.F. & Price, L.H. (1995) Risperidone addition in fluvoxamine-refractory obsessive-compulsive disorder: three cases. *J Clin Psychiatry* **56**, 526–8.

McDougle, C.J., Goodman, W.K. & Price, L.H. (1994) Dopamine antagonists in tic-related and psychotic spectrum obsessive-compulsive disorder. *J Clin Psychiatry Suppl* **55**, 24–31.

McGlashan, T., Carpenter, W.R. & J. (1976) An investigation of the postpsychotic depression syndrome. *Am J Psychiatry* **133**, 14–19.

Meltzer, H.Y. (1989) Clinical studies on the mechanism of action of clozapine: the dopamine-serotonin hypothesis of schizophrenia. *Psychopharmacology Berl* **99** (Suppl.) S18–S27.

Meltzer, H.Y. (1999) The role of serotonin in antipsychotic drug action. *Neuropsychopharmacology* **21** (Suppl. 2), S106–S115.

Meltzer, H.Y. & Okayli, T. (1995) Reduction of suicidality during clozapine treatment of neuroleptic-resistant schizophrenia: impact on risk-benefit assessment. *Am J Psychiatry* **152**, 183–190.

Meyer, H., Taiminen, T., Vuori, T., Aijala, A. & Helenius, H. (1999) Post-traumatic stress disorder symptoms related to psychosis and acute involuntary hospitalization in schizophrenic and delusional patients. *J Nerv Ment Dis* **187**(6), 343–52.

Mikkelsen, E.J., Detlor, J. & Cohen, D.J. (1981) School avoidance and social phobia triggered by haloperidol in patients with Tourette's disorder. *Am J Psychiatry* **138**, 1572–6.

Mueser, K.T., Goodman, L.B., Trumbetta, S.L. *et al.* (1998) Trauma and post-traumatic stress disorder in severe mental illness. *J Consult Clin Psychol* **66**(3), 493–9.

Muller, C. (1953) Der ubergomg von zwangsnervose in schizophrenia im licht der katamnese. *Arch Neurol* **72**, 218–25.

Norman, R.M. & Malla, A.K. (1994) Correlations over time between dysphoric mood and symptomatology in schizophrenia. *Compr Psychiatry* **35**(1), 34–8.

Nyberg, S., Nakashima, Y., Nordstrom, A.L., Halldin, C. & Farde, L. (1996) Positron emission tomography of *in-vivo* binding characteristics of atypical antipsychotic drugs. Review of D2 and 5-HT2 receptor occupancy studies and clinical response. *Br J Psychiatry Suppl* **29** 40–4.

O'Dwyer, A.-M. & Marks, I. (2000) Obsessive-compulsive disorder and delusions revisited. *Br J Psychiatry*, **176**, 281–4.

Ohuoha, D.C., Hyde, T.M. & Kleinman, J.E. (1993) The role of serotonin in schizophrenia: an overview of the nomenclature, distribution and alterations of serotonin receptors in the central nervous system. *Psychopharmacology Berl* **112** (Suppl. 1), S5–S15.

Pallanti, S., Quercioli, L., Rossi, A. & Pazzagli, A. (1999) The emergence of social phobia during clozapine treatment and its response to fluoxetine augmentation. *J Clin Psychiatry* **60**(12), 819–23.

Patel, B. & Tandon, R. (1993) Development of obsessive-compulsive symptoms during clozapine treatment [letter: comment]. *Am J Psychiatry* **150**(5), 836.

Patil, V.J. (1992) Development of transient obsessive-compulsive symptoms during treatment with clozapine [letter: comment]. *Am J Psychiatry* **149**(2), 272.

Penn, D.L., Hope, D.A., Spaulding, W. & Kucera, J. (1994) Social anxiety in schizophrenia. *Schizophr Res* **11**(3), 277–84.

Pittman, R.K. (1987) Pierre Janet on obsessive-compulsive disorder: review and commentary. *Arch Gen Psychiatry* **44**, 226–32.

Pollack, M.H. & Marzol, P.C. (2000) Panic: course, complications and treatment of panic disorder. *J Psychopharmacol* **14**(2) (Suppl. 1), S25–S30.

Pollit, J.D. (1957) Natural history of obsessional states. *Br Medical J*, **1**, 195–8.

Poyurovsky, M., Bergman, Y., Shoshani, D., Schneidman, M. & Weizman, A. (1998) Emergence of obsessive–compulsive symptoms and tics during clozapine withdrawal. *Clin Neuropharmacol* **21**(2), 97–100.

Poyurovsky, M., Fuchs, C. & Weizman, A. (1999) Obsessive-compulsive disorder in patients with first-episode schizophrenia. *Am J Psychiatry* **156**(12), 1998–2000.

Priebe, S., Broker, M. & Gunkel, S. (1998) Involuntary admission and post-traumatic stress disorder symptoms in schizophrenia patients. *Compr Psychiatry* **39**(4), 220–4.

Ravizza, L., Barzega, G., Bellino, S., Bogetto, F. & Maina, G. (1996) Therapeutic effect and safety of adjunctive risperidone in refractory obsessive-compulsive disorder. *Psychopharmacol Bull* **32**, 677–82.

Remington, G. & Adams, M. (1994) Risperidone and obsessive-compulsive symptoms. *J Clin Psychopharmacol* **14**, 358–9.

Remington, G. & Kapur, S. (1999) D2 and 5-HT2 receptor effects of antipsychotics: bridging basic and clinical findings using PET. *J Clin Psychiatry* **60** (Suppl. 10), 15–19.

Rosen, I. (1957) The clinical significance of obsessions in schizophrenia. *J Ment Sci* **103**, 778–85.

Rosenberg, C.M. (1968) Complications of obsessional neurosis. *Br J Psychiatry* **114**, 477–8.

Roy, A., Thompson, R. & Kennedy, S. (1983) Depression in chronic schizophrenia. *Br J Psychiatry* **142**, 465–70.

Rudin, G. (1953) Ein beitrag zur frage der zwangskrankheit. *Arch Psychiatr Nervenkr* **191**, 14–54.

Sandberg, L. & Siris, S.G. (1987) "Panic disorder" in schizophrenia. *J Nerv Ment Dis* **175**(10), 627–8.

Sautter, F.J., Brailey, K., Uddo, M.M., Hamilton, M.F., Beard, M.G. & Borges, A.H. (1999) PTSD and comorbid psychotic disorder: comparison with veterans diagnosed with PTSD or psychotic disorder. *J Trauma Stress* **12**(1), 73–88.

Saxena, S., Wang, D., Bystritsky, A., Baxter-L.R., J. (1996) Risperidone augmentation of SRI treatment for refractory obsessive-compulsive disorder [see comments]. *J Clin Psychiatry* **57**(7), 303–6.

Shaw, K., McFarlane, A. & Bookless, C. (1997) The phenomenology of traumatic reactions to psychotic illness. *J Nerv Ment Dis* **185**(7), 434–41.

Siris, S.G. (1991) Diagnosis of secondary depression in schizophrenia: implications for DSM-IV. *Schizophr Bull* **17**, 75–98.

Siris, S. (1993) Adjunctive medication in the maintenance treatment of schizophrenia and its conceptual implications. *Br J Psychiatry* **163** (Suppl. 22), 66–78.

Siris, S.G., Mason, S.E. & Shuwall, M.A. (1993) Histories of substance abuse, panic and suicidal ideation in schizophrenic patients with histories of post-psychotic depressions. *Prog Neuropsychopharmacol Biol Psychiatry* **17**(4), 609–17.

Snyder, S.H. (1972) Catecholamines in the brain as mediators of amphetamine psychosis. *Arch Gen Psychiatry* **27**, 169–79.

Snyder, S. (1976) The dopamine hypothesis of schizophrenia: focus on the dopamine receptor. *Am J Psychiatry* **133**, 197–202.

Sobin, C., Blundell, M.L., Weiller, F., Gavigan, C., Haiman, C. & Karayiorgou, M. (2000) Evidence of a schizotypy subtype in OCD. *J Psychiatr Res* **34**(1), 15–24.

Stampfer, H.G. (1990) Negative symptoms: a cumulative trauma stress disorder? *Aust N Z J Psychiatry* **24**(4), 516–28.

Stein, D.J., Bouwer, C.J., Hawkridge, S.M. & Emsley, R.A. (1997) Risperidone augmentation of serotonin reuptake inhibitors in obsessive-compulsive and related disorders. *J Clin Psychiatry* **58**, 119–22.

Stern, R.G., Frank, D. & Mera, H. (1999) High social phobia scale scores in schizophrenia do not correlate with psychosis symptom severity scores. In: *New Research Program and Abstracts of the 152nd Annual Meeting of the American Psychiatric Association; May 18, 1999; Washington, D.C.* Abstract NR239: 131.

Strakowski, S.M., Keck, P.E.J., McElroy, S.L., Lonczak, H.S. & West, S.A. (1995) Chronology of comorbid and principal syndromes in first-episode psychosis. *Compr Psychiatry* **36**(2), 106–12.

Strakowski, S.M., Tohen, M., Stoll, A.L. *et al.* (1993) Comorbidity in psychosis at first hospitalization. *Am J Psychiatry* **150**(5), 752–7.

Szechtman, H., Culver, K. & Eilam, D. (1999) Role of dopamine systems in obsessive-compulsive disorder (OCD): implications from a novel psychostimulant-induced animal model. *Pol J Pharmacol* **51**(1), 55–61.

Tibbo, P. & Warneke, L. (1999) Obsessive-compulsive disorder in schizophrenia: epidemiologic and biologic overlap. *J Psychiatry Neurosci* **24**(1), 15–24.

Tien, A.Y. & Eaton, W.W. (1992) Psychopathologic precursors and sociodemographic risk factors for the schizophrenia syndrome. *Arch Gen Psychiatry* **49**(1), 37–46.

Tollefson, G.D. & Sanger, T.M. (1999) Anxious-depressive symptoms in schizophrenia: a new treatment target for pharmacotherapy? *Schizophr Res* **35** (Suppl.), S13–S21.

Tollefson, G.D., Sanger, T.M., Beasley, C.M. & Tran, P.V. (1998) A double-blind, controlled comparison of the novel antipsychotic olanzapine versus haloperidol or placebo on anxious and depressive symptoms accompanying schizophrenia. *Biol Psychiatry* **43**(11), 803–10.

Van-Putten, T., May, P.R. & Marder, S.R. (1984) Akathisia with haloperidol and thiothixene. *Arch Gen Psychiatry* **41**(11), 1036–9.

Welner, A., Reich, T. & Robins, E. (1976) Obsessive-compulsive neurosis: record, family and follow-up studies. *Compr Psychiatry* **17**, 527–39.

Westphal, K. (1878) Ueber zwangvorstellungen. *Arch Psychiatr Nervenkr* **8**, 734–50.

Wolkowitz, O.M., Breier, A., Doran, A. *et al.* (1988) Alprazolam augmentation of the antipsychotic effects of fluphenazine in schizophrenic patients. Preliminary results. *Arch Gen Psychiatry* **45**, 664–71.

Yaryura-Tobias, J.A., Campisi, T.A., McKay, D. & Neziroglu, F.A. (1995) Schizophrenia and obsessive-compulsive disorder: shared aspects of pathology. *Neurology, Psychiatry and Brain Research* **3**, 1–6.

PART THREE

Mechanisms

11 Neurochemical Aspects of Anxiety

S.V. Argyropoulos & D.J. Nutt

Introduction

Most work in the field of the neurochemistry of anxiety has been conducted, so far, in relation to γ-aminobutyric acid (GABA) and the monoamine neurotransmitters, norepinephrine (noradrenaline) serotonin (5-hydroxy-tryptamine) and, to a lesser extent, dopamine. These transmitters became the focus of attention after the serendipitous discovery of compounds that were effective anxiolytics. These drugs were found to exert some of their behavioral effects by altering the function of the receptors upon which these transmitters naturally bound.

It was hoped that the identification of relevant receptors and the unravelling of the function of these neurotransmitters would give answers about the nature of anxiety and lead to better designed treatments. What emerged is an ever increasingly complex picture of the pathophysiology of anxiety, that has generated at least as many questions as it has answered. On the other hand, new compounds that act as agonists or antagonists at specific receptor sites have been developed, and some of them successfully tested. The behavioral effects of these drugs are studied with the experimental provocation and prevention of anxiety. This is usually achieved with the use of challenge tests (see Chapter 15). Some of them are not strictly speaking neurochemical challenges, but they affect the neurotransmitter systems all the same.

Of the anxiety syndromes, as they appear in the modern classification systems (American Psychiatric Association 1994), panic disorder has been the focus of most of the research so far. In recent years there is increasing interest in other anxiety states, such as social and generalized anxiety, both as independent conditions and in their relationship to panic. Data relating to post-traumatic stress disorder and obsessive-compulsive disorder are also accumulating. We will review some findings relevant to specific syndromes under each neurotransmitter system heading. Reference to animal work will be limited. Finally, new developments in other areas, like the neuropeptides, are covered in other chapters in this book and they will not be discussed here.

GABA-benzodiazepine receptor complex

GABA is the main inhibitory transmitter in the brain. It is synthesized from glutamate, through the Krebs cycle. There are two distinct types of GABA receptors. Of these, the $GABA_A$ receptor is the one linked with anxiety. The effector of the $GABA_A$ receptor is the Cl^- ion. The five protein subunits that make up the receptor complex are arranged, in a doughnut shape, around a chloride channel. The physiological functions of the $GABA_A$ extend well beyond anxiety and include memory acquisition, muscle relaxation and control of convulsions (Doble 1999; Nutt & Malizia 2001).

Direct measurement of the synaptic levels of GABA in the brain is not possible. Various indirect methods of assessment of central GABA function have been used in anxiety studies. These include the growth hormone and cortisol responses to the administration of benzodiazepines, the performance in specific cognitive tasks, or the measurement of the benzodiazepine effects on the electroencephalogram (EEG). However, these techniques rely on the measurement of phenomena that are not under the exclusive control of the GABA system. The most specific indirect estimate of central GABA function available is the study of the saccadic eye movement responses to intravenous midazolam (Potokar *et al.* 2000). Nowadays, the advent of neuroimaging allows for closer study of this system in health and disease, with the use of specific ligands that modify the receptor complex (see Chapter 12).

Drugs that work at the GABA$_A$ receptor have a long history of use and abuse in anxiety. Alcohol is the most widely used anxiolytic and is active at the GABA-chloride ionophore. Its use, in a self-medicating fashion, to treat normal and pathological anxiety is well recognized. One of the advantages of alcohol, along with barbiturates, benzodiazepines, and other compounds that act at the GABA$_A$ receptor, is that they have a fast anxiolytic action. However, it is possible that alcohol in general, and repeated withdrawal symptoms in particular, can also produce *de novo* anxiety disorders such as panic (George *et al.* 1990). After the clinical development of the benzodiazepines in the 1960s, interest was focused on their mode of action. They bind to the high affinity benzodiazepine site of the GABA$_A$ receptor. This site modulates allosterically the GABA-chloride ionophore complex (Braestrup & Squires 1978; Braestrup *et al.* 1983). Unlike alcohol and the barbiturates, the benzodiazepines have no direct action on the chloride ionophore itself. They exercise their effect by augmenting the function of the endogenous transmitter (GABA).

The GABA$_A$ receptor is unique in that it shows bi-directional agonism. Apart from agonists and antagonists of this receptor, there are also inverse agonists (Jackson & Nutt 1992). Agonists, such as the classical benzodiazepines, are anxiolytic. Antagonists, such as flumazenil, have little action of their own but block the actions of both agonists and inverse agonists. Inverse agonists, such as the β-carboline FG 7142 and the benzodiazepine Ro 15-3505, are anxiogenic in man (Dorow *et al.* 1983; Gentil *et al.* 1990).

This property of the GABA$_A$ receptor led to the idea that endogenous inverse agonists or endogenous agonists to this receptor may play a pivotal role in the regulation of anxiety. Initially, there was some interest in candidate inverse agonists that included tribulin (Clow *et al.* 1983) and diazepam-binding inhibitor (DBI) (Barbaccia *et al.* 1986). Tribulin was found in increased concentrations in the urine of patients with generalized anxiety, or after panic attacks induced with

sodium lactate (Clow *et al.* 1988a, 1988b). On the other hand, and contrary to predictions, DBI was increased in the cerebrospinal fluid (CSF) of depressed patients but not panic disorder patients (Barbaccia *et al.* 1986). Interest in endogenous inverse agonists waned in recent years, especially after it was shown that untreated panic patients experienced marked anxiety during a challenge with flumazenil (Nutt *et al.* 1990), a GABA$_A$ receptor antagonist that has very little effect on healthy controls. This finding pointed towards an endogenous agonist or a receptor abnormality, rather than a significant role for inverse agonists.

Endogenous agonists, called endozepines, have been isolated both from the rat and human brain (Rothstein *et al.* 1992a,b). Accumulation of the subtype endozepine-4 appears to be related to recurring idiopathic stupor, which is responsive to the benzodiazepine antagonist flumazenil, therefore supporting the notion of naturally occurring agonists (Lugaresi *et al.* 1998). However, their role in anxiety disorders is not clarified yet. Interest in the area of the endogenous agonists is mainly focused on another group of ligands, the neurosteroids. These substances act on the GABA$_A$ receptor, but at a different site from the benzodiazepines. They modulate allosterically the GABA receptor complex, but they also have an action on the N-methyl-D-aspartate (NMDA) receptors of the excitatory amino acids (Baulieu 1998). Indirect evidence for the importance of these compounds in the regulation of anxiety comes from the observation that pronounced natural fluctuations of the gonadal steroids (during the menstrual cycle, the pregnancy and the postpartum period) appear to affect anxiety levels (Wilson 1996). Animal studies indicate that progesterone, one of the naturally produced gonadal steroids, is metabolized to a neurosteroid that augments the function of GABA. However, other important gonadal steroids, the estrogens, do not appear to affect GABA function (Wilson 1996). Overall, the above indicate that some, at least, neurosteroids may play an endogenous anxiolytic role, which is mediated through the GABA receptor complex.

An alternative hypothesis is that an abnormality in the benzodiazepine receptor complex may underlie some anxiety phenomena. As mentioned earlier, flumazenil infusion precipitates panic attacks in panic patients (Nutt *et al.* 1990), while it has little or no anxiogenic effect on normal controls, social phobics (Coupland *et al.* 2000), or subjects in alcohol withdrawal (Nutt *et al.* 1993; Potokar *et al.* 1997). This suggested that panic patients might display a shift in the "set point" of their benzodiazepine receptors (Nutt *et al.* 1990). Similar change is known to occur after chronic benzodiazepine use and manifests at the withdrawal of the drug. It has been observed that during benzodiazepine withdrawal the effects of benzodiazepine agonists are attenuated, while those of the inverse agonists are enhanced (Nutt 1990) and antagonists become slightly inverse agonists (Little *et al.* 1987). Nutt and Lawson (1992) hypothesized that a similar shift of the receptor set point is present in panic patients, either as a state or trait phenomenon. However, the lack of any similar effect of flumazenil challenge in other anxiety disorders indicates that this receptor shift may be a phenomenon specific to panic but not anxiety as a whole.

Further evidence of abnormal benzodiazepine receptor function in panic, and possibly other anxiety disorders, derives from single photon emission computerized tomography (SPECT) and positron emission tomography (PET) neuroimaging studies (Malizia *et al.* 1996; Lingford-Hughes & Malizia 1999; see also Chapter 12). There is evidence from SPECT studies of decreased density of $GABA_A$ receptors in the right hippocampus and left temporal region (Kaschka *et al.* 1995) and the frontal, occipital and temporal cortices (Schlegel *et al.* 1994). However, this work is not without contradicting results. One study showed increased density in temporal regions (Kuikka *et al.* 1995). In a PET study, Malizia *et al.* (1998) demonstrated a global reduction of benzodiazepine binding in panic patients compared with controls. The differences were more pronounced in the orbitofrontal cortex and the insula. The above support the idea of $GABA_A$-benzodiazepine receptor down-regulation in anxiety. This would result in decreased function of the endogenous transmitter and it may underlie the clinical expression of some anxiety phenomena.

Norepinephrine

Norepinephrine (noradrenaline: NE), a catecholamine, is synthesized from dopamine through hydroxylation. In some tissues, NE is then converted (methylated) to epinephrine (adrenaline). While epinephrine in the periphery is playing a significant role in stress responses (see below), the main sympathetic transmitter in the central nervous system (CNS) is NE. Virtually all NE containing neurones originate in the brain stem, mainly the nucleus known as locus coeruleus, but they branch out extensively throughout the forebrain. Following release in the synaptic cleft, NE is actively transported back to the nerve terminal for reuse, but some spills over from the synapse and is taken up by glial cells. NE is catabolized in the neurones with the help of the enzyme monoamine oxidase inhibitor (MAO), and the end product is 3-methoxy-4-hydroxyphenylglycol (MHPG). The NE that diffuses to glia is catabolized to normetanephrine with the help of catechol-O-methyltransferase (COMT) (Nutt 1993).

Three distinct classes of adrenergic receptors have been identified. The α_1 type acts by stimulating the phosphoinositol (PI) cycle, while α_2 and β receptors are coupled with G proteins. The α_1 receptors are postsynaptic. They are involved in arousal and the regulation of blood pressure, but they have not been directly linked to anxiety. The α_2 receptors are both pre- and postsynaptic. The postsynaptic ones are involved in arousal, blood pressure regulation as well as the release of growth hormone. The latter property has been used in the study of depression and anxiety (see later). The presynaptic α_2 receptors are involved in the feedback control of the NE release. The role of the β receptors in the brain is not fully clarified yet. Their involvement in the stimulation of the production of melatonin in the pineal gland is exploited for neurochemical studies. The peripheral β receptors are not directly related to the mental experience of anxiety, though they mediate its autonomic/somatic aspects (Nutt 1993).

For over a century the sympathetic autonomic system has been linked to behavioral arousal. Arousal is mediated by the catecholamines, epinephrine in the periphery and NE in the CNS. A number of observations led support to the theory that excessive sympathetic activation may produce dysfunctional arousal and anxiety through increased catecholamine transmission. When Da Costa (1871) described the "irritable heart syndrome," a constellation of symptoms that would fall under the rubric of panic anxiety nowadays, he postulated increased function of the cardiac nerve centers. Somatic symptoms of acute anxiety, such as tachycardia, palpitations, tachypnoea, sweating, dry mouth, epigastric discomfort, etc., are indeed reminiscent of the peripheral effects of the sympathetic system at times of arousal and stress, when the organism is preparing to fight or flee.

In later years, the focus shifted from the periphery to sympathetic overactivity within the CNS. Klein and Fink (1962) reported that imipramine, a tricyclic antidepressant that acts partly by blocking the reuptake of NE, is effective in controlling panic attacks. Drugs that increase central NE availability, such as amphetamines and cocaine, are known to have an anxiogenic effect (Louie *et al.* 1989). Further, the sympathetic activity induced during various neurochemical challenge paradigms seems to correlate with the levels of anxiety that these challenges elicit (Ko *et al.* 1983; Charney *et al.* 1984). Animal studies showed that locus coeruleus, the main sympathetic nucleus of the brain, plays a central role in the control of arousal (Aston-Jones *et al.* 1994; Smith & Nutt 1996) and anxiety (Redmond & Huang 1979). Stressful events produce a marked elevation of NE release in a variety of regions of the rat brain, including the hypothalamus, the amygdala and the locus coeruleus (Tanaka *et al.* 2000). Changes in the activity of locus coeruleus appear to result in changes in central NE levels, which are reflected in changes in peripheral sympathetic activity (Kelly & Cooper 1998). Therefore, it comes as no surprise that NE, the main sympathetic transmitter in the brain, attracted a lot of attention in the study of pathological human anxiety.

Direct access and measurement of the central sympathetic activity is impossible. NE only crosses the blood–brain barrier to the periphery with great difficulty (Esler *et al.* 1995). On the other hand, the contribution of the adrenal glands to the circulating NE is thought to be minimal (Brown *et al.* 1981). Plasma NE is therefore considered to be the product of overspill from postganglionic terminals to the periphery (Frankenhauser 1971; Kopin 1984). Values of this indirect measure are thought to reflect central NE activity in humans, because plasma NE levels correlate closely with NE levels in the CSF (Ziegler *et al.* 1977). This view is supported further by animal studies showing a correlation between plasma NE and MHPG in the CSF (Elsworth *et al.* 1982). As a result, plasma NE assessments have been used as a proxy measure of central NE levels. MHPG levels measured in plasma, urine and CSF are also used as a proxy index of the NE turnover, although a substantial proportion of the metabolite is obviously peripheral in origin (Nutt 1993).

Studies of plasma NE levels in anxious patients at rest have been mostly negative (Kelly & Cooper 1998).

Starkman *et al.* (1990) found no difference between panic patients and healthy controls. Similar results were produced from a group of generalized anxiety patients (Munjack *et al.* 1990), and a mixed panic and generalized anxiety sample (Cameron *et al.* 1990). Kelly and Cooper (1998) compared patients with depression or generalized anxiety and healthy volunteers. Depressed patients, especially those with melancholic and/or psychotic illness, showed significant elevation of NE levels compared with the controls. NE levels of the anxious group were also elevated, but this was not statistically significant.

Another way of studying NE and its relation to anxiety is to examine the functional integrity of the sympathetic system. For this, subjects are challenged with various compounds that act upon the central or peripheral NE receptors (Table 11.1). The assumption is that while NE and sympathetic activity may be normal at rest, when the organism comes under stress and anxiety ensues, it can be abnormal. This, in turn, may be either the cause or the result of anxiety. This notion was supported by a study conducted by Wilkinson *et al.* (1998), who found that whole body and regional sympathetic activity was not increased at rest or during a mental stress task in panic patients compared with controls, but both epinephrine and NE release was elevated in the patient group shortly after a spontaneous panic attack. Of interest that this elevation of the catecholamines, resulting from sympathetic activation, was not global as previously thought, but confined to the heart rather than the musculature.

Epinephrine and isoprenaline, a selective agonist of β postsynaptic receptors, do not cross the blood–brain barrier (Schildkraut & Ketty 1967); therefore their neurochemical action is considered to be purely peripheral. It has been shown that, apart from inducing the somatic symptoms described earlier in this section, epinephrine and isoprenaline can also induce mental anxiety (Maranon 1924; Cantril & Hunt 1932; Frankenhauser *et al.* 1961), and even panic (Rainey *et al.* 1984; Pyke & Greenberg 1986) in populations with panic disorder. This was not the case in patients with social phobia, despite the presence of increased catecholamine levels and the presence of the expected peripheral physiologic effects (Papp *et al.* 1988). These findings led to speculation that peripheral β receptors may be hypersensitive, at least in panic (Rainey *et al.* 1984). However, there is also evidence of downregulation of β receptors in panic patients (Nesse

Table 11.1 Summary of the evidence for functional abnormality of norepinephrine receptors in anxiety conditions.

Receptor	Challenge test	Population tested	Results compared with controls	Postulated mechanism
α_2-presynaptic	Yohimbine (non-selective antagonist leads to increased locus coeruleus firing)	Healthy volunteers PD PTSD GAD OCD	Increases anxiety Increases anxiety, panic attacks and MHPG Increases anxiety, flashbacks and panic attacks No difference from controls	Increases locus coeruleus firing supersensitivity of α_2 receptors at locus coeruleus leads to anxiety/panic
	Idazoxan (non-selective antagonist)	Healthy volunteers	Increases anxiety	
	Ethoxy-idazoxan (highly selective antagonist)	Healthy volunteers	Anxiogenic in very high doses	Anxiogenic effects of yohimbine ? through other mechanism
	Clonidine (partial agonist leads to decreased firing of locus coeruleus)	Spontaneous and lactate-induced panic attacks PTSD OCD GAD, SAD	Decreased anxiety, panic attacks and MHPG, exaggerated hypotensive response Some efficacy Not effective ?Effect on anxiety	Supersensitivity of α_2 receptors at locus coeruleus leads to anxiety/panic
α_2 postsynaptic	Clonidine (partial agonist leads to GH release)	PD GAD OCD, SAD	Blunted GH response Mixed results	Hyposensitive postsynaptic α_2 receptors
β (peripheral)	Isoprenaline (agonist)	PD SAD	Increases anxiety and panic Increases catecholamines no difference in anxiety	? β receptor hypersensitivity No β receptor abnormality
	Epinephrine (agonist)	GAD	Increases anxiety and cardiovascular responses but no differential response in catecholamine levels	Cognitive misinterpretation of peripheral symptoms

GAD, generalized anxiety disorder; GH, growth hormone; MHPG, 3-methoxy-4-hydroxyphenylglycol; OCD, obsessive-compulsive disorder; PD, panic disorder; PTSD, post-traumatic stress disorder; SAD, social anxiety disorder.

et al. 1984), presumably secondary to paroxysms of increased NE activity. Further, environmental cues undoubtedly affect one's interpretation of the physiological/somatic sequelae of peripherally acting catecholamines (Schachter & Singer 1962). This led to the view that the physiological changes induced by peripherally acting drugs, such as epinephrine and isoproterenol, produce anxiety and panic through a secondary cognitive interpretation of these changes (Nutt & Lawson 1992). Further support for this hypothesis was produced by a study that compared patients with generalized anxiety and normal controls in their response to intramuscular injection of epinephrine (Mathew et al. 1982). Both patients and controls had a similar increase in plasma levels of epinephrine and NE after the injection. However, the patient group showed increased heart rate and anxiety response compared with the controls. The possibility of cognitive misinterpretation of the peripheral effects of catecholamines should also be taken into account when the anxiogenic quality of drugs acting both in the CNS and the periphery are studied (see later).

Studies of the CNS sympathetic function in anxiety have revolved around the regulatory role of α_2 autoreceptors in the locus coeruleus. Yohimbine, an α_2 receptor antagonist, causes anxiety in normal people (Goldberg *et al.* 1983). It is thought to exert its action by antagonizing the presynaptic α_2 receptors of NE neurones, especially those in the locus coeruleus. This antagonism results in disruption of the normal negative feedback loop from the synapse to the cell, leading to increased firing of the cell bodies in locus coeruleus, and increased synaptic availability of NE (Charney *et al.* 1984). Another α_2 receptor antagonist, idazoxan, produced results similar to those of yohimbine in healthy volunteers (Krystal *et al.* 1992). When yohimbine was given to panic patients, it led to an increase in anxiety and panic frequency (Charney *et al.* 1984). Plasma levels of MHPG were significantly increased in the patient group compared with the controls, suggesting an increased sensitivity to yohimbine in panic patients. This altered functional response of panic patients to yohimbine is normalized after successful treatment with tricyclic antidepressants, but not after cognitive therapy (Middleton 1990). In post-traumatic stress disorder (PTSD), patients showed a similar anxiogenic response to yohimbine. This response was associated with the characteristic flashbacks of the condition, as well as panic attacks (Southwick *et al.* 1993). Withdrawal states from opiates (Glue *et al.* 1992) and cocaine (McDougle *et al.* 1994), that are associated with sympathetic overactivity, also elicit an exaggerated response to yohimbine. On the other hand, yohimbine was not more anxiogenic in patients with obsessive-compulsive disorder (OCD) (Rasmussen *et al.* 1987) or generalized anxiety disorder (GAD) (Charney *et al.* 1989) compared with normal controls, thus indicating that individual anxiety syndromes may not share the same pathophysiology of the adrenergic system.

If the assumption that yohimbine increased anxiety by antagonizing the α_2 presynaptic autoreceptors were correct, one would expect that an agonist at this site should have an anxiolytic effect, by reducing locus coeruleus firing and the levels of available synaptic NE. Clonidine is such a centrally acting α_2 receptor partial agonist. It has been shown to reduce firing at the locus coeruleus, decrease the sympathetic outflow and reduce anxiety (Reid 1983). It is efficacious against both spontaneous and lactate induced panic attacks (Uhde *et al.* 1989; Coplan *et al.* 1992), although its use in clinical populations is restricted by its hypotensive and sedative side-effects (Hoehn-Saric *et al.* 1981; Uhde *et al.* 1989). Positive results have also been obtained in small studies with patients suffering PTSD. The therapeutic effect is, however, short-lived, due to development of tolerance (Friedman 1998). On the other hand, clonidine does not appear to be useful in reducing symptoms of OCD (Hewlett *et al.* 1992) while its status in GAD and social anxiety remains unclear (Argyropoulos *et al.* 2000). Panic patients also show a significantly greater decrease in plasma MHPG (Charney & Heninger 1986) and an exaggerated hypotensive response to clonidine (Nutt 1986) compared with normal controls, although these results are not universally replicated (Abelson *et al.* 1992). Overall, the above findings of the yohimbine and clonidine studies point towards an abnormal supersensitivity of presynaptic α_2 autoreceptors to both its antagonists and agonists, at least in some forms of anxiety. Such supersensitivity would make the sympathetic system much more reactive, unstable and prone to panic and anxiety reactions.

The exaggerated responsiveness of presynaptic α_2 autoreceptors in panic, led Nutt (1989) to propose a failure of control of the locus coeruleus as the neurochemical basis of pathological acute anxiety. He suggested that such an underlying phenomenon could explain wide swings in locus coeruleus activity, resulting in paroxysms of central and peripheral sympathetic activation, perhaps analogous to panic attacks (Redmond 1986). Animal studies show that α_2 receptors may also be altered by stress (Stone 1983; Stanford 1989) and conditioning (Rasmussen & Jacobs 1986). This, in turn, could explain the association between life events and panic attacks (Klein 1981; Roy-Byrne *et al.* 1986). Further, the system appears to be under the influence of corticotropin-releasing factor (CRF) neurones in locus coeruleus, thus indicating a putative neuroanatomical link between stress experiences and central catecholamine activity (Koob 1999).

While this model of presynaptic α_2 supersensitivity in panic is attractive, there are some inconsistencies.

The panic attacks induced by yohimbine may not be representative of what happens in clinical anxiety, because they are also associated with cortisol release (den Boer & Westenberg 1993), unlike the spontaneous ones. Ethoxy-idazoxan, a much more selective α_2 receptor antagonist than yohimbine or idazoxan caused significant increase in blood pressure, plasma NE and attention in a group of healthy volunteers thus indicating strong sympathetic activation, as expected. However, it was only anxiogenic at very high doses (Coupland et al. 1994). It may be the case that other effects of yohimbine, such as serotonergic ones, which extend beyond its α_2 antagonism and the sympathetic system at large, are responsible for its anxiogenic properties (Nutt & Lawson 1992). To our knowledge, there are no studies with ethoxy-idazoxan in patient populations.

The sensitivity of the postsynaptic α_2 receptors is measured by the growth hormone (GH) response to the clonidine challenge. Similar to what had already been observed in depression, this response is blunted in panic patients, thus indicating a hyposensitivity of the postsynaptic receptors in such patients (Charney & Heninger 1986; Nutt 1986). Although there has been at least one negative study (Gann et al. 1995), albeit with a small sample size, the blunting of GH has been reproduced in many studies before and after successful treatment (Coplan et al. 1995; Brambilla et al. 1995). The same blunted response was produced in generalized anxiety (Abelson et al. 1991). In OCD the results were mixed: one study (Brambilla et al. 1997a) produced a blunted GH response, while two others did not (Lee et al. 1990; Hollander et al. 1991). It should be noted though that this last study also reported a significant reduction of obsessions and compulsions with clonidine, a finding contrary to evidence from other studies (Hewlett et al. 1992). The situation in social phobia was also not clear with two studies from the same group reporting different results (Tancer et al. 1993, 1994/1995). There were two important differences in the design of these studies that may account for the discrepant results. In the first study, intravenous clonidine resulted in a blunted GH response in a mixed group consisting of both generalized and specific social phobia subjects. In the second study, oral clonidine did not show a blunted GH response in a patient sample with generalized social anxiety. Therefore the route of administration of the challenge may be crucial in eliciting the

functional abnormality in question or specific types of anxiety may or may not be related to α_2 postsynaptic hyposensitivity.

Apart from the chemical challenges described above, physiological challenges such as isometric exercise, Valsalva's maneuver and rapid elevation of the body from supine position have also been used to study the cardiovascular autonomic responses of anxious patients and normal subjects alike. These cardiovascular responses depend on sympathetic activity; hence they provide another indirect view on the functional integrity of the sympathetic system. The picture is still incomplete and the interpretation of these results is difficult. Orthostatic challenge, exercise and Valsalva's maneuver in panic patients did not result in differential cardiovascular response, or plasma NE levels, compared with controls (Stein et al. 1992). However, the picture was different in social anxiety. An exaggerated blood pressure response to Valsalva's maneuver and a smaller immediate fall in blood pressure upon standing, coupled with increased supine and standing NE levels were observed (Stein et al. 1994; Nutt et al. 1998). It is not clear yet whether these subtle changes are specific to social anxiety, or whether they depend on the strength of the challenge used. Yonidine, on the other hand, did produce an exaggerated cardiovascular response in panic patients, compared with controls (Nutt 1989).

A new method of enquiry that has emerged in recent years is that of catecholamine depletion of the CNS. This can be achieved by means of inhibiting tyrosine hydroxylase, with α-methyl-p-tyrosine (AMPT), therefore blocking the production of catecholamines in the brain. Although this method has been successfully used in depression (Delgado et al. 1993), it has not been adequately tested in anxiety, not least as much as the equivalent paradigm for serotonin transmission (tryptophan depletion). So far, only one double-blind, placebo-controlled study has been reported, in drug-free obsessive-compulsive patients (Longhurst et al. 1999). The acute decrease in catecholamine availability did not produce any changes in anxiety or obsessive measurements, when patients were compared with controls. While this is only the first study of its kind, it should be noted that, similar to the tryptophan depletion studies in anxiety, there might be a need to add a behavioral or chemical challenge in order to produce a measurable response with AMPT (Bell et al. 2001).

Serotonin

The substrate for the synthesis of the indoleamine 5-hydroxytryptamine (5-HT) or serotonin is the dietary amino acid L-tryptophan. The transmitter is synthesized in discrete brainstem nuclei, mainly the dorsal and the median raphe. From there, nerve axons travel throughout the forebrain. After release in the synaptic cleft, 5-HT is actively transported back into the nerve terminal. Serotonin is catabolized to 5-hydroxyindoleacetic acid (5-HIAA), which is cleared from the brain through the CSF and blood (Nutt 1993).

A whole host of serotonin receptors have been identified in recent years. While the function of some of these receptor groups remains speculative or even obscure, there is substantial evidence for the involvement of a number of them in anxiety. These include the G protein linked pre- and postsynaptic 5-HT1A (Olivier *et al.* 1999), the phosphoinositol (PI) linked 5-HT2 (Roth *et al.* 1998) and the Na^+ channel-linked 5-HT3 (Olivier *et al.* 2000) receptor classes. Animal studies have also implicated the terminal 5-HT1B/D autoreceptor (Moret & Briley 2000). Given the diffuse innervation that 5-HT neurones provide to the brain, it comes as no surprise that this transmitter is involved in the coordination of a variety of other functions, including impulse control and aggression, appetite, neuroendocrine regulation, sleep, sexual function and mood (Nutt 1993; Lucki 1998).

Serotonin has been implicated in the neurochemistry of anxiety for a long time, but interest in this field of research increased dramatically in recent years. This was the result of a combination of advances in clinical practice and research technology. Drugs that block the reuptake of 5-HT from the synaptic cleft back to the nerve terminal, the selective serotonin reuptake inhibitors (SSRIs), demonstrated clear efficacy across the board of different anxiety disorders (Argyropoulos *et al.* 2000). Not so long ago the measurement of the levels of 5-HIAA was used as a credible but proxy index of the central 5-HT turnover. Nowadays, the development of specific ligands allows the visualization and the study of the multiplicity of 5-HT receptors and their functional role in health and disease (Lucki 1996; Passchier & van Waarde 2001). Further, the use of the tryptophan depletion technique in humans (Bell *et al.* 2001), and molecular manipulations (Murphy *et al.* 1999; Zhuang *et al.* 1999) and microdialysis (Parent *et al.* 2001) studies in animals, allow for a more rigorous assessment of the integrity of the 5-HT systems in the CNS.

Although the case for the involvement of 5-HT in anxiety is an overwhelming one, it is not clear yet whether anxiety results from excessive or deficient central serotonin function (Table 11.2). Challenge paradigms that increase central 5-HT transmission have produced mixed results. The 5-HT agonist *m*-chlorophenylpiperizine (mCPP) is anxiogenic in patients with panic disorder (Charney *et al.* 1987), OCD (Zohar *et al.* 1987), generalized anxiety (Germine *et al.* 1992) and in normal controls at high enough doses (Charney *et al.* 1987). Fenfluramine, a drug that releases

Table 11.2 Evidence for excessive or deficient serotonin in the origin of anxiety.

5-HT excess	5-HT deficiency
mCPP (5-HT agonist) $\Rightarrow \uparrow$ anxiety in PD, OCD, healthy volunteers	Precursors of 5-HT (tryptophan, 5-HTP) $\Rightarrow$ anxiolytic or neutral (PD, healthy volunteers)
Fenfluramine (5-HT releaser) $\Rightarrow \uparrow$ anxiety in PD, SAD	Tryptophan depletion $\Rightarrow \uparrow$ anxiety (PD but not OCD)
mCPP and fenfluramine $\Rightarrow \uparrow$ and ritanserin (5-HT blocker) $\Rightarrow \downarrow$ of skin conductance in conditioned anxiety (loud noise) in healthy volunteers	Fenfluramine $\Rightarrow \downarrow$ and ritanserin $\Rightarrow \uparrow$ of unconditioned anxiety (public speaking) in healthy volunteers
	SSRIs $\Rightarrow \downarrow$ anxiety after down regulation of autoreceptors and $\uparrow$ 5-HT (microdialysis studies)

5-HT, 5-hydroxytryptamine (serotonin); 5-HTTP, 5-hydroxytryptophan; GAD, generalized anxiety disorder; MCPP, m-chlorophenylpiperazine; OCD, obsessive-compulsive disorder; PD, panic disorder; SAD, social anxiety disorder; SSRIs, selective serotonin reuptake inhibitors.

5-HT, is also anxiogenic in panic disorder and social anxiety (Targum 1990; Tancer *et al.* 1994/1995). The same is true for the intravenous administration of clomipramine, a tricyclic antidepressant with a strong serotonin reuptake inhibition, in panic patients (George *et al.* 1995). On the other hand, L-tryptophan and 5-hydroxytryptophan (5-HTP), the precursors of 5-HT, are known to cause sedation and anxiolysis or, at worst, to have no effect on anxiety (Westenberg & den Boer 1989; van Vliet *et al.* 1996). Further, the SSRIs are traditionally thought to exert their action by increasing the availability of the transmitter in the synaptic cleft.

A number of theories have been put forward in an attempt to explain this apparent contradiction. The anxiety response to the 5-HT agonists fenfluramine and mCPP could simply be a cognitive misinterpretation of the side-effects produced by these drugs (Kahn *et al.* 1988). However, mCPP and fenfluramine also produced enhanced prolactin and/or cortisol responses in most of the studies cited above, indicating that the anxiogenic effect is not merely an artefact.

A possible interpretation of the neuroendocrine activation by fenfluramine and mCPP is that the postsynaptic 5-HT receptors (especially 5-HT2) are hypersensitive in anxiety. This may also account for the exacerbation of anxiety that is sometimes observed at the initial stages of treatment with SSRIs, before their therapeutic effect becomes evident a few weeks into the administration of the drugs (Argyropoulos *et al.* 2000). Kahn *et al.* (1988) proposed that this is the result of initial stimulation of hypersensitive postsynaptic 5-HT receptors by an excess of the transmitter, which is followed by down-regulation of these receptors in response to chronic bombardment. If this were correct, then the SSRIs would eventually exert their action by reducing central 5-HT transmission. By inference then anxiety could be considered to be a state of increased global serotonin function.

This theory is contradicted by animal studies using microdialysis. With this technique it is possible to measure the overflow of 5-HT into the extracellular space. It is generally, but not universally, considered that this overflow represents an indirect measure of 5-HT release in the synaptic cleft (Parent *et al.* 2001). The microdialysis studies show that 5-HT is not increased in the synapse during the acute treatment with SSRIs, but only after there is down-regulation of the presynaptic 5-HT1A autoreceptors (Blier *et al.* 1990). This leads to the reduction of the negative feedback to the 5-HT cell and subsequent increase in cell firing and serotonin release. Buspirone, a drug that is effective in generalized anxiety, is thought to exert its action through these autoreceptors (Taylor *et al.* 1985).

Tryptophan depletion is another technique that can be used to explore the functional importance of serotonin in psychiatric syndromes. Through a combination of special diet and consumption of an amino acid drink, it is possible to reduce plasma tryptophan up to 80% acutely. This is then supposed to result in substantially reduced central serotonin synthesis during the experiment. Patient populations can be studied before or after treatment, with or without concomitant challenge tests that attempt to reproduce particular symptom sets in the laboratory (Bell *et al.* 2001). So far, few studies have been performed in anxiety patients. While obsessive-compulsive or panic unmedicated patients do not seem to become acutely anxious when they are depleted of tryptophan, panic patients treated with SSRIs experience significant increase in their anxiety, after a flumazenil challenge, on the day of the tryptophan depletion (Nutt *et al.* 1999). Although these results are still preliminary, they provide a very strong indication that increased, rather than decreased, 5-HT is a necessary condition for the SSRIs to exert their anxiolytic effect. A similar study has just been completed in social anxiety, and preliminary analysis suggests a similar relapse.

The answer to the conundrum of too much or too little serotonin in anxiety may lie in the complex anatomy of the central 5-HT innervation. There are two major serotonergic systems that have been implicated in anxiety. They originate from the medial raphe nuclei (MRN) and the dorsal raphe nuclei (DRN), respectively. The two systems are morphologically distinct, and have different afferent and efferent projections (Graeff 1990; Azmitia & Whitaker 1995), but they function in parallel (Tork *et al.* 1990). It may be that each system mediates distinct aspects of anxiety. According to Grove *et al.* (1997), the MRN projection is crucial for the modulation of fear and anticipatory anxiety, while the DRN modulates cognitive processes related to anxiety. Other authors have suggested that the pathway from MRN to the dorsal hippocampus mediates resistance to chronic unavoidable stress (Deakin & Graeff 1991). The failure of one or all these subsystems may be responsible for the phenomenologically different clinical syndromes of anxiety and depression (Deakin & Graeff 1991; Bell & Nutt 1998).

While an excess of serotonin may precipitate anxiety in one subsystem, it may be anxiolytic in another. According to Deakin and Graeff (1991), the role of 5-HT in the ascending pathway from DRN to the amygdala and the frontal cortex facilitates anxiety, and more specifically conditioned fear. On the other hand, 5-HT in the pathway from DRN to periaqueductal gray (PG) matter may inhibit unconditioned fear, inborn fight/flight reactions to impending danger and panic (Graeff et al. 1996). Some support for this anatomical/functional diversity of 5-HT systems in relation to anxiety is lent by experiments showing that 5-HT promoting agents (fenfluramine and mCPP) increase skin conductance in a paradigm of an aversive conditioned stimulus (loud tone) in healthy volunteers, while fenfluramine decreased the subjective anxiety induced by a paradigm of unconditioned stimulus (public speaking). On the other hand, a 5-HT blocking agent (ritanserin) had exactly the opposite effect in the above paradigms (Graeff et al. 1996; Guimaraes et al. 1997).

One may hypothesize that a combination of specific functional/anatomical pathways and different 5-HT receptor subtypes may be ultimately responsible for the clinical expression of distinct forms of anxiety. If this were true, not only could the contradictions be explained and accommodated in a comprehensive theory of 5-HT and anxiety, but pharmacological manipulations targeting the suspect brain loci/receptors could be possible. Most of the work in this field so far is done in animals, but it is very promising. For example, it appears that the enhancement of 5-HT2 transmission in the orbitofrontal cortex may be responsible for the therapeutic effect of the SSRIs in OCD (Martin et al. 1998; Blier & Abbott 2001). Early animal work suggests that a specific 5-HT2C agonist exerts its antipanic effect through the peri-acqueductal gray (PAG) (Jenck et al. 1998).

The advent of neuroimaging should also help in answering some of the questions raised above. Radioligands, like the [carbonyl-11C] Way-100635 compound, have become available in recent years for the study of 5-HT1A receptors. The finding that these receptors mainly localize in the limbic forebrain supports the long held view that they are implicated in the modulation of emotions (Passchier & van Waarde 2001). Attempts to study the 5-HT systems and receptors in the brain, before and after treatment, have mainly focused on depression so far, but one study in treated panic disorder patients has reported a decrease in 5-HT1A receptor density, similar to that seen in depression (Sargent et al. 2000). A systematic study of anxiety conditions, using positron emission tomography (PET) or single photon emission computerized tomography (SPECT), may yield valuable information towards the understanding of the precise role of 5-HT in these conditions.

Finally, evidence for the molecular/genetic processes involved in the regulation of the central 5-HT system, and their significance for anxiety, have just begun to emerge. A polymorphism of the 5-HT transporter (5-HTT) gene has been associated with anxiety personality traits (Lesch & Mossner 1998) (see Chapter 13). However, these data are still preliminary and they have not been yet integrated in the existing serotonin/anxiety framework. This framework should also take into account another potential source of heterogeneity and contradictory experimental results, namely the environmental factors (especially early ones) that may have long-term consequences and shape the 5-HT system sensitivity to stress (Chalouoff 2000).

Dopamine

The catecholamine dopamine (DA), as mentioned earlier, is the precursor of NE. It is synthesized from the dietary amino acid tyrosine. Similar to the other monoamine transmitters, following release in the synaptic cleft it is actively absorbed back to the nerve terminal, although some spills over to glial cells. DA is catabolized by MAO and COMT. The final product of both catabolic processes is homovanillic acid (HVA). Measurement of HVA in CSF and plasma has been used as a proxy measure of central DA turnover. The largest nucleus containing DA-secreting cells is substantia nigra in the mid-brain. From there DA is supplied mainly to the basal ganglia, nucleus accumbens, cingulate and prefrontal cortex. A number of G protein linked DA receptors have been characterized (D_{1-5}). The involvement of DA in movement disorders, schizophrenia, depression, reinforcement mechanisms (e.g., in drug dependence), and emesis is well researched and documented. Its role in anxiety though has not been as well established (Nutt 1993).

A number of clinical observations led to the hypothesis that DA dysfunction may play a role in social anxiety disorder (Argyropoulos *et al*. 2001b). However, the first study that attempted to elucidate the role of DA in this condition was negative. Patients were challenged with levodopa, but the resulting DA-mediated release of prolactin and the eye-blink response were not different from that of controls (Tancer *et al*. 1994/1995). A later SPECT study though showed a decrease in striatal DA reuptake sites in patients compared with controls (Tiihonen *et al*. 1997). Another SPECT study (Schneier *et al*. 2000) found that the mean D2 receptor binding potential in the striatum of patients was significantly lower than that of controls. The above support the idea that the number of dopaminergic synapses/neurones may be reduced in social anxiety, leading to DA hypoactivity in this syndrome. At present we cannot answer the question whether these changes are simply functional or whether they point towards structural abnormalities of similar nature to the ones seen in neurodegenerative conditions, albeit subtler. A magnetic resonance imaging (MRI) study (Potts *et al*. 1994) found no specific structural abnormalities in social phobia. It suggested, however, a greater age-related reduction in the volume of the putamen in social anxiety patients compared with controls. A way forward might be to challenge patients with a DA-releasing agent, such as an amphetamine, and then measure the displacement of the tracer from the receptors that the released transmitter will produce (Laruelle & Abi-Dargham 1999).

Information about the role of DA in other anxiety states is scarce. Levels of HVA in the CSF do not differ between untreated panic patients and controls (Eriksson *et al*. 1991). In another study, GH response was measured after apomorphine (DA receptor agonist) challenge in depressed and panic patients and normal controls. While the depressed group showed the well characterized blunting of GH response, the panic group did not differ from the controls, thus indicating no postsynaptic dopaminergic hypoactivity in this anxiety disorder (Pitchot *et al*. 1995). In PTSD, a role for DA dysfunction has been postulated in relation to the occurrence of paranoid/psychotic symptoms, impaired motivation and concentration, emotional numbing, dissociation and memory deficits in this population (Coupland 2000). However, this is still only a speculative possibility, neither confirmed nor disproved by experimental data. Some tentative evidence of involvement of DA in PTSD comes from a study measuring the urinary catecholamine concentrations

in a sample of Vietnam veterans (Yehuda *et al*. 1992). DA concentrations were higher in patients than controls and they correlated positively with the severity of symptoms.

In OCD the picture is also incomplete. Several lines of evidence point towards the involvement of DA in OCD, not least the brain circuitry of this disorder, which includes areas very rich in DA innervation (Insel 1992), and the clinical observation that neuroleptics are sometimes effective in obsessive-compulsive spectrum disorders, including tics (Goodman *et al*. 1992). Preliminary evidence from genetic studies suggests that polymorphisms in the D_4 (but not the D_2 or D_3) receptor gene may be associated with this disorder (Catalano *et al*. 1994; Novelli *et al*. 1994; Billet *et al*. 1998). As mentioned earlier, acute catecholamine depletion with AMPT failed to induce OCD symptoms in drug-free patients (Longhurst *et al*. 1999). It may well be though that, similar with the tryptophan depletion technique in anxiety described earlier, a challenge is needed in parallel with AMPT in order to produce measurable change in symptoms. The apomorphine challenge has been used in OCD with mixed results. It elicited a cortisol response similar to the control group (Brambilla *et al*. 2000), but the GH response was blunted and the emetic response was significantly stronger in patients than in controls (Brambilla *et al*. 1997b). Of note is that a smaller study failed to produce a blunted GH response (Pitchot *et al*. 1996).

Summary

Achieving a greater understanding of the nature and diversity of anxiety or "the anxieties" has perplexed psychologists for well over a century. In the last 30 years, neuroscientists have attempted to elucidate the neurobiological circuitry that underlies anxiety and hence shed light on the causes of pathological anxiety states. Early work on humans tended to look at the physiological and pharmacological provocation of anxiety in various patient and volunteer groups. More recently, with the advent of dynamic brain imaging techniques and the increasing availability of new ligands, work has focused on a more systematic "teasing out" of the pathways involved in the various forms of anxiety. Whilst noradrenergic, serotonergic and GABAergic systems have remained the focus of attention, other transmitters and modulators (e.g., DA, cholecystokinin) are becoming more prominent, while researchers also try to assess the importance of the balance between these systems (Ressler & Nemeroff 2000). More work needs to be done towards a truly robust and comprehensive neurobiological understanding of anxiety, with the hope that this will lead to even more effective and better tolerated treatments.

References

Abelson, J.L., Glitz, D., Cameron, O.G., Lee, M.A., Bronzo, M. & Curtis, G.C. (1991) Blunted growth hormone response to clonidine in patients with generalised anxiety disorder. *Arch Gen Psychiatry* 48, 157–62.

Abelson, J.L., Glitz, D., Cameron, O.G., Lee, M.A., Bronzo, M. & Curtis, G.C. (1992) Endocrine, cardiovascular, and behavioral responses to clonidine in patients with panic disorder. *Biol Psychiatry* 32, 18–25.

American Psychiatric Association (1994) *Diagnostic Statistical Manual of Mental Disorders*, 4th edn. American Psychiatric Association, Washington, D.C.

Argyropoulos, S.V., Abrams, J.K. & Nutt, D.J. (2001a) The tryptophan depletion technique in psychiatric research. In: *Anxiety Disorders: an Introduction to Clinical Management and Research*. (E.J.L. Griez, C. Faravelli, D.J. Nutt & J. Zohar (eds), pp. 359–69). John Wiley, Chichester.

Argyropoulos, S.V., Bell, C.J. & Nutt, D.J. (2001b) Brain function in social anxiety disorder. *Psychiatr Clin North Am* 24, 707–21.

Argyropoulos, S.V., Sandford, J.J. & Nutt, D.J. (2000) The psychobiology of anxiolytic drugs. Part 2. Pharmacological treatments of anxiety. *Pharmacol Ther* 88, 213–27.

Aston-Jones, G., Rajkowski, J., Kibiak, P. & Alexinsky, T. (1994) Locus coeruleus neurones in the monkey are selectively activated by attended stimuli in a vigilance task. *J Neurosci* 14, 4467–80.

Azmitia, E.C. & Whitaker, P.M. (1995) Anatomy, cell biology and plasticity of the serotonergic system. Neuropsychopharmacological implications for the actions of psychotropic drugs. In: *Psychopharmacology: the Fourth Generation of Progress* (F.E. Bloom & D.J. Kupfer (eds), pp. 443–90). Raven Press, New York.

Barbaccia, M.L., Costa, E., Ferrero, P. *et al.* (1986) Diazepam-binding inhibitor. *Arch Gen Psychiatry* 43, 1143–7.

Baulieu, E.E. (1998) Neurosteroids: a novel function of the brain. *Psychoneuroendocrinology* 23, 963–87.

Bell, C.J., Abrams, J.K. & Nutt, D.J. (2001) Tryptophan depletion and its implications for psychiatry. *Br J Psychiatry* 178, 399–405.

Bell, C.J. & Nutt, D.J. (1998) Serotonin and panic. *Br J Psychiatry* 172, 465–71.

Billet, E.A., Richter, M.A., Sam, F. *et al.* (1998) Investigation of dopamine system genes in obsessive-compulsive disorder. *Psychiatr Genet* 8, 163–9.

Blier, P. & Abbott, F.V. (2001) Putative mechanisms of action of antidepressant drugs in affective and anxiety disorders and pain. *J Psychiatry Neurosci* 26, 37–43.

Blier, P., de Montigny, C. & Chaput, Y. (1990) A role for the serotonergic system in the mechanism of action of antidepressant treatments: preclinical evidence. *J Clin Psychiatry* 6 (Suppl. 5), 5–12.

den Boer, J.A. & Westenberg, H.G.M. (1993) Critical notes on the locus coeruleus hypothesis of panic disorder. *Acta Neuropsychiat* 5, 48–54.

Braestrup, C., Nielsen, M., Honore, T., Jensen, L.H. & Petersen, E.N. (1983) Benzodiazepine receptor ligands with positive and negative efficacy. *Neuropharmacology* 22, 1451–7.

Braestrup, C. & Squires, R.F. (1978) Brain specific benzodiazepine receptors. *Br J Psychiatry* 133, 249–60.

Brambilla, F., Bellodi, L., Perna, G., Arancio, C. & Bertani, A. (1997b) Dopamine function in obsessive-compulsive disorder: growth hormone response to apomorphine stimulation. *Biol Psychiatry* 42, 889–97.

Brambilla, F., Perna, G., Bellodi, L. *et al.* (1997a) Noradrenergic receptor sensitivity in obsessive-compulsive disorders. I. Growth hormone response to clonidine stimulation. *Psychiatry Res* 69, 155–62.

Brambilla, F., Perna, G., Bussi, R. & Bellodi, L. (2000) Dopamine function in obsessive compulsive disorder: cortisol response to acute apomorphine stimulation. *Psychoneuroendocrinology* 25, 301–10.

Brambilla, F., Perna, G., Garberi, A., Nobile, P. & Bellodi, L. (1995) α_2-adrenergic receptor sensitivity in panic disorder. I. GH response to GHRH and clonidine stimulation in panic disorder. *Psychoneuroendocrinology* 20, 1–9.

Brown, M.J., Jenner, D.A., Allison, D.J. & Dollery, C.T. (1981) Variations in individual organ release of noradrenaline measured by an improved radioenzymatic technique: limitations of peripheral venous measurements in the assessment of sympathetic nervous activity. *Clin Sci* 61, 585–90.

Cameron, O.G., Smith, C.B., Lee, M.A., Hollingsworth, P.G., Hill, E.M. & Curtis, G.C. (1990) Adrenergic status in anxiety disorders: platelet α_2-adrenergic receptor binding, blood pressure, pulse and plasma catecholamines in panic and generalised anxiety disorder patients and normal subjects. *Biol Psychiatry* 28, 3–20.

Cantril, H. & Hunt, W.A. (1932) Emotional effects produced by the injection of adrenaline. *Am J Psychol* 44, 300–7.

Catalano, M., Sciuto, G., Di Bella, D., Novelli, E., Nobile, M. & Bellodi, L. (1994) Lack of association between obsessive-compulsive disorder and the dopamine D3 receptor gene: some preliminary considerations. *Am J Med Genet* 54, 253–5.

Chalouoff, F. (2000) Serotonin, stress and corticoids. *Journal of Psychopharm* **14**, 139–51.

Charney, D.S. & Heninger, G.R. (1986) Abnormal regulation of noradrenergic function in panic disorders. *Am J Psychiatry* **43**, 1042–54.

Charney, D.S., Heninger, G.R. & Breier, A. (1984) Noradrenergic function and panic anxiety effects of yohimbine in healthy subjects and patients with agoraphobia and panic disorder. *Arch Gen Psychiatry* **41**, 751–63.

Charney, D.S., Woods, S.W., Goodman, W.K. & Heninger, G.R. (1987) Serotonin function in anxiety. II. Effects of the serotonin agonist mCPP in panic disorder patients and healthy subjects. *Psychopharmacology* **92**, 14–24.

Charney, D.S., Woods, S.W. & Heninger, G.R. (1989) Noradrenergic function in generalized anxiety disorder: effects of yohimbine in healthy subjects and patients with generalized anxiety disorder. *Psychiatry Res* **27**, 173–82.

Clow, A., Glover, V., Armando, I. & Sandler, M. (1983) New endogenous benzodiazepine receptor ligand in human urine: identity with endogenous monoamine oxidase inhibitor? *Life Sci* **33**, 735–41.

Clow, A., Glover, V., Sandler, M. & Tiller, J. (1988a) Increased urinary tribulin output in generalised anxiety disorder. *Psychopharmacology* **95**, 378–80.

Clow, A., Glover, V., Weg, M.W. *et al.* (1988b) Urinary catecholamine metabolic and tribulin output during lactate infusion. *Br J Psychiaty* **152**, 122–6.

Coplan, J.D., Liebowitz, M.R., Gorman, J.M. *et al.* (1992) Noradrenergic function in panic disorder: effects of intravenous clonidine pretreatment on lactate induced panic. *Biol Psychiatry* **31**, 135–46.

Coplan, J.D., Papp, L.A., Martinez, J. *et al.* (1995) Persistence of blunted human hormone response to clonidine in fluoxetine-treated patients with panic disorder. *Am J Psychiatry* **152**, 619–22.

Coupland, N.J. (2000) Brain mechanisms and neurotransmitters. In: *Post-Traumatic Stress Disorder: Diagnosis, Management and Treatment* (D.J. Nutt, J.R.T. Davidson & J. Zohar (eds), pp. 69–99). Martin Dunitz, London.

Coupland, N.J., Bailey, E.J., Wilson, S.J., Potter, W.Z. & Nutt, D.J. (1994) A pharmacodynamic study of the α_2-antagonist, ethoxy-idazoxan, in healthy volunteers. *Clin Pharmacol Ther* **56**, 420–9.

Coupland, N.J., Bell, C.J., Potokar, J.P., Dorkins, E. & Nutt, D.J. (2000) Flumazenil challenge in social phobia. *Depress Anx* **11**, 27–30.

Da Costa, J.M. (1871) On irritable heart. *Am J Med Sci* **61**, 17–52.

Deakin, J.F.W. & Graeff, F.G. (1991) 5-HT and mechanisms of defense. *J Psychopharmacol* **5**, 305–15.

Delgado, P.L., Miller, H.L., Solomon, R.M. *et al.* (1993) Monoamines and the mechanism of antidepressant action: effects of catecholamine depletion on mood of patients treated with antidepressants. *Psychopharmacol Bull* **29**, 389–96.

Doble, A. (1999) New insights into the mechanism of action of hypnotics. *J Psychopharmacol* **13** (Suppl. 1), S11–S20.

Dorow, R., Horowski, R., Paschelke, G., Amin, M. & Braestrup, C. (1983) Severe anxiety induced by FG 7142. A β-carboline ligand for benzodiazepine receptors. *Lancet* **2**, 98–9.

Elsworth, J.D., Redmond, D.E. & Roth, R.H. (1982) Plasma and cerebrospinal fluid 3-methoxy-4-hydroxyphenylethylene glycol (MHPG) as indices of brain norepinephrine metabolism in primates. *Brain Res* **235**, 115–24.

Eriksson, E., Westberg, P., Alling, C., Thuresson, K. & Modigh, K. (1991) Cerebrospinal fluid levels of monoamine metabolites in panic disorder. *Psychiatry Res* **36**, 243–51.

Esler, M.D., Lambert, G.W., Ferrier, C. *et al.* (1995) Central nervous system noradrenergic control of sympathetic outflow in normotensive and hypertensive humans. *Clin Exp Hypertens* **17**, 409–23.

Frankenhauser, M. (1971) Behavior and circulating catecholamines. *Brain Res* **31**, 241–62.

Frankenhauser, M., Jarpe, G. & Matell, G. (1961) Effects of intravenous infusions of adrenaline and noradrenaline on certain psychological and physiological functions. *Acta Physiol Scand* **51**, 175–86.

Friedman, M.J. (1998) Current and future drug treatment for posttraumatic stress disorder patients. *Psychiatr Ann* **28**, 461–8.

Gann, H., Riemann, D., Stoll, S., Berger, M. & Muller, W.E. (1995) Growth-hormone to clonidine in panic disorder patients in comparison to patients with major depression and healthy controls. *Pharmacopsychiatry* **28**, 80–3.

Gentil, V., Tavares, S., Gorenstein, C., Bello, C., Mathias, L., Gronich, G. & Singer, J. (1990) Acute reversal of flunitrazepam effects by Ro 15-1788 and Ro 15-3505: inverse agonism, tolerance and rebound. *Psychopharmacology* **100**, 54–9.

George, D.T., Nutt, D.J., Dwyer, B.A. & Linnoila, M. (1990) Alcoholism and panic disorder: is the comorbidity more than coincidence? *Acta Psychiatr Scand* **81**, 97–107.

George, D.T., Nutt, D.J., Rawlings, R.R. *et al.* (1995) Behavioral and endocrine responses to clomipramine in panic disorder patients with and without alcoholism. *Biol Psychiatry* **37**, 112–19.

Germine, M., Goddard, A.W., Woods, S.W., Charney, D.S. & Heninger, G.R. (1992) Anger and anxiety responses to m-chlorophenylpiperazine in generalized anxiety disorder. *Biol Psychiatry* **32**, 457–61.

Glue, P., Nutt, D.J. & Linnoila, M. (1992) Adrenergic changes during alcohol and drug intoxication and withdrawal. In: *Adrenergic Dysfunction and Psychobiology American* (O.G. Cameron (ed.), pp. 467–509). Psychiatric Association Press, Washington, D.C.

Goldberg, M.R., Hollister, A.S. & Robertson, D. (1983) Influence of yohimbine on blood pressure, autonomic reflexes and plasma catecholamines in humans. *Hypertens* 5, 772–8.

Goodman, W.K., McDougle, C.J. & Price, L.H. (1992) The role of serotonin and dopamine in the pathophysiology of obsessive-compulsive disorder. *Int Clin Psychopharmacol* 7 (Suppl. 1), 35–8.

Graeff, F.G. (1990) Brain defence systems and anxiety. In: *Handbook of Anxiety*, Vol. 3 (M. Roth, G.D. Burrows & R. Noyes, Jr (eds), pp. 307–57). Elsevier Science Publishers, Amsterdam.

Graeff, F.G., Guimaraes, F.S., De Andrade, T.G. & Deakin, J.F. (1996) Role of 5-HT in stress, anxiety and depression. *Pharmacol Biochem Behav* 86, 334–8.

Grove, G., Coplan, J.D. & Hollander, E. (1997) The neuroanatomy of 5-HT dysregulation and panic disorder. *J Neuropsychiatry Clin Neurosci* 9, 198–207.

Guimaraes, F.S., Mbaya, P.S. & Deakin, J.F.W. (1997) Ritanserin facilitates anxiety in a simulated public-speaking paradigm. *J Psychopharmacol* 11, 225–31.

Hewlett, W.A., Vinogradov, S. & Agras, W.S. (1992) Clomipramine, clonazepam and clonidine treatment of obsessive-compulsive disorder. *J Clin Psychopharmacol* 12, 420–30.

Hoehn-Saric, R., Merchant, A.F., Keyser, M.C. & Smith, V.K. (1981) Effects of clonidine on anxiety disorders. *Arch Gen Psychiatry* 38, 1278–82.

Hollander, E., DeCaria, C., Nitescu, A. *et al.* (1991) Noradrenergic function in obsessive-compulsive disorder: behavioral and neuroendocrine responses to clonidine and comparison to healthy controls. *Psychiatry Res* 37, 161–77.

Insel, T.R. (1992) Toward a neuroanatomy of obsessive-compulsive disorder. *Arch Gen Psychiatry* 49, 739–44.

Jackson, H.C. & Nutt, D.J. (1992) Effects of benzodiazepine receptor inverse agonists on locomotor activity and exploration in mice. *Eur J Pharmacol* 221, 199–204.

Jenck, F., Moreau, J.L., Berendsen, H.H. *et al.* (1998) Anti-aversive effects of 5HT2C receptor agonists and fluoxetine in a model of panic-like anxiety in rats. *Eur Neuropsychopharmacol* 8, 161–8.

Kahn, R.S., Wetzler, S., van Praag, H.M., Asnis, G.M. & Strauman, T. (1988) Behavioral indications for receptor hypersensitivity in panic disorder. *Psychiatry Res* 25, 101–4.

Kaschka, W., Feistel, H. & Ebert, D. (1995) Reduced benzodiazepine receptor binding in panic disorders measured by iomazenil SPECT. *J Psychiatr Res* 29, 427–34.

Kelly, C.B. & Cooper, S.J. (1998) Differences and variability in plasma noradrenaline between depressive and anxiety disorders. *J Psychopharmacol* 12, 161–7.

Klein, D.F. (1981) Anxiety reconceptualized. In: *Anxiety: New Research and Changing Concepts* (D.F. Klein & J. Rabkin (eds), pp. 235–63). Raven Press, New York.

Klein, D.F. & Fink, M. (1962) Psychiatric reaction patterns to imipramine. *Am J Psychiatry* 119, 432–8.

Ko, G.N., Elsworth, J.D., Roth, R.H., Rifkin, B.G., Leigh, H. & Redmond, E. (1983) Panic-induced elevation of plasma MHPG levels in phobic-anxious patients, effects of clonidine and imipramine. *Arch Gen Psychiatry* 40, 425–30.

Koob, G.F. (1999) Corticotropin-releasing factor, norepinephrine and stress. *Biol Psychiatry* 46, 1167–80.

Kopin, I.J. (1984) Avenues of investigation for the role of catecholamines in anxiety. *Psychopathology* 17, 3–8.

Krystal, J.H., McDougle, C.J., Woods, S.W., Price, L.H., Heninger, G.R. & Charney, D.S. (1992) Dose–response relationship for oral idazoxan effects in healthy human subjects: comparison with oral yohimbine. *Psychopharmacology* 108, 313–19.

Kuikka, J.T., Pitkanen, A., Lepola, U. *et al.* (1995) Abnormal regional benzodiazepine receptor uptake in the prefrontal cortex in patients with panic disorder. *Nucleic Medical Communications* 16(4), 273–80.

Laruelle, M. & Abi-Dargham, A. (1999) Dopamine as the wind of the psychotic fire: new evidence from brain imaging studies. *J Psychopharmacol* 13, 358–71.

Lee, M.A., Cameron, O.G., Gurguis, G.N. *et al.* (1990) α_2 adrenoreceptor status in obsessive-compulsive disorder. *Biol Psychiatry* 27, 1083–93.

Lesch, K.P. & Mossner, R. (1998) Genetically driven variation of serotonin uptake: is there a link to affective spectrum, neurodevelopmental, and neurodegenerative disorders? *Biol Psychiatry* 44, 179–92.

Lingford-Hughes, A. & Malizia, A. (1999) Measurement of brain GABA-benzodiazepine receptor levels *in vivo* using emission tomography. *Meth Mol Biol* 106, 119–36.

Little, H.J., Nutt, D.J. & Taylor, S.C. (1987) Bidirectional effects of chronic treatment with agonists and inverse agonists at the benzodiazepine receptor. *Brain Res Bull* 19, 371–8.

Longhurst, J.G., Carpenter, L.L., Epperson, C.N., Price, L.H. & McDougle, C.J. (1999) Effects of catecholamine depletion with AMPT (alpha-methyl-para-tyrosine) in obsessive-compulsive disorder. *Biol Psychiatry* 46, 573–6.

Louie, A.K., Lannon, R.A. & Ketter, T.A. (1989) Treatment of cocaine-induced panic disorder. *Am J Psychiatry* 146, 40–4.

Lucki, I. (1996) Serotonin receptor specificity in anxiety disorders. *J Clin Psychiatry* 57 (Suppl. 6), 5–10.

Lucki, I. (1998) The spectrum of behaviors influenced by serotonin. *Biol Psychiatry* 44, 151–62.

Lugaresi, E., Montagna, P., Tinuper, P. *et al.* (1998) Endozepine stupor: recurring stupor linked to endozepine-4 accumulation. *Brain* 121, 127–33.

Malizia, A.L., Cunningham, V.J., Bell, C.J., Liddle, P.F., Jones, T. & Nutt, D.J. (1998) Decreased brain GABA-benzodiazepine receptor binding in panic disorder. *Arch Gen Psychiatry* 55, 715–20.

Malizia, A.L., Gunn, R.N., Wilson, S.J. *et al.* (1996) Benzodiazepine site pharmacokinetic/pharmacodynamic quantification in man: direct measurement of drug occupancy and effects on the human brain *in vivo*. *Neuropharmacology* **35**, 1483–91.

Maranon, G. (1924) Contribution a l'etude de l'action emotive de l'adrenaline. *Rev Franc Endocrinol* **2**, 301–25.

Martin, J.R., Boes, M., Jenck, F. *et al.* (1998) 5-HT2C receptor agonists: pharmacological characteristics and therapeutic potential. *J Pharmacol Exp Ther* **286**, 913–24.

Mathew, R.J., Ho, B.T., Francis, D.J., Taylor, D.L. & Weinman, M.L. (1982) Catecholamines and anxiety. *Acta Psychiatr Scand* **65**, 142–7.

McDougle, C.J., Black, J.E., Malison *et al.* (1994) Noradrenergic dysregulation during discontinuation of cocaine use in addicts. *Arch Gen Psychiatry* **51**, 713–19.

Middleton, H.C. (1990) Cardiovascular dystonia in recovered panic patients. *J Affect Disord* **19**, 229–36.

Moret, C. & Briley, M. (2000) The possible role of 5-HT (1B/D) receptors in psychiatric disorders and their potential as a target for therapy. *Eur J Pharmacol* **404**, 1–12.

Munjack, D.J., Baltazaar, P.L., De Quattro, V. *et al.* (1990) Generalised anxiety disorder: some biochemical aspects. *Psychiatry Res* **32**, 35–43.

Murphy, D.L., Wichems, C., Li, Q. & Heils, A. (1999) Molecular manipulations as tools for enhancing our understanding of 5-HT neurotransmission. *Tr Pharmacological Sience* **20**, 246–52.

Nesse, R.M., Cameron, O.G., Curtis, G.C., McCann, D.S. & Huber-Smith, M.J. (1984) Adrenergic function in patients with panic anxiety. *Arch Gen Psychiatry* **41**, 771–6.

Novelli, E., Nobile, M., Diaferia, G., Sciuto, G. & Catalano, M. (1994) A molecular investigation suggests no relationship between obsessive-compulsive disorder and the dopamine D2 receptor. *Neuropsychobiology* **29**, 61–3.

Nutt, D.J. (1986) Increased central α_2-adrenoceptor sensitivity in panic disorder. *Psychopharmacology* **90**, 268–9.

Nutt, D.J. (1989) Altered α_2-adrenoceptor sensitivity in panic disorder. *Arch Gen Psychiatry* **46**, 165–9.

Nutt, D.J. (1990) The pharmacology of human anxiety. *Pharmacol Ther* **47**, 233–66.

Nutt, D.J. (1993) Neurochemistry and neuropharmacoloy. In: *Seminars in Basic Neurosciences* (G. Morgan & S. Butler (eds), pp. 71–111). Gaskell, London.

Nutt, D.J., Bell, C.J. & Malizia, A.L. (1998) Brain mechanisms of social anxiety disorder. *J Clin Psychiatry* **59** (Suppl. 17), 4–9.

Nutt, D.J., Forashall, S., Bell, C.J. *et al.* (1999) Mechanisms of action of selective serotonin reuptake inhibitors in the treatment of psychiatric disorders. *Eur Neuropsychopharmacol* **9** (Suppl. 3), S81–S6.

Nutt, D.J., Glue, P., Lawson, C. & Wilson, S. (1990) Evidence for altered benzodiazepine receptor sensitivity in panic disorder: effects of the benzodiazepine receptor antagonist flumazenil. *Arch Gen Psychiatry* **47**, 917–25.

Nutt, D.J., Glue, P., Wilson, S.J., Groves, S., Coupland, N.J. & Bailey, J.E. (1993) Flumazenil in alcohol withdrawal. *Alcohol and Alcoholism* **2** (Suppl.), 337–41.

Nutt, D.J. & Lawson, C. (1992) Panic attacks: a neurochemical overview of models and mechanisms. *Br J Psychiatry* **160**, 165–78.

Nutt, D.J. & Malizia, A.L. (2001) New insights into the role of the GABA-A benzodiazepine receptor. *Br J Psychiatry* **179**, 390–6.

Olivier, B., Soudijn, W. & van Wijngaarden, I. (1999) The 5-HT1A receptor and its ligands: structure and function. *Prog Drug Res* **52**, 103–65.

Olivier, B., van Wijngaarden, I. & Soudijn, W. (2000) 5-HT (3) receptor antagonists and anxiety; a preclinical and clinical review. *Eur Neuropsychopharmacol* **10**, 77–95.

Papp, L.A., Gorman, J.M., Liebowitz, M.R., Fyer, A.J., Cohen, B. & Klein, D.F. (1988) Epinephrine infusions in patients with social phobia. *Am J Psychiatry* **145**, 733–6.

Parent, M., Bush, D., Rauw, G., Master, S., Vaccarino, F. & Baker, G. (2001) Analysis of amino acids and catacholamines, 5-hydroxytryptamine and their metabolites in brain areas in the rat using *in vivo* microdialysis. *Methods* **23**, 11–20.

Passchier, J. & van Waarde, A. (2001) Visualisation of serotonin-1A (5-HT1A) receptors in the central nervous system. *Eur J Nucl Med* **28**, 113–29.

Pitchot, W., Hansenne, M., Gonzalez-Moreno, A. & Ansseau, M. (1995) Growth hormone response to apomorphine in panic disorder: comparison with major depression and normal controls. *Eur Arch Psychiatry Clin Neurosci* **245**, 306–8.

Pitchot, W., Hansenne, M., Gonzalez-Moreno, A. & Ansseau, M. (1996) Growth hormone response to apomorphine in obsessive-compulsive disorder. *J Psychiatry Neurosci* **21**, 343–5.

Potokar, J., Coupland, N., Glue, P. *et al.* (1997) Flumazenil in alcohol withdrawal: a double-blind placebo-controlled study. *Alcohol and Alcoholism* **32**, 605–11.

Potokar, J., Nash, J., Sandford, J., Rich, A. & Nutt, D.J. (2000) GABA$_A$ benzodiazepine receptor (GBzR) sensitivity: test–retest reliability in normal volunteers. *Hum Psychopharmacol Clin Exp* **15**, 281–6.

Potts, N.L., Davidson, J.R., Krishnan, K.R. & Doraiswamy, P.M. (1994) Magnetic resonance imaging in patients with social phobia. *Psychiatry Res* **52**, 35–42.

Pyke, R.E. & Greenberg, H.S. (1986) Norepinephrine challenges in panic patients. *J Clin Pharmacol* **6**, 279–85.

Rainey, J.M., Pohl, R.B., Williams, Knitter, E., Freedman, R.R. & Ettedgui, E. (1984) A comparison of lactate and isoproterenol anxiety states. *Psychopathology* **17** (Suppl. 1), 74–82.

Rasmussen, S.A., Goodman, W.K., Woods, S.W., Heninger, G.R. & Charney, D.S. (1987) Effects of yohimbine in obsessive-compulsive disorder. *Psychopharmacology* **93**, 308–13.

Rasmussen, K. & Jacobs, B.L. (1986) Single unit activity of locus coeruleus neurons in freely moving cat. II. Conditioning and pharmacologic studies. *Brain Res* **371**, 335–44.

Redmond, D.E. (1986) The possible role of locus coeruleus noradrenergic activity in anxiety-panic. *Clin Neuropharmacol* **9**, 40–2.

Redmond, D.E. & Huang, Y. (1979) Current concepts. II. New evidence for a locus coeruleus-norepinephrine connection with anxiety. *Life Sci* **25**, 2149–62.

Reid, J.C. (1983) Central and peripheral autonomic control mechanisms. In: *Autonomic Failure* (R. Bannister (ed.), pp. 17–35). Oxford University Press, Oxford.

Ressler, K.J. & Nemeroff, C.B. (2000) Role of serotonergic and noradrenergic systems in the pathophysiology of depression and anxiety disorders. *Depress Anxiety* **12** (Suppl. 1), 2–19.

Roth, B.L., Willins, D.L., Kristiansen, K. & Kroese, W.K. (1998) 5-Hydroxytryptamine2-family receptors (5-hydroxytryptamine2A, 5-hydroxytryptamine2B, 5-hydroxytryptamine2C): where structure meets function. *Pharmacol Ther* **79**, 231–57.

Rothstein, J.D., Garland, W., Puia, G., Guidotti, A., Weber, R.J. & Costa, E. (1992a) Purfication and characterization of naturally occurring benzodiazepine receptor ligands in rat and human brain. *J Neurochem* **58**, 2102–15.

Rothstein, J.D., Guidottie, A. & Costa, E. (1992b) Release of endogenous benzodiazepine receptor ligands (endozepines) from cultured neurons. *Neurosci Lettt* **143**, 210–14.

Roy-Byrne, P.P., Geraci, M. & Uhde, T.W. (1986) Life events and the onset of panic disorder. *Am J Psychiatry* **143**, 1424–27.

Sargent, P.A., Nash, J., Hood, S. *et al.* (2000) 5-HT1A receptor binding in panic disorder; comparison with depressive disorder and healthy volunteers using PET and [11C]WAY-100635. *Neuroimage* **11**, 189.

Schachter, S. & Singer, J. (1962) Cognitive social and physiological determinants of emotional state. *Psychol Rev* **69**, 379–97.

Schildkraut, J.J. & Ketty, S.S. (1967) Biogenic amines and emotion. *Science* **156**, 21–30.

Schlegel, S., Steinert, H., Bockisch, A., Hahn, K., Schloesser, R. & Benkert, O. (1994) Decreased benzodiazepine receptor binding in panic disorder measured by iomazenil-SPECT. A preliminary report. *Eur Arch Psychiatry Clin Neurosci* **244**, 49–51.

Schneier, F.R., Liebowitz, M.R., Abi-Dargham, A., Zea-Ponce, Y., Lin, S.-H. & Laruelle, M. (2000) Low dopamine D2 receptor binding potential in social phobia. *Am J Psychiatry* **157**, 457–9.

Smith, A. & Nutt, D. (1996) Noradrenaline and attention lapses. *Nature* **380**, 291.

Southwick, S.M., Krystal, J.H., Morgan, A. *et al.* (1993) Abnormal noradrenergic function in post-traumatic stress disorder. *Arch Gen Psychiatry* **50**, 266–74.

Stanford, S.C. (1989) Central adrenoceptors in response and adaptation to stress. In: *The Pharmacology of Noradrenaline in the Central Nervous System* (C.A. Marsden & D.J. Heal (eds), pp. 379–422). Oxford University Press, Oxford.

Starkman, M.N., Cameron, O.G., Nesse, R.M. & Zebrik, T. (1990) Peripheral catecholamine levels and the symptoms of anxiety with and without phaeochromocytoma. *Psychosom Med* **652**, 129–42.

Stein, M.B., Asmundson, C.J. & Chartier, M. (1994) Autonomic responsivity in generalised social phobia. *J Affect Disord* **31**, 211–21.

Stein, M.B., Tancer, M.E. & Uhde, T.W. (1992) Heart rate and plasma norepinephrine responsivity to orthostatic challenge in anxiety disorders: comparison of patients with panic disorder and social phobia and normal control subjects. *Arch Gen Psychiatry* **49**, 311–17.

Stone, E.A. (1983) Problems with current catecholamine hypotheses of antidepressant agents: speculations leading to a new hypothesis. *Behav Brain Sci* **6**, 535–77.

Tanaka, M., Yoshida, M., Emoto, H. & Ishii, H. (2000) Noradrenaline systems in the hypothalamus, amygdala and locus coeruleus are involved in the provocation of anxiety: basic studies. *Eur J Pharmacol* **405**, 397–406.

Tancer, M.E., Mailman, R.B., Stein, M.B., Mason, G.A., Carson, S.W. & Golden, R.N. (1994/1995) Neuroendocrine responsivity to monoaminergic system probes in generalized social phobia. *Anxiety* **1**, 216–23.

Tancer, M.E., Stein, M.B. & Uhde, T.W. (1993) Growth hormone response to intravenous clonidine in social phobia: comparison to patients with panic disorder and healthy volunteers. *Biol Psychiatry* **34**, 591–5.

Targum, S. (1990) Differential responses to anxiogenic challenge studies in patients with major depressive disorder and panic disorder. *Biol Psychiatry* **28**, 21–34.

Taylor, D.P., Eison, M.S., Riblet, L.S. & Vandermaelen, C.P. (1985) Pharmacological and clinical effects of buspirone. *Pharmacol Biochem Behav* **23**, 687–94.

Tiihonen, J., Kuikka, J., Bergström, K., Lepola, U., Koponen, H. & Leinonen, E. (1997) Dopamine reuptake site densities in patients with social phobia. *Am J Psychiatry* **154**, 239–42.

Tork, I. & Hornung, J.P. (1990) *Raphe Nuclei and the Serotonergic System*. In: *The Human Nervous System* (G. Paxinos & F.L. Orlando (eds), pp. 1001–22). Academic Press, New York.

Uhde, T.W., Stein, M.B., Vittone, B.J. *et al.* (1989) Behavioral and physiologic effects of short-term and long-term administration of clonidine in panic disorder. *Arch Gen Psychiatry* **46**, 170–7.

van Vliet, I.M., Slaap, B.R., Westenberg, H.G. & den Boer, J.A. (1996) Behavioral, neuroendocrine and biochemical effects of different doses of 5-HTP in panic disorder. *Eur Neuropsychopharmacol* **6**, 103–10.

Westenberg, H. & den Boer, J. (1989) Serotonin function in panic disorder: effect of 1–5 hydroxytrptophan in patients and controls. *Psychopharmacology* **98**, 283–5.

Wilkinson, D.J.C., Thompson, J.M., Lambert, G.W. *et al.* (1998) Sympathetic activity in patients with panic disorder at rest, under laboratory mental stress, and during panic attacks. *Arch Gen Psychiatry* **55**, 511–20.

Wilson, M.A. (1996) GABA physiology: modulation by benzodiazepines and hormones. *Crit Rev Neurobiol* **10**, 1–37.

Yehuda, R., Southwick, S., Giller, E.L., Ma, X. & Mason, J.W. (1992) Urinary catecholamine excretion and severity of PTSD symptoms in Vietnam combat veterans. *J Nerv Ment Dis* **180**, 321–5.

Zhuang, X., Gross, C., Santarelli, L., Compan, V., Trillat, A.C. & Hen, R. (1999) Altered emotional states in knockout mice 5-HT1A or 5-HT1B receptors. *Neuropsychopharmacology* **21** (Suppl. 2), S52–S60.

Ziegler, M.G., Lake, L.R., Wood, J.H., Brooks, B.R. & Ebert, M.H. (1977) Relationship between norepinephrine in blood and cerebrospinal fluid in the presence of a blood cerebrospinal fluid barrier for norepinephrine. *J Neurochem* **28**, 677–9.

Zohar, J., Mueller, E.A., Insel, T.R., Zohar-Kadouch, R.C. & Murphy, D.L. (1987) Serotonergic responsiveness in obsessive compulsive disorder. *Arch Gen Psychiatry* **44**, 946–51.

12 Brain Imaging and Anxiety Disorders

A.L. Malizia

Introduction

Anxiety disorders are a collection of psychiatric conditions in which the prominent presence of severe and inappropriate anxiety or fear is part of the characterizing phenomenology of the individual disorder. At least 25% of people will experience one anxiety syndrome in their lifetime, and these disorders have great economic impact being responsible for approximately 10% of all working days lost through illness in the UK. Research on the biological, psychological and social brain substrates of these disorders, and of the "healthy" emotions of anxiety and fear is carried out in the belief that an improved understanding of the underlying mechanisms will lead to improved treatments for these disabling conditions. Tools used for this purpose have ranged from the molecular to the social and have been applied to animals and humans. At the cellular level, intracellular changes in specific neuronal populations of brains of animals subjected to anxiety provocation have been described. At the systems level the effects of human social situations on the expression of symptoms have also been elucidated.

Yet, the final common pathway of the expression of anxiety and anxiety disorders is dictated by the summed output of specific and separate regional brain activity at the time that the emotions or symptoms are experienced. Thus the most valid investigational and explanatory level is likely to be a description of the global and regional brain physiological changes associated with the expression of anxiety. This type of work has been carried out in rodents with exquisite detail, and has generated a considerable body of knowledge related to the neuroanatomical and neurochemical changes that map anxiety conditioning and innate fear (Davis *et al.* 1994; Davis 2000; LeDoux 2000). This knowledge, derived from animal experiments is thought to provide a solid basis for the understanding of human anxiety emotions and disorders. This consideration is based on the belief that, on the face of it, adaptive and pathological anxiety and fear are the emotive and cognitive brain functions that map best between animal models, humans, and human psychiatric disorders. This is because unlike elation, sadness, hallucinations, or thought disorder, the stimuli and the behavioral outputs are more congruent between species, as well as accessible to observation and thus more explicitly charted.

However, it is unlikely that these animal experimental paradigms alone will provide a robust understanding of anxiety and anxiety disorders in humans. This is due to three principal factors:

• *Species difference*—while the building blocks of the human central nervous system are shared with other animals, the human brain is very different in size and in the relative contribution of the frontal lobes. The frontal lobes account for about one-half of the human brain and this is disproportionate to all other species including primates that are closest to us in terms of phylogeny. There is a great deal of evidence which demonstrates that parts of the frontal lobe such as the dorsolateral prefrontal cortex and the orbitofrontal cortex greatly contribute to human cognitive and emotional processes, and these areas have extensive direct and indirect connections to all other parts of the human brain. It is hence not conceivable that a thorough understanding will be possible without elucidating the necessary, unique and modulatory inputs that these areas have on human anxiety.

• *Individual differences*—it is quite clear from animal experimentation that individual diversity such as genetic differences in colonies bred for contrasting character-istics (e.g. Maudsley reactive and nonreactive rats), variations in individual housing and disparity in early life events, including the intrauterine period, lead to unequal anxiety responses and to dissimilarities in pharmacological sensitivity. Similar factors also apply to humans and are probably not easily mapped between animals and humans because of the influence of genetic heterogeneity, species specific appetitive behaviors and untranslatable human events, such as child abuse, interpersonal and family strife and personal meaning of life events amongst many others.

• *Anxiety is only a part of anxiety disorders*—while anxiety is the common denominator of the disorders grouped together, it is neither exclusive to these disorders (e.g., anxiety symptoms occur commonly in depressive disorders) nor the most prominent symptom or cause of distress in all the anxiety disorders (e.g., rumina-tions in obsessive-compulsive disorder or flashbacks in post-traumatic stress disorder are as disruptive as anxiety symptoms).

The consequence of all the above is that the most appropriate level of investigation and analysis, which will allow to build a robust understanding of human anxiety disorders, is the topology of human brain functions associated with anxiety symptoms. A num-ber of experimental tools have been employed for this strategy over the last 50 years. However, none have the descriptive and investigational potential of the recently matured tools of brain imaging such as positron emis-sion tomography and magnetic resonance imaging. These neuroimaging techniques can provide charts of gray and white matter distribution and tracts as well as maps of receptor, enzyme, neurotransmitter and trans-porter density and metabolic activity in the human brain with a spatial resolution of the order of 4–10 nm. This information provides a unique opportunity of linking specific brain structures, regional neuropharmacology and observable behavioral or cognitive outputs in a manner that has not been possible up to recently. This chapter first reviews the imaging techniques that are available, their maturity, advantages and disadvant-ages. The second part then reviews the current state of knowledge in anxiety and anxiety disorders. The third part critically examines the current effort and discusses how imaging can be applied in the future in order to understand the anxiety disorders.

Brain imaging and anxiety disorders: the tools

Principles of human imaging

An understanding of the mechanisms of data acquisi-tion in imaging is essential in order to make sense of imaging studies. This section introduces the prin-cipal concepts for such an interpretation, focusing on X-ray computed tomography (CT), positron emission tomography (PET), single photon emission computed tomography (SPECT), various applications of mag-netic resonance imaging (MRI) such as functional MRI (fMRI), magnetic resonance spectroscopy (MRS) and diffusion tensor imaging (DTI). The electrical recording and electrical averaging techniques such as electroencephalography (EEG), computed multiarray EEG and magnetoencephalography (MEG) will not be discussed here. EEG has been in existence for 50 or so years during which it has provided some leads; however, it has not lived up to its initial promise and a comparison between EEG and the imaging modalities discussed here will be made in the concluding parts of the chapter. Dense EEG mapping and MEG are less mature techniques, so there is little volume of evidence. However it is likely that, in combination with the techniques discussed in this section, they will provide very useful information by adding temporal resolution not possible with the tools here described that, instead, have good spatial resolution.

Anatomical imaging
Anatomical images of the human brain can be pro-duced by the use CT or of MRI. CT maps the tomo-graphic attenuation of X-rays which are transmitted through the head in the camera. MRI uses a number of steps:

• a powerful magnetic field aligns all magnetic nuclei (in most cases water) parallel or antiparallel to the magnetic field;
• these molecules are excited by radiofrequency pulse protocols which are spatially varied in order to pro-vide spatial resolution;
• radio waves are turned off;
• signals are emitted from the brain;
• signals are received, recorded and reconstructed to obtain a map, spectrum or picture.

MRI has superseded CT for structural brain imaging as MRI provides better resolution of soft tissues and, by varying the parameters of acquisition, can reveal white matter lesions and areas of altered signal intensity which reflect nonspecific pathology. Further, MRI does not employ ionizing radiation and its use is therefore not restricted by radiation dose considerations. Many studies have been carried out with these techniques to assess volumetric changes in patients' brain structures as compared with healthy controls. Volumetric studies ought to have large numbers, ought to be blinded, to employ automatic parcellation in order to avoid observer bias and need careful matching of variables such as age, sex, handedness, intellectual ability and level of education in order to avoid intrinsic biases. Further, it is important that control sample scanning should be temporally interleaved with scans for the patient group in order to avoid bias effects from machine parameter drift. Most of the studies published fail to meet these very stringent criteria.

More recently it has been possible to image white matter tracts with DTI. This form of imaging uses MRI to produce pictures of water molecules alignment in the three separate spatial axes, thus allowing visualization of myelinated axonal direction. This should provide information about the physical connectivity of various areas of the brain and may be important in determining whether particular patient groups have abnormal connections. Further, it will be of use in exploring connections between activated areas in the brain (see below—fMRI, p. 205).

Paradoxically, many of the techniques that were developed to investigate neuroreceptor density can also provide information on brain shrinkage or abnormal gray matter in brain areas. This is because a decrease or a change in neuronal density will also result in a decrease or change in total receptor density unless the whole brain matrix also shrinks proportionally. It is therefore important, especially when head injury or alcohol or substance abuse are likely to be involved, that neuroreceptor studies should involve some anatomical imaging in order to control for the possibility of this shrinkage.

Functional imaging
Physiological and neurochemical images of brain processing can be obtained by the use of nuclear medicine techniques such PET and SPECT. These involve the recording of signals emitted by a radiolabeled compound which has been administered to the subject. The observed tomographic signal represents the total radioactive counts from a particular region and, thus, is the sum of radioactivity from parent compound and labeled metabolites (if present) both in blood and the various tissue compartments. PET and SPECT are used either to generate surrogate maps of brain activity associated with particular tasks or conditions or to measure neurochemical parameters such as receptor, transporter or enzyme density (see Table 12.1 for a list of commonly used PET tracers).

Table 12.1 Some commonly used brain PET radioligands.

Name of ligand	Label	Type of ligand	Measures
Raclopride	C-11	Dopamine D2 receptors antagonist	Dopamine D2 receptors
Flumazenil	C-11	Central benzodiazepine site antagonist (alpha 1,2,3,5)	Central benzodiazepine sites
Diprenorphine	C-11	Opiate antagonist	Opiate receptors (μ,κ,δ)
DOPA	F-18	Dopamine precursor	DOPA transport into presynaptic terminal
WAY 100635	C-11	5-HT1A antagonist	Serotonin 5-HT1A receptors
PK 11195	C-11	Peripheral benzodiazepine receptor antagonist	CNS microglia activation
Carfentanyl	C-11	Opiate (μ) agonist	Opiate receptors (mainly μ)
Setoperone	F-18	5-HT2 antagonist	Serotonin 5-HT2 receptors
N-methyl-spiperone	C-11	D2 and 5-HT2 antagonist	D2 or 5-HT2 receptors
RTI 55	C-11	Dopamine and serotonin transporter substrate	Dopamine transporters
MDL 100907	C-11	5-HT2A antagonist	Serotonin 5-HT2A receptor density
Ro 15-4513	C-11	Central benzodiazepine site antagonist (more selective for alpha 5)	Alpha 5 central benzodiazepine density (mainly)
Deprenyl	C-11	Monoamine oxidase B inhibitor	Monoamine B availability and glial density

Neuronal populations engaged by mental processes use energy. This consumption can usually be imaged directly by administering radiolabeled glucose or glucose analogs, or indirectly by imaging increased blood flow or perfusion to the region. This is because local blood flow is, usually, tightly coupled to variations in local oxygen requirements in the brain. Regional metabolism or blood flow maps thus produced represent changes in energy requirements at synaptic sites as synaptic neurotransmitter release and uptake is linked with the greatest proportion of brain energy expenditure. There is a debate on whether the location of the bulk of aerobic metabolism is in the neurone or the surrounding glia; this debate, however, is unlikely to influence mapping from imaging as the synapses and supporting glia are colocalized within the resolution of the techniques (Magistretti & Pellerin 1999). Blood flow maps can also be influenced globally by changes in carbon dioxide (CO_2) concentrations and regionally by neurotransmitters (norepinephrine [noradrenaline], acetylcholine, serotonin and a number of peptides) released in nerve endings that act on the cerebral vasculature.

The maps thus produced represent the summation of synaptic activity over hundreds of thousands of synapses. This is one of the factors which can lead to seemingly paradoxical effects. For instance, increasing inhibitory γ-aminobutyric acid (GABA)-ergic activity in "activated" cortex results in a decrease in local cerebral blood flow despite the increased synaptic work at inhibitory synapses; this occurs because this signal is overwhelmed by the decreased metabolism in excitatory neurone synapses (Roland & Friberg 1988). However both increases and decreases in metabolism can be observed by increasing GABAergic input to resting cortex or to other areas of the brain where the balance between excitatory and inhibitory cells may be different (Peyron *et al.* 1994; Tagamets & Horwitz 2001). Further, since the observed changes are in the synaptic fields rather than the cell bodies, the greatest activation may be in locations distal to the ones suggested by electrophysiology or lesion experiments. Finally, in the investigation of anxiety and anxiety disorders, the net result can be affected by other factors such as changes in respiration, noradrenergic activity, timing and complexity of task and of image acquisition (Mathew *et al.* 1997; Malizia 1999) so that the valence of perfusion change may change according to paradigm and timing of scans but still involve the same nodal brain structures.

Fluorine labeled deoxyglucose (^{18}FDG) and [^{11}C] labeled glucose have been used with PET for direct measure of glucose metabolism. ^{18}FDG has been used in preference as it accumulates in cells proportionally to the glucose transport rates and is not further metabolized (unlike [^{11}C] glucose). This feature results in less complex mathematical modeling in order to interpret the tomographic data and has been preferred as a method despite the fact that the transport and metabolic rate constants for fluorodeoxyglucose are different from pure glucose. ^{18}FDG produces a map of summed glucose transport into the cells dominated by activity over a period of approximately 30 min, 20 min after its intravenous injection. Therefore, it provides a map of energy consumption by any particular brain state which can be maintained for tens of minutes. Although only one or two scans per individual can be produced, the count statistics are very favorable and robust comparisons can be obtained with groups of 10–12 individuals per arm.

Blood flow (or more precisely perfusion) can be measured with PET using oxygen [^{15}O] labeled injected water or inhaled $C^{15}O_2$ (converted to water in the lung capillaries). ^{133}xenon (an inert gas which is fully diffusible) and ^{99}Tc-HMPAO (a ligand which is freely diffusible across the blood–brain barrier but gets trapped intracellularly by the changes in pH) have been used with SPECT for the same purposes. Oxygen PET maps blood flow over a period of up to 2 min postinjection, with most of the information being acquired in the first 60 s. The amount of radioactivity administered to produce good images with contemporary PET cameras allows up to 12–16 scans to be performed in a single individual at 8–10 min interval. Thus repeated "activation" experiments can be performed where statistically significant changes in regional radioactivity are interpreted as mapping the cerebral regions associated with particular tasks. Usually these studies have employed 10–20 subjects, thus producing 50–150 scans per specific experimental task. This technique has been very successful in delineating areas of the brain involved in particular motor, sensory, language, affective and memory tasks.

^{133}Xenon is a breathed in, freely diffusible inert gas used in the original nontomographic studies which measured brain metabolism. It has been employed tomographically by some investigators to quantify cerebral blood flow with SPECT. ^{99}Tc-HMPAO produces a "stationary" picture of cerebral blood flow over a period of 2 min after injection which, because of the slow decay of ^{99}technecium, can be imaged for some hours. This has been particularly useful when it has been advantageous to inject patients at sites (e.g., a ward) away from the camera in order to record transient events such as hallucinations. The technique, however, exposes subjects to large amounts of radiation as SPECT is poorly sensitive. Its use in research should therefore be restricted for the study of such transient events.

Much of the activation work, pioneered with nuclear medicine techniques, has been expanded using fMRI. fMRI images changes in deoxyhemoglobin/oxyhemoglobin associated with increased or decreased oxygen consumption. As metabolic demands increase, there is an overcompensation in the amount of oxyhemoglobin delivered to a particular brain area and this generates the change in signal. Some technical issues have not been fully resolved, such as susceptibility artefacts causing loss of signal at tissue interfaces such as the ventral orbito-frontal cortex. However, the advantages of the absence of ionizing radiation and better spatial and temporal resolution are so great that many research centers have enthusiastically embarked on research protocols with this technique. MRI scanners are like tunnels and can generate considerable anticipatory anxiety. Some patient populations such as people with anxiety disorders find it difficult to tolerate. This adds a further uncontrollable dimension to the experimental procedure and diminishes the value of this technology in the study of anxiety disorders.

MRS can also be used to produce spectra associated with particular compounds in the brain. In this sense it is a form of functional imaging and it produces information on the regional presence and concentration of chemicals of interest, such as lactate, glutamate and GABA. Further, analysis of the ratio of N-acetyl aspartate (NAA) to other compounds such as creatinine and choline is an index of neuronal integrity. This technique is being increasingly used to quantify regional neuronal loss.

PET and SPECT have also been used to image pharmacokinetic parameters related to receptors, transporters, enzymes and transmitters. Ligands appropriate for the system under study are labeled with a radiation emitting nuclei to produce maps of their brain distribution after injection. PET is far more versatile than SPECT for this purpose as it usually labels nuclei such as carbon which are universal in molecules with biological activity. However, finding compounds that have the ideal characteristics (e.g., very selective receptor/transporter binding, low nonspecific binding, easily cross the blood–brain barrier, no lypophyllic metabolites, rapid brain–blood equilibration, no physiological action) and which can be radiolabeled is extremely expensive in terms of time and resources. Further, with single scan protocols B_{max} and K_d cannot be separated and the pharmacokinetic parameters may also include tissue delivery effects and nonspecific binding. Whenever semiquantitative methods are applied (as most often in SPECT) errors may also arise by scanning too early after injection or by the inappropriate use of reference or comparison regions (Olsson & Farde 2001). This results in either the data being heavily influenced by delivery to the brain rather than binding to the receptors, or in inappropriate conclusions from areas where a secular equilibrium at the receptor site has not been reached. These methodological problems accompanied by unsophisticated experimental design, characteristic of new technology, have resulted in a relatively small number of adequate radioligand studies in the current brain research literature. Indeed, so far, very few centers worldwide have been able to meet the methodological challenges. However, these problems are likely to subside as researchers become more experienced in imaging methodology. An additional exciting development is that both SPET and PET may also be used to detect the endogenous release of neurotransmitters thus allowing the study of functional neurochemistry *in vivo* in humans and which would parallel *in vivo* microdialysis in animals (reviewed in Laruelle & Huang 2001).

Brain imaging and anxiety disorders: the evidence

Obsessive-compulsive disorder

Obsessive-compulsive disorder (OCD) is the anxiety disorder in which imaging has contributed most to current understanding of its neurobiology. The disorder seems to have two main components: the repetition of acts or thoughts which are involuntary and cause distress, and an increase in anxiety provoked by the occurrence of such acts or thoughts. While imaging has to date not been able to separate these two factors, a consensus has emerged on the circuits associated with the condition. The most consistent piece of evidence is abnormal metabolism in the orbito-frontal cortex, in the anterior cingulate and in the basal ganglia, most studies showing hypermetabolism in these structures. These areas seem to have abnormal metabolic or blood flow both at rest and on symptom provocation. In addition, successful treatment, whether psychological or pharmacological reverses these abnormalities. Structural imaging has on the whole been less definitive, although a considered view of the evidence would point to some damage in the caudate nuclei and in the thalamus. No progress has been made on the pharmacological imaging of this disorder.

Structural imaging

After early reports (Behar *et al.* 1984) of increased ventricle to brain ratio (VBR: a nonspecific measure of decreased brain parenchyma) in patients with OCD using X-ray CT, the first observation of specifically reduced caudate nucleus volume was reported by Luxenberg *et al.* (1988). This study also used X-ray CT and a sample of 10 male patients with severe OCD and 10 controls. The use of severely affected individuals may have provided a cleaner sample that emphasizes biological differences but results in reduced confidence in generalizing the results. Since then, the results of volumetric studies have been somewhat contradictory with one study (Scarone *et al.* 1992) showing an increased right caudate volume, four showing no differences (Aylward *et al.* 1996; Jenike *et al.* 1996; Stein *et al.* 1997; Bartha *et al.* 1998) and two showing a decrease in striatal volume (Robinson *et al.* 1995; Rosenberg *et al.* 1997). Factors affecting the presence or absence of reductions in caudate volume detectable by MRI seem to include gender (females show fewer differences), age of onset (earlier onset is more likely to be associated with volumetric reductions), and presence of soft neurological signs. These papers are complemented by MRS studies which have demonstrated reduced NAA and thus a degenerative process in the caudate nuclei (Ebert *et al.* 1997; Bartha *et al.* 1998).

Other reported differences include an increase in lobar white matter (Jenike *et al.* 1996), decreases in orbito-frontal gray matter and amygdala volume (Szeszko *et al.* 1999), increased MRI T1 relaxation time in the orbito-frontal cortex (Garber *et al.* 1989), and an abolition of amygdala-hippocampal left-to-right asymmetry (Szeszko *et al.* 1999). In addition studies in pediatric OCD have demonstrated an increase in myelinated callosal fibers (Rosenberg *et al.* 1997) and

a decrease in thalamic volume (Rosenberg *et al.* 2000), which the authors argued to be a consequence of the effects of paroxetine treatment (Rosenberg *et al.* 2000). However the observation that the medial thalamus of treatment naive patients with pediatric OCD has reduced NAA levels that correlate with symptom severity, indicates that thalamic abnormalities are probably a part of the essential brain pathology of this disorder (Fitzgerald *et al.* 2000).

Functional imaging

It can be argued that functional imaging has contributed more to our understanding of the brain circuits of OCD than of any other psychiatric condition. The resting metabolic changes often observed in the orbito-frontal cortex, the anterior cingulate and the caudate nucleus are consistent with the observations reported in activation studies, where these structures are activated by symptom experience. These observations are congruent with theories of frontal lobe function. Importantly, the resting metabolic differences normalize on treatment with the suggestion that treatment response is related to a lesser degree of abnormality. The anatomical findings of the various resting metabolic studies are reported in Table 12.2. Close inspection of the results indicates that the area most often involved is the orbito-frontal cortex where the majority of studies find an increase in resting metabolism. Most of the studies that find a decrease in this region utilize HMPAO SPECT rather than FDG PET. Significant differences in thalamic, caudate and other frontal metabolism are reported in about half the studies, but the polarity of the change is as much for decreases as for increases in metabolism. Additional areas include the parietal cortex and the cerebellum. As discussed in the section on imaging techniques (p. 204) the significance of increases or decreases in metabolism or blood flow is not as unambiguous as it first appears. Hence, for the time being, the observation of significant changes in a particular area, whatever the polarity may be, is likely to be more robust in helping researchers identify the likely networks engaged in pathological processes.

Activation studies have shown a similar pattern upon provocation of symptoms in the scanner. In these studies OCD symptoms are provoked while the patient is in the camera and the changes in blood flow compared with rest or with an appropriate control task. The comparison can be either categorical which employs

Table 12.2 Resting metabolic studies of OCD.

Author	Year	Method	OF	CN	ACC	Other frontal	Other	Notes
Mindus *et al.*	1986	[11]C glucose	+	−	0	0		Rx resistant
Baxter *et al.*	1987	FDG	+	+	0	0		
Baxter *et al.*	1988	FDG	+	+	0	0		
Nordhal *et al.*	1989	FDG	+	0	+	0		
Swedo *et al.*	1989	FDG	+	0	+	+		Children
Martinot *et al.*	1989	FDG	0	−	0	−		Some on Rx
Machlin *et al.*	1991	HMPAO	0	0	0	+		
Sawle *et al.*	1991	H_2O	+	0	0	+		
Rubin *et al.*	1992	Xenon	0	0	0	0		
Rubin *et al.*	1992	HMPAO	+	−	0	+	+Parietal	
Perani *et al.*	1995	FDG	+	0	+	0	+Thalamus	
Lucey *et al.*	1995	HMPAO	−	−	0	−	−Thalamus −Parietal	
Busatto *et al.*	2000	HMPAO	−	0	−	0	+Cerebellum	

+, increase in metabolism compared with controls; −, decrease in metabolism; 0, no difference found; ACC, anterior cingulate cortex; CN, caudate nucleus; OF, orbito-frontal cortex; Rx, treatment.

subtraction techniques or correlational whereby the changes in blood flow across the scans are related to changes in symptom scores. The first categorical study in this area was performed by the OCD group in Boston (Rauch *et al.* 1994) that found increases in the right caudate, bilaterally in the orbito-frontal cortex and in the anterior cingulate cortex with stimulus presentation. These findings were echoed in a correlation study of four patients (McGuire *et al.* 1994) where increases in the right inferior frontal gyrus, the caudate nuclei, putamen and globus pallidus, the thalamus, the left hippocampus, and the posterior cingulate were all found to correlate with symptom severity. Since then orbito-frontal cortical activation has been confirmed in three studies (Breiter *et al.* 1996; Cottraux *et al.* 1996; Adler *et al.* 2000) with additional foci in lateral frontal, anterior cingulate and anterior medial temporal (Breiter *et al.* 1996; Adler *et al.* 2000), and in caudate, insula and amygdala (Breiter *et al.* 1996). Cottraux *et al.* (1996) employed a complex experimental design presenting auditory stimulation to both patients and controls. The auditory stimulation could be of obsessive thoughts or neutral and was also compared with rest. They observed that both neutral and obsessive thought stimulation would increase caudate metabolism in patients and that obsessive thought provocation would increase orbito-frontal metabolism in both patients and controls. However the pattern differed in that patients also exhibited an increased correlation between superior temporal and orbito-frontal activity which was absent in control subjects. Other studies (Horwitz *et al.* 1991) have reported an increased correlation in metabolism between anterior structures (orbito-frontal cortex, caudate nuclei, anterior limbic cortex) that is reversed by successful treatment (Azari *et al.* 1993; Brody *et al.* 1998).

The latter finding is in keeping with the consistent pattern emerging from treatment studies (Table 12.3) where a decrease in orbito-frontal and caudate metabolism is associated with treatment response in about half the studies. These decreases are across all treatment modalities including behavior therapy, pharmacotherapy and neurosurgery. Where this has been recorded, lesser baseline abnormality in these areas is associated with better outcome. One study (Brody *et al.* 1998) suggests that a different basal abnormality pattern is associated with prediction of differential response to behavior therapy or pharmacotherapy. While good response to medication is, as in the other studies, associated with lower resting metabolism in orbito-frontal metabolism, better response to behavior therapy is related to higher resting metabolism in the orbito-frontal cortex. This issue will have to be further explored but it heralds an interesting line of enquiry that suggests

207

Table 12.3 Treatment induced changes in brain metabolism in OCD.

Author	Year	Method	Treatment	OF	CN	ACC	Other frontal	Other	Notes
Mindus et al.	1986	[11C] glucose	Surgery	–	0	0	0	0	Limited FOV
Baxter et al.	1987	FDG	Traxodone	0	+	0	0	0	?Comorbid
Benkelfat et al.	1990	FDG	Clomipramine	–	0	0	0	0	
Baxter et al.	1992	FDG	Fluoxetine/BT	0	–	0	0	0	
Swedo et al.	1992	FDG	Various	–	0	0	0	0	
Rubin et al.	1995	Xe	Clomipramine	0	0	0	0	0	
Rubin et al.	1995	HMPAO	Clomipramine	–	–	0	0	0	
Biver et al.	1995	FDG	Surgery	–	–	0	0	–	Thalamus Case report
Perani et al.	1995	FDG	SSRI	0	0	–	0	0	
Schwartz et al.	1996	FDG	BT	0	–	0	0	0	
Saxena et al.	1999	FDG	Paroxetine	–	–	0	0	0	

+, increase in metabolism; –, decrease in metabolism; 0, no difference found; ACC, anterior cingulate cortex; BT, behavior therapy; CN, caudate nucleus; FOV, field of view; OF, orbito-frontal cortex; SSRI, selective serotonin reuptake inhibitors.

that the different treatment efficacy can be predicted by diverse changes in brain function correlates.

Another line of enquiry which is likely to produce useful leads on patterns of brain processing in OCD is the exploration of changes in task related activations when compared with healthy volunteers. Such an approach has been pioneered by Rauch et al. (1997a) who have demonstrated that OCD patients do not activate the inferior striatum when performing an implicit learning task, while these patients activate abnormally the temporal cortices. This approach has been also utilized by Pujol et al. (1999) who have demonstrated that OCD patients activate the frontal cortex to a greater extent than controls during a verbal fluency task and that these activations are not suppressed efficiently during a control condition. The results of these experiments speak either to a difference in brain wiring in patients with OCD or to pathological processes occurring in the background while these patients perform other tasks. These possibilities need to be explored in further experiments detailing the similarities and differences in brain activation and mental processing between controls and patients.

Panic disorder

Initial functional results in panic disorder (PD) showed hippocampal and anterior temporal poles activation and asymmetry with the experience of anxiety in patients with PD. However, this signal had to be reinterpreted as a consequence of the reappraisal of the anatomical specificity of temporal lobe data collected on prototypical scanners. In these cameras it was difficult to distinguish between temporal lobe activations and extra-cranial muscular events; the latter were responsible for the large activations observed, hence discounting the original results.

Since then hippocampal metabolic asymmetry and parieto-temporal hypofunction at rest as well as anterior cingulate and orbito-frontal activation with anxiety experience are the most reproduced findings. Other major advances in understanding PD have come from pharmacological imaging where abnormalities in $GABA_A$-benzodiazepine binding and GABA brain concentrations have been demonstrated. Anatomical imaging has supported the notion of temporal lobe, but not hippocampal, abnormalities.

Structural imaging
Structural imaging has been used to investigate the notion that PD may be associated with temporal lobe abnormalities. The results thus far indicate that this may indeed be the case, since both an increased number of nonspecific lesions and shrinkage of the temporal lobes are documented in all the published studies. There is, however, no evidence that hippocampal volume is reduced in PD in contrast to post-traumatic stress disorder and depressive disorders.

In a study of 30 consecutive patients from their clinic with PD, Ontiveros *et al.* (1989) compared them with 20 healthy volunteers using structural MRI. Eleven patients and one control were thought to have significant brain abnormalities mainly in the right temporal lobe (mainly areas of white matter abnormality) while five patients and one control showed dilatation of the temporal horn of the lateral ventricle. Patients with the temporal lobe abnormalities were younger at onset of PD, had longer duration of illness and had more panic attacks (PAs). In a similar sample of patients, the same group found that 40% of patients with PD and 10% of healthy volunteers had medial temporal structural abnormalities (Fontaine *et al.* 1990). These findings are extended in a large study of 120 PD patients and 28 controls by Dantendorfer *et al.* (1996) which demonstrated an excess of temporal lobe abnormalities in patients when compared with controls (29% vs. 4%). The prevalence of these abnormalities increased to 61% in PD patients with "nonepileptic" EEG abnormalities, while they were present in 18% of the PD patients without EEG abnormalities. The authors commented that a high number of septo-hippocampal abnormalities were found. Hippocampal volume, however, was not different between PD patients and controls in a volumetric MRI study by Vythilingam *et al.* (2000) which compared 13 patients and 14 healthy volunteers. These researchers also found that both temporal lobes (excluding the hippocampus) were 10% smaller in PD patients even after controlling for the fact that these patients have smaller brains (7%) than healthy controls. Interestingly, this result was not due to the larger number of women in the PD group as males and females with PD have almost identical brain volumes.

Functional imaging
PD was investigated early in the development of neuroimaging research because of the clear definition of the disorder and because of the relative ease with which PAs could be induced. This would allow comparison of brain activity during an attack with activity in the resting state. Investigators, however, soon realized that it was very difficult to observe patients during a PA as patients would find it difficult to stay in the camera. Hence some experiments were focused on the resting state and by separating out subgroups of patients who were sensitive to anxiogenic challenges such as lactate infusion.

Initial work by one group produced three studies (Reiman *et al.* 1984, 1986, 1989). These initial results seemed congruent with activations provoked in healthy volunteers by fear conditioning (Reiman *et al.* 1984) and were therefore cited as evidence of a continuity between healthy and pathological anxiety whereby the same brain modules were engaged during any subjective experience of anxiety and whereby resting dysfunction in these modules may underlie the predisposition to PD.

This group showed that in fear conditioning there were large anterior temporal pole activations and that these areas showed elevated blood flow during PAs in the context of abnormal asymmetries (left less than right) in the hippocampi at rest in PD patients. In the first resting study (Reiman *et al.* 1984) 16 patients with PD (some being on medication) were compared with 25 controls and showed abnormally low left to right ratios of hippocampal blood flow at rest. This was particularly significant in the eight patients who were sensitive to lactate challenge. Other areas (hippocampus, amygdala, inferior parietal lobule, anterior cingulate, hypothalamus, orbito-insular gyri) had no significant left to right differences. Two years later another study which included many of the subjects from the first (Reiman *et al.* 1986) was published. This compared eight lactate sensitive PD patients with eight lactate insensitive PD patients and 25 controls at rest. The lactate sensitive patients had lower ratio of left to right parahippocampal blood flow, blood volume and metabolic rate for oxygen which the authors interpreted as an increase in metabolism in the right hippocampus. Finally in 1989 the third study (Reiman *et al.* 1989) compared 17 patients and 15 controls before and during lactate infusion. Lactate infusion seemed to produce small increases in blood flow in the superior colliculi bilaterally and the left anterior cerebellar vermis. Only patients who had a PA ($N = 8$) showed large bilateral increases in blood flow in the temporal poles, in the claustrum/pallidum/insula bilaterally, in the superior colliculi bilaterally and in the left anterior cerebellar vermis.

Later it was demonstrated that the most significant activations in conditioned fear were due to extracerebral signal secondary to teeth clenching (Drevets *et al.* 1992) and so all the temporal activations reported by this group at that time have to be considered cautiously. The use of modern scanners and of coregistration with anatomical images makes this sort of error difficult to repeat. However, a consequence is that there have been relatively few activation and resting studies in PD when compared with post-traumatic stress disorder, depression or OCD. While a pattern is starting to emerge the data is still scarce and a synthesis is difficult because of the variety of techniques and analyses used, with a particular paucity of pixel-based analyses.

Symptom provocation and ^{133}xenon SPECT was used by Stewart *et al.* (1988) when 10 patients with PD and five healthy controls were compared. Scans were carried out before and after either a lactate or a saline infusion. Six patients had a PA and were compared with nonpanickers and controls. Hemispheric blood flow was increased postlactate infusion in nonpanickers and controls. This change was greatest on the right but it did not reach statistical significance. People who experienced a PA did not show such a change, possibly due to hyperventilation which would in itself decrease blood flow. In addition, people who experienced a PA showed a significant increase in the occipital lobe blood flow normalized to hemispheric blood flow bilaterally, as well as a trend for a decrease in left prefrontal blood flow with PAs. More recently Fischer *et al.* (1998) reported data from a healthy volunteer who experienced a PA in an experimental setting within a PET camera. Panic in this woman was associated with activations in the right ventral and medial orbito-frontal cortex. Activations reported in the genual anterior cingulate and in the right temporal cortex show stereotactic co-ordinates which could be interpreted as being in the orbito-frontal cortex also. In summary there is little convergence between these reports indicating that more investigations are needed to understand the pattern of brain activity during a PA.

A consistent pattern is also difficult to establish in the five studies which have examined basal blood flow or metabolism in PD, although there is some convergence of observed decreases in resting metabolism in the parieto-temporal cortices and of lower left to right hippocampal ratios in some patients. Nordahl *et al.* (1990) reported the results of ^{18}FDG PET resting scans. He compared 12 medication-free patients with PD and 30 healthy volunteers. Ten patients had a history of lifetime comorbidity but none had other diagnoses at the time of examination. All subjects were scanned during an auditory continuous performance task (CPT) in order to control the environmental conditions. The investigators found a significantly lower left to right

hippocampal ratio, a lower metabolic rate in the left inferior parietal lobule, trends towards significant increases in the right hippocampal region, medial orbito-frontal cortex and towards significant decreases in the anterior cingulate. Anxiety measures did not correlate with metabolism in any particular area while depressed mood ratings and CPT performance correlated positively with medial orbito-frontal metabolism.

The same group (Nordahl *et al.* 1999) went on to report on nine PD patients successfully treated with imipramine and compared their resting cerebral metabolism measured with ^{18}FDG PET with healthy volunteers and untreated PD patients. Compared with healthy volunteers, treated PD patients had lower left to right hippocampal and prefrontal metabolic ratios (but no difference with untreated PD patients). Lower posterior orbito-frontal metabolism was found in treated patients when compared with healthy volunteers or untreated patients and this effect was ascribed to clomipramine since it was similar to effects observed with imipramine in OCD (Benkelfat *et al.* 1990). Post hoc comparisons revealed that treated patients were no different from controls in the left parietal and left Rolandic areas which were hypometabolic in untreated PD patients.

Malizia *et al.* (1997) compared resting PET ligand delivery (a measure indicative of regional cerebral blood flow) between 11 patients with PD on no medication and seven healthy controls. All subjects were being scanned for the first time. Patients had significant lower delivery in posterior temporal, inferior parietal and cerebellar cortex bilaterally. In patients but not in controls the Spielberger State Anxiety Inventory administered just prior to scanning covaried positively with anterior cingulate and negatively with middle temporal and cerebellar delivery. These observations indicate that the experience of anxiety in this group correlates with increases in blood flow in the anterior cingulate and with decreases in flow in posterior structures.

In a SPECT study, De Cristofaro *et al.* (1993) examined nine patients with PD and five controls at rest with ^{99}Tc-HMPAO. The results for the seven patients who were lactate sensitive were then reported. This group had significantly increased asymmetry (interpreted as increased right-sided flow) in the inferior orbito-frontal cortex, increased flow in the left occipital cortex and decreased flow in the hippocampal/amygdala bilaterally. These PD patients were treatment naive (although some of them had occasionally taken benzodiazepines), young, and had a mean duration of illness of 11 months. Bisaga *et al.* (1998) also compared the resting cerebral metabolism of six lactate sensitive, treatment free, female patients with PD with healthy volunteers using ^{18}FDG PET. They found significant decreases in metabolism in the right inferior parietal area, and the right superior temporal gyrus, with increases in metabolism in the left parahippocampal gyrus.

Two studies have been conducted using a pharmacological challenge. In the first (Woods *et al.* 1988) yohimbine provocation of panic in PD patients resulted in large decreases in HMPAO SPECT signal in the frontal cortex. The study has, however, not been described in more detail elsewhere and so detailed comment is not possible. The second (Meyer *et al.* 2000) used fenfluramine in a protocol which examined blood flow before and after this challenge in PD patients and volunteers. The scans were timed so that PAs, if present, would occur while the person was not being scanned. The investigators found that, at rest, PD patients had lower blood flow in the posterior parieto-temporal area. This area of cortex also had significantly greater increases in perfusion in PD patients after fenfluramine when compared with healthy volunteers; the data presented, however, does not explain whether any patients found the infusion panicogenic and, if so, whether this affected the later blood flow differentially. The authors argue that this area could be predicted to be activated as it was reported to elicit feelings of suffocation and nausea when stimulated during neurosurgical procedures in the 1950s. Further, validation for the significance of this area in PD comes from the fact that it is coterminous with the hypometabolic areas reported by other metabolic studies in these patients (Nordahl *et al.* 1990; Malizia *et al.* 1997; Nordahl *et al.* 1999).

In summary it is difficult at present to make complete sense of the data collected so far and to relate it to what is known about the functional anatomy of fear in animals. Three findings are, however, somewhat consistent:
- the presence of a left-to-right asymmetry in hippocampal metabolism which is mainly detected at rest, although the side which is predominant is in dispute.
- parieto-temporal hypometabolism which may rectify on treatment, and which is in the same location as fenfluramine activation.
- changes in anterior cingulate or orbito-frontal metabolism as in other affective or anxiety conditions.

In vivo neurochemistry

Receptor binding The only system which has been thus far investigated by more than one group is the $GABA_A$-benzodiazepine. Following the lead from psychopharmacology challenge findings (e.g., Nutt *et al.* 1990), six iomazenil SPECT studies of PD so far published have attempted to address the question of whether benzodiazepine site binding is decreased in particular cortical areas (Schlegel *et al.* 1994; Kaschka *et al.* 1995; Kuikka *et al.* 1995; Tokunaga *et al.* 1997; Brandt *et al.* 1998; Bremner *et al.* 2000). All but the last one have significant methodological problems (inappropriate control groups, relative quantification only, presence of medication, unclear diagnostic systems and, most importantly, too short an interval between injection and scanning to separate delivery effects from binding) which result in considerable difficulty in interpreting the data. At best these can only be regarded as pilot data.

Schlegel *et al.* (1994) was the first to report decreased benzodiazepine receptor binding in PD using iomazenil SPECT comparing, at 90–110 min postinjection, 10 patients with PD with 10 patients with epilepsy on carbamazepine. The decreases were significant in the occipital and frontal lobes and maximal in the temporal lobes. Kaschka *et al.* (1995) studied nine medicated patients with PD *and* depression compared with a matched group of medicated patients with dysthymia using iomazenil SPECT scans at 2 h after injection. Decreases in binding were seen in the inferior temporal lobes both medially and laterally and in the inferior medial and lateral frontal cortex. These changes were already detectable at 10 min postinjection reflecting changes dominated by delivery effects. All participants were on antidepressants. On the other hand Kuikka *et al.* (1995) using two different SPECT cameras (at 90 min postinjection) studied 17 unmedicated patients with PD and 17 healthy age and sex matched controls using iomazenil and found an increase in iomazenil signal bilaterally in the temporal cortex and in the right middle/inferior lateral frontal gyrus. Brandt *et al.* (1998) showed that patients with PD have a significant increase of benzodiazepine receptor binding in the right supraorbital cortex and a trend to an increased uptake in the right temporal cortex. Both studies are, however, very likely to be contaminated by signal dependant on ligand delivery. Tokunaga *et al.* (1997) followed a very rigorous scanning methodology in an excellent technical study but did not use a standard psychiatric

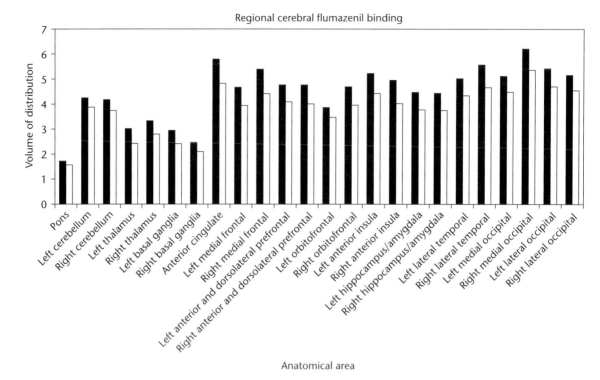

Fig. 12.1 Volume of distribution is a measure related to binding potential and proportional to B_{max}/K_d. Note that panic disorder patients show reduced flumazenil binding in all brain areas. For full data and discussion see Malizia *et al.* (1998). ■ Control, □ panic disorder.

classification which limits the generalization of his demonstration of global reduced benzodiazepine binding in patients with anxiety disorders. Bremner *et al.* (2000) carried out a very careful SPECT study with robust technological methodology. They showed a relative decrease in measures of benzodiazepine receptor binding in left hippocampus and precuneus in PD patients relative to controls. This group further observed that PD patients who had a PA had a decrease in benzodiazepine receptor binding in prefrontal cortex when compared with patients who did not have a PA at the time of the scan They also reported an increase in benzodiazepine binding in the right caudate, in the occipital lobes, in the middle temporal, and in the middle frontal cortex. However, although patients were drug free at the time of the scan none of them were benzodiazepine naive and therefore changes in receptor expression due to previous treatment cannot be excluded.

In the only fully quantitative study of benzodiazepine naive subjects, Malizia *et al.* (1998) employed [11C]flumazenil PET and found a global decrease in binding (20% decrease in volume of distribution) in benzodiazepine naive, drug-free patients with PD who had no comorbid conditions and did not abuse alcohol (Fig. 12.1). These changes were maximal in ventral basal ganglia, orbito-frontal and temporal cortex. Decreased binding in thalamus, dorso-lateral and medial prefrontal, medial temporal and cerebellar cortex, and vermis were accounted for by the global changes. One other study (Abadie *et al.* 1999) has examined [11C]flumazenil binding. This study compared patients with a number of anxiety disorders with healthy volunteers. Measures of binding were derived by using the pons as a reference region. However, since this measure is very noisy, it included negative values for some of the subjects and therefore a "pooled" reference region was used;

Table 12.4 Comparison of [^{11}C] flumazenil volumes of distribution values in the Malizia *et al.* (1998) PD study and in the Abadie *et al.* (1999) anxiety disorders study. Data redrawn from published tables.

	Medial frontal	Right lateral frontal	Left lateral frontal	Cingulate	Posterior occipital	Right lateral occipital	Left lateral occipital	Right lateral temporal	Left lateral temporal	Cerebellum
Abadie patients	4.8	4.1	4.3	5.1	5.3	4.1	4.6	4.2	4.1	2.9
Abadie controls	5.6	4.7	4.6	5.8	6.0	4.5	4.6	5.1	4.8	3.6
Malizia patients	4.2	4.0	4.1	4.8	4.9	4.5	4.7	4.7	4.3	3.8
Malizia controls	5.0	4.7	4.8	5.8	5.5	5.1	5.4	5.6	5.0	4.2

this resulted in an unusually high variance in binding measures. In the five patients and the five controls in whom an arterial input function was available, all areas examined had lower benzodiazepine binding in patients; however, these differences were not statistically significant with the methods employed by the authors. The data are presented in Table 12.4 alongside the results from Malizia *et al.* (1998), and show that UK and French brain-binding data *in vivo* are quite comparable (except perhaps in the cerebellum) and show a reduction in benzodiazepine binding.

Decreased benzodiazepine receptor binding is consistent with the idea that PD is due to a deficiency in brain inhibition that leads to, or allows, paroxysmal elevations in anxiety during PAs. The peak decreases in benzodiazepine binding are in anatomical areas (e.g. orbito-frontal cortex and insula) thought to be involved in the experience of anxiety in humans and could represent a primary pathology. The reduction in binding not only explains some of the known features of benzodiazepine receptor function in PD but is also congruent with animal data showing that chronic stress decreases benzodiazepine binding (Inoue *et al.* 1985; Weizman *et al.* 1989, 1990) and that animals with genetically decreased flumazenil binding experience more anxiety (Crestani *et al.* 1999). It is thus possible that this finding could be the result of experiencing repeated PAs, or the consequence of one or more of the etiological factors, such as genetic predisposition or life events.

These hypotheses can be further tested. If the genetic vulnerability is specific to PD, it is expected that polymorphisms for one of the GABA receptor subunits will be associated with the expression of this disorder in particular families; also, reduced binding would not be found in other anxiety disorders. If the vulnerability is for the experience of inappropriate anxiety, then the difference in binding should also be found in other anxiety disorders and polymorphisms, if present, will not be specific to PD. If the changes are secondary to environmental factors, then they may also be found after chronic stress and no association would be found between GABA subunit polymorphisms and anxiety disorders.

[^{11}C]WAY 100635 has been available as a useful PET radioligand to investigate 5-HT1A receptors and following the demonstration of global decreases in benzodiazepine binding, global decreases in cortical and subcortical 5-HT1A binding in PD patients when compared with controls have also been demonstrated by the same research group (Sargent *et al.* 2000). These patients were, however, on active selective serotonin reuptake inhibitor (SSRI) treatment when scanned and, therefore, the findings could be a consequence of the therapeutic interventions rather than a correlate of the psychopathology. In this light the findings of an inverse correlation between 5-HT1A binding and anxious personality (Tauscher *et al.* 2001) is of great interest, as it may indicate that low 5-HT1A receptor density predisposes to anxiety in humans. Further, reduced binding at benzodiazepine and 5-HT1A receptors may share a common etiology as demonstrated in the 5-HT1A knockout mice (Sibille *et al.* 2000).

Brain GABA concentrations One of the possible mechanisms by which GABA$_A$-benzodiazepine receptor subunit composition could be altered or down-regulated is via a change in brain GABAergic activity. Goddard *et al.* (2001) have demonstrated that patients with PD have a 22% reduction in total occipital cortex GABA

213

concentration (GABA plus homocarnosine) compared with controls. GABA concentration was measured by using MRS of occipital cortex *in vivo*; the selection of this area of the brain was dictated by current constraints in data acquisition using this method. This remarkable finding was present in 12 of the 14 patient–control pairs, but there were no significant correlations between occipital cortex GABA levels and measures of illness or state anxiety. Further studies will be needed to determine GABA concentration in areas more germane to the expression of anxiety, but these data provide an interesting model of pathophysiology in PD.

Response to challenge Finally, while lactate has been well-recognized as a panicogenic agent, the mechanism of action has been disputed. In particular, it was argued that since lactate could not cross the blood–brain barrier, its effects were likely to be peripheral. However, Dager *et al.* (1999), using whole brain MRS, have demonstrated that patients with PD who are lactate sensitive have a greater and more prolonged elevation in cerebral lactate after the infusion of l-lactate when compared with healthy controls or with patients who do not panic. This increase in lactate is not region specific and seems to occur throughout the brain correlating well with cerebrospinal fluid cisternal values.

Summary

Four main findings emerge from the biochemical imaging experiments in PD, although these conclusions are based on only a few experiments:
• There is reduced benzodiazepine binding in benzodiazepine naive PD patients.
• PD patients may show reduced 5-HT1A binding.
• PD patients have decreased GABA cerebral levels which at present have only been demonstrated in the occipital cortex.
• PD patients who experience the panicogenic effects of lactate have larger and more persistent increases in cerebral lactate after infusion than healthy controls or nonpanicking PD patients. This central effect may provide a link between CO_2 and lactate as panicogens, since both can lead to very similar metabolic changes in tissue.

Post-traumatic stress disorder

The main findings in post-traumatic stress disorder (PTSD) have come from structural studies with a consistent demonstration of small reduction in hippocampal volume in adult but not childhood PTSD. Findings from activation studies have been somewhat inconsistent and may reflect the disparity in symptom provocation methods as well as heterogeneity in the patient groups. Regional alterations in benzodiazepine binding and global changes in α_2-adrenergic metabolic responsivity have also been demonstrated.

Structural imaging

PTSD is a condition which by definition occurs after an unusually severe stressful event. Stress is known to result in a physiological response which is mediated by ascending monoaminergic systems in the short term and by the hypothalamic–pituitary–adrenal axis in the longer term whereby stress results in increased glucocorticoid (GC) concentration in plasma and brain. Recently, much attention has been devoted to the noxious effects of increased GC on neurones (Sapolsky 1996), particularly in the hippocampus, where it is thought that persistently high GC concentrations induce reversible atrophy of the dendritic spines. These observations lead to the conclusion that prolonged periods of stress, leading to increased GC concentration, result in hippocampal atrophy in humans, a theory supported by findings in depression (which is accompanied by hypothalamic-pituitary axis (HPA) abnormalities in many patients) where atrophy is correlated with total period of illness (Sheline *et al.* 1999).

In PTSD severe stress is experienced repeatedly over a period of months, first because of the incident itself and then through the re-experience of the traumatic events. It should therefore follow that a reduction in hippocampal volume should be observed in patients with this condition and that the greatest damage should be seen in patients with the longest history of PTSD. Four MRI studies (Table 12.5) of PTSD patients have been performed that have used volumetric MRI with manual segmentation of the hippocampus (Bremner *et al.* 1995; Gurvits *et al.* 1996; Bremner *et al.* 1997b; Stein *et al.* 1997). Each study had a different criterion for definition of the hippocampus since some investigators prefer to measure a clearly defined portion (e.g., middle) rather than increasing noise by including areas with poor boundary definition. All studies reported a small decrease in hippocampal volume (about 5%) except for Gurvits *et al.* (1996: about 25%) who, however, did not interleave measurements of patients and controls, thus being open to the possibility of scanner

Table 12.5 Studies of hippocampal and cortical volume in PTSD.

Author and method	PTSD patient group	Controls	Left hippocampus	Right hippocampus	Other
Bremner *et al.* (1995) Volumetric MRI	Veterans (*N* = 26) Males	Healthy volunteers (*N* = 22). Males Matched on many parameters	4% smaller (NS)	8% smaller (*p* = 0.03)	Right hippocampal volume correlates to Wechsler Verbal Memory Score
Bremner *et al.* (1997) Volumetric MRI	Child abuse (*N* = 17) 12 males	Healthy volunteers (*N* = 17). Males Matched on many parameters	12% smaller (*p* = 0.008)	5% smaller (NS)	Larger left temporal lobe and trend for larger amygdala in PTSD
Gurvits *et al.* (1996) Volumetric MRI	Veterans (*N* = 7) Males	NonPTDS veterans (*N* = 7) Healthy volunteers (*N* = 8) Matched on many parameters. Males	28% smaller (*p* < 0.001)	30% smaller (*p* < 0.001)	Subarachnoid space increased in all veterans. Total hippocampal volume decrease correlates to combat exposure
Stein *et al.* (1997) Volumetric MRI	Child sexual abuse (*N* = 21) Females	Healthy volunteers (*N* = 21). Female Matched for age and education	5% smaller (*p* < 0.05)	3% smaller (NS)	Left hippocampus volume decrease correlates to severity of dissociation

drift as an explanation for the large differences. Laterality is mixed as some report greater loss of volume on the left and some on the right but Bremner *et al.* (1995) report that right hippocampal volume correlates to the Wechsler Verbal Memory score and Stein *et al.* (1997) observe that left hippocampus volume decrease correlates to severity of dissociation.

While on the face of it, this converging evidence could be regarded as robust, a firm conclusion is made difficult by the usual problem of the unlikely reporting in the literature of equally small negative studies. In addition, as in all PTSD studies, interpretation is made more difficult by considerable clinical methodological problems such as psychiatric comorbidity, substance, and alcohol abuse. Some of these MR investigations attempted to minimize these problems by careful matching and the use of multiple linear regression; however, the direct effect of these factors cannot be definitely excluded.

The observation of mild hippocampal atrophy is, however, supported by the only published MRS study (Freeman *et al.* 1998). This study shows significantly reduced N acetyl aspartate/creatinine (NAA/Cr) proton

MRS ratios (an index of neuronal damage) in the right medial temporal lobe, and significant reduction in choline/creatinine (Cho/Cr) ratios (possibly an index of white matter damage) in the left medial temporal lobe in 21 veterans with PTSD compared with eight control veterans.

The significance of a decrease in hippocampal volume is difficult to interpret as it may be a predisposing factor to developing PTSD and not a consequence of the trauma. If mild hippocampal atrophy is a predisposing factor, then it may be possible to devise screening procedures to prevent vulnerable individuals from coming in contact with severe stressors as part of their jobs. The finding would be of great significance for biological psychiatry as it would link anatomical predisposition to psychological vulnerability to trauma. If, however, the hippocampal changes are secondary to the trauma, it would be important to determine the mediating factor. This is unlikely to be a plain increase in GC as PTSD patients have been demonstrated to have normal or low cortisol levels in the blood and a hyper-responsive pituitary (Yehuda *et al.* 1999). Therefore this area merits further close scrutiny and a study

215

of structural brain scans in trauma victims in the immediate aftermath of the accident and at follow-up comparing people who have developed PTSD with people who have not, should help resolve the question.

A different picture emerges from the study of children with PTSD where the whole brain volume is reduced when compared with healthy controls, while the hippocampus is not significantly different in volume (De Bellis *et al.* 1999). In this group of 44 maltreated children the reduction in whole brain volume was positively correlated with age of onset of trauma and negatively correlated with duration of abuse; these effects were more pronounced in males than females and resulted in a smaller corpus callosum and larger ventricular volume after correction for total brain volume reduction. Findings of lack of hippocampal or temporal atrophy have been confirmed by the same group in a longitudinal study (De Bellis *et al.* 2001) discounting the hypothesis that the original findings were due to the short time separating trauma and MR examination.

Functional imaging

Activation studies have involved the subtraction of relative regional blood flow between a resting or control condition and an activation condition congruent with the trauma. In many of these sophisticated controls were also included in order to ascertain whether the changes in cerebral blood flow were specific to PTSD patients or a general response to highly arousing stimuli in people subjected to trauma.

The psychiatry imaging group at Massachusetts General Hospital in Boston has performed the most comprehensive set of studies using $C^{15}O_2$ PET. In all these studies patients had been off medication for at least 2 weeks. A total of 31 patients were studied, one study being completely on childhood sexual abuse victims and one on war veterans. In all the studies the exposure to the trauma-related stimuli (either autobiographical memories or imagery/perception of trauma scenes) produced an increase in emotional cognitions and physiological signs of increased arousal; these changes were far greater in magnitude in PTSD patients than controls.

Two studies (Rauch *et al.* 1996; Shin *et al.* 1999) employed autobiographical scripts to induce emotion. In these studies the resting condition is listening to a script of neutral personal memories while the activated condition consists of listening to a script of memories of the traumatic event. Both studies showed a similar pattern of increased blood flow in the anterior cingulate, anterior insula, orbito-frontal cortex, and anterior temporal pole. Decreases in blood flow were observed in the left inferior frontal cortex. Anterior cingulate and anterior insula activations were thought to be nonspecific as they were induced by the experience of strongly emotionally laden memories irrespective of having developed PTSD. Volunteers re-experiencing traumatic events (but who had not developed PTSD) also had similar magnitudes of activation in these areas. Orbito-frontal and anterior temporal activations were greater in PTSD patients but not unique to the patient group, suggesting a quantitative rather than qualitative difference in the circuits subserving emotional responses to trauma memories. The left inferior frontal decreases were present only in the PTSD patients and could therefore represent a specific pathological response.

Another study (Shin *et al.* 1997) compared the activations produced by perception or imagery of war scenes with either negative or neutral stimuli. The study selected war veterans with and without PTSD. The pattern of regional blood flow change differed according to the modality of the subtraction paradigm employed and the only common pattern that emerged was of cingulate increases (albeit in different loci) and of left inferior frontal decreases.

Four other activation studies contribute to the current knowledge. One study documented a failure of parietal activation with an attentional task in PTSD patients when compared with controls (Semple *et al.* 1996) but little can be concluded from this study as the performance was also impaired; thus the difference in activation may be due to the subjects not performing the task equally well. One employed a similar strategy to the Boston group by investigating victims of childhood sexual abuse with and without PTSD using autobiographical scripts of trauma minus neutral scripts (Bremner *et al.* 1999a). This study showed a completely different pattern of regional blood flow change compared to the Boston group, with increases in perfusion in posterior insula, posterior cingulate, superior and middle frontal gyri and motor cortex, and decreases in perfusion in inferior temporal, supramarginal and fusiform gyri in PTSD, compared with controls. In seemingly common areas the changes differ either by exact location (e.g., increases in the posterior rather than anterior insula) or by valence (decreases rather than increases in anterior cingulate).

The other two studies are from the same group. One study set out to test the hypothesis of an increase in medial prefrontal blood flow in PTSD victims (medial prefrontal cortex is involved in extinction and had been activated in previous studies by the same group) when compared with healthy controls or veterans when listening to combat sounds compared with white noise (Zubieta *et al.* 1999), and indeed found such an increase. The other study (Liberzon *et al.* 1999) found an increase in anterior cingulate blood flow with exposure to combat sounds irrespective of diagnosis, as well as increases in left amygdala and a decrease in retrosplenial cortex particular to patients with PTSD. This same group also described the changes in brain metabolism in one patient observed during a flashback which occurred by chance during an HMPAO SPECT study (Liberzon *et al.* 1997). In this paradigm the images obtained by scanning represent the sum of the regional brain blood flow occurring in the first few minutes after injection of the ligand when, having listened to a tape of combat sounds, the subject experienced feeling "back in Vietnam" and extreme distress. The scan demonstrated an alteration in perfusion ratio between the thalamus and the cortex so that during the flashback the ratio of thalamic/cortical-basal ganglia metabolism was increased by 15%. This change in cortico-thalamic ratio could not be explained by changes due to hyperventilation and the authors interpreted it as representing a dissociative change in state of consciousness.

No consistent picture seems to emerge from the imaging studies thus far conducted in PTSD. In particular the total dissonance of two studies which at face value are very similar (Bremner *et al.* 1999b; Shin *et al.* 1999) could be a cause for concern. Because of the differences in the laboratories, of the detail of the paradigms employed, and of the relatively small numbers it is perhaps not surprising that differences are more striking than similarities. Hence it should not be seen as a failure or as something which is peculiar to human research, as recently demonstrated by the differences in behavioral observations of genetically identical mice put in ostensibly identical equipment in different laboratories (Crabbe *et al.* 1999). However the message is clear: large studies employing comparable techniques in different laboratories are needed in order to generate robust analyses of a generalizable nature. The current work has been successful in generating testable hypotheses:

- Decreased activity in left inferior frontal lobe when exposed to emotionally arousing material may be a marker of PTSD. This area is contiguous with areas involved in speech generation and in working memory that may be essential in the cognitive restructuring necessary to decrease the emotional impact of re-experiencing features of trauma.
- The orbito-frontal cortex, anterior cingulate, anterior temporal pole and anterior insula are also activated in other anxiety disorders (Rauch *et al.* 1996; Malizia 1999) and may represent a nodal circuit driving the somatic expression of anxious cognitions.
- Altered thalamo-cortical metabolic ratios may be the process that allows memory-driven experiences to dominate over actual input from the sensorium.

In vivo neurochemistry

Alterations of noradrenergic and serotonergic function have been observed in patients with PTSD, possible CCK-B involvement has been postulated from animal experiments, while, contrary to PD, only one experiment has postulated $GABA_A$-benzodiazepine dysregulation in this disorder (Coupland *et al.* 1997), yet human imaging has demonstrated changes in iomazenil binding in PTSD patients. Other imaging studies of receptor binding in PTSD are absent, partly because of the absence of relevant ligands.

Radioligand binding

The Yale group (Bremner *et al.* 2000) investigated Vietnam veterans with PTSD using iomazenil SPECT and found that there was a significant decrease in the volume of distribution of benzodiazepine $GABA_A$ receptors in the frontal cortex of these patients in an area which corresponds to Brodmann area 9. The authors argue that, despite the lack of human pharmacological data to indicate that GABA receptors are dysfunctional in PTSD, this finding is consistent with the preclinical observations which suggest that exposure to chronic stress decreases benzodiazepine binding maximally in the frontal cortex (Weizmann *et al.* 1989). This finding may be of particular significance as this area is involved in extinction of conditioned responses, thus misfunction of local inhibitory circuits could be either a consequence or a predispositon to developing inappropriate responses to trauma.

Activation studies

Another investigation by the Yale group (Bremner

et al. 1997a) examined the differences in regional metabolic rate after the administration of yohimbine to patients with PTSD and healthy volunteers. Yohimbine is an α_2 noradrenergic antagonist which increases norepinephrine release by blocking the presynaptic autoreceptors.

The study employed [18]FDG PET as the measure of metabolism. The metabolic effects of norepinephrine are inhibitory on postsynaptic neurones; however, the overall metabolic effects for a cortical volume depend on the extent of noradrenergic activation. Low levels of norepinephrine release are postulated to increase regional metabolism through an increase in local synaptic work that is responsible for a large proportion of the local metabolic requirements. At higher levels of noradrenergic activity, however, a net decrease in local metabolism is observed. This occurs, presumably, because the reduction in the number of active local interneurones becomes predominant in comparison to the increase synaptic transmission at noradrenergic synapses. Although noradrenergic modulation affects vascular responsivity, this can be corrected for in [18]FDG PET and is therefore not a confounding factor.

This study demonstrated that yohimbine generates a global small increase in gray matter metabolism in healthy volunteers consistent with a small increase in norepinephrine release, while patients with PTSD respond with a moderate global decrease in gray matter metabolism. These effects were maximal in the orbito-frontal cortex and significant in the prefrontal, parietal and temporal cortices and were accompanied by significant behavioral activation in PTSD patients. The authors interpreted this observation as evidence of increased sensitivity to the noradrenergic releasing properties of yohimbine in PTSD, in line with their previous pharmacological observations in this patient group.

Social anxiety disorder (social phobia)

Social anxiety disorder has only more recently been studied with imaging. Two main findings have been demonstrated: an abnormality in the dopaminergic system and a, possibly inappropriate, involvement of the amygdala in anxiety provocation, in conditioning, and in the perception of nonthreatening visual cues. A finding of increased relative cortical concentrations of myoinositol and choline has been replicated but is of uncertain significance.

Structural imaging

Only one volumetric study using MRI has reported on the comparison of anatomical brain structures between healthy volunteers and patients. Potts *et al.* (1994) using a 1.5 Tesla camera showed that there were no differences in brain structure volumes; however, the age-related decrease in putamen volume was more marked in patients with the disorder than in healthy controls. This reduction was not correlated to symptom severity but is of interest given the changes in dopaminergic function reported below.

Functional imaging

The first study that compared resting metabolism between healthy volunteers and controls used HMPAO SPECT with a single headed rotating gamma camera and showed no difference between 11 patients and 11 controls (Stein & Leslie 1996). Since then a treatment study by Van der Linden *et al.* (2000) using the same technique, showed that an 8 week course of citalopram reduced metabolism in the left temporal and frontal cortices and in the left cingulum. This reduction was not observed in nonresponders who had higher baseline metabolism in these regions when compared with responders. There was no healthy volunteer group in this study.

Activation studies

Two groups have examined whole brain changes in blood flow with anxiety provocation in patients with social anxiety disorder using $H_2^{15}O$ PET. Tillfors *et al.* (2001) compared 18 patients with social phobia with 6 healthy volunteers during the private or public performance of a prepared 2.5 min speech about a travel experience or a holiday. When the public performance was subtracted with the private performance, patients with social phobia (who experienced significant changes in anxiety ratings and psychophysiological measures) showed significant relative increases in the right amygdala and relative decreases in the right and left insula, right and left retrosplenial cortex, right and left perirhinal cortex, right temporal pole, right secondary visual cortex and right parietal cortex. Significant activation in all these areas was demonstrated on the basis of predictions made by analysis of previous imaging studies in anxiety disorders.

Malizia (2001) investigated seven patients with social phobia using an autobiographical scripts paradigm; there was no comparison with healthy volunteers. In this, scans acquired during listening to different auto-biographical scripts of recent social anxiety and positive affect generating events, were compared. During the anxiogenic scripts, self-reported and psychophysiological measures of anxiety were increased and blood flow increases were noted in the right anterior insula, right anterior prefrontal cortex, left thalamus, left anterior cingulate and decreases in the left amygdala with a trend for decrease in the right amygdala.

Direct comparison of the two studies is difficult because of the different methods employed, the different thresholds accepted for significance($z = 2.6$ in Uppsala and $z = 3.1$ in Bristol) and the lack of a comparison with healthy volunteers in the second study. However, alterations in essential limbic structures such as the amygdalae and anterior insula were present in both studies, albeit in a reciprocal fashion in terms of direction of change. The amygdala was also implicated in two other studies which employed fMRI to test specific hypotheses about brain processing in social phobia. Birbaumer et al. (1998) elegantly demonstrated that patients with social phobia activate the amygdala when exposed to slides of neutral faces while controls do not. The same group also demonstrated (Schneider et al. 1999) that these differences are exacerbated when neutral faces are paired with a negative odor thus becoming a conditioned negative stimulus. In this experiment, controls decreased perfusion in the amygdala in the presence of the conditioned stimulus while patients with social phobia increased it; no significant statistical differences were, however, observed in the habituation or extinction phases.

All four of these experiments seem to indicate that the amygdala is an essential part of the malfunctioning networks in social anxiety disorder and confirm that the exact direction of perfusion change is changeable according to the paradigm used.

In vivo neurochemistry
Dopaminergic underactivity and social anxiety have been postulated to be related from animal models, human diseases, such as Parkinson's disease, and the effects of dopamine modulating agents (reviewed in Bell et al. 1999). Two studies have provided evidence for dopaminergic dysfunction in social phobia by measuring the density of dopamine tansporters and D2 (mainly postsynaptic) receptors in the basal ganglia of patients with this condition and controls, using SPECT. The first study, using ^{123}I β CIT, demonstrated that 11

Finnish social phobia patients had decreased binding potential for the dopamine transporter in the striatum (Tiihonen et al. 1997a). This was followed by a study by Schneier et al. (2000) who demonstrated that 10 New York patients with social phobia had lower D2 binding potential than controls. These data suggest three possibilities:
• Down regulation of both sites as a trait associated with possible dopaminergic hypofunction.
• Increased dopaminergic tonic release, which would decrease the proportion of sites available for radioligand binding.
• Mild atrophy of the basal ganglia.

Spectroscopy
Two studies (Davidson et al. 1993; Tupler et al. 1997) have examined creatinine, NAA, choline and myoinositol spectra in patients with social anxiety disorder. The measures have all been relative and the second study allowed separation of cortical and subcortical gray and white matter. The authors find a number of significant differences in spectra between patients and controls which they interpret as cortical increases in myoinositol and choline concentrations in patients that were not altered by 8-week treatment with benzodiazepines. The biological significance of this altered signal is, however, uncertain. Thus these findings do not, as yet, contribute to a biological understanding of this disorder.

Generalized anxiety disorder

Generalized anxiety disorder (GAD) has been little studied with imaging. This is in keeping with the fact that there is a dearth of biological investigations in this disorder, possibly because its pure form does not come to the attention of secondary services and therefore recruiting into laboratory based studies is additionally difficult. No conclusion can be drawn from any of the published studies in anxiety disorders, except that benzodiazepines reduce global and regional brain metabolism in a manner similar to healthy volunteers. The nonspecific effects of benzodiazepines are larger than any specific ones related to decreased anxiety.

Three studies have investigated the effect of benzodiazepines in GAD (Buchsbaum et al. 1987; Mathew & Wilson 1991; Wu et al. 1991). In all three studies the administration of diazepam resulted in decreases in global and regional metabolism which was gretaest in the areas with the greatest density of benzodiazepine binding sites. Changes in anxiety score on benzodiazepines did not correlate with any of the regional changes, while changes in anxiety score during placebo administration correlated with reductions in limbic and basal ganglia metabolism. Wu *et al.* (1991) also observed that GAD patients did not exhibit the usual left-to-right asymmetry in hippocampal metabolism.

Two further studies contribute to the meagre information available for this disorder: Tiihonen *et al.* (1997b) demonstrated a significant decrease in left temporal pole benzodiazepine binding using ^{123}I NNC 13-8241 SPECT. This was accompanied by a decrease in variability in binding (as assessed by fractal analysis), which the authors interpreted as being pathological. More recently larger bilateral amygdala volumes have been described with MRI in children with GAD when compared with controls (De Bellis *et al.* 2000).

Specific phobias

Initial studies showed no change in perfusion with exposure to feared objects (Mountz *et al.* 1989); however, this was probably due to technical limitations as Rauch *et al.* (1995) demonstrated increases in perfusion of the anterior cingulate, insula, anterior temporal and somatosensory cortex, posterior medial orbitofrontal cortex and thalamus when subtracting control condition from exposure to feared objects; these findings are consistent with the idea that all anxiety disorders would share some common activations related to the experience of this emotion. O'Carroll *et al.* (1993), however, using SPECT reported decreased HMPAO uptake in the occipital cortex while patients with specific phobias listened to a 4-min recording recounting exposure to phobic stimulus when this was compared with a relaxation tape. The findings may be related to the visual salience of the imagined stimuli but no activations in common anxiety related brain areas were reported, possibly because of the low statistical power of the technique. No other studies have been conducted since these three were reported.

Commonalities among anxiety disorders

There are three groups who have done similar anxiety provocation studies in more than one group of volunteers. Rauch and colleagues (Rauch *et al.* 1994, 1995, 1996) in Boston studied patients with OCD, with simple phobia and with PTSD, and have subsequently reported a formal comparison (Rauch *et al.* 1997b). Fredrikson and colleagues (Fredrikson *et al.* 1993, 1995; Wik

et al. 1993, 1996, 1997; Fischer *et al.* 1996; Tillfors *et al.* 2001) have investigated two separate groups of patients with simple phobia, a group with social anxiety disorder and a group of bank clerks re-experiencing a robbery, as well as the neural networks of conditioning by pairing a snake video with the delivery of electric shocks to the hand. This group published a comparison between the phobic provocation and the re-experience of the bank robbery, but without formal statistical comparison. Malizia and colleagues (Malizia 2001) examined patients with social phobia and healthy volunteers taking part in a conditioned anticipatory anxiety paradigm and conducted a formal comparison of these groups (Malizia 1997: Fig. 12.2).

Altogether, these data have to be interpreted in the light of comparative findings in studies of anxiety provocation in healthy volunteers (Benkelfat *et al.* 1995; Parekh *et al.* 1995; Malizia *et al.* 1996; Servan-Schreiber *et al.* 1998; Chua *et al.* 1999; Javanmard *et al.* 1999; Cameron *et al.* 2000; Simpson *et al.* 2001). In general two sets of areas seem to be activated in anxiety and anxiety disorders whether at rest or after a challenge. The first set comprises the supragenual anterior cingulate, the orbito-frontal cortex, the insulae, the cerebellum, a pontine locus variously described as superior colliculi or periaqueductal gray (PAG) matter, and often, but not always, medial temporal structures (amygdala, parahippocampal gyrus), especially on the left. All of these (except the cerebellum) are areas that are directly involved with the evaluation of noxious stimuli and which produce autonomic responses when stimulated. In essence they may represent the essential circuits of the anxiety responses. The surprising element here is the activation of the cerebellum which speaks to its hitherto unsuspected involvement in processes which do not have a primary motor component. This finding is not specific to anxiety as it has been observed in cognitive manipulations where movement components have been controlled for (e.g., Kim *et al.* 1994).

The second set of activations represents areas of sensory or polymodal association cortices which may represent the processing of relevant anxiogenic stimuli or their imagery.

Other activations seem to be congruent with particular aspects of the anxiety disorder; basal ganglia activation fits well with the theory of cortico-striatal involvement in the obsessive-compulsive aspects of this disorder (Saxena & Rauch 2000), and amygdala is consistently involved in studies of social anxiety

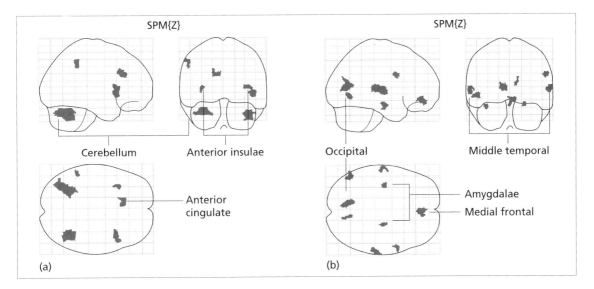

Fig. 12.2 Common increases (a) and common decreases (b) in perfusion in anxiety provocation in healthy volunteers and patients with social anxiety disorder. Brain areas are labeled on the statistical parametric maps showing corrected significance at $P < 0.05$ using conjunction analyses.

disorder and decreased activations in the inferior frontal lobes in PTSD.

Overall this set of data has to be considered as pilot data to be used to guide hypothesis generation. This is because a direct comparison (and therefore an assessment of the robustness of the findings) is not possible as paradigms, technology, analysis and reporting were very different between the different centers.

Brain imaging and anxiety disorders: conclusions

The impact of the last 10 years of imaging on the understanding of anxiety disorders is difficult to assess. This is not because there has been a shortage of findings but because, as the studies have informed contemporary thinking, it is difficult to retrace a time when this data was not available.

In general the main findings are:
• Anxiety experience, whether "healthy" or pathological, whether behaviorally or pharmacologically induced, provokes regional brain metabolic changes that can be mapped. Some of these regions are consistently activated *across* anxiety disorders and conditions. Within these regions, some, such as anterior cingulate, orbito-frontal cortex, medial temporal structures and

anterior insula, could be predicted a *priori*. Some, such as the cerebellum, could not.
• Resting brain metabolism in the scanner is altered in anxiety disorders patients when compared with healthy volunteers. Areas of hyper- or hypometabolism often correspond to areas activated by the experience of pathological emotions as exemplified by OCD and possibly PD.

The above findings support a notion of a network in which some global processes are tapped by diverse tasks and local regions, which are consistently by particular disease or emotional domains. For instance, while activations of the anterior cingulate cortex may be considered to be common to many activation studies in all types of cognitive domains other than emotions, orbito-frontal cortex involvement is likely to be common with other affective domains (including affective decision making) but not with many other cognitive domains. Further, increased correlations between orbito-frontal, thalamic and caudate metabolism is likely to be specific to OCD. These observations support the theory of a modular model of brain function where individual components are responsible for particular tasks but also affect and change the function of other components of the network. These ideas are discussed in detail in Malizia (1999) and Cabeza and Nyberg (2000).

Hypotheses that specific processing dysfunction are associated with particular disorders can start to be generated and therefore tested. These patterns of dysfunction may be predictive of treatment response as early data in OCD suggest.

Finally, specific neurochemical abnormalities can be detected and these may inform future therapeutic developments and pharmacogenomic investigations. For example investigation of $GABA_A$ α_1, α_2 and γ_2 polymorphisms (if they exist in humans) and selective agonists may lead to a better understanding of the pathophysiology and treatment of PD.

Brain imaging and anxiety disorders: the future

The same enthusiasm now witnessed for MR and nuclear brain imaging was apparent in the early days of EEG; however, this technique failed to deliver its promise. This was due to a number of factors including poor localization and identification of the signals and large interindividual variability in signal and signal modulation. The future of brain imaging in the investigation of anxiety disorders will depend upon a number of factors, some of which have already been mentioned in this chapter:

- Standardization of technical methods, analysis techniques and experimental protocols.
- Increased signal to noise to allow individual subject experiments to produce maps of function.
- Involvement of large numbers of experimental subjects.
- Combination of naturalistic experiments and experiments designed to test specific aspects of brain function.
- Combining techniques with good spatial resolution with techniques which have superior temporal resolution such as magnetoencephalography (MEG).
- Production of new radioligands that will allow definition of the various neurochemical systems in health and disease.
- Combined approaches where other information, e.g., genomics is used to select samples of patients or healthy volunteers.
- Synergy with preclinical science whereby human imaging results are used as starting hypotheses for testing in animal and *in vitro* models.

Many of these are being worked on at present and these efforts should result in robust and effective investigational tools.

Acknowledgements

The author was supported by grants from the Psychopharmacology Unit, the Institute of Clinical Neuroscience, and the Department Of Old Age Medicine of the University of Bristol while writing this chapter.

References

Abadie, P., Boulenger, J.P., Benali, K., Barre, L., Zarifian, E. & Baron, J.C. (1999) Relationships between trait and state anxiety and the central benzodiazepine receptor: a PET study. *Eur J Neurosci* **11**, 1470–8.

Adler, C.M., McDonough-Ryan, P., Sax, K.W., Holland, S.K., Arndt, S. & Strakowski, S.M. (2000) fMRI of neuronal activation with symptom provocation in unmedicated patients with obsessive-compulsive disorder. *J Psychiatr Res* **34**(4–5), 317–24.

Aylward, E.H., Harris, G.J., Hoehn-Saric, R., Barta, P.E., Machlin, S.R. & Pearlson, G.D. (1996) Normal caudate nucleus in obsessive-compulsive disorder assessed by quantitative neuroimaging. *Arch Gen Psychiatry* **53**(7), 577–584.

Azari, N.P., Pietrini, P., Horwitz, B. *et al.* (1993) Individual differences in cerebral metabolic patterns during pharmacotherapy in obsessive-compulsive disorder: a multiple regression/discriminant analysis of positron emission tomographic data. *Biol Psychiatry* **34**(11), 798–809.

Bartha, R., Stein, M.B., Williamson, P.C. *et al.* (1998) A short echo 1H spectroscopy and volumetric MRI study of the corpus striatum in patients with obsessive-compulsive disorder and comparison subjects. *Am J Psychiatry* **155**(11), 1584–91.

Baxter, L.R., Jr, Phelps, M.E., Mazziotta, J.C., Guze, B.H., Schwartz, J.M. & Selin, C.E. (1987) Local cerebral glucose metabolic rates in obsessive-compulsive disorder: a comparison with rates in unipolar depression and in normal controls. *Arch Gen Psychiatry* **44**(3), 211–18.

Baxter, L.R., Jr, Schwartz, J.M., Bergman, K.S. *et al.* (1992) Caudate glucose metabolic rate changes with both drug and behavior therapy for obsessive-compulsive disorder. *Arch Gen Psychiatry* **49**(9), 681–9.

Baxter, L.R., Jr, Schwartz, J.M., Mazziotta, J.C. *et al.* (1988) Cerebral glucose metabolic rates in nondepressed patients with obsessive-compulsive disorder. *Am J Psychiatry* **145**, 1560–3.

Behar, D., Rapoport, J.L., Berg, C.J. *et al.* (1984) Computerized tomography and neuropsychological test measures in adolescents with obsessive-compulsive disorder. *Am J Psychiatry* **141**(3), 363–9.

Bell, C.J., Malizia, A.L. & Nutt, D.J. (1999) The neurobiology of social phobia. *Eur Arch Psychiatry Clin Neurosci* **249** (Suppl. 1), S11–S18.

Benkelfat, C., Bradwein, J., Meyer, E. *et al.* (1995) Functional neuroanatomy of CCK-4-induced anxiety in normal healthy volunteers. *Am J Psychiatry* **152**, 1180–4.

Benkelfat, C., Nordahl, T.E., Semple, W.E., King, A.C., Murphy, D.L. & Cohen, R.M. (1990) Local cerebral glucose metabolic rates in obsessive-compulsive disorder. Patients treated with clomipramine. *Arch Gen Psychiatry* **47**(9), 840–8.

Birbaumer, N., Grodd, W., Diedrich, O. *et al.* (1998) fMRI reveals amygdala activation to human faces in social phobics. *Neuroreport* **9**(6), 1223–6.

Bisaga, A., Katz, J.L., Antonini, A. *et al.* (1998) Cerebral glucose metabolism in women with panic disorder. *Am J Psychiatry* **155**(9), 1178–83.

Biver, F., Goldman, S., Francois, A. *et al.* (1995) Changes in metabolism of cerebral glucose after stereotactic leukotomy for refractory obsessive-compulsive disorder: a case report. *J Neurol Neurosurg Psychiatry* **58**(4), 502–5.

Brandt, C.A., Meller, J., Keweloh, L. *et al.* (1998) Increased benzodiazepine receptor density in the prefrontal cortex in patients with panic disorder. *J Neural Transm* **105**(10–12), 1325–33.

Breiter, H.C., Rauch, S.L., Kwong, K.K. *et al.* (1996) Functional magnetic resonance imaging of symptom provocation in obsessive-compulsive disorder. *Arch Gen Psychiatry* **53**(7), 595–606.

Bremner, J.D., Innis, R.B., Ng, C.K. *et al.* (1997a) Positron emission tomography measurement of cerebral metabolic correlates of yohimbine administration in combat-related post-traumatic stress disorder. *Arch Gen Psychiatry* **54**(3), 246–54.

Bremner, J.D., Innis, R.B., White, T. *et al.* (2000) SPECT [I-123]iomazenil measurement of the benzodiazepine receptor in panic disorder. *Biol Psychiatry* **47**(2), 96–106.

Bremner, J.D., Narayan, M., Staib, L.H., Southwick, S.M., McGlashan, T. & Charney, D.S. (1999a) Neural correlates of memories of childhood sexual abuse in women with and without post-traumatic stress disorder. *Am J Psychiatry* **156**, 1787–95.

Bremner, J.D., Randall, P., Scott, T.M. *et al.* (1995) MRI-based measurement of hippocampal volume in patients with combat-related post-traumatic stress disorder. *Am J Psychiatry* **152**(7), 973–81.

Bremner, J.D., Randall, P., Vermetten, E. *et al.* (1997b) Magnetic resonance imaging-based measurement of hippocampal volume in post-traumatic stress disorder related to childhood physical and sexual abuse—a preliminary report. *Biol Psychiatry* **41**, 23–32.

Bremner, J.D., Staib, L.H., Kaloupek, D., Southwick, S.M., Soufer, R. & Charney, D.S. (1999b) Neural correlates of exposure to traumatic pictures and sound in Vietnam combat veterans with and without post-traumatic stress

disorder: a positron emission tomography study. *Biol Psychiatry* **45**(7), 806–16.

Brody, A.L., Saxena, S., Schwartz, J.M. *et al.* (1998) FDG PET predictors of response to behavioral therapy versus pharmacotherapy in obsessive-compulsive disorder. *Psychiatry Res: Neuroimaging* **84**(1), 1–6.

Buchsbaum, M.S., Wu, J., Haier, R. *et al.* (1987) Positron emission tomography assessment of effects of benzodiazepines on regional glucose metabolic rate in patients with anxiety disorder. *Life Sci* **40**(25), 2393–400.

Busatto, G.F., Zamignani, D.R., Buchpiguel, C.A. *et al.* (2000) A voxel-based investigation of regional cerebral blood flow abnormalities in obsessive-compulsive disorder using single photon emission computed tomography (SPECT). *Psychiatry Res* **99**(1), 15–27.

Cabeza, R. & Nyberg, L. (2000) Neural bases of learning and memory: functional neuroimaging evidence. *Curr Opin Neurol* **13**(4), 415–21.

Cameron, O.G., Zubieta, J.K., Grunhaus, L. & Minoshima, S. (2000) Effects of yohimbine on cerebral blood flow, symptoms, and physiological functions in humans. *Psychosom Med* **62**(4), 549–59.

Chua, P., Krams, M., Toni, I., Passingham, R. & Dolan, R. (1999) A functional anatomy of anticipatory anxiety. *Neuroimage* **9**, 563–71.

Cottraux, J., Gerard, D., Cinotti, L. *et al.* (1996) A controlled positron emission tomography study of obsessive and neutral auditory stimulation in obsessive-compulsive disorder with checking rituals. *Psychiatry Res* **60**(2–3), 101–12.

Coupland, N., Lillywhite, A., Bell, C.E., Potokar, J.P. & Nutt, D.J. (1997) A pilot controlled study of the effects of flumazenil in post-traumatic stress disorder. *Biol Psychiatry* **41**(9), 988–90.

Crabbe, J.C., Wahlsten, D. & Dudek, B.C. (1999) Genetics of mouse behavior: interactions with laboratory environment. *Science* **284**, 1670–2.

Crestani, F., Lorez, M., Baer, K. & Mohler, H. (1999) Decreased $GABA_A$-receptor clustering results in enhanced anxiety and a bias for threat cues. *Nat Neurosci* **2**, 833–9.

Dager, S.R., Friedman, S.D., Heide, A. *et al.* (1999) Two-dimensional proton echo-planar spectroscopic imaging of brain metabolic changes during lactate-induced panic. *Arch Gen Psychiatry* **56**(1), 70–7.

Dantendorfer, K., Prayer, D., Kramer, J. *et al.* (1996) High frequency of EEG and MRI brain abnormalities in panic disorder. *Psychiatry Res* **68**(1), 41–53.

Davidson, J.R., Krishnan, K.R., Charles, H.C. *et al.* (1993) Magnetic resonance spectroscopy in social phobia: preliminary findings. *J Clin Psychiatry* **54** (Suppl.) 19–25.

Davis, M. (2000) The role of the amygdala in conditioned and unconditioned fear and anxiety. In: *The Amygdala: a Functional Analysis*, 2nd edn (J.P. Aggleton (ed.), pp. 213–87. Oxford University Press, New York.

Davis, M., Rainnie, D. & Cassell, M. (1994) Neurotransmission in the rat amygdala related to fear and anxiety. *Trends Neurosci* **17**, 208–14.

De Bellis, M.D., Casey, B.J., Dahl, R.E. *et al.* (2000) A pilot study of amygdala volumes in pediatric generalized anxiety disorder. *Biol Psychiatry* **48**(1), 51–7.

De Bellis, M.D., Hall, J., Boring, A.M., Frustaci, K. & Moritz, G. (2001) A pilot longitudinal study of hippocampal volumes in pediatric maltreatment-related post-traumatic stress disorder. *Biol Psychiatry* **50**(4), 305–9.

De Bellis, M.D., Keshavan, M.S. Clark, D.B. *et al.* (1999) Developmental traumatology part III. *Biol Psych* **45**(10), 1271–84.

De Cristofaro, M.T., Sessarego, A., Pupi, A., Biondi, F. & Faravelli, C. (1993) Brain perfusion abnormalities in drug-naive, lactate-sensitive panic patients: a SPECT study. *Biol Psychiatry* **33**, 505–12.

Drevets, W.C., Videen, T.Q., MacLeod, A.K., Haller, J.W. & Raichle, M.E. (1992) PET images of blood flow changes during anxiety: correction. *Science* **256**(5064), 1696.

Ebert, D., Speck, O., Konig, A., Berger, M., Hennig, J. & Hohagen, F. (1997) 1H-magnetic resonance spectroscopy in obsessive-compulsive disorder: evidence for neuronal loss in the cingulate gyrus and the right striatum. *Psychiatry Res* **74**(3), 173–6.

Fischer, H., Andersson, J.L., Furmark, T. & Fredrikson, M. (1998) Brain correlates of an unexpected panic attack: a human positron emission tomographic study. *Neurosci Lett* **251**(2), 137–40.

Fischer, H., Wik, G. & Fredrikson, M. (1996) Functional neuroanatomy of robbery re-experience: affective memories studied with PET. *Neuroreport* **7**, 2081–6.

Fitzgerald, K.D., Moore, G.J., Paulson, L.A., Stewart, C.M. & Rosenberg, D.R. (2000) Proton spectroscopic imaging of the thalamus in treatment-naive pediatric obsessive-compulsive disorder. *Biol Psychiatry* **47**(3), 174–82.

Fontaine, R., Breton, G., Dery, R., Fontaine, S. & Elie, R. (1990) Temporal lobe abnormalities in panic disorder: an MRI study. *Biol Psychiatry* **27**(3), 304–10.

Fredrikson, M., Wik, G., Fischer, H. & Andersson, J. (1995) Affective and attentive neural networks in humans: a PET study of Pavlovian conditioning. *Neuroreport* **7**, 97–101.

Fredrikson, M., Wik, G., Greitz, T. *et al.* (1993) Regional cerebral blood flow during experimental phobic fear. *Psychophysiology* **30**, 126–130.

Freeman, T.W., Cardwell, D., Karson, C.N. & Komoroski, R.A. (1998) *In vivo* proton magnetic resonance spectroscopy of the medial temporal lobes of subjects with combat-related post-traumatic stress disorder. *Magn Reson Med* **40**(1), 66–71.

Garber, H.J., Ananth, J.V., Chiu, L.C., Griswold, V.J. & Oldendorf, W.H. (1989) Nuclear magnetic resonance study of obsessive-compulsive disorder. *Am J Psychiatry* **146**(8), 1001–5.

Goddard, A.W., Mason, G.F., Almai, A. *et al.* (2001) Reductions in occipital cortex GABA levels in panic disorder detected with 1H-magnetic resonance spectroscopy. *Arch Gen Psychiatry* **58**(6), 556–61.

Gurvits, T.V., Shenton, M.E., Hokama, H. *et al.* (1996) Magnetic resonance imaging study of hippocampal volume in chronic, combat-related post-traumatic stress disorder. *Biol Psychiatry* **40**(11), 1091–9.

Horwitz, B., Swedo, S.E., Grady, C.L. *et al.* (1991) Cerebral metabolic pattern in obsessive-compulsive disorder: altered intercorrelations between regional rates of glucose utilization. *Psychiatry Res* **40**(4), 221–37.

Inoue, O., Akimoto, Y., Hashimoto, K. & Yamasaki, T. (1985) Alterations in biodistribution of [3H]Ro 15 1788 in mice by acute stress: possible changes *in vivo* binding availability of brain benzodiazepine receptor. *Int J Nucl Med Biol* **12**, 369–74.

Javanmard, M., Shlik, J., Kennedy, S.H., Vaccarino, F.J., Houle, S. & Bradwejn, J. (1999) Neuroanatomic correlates of CCK-4-induced panic attacks in healthy humans: a comparison of two time points. *Biol Psychiatry* **45**, 872–82.

Jenike, M.A., Breiter, H.C., Baer, L. *et al.* (1996) Cerebral structural abnormalities in obsessive-compulsive disorder: a quantitative morphometric magnetic resonance imaging study. *Arch Gen Psychiatry* **53**(7), 625–32.

Kaschka, W., Feistel, H. & Ebert, D. (1995) Reduced benzodiazepine receptor binding in panic disorders measured by iomazenil SPECT. *J Psychiatr Res* **29**, 427–433.

Kim, S.G., Ugurbil, K. & Strick, P.L. (1994) Activation of a cerebellar output nucleus during cognitive processing. *Science* **265**, 949–51.

Kuikka, J.T., Pitkanen, A., Lepola, U. *et al.* (1995) Abnormal regional benzodiazepine receptor uptake in the prefrontal cortex in patients with panic disorder. *Nucl Med Commun* **16**, 273–80.

Laruelle, M. & Huang, Y. (2001) Vulnerability of positron emission tomography radiotracers to endogenous competition. New insights. *Quarterly Journal of Nucleic Medicine* **45**(2), 124–38.

LeDoux, J.E. (2000) Emotion circuits in the brain. *Annals of Review of Neuroscience* **23**, 155–84.

Liberzon, I., Taylor, S.F., Amdur, R. *et al.* (1999) Brain activation in PTSD in response to trauma-related stimuli. *Biol Psychiatry* **45**, 817–26.

Liberzon, I., Taylor, S.F., Fig, L.M. & Koeppe, R.A. (1997) Alteration of corticothalamic perfusion ratios during a PTSD flashback. *Depress Anxiety* **4**(3), 146–50.

Lucey, J.V., Costa, D.C., Busatto, G. *et al.* (1995) Caudate regional cerebral blood flow in obsessive-compulsive disorder, panic disorder and healthy controls on single photon emission computerized tomography. *Psychiatry Res* **74**(1), 25–33.

Luxenberg, J.S., Swedo, S.E., Flament, M.F., Friedland, R.P., Rapoport, J. & Rapoport, S.I. (1988) Neuroanatomical abnormalities in obsessive-compulsive disorder detected with quantitative X-ray computed tomography. *Am J Psychiatry* **145**(9), 1089–93.

Machlin, S.R., Harris, G.J., Pearlson, G.D., Hoehn-Saric, R., Jeffery, P. & Camargo, E.E. (1991) Elevated medial-frontal cerebral blood flow in obsessive-compulsive patients: a SPECT study. *Am J Psychiatry* **148**, 1240–42.

Magistretti, P.J. & Pellerin, L. (1999) Cellular mechanisms of brain energy metabolism and their relevance to functional brain imaging. *Philos Trans R Soc Lond B Biol Sci* **354**, 1155–63.

Malizia, A.L. (1997) PET studies in experimental and pathological anxiety. *J Psychopharmacol* **11**(3), A88.

Malizia, A.L. (1999) What do imaging studies tell us about anxiety disorders? *J Psychopharmacol* **13**(4), 372–8.

Malizia, A.L. (2001) Positron emitting ligands in the study of the clinical psychopharmacology of anxiety and anxiety disorders. MD Thesis. University of Bristol.

Malizia, A.L., Cunningham, V.J., Bell, C.J., Liddle, P.F., Jones, T. & Nutt, D.J. (1998) Decreased brain GABA$_A$-benzodiazepine receptor binding in panic disorder: preliminary results from a quantitative PET study. *Arch Gen Psychiatry* **55**(8), 715–20.

Malizia, A.L., Cunningham, V.J. & Nutt, D.J. (1997) Flumazenil delivery changes in panic disorder at rest. *Neuroimage* **5**(4, Part 2), S302.

Malizia, A.L., Wilson, S.J., Nutt, D.J. & Grasby, P.M. (1996) Brain networks in conditioned anticipatory anxiety in normal volunteers. *J Psychopharmacol* **10**(3), A42.

Martinot, J.L., Allilaire, J.F., Mazoyer, B.M. et al. (1989) Obsessive-compulsive disorder: a clinical, neuropsychological and positron emission tomography study. *Acta Psychiatr Scand* **82**(3), 233–42.

Mathew, R.J. & Wilson, W.H. (1991) Evaluation of the effects of diazepam and an experimental antianxiety drug on cerebral blood flow. *Psychiatry Res* **40**, 125–34.

Mathew, R.J., Wilson, W.H., Humphreys, D., Lowe, J.V. & Wiethe, K.E. (1997) Cerebral vasodilation and vasoconstriction associated with acute anxiety. *Biol Psychiatry* **41**(7), 782–95.

McGuire, P.K., Bench, C.J., Frith, C.D., Marks, I.M., Frackowiak, R.S. & Dolan, R.J. (1994) Functional anatomy of obsessive-compulsive phenomena. *Br J Psychiatry* **164**, 459–68.

Meyer, J.H., Swinson, R., Kennedy, S.H., Houle, S. & Brown, G.M. (2000) Increased left posterior parietal-temporal cortex activation after D-fenfluramine in women with panic disorder. *Psychiatry Res* **98**(3), 133–43.

Mindus, P., Ericson, K., Greitz, T., Meyerson, B.A., Nyman, H. & Sjogren, I. (1986) Regional cerebral glucose metabolism in anxiety disorders studied with positron emission tomography before and after psychosurgical intervention. A preliminary report. *Acta Radiol Suppl* **369**, 444–8.

Mountz, J.M., Modell, J.G., Wilson, M.W. et al. (1989) Positron emission tomographic evaluation of cerebral blood flow during state anxiety in simple phobia. *Arch Gen Psychiatry* **46**, 501–4.

Nordahl, T.E., Benkelfat, C., Semple, W.E., Gross, M., King, A.C. & Cohen, R.M. (1989) Cerebral glucose metabolic rates in obsessive-compulsive disorder. *Neuropsychopharmacology* **2**, 23–8.

Nordahl, T.E., Semple, W.E., Gross, M. et al. (1990) Cerebral glucose metabolic differences in patients with panic disorder. *Neuropsychopharmacology* **3**, 261–72.

Nordahl, T.E., Stein, M.B., Benkelfat, C. et al. (1999) Regional cerebral metabolic asymmetries replicated in an independent group of patients with panic disorders. *Biol Psychiatry* **44**(10), 998–1006.

Nutt, D.J., Glue, P., Lawson, C. & Wilson, S. (1990) Flumazenil provocation of panic attacks. *Arch Gen Psychiatry* **47**, 917–25.

O'Carroll, R.E., Moffoot, A.P., van Beck, M. et al. (1993) The effect of anxiety induction on the regional uptake of ^{99}Tc-exametazime in simple phobia as shown by single photon emission tomography (SPET). *J Affect Disord* **28**, 203–10.

Olsson, H. & Farde, L. (2001) Potentials and pitfalls using high affinity radioligands in PET and SPET determinations on regional drug induced D2 receptor occupancy-a simulation study based on experimental data. *Neuroimage* **14**(4), 936–45.

Ontiveros, A., Fontaine, R., Breton, G., Elie, R., Fontaine, S. & Dery, R. (1989) Correlation of severity of panic disorder and neuroanatomical changes on magnetic resonance imaging. *J Neuropsychiatry Clin Neurosci* **1**(4), 404–8.

Parekh, P.I., Spencer, J.W., George, M.S. et al. (1995) Procaine-induced increases in limbic rCBF correlate positively with increases in occipital and temporal EEG fast activity. *Brain Topogr* **7**(3), 209–16.

Perani, D., Colombo, C., Bressi, S. et al. (1995) FDG PET study in obsessive-compulsive disorder: a clinical metabolic correlation study after treatment. *Br J Psychiatry* **166**, 244–50.

Peyron, R., Le Bars, D., Cinotti, L. et al. (1994) Effects of GABA$_A$ receptors activation on brain glucose metabolism in normal subjects and temporal lobe epilepsy (TLE) patients. A positron emission tomography (PET) study. Part I: brain glucose metabolism is increased after GABA$_A$ receptors activation. *Epilepsy Res* **19**(1), 45–54.

Potts, N.L., Davidson, J.R., Krishnan, K.R. & Doraiswamy, P.M. (1994) Magnetic resonance imaging in social phobia. *Psychiatry Res* **52**(1), 35–42.

225

Pujol, J., Torres, L., Deus, J. *et al.* (1999) Functional magnetic resonance imaging study of frontal lobe activation during word generation in obsessive-compulsive disorder. *Biol Psychiatry* **45**(7), 891–7.

Rauch, S.L., Jenike, M.A., Alpert, N.M. *et al.* (1994) Regional cerebral blood flow measured during symptom provocation in obsessive-compulsive disorder using ^{15}O-labeled CO_2 and positron emission tomography. *Arch Gen Psychiatry* **51**, 62–70.

Rauch, S.L., Savage, C.R., Alpert, N.M. *et al.* (1997a) Probing striatal function in obsessive-compulsive disorder: a PET study of implicit sequence learning. *J Neuropsychiatry* **9**, 568–73.

Rauch, S.L., Savage, C.R., Alpert, N.M., Fischman, A.J. & Jenike, M.A. (1997b) The functional neuroanatomy of anxiety: a study of three disorders using positron emission tomography and symptom provocation. *Biol Psychiatry* **42**(6), 446–52.

Rauch, S.L., Savage, C.R., Alpert, N.M. *et al.* (1995) A positron emission tomographic study of simple phobic symptom provocation. *Arch Gen Psychiatry* **52**, 20–8.

Rauch, S.L., van der Kolk, B.A., Fisler, R.E. *et al.* (1996) A symptom provocation study of post-traumatic stress disorder using positron emission tomography and script-driven imagery. *Arch Gen Psychiatry* **53**, 380–7.

Reiman, E.M., Raichle, M.E., Butler, F.K., Herscovitch, P. & Robins, E. (1984) A focal brain abnormality in panic disorder, a severe form of anxiety. *Nature* **310**(5979), 683–5.

Reiman, E.M., Raichle, M.E., Robins, E. *et al.* (1986) The application of positron emission tomography to the study of panic disorder. *Am J Psychiatry* **143**, 469–77.

Reiman, E.M., Raichle, M.E., Robins, E. *et al.* (1989) Neuroanatomical correlates of a lactate-induced anxiety attack. *Arch Gen Psychiatry* **46**, 493–500.

Robinson, D., Wu, H., Munne, R.A. *et al.* (1995) Reduced caudate nucleus volume in obsessive-compulsive disorder. *Arch Gen Psychiatry* **52**, 393–8.

Roland, P.E. & Friberg, L. (1988) The effect of the $GABA_A$ agonist THIP on regional cortical blood flow in humans. A new test of hemispheric dominance. *J Cereb Blood Flow Metab* **8**(3), 314–23.

Rosenberg, D.R., Keshavan, M.S., O'Hearn, K.M. *et al.* (1997) Frontostriatal measurement in treatment-naive children with obsessive-compulsive disorder. *Arch Gen Psychiatry* **554**, 824–30.

Rosenberg, D.R., MacMaster, F.P., Keshavan, M.S., Fitzgerald, K.D., Stewart, C.M. & Moore, G.J. (2000) Decrease in caudate glutamatergic concentrations in pediatric obsessive-compulsive disorder patients taking paroxetine. *J Am Acad Child Adolesc Psychiatry* **39**(9), 1096–103.

Rubin, R.T., Ananth, J., Villanueva-Meyer, J., Trajmar, P.G. & Mena, I. (1995) Regional ^{133}xenon cerebral blood flow and cerebral ^{99m}Tc-HMPAO uptake in patients with obsessive-compulsive disorder before and during treatment. *Biol Psychiatry* **38**(7), 429–37.

Rubin, R.T., Villaneuva-Myer, J., Ananth, J., Trajmar, P.G. & Mena, I. (1992) Regional ^{133}xenon cerebral blood flow and cerebral ^{99m}Technetium-HMPAO uptake in unmedicated patients with obsessive-compulsive disorder and matched normal control subjects. *Arch Gen Psychiatry* **49**, 695–702.

Sapolsky, R.M. (1996) Why stress is bad for your brain. *Science* **273**, 749–50.

Sargent, P.A., Nash, J., Hood, S. *et al.* (2000) 5-HT1A receptor binding in panic disorder: comparison with depressive disorder and healthy volunteers using PET and [11C] WAY 100635. *Neuroimage* **11**(5), S189.

Sawle, G.V., Hymas, N.F., Lees, A.J. & Frackowiak, R.S. (1991) Obsessional slowness. Functional studies with positron emission tomography. *Brain* **114**(5), 2191–202.

Saxena, S., Brody, A.L., Maidment, K.M. *et al.* (1999) Localized orbito-frontal and subcortical metabolic changes and predictors of response to paroxetine treatment in obsessive-compulsive disorder. *Neuropsychopharmacology* **21**(6), 683–93.

Saxena, S. & Rauch, S.L. (2000) Functional neuroimaging and the neuroanatomy of obsessive-compulsive disorder. *Psychiatr Clin North Am* **23**(3), 563–86.

Scarone, S., Colombo, C., Livian, S. *et al.* (1992) Increased right caudate nucleus size in obsessive-compulsive disorder: detection with magnetic resonance imaging. *Psychiatry Res: Neuroimaging* **45**, 115–21.

Schlegel, S., Steinert, H., Bockisch, A., Hahn, K., Schloesser, R. & Benkert, O. (1994) Decreased benzodiazepine receptor binding in panic disorder measured by iomazenil SPECT. A preliminary report. *Eur Arch Psychiatry Clin Neurosci* **244**, 49–51.

Schneider, F., Weiss, U., Kessler, C. *et al.* (1999) Subcortical correlates of differential classical conditioning of aversive emotional reactions in social phobia. *Biol Psychiatry* **45**, 863–71.

Schneier, F.R., Liebowitz, M.R., Abi-Dargham, A., Zea-Ponce, Y., Lin, S.H. & Laruelle, M. (2000) Low dopamine D2 receptor binding potential in social phobia. *Am J Psychiatry* **157**(3), 457–9.

Schwartz, J.M., Stoessel, P.W., Baxter, L.R., Jr, Martin, K.M. & Phelps, M.E. (1996) Systematic changes in cerebral glucose metabolic rate after successful behavior modification. *Arch Gen Psychiatry* **53**, 109–13.

Semple, W.E., Goyer, P., McCormick, R. *et al.* (1996) Preliminary report: brain blood flow using PET in patients with post-traumatic stress disorder and substance-abuse histories. *Biol Psychiatry* **34**, 115–18.

Servan-Schreiber, D., Perlstein, W.M., Cohen, J.D. & Mintun, M. (1998) Selective pharmacological activation of limbic structures in human volunteers: a positron emission tomography study. *J Neuropsychiatry Clin Neurosci* **10**, 148–59.

Sheline, Y.I., Sanghavi, M., Mintun, M.A. & Gado, M.H. (1999) Depression duration but not age predicts hippocampal volume loss in medically healthy women with recurrent major depression. *J Neurosci* **19**, 5034–43.

Shin, L.M., Kosslyn, S.M., McNally, R.J. *et al.* (1997) Visual imagery and perception in post-traumatic stress disorder: a positron emission tomographic investigation. *Arch Gen Psychiatry* **54**, 233–41.

Shin, L.M., McNally, R.J., Kosslyn, S.M. *et al.* (1999) Regional cerebral blood flow during script-driven imagery in childhood sexual abuse-related post-traumatic stress disorder: a PET investigation. *Am J Psychiatry* **156**, 575–84.

Sibille, E., Pavlides, C., Benke, D. & Toth, M. (2000) Genetic inactivation of the Serotonin 1A receptor in mice results in downregulation of major GABA$_A$ receptor alpha subunits, reduction of GABA$_A$ receptor binding, and benzodiazepine-resistant anxiety. *J Neurosci* **20**(8), 2758–65.

Simpson, J.R., Jr, Drevets, W.C., Snyder, A.Z., Gusnard, D.A. & Raichle, M.E. (2001) Emotion-induced changes in human medial prefrontal cortex. II. During anticipatory anxiety. *Proc Natl Acad Sci U S A* **98**(2), 688–93.

Stein, M.B., Koverola, C., Hanna, C., Torchia, M.G. & McClarty, B. (1997) Hippocampal volume in women victimized by childhood sexual abuse. *Psychological Medicine* **27**, 951–60.

Stein, M.B. & Leslie, W.D. (1996) A brain SPECT study of generalized social phobia. *Biol Psychiatry* **39**, 825–8.

Stewart, R.S., Devous, M.D., Sr, Rush, A.J., Lane, L. & Bonte, F.J. (1988) Cerebral blood flow changes during sodium-lactate-induced panic attacks. *Am J Psychiatry* **145**(4), 442–9.

Swedo, S.E., Pietrini, P., Leonard, H.L. *et al.* (1992) Cerebral glucose metabolism in childhood-onset obsessive-compulsive disorder: revisualization during pharmacotherapy. *Arch Gen Psychiatry* **49**, 690–4.

Swedo, S.E., Schapiro, M.B., Grady, C.L. *et al.* (1989) Cerebral glucose metabolism in childhood-onset obsessive-compulsive disorder. *Arch Gen Psychiatry* **46**, 518–23.

Szeszko, P.R., Robinson, D., Alvir, J.M. *et al.* (1999) Orbital frontal and amygdala volume reductions in obsessive-compulsive disorder. *Arch Gen Psychiatry* **56**(10), 913–19.

Tagamets, M.A. & Horwitz, B. (2001) Interpreting PET and fMRI measures of functional neural activity: the effects of synaptic inhibition on cortical activation in human imaging studies. *Brain Res Bull* **54**(3), 267–73.

Tauscher, J., Bagby, R.M., Javanmard, M., Christensen, B.K., Kasper, S. & Kapur, S. (2001) Inverse relationship between serotonin 5-HT1A receptor binding and anxiety: a [11C] WAY 100635 PET investigation in healthy volunteers. *Am J Psychiatry* **158**(8), 1326–8.

Tiihonen, J., Kuikka, J., Bergstrom, K., Lepola, U., Koponen, H. & Leinonen, E. (1997a) Dopamine reuptake site densities in patients with social phobia. *Am J Psychiatry* **154**(2), 239–242.

Tiihonen, J., Kuikka, J., Rasanen, P. *et al.* (1997b) Cerebral benzodiazepine receptor binding and distribution in generalized anxiety disorder: a fractal analysis. *Mol Psychiatry* **2**(6), 463–71.

Tillfors, M., Furmark, T., Marteinsdottir, I. *et al.* (2001) Cerebral blood flow in subjects with social phobia during stressful speaking tasks: a PET study. *Am J Psychiatry* **158**(8), 1220–6.

Tokunaga, M., Ida, I., Higuchi, T. & Mikuni, M. (1997) Alterations of benzodiazepine receptor binding potential in anxiety and somatoform disorders measured by [123I]iomazenil SPECT. *Radiat Med* **15**(3), 163–9.

Tupler, L.A., Davidson, J.R., Smith, R.D., Lazeyras, F., Charles, H.C. & Krishnan, K.R. (1997) A repeat proton magnetic resonance spectroscopy study in social phobia. *Biol Psychiatry* **42**(6), 419–24.

Van der Linden, G., van Heerden, B., Warwick, J. *et al.* (2000) Functional brain imaging and pharmacotherapy in social phobia: single photon emission computed tomography before and after treatment with the selective serotonin reuptake inhibitor citalopram. *Prog Neuropsychopharmacol Biol Psychiatry* **24**(3), 419–38.

Vythilingam, M., Anderson, E.R., Goddard, A. *et al.* (2000) Temporal lobe volume in panic disorder—a quantitative magnetic resonance imaging study. *Psychiatry Res* **99**(2), 75–82.

Weizman, R., Weizman, A., Kook, K.A., Vocci, F., Deutsch, S.I. & Paul, S.M. (1989) Repeated swim stress alters brain benzodiazepine receptors measured *in vivo*. *J Pharmacol Exp Ther* **249**, 701–7.

Weizman, A., Weizman, R., Kook, K.A., Vocci, F., Deutsch, S.I. & Paul, S.M. (1990) Adrenalectomy prevents the stress induced decrease *in vivo* [3H]Ro 15 1788 binding to GABA$_A$ benzodiazepine receptors in the mouse. *Brain Res* **519**, 347–50.

Wik, G., Fredrikson, M., Ericson, K., Eriksson, L., Stone-Elander, S. & Greitz, T. (1993) A functional cerebral response to frightening visual stimulation. *Psychiatry Res: Neuroimaging* **50**, 15–24.

Wik, G., Fredrikson, M. & Fischer, H. (1996) Cerebral correlates of anticipated fear: a PET study of specific phobia. *Int J Neurosci* **87**(3–4), 267–76.

Wik, G., Fredrikson, M. & Fischer, H. (1997) Evidence of altered cerebral blood-flow relationships in acute phobia. *Int J Neurosci* **91**, 253–63.

Woods, S.W., Koster, K., Krystal, J.K. *et al.* (1988) Yohimbine alters regional cerebral blood flow in panic disorder. *Lancet* **2**, 678.

Wu, J.C., Buchsbaum, M.S., Hershey, T.G., Hazlett, E., Sicotte, N. & Johnson, J.C. (1991) PET in generalized anxiety disorder. *Biol Psychiatry* **29**(12), 1181–99.

Yehuda, R., Levengood, R.A., Schmeidler, J., Wilson, S., Guo, L.S. & Gerber, D. (1999) Increased pituitary activation following metyrapone administration in post-traumatic stress disorder. *Psychoneuroendocrinology* **21**(1), 1–16.

Zubieta, J.K., Chinitz, J.A., Lombardi, U., Fig, L.M., Cameron, O.G. & Liberzon, I. (1999) Medial frontal cortex involvement in PTSD symptoms: a SPECT study. *J Psychiatr Res* **33**(3), 259–64.

Genetic Dissection of Anxiety and Related Disorders

K.P. Lesch

Introduction

Genetic research in psychobiology and psychiatry has traditionally taken an epidemiologic approach since etiopathogenetic mechanisms continue to be inadequately understood at the molecular level. A large body of evidence from family, twin, and adoptee studies has been accumulated that a complex genetic component is involved in anxiety-related traits, and in the liability to anxiety spectrum disorders. While genetic research has typically focused either on normal personality characteristics or on psychiatric disorders, with few investigations evaluating the genetic and environmental relationship between the two, it is of critical importance to answer the questions whether a certain quantitative trait etiopathogenetically influences the disorder, or whether the trait is a syndromal dimension of the disorder. After all, it is no longer about whether nature or nuture shapes human development but about how complex genetic and environmental factors interact in the formation and expression of a behavioral phenotype. Behaviorial genetics is indeed progressing rapidly in great strides towards an evidence-based demonstration of the relevance of both genetic *and* environmental factors for anxiety-related traits as well as anxiety disorders.

A complementary approach to genetic studies of anxiety and related disorders in humans involves the investigation of genes (i.e. construction of transcriptome maps) and their protein products (i.e. application of proteomics) implicated in the brain neurocircuitry of fear and anxiety in animal models. Based on an increasing body of evidence that genetically driven variability of expression and function of proteins that regulate the function of brain neurotransmitter systems (e.g. receptors, ion channels, transporters, and enzymes) are associated with complex behavioral traits, research is also giving strong emphasis to the molecular psychobiological basis of anxiety-related behaviors in rodents and, increasingly, nonhuman primates. Conditioning of fear and anxiety involves pathways transmitting information to and from the amygdala to various neural networks that control the expression of aggressive or defensive reactions, including behavioral, autonomic nervous system, and stress hormone responses. While pathways from the thalamus and cortex (sensory and prefrontal) project to the amygdala, inputs are processed within intra-amygdaloid circuitries and out-puts are directed to the hippocampus, brainstem, hypothalamus, and other regions. Thus, the amygdala-associated neural network is critical to integration of the "fight or flight" response. Identification of molecular components of neural circuits involved in fear and anxiety are currently leading to new candidate genes of presumed pathophysiologic pathways in addition to candidates that are generally derived from hypothesized pathogenetic mechanisms of the disorder, or from clinical observations of therapeutic response.

This review describes fundamental aspects of the genetics of anxiety-related traits and anxiety disorders and provides an appraisal of quantitative genetic research, both humans (twin and adoption studies) and rodents (inbred strain, selection, and knockout studies). Conceptual and methodological issues in the search for candidate genes for anxiety and for the development of mouse models of human fearfulness and anxiety will also be considered.

Anxiety-related traits

The behavioral predisposition of an individual is commonly referred to as his or her temperament or personality. Systematic research attempts to characterize the dimensional structure of personality traits including the anxiety-related cluster comprising fearfulness, emotional instability, and stress reactivity. Individual differences in anxiety-related traits, and the ultimate behavioral consequences of the "fight or flight" response, are relatively enduring, continuously distributed, as well as substantially heritable, although they seem to result from additive or nonadditive interaction of genetic variations with environmental influences (Loehlin 1992). This is convincingly illustrated by the striking similarity of identical twins adopted out and reared apart (Minnesota Twin Study), some of whom had not known each other prior to the study (Bouchard 1994). Twin studies take advantage of the experiment of nature in which some twins are genetically identical (monozygotic twins) and others share, on average, only half their genes (dizygotic twins). On measures of interests, skills, and personality traits, monozygotic twins had correlations between 34% and 78%, whereas fraternal twins showed correlations between 7% and 39% (Tellegen et al. 1988). Twin studies of self-reported symptoms of anxiety, often called negative emotionality or neuroticism, consistently indicate that approximately 40–60% of the variance can be attributed to genetic factors. While studies of the patterns of inheritance of personality indicate that various dimensions are likely to be influenced by many genes making it polygenic or *quantitative* traits, they likewise document the significance of environmental factors. However, contrary to expectation, the relevant environmental cues appear to be those that are not shared by relatives reared together (McGue & Bouchard 1998). The relative influence of genetic and environmental factors on temperamental and behavioral differences is, however, among the most contentious controversies. While current views emphasize the joint influence of genes and environmental sources, the complexities of gene–gene and gene–environment interactions (genotypes may *respond* differentially to different environments) as well as gene–environment correlations (genotypes may be *exposed* differentially to environments) represent research areas in their infancy.

"Fight or flight" responses which are the consequence of predominance of either aggression or anxiety seem to delineate a biologically based model of dispositions to both normal and pathological functioning, with a continuum of genetic risk underlying personality and behavioral dimensions that extend from normal to abnormal. Thus, the analysis of genetic contributions to anxiety-related or aggressive behavior is both conceptually and methodologically difficult, so that consistent findings remain sparse. The documented heterogeneity of both genetic and environmental determinants suggests the futility of searching for unitary causes. This vista has therefore increasingly encouraged the pursuit of dimensional and quantitative approaches to behaviorial genetics, in addition to the traditional strategy of studying individuals with categorically defined psychiatric entities (Plomin et al. 1994). While quantitative genetics has focused on complex, quantitatively distributed traits and their origins in naturally occurring variation caused by multiple genetic and environmental factors, molecular genetics has begun to identify specific genes for quantitative traits, called quantitative trait loci (QTLs) (Eley & Plomin 1997). This perspective suggests that it may be less difficult to identify genes for psychopathology by searching for genes influencing personality, and that complex traits are not attributable to single genes necessary or sufficient to cause a disorder. The QTL concept thus implies that there may not be genes for psychiatric disorders, just genes for behavioral dimensions.

Because the power of linkage analysis to detect small gene effects is quite limited, at least with realistic samples, QTL research in humans has relied on association analysis using DNA variants in or near candidate genes that are functional. Gene variants with a significant impact on the functionality of components of brain monoamine neurotransmission, such as the serotonin (5-hydroxtryptamine; 5-HT) system, are a rational beginning. Based on converging lines of evidence that the 5-HT and serotonergic gene expression are involved in a myriad of processes during brain development as well as synaptic plasticity in adulthood, temperamental predispositions and complex behavior is likely to be influenced by genetically driven variability of 5-HT function. Consequently, the contribution of a polymorphism in the 5′-flanking regulatory region of the 5-HT tranporter gene (5-HTTLPR) to individual phenotypic differences in personality traits was explored in independent population- and family-based genetic studies (for review see Lesch et al. 2001). Evidence is accumulating that 5-HT transporter gene variability results in

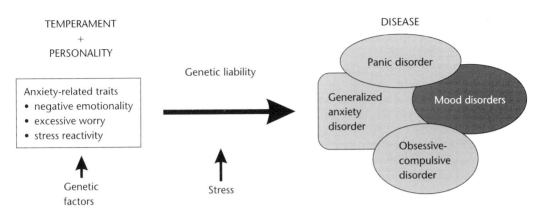

TEMPERAMENT
+
PERSONALITY

Anxiety-related traits
• negative emotionality
• excessive worry
• stress reactivity

Genetic
factors

Genetic liability

Stress

DISEASE

Panic disorder

Generalized anxiety disorder

Mood disorders

Obsessive-compulsive disorder

Fig. 13.1 Structural relationship of the dimensions comprising anxiety-related personality traits and various anxiety and mood disorders. Anxiety-related personality traits and generalized anxiety disorder (GAD)-associated negative affect and worry are conceptionalized as dispositional traits common to both anxiety and mood disorders including depression.

allelic variation of 5-HT transporter expression and function, is associated with personality traits of negative emotionality including anxiety, depression, and aggressiveness (neuroticism and agreeableness). In addition, a within-family analysis of sibling pairs discordant for the 5-HTTLPR genotype confirmed this association, in that the sibling with the short-form allele had higher neuroticism scores than their siblings homozygous for the long variant. The 5-HTTLPR was not associated with other major dimensions of personality (extraversion, openness, and conscientiousness).

The effect sizes for the 5-HTTLPR personality associations indicate that this polymorphism has a moderate influence on these behavioral predispositions that corresponds to 3–4% of the total variance and 7–9% of the genetic variance, based on estimates from twin studies using these and related measures which have consistently demonstrated that genetic factors contribute 40–60% of the variance in neuroticism and other related personality traits. The associations represent only a small portion of the genetic contribution to anxiety-related traits. If additional genes were hypothesized to contribute similar gene–dose effects to anxiety, at least 10 genes are predicted to be involved. Additive contribution of comparable size or epistatic interaction have, in fact, been found in studies of other quantitative traits. Thus, the results are consistent with the view that the influence of a single, common polymorphism on continuously distributed traits is likely to be very modest in humans, and that this is likely to hold true also for miscellaneous quantitative characteristics in other

species (Plomin *et al.* 1994). From the evolutionary psychological perspective, anxiety is a pervasive and innately driven form of distress that arises in response to actual or threatened exclusion from social groups (Baumeister & Tice 1990; Buss 1991). Notably, Nakamura *et al.* (1997) have discussed the higher prevalence of the anxiety and depression-related l/s and s/s genotypes in the context of notable emotional restraint and interpersonal sensitivity in Japanese people as a possible population-typical adaptation to prevent social exclusion (Ono *et al.* 1996).

A growing body of evidence implicates personality traits, such as neuroticism or negative emotionality, in the comorbidity of affective spectrum disorders (Kendler *et al.* 1993a; Livesley *et al.* 1998) (Fig. 13.1). Separation of mental illness from personality disorders in current consensual diagnostic systems, has remarkably enhanced interest in the link between temperament, personality, and psychiatric disorders as well as the impact of this inter-relationship on the heterogeneity within diagnostic entities, prediction of long-term course, and treatment response (Mulder *et al.* 1994). Based on multivariate genetic analyses of comorbidity, generalized anxiety disorder and major depression have common genetic origins and the phenotypic differences between anxiety and depression are dependent upon the environment (Kendler *et al.* 1992b; Kendler 1996). Moreover, indexed by the personality scale of neuroticism, general vulnerability overlaps genetically to a substantial extent with both anxiety and depression (Kendler *et al.* 1993a,b). These results predicted that when a QTL, such as the 5-HTTLPR, is found for neuroticism, the same QTL should be associated with symptoms of anxiety and depression. Anxiety and mood disorders are therefore likely to represent the extreme end of variation in negative emotionality (Eley & Plomin 1997; Eley & Stevenson 1999). The genetic factor contributing to the extreme ends of dimensions of variation commonly recognized as a disorder may be quantitatively, not qualitatively, different from the rest of the distribution. This vista has important implications for identifying genes for complex traits related to a distinct disorders. An association of the 5-HTTLPR and affective illness including unipolar depression and bipolar disorder has been reported by Collier *et al.* (1996), although subsequent studies did not consistently replicate these results. Possible reasons for these conflicting results have recently been discussed in detail by Greenberg *et al.* (2000).

Anxiety spectrum disorders

Generalized anxiety disorder

Generalized anxiety disorder (GAD) is defined by excessive and uncontrollable worry about a number of life events or activities for at least 6 months, accompanied by at least three of six associated symptoms of negative affect or tension, such as restlessness, fatigability, concentration difficulties, irritability, muscle tension, or sleep disturbance (Brown 1997). Studies of the lifetime prevalence for GAD in the general population have provided estimates ranging from 1.6% to 5.1% and indicated a female : male preponderance of 2 : 1 (Torgersen 1983; Weissman 1990; Kendler *et al.* 1992a; Lyons *et al.* 2000). Relative to other anxiety and mood disorders, GAD is more likely to show a gradual onset and/or life-long history of symptoms. While early ages of onset are common, the syndrome itself may emerge only later in life and a considerable number of patients with GAD report an onset in adulthood that is usually in response to psychosocial and emotional stress. Research has consistently shown that GAD is associated with high comorbidity rates for other psychiatric disorders, including panic disorder, major depression, dysthymia, social phobia, and specific phobia (Kendler *et al.* 1992a; Weissman 1993; Skre *et al.* 1994; Kendler *et al.* 1995b; Roy *et al.* 1995). Moreover, patients with GAD frequently undergo treatment for stress-associated

physical conditions (e.g. irritable bowel syndrome, chronic pain syndromes).

Based on inadequate diagnostic reliability and high comorbidity the discriminant validity of GAD is controversial. Studies have begun to address the structural relationship of the dimensions comprising various anxiety disorders and there is an increasing body of evidence that GAD-associated negative affect and worry are dispositional traits common to both anxiety and mood disorders including depression (Fig. 13.1). GAD may therefore be conceptionalized as a trait or vulnerability dimension predisposing to other disorders, and etiological models of GAD integrate both psychosocial and biological factors.

Twin and family based studies indicate a clear genetic influence in GAD with a heritability of approximately 30%. GAD-associated genetic factors are completely shared with depression, while environmental determinants seem to be distinct (Kendler *et al.* 1992b; Kendler 1996). This notion is consistent with recent models of emotional disorders that view anxiety and mood disorders as sharing common vulnerabilities but differing on dimensions including, for instance, focus of attention or psychosocial liability.

Panic disorder

Panic disorder (PD) typically has its onset between late adolescence and the mid-30s. PD is strikingly different from other types of anxiety in that panic attacks are sudden, appear to be unprovoked, and are often disabling. They may include intense fear, fear of dying, a sense that something unimaginably horrible is about to occur and one is powerless to prevent it, or discomfort accompanied by several physiological symptoms, including palpitations, chest pain, choking sensations, sweating, trembling or shaking, dizziness, lightheadedness or nausea, flushes or chills, tingling or numbness in the hands, fear of losing control and doing something embarrassing, dreamlike sensations or perceptual distortions. A panic attack typically lasts from several minutes to hours, and may be one of the most distressing experiences that someone has suffered. Panic attacks are followed by persistent concerns about having additional attacks, worry about the implications of the attack or its consequences, and significant changes in behavior related to the attacks.

With one or more repeated panic attacks, for instance while driving, shopping in a crowded store, or riding in an elevator, patients may develop an irrational fear, or phobia, about these situations and begin to avoid them. Ultimately, the pattern of avoidance and level of anxiety about another attack may reach a point where a PD patient may be incapable of driving or even leaving home. At this stage, PD is complicated by agoraphobia. PD, agoraphobia, and depression display significant comorbidity (Wittchen *et al.* 1991). The first attacks are frequently triggered by physical illnesses, psychosocial stress, or certain drug treatments, or drugs of abuse that increase activity of neural systems involved in fear and anxiety responses. Attacks can be pharmacologically precipitated by carbon dioxide, caffeine, lactate, cholecystokinin tetrapeptide (Bradwejn & Koszycki 1991), and serotonergic compounds (Kahn & Wetzler 1991). Sensitivity to carbon dioxide and lactate may indicate a distinct genetic liability (Balon *et al.* 1989; Reschke *et al.* 1995; Perna *et al.* 1996).

Independently conducted epidemiologic studies in several countries revealed lifetime prevalences from 0.4% to 3.5%, with female : male ratios ranging from 0.2 to 2.5 (Eaton *et al.* 1994; Kessler *et al.* 1994; Weissman *et al.* 1997). Relative risks for the co-occurrence of PD with agoraphobia and major depression range from 7.5 to 21.4 and from 3.8 to 20.1, respectively (Weissman *et al.* 1997). Twin studies yielded a population prevalence of 6.0–14.1% (Kendler *et al.* 1993c; Perna *et al.* 1997). The ratios of risk in first-degree relatives of patients with PD versus relatives of normal controls ranged from 3.4 to 14.7. Interestingly, a subdivision of PD patients according to age at onset before or after 20 years of age led to remarkable differences in risk of 22% and 8%, respectively (Goldstein *et al.* 1997). Lifetime risk in second-degree relatives of patients with PD extends to 12.5% (Moran & Andrews 1985; Hopper *et al.* 1987; Battaglia *et al.* 1995). Familial patterns of aggregation also suggest that PD, GAD, depression, and agoraphobia may co-occur but it is still a matter of considerable debate whether they have related or different genetic etiologies (Weissman 1993; Woodman 1993; Maier *et al.* 1995).

Twin study designs compare the similarity of monozygotic twins (MZ) with that of dizygotic twins (DZ). A higher correlation for MZ than for DZ indicates a genetic influence on the trait under investigation. Two twin studies reported MZ : DZ pair-wise concordance rates of 22 : 0 and 24 : 11, with respective heritability estimates of 35% and 46% for a narrow

phenotype and a multiple threshold model (Torgersen 1990; Kendler *et al.* 1993c). However, models for the mode of inheritance of PD remain highly speculative. Logistic regression analysis of PD family data yielded evidence of vertical transmission and the effect of sibship environment, whereas segregation analysis of family data resulted in moderate evidence of an incompletely penetrant dominant or recessive major gene (Bonney 1986; Hopper *et al.* 1990). Twin data indicate nonadditive genetic (dominant or epistatic) and unique environmental effects, but little impact of shared environment (Martin *et al.* 1988). Model fitting in a large twin sample found evidence that the familial transmission of panic-phobia was influenced by sex-dependent additive genetic effects, dominant genetic factors, individual-specific environmental factors, and a shared environmental effect for women only (16% vs. 1%), while higher heritability in males (38%) compared to females (16%) was predicted (Kendler *et al.* 1995c).

Two complete genome-wide linkage scans for PD liability genes have recently been published (Knowles *et al.* 1998; Crowe *et al.* 2001). Linkage analyses are based on the identification of large, densely affected families so that the inheritance patterns of known sections of DNA, such as polymorphic repetitive elements, can be compared to the family's transmission of the disorder. Linkage of a particular allele to the presence or absence of a phenotype which breeds true allows us to define and to narrow down the location of the suspect gene. Although none of the findings based on lod scores or the proportion of allele sharing reached a level of statistical confidence according to the stringent Lander–Kruglyak criteria, a region suggestive of a susceptibility locus for PD on chromosome 7p15 was independently identified in both studies. Crowe and associates (Crowe *et al.* 2001) detected the highest lod score of 2.23 at the D7S2846 locus, located at 57.8 cm on chromosome 7, in a region that lies within 15 cm from the D7S435 locus reported by Knowles *et al.* (1998). Linkage to numerous other markers over a substantial proportion of the human genome had previously been excluded under various parametric models in different sets of pedigrees (Crowe 1990; Crowe *et al.* 1990; Mutchler *et al.* 1990; Wang *et al.* 1992; Kato *et al.* 1996). Some of the conflicting results of linkage analyses in PD may be ascribed to methodological differences in family ascertainment, phenotype definition, diagnostic assessment, and approaches to data analysis. Even more likely, they may represent true etiologic differences due to locus heterogeneity. Susceptibility to PD may thus be influenced either by an incompletely penetrant major gene in some families, or by multiple genes of weak and varying effect in others.

Since evidence for a genetic liability in PD is persuasive, a small number of putative vulnerability genes have been assessed in association studies. Candidate genes were selected in consideration of components of neurotransmitter systems involved in anxiogenic responses or therapeutic action of anxiolytic drugs. Studies of genetic association compare the frequency of a particular polymorphism in patients with controls, or compare scores on a continuous measure for two groups with a genetic marker of interest. While linkage analysis is systematic but not powerful, association studies are powerful but not systematic. Since quantitative traits are influenced by multiple genes of varying effect size and by environmental factors, QTLs for complex traits are likely to be of very modest, if not minimal, effect size and thus account for only a small proportion of the variance in the population.

A role of monoamine neurotransmitters in the etiology of PD has been suggested by the observations that increased serotonergic neurotransmission provokes anxiety even up to the level of panic attacks in PD patients (Kahn & Wetzler 1991) and that decreased 5-HT uptake is found in patients with anxiety disorders (Iny et al. 1994). This corresponds well to the observation that in rodent models increased serotonergic function is anxiogenic while a decrease is anxiolytic. Although it may be hypothesized that enhanced serotonergic neurotransmission in PD is due to decreased 5-HT uptake, no association with 5-HTTLPR-dependent variation in 5-HT transporter expression and PD was detected in different populations (Deckert et al. 1997; Ishiguro et al. 1997; Matsushita et al. 1997; Hamilton et al. 1999). These negative findings are compatible with the assumption that additional or alternative cellular pathways and neural circuits are involved in panic anxiety (Charney & Deutch 1996). Monoamine oxidase A (MAOA), an enzyme involved in the degradation of 5-HT and norepinephrine (noradrenaline) and thus positioned at the crossroads of two monoaminergic systems, is another plausible candidate gene. A 30-bp repeat polymorphism was recently identified in the promoter region of the MAOA gene that differentially modulates gene transcription (Deckert et al.

1997). Variation in the number of repeats (3–5) of this MAOA gene-linked polymorphic region (MAOALPR) displayed allele-dependent transcriptional efficiency. The effectiveness of the 3-repeat allele was two-fold lower than those with longer repeats. Assessment of the MAOALPR for association with PD in two independent samples (combined $N = 209$) showed that the longer alleles were significantly more frequent in female patients than in females of the corresponding control populations (Deckert et al. 1997). Together with the observation that inhibition of MAOA is clinically effective in the treatment of PD, particularly in women, these findings suggest that altered MAOA activity may be a gender-specific risk factor for PD.

Notably, no consistently significant associations between PD and alleles of the γ-aminobutyric acid type A (GABA-A), dopamine D2 and D4, cholecystokinin B as well as the adenosine A1 and A2a receptor genes have been detected (Crawford et al. 1995; Kato et al. 1996; Crowe et al. 1997; Deckert et al. 1998; Wang et al. 1998; Kennedy et al. 1999). Population-based studies also found no evidence for an association between PD and the gene for the dopamine transporter (Hamilton et al. 2000).

Phobias

Phobias occur in several forms and specific phobias are linked to a particular object or situation. Social phobia as an example is an intense fear of becoming humiliated in a social setting, or being painfully embarrassed in front of other people. Lifetime prevalence of social phobia was 9.5% in females and 4.9% in males, with about one-third being classified as individuals with generalized social phobia (Wittchen et al. 2000). Little is known about the psychobiology and heritability of specific phobias, although twin studies of common phobias and fears in unselected samples point toward a genetic influence (Stein 1998).

Assessment of lifetime history of five unreasonable fears and phobias, including agoraphobia and social, situational, animal, and blood-injury phobia, in female twins resulted in heritability between 46% and 67% (Kendler et al. 1999). Correcting for unreliability of ascertainment, the liability to fears and their associated phobias is moderately heritable. Individual-specific environmental experiences play an important role in the development of phobias, while familial and other environmental factors appear to be of little etiological significance.

Only few population-based association and linkage-disequilibrium studies have been conducted in phobias. Linkage-disequilibrium studies in a population capitalize on the likelihood that the susceptibility genes for a particular disorder probably came from one or a few founding members. Stein *et al.* (1998) excluded linkage between generalized social phobia and the 5-HT transporter and 5-HT2A receptor, although modifier effects could not be ruled out.

Obsessive-compulsive disorder

Obsessive-compulsive disorder (OCD) is a relatively common condition, usually begins in adolescence or early adulthood, and is characterized by persistent ideas, unwanted thoughts, and repetitive or ritualistic behaviors performed to neutralize or prevent discomfort, or some dreaded event. These thoughts and behaviors cause marked distress and are time-consuming or significantly interfere with a patient's normal functioning. OCD and related disorders may be heterogenous conditions, and the neurobiology of many putative OCD spectrum disorders has not been well studied (Stein 2000). Comorbidity with depression, anorexia nervosa, and Tourette's syndrome is considerable. The prevalence of OCD may range from 0.7% to 2.1%, with no difference between men and women (Bebbington 1998). Based on the results of family and twin studies, the involvement of a genetic factor in OCD is likely (Rasmussen 1993; Alsobrook *et al.* 1999). In a large set of studies using operationalized criteria the risk to first-degree relatives ranged from 3% to 35% for narrowly defined OCD (Lenane *et al.* 1990; Riddle *et al.* 1990; Bellodi *et al.* 1992; Black *et al.* 1992; Leonard *et al.* 1992; Pauls *et al.* 1995; Sciuto *et al.* 1995). Pooling age-corrected data across studies resulted in a lifetime risk of 9.2% for relatives of OCD patients and a lifetime risk of 2.2% in controls. The use of broader criteria including subthreshold OCD as affected revealed a lifetime risk of 28.1% in relatives of OCD patients and 15.0% in controls (Lenane *et al.* 1990; Black *et al.* 1992). The twin data are conflicting with respect to MZ and DZ pairwise concordance rates of 7–33% and a heritability of 68% (Torgersen 1983; Andrews *et al.* 1990). Analysis of obsessiveness/compulsiveness as a quantitative trait resulted in a heritability estimate of 47% (Clifford *et al.* 1984).

Although the pattern of inheritance in OCD does not appear to be straightforward, molecular studies may provide valuable clues as to the contribution of genetic factors in the disorder (Cavallini *et al.* 2000). Prompted by the accumulating body of research pointing to the importance of the 5-HT transporter in this disorder, mutation screening of the gene coding region in two samples of patients with OCD detected no variants associated with the disorder (Altemus *et al.* 1996; Di Bella *et al.* 1996). Analysis of allele frequencies of the 5-HT transporter gene promoter polymorphism (5-HTTLPR) in 72 patients with OCD and 72 matched controls failed to detect a significant difference between the two groups; however, patients tended to be homozygous more often than controls (Billett *et al.* 1997). This trend became significant in a smaller sample, which consisted of the subset of controls who had Structured Clinical Interview for DSM-IV (SCID) diagnostic interviews. In this analysis, patients were more likely to be homozygous than controls. If this trend is indeed representative of an actual genetic difference in OCD patients, it may point to genetic heterogeneity of OCD. The possibility that OCD patients are homozygous more often than controls is noteworthy, given the finding that the long 5-HTTLPR allele leads to higher 5-HT transporter expression compared to the short allele. Since homozygotes have only one version of the allele they would maintain either high or low levels of transporter expression. The presence of both alleles may provide 5-HT system-dependent neuronal communication with more adaptability and therefore moderate levels of expression that result from having both allelic variants may be protective against OCD. In line with this thinking, two more recent studies, one using a family-based design, revealed an increased prevalence of homozygosity for the long variant in OCD patients (McDougle *et al.* 1998; Bengel *et al.* 1999).

Other population-based studies including the genes for 5-HT2A receptor, dopamine D2, D3, D4 receptor, dopamine transporter, catechol-*O*-methyltransferase (COMT), and MAOA have had variable, but generally negative results (Billett *et al.* 1998; Ohara *et al.* 1998; Rowe *et al.* 1998; Karayiorgou *et al.* 1999). Interpretation of these studies is complicated by their use of relatively small samples, which greatly increases the risk of type II error, of heterogeneous subject populations, and the lack of within-family designs to control for population stratification artifacts.

235

Mouse models

Quantitative genetic research on animal models consists primarily of inbred strain and selection studies. While comparisons between different inbred strains of mice expose remarkable differences in measures of anxiety-related behavior, such as performance in the Open Field or Elevated Plus Maze paradigm, differences within strains can be attributed to environmental influences. Inbred and recombinant inbred strain studies are highly efficient in dissecting genetic influences, for investigating interactions between genotype and environment, and for testing the disposition–stress model.

Selective breeding of mice for many generations produces difference between high- and low-anxiety lines that steadily increase each generation. Selection studies of behavioral traits strongly suggest a genetic influence and that many genes contribute to variation in behavior. Mice strains that have been selectively bred to display a phenotype of interest are currently being used to identify genetic loci that contribute to behavioral traits. The QTL approach has been applied with some success to a trait in mice called "emotionality" (Flint *et al.* 1995). Crosses between the high- and low-activity selected mouse lines yielded three QTL regions that appear to be related to various measures of fearfulness. A modified QTL strategy that uses recombinant inbred mouse strains produced candidate QTLs for Open Field fearfulness (Phillips *et al.* 1995).

However, such linkage analyses provide only a rough chromosomal localization, whereas the next step, identifying the relevant genes by positional cloning, remains a challenging task (Tecott & Barondes 1996). Since mice and humans share many orthologous genes mapped to syntenic chromosomal regions, it is conceivable that individual genes identified for one or more types of murine anxiety-related behavior may be developed as animal models for human anxiety. Following chromosomal mapping of polymorphic genes and evaluation of gene function using knockout mutants, behavioral parameters, including the type of anxiety, measure of anxiety, test situation and opponent type are investigated. Thus, the combination of elaborate genetic and behavioral analyses results in the identification of many genes with effects on variation and development of murine anxiety-related behavior and, ultimately, mouse QTL research is likely to generate candidate QTL for human anxiety disorders.

Recent advances in gene targeting (constitutive or conditional knockout and knockin techniques) is increasingly impacting upon our understanding of the neurobiologic basis of anxiety-related behavior in mice (Lesch & Mössner 1999; Rudolph & Mohler 1999). However, the majority of neural substrates and circuitries that regulate emotional processes or cause anxiety disorders remain remarkably elusive. Among the reasons for the lack of progress are several conceptional deficiencies regarding the psychobiology of fear and anxiety, which make it difficult to develop and validate reliable models. The clinical presentation of anxiety disorders and the lack of consensus on clinical categories further complicates the development of mouse models for specific anxiety disorders. The dilemma that no single paradigm mimics the diagnostic entities or treatment response of anxiety disorders may reflect the inadequacy of classification rather than failure to develop valid mouse models.

Various approaches have been employed to study anxiety-related traits in mice and the majority postulate that aversive stimuli, such as novelty or potentially harmful environments, induce a central state of fear and defensive reactions which can be assessed and quantified through physiologic and behavioral paradigms (Crawley & Paylor 1997; Crawley 1999). While substantial similarities between human and murine avoidance, defense or escape response exist, it remains obscure whether mice also experience subjective anxiety and associated cognitive processes similar to humans or whether defense responses represent pathological forms of anxiety in humans. In general, pathological anxiety may reflect an inappropriate activation of normally adaptive, evolutionarily conserved defense reaction. It should therefore be practicable to elucidate both physiologic and pathologic anxiety by studying avoidant and defensive behavior in mice using a broad range of anxiety models to ensure comprehensive characterization of the behavioral phenotype.

The design of a mouse model partially or completely lacking a gene of interest during all stages of development (constitutive knockout) is among the prime strategies directed at elucidating the role of genetic factors in fear and anxiety. Following the landmark studies by Mohler and coworkers (Crestani *et al.* 1999) who generated mice lacking the γ_2 subunit of the GABA-A receptor, a notable body of evidence has been accumulated that GABA-A function is compromised in anxiety disorders (for review see Nutt & Malizia 2001, in press). Heterozygous GABA-A γ_2 subunit knockout mice are less sensitive to benzodiazepines, display hypervigilance and anxiety, and show decreases in ligand binding throughout the brain. These mice may represent a genetically defined model of trait anxiety that closely mimics pharmacological, morphological, and behavioral phenotype of human anxiety disorders (Crestani *et al.* 1999). Various other types of GABA-A subunits, including α_1, α_2, α_3, and β_3, have been genetically altered in mice by introducing a defined mutation (constitutive knockin) (Rudolph *et al.* 1999; Low *et al.* 2000). While mice with a mutated α_1 subtype gene are insensitive to the sedative actions of benzodiazepines but still responsive to GABA, the anxiolytic effect is lost if the α_2 but not the α_3 subtype is modified. The localization of the α_2 subtype in the limbic system further supports a role of this neurocircuit in anxiety (Nutt & Malizia 2001).

A possible role for the 5-HT1A receptor in the modulation of anxiety (and depression) as well as in the mode of action of anxiolytic and antidepressant drugs has been suspected for many years. 5-HT1A receptors operate both as somatodendritic autoreceptors and as postsynaptic receptors. Somatodendritic 5-HT1A autoreceptors are predominantly located on 5-HT neurones and dendrites in the midbrain raphe complex, and their activation by 5-HT or 5-HT1A agonists decreases the firing rate of serotonergic neurones and subsequently reduces the release of 5-HT from nerve terminals (Fig. 13.2). Postsynaptic 5-HT1A receptors are widely distributed in forebrain regions that receive serotonergic input, notably in the cortex, hippocampus, and hypothalamus. Their activation results in neuronal inhibition, the consequences of which are not well understood, and in physiological responses that depend upon the function of the target cells (e.g. activation of the

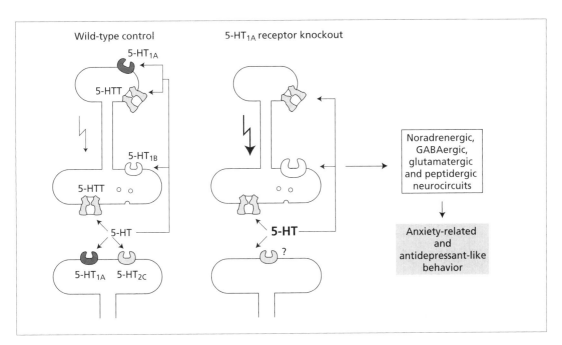

Fig. 13.2 Hypothetical mechanism of physiological and behavioral consequences of targeted inactivation of the 5-HT1A receptor gene in mice. Anxiety-related and antidepressant-like behavior in 5-HT1A receptor knockout mice may represent a consequence of increased terminal 5-HT availability resulting from the lack or reduction in presynaptic somatodendritic 5-HT1A autoreceptor negative feedback function. Indirect evidence for increased presynaptic serotonergic activity is provided by the compensatory up-regulation of terminal 5-HT1B receptors. While increased 5-HT availability and activation of other serotonergic receptor subtypes that have been shown to mediate anxiety (e.g. 5-HT2C receptor) may contribute to increased anxiety in rodent model, multiple downstream neurotransmitter pathways or neurocircuits, including noradrenergic, GABAergic, glutamatergic, and peptidergic transmission, are likely to participate in the processing of this complex behavioral trait.

Table 13.1 Behavioral phenotype of 5-HT1A knockout mice.

	Genetic background	Anxiety-related behavior[a]	Antidepressant-like behavior[b]	Locomotor activity	Motor coordination[c]
Parks et al. (1998)	129Sv into Swiss-Webster	OF: ↑↑m, ↑f	FS: ↑↑	↑f	–
Ramboz et al. (1998)	129Sv	OF: ↑↑m, ↑f EPM: ↑	FS: ↑	–	nd
Heisler et al. (1998)	129Sv into C57BL/63 J	OF: ↑ (+/– < –/–) EZM: ↑ NO: ↑↑ (+/– < –/–)	TS: ↑↑ (+/– < –/–)	–	–

[a] OF, Open Field; EZM, Elevated Zero Maze; EPM, Elevated Plus Maze; NO, Novel Objects. [b] FS, Forced Swim; TS, Tail Suspension. [c] Rotorod. f, female; m, male; –, no change; nd, not done; +/– < –/–, gene/dose-effect

hypothalamic pituitary adrenocortical system). At the end of 1998 a series of three papers reported the generation of mice with a targeted inactivation of the 5-HT1A receptor (Heisler et al. 1998; Parks et al. 1998; Ramboz et al. 1998). Functional 5-HT1A receptor knockout was confirmed by a complete lack of 5-HT1A receptor binding in brain of null-mutant mice, with intermediate binding in heterozygote mice.

Mice with a targeted inactivation of the 5-HT1A receptor consistently display a spontaneous phenotype that is associated with a gender-modulated and gene/dose-dependent increase of anxiety-related behaviors (Table 13.1). With the exception of an enhanced sensitivity of terminal 5-HT1B receptors and down-regulation of GABA-A receptors (Sibille et al. 2000), no major neuroadaptational changes were detected. Noteworthy is that this behavioral phenotype was observed in animals in which the mutation was bred into mice of Swiss-Webster, C57BL/6 J and 129/Sv backgrounds, solidly substantiating the assumption that this behavior is an authentic consequence of reduced or absent 5-HT1A receptors. While all research groups used Open Field exploratory behavior as a model for assessing anxiety, two groups confirmed that 5-HT1A knockout mice had increased anxiety by using other models, the Elevated Zero Maze or Elevated Plus Maze test. These ethologically based conflict models test fear and anxiety-related behaviors based on the natural tendencies for rodents to prefer enclosed, dark spaces versus their interest in exploring novel environments.

Activation of presynaptic 5-HT1A receptors provide the brain with an autoinhibitory feedback system controlling 5-HT neurotransmission. Thus, enhanced anxiety-related behavior most likely represents a consequence of increased terminal 5-HT availability resulting from the lack or reduction in presynaptic somatodendritic 5-HT1A autoreceptor negative feedback function. Indirect evidence for increased presynaptic serotonergic activity is provided by the compensatory up-regulation of terminal 5-HT1B receptors. This mechanism is also consistent with recent theoretical models of fear and anxiety that are primarily based upon pharmacologically derived data. The cumulative reduction in serotonergic impulse flow to septohippocampal and other limbic and cortical areas involved in the control of anxiety is believed to explain the anxiolytic effects of ligands with selective affinity for the 5-HT1A receptor in some animal models of anxiety-related behavior. This notion is based, in part, on evidence that 5-HT1A agonists (e.g. 8-OH-DPAT [8-hydroxy-2-(di-n-propylamino)tetralin]) and antagonists (e.g. WAY 100635) have anxiolytic or anxiogenic effects, respectively. However, to complicate matters further, 8-OH-DPAT has anxiolytic effects when injected in the raphe nucleus, whereas it is anxiogenic when applied to the hippocampus. Thus, stimulation of postsynaptic 5-HT1A receptors has been proposed to elicit anxiogenic effects, while activation of 5-HT1A autoreceptors is thought to induce anxiolytic effects via suppression of serotonergic neuronal firing resulting in attenuated 5-HT release in limbic terminal fields.

Excess serotonergic neurotransmission may also be implicated in increased anxiety-related behaviors recently found in 5-HT tranporter-deficient mice (Wichems *et al.* 2000). These findings are consistent with other evidence suggesting that increased 5-HT availability may contribute to increased anxiety in rodents, and the studies reporting that anxiety-related traits in humans are associated with allelic variation of 5-HT transporter function (Lesch *et al.* 1996). Mice with a disrupted 5-HT transporter gene have been suggested as an alternative model to pharmacological studies of selective serotonin reuptake inhibitor (SSRI)-evoked antidepressant and anxiolytic mechanisms to assess the hypothesized association between 5-HT uptake function and 5-HT1A receptor desensitization (Bengel *et al.* 1998). Excess serotonergic neurotransmission in mice lacking 5-HT transport results in desensitized and, unlike observations following SSRI administration, down-regulated 5-HT1A receptors in the mid-brain raphe complex but not in the hippocampus (Li *et al.* 2000), and is suspected to play a role in the increased anxiety-related and antidepressant-like behaviors in these mice using the Light-Dark and Elevated Zero Maze paradigms, and Tail Suspension paradigms. In contrast to 5-HT1A-deficient mice, anxiety-related behavior that can be reversed by anxiolytics of the diazepam type is more pronounced in female 5-HT transporter null mutants.

Morphological analyses of cortical and subcortical structures where 5-HT has been suggested to act as a differentiation signal in cortical development revealed an impact of 5-HT transporter inactivation on the formation and plasticity of brain structures. Inactivation of the 5-HT transporter gene profoundly disturbs formation of the somatosensory cortex (SSC) with altered cytoarchitecture of cortical layer IV, the layer that contains synapses between thalamocortical terminals and their postsynaptic target neurones (Persico *et al.* 1999). These findings demonstrate that excessive amounts of extracellular 5-HT are detrimental to SSC development and suggest that transient 5-HT transporter expression in thalamocortical neurones is responsible for barrel patterns in neonatal rodents, and its permissive action is required for barrel pattern formation, presumably by maintaining extracellular 5-HT concentrations below a critical threshold (Salichon *et al.* 2001). Since the gene-dose dependent reduction

in 5-HT transporter availability in heterozygous mice, that leads to a modest delay in 5-HT uptake but distinctive irregularities in barrel and septum shape, is similar to those reported in humans carrying low activity allele of the 5-HTTLPR, it may be speculated that allelic variation in 5-HT transporter function also affects the human brain during development with due consequences for personality, disease liability, and therapeutic response. Preliminary data suggest that other sensory cortices such as the visual system (Upton *et al.* 2001) as well as in hippocampal neurogenesis (A. Schmitt & K.P. Lesch, pers. comm.) are altered in 5-HT transporter knockout mice. In line with these findings, it has recently been shown that electrical substrates of the execution and the inhibition of motor response elicited by the Continuous Performance (CPT) Task test is associated with the 5-HTTLPR genotype in healthy subjects, thus indicating a role of 5-HT transporter function in neurophysiologically assessed topography of inhibitory motor control located in human prefrontal cortex (Fallgatter *et al.* 1999).

The evidence that changes in 5-HT system homeostasis exerts long-term effects on cortical development and adult brain plasticity may be an important step forward in establishing the psychobiological groundwork for a neurodevelopmental hypothesis of neuroticism, negative emotionality, and anxiety disorders. Although there is converging evidence that serotonergic dysfunction contributes to anxiety-related behavior, the precise mechanism that renders 5-HT1A receptor and 5-HT transporter-deficient mice more anxious remains to be elucidated. While increased 5-HT availability and activation of other serotonergic receptor subtypes that have been shown to mediate anxiety (e.g. 5-HT2C receptor) may contribute to increased anxiety in rodent model, multiple downstream cellular pathways or neurocircuits, including noradrenergic, GABAergic, glutamatergic, and peptidergic transmission, as suggested by overexpression or targeted inactivation of critical genes within these systems, have been implicated to participate in the processing of this complex behavioral trait. Recent work has therefore been focused on a large number of genes that have known relevance in the neurocircuitries of fear and anxiety, although the knockout of some genes that appear to not be directly involved in anxiety may also lead to an anxiety related phenotype (Table 13.2).

Table 13.2 Knockout mice displaying an anxiety-related phenotype and behavior.

Knockout	Effect of anxiety-related behavior	Additional behavioral phenotypes, special features	Author
GABA			
GABA-A receptor subunit γ₂	↑	Synaptic clustering of GABA-A	Crestani *et al.* (1999)
GAD65	↑	Aggression ↓, depression ↓	Kash *et al.* (1999) Stork *et al.* (2000)
Serotonin (5-HT)			
5-HT receptor 1 A	↑	Consistent in different	Heisler *et al.* (1998)
	–	genetic backgrounds	Ramboz *et al.* (1998)
	–	(Table 13.1)	Parks *et al.* (1998) Sibille *et al.* (2000)
5-HT receptor 1B	↓	Aggression ↑ GABA-A receptor ↓	Brunner *et al.* (1999)
5-HT receptor 2C	↑	Hyperphagia/weight gain Spatial learning ↓	Tecott & Barondes (1996)
5-HT transporter	↑	Depression ↓	Wichems *et al.* (2000)
MAOA	↓	Aggression ↑	Cases *et al.* (1995)
Catecholamines			
Dopamine receptor D3	↓		Steiner *et al.* (1997)
Dopamine receptor D4	↑ (Small)	Exploration ↓	Dulawa *et al.* (1999)
COMT	↓	Aggression ↑	Gogos *et al.* (1998)
Adenosine			
Receptor A2a	↑	Aggression ↑	Ledent *et al.* (1997)
Opioid			
δ	↑	Depression ↑	Filliol *et al.* (2000)
μ	↓	Depression ↓	
Nociceptin	↑	Stress response ↑	Koster *et al.* (1999)
Signal transduction			
AC VIII	↑		Schaefer *et al.* (2000)
CamKII	↓	Offensive aggression ↑	Chen *et al.* (1994)
CREM	↓		Maldonado *et al.* (1999)
Stress system			
CRH1 receptor	↓	Stress response ↓	Timpl *et al.* (1998) Contarino *et al.* (1999)
CRH2 receptor	↑	Stress response ↑	Bale *et al.* (2000) Kishomoto *et al.* (2000)
Glucocorticoid receptor	↓	Stress response ↓	Tronche *et al.* (1999)

(Continued)

Table 13.2 (cont'd)

Knockout	Effect of anxiety-related behavior	Additional behavioral phenotypes, special features	Author
Miscellaneous			
Neuropeptide Y	↑	Food intake ↓	Bannon *et al.* (2000)
Interferon-γ	↑		Kustova *et al.* (1998)
Midkine	↑		Nakamura *et al.* (1998)
Neurokinine 1 receptor	↑	Serotonergic function ↑	Santarelli *et al.* (2001)
ApoE	↑		Raber *et al.* (2000)
NCAM	↑	5-HT1A receptor ↑	Stork *et al.* (1999)
FMR1	↓		Peier *et al.* (2000)

↑/↓, increase/decrease in anxiety-related behavior; AC VIII, adenylyl cyclase type VIII; ApoE, apolipoprotein E; CamKII, calcium–calmodulin kinase II; COMT, catechol-O-methyltransferase; CREM, cAMP-responsive element modulator; CRH corticotropin- releasing hormone; FMR1, fragile X syndrome gene; GABA, γ-amino butyric acid; GAD65, 65-kDa isoform of glutamic acid decarboxylase; MAOA, monoamine oxidase A; NCAM, neural cell adhesion molecule.

Towards resolution of gene–gene and gene–environment interactions

Although still in its infancy, investigation of gene–gene and gene–environment interactions in nonhuman primates and humans support the view that genetic factors influence brain development, neuroplasticity, and complex behavior. Despite evidence for a substantial contribution of the genetic "blueprint" to the formation of synaptic connections in the mammalian brain during development, adult life, and old age, detailed knowledge of the molecular mechanisms involved in these fine-tuning processes is only beginning to accumulate. Integration of advanced strategies of complex genetic analysis with behavioral traits such as anxiety-related phenotypes, and techniques that alter or inactivate gene expression, will eventually elucidate the role of the genetics in development of complex behavioral traits and anxiety disorders.

The resolution of epistatic gene–gene interaction in the development of personality and behavior is among the last frontiers of genetic research. In the evaluation of complex genetic effects it seems to be essential to control for environmental factors. Recent studies have therefore focused on the neonatal period, a time in early development when environmental influences are minimal and least likely to confound associations between temperament and genes. In this context the term temperament is used to refer to the psychological qualities of infants that display considerable variation and have a relatively, but not indefinitely, stable biological basis in the individual's genotype, even though different phenotypes may emerge as the child grows (Kagan *et al.* 1988; Kagan 1989).

Ebstein *et al.* (1998) investigated the behavioral effects of variable number of tandem repeats (VNTR) polymorphism in exon 3 of the dopamine D4 receptor (D4DR), which had previously been linked to the personality trait of novelty seeking, and the 5-HTTLPR, which seems to influence negative emotionality and anxiety, in 2-week-old neonates ($N = 81$). In addition to a significant association of the D4DR polymorphism across four behavioral clusters relevant to temperament including orientation, motor organization, range of state and regulation of state, an interaction was also observed between the D4DR polymorphism and 5-HTTLPR. The presence of two short alleles of the 5-HTTLPR decreased the orientation score for the group of neonates lacking the long variant of D4DR. The D4DR polymorphism–5-HTTLPR interaction was also assessed in a sample of adult subjects. Interestingly, there was no significant effect of long allele of D4DR (6–8 repeats) in those subjects homozygous for the 5-HTTLPR s form when they were grouped by the 5-HTTLPR, whereas in the group without the homozygous genotype the effect of long D4DR variant was significant and represented 13% of the variance in novelty seeking scores between groups. Temperament and behavior of these infants were reexamined at 2 months using Rothbart's Infant Behavior Questionnaire (IBQ) (Auerbach *et al.* 1999). There were significant negative correlations between neonatal orientation and motor organization as measured by the Neonatal Behavioral Assessment Scale (NBAS) at 2 weeks and negative emotionality, especially distress in daily situations, at 2 months of age. Furthermore, grouping of the infants by D4DR polymorphism and 5-HTTLPR revealed significant main effects for negative emotionality and distress. Infants with long D4DR alleles had lower scores on Negative Emotionality and Distress to Limitations than infants with short D4DR alleles. In contrast, infants homozygous for the 5-HTTLPR's allele had higher scores on Negative Emotionality and Distress than infants with the l/s or l/l genotypes. Infants with the s/s genotype who also were lacking the novelty seeking-associated long D4DR alleles showed most negative emotionality and distress, temperament traits that possibly contribute to the predisposition for adult negative emotionality and anxiety.

The relationship between emotional reactions to stress (emotionality) and psychiatric disorders is also central to the disposition–stress model of syndromal dimensions of affective spectrum disorders, such as anxiety and depression, in which the expression of genetic vulnerability is triggered by stress (Eley and Plomin 1997; Paris 1998; Ramos & Mormede 1998). In line with this notion, a twin study suggests that genetic liability to depression interacts with the presence of stressful life events in producing the outcome of depression (Kendler *et al.* 1995a). Additional, although preliminary, evidence comes from studies of rhesus macaques, a higher nonhuman primate species that, like humans, carries the 5-HT transporter gene-associated polymorphism (rh5-HTTLPR).

Previous work in rhesus monkeys has shown that early adverse experiences have long-term consequences for the functioning of the central 5-HT system, as indicated by robustly altered cerebrospinal fluid (CSF) 5HIAA levels as well as anxiety and depression-related behavior, in monkeys deprived of their parents at birth and raised only with peers (Higley *et al.* 1991; Higley *et al.* 1992). Accumulating evidence demonstrates the complex interplay between individual differences in the central 5-HT system and social success. In monkeys, lowered 5-HT functioning, as indicated by decreased CSF 5HIAA levels, is associated with lower rank within a social group, less competent social behavior, and greater impulsive aggression. Association between central 5-HT turnover and rh5-HTTLPR genotype was tested in rhesus monkeys with well-characterized environmental histories (Bennett *et al.* 2001). The monkeys' rearing fell into one of the following categories: mother-reared, either reared with the biological mother or cross-fostered; or peer-reared, either with a peer group of 3–4 monkeys or with an inanimate surrogate and daily contact with a playgroup of peers. Peer-reared monkeys were separated from their mothers, placed in the nursery at birth, and given access to peers at 30 days of age either continuously or during daily play sessions. Mother-reared and cross-fostered monkeys remained with the mother, typically within a social group. At roughly 7 months of age, mother-reared monkeys were weaned and placed together with their peer-reared cohort in large, mixed-gender social groups.

Since the monkey population comprised two groups that received dramatically different social and rearing experience early in life, the interactive effects of environmental experience and the rh5-HTTLPR on cisternal CSF 5HIAA levels and 5-HT-related behavior was assessed. CSF 5HIAA concentrations were significantly influenced by genotype for peer-reared, but not for mother-reared subjects. Peer-reared rhesus monkeys with the low-activity rh5-HTTLPR s allele had significantly lower concentrations of CSF 5HIAA than their homozygous l/l counterparts Low 5-HT turnover in monkeys with the s allele is congruent with *in vitro* studies that show reduced binding and transcriptional efficiency of the 5-HT tranporter gene associated with the short 5-HTTLPR allele (Lesch *et al.* 1996). This suggests that the rh5-HTTLPR genotype is predictive of CSF 5HIAA concentrations, but that early experiences make unique contributions to variation in later 5-HT functioning. This finding is the first to provide evidence of an environment–dependent association between a polymorphism in the 5′-regulatory region of the 5-HT transporter gene and a direct measure of 5-HT functioning, cisternal CSF 5HIAA concentration, thus revealing an interaction between rearing environment and rhHTTLPR genotype. Similar to the 5-HTTLPR's influence on anxiety-related traits in humans, however, the effect size is small, with 4.7% of variance in CSF 5HIAA accounted for by the rh5-HTTLPR–rearing environment interaction.

As the scope of human studies has also been extended to the neonatal period, a time in early development when environmental influences are modest and least likely to confound gene–temperament associations, complementary approaches have recently been applied to nonhuman primate behavioral genetics to facilitate investigation of the contribution of genotype and early rearing environment to the development of behavioral traits. Rhesus macaque infants heterozygous for the short and long variant of the rhHTTLPR displayed higher behavioral stress-reactivity compared to infants homozygous for the long variant of the allele (Champoux *et al.* 1999). Mother-reared and peer-reared monkeys were assessed on days 7, 14, 21, and 30 of life, on a standardized primate neurobehavioral test designed to measure orienting, motor maturity, reflex functioning, and temperament. The main effects of genotype and, in some cases, interactions between rearing condition and genotype, were demonstrated for items indicative of orienting, attention, and temperament. In general, heterozygote animals demonstrated diminished orientation, lower attentional capabilities, and increased affective responding relative to l/l homozygotes. However, the genotype effects were more pronounced for animals raised in the neonatal nursery than for animals reared by their mothers. These results demonstrate the contributions of rearing environment and genetic background, and their interaction, in a nonhuman primate model of behavioral development.

Taken together, these findings provide evidence of an environment–dependent association between allelic variation of 5-HT transporter expression and central 5-HT function, and illustrate the possibility that specific genetic factors play in social competence and related traits. The objective of further studies will be the elucidation of the relationship between the genotypes and sociality in monkeys as this behavior is expressed with characteristic individual differences both in daily life and in response to challenge. Because rhesus monkeys exhibit temperamental and behavioral traits that parallel anxiety, depression, and aggression-related personality dimensions associated in humans with the low-actitvity 5-HTTLPR variant, it may be possible to search for evolutionary continuity in this genetic mechanism for individual differences.

The biobehavioral results of deleterious early experiences of social separation are consistent with the notion that the 5-HTTLPR may influence the risk for affective spectrum disorders. Evolutionary preservation of two prevalent 5-HTTLPR variants and the resulting allelic variation in 5-HT transporter expression may be part of the genetic mechanism resulting in the emergence of temperamental traits that facilitate adaptive functioning in the complex social worlds most primates inhabit. The uniqueness of the 5-HTTLPR among humans and simian nonhuman primates, but not among prosimians or other mammals, along with the role 5-HT plays in complex primate sociality, form the basis for the hypothesized relationship between the 5-HT transporter function and personality traits that mediate individual differences in social behavior. Nonhuman primate studies may therefore be useful to help identify environmental factors that either compound the vulnerability conferred by a particular genetic makeup or, conversely, act to improve the behavioral outcome associated with that genotype.

Outlook

Progress in behaviorial genetics will eventually be accelerated by closer integration of neuroscience and genetic approaches. Integration of emerging tools and technologies for genetic analysis will provide the groundwork for an advanced stage of gene identification and functional studies in anxiety and related disorders.

However, several conceptual refinements need to be adopted in behavioral and psychiatric genetics. First, to detect small gene effects, a dimensional, semiquantitative approach to behavioral phenotypes arising from psychometric research and standardized trait assessment is needed. Established are two parallel definitions of anxiety phenotypes: categorical diagnoses (i.e., PD, social phobia, etc.) and dimensional traits (e.g., anxious temperament, behavioral inhibition, negative emotionality). Given the limitation of the diagnostic approach, future studies will require extended, homogeneous, and ethnically matched samples. With recent advances in molecular genetics, the rate-limiting step in identifying susceptibility genes has become definition of phenotype or endophenotypes. Thus, investigation of genetic differences associated with variation along behavioral dimensions within diagnoses will be a useful complement to the traditional strategy of looking for genetic differences between categorically defined diagnostic entities.

Second, more functionally relevant polymorphisms in genes within a single neurotransmitter system, or in genes that comprise a functional unit in their concerted actions, need to be identified and assessed in both large population and family-based association studies to avoid stratification artifacts, and to elucidate complex epigenetic interactions of multiple loci. Further studies of the genetics of anxiety-related traits using refined linkage strategies, association techniques, and newer but well advanced methods such as single nucleotide polymorphism (SNP) analysis, will be especially useful in the characterization of the heritable components of anxiety disorders. Based on the first draft sequence of the human genome, more than 1.4 million SNPs in the human genome have been identified (Consortium 2001). Large-scale association studies that couple the genotyping of functional SNPs with linkage disequilibrium mapping in chromosomal regions implicated in linkage studies is an approach complementary to linkage analyses. Its success will depend on the availability of SNPs in the coding or regulatory regions of a large number of candidate genes, as well as knowledge of the average extent of linkage disequilibrium between SNPs, the development of high-throughput technologies for genotyping SNPs, identification of protein-altering SNPs by DNA, and protein microarray-assisted expression analysis, and collection of DNA from well-phenotyped patients.

Third, genetic influences are not the only pathway that lead to individual differences in personality dimensions, behavior, and psychopathology. Complex traits are most likely to be generated by a complex interaction of environmental and experiental factors with a number of genes and their products. Even pivotal regulatory proteins of cellular pathways and neurocircuits, will have a modest impact, while noise from nongenetic mechanisms obstructs identification of relevant gene variants. Although current methods for the detection of gene–environment interaction in behaviorial genetics are largely indirect, the most relevant consequence of gene identification for personality and behavioral traits may be that it will provide the tools required to systematically clarify the effects of gene–environment interaction.

Finally, future benefits will stem from the potential development of techniques involving molecular cell biology, transgenics, and gene transfer technology that could facilitate novel drug design. Paralleling the resolution of gene–gene and gene–environment interactions

and the fading dogma that neurones are highly vulnerable and their capacity for regeneration, reproducibility, and plasticity is limited, it is being realized that gene transfer strategies may eventually be applicable to genetic factors associated with complex disorders. While targeting gene regulation or gene transfer approaches are quite appealing, no presently available technique meets the rigorous requirements obligatory for human trials, but the technical prerequisites are being developed at an incredible pace, thus raising hopes for a beneficial application of these treatment strategies in some forms of chronic and treatment-resistant anxiety disorders.

Summary

Genetic epidemiology has assembled convincing evidence that anxiety and related disorders are influenced by genetic factors and that the genetic component is highly complex, polygenic, and epistatic. Although several genes that may contribute to the genetic variance of anxiety-related traits, or may modify the phenotypic expression of pathologic anxiety are currently under investigation, molecular genetics has so far failed to identify a genomic variation that can consistently contribute susceptibility of anxiety disorders. Investigation of gene–gene and gene–environment interactions in humans and nonhuman primates as well as gene inactivation studies in mice further intensify the identification of genes that are essential for development and adult plasticity of the brain related to complex anxiety responses. Because the modes of inheritance of anxiety disorders are complex, it has been concluded that multiple genes of modest effect, in interaction with each other and in conjunction with nongenetic neurodevelopmental events, produce vulnerability to the disorder. Future research strategies will take advantage of the completion of the sequencing of the human and mouse genome coinciding with the revolution in bioinformatics. More than 1.4 million SNPs in the human genome have been identified. This collection should allow the initiation of genome-wide linkage disequilibrium mapping of the genes influencing anxiety in the human population. Integration of these emerging tools and technologies for genetic analysis will provide the groundwork for an advanced stage of gene identification and functional studies in anxiety and related disorders.

References

Alsobrook, I.J., Leckman, J.F., Goodman, W.K., Rasmussen, S.A. & Pauls, D.L. (1999) Segregation analysis of obsessive-compulsive disorder using symptom-based factor scores. *Am J Med Genet* **88**, 669–75.

Altemus, M., Murphy, D.L., Greenberg, B. & Lesch, K.P. (1996) Intact coding region of the serotonin transporter in obsessive-compulsive disorder. *Am J Med Genet* **67**, 104–9.

Andrews, G., Stewart, G., Allen, R. & Henderson, A.S. (1990) The genetics of six neurotic disorders: a twin study. *J Affect Disord* **19**, 23–9.

Auerbach, J., Geller, V., Lezer, S. *et al.* (1999) Dopamine D4 receptor (D4DR) and serotonin transporter promoter (5-HTTLPR) polymorphisms in the determination of temperament in 2-month-old infants. *Mol Psychiatry* **4**, 369–73.

Bale, T.L., Contarino, A., Smith, G.W. *et al.* (2000) Mice deficient for corticotropin-releasing hormone receptor-2 display anxiety-like behavior and are hypersensitive to stress. *Nat Genet* **24**, 410–14.

Balon, R., Jordan, M., Pohl, R. & Yeragani, V.K. (1989) Family history of anxiety disorders in control subjects with lactate-induced panic attacks. *Am J Psychiatry* **146**, 1304–6.

Bannon, A.W., Seda, J., Carmouche, M. *et al.* (2000) Behavioral characterization of neuropeptide Y Knockout mice. *Brain Res* **868**(1), 79–87.

Battaglia, M., Bertella, S., Politi, E. *et al.* (1995) Age at onset of panic disorder: influence of familial liability to the disease and of childhood separation anxiety disorder. *Am J Psychiatry* **152**, 1362–4.

Baumeister, R.F. & Tice, D.M. (1990) Anxiety and social exclusion. *J Clin Psychol* **9**, 165–95.

Bebbington, P.E. (1998) Epidemiology of obsessive-compulsive disorder. *Br J Psychiatry Suppl* **35**, 2–6.

Bellodi, L., Sciuto, G., Diaferia, G., Ronchi, P. & Smeraldi, E. (1992) Psychiatric disorders in the families of patients with obsessive-compulsive disorder. *Psychiatry Res* **42**, 111–20.

Bengel, D., Greenberg, B., Cora-Locatelli, G. *et al.* (1999) Association of the serotonin transporter promoter regulatory region polymorphism and obsessive-compulsive disorder. *Mol Psychiatry* **4**, 463–6.

Bengel, D., Murphy, D.L., Andrews, A.M. *et al.* (1998) Altered brain serotonin homeostasis and locomotor insensitivity to 3,4-methylenedioxymethamphetamine ("Ecstasy") in serotonin transporter-deficient mice. *Mol Pharmacol* **53**, 649–55.

Bennett, A.J., Lesch, K.P., Heils, A. *et al.* (2001) Early experience and serotonin transporter gene variation interact to influence primate CNS function. *Mol Psychiatry* **7**, 118–22.

Billett, E.A., Richter, M.A., King, N., Heils, A., Lesch, K.P. & Kennedy, J.L. (1997) Obsessive-compulsive disorder: response to serotonin reuptake inhibitors and the serotonin transporter gene. *Mol Psychiatry* **2**, 403–6.

Billett, E.A., Richter, M.A., Sam, F. *et al.* (1998) Investigation of dopamine system genes in obsessive-compulsive disorder. *Psychiatr Genet* **8**, 163–9.

Black, D.W., Noyes, R. Jr, Goldstein, R.B. & Blum, N. (1992) A family study of obsessive-compulsive disorder. *Arch Gen Psychiatry* **49**, 362–8.

Bonney, G.E. (1986) Regressive logistic models for familial disease and other binary traits. *Biometrics* **42**, 611–25.

Bouchard, T.J. (1994) Genes, environment and personality. *Science* **264**, 1700–1.

Bradwejn, J. & Koszycki, D. (1991) Comparison of the panicogenic effect of cholecystokinin 30–33 and carbon dioxide in panic disorder. *Prog Neuropsychopharmacol Biol Psychiatry* **15**, 237–9.

Brown, T.A. (1997) The nature of generalized anxiety disorder and pathological worry: current evidence and conceptual models. *Can J Psychiatry* **42**, 817–25.

Brunner, D., Buhot, M.C., Hen, R. & Hofer, M. (1999) Anxiety, motor activation, and maternal–infant interactions in 5-HT1B knockout mice. *Behav Neurosci* **113**, 587–601.

Buss, D.M. (1991) Evolutionary personality psychology. *Annu Rev Psychol* **42**, 459–91.

Cases, O., Seif, I., Grimsby, J. *et al.* (1995) Aggressive behavior and altered amounts of brain serotonin and norepinephrine in mice lacking MAOA [see comments]. *Science* **268**, 1763–6.

Cavallini, M.C., Bertelli, S., Chiapparino, D., Riboldi, S. & Bellodi, L. (2000) Complex segregation analysis of obsessive-compulsive disorder in 141 families of eating disorder probands, with and without obsessive-compulsive disorder. *Am J Med Genet* **96**, 384–91.

Champoux, M., Bennett, A., Lesch, K.P. *et al.* (1999) Serotonin transporter gene polymorphism and neurobehavioral development in rhesus monkey neonates. *Soc Neurosci Abstr* **25**, 69.

Charney, D.S. & Deutch, A. (1996) A functional neuroanatomy of anxiety and fear: implications for the pathophysiology and treatment of anxiety disorders. *Crit Rev Neurobiol* **10**, 419–46.

Chen, C., Rainnie, D.G., Greene, R.W. & Tonegawa, S. (1994) Abnormal fear response and aggressive behavior in mutant mice deficient for alpha-calcium-calmodulin kinase II. *Science* **266**, 291–4.

Clifford, C.A., Murray, R.M. & Fulker, D.W. (1984) Genetic and environmental influences on obsessional traits and symptoms. *Psychol Med* **14**, 791–800.

Collier, D.A., Stöber, G., Li, T. *et al.* (1996) A novel functional polymorphism within the promoter of the serotonin transporter gene: possible role in susceptibility to affective disorders. *Mol Psychiatry* **1**, 453–60.

Consortium, I.H.G.S. (2001) Initial sequencing and analysis of the human genome. *Nature* **409**, 860–921.

Contarino, A., Dellu, F., Koob, G.F. *et al.* (1999) Reduced anxiety-like and cognitive performance in mice lacking the corticotropin-releasing factor receptor 1. *Brain Res* **835**, 1–9.

Crawford, F., Hoyne, J., Diaz, P. *et al.* (1995) Occurrence of the Cys311 DRD2 variant in a pedigree multiply affected with panic disorder. *Am J Med Genet* **60**, 332–4.

Crawley, J.N. (1999) Behavioral phenotyping of transgenic and knockout mice: experimental design and evaluation of general health, sensory functions, motor abilities, and specific behavioral tests. *Brain Res* **835**, 18–26.

Crawley, J.N. & Paylor, R. (1997) A proposed test battery and constellations of specific behavioral paradigms to investigate the behavioral phenotypes of transgenic and knockout mice. *Horm Behav* **31**, 197–211.

Crestani, F., Lorez, M., Baer, K. *et al.* (1999) Decreased GABAA-receptor clustering results in enhanced anxiety and a bias for threat cues. *Nat Neurosci* **2**, 833–9.

Crowe, R.R. (1990) Panic disorder: genetic considerations. *J Psychiatr Res* **24**, 129–34.

Crowe, R.R., Goedken, R., Samuelson, S., Wilson, R., Nelson, J. & Noyes, R.J. (2001) Genomewide survey of panic disorder. *Am J Med Genet* **105**, 105–9.

Crowe, R.R., Noyes, R. Jr, Samuelson, S., Wesner, R. & Wilson, R. (1990) Close linkage between panic disorder and alpha-haptoglobin excluded in 10 families. *Arch Gen Psychiatry* **47**, 377–80.

Crowe, R.R., Wang, Z., Noyes, R., Jr, *et al.* (1997) Candidate gene study of eight GABAA receptor subunits in panic disorder. *Am J Psychiatry* **154**, 1096–100.

Deckert, J., Catalano, M., Heils, A. *et al.* (1997) Functional promoter polymorphism of the human serotonin transporter: lack of association with panic disorder. *Psychiatr Genet* **7**, 45–7.

Deckert, J., Nothen, M.M., Franke, P. *et al.* (1998) Systematic mutation screening and association study of the A1 and A2a adenosine receptor genes in panic disorder suggest a contribution of the A2a gene to the development of disease. *Mol Psychiatry* **3**, 81–5.

Di Bella, D., Catalano, M., Balling, U., Smeraldi, E. & Lesch, K.P. (1996) Systematic screening for mutations in the coding region of the 5-HTT gene using PCR and DGGE. *Am J Med Genet* **67**, 541–5.

Dulawa, S.C., Grandy, D.K., Low, M.J., Paulus, M.P. & Geyer, M.A. (1999) Dopamine D4 receptor-knockout mice exhibit reduced exploration of novel stimuli. *J Neurosci* **19**, 9550–6.

Eaton, W.W., Kessler, R.C., Wittchen, H.U. & Magee, W.J. (1994) Panic and panic disorder in the United States. *Am J Psychiatry* **151**, 413–20.

Ebstein, R.P., Levine, J., Geller, V., Auerbach, J., Gritsenko, I. & Belmaker, R.H. (1998) Dopamine D4 receptor and serotonin transporter promoter in the determination of neonatal temperament. *Mol Psychiatry* **3**, 238–46.

Eley, T.C. & Plomin, R. (1997) Genetic analyses of emotionality. *Curr Opin Neurobiol* **7**, 279–84.

Eley, T.C. & Stevenson, J. (1999) Exploring the covariation between anxiety and depression symptoms: a genetic analysis of the effects of age and sex. *J Child Psychol Psychiatry* **40**, 1273–82.

Fallgatter, A., Jatzke, S., Bartsch, A., Hamelbeck, B. & Lesch, K. (1999) Serotonin transporter promoter polymorphism influences topography of inhibitory motor control. *Int J Neuropsychopharm* **2**, 115–20.

Filliol, D., Ghozland, S., Chluba, J. *et al.* (2000) Mice deficient for delta- and mu-opioid receptors exhibit opposing alterations of emotional responses. *Nat Genet* **25**, 195–200.

Flint, J., Corley, R., DeFries, J.C. *et al.* (1995) A simple genetic basis for a complex psychological trait in laboratory mice. *Science* **269**, 1432–5.

Gogos, J.A., Morgan, M., Luine, V. *et al.* (1998) Catechol-O-methyltransferase-deficient mice exhibit sexually dimorphic changes in catecholamine levels and behavior. *Proc Natl Acad Sci USA* **95**, 9991–6.

Goldstein, R.B., Wickramaratne, P.J., Horwath, E. & Weissman, M.M. (1997) Familial aggregation and phenomenology of "early"-onset (at or before age 20 years) panic disorder. *Arch Gen Psychiatry* **54**, 271–8.

Gorman, J.M., Kent, J.M., Sullivan, G.M. & Coplan, J.D. (2000) Neuroanatomical hypothesis of panic disorder, revised. *Am J Psychiatry* **157**, 493–505.

Greenberg, B.D., Li, Q., Lucas, F.R. *et al.* (2000) Association between the serotonin transporter promoter polymorphism and personality traits in a primarily female population sample. *Am J Med Genet* **96**, 202–16.

Hamilton, S.P., Haghighi, F., Heiman, G.A. *et al.* (2000) Investigation of dopamine receptor (DRD4) and dopamine transporter (DAT) polymorphisms for genetic linkage or association to panic disorder. *Am J Med Genet* **96**, 324–30.

Hamilton, S.P., Heiman, G.A., Haghighi, F. *et al.* (1999) Lack of genetic linkage or association between a functional serotonin transporter polymorphism and panic disorder. *Psychiatr Genet* **9**, 1–6.

Heisler, L.K., Chu, H.M., Brennan, T.J. *et al.* (1998) Elevated anxiety and antidepressant-like responses in serotonin 5-HT1A receptor mutant mice [see comments]. *Proc Natl Acad Sci USA* **95**, 15 049–54.

Higley, J.D., Suomi, S.J. & Linnoila, M. (1991) CSF monoamine metabolite concentrations vary according to age, rearing, and sex, and are influenced by the stressor of social separation in rhesus monkeys. *Psychopharmacology* **103**, 551–6.

Higley, J.D., Suomi, S.J. & Linnoila, M. (1992) A longitudinal assessment of CSF monoamine metabolite and plasma cortisol concentrations in young rhesus monkeys. *Biol Psychiatry* **32**, 127–45.

Hopper, J.L., Judd, F.K., Derrick, P.L. & Burrows, G.D. (1987) A family study of panic disorder. *Genet Epidemiol* **4**, 33–41.

Hopper, J.L., Judd, F.K., Derrick, P.L., Macaskill, G.T. & Burrows, G.D. (1990) A family study of panic disorder: reanalysis using a regressive logistic model that incorporates a sibship environment. *Genet Epidemiol* **7**, 151–61.

Iny, L.J., Pecknold, J., Suranyi-Cadotte, B.E. *et al.* (1994) Studies of a neurochemical link between depression, anxiety, and stress from (3H) imipramine (3H) paroxetine binding on human platelets. *Biol Psychiatry* **36**, 281–91.

Ishiguro, H., Arinami, T., Yamada, K., Otsuka, Y., Toru, M. & Shibuya, H. (1997) An association study between a transcriptional polymorphism in the serotonin transporter gene and panic disorder in a Japanese population. *Psychiatry Clin Neurosci* **51**, 333–5.

Kagan, J. (1989) Temperamental contributions to social behavior. *American Psychologist* **44**, 664–8.

Kagan, J., Reznick, J.S. & Snidman, N. (1988) Biological bases of childhood shyness. *Science* **240**, 167–71.

Kahn, R.S. & Wetzler, S. (1991) m-Chlorophenylpiperazine as a probe of serotonin function. *Biol Psychiatry* **30**, 1139–66.

Karayiorgou, M., Sobin, C., Blundell, M.L. *et al.* (1999) Family-based association studies support a sexually dimorphic effect of COMT and MAOA on genetic susceptibility to obsessive-compulsive disorder. *Biol Psychiatry* **45**, 1178–89.

Kash, S.F., Tecott, L.H., Hodge, C. & Baekkeskov, S. (1999) Increased anxiety and altered responses to anxiolytics in mice deficient in the 65-kDa isoform of glutamic acid decarboxylase. *Proc Natl Acad Sci USA* **96**, 1698–703.

Kato, T., Wang, Z.W., Zoega, T. & Crowe, R.R. (1996) Missense mutation of the cholecystokinin B receptor gene: lack of association with panic disorder. *Am J Med Genet* **67**, 401–5.

Kendler, K.S. (1996) Major depression and generalised anxiety disorder. Same genes, (partly) different environments—revisited. *Br J Psychiatry Suppl* **30**, 68–75.

Kendler, K.S., Karkowski, L.M. & Prescott, C.A. (1999) Fears and phobias: reliability and heritability. *Psychol Med* **29**, 539–53.

Kendler, K.S., Kessler, R.C., Neale, M.C., Heath, A.C. & Eaves, L.J. (1993a) The prediction of major depression in women: toward an integrated etiologic model. *Am J Psychiatry* **150**, 1139–48.

Kendler, K.S., Kessler, R.C., Walters, E.E. *et al.* (1995a) Stressful life events, genetic liability, and onset of an episode of major depression in women. *Am J Psychiatry* **152**, 833–42.

Kendler, K.S., Neale, M.C., Kessler, R.C., Heath, A.C. & Eaves, L.J. (1992a) Generalized anxiety disorder in women. A population-based twin study [see comments]. *Arch Gen Psychiatry* **49**, 267–72.

Kendler, K.S., Neale, M.C., Kessler, R.C., Heath, A.C. & Eaves, L.J. (1992b) Major depression and generalized anxiety disorder. Same genes, (partly) different environments? *Arch Gen Psychiatry* **49**, 716–22.

Kendler, K.S., Neale, M.C., Kessler, R.C., Heath, A.C. & Eaves, L.J. (1993b) A longitudinal twin study of personality and major depression in women. *Arch Gen Psychiatry* **50**, 853–62.

Kendler, K.S., Neale, M.C., Kessler, R.C., Heath, A.C. & Eaves, L.J. (1993c) Panic disorder in women: a population-based twin study [see comments]. *Psychol Med* **23**, 397–406.

Kendler, K.S., Walters, E.E., Neale, M.C., Kessler, R.C., Heath, A.C. & Eaves, L.J. (1995b) The structure of the genetic and environmental risk factors for six major psychiatric disorders in women. Phobia, generalized anxiety disorder, panic disorder, bulimia, major depression, and alcoholism. *Arch Gen Psychiatry* **52**, 374–83.

Kendler, K.S., Walters, E.E., Truett, K.R. *et al.* (1995c) A twin-family study of self-report symptoms of panic-phobia and somatization. *Behav Genet* **25**, 499–515.

Kennedy, J.L., Bradwejn, J., Koszycki, D. *et al.* (1999) Investigation of cholecystokinin system genes in panic disorder. *Mol Psychiatry* **4**, 284–5.

Kessler, R.C., McGonagle, K.A., Zhao, S. *et al.* (1994) Lifetime and 12-month prevalence of DSM-III-R psychiatric disorders in the United States. Results from the National Comorbidity Survey. *Arch Gen Psychiatry* **51**, 8–19.

Kishimoto, T., Radulovic, J., Radulovic, M. *et al.* (2000) Deletion of CRHR2 reveals an anxiolytic role for corticotropin-releasing hormone receptor-2. *Nat Genet* **24**, 415–19.

Knowles, J.A., Fyer, A.J., Vieland, V.J. *et al.* (1998) Results of a genome-wide genetic screen for panic disorder. *Am J Med Genet* **81**, 139–47.

Koster, A., Montkowski, A., Schulz, S. *et al.* (1999) Targeted disruption of the orphanin FQ/nociceptin gene increases stress susceptibility and impairs stress adaptation in mice. *Proc Natl Acad Sci USA* **96**, 10 444–9.

Kustova, Y., Sei, Y., Morse, H.C. & Basile, A.S. (1998) The influence of a targeted deletion of the IFNγ gene on emotional behaviors. *Brain Behav Immun* **12**, 308–24.

Ledent, C., Vaugeois, J.M., Schiffmann, S.N. *et al.* (1997) Aggressiveness, hypoalgesia and high blood pressure in mice lacking the adenosine A2a receptor [see comments]. *Nature* **388**, 674–8.

Lenane, M.C., Swedo, S.E., Leonard, H., Pauls, D.L., Sceery, W. & Rapoport, J.L. (1990) Psychiatric disorders in first degree relatives of children and adolescents with obsessive compulsive disorder. *J Am Acad Child Adolesc Psychiatry* **29**, 407–12.

Leonard, H.L., Lenane, M.C., Swedo, S.E., Rettew, D.C., Gershon, E.S. & Rapoport, J.L. (1992) Tics and Tourette's disorder: a 2- to 7-year follow-up of 54 obsessive-compulsive children. *Am J Psychiatry* **149**, 1244–51.

Lesch, K.P., Bengel, D., Heils, A. *et al.* (1996) Association of anxiety-related traits with a polymorphism in the serotonin transporter gene regulatory region. *Science* **274**, 1527–31.

Lesch, K.P., Greenberg, B.D., Bennett, A., Higley, J.D. & Murphy, D.L. (2002) Serotonin transporter, personality, and behavior: toward dissection of gene–gene and gene–environment interaction. In: *Molecular Genetics and the Human Personality* (J. Benjamin, R. Ebstein & R.H. Belmaker (eds)) American Psychiatric Press, Washington, D.C., 109–35.

Lesch, K.P. & Mössner, R. (1999) 5-HT1A receptor inactivation: anxiety or depression as a murine experience. *Int J Neuropsychopharmacology* **2**, 327–31.

Li, Q., Wichems, C., Heils, A., Lesch, K.P. & Murphy, D.L. (2000) Reduction in the density and expression, but not G-protein coupling, of serotonin receptors (5-HT1A) in 5-HT transporter knock-out mice: gender and brain region differences. *J Neurosci* **20**, 7888–95.

Livesley, W.J., Jang, K.L. & Vernon, P.A. (1998) Phenotypic and genetic structure of traits delineating personality disorder. *Arch Gen Psychiatry* **55**, 941–8.

Loehlin, J.C. (1992) *Genes and Environment in Personality Development*. Newburg Park, CA.

Low, K., Crestani, F., Keist, R. *et al.* (2000). Molecular and neuronal substrate for the selective attenuation of anxiety. *Science* **290**(5489), 131–4.

Lyons, M.J., Huppert, J., Toomey, R. *et al.* (2000) Lifetime prevalence of mood and anxiety disorders in twin pairs discordant for schizophrenia. *Twin Res* **3**, 28–32.

Maier, W., Minges, J. & Lichtermann, D. (1995) The familial relationship between panic disorder and unipolar depression. *J Psychiatr Res* **29**, 375–88.

Maldonado, R., Smadja, C., Mazzucchelli, C., Sassone-Corsi, P. & Mazucchelli, C. (1999) Altered emotional and locomotor responses in mice deficient in the transcription factor CREM. *Proc Natl Acad Sci USA* **96**, 14 094–9.

Martin, N.G., Jardine, R., Andrews, G. & Heath, A.C. (1988) Anxiety disorders and neuroticism: are there genetic factors specific to panic? *Acta Psychiatr Scand* **77**, 698–706.

Matsushita, S., Muramatsu, T., Kimura, M. *et al.* (1997) Serotonin transporter gene regulatory region polymorphism and panic disorder [letter]. *Mol Psychiatry* **2**, 390–2.

McDougle, C.J., Epperson, C.N., Price, L.H. & Gelernter, J. (1998) Evidence for linkage disequilibrium between serotonin transporter protein gene (SLC6A4) and obsessive-compulsive disorder. *Mol Psychiatry* **3**, 270–3.

McGue, M. & Bouchard, T.J. (1998) Genetic and environmental influences on human behavioral differences. *Annu Rev Neurosci* **21**, 1–24.

Moran, C. & Andrews, G. (1985) The familial occurrence of agoraphobia. *Br J Psychiatry* **146**, 262–7.

Mulder, R., Joyce, P. & Cloninger, C. (1994) Temperament and early environment influence comorbidity and personality disorders in major depression. *Compr Psychiatry* **35**, 225–33.

Mutchler, K., Crowe, R.R., Noyes, R., Jr & Wesner, R.W. (1990) Exclusion of the tyrosine hydroxylase gene in fourteen panic disorder pedigrees. *Am J Psychiatry* **147**, 1367–9.

Nakamura, E., Kadomatsu, K., Yuasa, S. *et al.* (1998) Disruption of the midkine gene (Mdk) resulted in altered expression of a calcium binding protein in the hippocampus of infant mice and their abnormal behavior. *Genes Cells* **3**, 811–22.

Nakamura, T., Muramatsu, T., Ono, Y. (1997) Serotonin transporter gene regulatory region polymorphism and anxiety-related traits in the Japanese. *Am J Med Genet* **74**, 544–5.

Ohara, K., Nagai, M., Suzuki, Y. & Ochiai, M. (1998) No association between anxiety disorders and catechol-O-methyltransferase polymorphism. *Psychiatry Res* **80**, 145–8.

Ono, Y., Yoshimura, K., Sueoka, R. *et al.* (1996) Avoidant personality disorder and taijin kyoufu: sociocultural implications of the WHO/ADAMHA international study of personality disorders in Japan. *Acta Psychiatr Scand* **93**, 172–6.

Paris, J. (1998) Anxious traits, anxious attachment, and anxious-cluster personality disorders. *Harv Rev Psychiatry* **6**, 142–8.

Parks, C.L., Robinson, P.S., Sibille, E., Shenk, T. & Toth, M. (1998) Increased anxiety of mice lacking the serotonin 1A receptor. *Proc Natl Acad Sci USA* **95**, 10 734–9.

Pauls, D.L., Alsobrook, J.P., 2nd, Goodman, W., Rasmussen, S. & Leckman, J.F. (1995) A family study of obsessive-compulsive disorder. *Am J Psychiatry* **152**, 76–84.

Peier, A.M., McIlwain, K.L., Kenneson, A., Warren, S.T., Paylor, R. & Nelson, D.L. (2000) (Over) correction of FMR1 deficiency with YAC transgenics: behavioral and physical features. *Hum Mol Genet* **9**, 1145–1159.

Perna, G., Bertani, A., Caldirola, D. & Bellodi, L. (1996) Family history of panic disorder and hypersensitivity to CO_2 in patients with panic disorder. *Am J Psychiatry* **153**, 1060–4.

Perna, G., Caldirola, D., Arancio, C. & Bellodi, L. (1997) Panic attacks: a twin study. *Psychiatry Res* **66**, 69–71.

Persico, A.M., Revay, R.S., Mössner, R. *et al.* (1999) Barrel pattern formation in somatosensory cortical layer IV requires serotonin uptake by thalamocortical endings, while vesicular monoamine release is necessary for development of supragranular layers. *J Neurosci* in press.

Phillips, T.J., Huson, M., Gwiazdon, C., Burkhart-Kasch, S. & Shen, E.H. (1995) Effects of acute and repeated ethanol exposures on the locomotor activity of BXD recombinant inbred mice. *Alcohol Clin Exp Res* **19**, 269–78.

Plomin, R., Owen, M.J. & McGuffin, P. (1994) The genetic basis of complex human behaviors. *Science* **264**, 1733–9.

Raber, J., Akana, S.F., Bhatnagar, S., Dallman, M.F., Wong, D. & Mucke, L. (2000) Hypothalamic–pituitary–adrenal dysfunction in Apoe (-/-) mice: possible role in behavioral and metabolic alterations. *J Neurosci* **20**, 2064–71.

Ramboz, S., Oosting, R., Amara, D.A. *et al.* (1998) Serotonin receptor 1A knockout: an animal model of anxiety-related disorder [see comments]. *Proc Natl Acad Sci USA* **95**, 14476–81.

Ramos, A. & Mormede, P. (1998) Stress and emotionality: a multidimensional and genetic approach. *Neurosci Biobehav Rev* **22**, 33–57.

Rasmussen, S. (1993) Genetic studies of obsessive-compulsive disorder. *Ann Clin Psychiatry* **5**, 241–7.

Reschke, A.H., Mannuzza, S., Chapman, T.F. *et al.* (1995) Sodium lactate response and familial risk for panic disorder. *Am J Psychiatry* **152**, 277–9.

Riddle, M.A., Scahill, L., King, R. *et al.* (1990) Obsessive-compulsive disorder in children and adolescents: phenomenology and family history. *J Am Acad Child Adolesc Psychiatry* **29**, 766–72.

Rowe, D.C., Stever, C., Gard, J.M. *et al.* (1998) The relation of the dopamine transporter gene (DAT1) to symptoms of internalizing disorders in children. *Behav Genet* **28**, 215–25.

Roy, M.A., Neale, M.C., Pedersen, N.L., Mathe, A.A. & Kendler, K.S. (1995) A twin study of generalized anxiety disorder and major depression. *Psychol Med* **25**, 1037–49.

Rudolph, U., Crestani, F., Benke, D. *et al.* (1999) Benzodiazepine actions mediated by specific gamma-aminobutyric acid(A) receptor subtypes. *Nature* **401**(6755), 796–800.

Rudolph, U. & Mohler, H. (1999) Genetically modified animals in pharmacological research: future trends. *Eur J Pharmacol* **375**(1–3), 327–37.

Salichon, N., Gaspar, P., Upton, A.L. *et al.* (2001) Excessive activation of serotonin (5-HT) 1B receptors disrupts the formation of sensory maps in monoamine oxidase A and 5-HT transporter knockout mice. *J Neurosci* **21**, 884–96.

Santarelli, L., Gobbi, G., Debs, P.C. *et al.* (2001) Genetic and pharmacological disruption of neurokinin 1 receptor function decreases anxiety-related behaviors and increases serotonergic function. *Proc Natl Acad Sci USA* **98** 1912–17.

Schaefer, M.L., Wong, S.T., Wozniak, D.F. *et al.* (2000) Altered stress-induced anxiety in adenylyl cyclase type VIII-deficient mice. *J Neurosci* **20**, 4809–20.

Sciuto, G., Pasquale, L. & Bellodi, L. (1995) Obsessive-compulsive disorder and mood disorders: a family study. *Am J Med Genet* **60**, 475–9.

Sibille, E., Pavlides, C., Benke, D. & Toth, M. (2000) Genetic inactivation of the Serotonin (1A) receptor in mice results in downregulation of major GABA (A) receptor alpha subunits, reduction of GABA (A) receptor binding, and benzodiazepine-resistant anxiety. *J Neurosci* **20**, 2758–65.

Skre, I., Onstad, S., Edvardsen, J., Torgersen, S. & Kringlen, E. (1994) A family study of anxiety disorders: familial transmission and relationship to mood disorder and psychoactive substance use disorder. *Acta Psychiatr Scand* **90**, 366–74.

Stein, M.B. (1998) Neurobiological perspectives on social phobia: from affiliation to zoology. *Biol Psychiatry* **44**, 1277–85.

Stein, D.J. (2000) Neurobiology of the obsessive-compulsive spectrum disorders. *Biol Psychiatry* **47**, 296–304.

Stein, M.B., Chartier, M.J., Kozak, M.V., King, N. & Kennedy, J.L. (1998) Genetic linkage to the serotonin transporter protein and 5-HT2A receptor genes excluded in generalized social phobia. *Psychiatry Res* **81**, 283–91.

Steiner, H., Fuchs, S. & Accili, D. (1997) D3 dopamine receptor-deficient mouse: evidence for reduced anxiety. *Physiol Behav* **63**, 137–41.

Stork, O., Ji, F.Y., Kaneko, K. *et al.* (2000) Postnatal development of a GABA deficit and disturbance of neural functions in mice lacking GAD65. *Brain Res* **865**, 45–58.

Stork, O., Welzl, H., Wotjak, C.T. *et al.* (1999) Anxiety and increased 5-HT1A receptor response in NCAM null mutant mice. *J Neurobiol* **40**, 343–55.

Tecott, L.H. & Barondes, S.H. (1996) Genes and aggressiveness. Behaviorial genetics. *Curr Biol* **6**, 238–40.

Tellegen, A., Lykken, D., Bouchard, T. *et al.* (1988) Personality similarity in twins reared apart and together. *J Personal Soc Psychol* **54**, 1031–9.

Timpl, P., Spanagel, R., Sillaber, I. *et al.* (1998) Impaired stress response and reduced anxiety in mice lacking a functional corticotropin-releasing hormone receptor 1. *Nat Genet* **19**, 162–6.

Torgersen, S. (1983) Genetic factors in anxiety disorders. *Arch Gen Psychiatry* **40**, 1085–9.

Torgersen, S. (1990) Comorbidity of major Depress Anxiety disorders in twin pairs [see comments]. *Am J Psychiatry* **147**, 1199–202.

Tronche, F., Kellendonk, C., Kretz, O. *et al.* (1999) Disruption of the glucocorticoid receptor gene in the nervous system results in reduced anxiety. *Nat Genet* **23**, 99–103.

Upton, A.L., Salichon, N., Mössner, R. *et al.* (2002) Role of the 5-HT transporter and the 5-HT1B receptor on the patterning of retinal fibres in the lateral geniculate nucleus and the superior colliculus. *Neuroscience* 597–670.

Wang, Z.W., Crowe, R.R. & Noyes, R. Jr (1992) Adrenergic receptor genes as candidate genes for panic disorder: a linkage study. *Am J Psychiatry* **149**, 470–4.

Wang, Z., Valdes, J., Noyes, R., Zoega, T. & Crowe, R.R. (1998) Possible association of a cholecystokinin promotor polymorphism (CCK-36CT) with panic disorder. *Am J Med Genet* **81**, 228–34.

Weissman, M.M. (1990) Panic and generalized anxiety: are they separate disorders? *J Psychiatr Res* **24**, 157–62.

Weissman, M.M. (1993) Family genetic studies of panic disorder. *J Psychiatr Res* **27**, 69–78.

Weissman, M.M., Bland, R.C., Canino, G.J. *et al.* (1997) The cross-national epidemiology of panic disorder. *Arch Gen Psychiatry* **54**, 305–9.

Wichems, C.H., Li, Q., Holmes, A. *et al.* (2000) Mechanisms mediating the increased anxiety-like behavior and excessive responses to stress in mice lacking the sero-tonin transporter. *Society of Neuroscience Abstract* **26**, 400.

Wittchen, H.U., Essau, C.A. & Krieg, J.C. (1991) Anxiety disorders: similarities and differences of comorbidity in treated and untreated groups. *Br J Psychiatry Suppl* **12**, 23–33.

Wittchen, H.U., Fuetsch, M., Sonntag, H., Muller, N. & Liebowitz, M. (2000) Disability and quality of life in pure and comorbid social phobia. Findings from a controlled study. *Eur Psychiatry* **15**, 46–58.

Woodman, C.L. (1993) The genetics of panic disorder and generalized anxiety disorder. *Ann Clin Psychiatry* **5**, 231–9.

14 Respiration and Anxiety

E. Griez & G. Perna

Introduction

In the last two decades it has become clear that respiration and its control mechanisms may represent a main system involved in abnormal anxiety, particularly panic disorder (Bellodi & Perna 1998). As early as in the late XIX century an association between shortness of breath and acute anxiety attacks was noted (Freud 1963), and the origin of a long research tradition may be traced back to Drury's first report on carbon dioxide intolerance in patients with the irritable heart syndrome (Drury 1918). However, analyses putting respiratory disturbances at the core of the concept of panic attacks are quite recent (Anderson *et al.* 1984; Ley 1985; Klein 1993). Since then the amount of data supporting and deepening the understanding of a connection between the vital function of breathing and (panic) anxiety has accumulated.

This chapter is an attempt to summarize the evidence on the association between respiration, from physiology to pathology, and panic anxiety, with an eye on future perspectives. The authors have chosen to organize the facts and conduct the discussion around a number of themes, keeping in mind old explanations as well as new hypotheses, rather than trying to assemble a complete catalogue of all experiments published in recent literature.

Panic-anxiety and hyperventilation

Patients reporting shocking sensations and other breathing problems during panic attacks is a common clinical experience. Accordingly, there has been a sustained interest into a possible link between malfunction of the respiratory system and anxiety. A first hypothesis that became quite popular in the 1970s was that a disordered respiratory pattern may cause anxiety. Clinician delineated a so-called hyperventilation syndrome affecting people who were believed to be either chronic or acute hyperventilators (Magarian 1982). In this conceptual model "bad breathing habits" are supposed to cause bursts of hyperventilation and respiratory alkalosis, eliciting various somatic symptoms, such as dizziness, shaking, and palpitations. These in turn were thought to precipitate fear and anxiety.

It is true that hyperventilation, i.e., breathing in excess to the metabolic requests, is often found in association with panic (Cowley & Roy-Byrne 1987; Kenardy *et al.* 1990). Starting from this observation, and reasoning along the lines of the hyperventilation syndrome concept, some authors supported the causal role of hyperventilation in the development of panic attacks: panic patients might be chronic hyperventilators that do shift toward a hypocapnic alkaloses as a consequence of stress induced acute hyperventilation, leading to panic attacks. This hypothesis has been built over three main experimental evidences. First, panic attacks and the "hyperventilation–n syndrome" show common symptomatology (Kerr *et al.* 1937; Cowley & Roy-Byrne 1987) with dyspnea, palpitations, tremors, paresthesias, and faintness. Second, the hyperventilation syndrome has been reported to overlap with panic disorder in up to 40% of patients (Garssen *et al.* 1983; Cowley & Roy-Byrne 1987; Hoes *et al.* 1987; de Ruiter *et al.* 1989). Finally, the acute hyperventilation challenge reproduces panic-like symptomatology in a significant rate of panic patients (Garssen *et al.* 1983;

Bass *et al.* 1989; Maddock & Carter 1991; Rapee *et al.* 1992; Nardi *et al.* 1999a). Although these data seem to support the idea of a causal role of hyperventilation, several pieces of evidence argue against it. A growing number of studies question the ability of acute hyperventilation to induce panic attacks (Gorman *et al.* 1984, 1988, 1994; Rapee 1986; Griez *et al.* 1988; Zandbergen *et al.* 1990; Spinhoven *et al.* 1992, 1993; van den Hout *et al.* 1992; Asmundson *et al.* 1994; Antony *et al.* 1997) and suggest that even though it is able to induce some anxiety, hyperventilation cannot induce a reaction similar to spontaneous panic attacks in patients with panic disorder (Lindsay *et al.* 1991). Moreover, spontaneous panic attacks as a rule are not associated with a decrease of Pco_2 levels (Hibbert & Pilsbury 1988, 1989; Buikhuisen & Garssen 1990) and several studies reported the absence of baseline chronic hyperventilation in panic patients (Woods *et al.* 1986; Holt & Andrews 1989; Zandbergen *et al.* 1993). The studies that did report signs of chronic respiratory alkalosis were somewhat inconclusive, as far as these signs were not documented in more than 50% of the patients (Liebowitz *et al.* 1985; Gorman *et al.* 1986; Salkovskis *et al.* 1986). Also, if present, chronic hyperventilation seems far from being specific for panic disorders subjects: it was found as often in patients with other anxiety disorders (van den Hout *et al.* 1992). Finally, almost all studies (Zandbergen *et al.* 1990; Gorman *et al.* 1994; Antony *et al.* 1997) although not all (Schmidt *et al.* 1996) show that hypercapnia is definitely a stronger panicogenic challenge than hyperventilation. It is worth noting that the analysis of challenge studies shows that induced panic precede hyperventilation and hypocapnia (Gorman & Papp 1990).

In conclusion, experimental evidence suggests that hyperventilation is a significant component of panic disorder, but question the idea of a putative causal role. It is, however, unquestionable that some panic patients show symptoms related to hyperventilation as also suggested by the evidence of a relationship between the severity of hyperventilation-induced anxiety symptoms and an exaggerated decrease of cerebral flow in response to hypercapnia (Gibbs 1992; Dager *et al.* 1995).

Panic disorder and respiratory diseases

Another strong line of evidence in favor of a relationship between panic disorder (PD) and a malfunction of

the respiratory system is the fact that patients with respiratory disorders often report panic-like experiences. Several studies have suggested an association between PD and asthma (Smoller & Otto 1998; Carr 1999). Kinsman *et al.* (1973) showed that panic sensation occurred frequently (42%) in a group of asthma patients. Subsequent studies reported an increased prevalence of panic attacks and PD in patients suffering with asthma compared to rates in the general population. Yellowlees *et al.* (1988) compared 13 patients who had suffered a near-miss death of asthma with 36 other asthma patients. All asthma patients had a higher than expected level of psychiatric morbidity but no difference was found when comparing the near-miss death group and the others, suggesting that it was not the simple near death experience that led to the development of panic. Shavitt *et al.* (1992) found that 13.1% and 6.1% of a sample of 107 outpatients with asthma were, respectively, agoraphobics and sufferers of PD. Perna *et al.* (1997b) found that patients with asthma have significantly higher lifetime prevalence of both PD (20%) and of sporadic unexpected panic attacks (26%) than those of the general population with a higher prevalence in women. In this study, in nine asthmatics (90%) with PD, the onset of asthma had preceded the onset of panic, and since only asthmatic patients with PD had higher familial vulnerability to PD, the authors excluded the existence of a common underlying familial vulnerability between PD and asthma.

There are arguments to believe that the relationship between PD and asthma, among respiratory diseases, is not specific. Van Peski-Oosterbaan *et al.* (1996) reported an increased rate of PD (9%) in all subjects referred for pulmonary function tests, regardless of pulmonary diagnosis. Despite very comparable results on the lung function tests, patients who had a comorbid PD perceived higher levels of breathlessness. This confirms findings (Porzelius *et al.* 1992; Carr *et al.* 1994) that patients with chronic obstructive pulmonary disease (COPD) and comorbid PD have more negative cognitions than patients without a comorbid PD, although their lung functions are equally impaired. Patients with COPD also show a high prevalence of anxiety disorders. Several studies have reported a higher prevalence of PD (8–24%) among patients with COPD compared to controls (Yellowlees *et al.* 1987; Karajgi *et al.* 1990). Conversely, repeated investigations (Zandbergen *et al.* 1991a; Perna *et al.* 1994b; Spinhoven *et al.* 1994; Verburg *et al.* 1995b) showed lifetime prevalence of respiratory diseases up to 50% in samples of patients with PD. This was definitely higher than usual lifetime prevalence observed among healthy controls and those occurring in the comparison groups, consisting of patients with other psychiatric disorders (obsessive compulsive, depressive and eating disorders). Since acute respiratory diseases are rarely seen in anxiety clinics, Zandbergen *et al.* (1991a) more specifically investigated whether PD patients show an increased prevalence of respiratory pathology before they develop PD. The results showed that while point prevalence of respiratory disorders was equal to the controls, childhood prevalence was significantly higher in PD patients. Other studies confirmed this finding. Perna *et al.* (1994b) found a lifetime prevalence of respiratory diseases of 29% in 102 PD patients, compared to 14% in a group of 101 patients with obsessive-compulsive disorder. Spinhoven *et al.* (1994) found relatively low rates of 16% in 100 PD patients, although clearly higher than the 5% observed in the control group of 100 Diagnostic Statistical Manual, third revised edition (DSM-III-R: American Psychiatric Association 1987), "V-codes" patients. In this latter study, a comparison group of depressive patients had an intermediate score of 9%. However, a hidden lifetime comorbidity between depression and PD may have influenced the results, increasing the rate of respiratory disorders in the depression group. The childhood prevalence of respiratory disorders in PD subjects was re-examined in a second study of the Maastricht team. Eighty-two PD patients and 68 other anxiety disorder patients (Verburg *et al.* 1995b) were included. The rates of respiratory disorders before the onset of the anxiety disorder were 42.7% and 16.2%, respectively. This study also showed that PD patients most frequently report a childhood history of chronic bronchitis. PD patients with more severe respiratory symptoms during their panic attacks reported significantly more often bronchitis than PD patients with less severe respiratory-like panic symptoms. In all the studies described there appear to be a time gap between the respiratory disease and the onset of the PD. Pollack *et al.* (1996) examined more than 100 patients who were referred for pulmonary function testing. Forty-one percent of these patients reported panic attacks and 17% met the screening criteria for PD. Patients with COPD had the highest rate of PD. All these studies confirm that respiratory diseases increase the risk of developing PD

later in life (OR = 3.9[21]). They suggest that in up to 40% of PD patients respiratory mechanisms could be a contributing factor.

Apparently, having suffered with a respiratory disease early in life increases the risk of developing panic symptoms in subjects at risk for PD (Perna *et al.* 1997b). However, this risk is not related to the objective severity of the respiratory pathology, even though patients who develop panic do perceive their respiratory symptoms as being more severe. In daily care the relationship between PD and diseases of the respiratory system is not very obvious. Virtually none of the patients referred to anxiety clinics have clinically evidences of impairment in their pulmonary functions and this aspect is confirmed by studies showing, if any, only subclinical anomalies in the lung functions of PD patients (Perna *et al.* 1994d). Other studies have reported normal lung functions (Carr *et al.* 1992; Verburg *et al.* 1997). Carr *et al.* (1996) reported that the airways of PD patients, either with or without asthma, are chronically more dilated in both stressful and nonstressful conditions.

To summarize, a relevant proportion, up to 40%, of adults who develop PD have a childhood history of respiratory disease, mainly bronchitis and asthma. Conversely, a higher than expected rate of PD has been reported amongst people with chronic respiratory diseases. The latter may be quite trivial: an increased prevalence of PD and affective pathology in general has been reported in other populations with severe somatic pathology (Chignon *et al.* 1993; Griez *et al.* 2000). However, the former observation may be specific, since, to-date, there are no reports on an increased childhood prevalence of other pathology in subjects with PD.

Respiration and panic provocation procedures

The symptomatological overlap between PD and hyperventilation syndrome prompted Gorman *et al.* (1984) to investigate the effects of provoked hyperventilation in PD patients. They wanted to know whether hyperventilation-induced hypocapnia contributes to the development of panic attacks. A group of subjects with a PD diagnosis voluntarily hyperventilated in a laboratory environment. To prevent hypocapnia and respiratory alkalosis in the control condition the authors administered a mixture of 5% carbon dioxide (CO_2), which was intended to allow hyperapnea without hypocapnia. To the authors surprise, not the hyperventilation but the control condition triggered panic attacks. In subsequent studies, similar findings were obtained in other laboratories. For instance, in their study comparing hyperventilation and hypercapnia, Zandbergen et al. (1990) reported that a group of PD patients who obviously were not affected by voluntary hyperventilation, displayed an increase in anxiety when administered a single breath of 35% CO_2 mixture. Hence, after Gorman's and coworkers unexpected finding, it was repeatedly confirmed that subjects with PD, in contrast with healthy controls, develop a panic like reaction after minutes after starting breathing a mixture which is 5% hypercapnic. Reviewing the issue, Sanderson and Wetzler (1990) conclude that, despite big methodological differences across different studies, it has been established beyond any doubt that subjects with PD are hypersensitive to hypercapnic gas mixtures. A different method of administering CO_2 challenges has also been developed, consisting of one single vital capacity breath of a 35% CO_2 and 65% oxygen (O_2) mixture (Griez et al. 1987). When given to healthy subjects, this type of challenge results in a brief but strong respiratory stimulation accompanied by neurovegetative symptoms that overlap largely with panic symptomatology (Griez et al. 1982; van den Hout & Griez 1984). In PD patients, however, the same intervention induces a sharp, though transitory rise in anxiety which has been equated with a real life panic attacks (Griez et al. 1987; Perna et al. 1994a). Administered in a controlled laboratory environment, the single breath 35% CO_2 challenge is a brief test the effects of which are completely reversible in a matter of seconds. Repeated studies have demonstrated that the procedure is safe and devoid of unwanted consequences both in the short and the long term (Perna et al. 1999). Thus, using this procedure, our two laboratories have thoroughly investigated whether CO_2 vulnerability must be regarded as the expression of a specific underlying mechanism in PD.

It has been established that CO_2 triggered anxiety is not merely a startle reaction generated by a strong physiological stimulus in overaroused individuals. When administered to a mixed group of patients with various anxiety disorders, who all had comparable ratings on arousal and anticipatory anxiety, the CO_2 test affected only those with a diagnosis of PD (Griez

et al. 1990b). Specifically, patients with obsessive-compulsive disorder failed to show any significant anxiety response to the inhalation of 35% CO_2 (Griez et al. 1990a; Perna et al. 1995b). Similarly, patients with a generalized anxiety disorder had little increase in subjective anxiety after a CO_2 breath (Verburg et al. 1995a; Perna et al. 1999). Among patients with a specific phobia, making a clear cut-distinction between animal and situational phobics, the 35% CO_2 challenge did not affect animal phobics while situational phobics had a CO_2 induced reaction which tended to resemble that of PD subjects (Verburg et al. 1994). Since situational phobias are closely related to agoraphobia, the different pattern in both types of phobias is striking. The case of social phobia is less clear as contrasting results have been reported. According to Caldirola et al. (1997) social phobics may be CO_2 sensitive while Verburg and coworkers (unpublished manuscript) were unable to confirm these findings. In conclusion, it is strongly suggested that amongst DSM-IV (American Psychiatric Association 1994) anxiety disorders, only patients suffering from panic type anxiety, or with disorders belonging to the panic spectrum, are vulnerable to CO_2. An analysis of 135 patients using receiver operating characteristics showed that the 35% CO_2 challenge discriminates between PD and normals with an 86% probability of classifying them correctly depending on the anxiety reaction triggered by CO_2 (Battaglia & Perna 1995). The high discriminatory power of a test with 35% CO_2 was recently confirmed in a larger sample of normal controls and patients suffering from various types of anxiety disorders (Verburg et al. 1998). As far as other psychiatric disorders are concerned, additional studies have shown that depressive patients who have no comorbid panic have no hypersensitivity to CO_2 (Perna et al. 1995a; Kent et al. 2001). The same applies to patients with eating disorders (Arancio et al. 1997). In contrast, females with late luteal phase disorder, a condition that is thought to belong to the panic spectrum, may be CO_2 vulnerable (Harrison et al. 1989; Kent et al. 2001).

A recent interesting finding suggests that not only hypercapnia but also hypoxia may yield panicogenic properties. Beck et al. (1999, 2000) examined respiratory response and anxiety while breathing a mixture that was 5% CO_2 and 12% O_2. Fourteen PD patients and 14 matched controls underwent the test. Results demonstrate PD patients respond with increased anxiety compared to healthy controls. If confirmed these results might suggest that PD is associated with a general sensitivity to abnormal respiratory signals rather than with a specific sensitivity to hypercapnia.

Other experimental procedures used to induce panic might be explained in the light of a panic-respiration connection. It was already known that lactate infusion produces unexpected respiratory effects, paradoxically inducing an increase in ventilation, while it is known to cause a systemic alkalosis (Liebowitz *et al.* 1984). In fact it was the lactate induced hyperventilation that prompted Gorman *et al.* (1984) to start studying the effects of respiration in experimental panic/anxiety. Similarly, also the other panicogenic compounds have significant effects on the respiratory system. The symptomatologies induced by both a 35% CO_2 challenge and a cholecystokinin-tetrapeptide (CCK-4) injection have been found to be very similar, both interventions yielding prominent respiratory symptoms (Bradwejn & Koszycki 1991). Most interestingly, CCK-4 injected to healthy volunteers produced a noticeable respiratory stimulation (Bradwejn *et al.* 1998). CCK receptors have been identified in the brain, and some of these receptors have been associated to respiratory control (Bourin *et al.* 1996). Caffeine increases chemosensitivity to CO_2 (D'Urzo *et al.* 1990) and caffeine-induced anxiety is associated with high levels of lactate possibly related to hyperventilation (Uhde 1990). Cathecolaminergic agents that have been reported to induce acute anxiety; i.e., isoproterenol and epinephrine (adrenaline) are known to stimulate respiration (Whelan & Young 1953; Keltz *et al.* 1972).

In summary, a bulk of facts based on the experimental approach of panic in the laboratory supports a close link between respiratory control mechanisms and PD. These data rely mainly on CO_2 vulnerability in PD subjects, but also on studies with lactate, CCK and other substances thought to be panicogenic.

Central respiratory chemosensitivity

Two lines of evidence suggest that panic attacks may originate in the brainstem (Gorman *et al.* 1989). The first is the nature of the symptoms that characterize panic attacks: all clinical signs of a panic attack can be explained by a surge of impulses from the autonomic nervous system. The second line of evidence is the CO_2 mediated experimental provocation of panic attacks itself. CO_2 primarily acts on the brainstem, specifically

on the respiratory center, located in the reticular substance of the medulla oblongata and the pons (Guyton 1985). Considering the hyperoxic mixtures that are used in the CO_2 challenges, any influence of the peripheral chemosensitive areas is as good as turned off. Accordingly, a number of studies were directed towards a possible dysfunction at the level of the central chemosensitive areas.

It appeared straightforward to attribute CO_2 induced panic attacks to a hypersensitive respiratory center. To explore CO_2 chemosensitivity in panic patients the ventilatory response to increasing CO_2 concentrations was monitored, under the hypothesis that an exaggerated response would testify some oversensitivity. Other experiments attempted to evaluate the effect of CO_2 accumulation on the central nervous system (CNS) by use of a simple breath-holding test.

Studies on the ventilatory response to CO_2, i.e., the increase in ventilation due to inhalation of increasing concentrations of CO_2, have yielded contradictory results. This may in part be explained by a possible lack of control of disturbing variables, and the well-known wide inter individual variability of CO_2 chemosensitivity. Two main methods have been used: the "steady-state canopy method" and Read's rebreathing technique. Using the first procedure, the Columbia team reported that patients susceptible to CO_2 reached the maximum minute ventilation quicker than those who failed to panic under CO_2. In addition, they found an enhanced "inspiratory drive" in panic patients compared to subjects without PD (Gorman *et al.* 1988). The same team reported an increased ventilatory response to different levels of inspired CO_2 in panic patients compared to healthy controls (Papp *et al.* 1989). As far as Read's rebreathing technique is concerned, several studies have been reported with contrasting results. This method measures increase in ventilation against increase in CO_2 concentration while the subject is breathing in a closed system. Three studies showed an enhanced respiratory response to accumulating CO_2 (Lousberg *et al.* 1988; Fishman *et al.* 1994; Bocola *et al.* 1998). Pain *et al.* (1988) did find a difference in respiratory patterns, PD patients having a higher frequency of breathing and a lower tidal volume. However, three other studies were unable to find significant differences between PD patients and controls (Woods *et al.* 1986; Zandbergen *et al.* 1991b; Papp *et al.* 1995).

Breath-holding induces an increase of P_{CO_2} and a decrease of P_{O_2}, resulting in chemoreceptor stimulation and a strong drive to restart breathing. Using this procedure, results have been disappointing: two studies reported a shorter breath-holding time in panic patients than in controls (Zandbergen *et al.* 1992; Asmundson & Stein 1994) while one did not (Van der Does 1997) and yet another failed to find differences between patients with PD and patients with generalized anxiety disorder (Roth *et al.* 1998).

In conclusion, despite the supposition that the brainstem respiratory center is involved in PD, data reported in the literature are far from being conclusive. The contradictory results suggest that the crude methods used so far are in need of methodological refinement and, possibly, call for technical improvement. For instance, it should be noted that Berkenbosch *et al.* (1989) compared Read's rebreathing method with the steady-state method to asses the ventilatory CO_2 sensitivity. They found that the two methods may produce different results in the same subject. They argue that in Read's rebreathing method, the increase in ventilation is a direct function of the brain tissues P_{CO_2}. That may sound attractive because it makes the method very suitable for the investigation of the effects of CO_2 on the CNS. Unfortunately matters are not that simple, Berkenbosch and coworkers attribute the differences between the two methods to changes in arterial blood flow. Considering that arterial blood flow has a marked influence on the results of these experiments, and that PD patients, compared to normal controls, show a different response in cerebral blood flow on changes in arterial P_{CO_2} (Gibbs 1992), close monitoring of cerebral blood flow may be a prerequisite for studies on the ventilatory response to CO_2 in PD patients. Alternatively, subjects should be used as their own control. Yet, possible adaptive changes in the peripheral respiratory system (Carr *et al.* 1996) should also be taken into account. In addition, other factors have to be considered. Ideally, the subject undergoing an assessment of his or her central chemosensitivity should be nonanxious and have a regular breathing pattern. PD patients are, by definition, anxious—especially when exposed to CO_2—and may display a usual pattern of irregular breathing.

Respiration physiology

Breathing pattern at rest may reveal some anomalies in ventilatory control. Accordingly, several studies investigated PD subjects focusing on baseline respiratory physiology between panic attacks. However, caution is needed when interpreting these results, since several measures were obtained immediately before panicogenic challenges and procedures used to obtain these measurements are heterogeneous. Often, data obtained are hardly comparable. For the aforementioned reasons, data reported in the literature are sometimes discordant. In general, most of the studies performed to-date have failed to find significant differences in mean values of respiratory rate, tidal volume, minute ventilation and respiratory gases between patients with PD, healthy controls, or patients with other anxiety disorders (Bellodi & Perna 1998). The two main positive findings that have been replicated are the evidence that patients with PD have a thoracic pattern of respiration (Beck & Scott 1988) with a strong muscular thoracic effort and the evidence that patients with PD show an abnormal variability and irregularity in breathing both during daytime (Bystritsky & Shapiro 1992; Schwartz *et al.* 1996; Papp *et al.* 1997; Bystritsky *et al.* 2000) and during sleep (Stein *et al.* 1995).

Since respiration is a complex physiological function with multiple central and peripheral inputs, abnormalities in its function could be more accurately investigated by the analysis of the complexity of the respiratory tracing rather than simply measuring the absolute values of the parameters. Consistent and specific respiratory abnormalities were found when the breathing pattern of PD patients was studied. Patients with PD show a greater breath-to-breath variability during a rebreathing test than what is usually observed in controls (Papp *et al.* 1995). Compared with healthy subjects, patients with PD showed an increased irregularity in tidal volume and minute ventilation and an increased rate of pauses in breathing during sleep (Stein *et al.* 1995; Martinez *et al.* 1996). In awake PD patients, baseline respiratory frequency and tidal volume were more irregular than in healthy controls (Gorman *et al.* 1988; Bystritsky & Shapiro 1992; Bystritsky *et al.* 2000). Patients with PD showed excessive sighing and they also reported tidal volume irregularity significantly greater than in healthy controls (Abelson *et al.* 2000, 2001) and in patients with generalized anxiety disorder (Wilhelm *et al.* 2001). Finally, the tidal volume irregularity persisted after both doxapram-induced hyperventilation and cognitive intervention, suggesting that it might be an intrinsic and stable feature of patients with PD (Abelson *et al.* 2001).

The importance of this finding for the understanding of panic etiopathogenesis is supported by the evidence of a higher variability in respiratory pattern in response to 5% CO_2 inhalation in relatives of panic patients compared to relatives of healthy controls and of affective patients (Coryell *et al.* 2001). Pine *et al.* (1998, 2000) reported more irregularities in respiratory rate in children with childhood anxiety disorders who developed panic symptoms after CO_2 inhalation. Finally, preliminary data from Perna *et al.* (2002) suggest that variability in respiration might be higher in children of patients with PD than in children of healthy controls. Respiratory irregularities and pattern variability could be a physiological trait marker of panic vulnerability able to identify subjects at risk for panic and to promote formal and molecular genetic studies in PD. Finally, this evidence has led researchers (Bellodi, pers. comm.) to the formulation of new hypotheses on the pathophysiology of PD. Normal respiration is characterized by a synchronized action of inspiratory and expiratory neurones and thus the high variability observed, together with the unpleasant respiratory sensations that ensue in patients with PD, could be the results of a mismatch of the activity of inspiratory and respiratory neurones. The abnormal responses to respiratory challenges might be the expression of a deranged adaptation mechanism related to this disregulation.

Antipanic drugs and respiration

More than 15 years ago, Gorman *et al.* (1985) showed that successful drug treatment of patients with PD led to a normalization of some respiratory biochemical parameters (pH, $P\text{CO}_2$ and bicarbonate). Thereafter several studies reported data supporting the relationship between respiration and antipanic medications. Subsequently, two main lines of research have been developed: the first investigated changes in the respiratory response to the inhalation of CO_2 before and after antipanic treatment, while the second investigated the modulation of CO_2 induced panic/anxiety by psychotropic drugs.

Some studies suggest that antipanic medication does modulate respiration physiology. Twelve weeks of antipanic treatment with tricyclic antidepressants decreased significantly CO_2 sensitivity (expressed by minute ventilation and end-tidal CO_2) in patients with PD, whereas there were no significant changes in the control group with healthy subjects (Gorman *et al.* 1997). Similarly, clomipramine reduced the ventilatory response (expressed by the respiratory frequency and the tidal volume) in patients with PD after 10 weeks of treatment (Pols *et al.* 1993) as well as fluoxetine after 1 month of treatment (Bocola *et al.* 1998).

The ability of antipanic medications to decrease panic/anxiety responses to CO_2 is clearly supported in the literature. High potency benzodiazepines have been repeatedly shown to decrease panic/anxiety responses to hypercapnic gas mixtures. An acute dose of (Nardi *et al.* 2000), a very short treatment (10 days) (Nardi *et al.* 1999b), and a short treatment (4–8 weeks) with clonazepam (Beckett *et al.* 1986; Pols *et al.* 1991) and alprazolam (Woods *et al.* 1986, 1989; Fishman *et al.* 1994) were able to decrease CO_2 induced anxiety while conflicting results have been found on the effect of an acute dose of alprazolam on 35% CO_2 reactivity (Sanderson *et al.* 1994; Pols *et al.* 1996a). Monoamino oxidase inhibitors, tricyclic antidepressants and selective serotonin reuptake inhibitors are also able to reduce CO_2 reactivity. The anxious response to 35% CO_2 was significantly reduced already after 1 week of treatment with toloxatone (Perna *et al.* 1994c), with clomipramine and fluvoxamine (Perna *et al.* 1997a), with imipramine, sertraline and paroxetine (Bertani *et al.* 1997), and with citalopram (Bertani *et al.* 2001). Six weeks of treatment with fluvoxamine (Pols *et al.* 1996b), and 1 month of treatment with imipramine and paroxetine (Woods *et al.* 1990; Bertani *et al.* 1995) as well significantly decreased the response to 35% CO_2 in patients with PD. A recent work (Perna *et al.* in press) emphasized the ability of five different antipanic medications (imipramine, clomipramine, sertraline, paroxetine, fluvoxamine) in reducing CO_2 hyper-reactivity. The same study reported that the reduction of CO_2 hyper-reactivity during the 1st week of treatment was able to predict clinical response in the long term.

Finally, some researchers investigated the effects of manipulations of the function of neurotransmitters on CO_2 reactivity. Tryptophan depletion, decreasing serotonergic tone, increases ventilation in panic patients during room air breathing but not in healthy subjects (Kent *et al.* 1996). Tryptophan depletion provokes increased anxiety after hypercapnic inhalation in healthy subjects (Klaassen *et al.* 1998) and in patients with PD (Miller *et al.* 2000; Schruers *et al.* 2000). In contrast, the administration of a balanced amino-acid mixture containing tryptophan has a protective effect against panic provocation in patients with PD (Schruers *et al.* 2000), while metergoline, a serotonin antagonist, enhances CO_2 induced anxiety in healthy volunteers (Ben-Zion *et al.* 1999).

The genetic relationship between PD and respiration

Genetic factors are important in the etiology of PD and thus, given the validity of CO_2 hypersensitivity as a biological marker of PD, it was an obvious step to investigate the genetic relationships between panic and respiration. Studies from three different teams suggested that there is a familial association between PD and CO_2 hypersensitivity (Perna *et al.* 1995d; Coryell 1997; Coryell & Arndt 1999; van Beek & Griez 2000). Perna *et al.* (1995d) tested the reactivity to the 35% CO_2 test in a group of healthy first-degree relatives of patients with PD that had never experienced panic attacks during their lifetime: healthy relatives reacted significantly more than healthy subjects without a familial history of PD, with rates of CO_2 induced panic-attacks of 22% in the first group and of 2% in the second group. These results, suggesting an association between hypersensitivity to hypercapnia and familial vulnerability to PD, was confirmed by Coryell (1997) who investigated reactivity to 35% CO_2 in groups of healthy subjects with a familial vulnerability to PD, to depressive disorders, and without a family history of panic or depressive disorders. CO_2 induced panic attacks were reported in 45.5% of the subjects with positive family history for PD but none in the other two groups. Finally, van Beek and Griez (2000) confirmed these data comparing an age–sex matched sample of 50 healthy first degree relatives and 50 healthy controls. The association between familial vulnerability to PD and respiration has been further confirmed by a study investigating the relationships between CO_2 hypersensitivity in patients with PD and familial-genetic risk for PD. Patients hyper-reactive to the CO_2 showed a morbidity risk for PD (14.4%) significantly higher than that found in patients with a normal reactivity to CO_2 (3.9%) suggesting that CO_2 hyper-reactivity might be associated with a subtype of

PD specifically related to a greater familial loading. (Perna *et al.* 1996). A familial association between respiration and PD has been also supported by a recent study of the Columbia team (Horwath *et al.* 1997). The results showed that relatives of patients with PD with respiratory symptoms had an almost three-fold higher risk for panic and an almost six-fold higher risk for panic with smothering symptoms as compared with relatives of patients without respiratory symptoms. The authors concluded that PD with smothering symptoms might be a subtype of PD associated with an increased familial risk, thus a group of interest for genetic studies. Finally, a recent study by Coryell *et al.* (2001) found an abnormal physiologic regulation of the respiratory function in adult first-degree relatives of patients with PD.

If the etiology of PD is strongly related to genetic factors and if CO_2 hypersensitivity is related to the pathogenesis of PD, it can be thought that CO_2 hypersensitivity is modulated by genetic influences. This idea has been confirmed by a recent twin study (Bellodi *et al.* 1998) showing that a proband-wise significantly different concordance rate for CO_2 induced panic attacks in MZ pairs (55.6%) than in DZ pairs (12.5%).

Finally, the role of familial-genetic factors in the panic–respiration connection is also supported by some preliminary results in children of panic patients. Perna and coworkers (unpublished) have shown that children of panic patients have higher variability of several physiological respiratory parameters compared to children of healthy controls.

Taken together, these studies support the idea that the panic–respiration connection might help for a further step trying to find out a valid "gold standard" phenotype for genetic research. CO_2 hypersensitivity has a relevant genetic component and seems to be significantly related to a familial vulnerability to PD. CO_2 hypersensitivity might be a phenotypical expression of a genetic vulnerability to PD even in the absence of PD, thus, subjects hyper-reactive to hypercapnia or with respiration abnormalities might be considered "affected" members in formal and molecular genetic studies. Alternatively, hypersensitivity to CO_2 might be considered the phenotypic expression of one of the genes involved in the "respiratory panic disease" and thus, only the presence of both clinical panics and CO_2 hypersensitivity could define the "true" phenotype for genetic studies.

Respiration and panic: conjectures and perspectives

In an interesting attempt that integrates a large amount of the above data, Klein (1993) has proposed that panic attacks result from the dysregulation of a phylogenetically evolved alarm system, directed to monitor suffocation signals in the organism. This alarm system has been evolutionarily programmed to fire when it senses metabolic signs of asphyxia and impending death. As a survival alert system this physiological suffocation monitor most likely serves a deeply rooted adaptive function: its activation only occurs in extreme life threatening circumstances. The crux of Klein's hypothesis is that PD represents an instance of repetitive misfiring in an oversensitive suffocation monitor.

Are animals or humans equipped with an inborn suffocation monitor? In this respect, Klein points to the existence of the congenital central hypoventilation syndrome. This rare condition affects infants who apparently are born with an aberrant sensitivity to signals of hypercapnia and hypoxia. Most of these children breathe while awake, but tend to hypoventilate and eventually stop breathing when falling asleep. They only survive with ventilatory support measures. If it is correct to consider the underlying physiological dysfunction in these children as a lack of sensitivity to normal suffocation signals, the existence of a biological suffocation monitor in humans is implicitly posited.

The idea that pathological panic attacks are erroneous survival alerts in an inborn suffocation alarm system opens interesting perspectives and may help to shed light on some crucial issues that have been discussed in the present chapter. For instance, it may help in understanding the preeminence of respiratory symptoms in panic attacks; it may help in explaining why patients with panic, in contrast to other types of anxiety, against any medical evidence, and despite repeated reassurance, invariably feel an overwhelming fear of dying and loosing control during their attacks. Supposing that the suffocation monitor continuously senses metabolic signs of asphyxia, an abnormal accumulation of either aerobic or anaerobic end products, such as CO_2 and lactate, may be expected to trigger the alarm. If the system becomes oversensitive the slightest fluctuation of lactate or CO_2 will induce a false alarm, i.e. real-life panic. It is then readily understandable

that administration of exogenous lactate or inhalation of CO_2 triggers panic in PD subjects. Further arguments have been discussed by Klein in several formulations of his hypothesis (Klein 1994, 1996a,b; Preter & Klein 1998). The most interesting point, however, is the suggestion that the congenital hypoventilation syndrome may be the pathophysiological mirror picture of PD. If some physiological functions implicated in the congenital hypoventilation syndrome are hyposensitive, why could they not be hypersensitive in other pathological conditions? Pine and coworkers have tried to verify the hypothesis that the congenital hypoventilation syndrome and PD are mirror pictures of each other. The alleged suffocation monitoring system being evolutionarily linked to the production of unconditional anxiety, one might expect that a hypoactive suffocation monitor decreases vulnerability to anxiety in general. With this idea in mind, Pine et al. (1994) investigated the presence of anxiety symptoms in 13 children with a congenital hypoventilation syndrome. They were compared with a large community sample, that included children with asthma and other chronic medical illnesses. As predicted, children with the congenital central hypoventilation syndrome had the lowest rate of anxiety, and, worth noting, children with asthma the highest.

A key argument in questioning Klein's hypothesis is that, to-date, no suffocation alarm system has been anatomically or functionally identified as such within the nervous system. However, as shown in this chapter, ample evidence does exist in favor of a connection between respiration and panic. One of the strongest pieces among this evidence is the vulnerability of panic prone individuals to CO_2 exposure. Consistently, the search for a panic circuitry in the brain should include those areas of the CNS that have chemosensitive properties. These structures should logically be considered as the best candidates to fulfil the function of suffocation detector.

For a long time it has been considered that central respiratory chemosensitivity is specifically and exclusively located at the ventral surface of the medulla. This view may now be superseded. Recent findings support the idea that CNS chemosensitive areas extend to several brainstem nuclei including the nucleus tractus solitarius (NTS), the locus ceruleus (LC) and the raphe nuclei, all of these structures being part of a broad brainstem respiratory network (Coates et al. 1993; Nattie 1999).

The ventral medulla, the NTS and the LC are intimately interconnected. Electrical stimulation of the ventrolateral medulla causes increased firing in the LC (Saper 1987), which is under afferent control originating in the brainstem. Indeed, the vast majority of the impulses to the LC comes from two nuclei in the rostral medulla, the nucleus prepositus hypoglossi and the nucleus paragigantocellularis, of which the latter is a crossroad for autonomic integration, namely cardiorespiratory functions(Aston Jones *et al.* 1986).

The LC, a small bilateral nucleus located in the rostral pons, contains the highest density of noradrenergic cells in the CNS, accounting for more than half of all central noradrenergic neurones (Svensson 1987). In a series of experiments conducted in the 1980s, Elam and coworkers showed that changes in internal state such as hypercapnia, hypoxia, blood volume loss, or dilatation of the digestive tract is followed by LC activation (Elam *et al.* 1981, 1984, 1985, 1986a,b). Changes that represent a vital threat to the organism, i.e. hypercapnia, hypoxia and blood loss, induce the most dramatic LC activation (Elam *et al.* 1986b). Accordingly there are grounds for considering the LC and the above chemosensitive brainstem structures as a system that monitors vital functions in the organism.

Finally, the raphe nuclei represents another major chemosensitive area. This is no real surprise: both the metabolism (De Yebenes Prous *et al.* 1997) and the reuptake of 5-HT (Mueller *et al.* 1982) are known to be influenced by hypercapnia, and the raphe represents the major serotonergic structure in the CNS. Also, the stimulation of the serotonergic pathways has been known for years to depress ventilation (Lundberg *et al.* 1980), possibly reducing the ventilatory response to CO_2 (Muller *et al.* 1982; Eriksson & Humble 1990). Within, or at least near, the raphe nuclei (Bernard & Li 1996; Veasey *et al.* 1997) there are neurones with specific chemosensitive function and some authors have recently suggested that they might be essential for a full expression of the ventilatory response to hypercapnia (Dreshaj *et al.* 1998). The two main rostral nuclei, the medial raphe nucleus (MRN) and the dorsal raphe nuclei (DRN), may play a crucial modulating role in the panic neuroanatomical circuitry. In respect to the LC, the DRN receives excitatory projections and itself inhibits the firing of the LC in a mutually regulatory feedback mechanism. The MRN simply receives inhibitory projections from the LC and the lateral hypothalamus (Grove *et al.* 1997). Thus the serotonergic system may largely influence the above suggested monitoring system of vital functions.

LC stimulation, however, produces activation in other brain areas. Specifically, there is a rich efferent network from the LC to the limbic structures connecting the putative vital monitoring system to the panic/anxiety circuitries that have recently been reviewed by others (see Coplan & Lydiard 1998). Noteworthy, also at a limbic level, structures such as the amygdala, hypothalamus, thalamus and the limbic circuit in general may reportedly become activated by hypercapnia and hypoxia (Corfield *et al.* 1995; Dempsey & Pack 1995).

An additional note is worth mentioning. The potential role of hypoxia as a signal of asphyxia, and the suggested sensitivity of PD patients to anoxia have been briefly evoked elsewhere in this chapter. There is some evidence from animal studies that the amygdala and the hippocampus are particularly sensitive to anoxic stimulation. Together with evidence of strong connections between the amygdala and the carotid body, the direct sensitivity of amygdala to acid-base changes, and the interconnections between the amygdala and the parabrachial nucleus (Takeuchi *et al.* 1982) this may delineate another pathway, a so called anoxia pathway, linking respiratory signals and panic (Coplan & Lydiard 1998).

Finally, since basic physiological functions in the organism are strictly interrelated in a neural network with reciprocal modulations, abnormal function of the respiratory system does not necessary imply an intrinsic instability in the control of that system but might be the expression of perturbations of other systems, or from a more general dysfunction of the homeostatic brain. The latter possibility seems to be supported by studies reporting evidences for a disregulation of the cardiovascular and the balance systems in PD patients. Cardiovascular and respiratory functions are highly interconnected and fluctuations in cardiac output or in cerebral blood flow could influence the entity and the time-course of the chemoreflex response by inducing variations in gas exchanges and in circulatory function (Khoo 2000). PD patients show a decrease in cardiac vagal function and a relative increase in sympathetic activity, with a decreased global heart rate variability, leading to a reduced and abnormal flexibility and adaptability to external/internal inputs. The brainstem respiratory network is also highly interconnected with the vestibular nuclei to maintain blood gas homeostasis during movement and changes in posture (Balaban & Thayer 2001). Recently, we found that many PD patients have subclinical abnormalities in their balance system function and that symptomatological reactivity to CO_2 is correlated to some static posturography parameters (Perna *et al.* 2001). Therefore, the connection between disordered respiration and panic, as discussed in the present chapter, might arise from a more global and complex abnormality in the integration of the brainstem neuronal circuits that regulate physiological homeostasis in general.

References

Abelson, J.L., Weg, J.G. & Curtis, G.C. (2000) Respiratory irregularity in panic patients may reflect excessive sighing. *Biol Psychiatry* **47** (Suppl. 1), 157–8.

Abelson, J.L., Weg, J.G., Nesse, R.M. & Curtis, G.C. (2001) Persistent respiratory irregularity in patients with panic disorder. *Biol Psychiatry* **49**, 588–95.

American Psychiatric Association (1987) *Diagnostic Statistical Manual of Mental Disorders*, 3rd edn revised. American Psychiatric Association, Washington, D.C.

American Psychiatric Association (APA) (1994) *Diagnostic Statistical Manual of Mental Disorders*, 4th edn. American Psychiatric Association, Washington, D.C.

Anderson, D.J., Noyes, R. & Crowe, R.R. (1984) A comparison between panic disorder and generalized anxiety disorder. *Am J Psychiatry* **141**, 572–5.

Antony, M.M., Brown, T.A. & Barlow, D.H. (1997) Response to hyperventilation and 5.5% CO_2 inhalation of subjects with types of specific phobia, panic disorder, or no mental disorder. *Am J Psychiatry* **154**, 1089–95.

Arancio, C., Casolari, A., Torres, V. *et al.* (1997) The 35% CO_2 challenge in women with eating disorders: preliminary results. *Eur Neuropsychopharmacol* **7**, S265.

Asmundson, G.J., Norton, G.R., Wilson, K.G. & Sandler, L.S. (1994) Subjective symptoms and cardiac reactivity to brief hyperventilation in individuals with high anxiety sensitivity. *Behav Res Ther* **32**, 237–41.

Asmundson, G.J. & Stein, M.B. (1994) Triggering the false suffocation alarm in panic disorder patients by using a voluntary breath-holding procedure. *Am J Psychiatry* **151**, 264–6.

Aston Jones, G., Ennis, M., Pieribone, V.A., Thompson Nicell, W. & Shipley, M.T. (1986) The brain nucleus locus coeruleus: restricted afferent control of a broad efferent network. *Science* **234**, 734–7.

Balaban, C.D. & Thayer, J.F. (2001) Neurological bases for balance–anxiety links. *J Anxiety Disord* **15**, 53–79.

Bass, C., Lelliott, P. & Marks, I. (1989) Fear talk versus voluntary hyperventilation in agoraphobics and normals: a controlled study. *Psychol Med* **19**, 669–76.

Battaglia, M. & Perna, G. (1995) The 35% CO_2 challenge in panic disorder: optimization by receiver operating characteristic (ROC) analysis. *J Psychiatr Res* **29**, 111–19.

Beck, J.G., Ohtake, P.J. & Shipherd, J.C. (1999) Exaggerated anxiety is not unique to CO_2 in panic disorder: a comparison of hypercapnic and hypoxic challenges. *J Abnorm Psychol* **108**, 473–82.

Beck, J.G. & Scott, S.K. (1988) Physiological and symptom responses to hyperventilation: a comparison of frequent and infrequent panickers. *J Psychopath and Behav Assessm* **10**, 117–27.

Beck, J.G., Shipherd, J.C. & Ohtake, P. (2000) Do panic symptom profiles influence response to a hypoxic challenge in patients with panic disorder? A preliminary report [in process citation]. *Psychosom Med* **62**, 678–83.

Beckett, A., Fishman, S.M. & Rosenbaum, J.F. (1986) Clonazepam blockade of spontaneous and CO_2 inhalation-provoked panic in a patient with panic disorder. *J Clin Psychiatry* **47**, 475–6.

van Beek, N. & Griez, E. (2000) Reactivity to a 35% CO_2 challenge in healthy first-degree relatives of patients with panic disorder. *Biol Psychiatry* **47**, 830–5.

Bellodi, L. & Perna, G. (eds) (1998) *The Panic Respiration Connection*. MDM Medical Media, Milan.

Bellodi, L., Perna, G., Caldirola, D., Arancio, C., Bertani, A. & Di Bella, D. (1998) CO_2 induced panic attacks: a twin study. *Am J Psychiatry* **155**, 1184–8.

Ben-Zion, I.Z., Meiri, G., Greenberg, B.D., Murphy, D.L. & Benjamin, J. (1999) Enhancement of CO_2 induced anxiety in healthy volunteers with serotonin antagonist metergoline. *Am J Psychiatry* **156**, 1635–7.

Berkenbosch, A., Bovill, J.G., Dahan, A., DeGoede, J. & Olievier, I.C.W. (1989) The ventilatory CO_2 sensitivities from Read's rebreathing method and the steady-state method are not equal in man. *J Physiol* **411**, 367–77.

Bernard, D.G., Li, A. & Nattie, E.E. (1996) Evidence for central chemoreception in the midline raphe. *J Appl Physiol* **80**, 108–15.

Bertani, A., Caldirola, D., Bussi, R., Bellodi, L. & Perna, G. (2001) 35% CO_2 hyper-reactivity and clinical symptomatology in patients with panic disorder after 1 week treatment with citalopram: an open study. *J Clin Psychopharmacol* **21**, 262–7.

Bertani, A., Perna, G., Arancio, C., Caldirola, D., & Bellodi, L. (1997) Pharmacologic effect of imipramine, paroxetine, and sertraline on 35% carbon dioxide hypersensitivity in panic patients: a double-blind, random, placebo-controlled study. *J Clin Psychopharmacol* **17**, 97–101.

Bertani, A., Perna, G., Cocchi, S., Gabriele, A. & Bellodi, L. (1995) The effects of paroxetine and imipramine treatments on 35% CO_2 sensitivity in panic patients. *Eur Neuropsychopharmacol* **5**, 356.

Bocola, V., Trecco, M.D., Fabbrini, G., Paladini, C., Sollecito, A. & Martucci, N. (1998) Antipanic effect of fluoxetine measured by CO_2 challenge test. *Biol Psychiatry* **43**, 612–15.

Bourin, M., Malinge, M., Vasar, E. & Bradwejn, J. (1996) Two faces of cholecystokinin: anxiety and schizofrenia. *Fundam Clin Pharmacol* **10**, 116–26.

Bradwejn, J. & Koszycki, D. (1991) Comparison of the panicogenic effect of cholecystokinin 30–33 and carbon dioxide in panic disorder. *Prog Neuropsychopharmacol Biol Psychiatry* **15**, 237–9.

Bradwejn, J., LeGrand, J.M., Koszycki, D., Bates, J.H. & Bourin, M. (1998) Effects of cholecystokinin tetrapeptide on respiratory function in healthy volunteers. *Am J Psychiatry* **155**, 280–2.

Buikhuisen, M. & Garssen, B. (1990) Hyperventilation and panic attacks. *Biol Psychol* **31**, 280.

Bystritsky, A., Craske, M., Maidenberg, E., Vapnik, T. & Shapiro, D. (2000) Autonomic reactivity of panic patients during a CO_2 inhalation procedure. *Depress Anxiety* **11**, 15–26.

Bystritsky, A. & Shapiro, D. (1992) Continuous physiological changes and subjective reports in panic patients: a preliminary methodological report. *Biol Psychiatry* **32**, 766–77.

Caldirola, D., Perna, G., Arancio, C., Bertani, A. & Bellodi, L. (1997) The 35% CO_2 challenge test in patients with social phobia. *Psychiatry Res* **71**, 41–8.

Carr, R.E. (1999) Panic disorder and asthma. *J Asthma* **36**, 143–52.

Carr, R.E., Lehrer, P.M. & Hochron, S.M. (1992) Panic symptoms in asthma and panic disorder: a preliminary test of the dyspnea-fear theory. *Behav Res Ther* **30**, 251–61.

Carr, R.E., Lehrer, P.M., Hochron, S.M. & Jackson, A. (1996) Effect of psychological stress on airway impedance in individuals with asthma and panic disorder. *J Abnorm Psychol* **105**, 137–41.

Carr, R.E., Lehrer, P.M., Rausch, L.L. & Hochron, S.M. (1994) Anxiety sensitivity and panic attacks in an asthmatic population. *Behav Res Ther* **32**, 411–18.

Chignon, J.M., Lépine, J.P. & Adès, J. (1993) Panic disorder in cardiac outpatients. *Am J Psychiatry* **150**(5), 780–5.

Coates, B.L., Li, A. & Nattie, E. (1993) Widespread sites of brainstem ventilatory chemoreceptors. *J Appl Physiol* **75**, 5–14.

Coplan, J.D. & Lydiard, R.B. (1998) Brain circuits in panic disorder. *Biol Psychiatry* **44**, 1264–76.

Corfield, D.R., Fink, G.R., Ramsay, S.C. *et al.* (1995) Evidence for the lymbic system activation during CO_2-stimulated breathing in man. *J Physiol* **488**, 77–84.

Coryell, W. (1997) Hypersensitivity to carbon dioxide as a disease-specific trait marker. *Biol Psychiatry* **41**, 259–63.

Coryell, W. & Arndt, S. (1999) The 35% CO_2 inhalation procedure: test–retest reliability. *Biol Psychiatry* **45**, 923–7.

Coryell, W., Fyer, A., Pine, D., Martinez, J. & Arndt, S. (2001) Aberrant respiratory sensitivity to CO_2 as a trait of familial panic disorder. *Biol Psychiatry* **49**, 582–7.

Cowley, D.S. & Roy-Byrne, P.P. (1987) Hyperventilation and panic disorder. *Am J Med* **83**, 929–37.

D'Urzo, A.D., Jhirad, R., Jenne, H. *et al.* (1990) Effect of caffeine on ventilatory response to hypercapnia, hypoxia, and exercise in humans. *J Appl Physiol* **68**, 322–8.

Dager, S.R., Strauss, W.L., Marro, K.I., Richards, T.L., Metzger, G.D. & Artru, A.A. (1995) Proton magnetic resonance spectroscopy investigation of hyperventilation in panic and comparison subjects. *Am J Psychiatry* **152**, 666–72.

De Yebenes Prous, J.G., Carlsson, A. & Mena Gomez, M.A. (1997) The effect of CO_2 on monamine metabolism in rat brain. *Arch Pharmachol* **301**, 11–15.

Dempsey, J.A. & Pack, A.I. (1995) *Regulation of Breathing*, 2nd edn. Marcell Dekker, New York.

Dreshaj, I.A., Haxhiu, M.A. & Martin, R.J. (1998) Role of the medullary raphe nuclei in the respiratory response to CO_2. *Resp Physiol* **111**, 15–23.

Drury, A.N. (1918) The percentage of carbon dioxide in the alveolar air, and the tolerance to accumulating carbon dioxide in cases of so-called "irritable heart." *Heart* **7**, 20.

Elam, M., Clark, D. & Svensson, T.H. (1986a) Electrophysiological effects of the enantiomers of 3-PPP on neurons in the locus coeruleus of the rat. *Neuropharmacology* **25**, 1003–8.

Elam, M., Svensson, T.H. & Thoren, P. (1985) Differentiated cardiovascular afferent regulation of locus coeruleus neurons and sympathetic nerves. *Brain Res* **358**, 77–84.

Elam, M., Thoren, P. & Svensson, T.H. (1986b) Locus coeruleus neurons and sympathetic nerves: activation by visceral afferents. *Brain Res* **375**, 117–25.

Elam, M., Yao, T., Svensson, T.H. & Thoren, P. (1984) Regulation of locus coeruleus neurons and splanchnic, sympathetic nerves by cardiovascular afferents. *Brain Res* **290**, 281–7.

Elam, M., Yao, T., Thoren, P. & Svensson, T.H. (1981) Hypercapnia and hypoxia. Chemoreceptor-mediated control of locus coeruleus neurons and splanchnic, sympathetic nerves. *Brain Res* **222**, 373–81.

Eriksson, E. & Humble, M. (1990) Serotonin in psychiatric pathophysiology. Review of data from experimental and clinical research. In: *The Biological Basis of Psychiatric Treatment: Progress in Basic and Clinical Pharmachology.*

(R. Pohl & S. Gerhon (eds), pp. 66–119). Karger, Basel, Switzerland.

Fishman, S.M., Carr, D.B., Beckett, A. & Rosenbaum, J.F. (1994) Hypercapneic ventilatory response in patients with panic disorder before and after alprazolam treatment and in pre- and postmenstrual women. *J Psychiatr Res* **28**, 165–70.

Freud, S. (1963) The introductory lectures on psychoanalysis, part III. In: *The Standard Edition of the Complete Psychological Works of Sigmund Freud* (J. Strachey (ed.), pp. 396–7). Hogarth Press and the Institute of Psycho-Analysis, London.

Garssen, B., van Veenendaal, W. & Bloemink, R. (1983) Agoraphobia and the hyperventilation syndrome. *Behav Res Ther* **21**, 643–9.

Gibbs, D.M. (1992) Hyperventilation-induced cerebral ischemia in panic disorder and effect of nimodipine. *Am J Psychiatry* **149**, 1589–91.

Gorman, J.M., Askanazi, J., Liebowitz, M.R. *et al.* (1984) Response to hyperventilation in a group of patients with panic disorder. *Am J Psychiatry* **141**, 857–61.

Gorman, J.M., Browne, S.T., Papp, L.A. *et al.* (1997) Effect of antipanic treatment on response to carbon dioxide. *Biol Psychiatry* **42**, 982–91.

Gorman, J.M., Cohen, B.S., Liebowitz, M.R. *et al.* (1986) Blood gas changes and hypophosphatemia in lactate-induced panic. *Arch Gen Psychiatry* **43**, 1067–71.

Gorman, J.M., Fyer, M.R., Goetz, R. *et al.* (1988) Ventilatory physiology of patients with panic disorder [published erratum appears in *Arch General Psychiatry* 48(2), 181]. *Arch Gen Psychiatry* **45**, 31–9.

Gorman, J.M., Fyer, A.J., Ross, D.C. *et al.* (1985) Normalization of venous pH, Pco_2, and bicarbonate levels after blockade of panic attacks. *Psychiatry Res* **14**, 57–65.

Gorman, J.M., Liebowitz, M.R., Fyer, A.J. & Stein, J. (1989) A neuroanatomical hypothesis for panic disorder. *Am J Psychiatry* **146**, 148–61.

Gorman, J.M. & Papp, L.A. (1990) Respiratory physiology of panic. In: *Neurobiology of Panic Disorder* (J.C. Ballanger (ed.), pp. 187–203). Alan R. Liss, New York.

Gorman, J.M., Papp, L.A., Coplan, J.D. *et al.* (1994) Anxiogenic effects of CO_2 and hyperventilation in patients with panic disorder. *Am J Psychiatry* **151**, 547–53.

Griez, E. & van den Hout, M.A. (1982) Effects of carbon dioxide–oxygen inhalations on subjective anxiety and some neurovegetative parameters. *J Behav Ther Exper Psychiatry* **13**, 27–32.

Griez, E., de Loof, C., Pols, H., Zandbergen, J. & Lousberg, H. (1990a) Specific sensitivity of patients with panic attacks to carbon dioxide inhalation. *Psychiatry Res* **31**, 193–9.

Griez, E.J., Lousberg, H., van den Hout, M.A. & van der Molen, G.M. (1987) CO_2 vulnerability in panic disorder. *Psychiatry Res* **20**, 87–95.

Griez, E., Mammar, N., Loirat, J.C., Djega, N., Trochut, C., Bouhour, J. (2000) Panic disorder and idiopathic cardiomyopathy. *J Psychosom Res* **48**, 585–7.

Griez, E., Zandbergen, J., Lousberg, H. & van den Hout, M. (1988) Effects of low pulmonary CO_2 on panic anxiety. *Compr Psychiatry* **29**, 490–7.

Griez, E., Zandbergen, J., Pols, H. & de Loof, C. (1990b) Response to 35% CO_2 as a marker of panic in severe anxiety. *Am J Psychiatry* **147**, 796–7.

Grove, G., Coplan, J.D. & Hollander, E. (1997) The neuroanatomy of 5-HT dysregulation and panic disorder. *J Neuropsychiatry Clin Neurosci* **9**, 198–207.

Guyton, A.C. (1985) *Textbook of Medical Physiology*. W.B. Saunders Co., Philadelphia.

Harrison, W.M., Sandberg, D., Gorman, J.M. *et al.* (1989) Provocation of panic with carbon dioxide inhalation in patients with premenstrual dysphoria. *Psychiatry Res* **27**, 183–92.

Hibbert, G. & Pilsbury, D. (1988) Hyperventilation in panic attacks. Ambulant monitoring of transcutaneous carbon dioxide. *Br J Psychiatry* **153**, 76–80.

Hibbert, G. & Pilsbury, D. (1989) Hyperventilation: is it a cause of panic attacks? *Br J Psychiatry* **155**, 805–9.

Hoes, M.J., Colla, P., van Doorn, P., Folgering, H. & de Swart, J. (1987) Hyperventilation and panic attacks. *J Clin Psychiatry* **48**, 435–7.

Holt, P.E. & Andrews, G. (1989) Hyperventilation and anxiety in panic disorder, social phobia, GAD and normal controls. *Behav Res Ther* **27**, 453–60.

Horwath, E., Adams, P., Wickramaratne, P., Pine, D. & Weissman, M.M. (1997) Panic disorder with smothering symptoms: evidence for increased risk in first-degree relatives. *Depress Anxiety* **6**, 147–53.

van den Hout, M.A., Hoekstra, R., Arntz, A., Christiaanse, M., Ranschaert, W. & Schouten, E. (1992) Hyperventilation is not diagnostically specific to panic patients. *Psychosom Med* **54**, 182–91.

Karajgi, B., Rifkin, A., Doddi, S. & Kolli, R. (1990) The prevalence of anxiety disorders in patients with chronic obstructive pulmonary disease. *Am J Psychiatry* **147**, 200–1.

Keltz, H., Samortin, T. & Stone, D.J. (1972) Hyperventilation: a manifestation of exogenous β-adrenergic stimulation. *Am Rev Resp Dis* **105**, 637–40.

Kenardy, J., Oei, T.P. & Evans, L. (1990) Hyperventilation and panic attacks. *Aust N Z J Psychiatry* **24**, 261–7.

Kent, J.M., Coplan, J.D., Martinez, J., Karmally, W., Papp, L.A. & Gorman, J.M. (1996) Ventilatory effects of tryptophan depletion in panic disorder: a preliminary report. *Psychiatry Res* **64**, 83–90.

Kent, J.M., Papp, L.A., Martinez, J.M. *et al.* (2001) Specificity of panic response to CO_2 inhalation in panic disorder: a comparison with major depression and premenstrual dysphoric disorder [in process citation]. *Am J Psychiatry* **158**, 58–67.

Kerr, W.J., Dalton, J.W. & Gliebe, P.A. (1937) Some physical phenomena associated with the anxiety states and their relation to hyperventilation. *Ann Intern Med* **11**, 961–92.

Khoo, M.C.K. (2000) Determinants of ventilatory instability and variability. *Respir Physiol* **122**, 167–82.

Kinsman, R.A., Luparello, T., O'Banion, K. & Spector, S. (1973) Multidimensional analysis of the subjective symptomatology of asthma. *Psychosom Med* **35**, 250–67.

Klaassen, T., Klumperbeek, J., Deutz, N.E., van Praag, H.M. & Griez, E. (1998) Effects of tryptophan depletion on anxiety and on panic provoked by carbon dioxide challenge. *Psychiatry Res* **77**, 167–74.

Klein, D.F. (1993) False suffocation alarms, spontaneous panics, and related conditions. An integrative hypothesis [see comments]. *Arch Gen Psychiatry* **50**, 306–17.

Klein, D.F. (1994) Testing the suffocation false alarm theory of panic disorder [see comments]. *Anxiety* **1**, 1–7.

Klein, D.F. (1996a) In reply to Ley. *Arch Gen Psychiatry* **53**, 83–5.

Klein, D.F. (1996b) Panic disorder and agoraphobia: hypothesis hothouse. *J Clin Psychiatry* **57**, 21–7.

Ley, R. (1985) Agoraphobia, the panic attacks and the hyperventilation syndrome. *Behav Res Ther* **23**, 79–81.

Liebowitz, M.R., Gorman, J. & Fyer, M. (1984) Lactate provocation of panic attacks. *Arch Gen Psychiatry* **41**, 764–70.

Liebowitz, M.R., Gorman, J.M., Fyer, M. *et al.* (1985) Lactate provocation of panic attacks. II. Biochemical and physiological findings. *Arch Gen Psychiatry* **42**, 709–19.

Lindsay, S., Saqi, S. & Bass, C. (1991) The test–retest reliability of the hyperventilation provocation test. *J Psychosom Res* **35**, 155–62.

Lousberg, H., Griez, E. & van den Hout, M.A. (1988) Carbon dioxide chemosensitivity in panic disorder. *Acta Psychiatr Scand* **77**, 214–18.

Lundberg, D.B., Mueller, A.R. & Breese, G.R. (1980) An evaluation of the mechanism by which serotonergic activation depresses respiration. *Journal of Pharmachological Experimental Therapy* **212**, 397–404.

Maddock, R.J. & Carter, C.S. (1991) Hyperventilation-induced panic attacks in panic disorder with agoraphobia. *Biol Psychiatry* **29**, 843–54.

Magarian, G.J. (1982) Hyperventilation syndromes: infrequently recognized common expressions of anxiety and stress. *Medicine (Baltimore)* **61**, 219–36.

Martinez, J.M., Papp, L.M., Coplan, J.D. *et al.* (1996) Ambulatory monitoring of respiration in anxiety. *Anxiety* **2**, 296–302.

Miller, H.E., Deakin, J.F. & Anderson, I.M. (2000) Effect of acute tryptophan depletion on CO_2 induced anxiety in patients with panic disorder and normal volunteers. *Br J Psychiatry* **176**, 182–8.

Mueller, A.R., Lundberg, D.B.A., Breese, G.R., Hedner, J., Hedner, T. & Jonason, C. (1982) The neuropharmachology of respiration control. *Pharmachol Rev* **34**, 255–79.

Nardi, A.E., Valenca, A.M., Nascimento, I., Mezzasalma, M.A. & Zin, W. (1999a) Panic disorder and hyperventilation. *Arq Neuropsiquiatrics* **57**, 932–6.

Nardi, A.E., Valenca, A.M., Nascimento, I., Mezzasalma, M.A. & Zin, W.A. (2000) Double-blind acute clonazepam versus placebo in carbon dioxide induced panic attacks. *Psychiatry Res* **94**, 179–84.

Nardi, A.E., Valenca, A.M., Zin, W. & Nascimento, I. (1999b) Carbon dioxide induced panic attacks and short term clonazepam treatment. Preliminary study. *Arq Neuropsiquiatrics* **57**, 361–5.

Nattie, E. (1999) CO_2 brainstem chemoreceptors and breathing. *Prog Neurobiol* **59**, 299–331.

Pain, M.C., Biddle, N. & Tiller, J.W. (1988) Panic disorder, the ventilatory response to carbon dioxide and respiratory variables. *Psychosom Med* **50**, 541–8.

Papp, L.A., Goetz, R., Cole, R. *et al.* (1989) Hypersensitivity to carbon dioxide in panic disorder. *Am J Psychiatry* **146**, 779–81.

Papp, L.A., Martinez, J.M., Klein, D.F., Coplan, J.D. & Gorman, J.M. (1995) Rebreathing tests in panic disorder. *Biol Psychiatry* **38**, 240–5.

Papp, L.A., Martinez, J.M., Klein, D.F. *et al.* (1997) Respiratory psychophysiology of panic disorder: three respiratory challenges in 98 subjects [see comments]. *Am J Psychiatry* **154**, 1557–65.

Perna, G., Alpini, D., Caldirola, D., Barozzi, S., Cesarani, A. & Bellodi, L. (2001) Panic disorder: the role of the balance system. *J Psychiatr Res* **35**, 279–86.

Perna, G., Barbini, B., Cocchi, S., Bertani, A. & Gasperini, M. (1995a) Thirty-five percent CO_2 challenge in panic and mood disorders. *J Affect Disord* **33**, 189–94.

Perna, G., Battaglia, M., Garberi, A., Arancio, C., Bertani, A. & Bellodi, L. (1994a) Carbon dioxide/oxygen challenge test in panic disorder. *Psychiatry Res* **52**, 159–71.

Perna, G., Bertani, A., Arancio, C., Ronchi, P. & Bellodi, L. (1995b) Laboratory response of patients with panic and obsessive-compulsive disorders to 35% CO_2 challenges. *Am J Psychiatry* **152**, 85–9.

Perna, G., Bertani, A., Caldirola, D. & Bellodi, L. (1996) Family history of panic disorder and hypersensitivity to CO_2 in patients with panic disorder. *Am J Psychiatry* **153**, 1060–4.

Perna, G., Bertani, A., Caldirola, D., Gabriele, A., Cocchi, S. & Bellodi, L. (in press) Antipanic drug modulation of 35% CO_2 hyper-reactivity and short-term treatment outcome. *J Clin Psychopharmacol.*

Perna, G., Bertani, A., Diaferia, G., Arancio, C. & Bellodi, L. (1994b) Prevalence of respiratory diseases in patients with panic and obsessive compulsive disorders. *Anxiety* **1**, 100–1.

Perna, G., Bertani, A., Gabriele, A., Politi, E. & Bellodi, L. (1997a) Modification of 35% carbon dioxide hyper-sensitivity across 1 week of treatment with clomipramine and fluvoxamine: a double-blind, randomized, placebo-controlled study. *J Clin Psychopharmacol* **17**, 173–8.

Perna, G., Bertani, A., Politi, E., Colombo, G. & Bellodi, L. (1997b) Asthma and panic attacks. *Biol Psychiatry* **42**, 625–30.

Perna, G., Cocchi, S., Allevi, L., Bussi, R. & Bellodi, L. (1999) A long-term prospective evaluation of first-degree relatives of panic patients who underwent the 35% CO_2 challenge. *Biol Psychiatry* **45**, 365–7.

Perna, G., Cocchi, S., Bertani, A., Arancio, C. & Bellodi, L. (1994c) Pharmacologic effect of toloxatone on reactivity to the 35% carbon dioxide challenge: a single-blind, random, placebo-controlled study. *J Clin Psychopharmacol* **14**, 414–18.

Perna, G., Cocchi, S., Bertani, A., Arancio, C. & Bellodi, L. (1995d) Sensitivity to 35% CO_2 in healthy first-degree relatives of patients with panic disorder. *Am J Psychiatry* **152**, 623–5.

Perna, G., Ieva, A., Caldirola, D., Bertani, A. & Bellodi, L. (2002) Respiration in children at risk for panic disorder. *Arch Gen Psychiatry* **59**, 185–6.

Perna, G., Marconi, C., Battaglia, M., Bertani, A., Panzacchi, A. & Bellodi, L. (1994d) Subclinical impairment of lung airways in patients with panic disorder. *Biol Psychiatry* **36**, 601–5.

Pine, D.S., Coplan, J.D., Papp, L.A. *et al.* (1998) Ventilatory physiology of children and adolescents with anxiety disorders. *Arch Gen Psychiatry* **55**, 123–9.

Pine, D.S., Klein, R.G., Coplan, J.D. *et al.* (2000) Differential carbon dioxide sensitivity in childhood anxiety disorders and nonill comparison group. *Arch Gen Psychiatry* **57**, 960–7.

Pine, D.S., Weese-Mayer, D.E., Silvestri, J.M., Davies, M., Whitaker, A.H. & Klein, D.F. (1994) Anxiety and congenital central hypoventilation syndrome. *Am J Psychiatry* **151**, 864–70.

Pollack, M.H., Kradin, R., Otto, M.W. *et al.* (1996) Prevalence of panic in patients referred for pulmonary function testing at a major medical center. *Am J Psychiatry* **153**, 110–13.

Pols, H.J., Hauzer, R.C., Meijer, J.A., Verburg, K. & Griez, E.J. (1996b) Fluvoxamine attenuates panic induced by 35% CO_2 challenge. *J Clin Psychiatry* **57**, 539–42.

Pols, H., Lousberg, H., Zandbergen, J. & Griez, E. (1993) Panic disorder patients show decrease in ventilatory response to CO_2 after clomipramine treatment [letter]. *Psychiatry Res* **47**, 295–6.

Pols, H., Verburg, K., Hauzer, R., Meijer, J. & Griez, E. (1996a) Alprazolam premedication and 35% carbon dioxide vulnerability in panic patients. *Biol Psychiatry* **40**, 913–17.

Pols, H., Zandbergen, J., de Loof, C. & Griez, E. (1991) Attenuation of carbon dioxide induced panic after clonazepam treatment. *Acta Psychiatr Scand* **84**, 585–6.

Porzelius, J., Vest, M. & Nochomovitz, M. (1992) Respiratory function, cognitions, and panic in chronic obstructive pulmonary patients. *Behav Res Ther* **30**, 75–7.

Preter, M. & Klein, D.F. (1998) Panic disorder and the suffocation false alarm theory: current state of knowledge and further implications for neurobiologic theory testing. In: *The Panic Respiration Connection* (L. Bellodi & G. Perna (eds)). MDM Medical Media, Milan.

Rapee, R. (1986) Differential response to hyperventilation in panic disorder and generalized anxiety disorder. *J Abnorm Psychol* **95**, 24–8.

Rapee, R.M., Brown, T.A., Antony, M.M. & Barlow, D.H. (1992) Response to hyperventilation and inhalation of 5.5% carbon dioxide-enriched air across the DSM-III-R anxiety disorders. *J Abnorm Psychol* **101**, 538–52.

Roth, W.T., Wilhelm, F.H. & Trabert, W. (1998) Voluntary breath holding in panic and generalized anxiety disorders [see comments]. *Psychosom Med* **60**, 671–9.

de Ruiter, C., Garssen, B., Rijken, H. & Kraaimaat, F. (1989) The hyperventilation syndrome in panic disorder, agoraphobia and generalized anxiety disorder. *Behav Res Ther* **27**, 447–52.

Salkovskis, P.M., Jones, D.R. & Clark, D.M. (1986) Respiratory control in the treatment of panic attacks. Replication and extension with concurrent measurement of behaviour and P_{CO_2}. *Br J Psychiatry* **148**, 526–32.

Sanderson, W.C. & Wetzler, S. (1990) Five percent carbon dioxide challenge: valid analogue and marker of panic disorder? *Biol Psychiatry* **27**, 689–701.

Sanderson, W.C., Wetzler, S. & Asnis, G.M. (1994) Alprazolam blockade of CO_2-provoked panic in patients with panic disorder. *Am J Psychiatry* **151**, 1220–2.

Saper, C.B. (1987) Function of the locus coeruleus. *TINS* **10**(9), 343–4.

Schmidt, N.B., Telch, M.J. & Jaimez, T.L. (1996) Biological challenge manipulation of P_{CO_2} levels: a test of Klein's (1993) suffocation alarm theory of panic. *J Abnorm Psychol* **105**, 446–54.

Schruers, K., Klaassen, T., Pols, H., Overbeek, T., Deutz, N.E. & Griez, E. (2000) Effects of tryptophan depletion on carbon dioxide provoked panic in panic disorder patients. *Psychiatry Res* **93**, 179–87.

Schwartz, G.E., Goetz, R.R., Klein, D.F., Endicott, J. & Gorman, J.M. (1996) Tidal volume of respiration and "sighing" as indicators of breathing irregularities in panic disorder patients. *Anxiety* **2**, 145–8.

Shavitt, R.G., Gentil, V. & Mandetta, R. (1992) The association of panic/agoraphobia and asthma. Contributing factors and clinical implications. *Gen Hosp Psychiatry* **14**, 420–3.

Smoller, J.W. & Otto, M.W. (1998) Panic, dyspnea, and asthma. *Curr Opin Pulm Med* **4**, 40–5.

Spinhoven, P., Onstein, E.J. & Sterk, P.J. (1993) Hyperventilation: not a cause of panic attacks [see comments]. *Ned Tijdschr Geneeskd* **137**, 2315–18.

Spinhoven, P., Onstein, E.J., Sterk, P.J. & Le Haen-Versteijnen, D. (1992) The hyperventilation provocation test in panic disorder [published erratum appears in *Behav Res Ther* **31**(2), 237]. *Behav Res Ther* **30**, 453–61.

Spinhoven, P., Ros, M., Westgeest, A. & Van der Does, A.J. (1994) The prevalence of respiratory disorders in panic disorder, major depressive disorder and V-code patients. *Behav Res Ther* **32**, 647–9.

Stein, M.B., Millar, T.W., Larsen, D.K. & Kryger, M.H. (1995) Irregular breathing during sleep in patients with panic disorder. *Am J Psychiatry* **152**, 1168–73.

Svensson, T.H. (1987) Brain norepinephrine neurons in the locus coeruleus and the control of arousal and respiration: implications for sudden infant death syndrome. In: *Neurobiology of the Control of Breathing*. (C. van Euler & H. Lagercrantz (eds), pp. 297–301). Karolinska Institute Nobel Conference Series, Raven Press, New York.

Takeuchi, Y., McLean, J.H. & Hopkins, D.A. (1982) Reciprocal connections between the amygdala and parabrachial nuclei: ultrastructural demonstration by degeneration and axonal transport of horse radish peroxidase in the cat. *Brain Res* **239**, 583–8.

Uhde, T.W. (1990) Caffeine provocation of panic. Focus on biological mechanisms. In: *Neurobiology of Panic Disorder* (J.C. Ballanger (ed.)) Alan. R. Liss, New York.

Van den Hout, M.A. & Griez, E. (1984) Panic symptoms after inhalation of carbon dioxide. *Br J Psychiatry* **144**, 503–7.

Van Peski-Oosterbaan, A.S., Spinhoven, P., Van der Does, A.J., Willems, L.N. & Sterk, P.J. (1996) Is there a specific relationship between asthma and panic disorder? *Behav Res Ther* **34**, 333–40.

Veasey, S.C., Fornal, C.A., Metzler, C.W. & Jacob, B.L. (1997) Single unit responses of serotoninergic dorsal raphe neurons to specific motor challenges in freely moving cats. *Neuroscience* **75**, 161–9.

Verburg, K., de Leeuw, M., Pols, H., Griez, E. (1997) No dynamic lung function abnormalities in panic disorder patients. *Biol Psychiatry* **41**, 834–6.

Verburg, C., Griez, E. & Meijer, J. (1994) A 35% carbon dioxide challenge in simple phobias. *Acta Psychiatr Scand* **90**, 420–3.

Verburg, K., Griez, E., Meijer, J. & Pols, H. (1995a) Discrimination between panic disorder and generalized anxiety disorder by 35% carbon dioxide challenge. *Am J Psychiatry* **152**, 1081–3.

Verburg, K., Griez, E., Meijer, J. & Pols, H. (1995b) Respiratory disorders as a possible predisposing factor for panic disorder. *J Affect Disord* **33**, 129–34.

Whelan, R.F. & Young, I.M. (1953) The effect of adrenaline and noradrenaline infusions on respiration in man. *Br J Pharmacol* **8**, 98–102.

Wilhelm, F.H., Trabert, W. & Roth, W.T. (2001) Physiologic instability in panic disorder and generalized anxiety disorder. *Biol Psychiatry* **49**, 596–605.

Woods, S.W., Charney, D.S., Delgado, P.L. & Heninger, G.R. (1990) The effect of long-term imipramine treatment on carbon dioxide induced anxiety in panic disorder patients. *J Clin Psychiatry* **51**, 505–7.

Woods, S.W., Charney, D.S., Loke, J., Goodman, W.K., Redmond, D.E., Jr & Heninger, G.R. (1986) Carbon dioxide sensitivity in panic anxiety. Ventilatory and anxiogenic response to carbon dioxide in healthy subjects and patients with panic anxiety before and after alprazolam treatment. *Arch Gen Psychiatry* **43**, 900–9.

Woods, S.W., Krystal, J.H., Heninger, G.R. & Charney, D.S. (1989) Effects of alprazolam and clonidine on carbon dioxide induced increases in anxiety ratings in healthy human subjects. *Life Sci* **45**, 233–42.

Yellowlees, P.M., Alpers, J.H., Bowden, J.J., Bryant, G.D. & Ruffin, R.E. (1987) Psychiatric morbidity in patients with chronic airflow obstruction. *Med J Aust* **146**, 305–7.

Yellowlees, P.M., Haynes, S., Potts, N. & Ruffin, R.E. (1988) Psychiatric morbidity in patients with life-threatening asthma: initial report of a controlled study. *Med J Aust* **149**, 246–9.

Zandbergen, J., Bright, M., Pols, H., Fernandez, I., de Loof, C. & Griez, E.J. (1991a) Higher lifetime prevalence of respiratory diseases in panic disorder? *Am J Psychiatry* **148**, 1583–5.

Zandbergen, J., Lousberg, H.H., Pols, H., de Loof, C. & Griez, E.J. (1990) Hypercarbia versus hypocarbia in panic disorder. *J Affect Disord* **18**, 75–81.

Zandbergen, J., Pols, H., de Loof, C. & Griez, E.J. (1991b) Ventilatory response to CO_2 in panic disorder. *Psychiatry Res* **39**, 13–19.

Zandbergen, J., Strahm, M., Pols, H. & Griez, E.J. (1992) Breath-holding in panic disorder. *Compr Psychiatry* **33**, 47–51.

Zandbergen, J., van Aalst, V., de Loof, C., Pols, H. & Griez, E. (1993) No chronic hyperventilation in panic disorder patients. *Psychiatry Res* **47**, 1–6.

15 Pharmacological Challenge Agents In Anxiety

J. Swain, D. Koszycki, J. Shlik & J. Bradwejn

Introduction

The pharmacological induction of anxiety has been used experimentally to study adaptive and pathological anxiety under controlled conditions. Pharmacological models of anxiety have a number of potential uses; they can provide insight into the underlying pathophysiology of various anxiety disorders, they serve as tests to evaluate putative anxiolytic/antipanic compounds, they are a method for identifying at risk individuals, and they can be used as a diagnostic tool (Guttmacher *et al.* 1983). As pharmacological models of anxiety are an artificial representation of naturally occurring phenomena, they are useful only to the extent that they elicit features that reflect the diverse behavioral and neurochemical concomitants of clinical anxiety. Empirical validation of chemical models of anxiety using established criteria, such as those outlined by Guttmacher *et al.* (1983), represents an important step in the development of empirically valid chemical models of human anxiety.

By far the most extensively studied anxiety phenomenon is panic attacks, and the pharmacological probes that are used are called panicogens. Experimental limitations to the access of pathophysiological changes in the human brain during panic, along with its episodic and complex nature, have historically plagued scientific investigation into their nature. Pharmacological models of panic can provide researchers with insight into the endogenous neurocircuitry instrumental to the expression of panic attacks and stimulate the development of pharmacological interventions. The goal of this chapter is to review some of the best studied panicogens. We will first review existing criteria that

have been used to evaluate panicogens, and then propose modifications to these criteria against which panicogens are evaluated as models of panic. Against these modified criteria, we will then evaluate each panicogen.

Criteria for a panicogenic agent

Existing criteria for a panicogenic agent

According to the criteria outlined by Guttmacher *et al.* (1983) and Gorman *et al.* (1987) an ideal panicogenic agent should have the following properties:

1 The agent should be safe for routine administration to humans.

2 The agent should induce a sudden crescendo increase in both affective (e.g. anxiety, fear, apprehension) and somatic (e.g. dyspnea, palpitations, choking, sweating) symptoms of panic.

3 The agent should provoke panic attacks which approximate naturalistic ones. Rather than producing a stereotypical panic attack or one that is much different from a patient's usual experience, an ideal panicogen should elicit panic attacks that are identical or very similar to those normally experienced.

4 The agent should be specific to panic disorder (PD) patients: this can be expressed in one of two ways: *either* the induced attack occurs exclusively in PD patients (absolute specificity), *or* the induced attack occurs in PD patients at a lower dose relative to other subjects (threshold specificity).

5 Reactivity to the agent should be reliable on retesting without desensitization.

6 Reactivity to the agent should be blocked by antipanic drugs.

7 Reactivity to the agent should not be blocked by inert/nonantipanic drugs.

Expanded criteria for a panicogenic agent

In this chapter we propose the following modifications of these criteria. First, we have grouped the criteria in order to more easily breakdown discussion of each panicogen. Next we have made some amendments in order to include our increasingly sophisticated knowledge of how panicogens work, and how the brain works in health and mental illness.

Basic properties
1 The agent should be safe for routine administration to humans
2 The agent should induce a sudden crescendo increase in both affective (e.g. anxiety, fear, apprehension) and somatic (e.g. dyspnea, palpitations, choking, sweating) symptoms of panic.
3 The agent should provoke panic attacks that approximate naturalistic ones. Rather than producing a stereotypical panic attack or one that is much different from a patient's usual experience, an ideal panicogen should elicit panic attacks that are *identical or very similar* to those normally experienced.
4 Reactivity to the agent should be reliable on retesting without desensitization.

Specificity
5a *Syndrome specificity.* The agent should be *relatively* specific to PD versus normal controls and other psychiatric syndromes. That is, the threshold to panic should be lower in PD versus other diagnostic groups.
5b *Symptom specificity.* The agent should trigger mechanisms which are specific to panic attacks and not elicit core symptoms of other anxiety syndromes (e.g. flashbacks in post-traumatic stress disorder (PTSD)).

Clinical validation
6 Reactivity to the agent should be blocked by antipanic drugs.
7 Reactivity to the agent should not be blocked by inert/nonantipanic agents.

Physiology
8 Behavioral response to the agent should be accompanied by broad cardiorespiratory activation.
9 Behavioral response to the agent should be accompanied by activation of the hypothalamic–pituitary–adrenal (HPA) axis.

Explanation of the expansion
In addition to the basic properties that a panicogen might possess in order to make it a useful investigative tool, ongoing research has revealed much regarding the symptoms and disease specificity as well as physiological mechanism. Most panicogens show relative specificity to elicit panic attacks in PD patients over control subjects rather than the absolute specificity, or provocation of panic only in PD patients, which was previously expected. In addition, panicogens have been shown to have a differential effectiveness to elicit panic attacks in patients with different anxiety disorders. This may suggest differential involvement of different neuroanatomical substrates and different organ systems in different anxiety disorders, and further that these brain circuits are present in normal healthy volunteers. Perhaps panic attacks do not involve the expression of a totally different brain circuitry, but rather a differential homeostasis of the same circuits that operate in health and different anxiety disorders. Further delineation and analysis of these critical systems will lead to a better understanding of panic as it occurs in different illnesses.

On the other side of syndrome selectivity of panicogenic agents is the issue of symptom selectivity of the agent. Investigators have explored whether panicogens could elicit core symptoms of other anxiety disorders, such as flashbacks in PTSD, blushing and a sense of being scrutinized in social anxiety disorder (SAD), obsessions and compulsions in obsessive-compulsive disorder (OCD), and persistent uncontrollable worry in generalized anxiety disorder (GAD) with some positive results. Although it is tantalizing to consider the possibility that there might be pharmacological challenges that can provoke symptoms of other anxiety syndromes besides panic attacks and allow study of these phenomena, such properties would not be in keeping with the idea of an "ideal" panicogen. The interpretation of these data is complex as the elicitation of nonpanic anxiety by a panicogen may mean that panic circuits have been rewired to cause other symptoms in a diseased brain, that the same circuits used in panic are being reused in different anxiety phenomena, or that the challenge agent is simply nonspecific. When a panicogen does elicit core symptoms of other anxiety syndromes it may not be "ideal," but the results do provoke interesting discussion of the biological underpinnings of these varied experiences.

We have also added criteria of physiological activation in order to help distinguish mechanisms at work in panic. Studies of "placebo" provoked panic attacks with no active chemical provocation have yielded much information about the basic properties of panic anxiety. These situationally provoked panic attacks are associated with increased cardiorespiratory activation such as heart rate, blood pressure, and minute ventilation beginning immediately before subjective symptoms of a panic attack (Goetz *et al.* 1993). We contend that panicogens should ideally activate the cardiorespiratory axis. In addition to the more obvious cardiorespiratory activation in panic, there is emerging recognition of the involvement of the HPA axis in the mediation of many forms of anxiety including panic (Charney & Bremner 1999). These differences in hormonal profile are starting to contribute significantly to discussions of the etiology of all anxiety disorders. In situational panic attacks there is evidence of the activation of the HPA axis with increases in serum cortisol and growth hormone (Woods *et al.* 1987). In addition, there is increased plasma prolactin and changes in cortisol and growth hormone (Cameron *et al.* 1987) as well as increases in salivary cortisol (Bandelow *et al.* 2000) with spontaneous panic attacks.

It is exciting that our definition of "core" anxiety symptoms of each anxiety disorder is still evolving and may be increasingly biologically orientated. So far, nosology has been largely driven by externally observed or reported phenomenology rather than direct brain activity measures. Challenge studies will continue to help determine future classification of anxiety. As brain imaging improves, it may be possible to use an array of pharmacological challenge agents with different profiles of anxiety elicitation to correlate signs and symptoms of different disorders with brain activity and perhaps even tailor treatments according to brain responses to challenges.

Agent-by-agent review of panicogens

Table 15.1 lists the panicogens that will be reviewed in this chapter, grouped according to their putative mechanism of action.

Sodium lactate

Sodium lactate is one of the most extensively studied panicogens, having been discussed in relation to anxiety since the 1940s. It was found that patients with the old diagnosis of "anxiety neurosis" developed higher levels of blood lactate with a standard exercise challenge (Cohen & White 1951), suggesting that it is associated with anxiety. This led to the first intravenous infusion of lactate in patients with anxiety neurosis to provoke anxiety attacks in 1967 (Pitts & McClure 1967). As a putative panicogen, this agent fulfils basic panicogen criteria and shows relative specificity, but it elicits other core anxiety symptoms and its physiological effects are inconsistent.

Basic properties

Detailed phenomenological work has shown that standard infusions (about 0.5 M sodium lactate solution at 10 mL/kg over about 20 min) of sodium lactate safely provokes panic attacks which include both affective and somatic symptoms of panic and which resemble patients' naturally occurring attacks (Liebowitz *et al.* 1984; Rainey *et al.* 1984a; Goetz *et al.* 1996). The reliability of lactate to produce panic attacks on repeated testing has not been studied, and in fact may be in question. Bonn *et al.* (1971) noted a decrease in anxiety with 3 weeks of twice-weekly lactate provocations, suggesting a possible therapeutic use of lactate to decrease anxiety. However, more recent work showed only a decrease in preinfusion anxiety on three serial infusions at 1-week intervals with essentially no change in panic attack frequency in PD patients (Yeragani *et al.* 1988).

Specificity

It has been consistently shown that PD patients are more vulnerable to lactate-induced panic than normal controls (Liebowitz *et al.* 1984; Rainey *et al.* 1984a; Balon *et al.* 1988; Aronson *et al.* 1989; Den Boer *et al.* 1989; Cowley & Arana 1990). Lactate hypersensitivity is also evident in other conditions. Patients with

Agent	Putative mechanism
Metabolic/respiratory (nonspecific) stimulants	
Sodium lactate	Metabolic or direct
Sodium bicarbonate	Induces metabolic alkalosis
CO_2	Stimulant of medullary chemoreceptors
Doxapram	Stimulant of carotid chemoreceptors
Caffeine	Intracellular modulator
Noradrenergic	
Norepinephrine*	Adrenergic agonist
Yohimbine	Adrenergic α_2-receptor antagonist
Isoproterenol	Peripheral β-receptor agonist
Serotonergic	
Fenfluramine	5-HT releaser + reuptake inhibitor
mCPP	Nonselective agonist of 5-HT receptors
GABAergic	
Flumazenil	GABA antagonist/inverse agonist
Peptidergic	
CCK-4	Agonist of CCK-B receptor
Pentagastrin	Agonist of CCK-B receptor

Table 15.1 Panicogens reviewed in this chapter grouped according to their putative mechanism of action.

*Noradrenaline.

CCK, cholecystokinin; CCK-4, cholecystokinin-tetrapeptide; CO_2, carbon dioxide; GABA, γ-aminobutyric acid; 5-HT, 5-hydroxtryptamine; mCPP, *m*-chlorophenylpiperazine.

GAD panicked at higher rates than controls, but not as high as PD patients (Cowley *et al.* 1988), suggesting that there may be some shared mechanisms involved in the panic of GAD and PD, but perhaps some important differences as well. Patients with premenstrual dysphoric disorder (PMDD) (Facchinetti *et al.* 1992; Sandberg *et al.* 1993) and fibromyalgia (Tanum & Malt 1995) are also more prone to panic with lactate infusion than normal controls. Bulimic patients demonstrated an enhanced sensitivity to lactate-induced anxiety but not panic than controls (George *et al.* 1987; Pohl *et al.* 1989), but in another study, lactate-induced panic was less in bulimics than controls (Lindy *et al.* 1988). Patients with SAD and OCD have been found to respond very similarly to lactate as healthy controls (Gorman *et al.* 1985; Liebowitz *et al.* 1985a). In addition, there appears to be no significant effect of depression on lactate-induced panic among panic patients (Cowley *et al.* 1986; Buller *et al.* 1989; Targum 1990), or nonpanic patients (Cowley *et al.* 1987). Overall, the data suggest that patients with PD, GAD, PMDD,

fibromyalgia and possibly bulimia may share some neurobiological characteristics that render them all the more sensitive to lactate-induced panic that differentiate them from patients with SAD, OCD and depression.

As for the symptom-specificity of lactate, one study found flashbacks associated with panic attacks induced by lactate in combat veterans with PTSD and comorbid PD (Rainey *et al.* 1987), and another study demonstrated flashbacks in noncombat-related PTSD patients (Jensen *et al.* 1997). This work suggests that lactate may be a useful probe to study flashbacks and perhaps other dissociative phenomena, but it renders lactate a less than ideal panicogen according to our criteria as it elicits more than just panic. In addition, lactate has been shown to elicit rage symptoms in perpetrators of domestic violence (George *et al.* 2000), further clouding its specificity.

Clinical validation

Various antipanic agents have been tested as to their ability to block lactate-induced panic. Acute treatment with the benzodiazepines alprazolam (Cowley *et al.* 1991) and diazepam (Liebowitz *et al.* 1995), and the adrenergic antagonist clonidine (Coplan *et al.* 1992a), as well as long-term treatment with tricyclic antidepressants (Rifkin *et al.* 1981; Yeragani *et al.* 1988), monoamine oxidase (MAO) inhibitors (Kelly *et al.* 1971), and benzodiazepines (Carr *et al.* 1986; Pohl *et al.* 1994) all partially reduce sensitivity to lactate-induced anxiety in PD patients. However, acute administration of the β-adrenergic blocker, propranolol, was ineffective at blocking or modulating lactate-induced panic in PD and control subjects (Gorman *et al.* 1983). Since there is no identified lactate receptor no specific lactate blocker has been studied. Placebo nonblocking has been demonstrated in the above studies.

Physiology

Increases in heart rate, blood pressure and hyperventilation have been found to accompany lactate-induced panic (Liebowitz *et al.* 1985b; Gorman *et al.* 1988a; Cowley & Arana 1990). It is interesting that no consistent correlation between lactate challenge and plasma HPA-axis hormones, including cortisol, prolactin, luteinizing hormone and growth hormone, has been demonstrated (Liebowitz *et al.* 1985b, 1986; Carr *et al.* 1986; Levin *et al.* 1987; Hollander *et al.* 1989; Targum 1992). However, an analysis of 10 years of lactate studies at one institution suggested that high plasma cortisol is a factor in the preinfusion period that predisposes subjects to lactate-induced panic (Coplan *et al.* 1998). The authors of this study postulated that HPA-axis activation may be specific to anticipatory anxiety rather than to acute panic itself. One possible explanation of HPA axis nonresponsiveness in lactate-induced panic has been offered by Kellner *et al.* (1995, 1998). They relate that lactate increases atrial naturetic factor (ANF) by increasing cardiac output. Apparently ANF suppresses cortisol release. On the other hand, however, other panicogens also increase cardiac output, yet do cause a cortisol response. Prolactin is the one pituitary hormone that increases with lactate infusion, but it occurs in subjects whether or not they panic, possibly reflecting a response to the osmotic stress of the infusion (Hollander *et al.* 1989).

Mechanisms

Several hypothetical mechanisms of sodium lactate-induced panic have been proposed and debated. They range from nonspecific metabolic or neurovascular mechanisms to indirect mechanisms involving neurohormones, to stimulation of a specific receptor or the anatomically susceptible brain region.

After it was discovered that the inhalation of 5% carbon dioxide (CO_2) induced panic, it was proposed that both lactate infusion and CO_2 inhalation caused increasing P_{CO_2}, which acted on central (medullary) chemoreceptors to cause panic. However, intravenous lactate in nonhuman primates did not change cisternal P_{CO_2} during or after lactate infusion (Dager *et al.* 1990). In addition, there was poor correlation between lactate-induced panic and depression of plasma ionized calcium or phosphate, epinephrine (adrenaline), norepinephrine (noradrenaline), or cortisol increase (Liebowitz *et al.* 1985b, 1986). Finally, glucose, but not chloride, co-administration with lactate reduced the sensitivity of both healthy volunteers and PD patients to panic with lactate infusion, perhaps due to sympathetic attenuation (George *et al.* 1995).

As for the possibility of a lactate receptor, none have been found and infusion of the supposedly inactive enantiomer of L-lactate, D-lactate, is actually similarly panicogenic (Gorman *et al.* 1990a), further confirming the need for lactate metabolism for lactate-induced panic, and requiring any possible lactate receptor to be similarly stimulated by the two enantiomers. A simpler explanation of these data is that both lactate enantiomers act by causing alkalosis, which in turn, activates a panic circuit. However, PD patients who panicked with lactate did not develop greater plasma alkalosis than nonpanicking patients (Liebowitz *et al.* 1986), suggesting that no absolute pH threshold exists for panic to occur in vulnerable patients. In addition, alkalosis induction by hyperventilation (Gorman *et al.* 1984) or bicarbonate infusion (Gorman *et al.* 1989) has been less effective than lactate infusion to cause panic.

Brain imaging work with lactate has focused on finding specific neuroanatomical regions of differential activity with lactate-induced panic. Work with positron emission tomography (PET) and proton magnetic resonance spectroscopy (MRS) has raised the question of increased uptake of lactate in temporoparietal cortex in lactate-induced panic (Reiman *et al.* 1986, 1989), but methodological difficulties have forced retraction (Drevets *et al.* 1992). Shekhar and Keim (1997) suggest a circumventricular brain region (the organum vasculosum lamina terminalis) which is not well-protected by the blood–brain barrier, as a lactate-sensitive site whose activation leads to autonomic activation and panic when γ-aminobutyric acid (GABA) neurotransmission is inhibited in the dorsomedial hypothalamus. These investigators propose a mechanism for the panicogenesis of lactate that involves direct stimulation of this brain region by lactate, resulting in activation of a compromised panic-generating circuit such as the dorsomedial hypothalamus or amygdala. However, this hypothesis is contradicted by Dager *et al.* (1999), who failed to find any distinct regional patterns of brain lactate rise to support any specific neuroanatomical substrate of lactate-induced panic. This result brings us back to the concept of lactate as a relatively nonspecific metabolic or neurovascular panic-inducing irritant.

The neurotransmitter mechanisms involved in lactate-induced panic are not fully understood. The apparent lack of effect of intravenous propranolol on lactate-induced panic suggests that this agent does not produce its effects via β-adrenergic mechanisms (Gorman *et al.* 1983). However, lactate vulnerability is decreased with clonidine, implicating the α-adrenergic system as a possible mechanism. GABAergic mechanisms may also play a role in lactate-panic. Pretreatment with benzodiazepines (e.g. Cowley *et al.* 1991) and the mood stabilizer valproate (which enhances GABA neurotransmission) (Keck *et al.* 1993) block lactate-panic, and lactate infusion decreases serum GABA (Balon *et al.* 1993). Lactate-blockade with tricyclic anti-depressants (Yeragani *et al.* 1988) and MAOIs (Kelly *et al.* 1971) also suggest that serotonin and noradrenergic mechanisms are important in some aspects of lactate-induced panic.

Other possible mechanisms of lactate vulnerability include psychological factors, such as cognitive and behavioral reactivity (Shear 1986), and genetics. Shear *et al.* (1991) reported that cognitive behavior therapy partially decreased lactate sensitivity, presumably by altering the tendency of patients to catastrophically misinterpret arousal symptoms. Evidence for a genetic influence on lactate vulnerability is supported by findings that patients whose lactate-induced panic resembled their clinical panic had a greater familial risk for panic attacks than relatives of those who responded to lactate in a nonnaturalistic way, or had no response (Cowley & Dunner 1988). Another study found that relatives of healthy volunteers who panicked in response to lactate had a higher rate of anxiety disorders than did relatives of nonpanicking healthy volunteers (Balon

et al. 1989). However, comparing first-degree relatives of PD patients who responded to lactate to nonresponders failed to find any differences in lactate sensitivity (Reschke *et al.* 1995). This work is still unclear because of methodological difficulties such as small sample sizes, and further work is required to show any genetic aspect to lactate sensitivity or define a genotypically distinct PD subtype that is more lactate-sensitive.

In summary, lactate is a safe and effective panicogen but appears to be a nonspecific brain irritant that may affect a number of brain areas, apparently without activating hormonal systems.

Hypertonic saline

Acute increases in serum sodium or osmolarity by hypertonic saline can produce panic without alkalosis (Jensen *et al.* 1991), but there is little detailed work using this challenge agent in the literature. Various specific explanatory hypotheses have been proposed but not yet studied. Hypertonic saline is equivalent to lactate in inducing panic and increases in serum sodium, and plasma vasopressin in PD patients, with no normal controls experiencing panic (Peskind *et al.* 1998). Likely, hypertonic saline may present a relatively nonspecific stressor like lactate with some differential sensitivity seen in PD.

Carbon dioxide

Like sodium lactate, CO_2 has received considerable empirical attention in relation to its panicogenic properties (see also Chapter 14). This agent fulfils basic criteria and shows relative specificity but its physiological effects are inconsistent.

Basic properties

Inhalation of CO_2-enriched air has been shown to cause safe (Harrington *et al.* 1996), dose-related panic attacks in adults (Woods *et al.* 1988a,b,c). Methods include continuous breathing of 5% or 7.5% CO_2 to a point of panic (Gorman *et al.* 1984), as well as single-breath inhalation of 35% CO_2 (van den Hout & Griez 1984). Inhalation of low concentrations of CO_2 has also been shown to safely provoke anxiety and panic attacks in children with anxiety disorders (Pine *et al.* 1998, 2000). The CO_2 challenge provokes crescendo increases in affective and somatic symptoms of panic in an apparently naturalistic fashion. Test–retest reliability of CO_2-induced anxiety has been demonstrated in patients with PD (Perna *et al.* 1994; Bertani *et al.* 1997; Verburg *et al.* 1998), although desensitization to frequent repeated administration of CO_2 has also been reported (Griez & van den Hout 1986). CO_2 has not been found to reliably induce panic attacks in healthy volunteers (Coryell & Arndt 1999), but this may be due to variability in inhalation patterns of subjects across trials.

Specificity

It has been consistently demonstrated that vulnerability to CO_2-induced panic is enhanced in PD patients versus normal controls (Woods *et al.* 1986; Papp *et al.* 1989). In addition, subjects who experience sporadic panic attacks but who do not meet criteria for PD react similarly to CO_2 as patients with PD but more intensely than healthy controls, suggesting that CO_2 sensitivity may be a trait marker of panic attacks rather than PD (Perna *et al.* 1995a). Exaggerated response to CO_2 is not limited to PD since individuals suffering from SAD (Papp *et al.* 1993; Caldirola *et al.* 1997), specific phobias (Verburg *et al.* 1994; Antony *et al.* 1997) and PMDD (Kent *et al.* 2001) are more likely to panic with CO_2 than normal controls. However, the threshold of panic vulnerability appears to be lower in PD relative to these other disorders (Caldirola *et al.* 1997; Kent *et al.* 2001). Enhanced vulnerability to CO_2-induced panic has not been observed in patients with GAD (Verburg *et al.* 1995; Perna *et al.* 1999a), although one study (Verburg *et al.* 1995) noted that GAD and PD patients exhibited comparable increases in somatic symptoms of panic, suggesting some common characteristics in these illnesses. Patients with OCD (Perna *et al.* 1995b) and major depression (Perna *et al.* 1995c; Kent *et al.* 2001) react similarly to CO_2 as healthy controls. These data suggest that there is a spectrum of CO_2 vulnerability, with sensitivity being lowest in OCD, major depression and normal control subjects and highest in PD. So far, CO_2 inhalation is not known to elicit core symptoms of other anxiety disorders.

Clinical validation

Several antipanic drugs have been shown to attenuate vulnerability to CO_2-panic in PD patients. CO_2-blockade has been demonstrated with long-term treatment with imipramine (Woods *et al.* 1990), fluvoxamine (Pols *et al.* 1996a), alprazolam (Woods *et al.* 1986) and clonazepam (Pols *et al.* 1991). Reactivity to CO_2 is

also diminished following 1-week treatment with the reversible MAOI toloxatone, the tricyclic antidepressants imipramine and clomipramine, and the selective serotonin reuptake inhibitors (SSRIs) paroxetine, fluvoxamine and sertraline (Perna *et al.* 1994; Bertani *et al.* 1997; Perna *et al.* 1997). Blockade of CO_2-induced panic following acute alprazolam treatment has been demonstrated in some (Woods *et al.* 1989; Sanderson *et al.* 1994; Nardi *et al.* 2000) but not all studies (Pols *et al.* 1996b). Methodological differences may account for variable results. It is also notable that consumption of alcohol diminishes sensitivity to CO_2 in PD patients (Kushner *et al.* 1996), a finding that sheds light on the mechanisms which contribute to high rates of alcohol abuse in PD. Placebo nonblocking has been shown in the above studies.

Physiology

CO_2-induced panic is associated with cardiorespiratory activation including increased respiratory rate and blunted tidal volume response, tachycardia, and increased blood pressure (Gorman *et al.* 1988b; Papp *et al.* 1997; Bystritsky *et al.* 2000; Bailey *et al.* 2001). Surprisingly, the effect of CO_2 challenge on HPA-axis activity has not been extensively studied and existing studies have produced disparate results. Sinha *et al.* (1999) found that inhalation of low doses of CO_2 (5% or 7%) did not produce significant increases in cortisol release in either PD patients or normal controls, suggesting that this panicogen does not activate the HPA axis. However, Bailey *et al.* (2001) recently found that inhalation of 35% CO_2 increased cortisol release in normal controls. Methodological differences may account for disparate findings. Clearly, further research is needed to clarify CO_2's effect on the HPA axis.

Mechanisms

The mechanisms of CO_2-induced panic have been the subject of much attention and debate with much comparison to lactate. It makes sense that inhalation of CO_2 and the resultant acidosis might be associated with compensatory hyperventilation as in a panic attack (Gorman *et al.* 1990b). However, the body's normal homeostatic response to a metabolic alkalosis, which also occurs with lactate challenge, is hypoventilation, as a compensatory measure, resulting in normalizing an elevated blood pH. Yet during naturally occurring panic attacks PD patients paradoxically hyperventilate, suggesting that the attacks (whether they are associated with the respiratory acidosis of CO_2 inhalation, the metabolic alkalosis of lactate, or PD with a normal serum pH) involve hyperventilation—even when it might result in an abnormal serum pH.

It has been hypothesized that PD patients are prone to hyperventilate because of a hypersensitive "suffocation alarm" (Klein 1993) system whereby increasing P_{CO_2} and brain lactate concentrations prematurely activates a physiological asphyxia monitor. A number of groups have tried to test this hypothesis. Asmundson and Stein (1994) attempted to test the "suffocation alarm theory" of panic by examining the length of time patients with PD could hold their breath. Indeed, they found that these patients could hold their breath for significantly less time than controls despite no end-tidal CO_2 differences. Along these lines, Pine and associates (Pine et al. 1994) demonstrated that subjects who are unable to perceive hypercapnia because of a congenital central hypoventilation syndrome (CCHS) exhibited a trend towards decreased rates of anxiety disorders compared to children with asthma, and also significantly fewer anxiety symptoms than controls. In addition, Biber and Alkin (1999) found that panic patients with prominent respiratory symptoms were more sensitive to CO_2 challenge. This suggests that CO_2 may differentiate a possible respiratory versus nonrespiratory type of PD.

Other studies do not support the universality of the "suffocation alarm" theory of panic attacks. Schmidt and associates (Schmidt et al. 1996) found significant numbers of PD patients who did not experience panic attacks despite inspired P_{CO_2} levels in excess of 100 times room air. They argue that response to CO_2 can be explained cognitively, as do many others (e.g., Salkovskis & Clark 1990). Many have proposed that a wide range of biochemical panicogens, including CO_2, work by creating physical sensations associated with panic which may be overinterpreted by the brains of PD patients and lead to the activation of panic circuits, rather than via the stimulation of some specific biochemical pathway. However, the mitigating effect of cognitive mediational variables on CO_2 vulnerability has not been supported in all studies (reviewed by Nutt & Lawson 1992; Koszycki & Bradwejn 2001).

Another possible explanatory theory is that hyperventilation leads to local relative vasoconstriction in the brains of PD patients (Mathew & Wilson 1988), presumably leading to "panic circuit" activation, which would be more sensitive than controls to blood flow changes.

Others have looked for differences in neurotransmission to explain sensitivity to CO_2-induced panic. Panicogenicity to CO_2 inhalation is increased with serotonin antagonism with metergoline (Ben-Zion et al. 1999) and tryptophan depletion (Miller et al. 2000; Schruers et al. 2000) and decreased with SSRIs (Pols et al. 1996a; Bertani et al. 1997; Perna et al. 1997). These data, in addition to studies demonstrating blockade of CO_2-panic with benzodiazepines and tricyclics antidepressants, suggest that serotonin, GABA and noradrenergic neurotransmission are important in some aspect of CO_2-induced panic.

The influence of genetics on CO_2-induced panic has also been considered. An Italian group has amassed fascinating evidence that CO_2 sensitivity reflects a trait marker that runs in families (Perna et al. 1995d, 1999b; Bellodi et al. 1998). These researchers suggest that CO_2 sensitivity may be considered a phenotypic expression of an underlying genetic vulnerability that may exist before the clinical onset of PD (Cavallini et al. 1999). Genetic mechanisms proposed include differential expression of chemoreceptors and neurotransmitter system activation. The ultimate isolation of genetic markers could lead to preventative measures for vulnerable individuals.

In summary, CO_2 is another safe and effective panicogen that has been considered to work primarily by stimulating hyperventilation. It remains to be understood whether sensitivity to CO_2 and the associated hyperventilation is a characteristic of all normal subjects and PD patients when they have panic attacks (part of standard "panic circuits," for instance). It is possible that CO_2 sensitivity is associated with a specific subtype of PD, a hypersensitive homeostatic response ("suffocation alarm"), or simply an indirect cause of panic through nonspecific irritation of any number of chemical or mechanical receptors.

Caffeine

Caffeine is a xanthine derivative that is widely used as a psychostimulant. The results of a self-report survey demonstrating that PD patients are more reactive to caffeine than normal controls and affectively ill patients (Boulenger et al. 1984), suggested that the caffeine challenge might be a useful biological model of panic. This agent fulfils some basic criteria, but is unreliable and has a complex physiology.

Basic properties

Large amounts (e.g., 480–720 mg) of oral or intravenous administration of caffeine safely produces symptoms of anxiety and panic attacks in humans with only the complication of a mild headache. Caffeine-induced panic attacks include both somatic and affective aspects of panic (Uhde *et al*. 1984; Charney *et al*. 1985). The extent to which the panic attacks induced by caffeine may be naturalistic has not been systematically examined. The core signs of caffeine-induced anxiety include a number of nonpanic symptoms, including restlessness, excitement, insomnia and diuresis. Also, unlike other panicogens which may elicit discrete attacks which resolve over minutes, caffeine-provoked panic is associated with longer lasting anxiety symptoms that last many hours beyond the panic attack that may be more akin to GAD. A dose dependence of caffeine-induced anxiety was shown in healthy volunteers, but only one of 10 subjects experienced a panic attack (Nickell & Uhde 1995). Tolerance has been demonstrated (reviewed by Nehlig *et al*. 1992) making it an unreliable challenge agent.

Specificity

Caffeine-induced panic attacks are relatively specific to PD (Charney *et al*. 1985; Uhde 1990; Beck & Berisford 1992) as healthy volunteers rarely panic with this agent (Nickell & Uhde 1995). In addition to panic attacks, longer-lasting anxiety induced by caffeine including insomnia and increased blood pressure occur at an increased rate and intensity in PD patients than healthy volunteers (Charney *et al*. 1985; Uhde 1990). This suggests PD patients are differentially sensitive to experience both long- and short-term anxiety caused by caffeine, such that the brain circuits used for panic, as well as experiences of anxiety that are subthreshold to panic, are both altered in PD.

Other anxiety disorders have been studied to determine whether caffeine-induced panic is specific to PD. Patients with GAD appear to be even more sensitive to caffeine than PD patients in the elicitation of anxiety symptoms (Bruce *et al*. 1992). However, caffeine-induced panic anxiety does not appear to be different between SAD and normal control subjects, and the symptoms induced in the SAD group did not mimic their naturally occurring symptoms (Tancer *et al*. 1991). Finally, no hypersensitivity to caffeine was detected in patients with depersonalization disorder (Stein & Uhde 1989). There is a great deal of work on the possible

association of caffeine intake to agitated depression, but it is unclear whether excess caffeine intake and anxiety is a cause or result of depression (reviewed by Nehlig *et al*. 1992). In addition, caffeine may cause exacerbation of psychosis, psychosis *de novo*, aggravate schizophrenia, and induce olfactory hallucinations (Lucas *et al*. 1990; Nickell & Uhde 1995). These findings point to less specific actions of caffeine.

Clinical validation

So far, no antipanic drugs have been tested as to their ability to block caffeine-induced panic, nor has placebo nonblocking been shown.

Physiology

Interestingly, although caffeine does increase the cardiorespiratory parameter of blood pressure, it has inconsistent effects on pulse, including one report of a decreased pulse (Charney *et al*. 1984a; Uhde 1990). There is little mention of respiratory changes in the literature. The caffeine challenge (480 mg) has been shown to increase plasma cortisol but not prolactin (Klein *et al*. 1991; Lovallo *et al*. 1996). Thus caffeine does appear to partially activate the HPA axis.

Mechanism

The highly complex mechanisms of caffeine action have been the subject of much investigation. It appears to act via multifaceted mechanisms including mobilization of intracellular calcium, phosphodiesterase inhibition (leading to increased intracellular cAMP), antagonism of adenosine receptors, and benzodiazepine receptor antagonism (reviewed by Nehlig *et al*. 1992). In addition, caffeine increases plasma levels of the tryptophan metabolite kynurenine (a neuroactive metabolite of tryptophan which is a precursor of 5-hydroxytryptamine [5-HT]) in healthy volunteers (Orlikov & Ryzov 1991), suggesting involvement of 5-HT systems in caffeine action. Imaging studies of cerebral blood flow using PET show significant decreases with caffeine infusion in healthy subjects as well as PD patients, but associated increases in glucose utilization (Cameron *et al*. 1990). These studies suggest that decreased cerebral blood flow is a relatively nonspecific effect, not solely responsible for caffeine-induced panic.

In summary, caffeine is a complex agent that produces anxiety symptoms and panic attacks. Caffeine vulnerability is higher in PD and GAD patients than normal controls, with the highest sensitivity in GAD. Its mechanism of action is complex and includes multiple neurotransmitter system involvement. Unfortunately, its complex modes of action limits the interpretation of results and its usefulness in research.

Doxapram

Doxapram is a central nervous system chemoreceptor stimulant that can activate the cerebrospinal axis at all levels depending on concentration (Calverley *et al.* 1983). At low intravenous doses it is a respiratory stimulant and panicogen (Lee *et al.* 1993) without affecting growth hormone, adrenocorticotrophic hormone or cortisol (Abelson *et al.* 1996). Unfortunately, its use is limited by risk of seizures.

Norepinephrine/epinephrine

It is well established that abnormalities in the autonomic nervous system are involved in mediating anxiety and there is a literature describing the use of epinephrine and norepinephrine to induce panic. As a putative panicogen, these agents fulfil the basic criteria but are still not well studied and the physiology is complex.

Basic properties
When infused intravenously to produce an artificial adrenergic signal, anxiety symptoms including panic attacks may be safely elicited. Panic attacks caused by norepinephrine (Pyke & Greenberg 1986) and epinephrine (Veltman *et al.* 1996, 1998; van Zijderveld *et al.* 1997) infusion include idiosyncratic symptoms closely resembling patients' spontaneous panic attacks, which include affective and somatic symptoms. The test–retest reliability of norepinephrine/epinephrine-induced panic has not been systematically studied.

Specificity
Epinephrine elicits anxiety but not panic attacks in healthy controls (van Zijderveld *et al.* 1992). Patients with PD are more likely to experience a panic attack with epinephrine infusion than normal controls (Veltman *et al.* 1996). This hypersensitivity does not appear to be related to preinfusion anxiety (Veltman *et al.* 1998). Infusion of epinephrine to patients with SAD provoked a panic attack in only one of 11 patients, suggesting that epinephrine-induced panic is specific to PD.

Clinical validation
Although it might be expected that norepinephrine blockers would attenuate the panicogenic effects of norepinephrine, this has not yet been studied. Possible placebo blocking has not been studied either.

Physiology
Panic attacks induced by norepinephrine were associated with cardiorespiratory activation, though some inconsistency was reported (Pyke & Greenberg 1986). Blood pressure increased, but heart rate decreased despite subjective reports of palpitations. With epinephrine infusion, increases in heart rate, blood pressure, and respiration as noted by decreased P_{CO_2} have been observed (Veltman *et al.* 1996). The association of epinephrine-induced panic attacks and the HPA axis has not been directly studied.

Mechanisms
Considerable preclinical and clinical data suggest that abnormal brain adrenergic and noradrenergic function is associated with the development of anxiety and fear (reviewed by Charney *et al.* 1990; Abelson *et al.* 1992). It is a central mediator of sympathetic ("fight or flight") activation and is associated with natural states of anxiety. However, epinephrine preferentially activates different β-adrenoreceptors, while norepinephrine preferentially activates α-receptors, and these pharmacological agents do not cross the blood–brain barrier, limiting their use as panicogens. There is little support for the role of cognitive mechanisms in epinephrine-induced panic. van Zijderveld *et al.* (1999) found that increased respiration and associated fall in transcutaneous P_{CO_2} correlated with the frequency of anxiety symptoms and not the fear of these symptoms. This finding suggests that the basis of epinephrine-induced panic is likely based on biological supersensitivity to the panicogen rather than cognitive distortions of bodily sensations.

Other adrenergic agents

Certain other adrenergic agents have been used to study the phenomenon of panic and the possible dysregulation of noradrenergic pathways in anxiety disorders. Both agonists and antagonists may induce anxiety likely by virtue of differential effects on pre- and postsynaptic central and peripheral receptors.

Yohimbine

This agent fulfills basic criteria for an ideal panicogen but elicits other core anxiety symptoms and is only partly blockable by antipanic drugs.

Basic properties

Yohimbine is an α_2-receptor antagonist that has been shown to safely induce panic attacks when administered by mouth (<20 mg) or intravenously (<0.8 mg/kg). It provokes affective and somatic components of panic attacks in adults and children (Charney et al. 1984b; Sallee et al. 2000). The question of naturalism of yohimbine-induced panic has been raised as its effects include nonpanic symptoms such as euphoria, lacrimation and rhinnorhea. Thus far, test–retest reliability has not been systematically examined.

Specificity

PD patients respond with panic attacks to yohimbine challenge with a much higher frequency than healthy controls. Further, sensitivity to yohimine is not enhanced in patients with depression, schizophrenia, GAD and OCD (Charney et al. 1987a; Rasmussen et al. 1987; Heninger et al. 1988; Charney et al. 1989; Guthrie et al. 1993). However, specificity of yohimbine is not limited to PD as individuals suffering from PTSD are more likely to panic with yohimbine than controls (Southwick et al. 1997). This suggests more severe abnormalities in catecholamine hormone regulation shared by PD and PTSD, perhaps related to the similarly episodic nature of both core symptoms of panic attacks and flashbacks. Yohimbine causes a heightened anxiety (though not panic per se) in children with anxiety disorders, primarily separation anxiety disorder (Sallee et al. 2000). In addition to panic, yohimbine administration has been shown to elicit flashback phenomena in combat-related as well as noncombat-related PTSD patients (Southwick et al. 1999). However, yohimbine was not found to elicit core symptoms of OCD (Rasmussen et al. 1987). Overall, yohimbine does not meet the ideal panicogenic criteria of specificity to elicit core symptoms of panic only. It is perhaps not surprising that the adrenergic system is important in the experience of different anxiety symptoms besides panic (Sullivan et al. 1999).

Clinical validation

Studies with anxiety blocking agents have shown that yohimbine-induced panic is reduced by long-term alprazolam (Charney & Heninger 1985a) and fluvoxamine treatment (Goddard et al. 1993) in patients with PD. In contrast, imipramine failed to decrease yohimbine-induced panic in PD (Charney & Heninger 1985b). Alprazolam (Charney et al. 1986) and diazepam (Charney et al. 1983) pretreatment have also been reported to reduce yohimbine-induced anxiety in healthy volunteers.

Physiology

Yohimbine-induced panic attacks are associated with cardiorespiratory and HPA-axis activation including increased blood pressure and pulse rate (Charney et al. 1984b), and plasma cortisol and prolactin release (Charney et al. 1987a; Matilla et al. 1988; Gurguis & Uhde 1990; Albus et al. 1992; Gurguis et al. 1997). In addition, yohimbine is associated with a blunted growth hormone response in PD (Uhde et al. 1992).

Mechanism

Yohimbine is a panicogen that has α_2-antagonistic effects. It is thought to increase noradrenergic function in the locus ceruleus to cause anxiety by blocking presynaptic negative feedback (Redmond 1977). The effects of yohimbine, however, are complicated by its other properties including blockade of both pre- and postsynaptic receptors in the hypothalamus along with some dopamine D2 autoreceptor agonism in the pituitary. In normal controls, there was a relationship between yohimbine effect on plasma MHPG and opposition by the α_2-agonist clonidine (Charney et al. 1992). This relationship was not seen in PD patients, suggesting a dysregulation of noradrenergic metabolism or difference in receptor subtype distribution, metabolism, or sensitivity in a subgroup of PD patients. The preferential effect of SSRI antidepressants versus tricyclic antidepressants in blocking yohimbine-induced panic suggests a point of possible further pharmacological dissection of the properties of this panicogen. Perhaps serotonin is a particularly important neurotransmitter in mediating yohimbine-induced panic.

The effects of yohimbine on brain blood flow have been studied with PET imaging with conflicting results. Woods et al. (1988b) found that panic patients showed decreased frontal cerebral blood flow compared to controls. Unfortunately only one of six controls experienced panic while six out of six PD patients experienced panic so it is unclear if the decreased blood flow is a cause or effect of yohimbine-induced panic. On the other hand, Cameron *et al.* (2000) found medial frontal, thalamic, and insular hyperperfusion with yohimbine, and over-all increased cerebral blood flow with the one patient that reported a panic attack.

Isoproterenol

Isoproterenol is a nonspecific, largely peripheral β-adrenergic agonist. This agent fulfils a number of criteria for an ideal panicogen. However, its physiological effects are inconsistent.

Basic properties
Isoproterenol safely elicits panic attacks in humans. The induced attacks encompass both affective and somatic symptoms of panic and are appraised by patients as being similar to naturally occurring panic (Rainey *et al.* 1984b, 1984c; Balon *et al.* 1990). The test–retest reliability of isoproterenol has not been studied.

Specificity
Isoproterenol evokes panic attacks preferentially in PD patients (Rainey *et al.* 1984b; Pohl *et al.* 1988a) compared to normal controls. Isoproterenol sensitivity across different anxiety disorders has not been studied, but bulimic patients have been shown to be more sensitive to isoproterenol-induced panic than controls (Pohl *et al.* 1989). The ability of isoproterenol to elicit core symptoms of other anxiety syndromes has not been evaluated.

Clinical validation
Panic attacks elicited by isoproterenol are blockable by imipramine (Rainey *et al.* 1984b) and desipram-ine (Pohl *et al.* 1993, 1990), perhaps because they decrease β-receptor number and function. Placebo nonblocking of isoproterenol were noted in the above studies.

Physiology
Cardiorespiratory activation with isoproterenol includes prominent dyspnea and cardiac activation including increased heart rate variability (Yeragani *et al.* 1995). Studies of possible HPA activation revealed that isoproterenol-induced panic is accompanied by growth hormone and cortisol release (Nesse *et al.* 1984).

Mechanism
It may be that peripheral β-adrenergic agonism by iso-proterenol elicits panic peripherally, without affecting "central panic circuits," which may be activated during panic elicited by other agents or during natural panic.

Serotonin

The role of serotonin in anxiety disorders has been a focus of attention because of the efficacy of serotonin modulators such as SSRI antidepressants in relieving anxiety symptoms including panic attacks (Bell & Nutt 1998). In contrast, however, a regular phenomenon early in pharmacological treatment using serotonergic medications is a "jittery" syndrome that is characterized by motor restlessness, insomnia, heightened anxiety and irritability (Pohl *et al.* 1988b). The role of serotonin in anxiety has been studied in a limited fashion using the releasing/reuptake inhibitor fenfluramine and the serotonin receptor agonist *m*-chlorophenylpiperazine (mCPP).

Fenfluramine

This agent does not fulfil basic criteria, and has incon-sistent physiology, but is specific and blockable.

Basic properties
Fenfluramine administration by mouth has complex behavioral effects with both anxiogenic and anxiolytic properties. At an oral dose of up to 60 mg, it evokes anxiety symptoms including panic (Targum *et al.* 1989; Targum 1990) in PD patients. Apparently, the experience of fenfluramine-induced anxiety is quite heterogenous, including "waves" of anxiety persisting for hours. Other investigators have commented that fenfluramine-stimulated anxiety is more similar to generalized anxiety than panic (Hollander *et al.* 1990; Coplan *et al.* 1992b). Perhaps this response may be akin to the increased anxiety sometimes observed in patients during the initial phases of treatment with SSRIs (Den Boer & Westenberg 1988). On the other hand, fenfluramine has been reported to cause a mild sedating and anxiolytic effect (Bond *et al.* 1995), and attenuated anxiety provoked by a public speaking test in healthy volunteers (Hetem *et al.* 1996). Possible toxicity of fenfluramine related to chronic administra-tion to cause valvular cardiac lesions and neuronal damage has raised concerns about the safety of fenflura-

mine use in panic research, even for short-term administration (McCann *et al.* 1998). Test–retest reliability of fenfluramine has not been systematically studied.

Specificity
Fenfluramine provokes symptoms of anxiety and panic attacks preferentially in PD patients compared to control subjects and patients with major depression (Targum *et al.* 1989; Targum 1990). Patients with major depression and normal controls react similarly to fenfluramine (Targum 1990). Interestingly, fenfluramine challenge was associated with a decline in obsessive symptoms in OCD patients. However, the results are difficult to interpret because initial severity ratings of obsessions were higher on the fenfluramine versus the placebo challenge day.

Clinical validation
The blockability of fenfluramine-provoked anxiety by antipanic drugs has not been studied.

Physiology
Surprisingly, the effects of fenfluramine challenge on cardiorespiratory activation has not been evaluated. With respect to HPA-axis activation, fenfluramine-induced panic is associated with increases in cortisol and prolactin (Lucey *et al.* 1992; Davis *et al.* 1999). Moreover, HPA-axis activation is greater in PD patients versus patients with major depression and normal controls (Targum & Marshall 1989; Targum 1990).

Mechanisms
Fenfluramine potently increases 5-HT release and inhibits reuptake (Rowland & Carlton 1986). Possible mechanisms of action are extremely speculative and troubled by complex effects and compensatory changes. In a recent study, fenfluramine increased anxiety and arousal but tended to reduce CO_2-induced anxiety and panic attacks in patients with PD (Mortimore & Anderson 2000). This paradoxical two-fold effect of fenfluramine is in line with the complexity of the role of serotonin neurotransmission in anxiety and panic attacks (Deakin & Graeff 1991).

m-Chlorophenylpiperazine

m-Chlorophenylpiperazine (mCPP) is a mixed agonist of 5-HT1/5-HT2 and antagonist of 5-HT2a, 5-HT3 and α-adrenergic receptors (Barnes & Sharp 1999). As a panicogen this agent has disputed basic properties and complex physiology, but is specific to PD.

Basic properties
mCPP effectively induces a variety of anxiety symptoms which sometimes include panic attacks (reviewed by Kahn & Wetzler 1991) peaking 90–120 min after intravenous infusion (although it may also be given orally). When attacks do occur, mCPP-induced panic does include affective and somatic components which appear naturalistic. The panicogenic effect of mCPP may be more clear-cut after rapid intravenous administration (Van der Wee *et al.* 1999). However, mCPP may be unsafe as there have been three reported cases of serotonin syndrome with single oral doses (Klaassen *et al.* 1998). The test–retest reliability of mCPP has not been studied.

Specificity
mCPP induces anxiety, dysphoria and panic attacks in PD patients more than in normal controls or depressed patients (Charney *et al.* 1987b; Kahn *et al.* 1988). One-third of patients with PTSD experienced mCPP-induced panic attacks and had significantly greater increases in symptoms of anxiety (Southwick *et al.* 1997). In some studies, mCPP challenge resulted in a transient exacerbation of OCD symptoms in the majority of patients (Zohar *et al.* 1987). This effect was absent on rechallenge after chronic treatment with clomipramine (Zohar *et al.* 1988), and diminished with fluoxetine treatment (Hollander *et al.* 1991). However, other studies failed to detect a mCPP-induced exacerbation of OCD phenomena (Charney *et al.* 1988; Goodman *et al.* 1995; Khanna *et al.* 2001). There is recent evid-ence that a lower dose of mCPP (0.25 mg/kg) may actually worsen obsessive-compulsive symptoms, while the standard dose (0.5 mg/kg) has general anxiogenic effects (Erzegovesi *et al.* 2001). Finally, mCPP increases anger ratings in GAD patients (Germine *et al.* 1992). Thus, the anxiogenic effects of mCPP may include syndrome-specific symptoms across a wide spectrum of anxiety disorders.

Clinical validation
There is limited data on the effect of antipanic drugs on mCPP-induced panic anxiety. One study demonstrated that alprazolam was more effectively than placebo in attenuating mCPP-induced anxiety and increases in cortisol and growth hormone in healthy volunteers (Sevy *et al.* 1994).

Physiology

mCPP-induced panic was not reported to be accompanied by increases in blood pressure and heart rate (Charney *et al.* 1987b). The mCPP-induced HPA-axis activation in PD patients has been found to be of similar extent to that observed in healthy controls (Charney *et al.* 1987b; Wetzler *et al.* 1996). However, findings of an augmented cortisol response (Broocks *et al.* 2000) and increased adrenocorticotrophic hormone (ACTH) and prolactin release as well as blunted prolactin response in women with PD have also been reported (Germine *et al.* 1994).

Mechanisms

mCPP-induced anxiety is associated with different patterns of neuroendocrine activation with more augmentation in PD and social phobia versus blunting in OCD. The behavioral and neuroendocrine properties of mCPP have been rather discrepant and serotonin 5-hydroxytryptophan does not elicit panic attacks (Westenberg & den Boer 1989). The involvement of serotonin in different circuits of anxiety appears to be complex and perhaps requires some differential stimulation of serotonin receptor subtypes to elicit anxiety. In addition, the properties of a modulator like mCPP are complex (Murphy *et al.* 1996) and there is a large pharmacokinetic variability after its oral administration (Gijsman *et al.* 1998) that renders interpretation of data difficult.

Other serotonergic modulators

Other serotonin agonists appear to be of limited use as a pharmacological model of panic. Although ipsapirone, a partial agonist of 5-HT1A receptors can induce panic attacks in patient with PD (Lesch *et al.* 1992; Broocks *et al.* 2000), other agents such as buspirone, sumatriptan, zolmitriptan, L-tryptophan and 5-hydroxytryptophan have no panicogenic activity (Charney & Heninger 1986; Goddard *et al.* 1994; Norman *et al.* 1994; van Vliet *et al.* 1996; Stein *et al.* 1999).

γ-aminobutyric acid

Modulation of GABA receptors using benzodiazepines (GABA-A agonists) is well established. It has been proposed that abnormalities in GABA receptor function underlie some anxiety disorders including PD. There is significant preclinical evidence for GABA dysfunction

in anxiety, but this review will focus on clinical work using the GABA antagonist flumazenil. There is one preliminary report on the anxiogenic effects of the inverse benzodiazepine receptor agonist, FG 7142, in healthy humans (Dorow *et al.* 1983). However, no other studies have been conducted with this agent.

Flumazenil

Flumazenil is a specific benzodiazepine ligand that has little intrinsic activity but blocks the pharmacological effects of benzodiazepine agonists (e.g. benzodiazepines) and inverse agonists (e.g. β-carbolines). So far, the data suggest that flumazenil may not be an ideal model of panic.

Basic properties

Intravenous infusion of flumazenil has been found to safely evoke anxiety including panic attacks in humans (Nutt *et al.* 1990). The induced panic attacks include both affective and somatic symptoms of panic that are naturalistic according to Woods *et al.* (1991). However, recent studies failed to confirm flumazenil's panicogenicity (Ströhle *et al.* 1998; Ströhle *et al.* 2000), raising questions about its validity as a model of panic. So far, test–retest reliability has not been studied.

Specificity

Flumazenil is panicogenic in patients with PD but not in normal controls, suggesting absolute specificity in PD (Nutt *et al.* 1990; Woods *et al.* 1991). Patients with PTSD and SAD have also been found to react similarly to flumazenil as healthy controls (Coupland *et al.* 1997, 2000), suggesting that abnormal GABA function may not be relevant in these disorders. On the other hand, similar to findings with lactate infusion and CO_2 inhalation, women with PMDD were more likely to panic with flumazenil than controls (Le Mellédo *et al.* 2000).

Clinical validation

Blockade of flumazenil-induced panic with the SSRI paroxetine was recently demonstrated by Bell and associates (Bell *et al.* 2002). This effect was partially reversed by lowering brain serotonin levels with tryptophan depletion.

Physiology

PD patients who panicked with flumazenil experienced increases in heart rate and blood pressure but not in respiratory symptoms (Nutt *et al.* 1990). It is unknown whether flumazenil-induced panic is accompanied by HPA-axis activation.

Mechanisms

Several theories may explain flumazenil's panicogenicity (Coplan & Klein 1996). It has been posited that PD patients suffer from underproduction of endogenous GABA agonists, such as desmethyldiazepam, leaving them more vulnerable to GABA antagonism. Alternatively, panic patients may secrete more endogenous anxiolytic to deal with their hyperactive "anxiety circuits," or hypoactive anxiolytic circuits (Roy-Byrne *et al.* 1990) which might be preferentially unmasked by flumazenil. Flumazenil might thus alter the GABAergic "set point" of anxiety/anxiolytic threshold. The concept of a "set point" has also been discussed to explain GABA tolerance. The proposal that PD is associated with alterations of GABAergic function is supported by findings of widespread reduction in $GABA_A$ receptor binding in PD (Malizia *et al.* 1998). Studies of disease specificity suggest the possibility of an abnormal set point in PD and PMDD but not in social phobia or PTSD.

Cholecystokinin

Cholecystokinin (CCK) is a gut-brain hormone found in high concentrations in brain regions implicated in the regulation of fear and anxiety. The central CCK-B (recently reclassifed as CCK-2) receptor agonists, CCK-tetrapeptide (CCK-4) and the synthetic analogue pentagastrin have become standard agents for inducing panic attacks in humans. Systematic evaluation of the validity of CCK-B receptor agonists as a model of panic indicates that CCK fulfils most criteria of an ideal panicogenic agent. At present, CCK is the only valid panicogen that also fulfils criteria for a neurotransmitter.

Basic properties

CCK safety is well established with a long track record devoid of any medically significant side-effects. About 5% of subjects experience a brief vasovagal reaction but this has been a mild and brief phenomenon which has never led to health problems. Panic attacks induced by CCK agonists include both somatic and affective symptoms and are appraised by patients as being identical or very similar to their spontaneous attacks (Bradwejn *et al.* 1990; Bradwejn & Koszycki 1991;

van Megen *et al.* 1994). Studies in PD patients have demonstrated that the panicogenic effects of CCK-4 are dose-dependent and undiminished with repeated challenge (Bradwejn *et al.* 1991a, 1992a,b).

Specificity

Response to CCK-4 and pentagastrin reliably differentiates PD patients from healthy controls with no personal of family history of panic (Bradwejn *et al.* 1991b; van Megen *et al.* 1994). This suggests that there may be abnormalities in the CCK receptor system in PD patients. Studies evaluating the specificity of CCK suggests that its paniocogencity is not limited to PD. Individuals suffering from PTSD (Kellner *et al.* 2000), SAD (McCann *et al.* 1997), OCD (De Leeuw *et al.* 1996), GAD (Brawman-Mintzer *et al.* 1997) and PMDD (Le Mellédo *et al.* 1999) all exhibit an augmented behavioral response to CCK compared to controls. However, the threshold of vulnerability to CCK panic appears to be lower in PD relative to other psychopathologies. The finding that CCK-induced panic is not peculiar to PD suggest that CCK activity is a common factor involved across a wide range of psychiatric conditions. Further work with differential specificity and brain imaging might help in understanding how CCK might have a role in all these disorders. Possible provocation of core anxiety symptoms of other disorders besides panic has not been extensively studied. So far, however, CCK does not elicit flashbacks in PTSD patients (Kellner *et al.* 2000), or obsessions or compulsions in OCD (De Leeuw *et al.* 1996), maintaining its relatively specific panicogenic properties.

Clinical validation

CCK-induced panic is blockable with antipanic drugs. Long-term treatment with the antidepressants imipramine (Bradwejn & Koszycki 1994), fluvoxamine (van Megen *et al.* 1997), and citalopram (Shlik *et al.* 1997a) significantly attenuate response to CCK-4 in patients with PD. Also, acute pretreatment with the benzodiazepine lorazepam (de Montigny 1989), the β-adrenergic blocker propranolol (Le Mellédo *et al.* 1998), and the 5-HT3 receptor antagonist ondansetron (Dépôt *et al.* 1998) were all effective in attenuating CCK-induced panic in healthy volunteers, although ondansetron did not antagonize pentagastrin-induced panic in PD patients (McCann *et al.* 1997). CCK-4 panic is not blocked by clonidine in either PD patients or healthy volunteers (Kellner *et al.* 1997; Shlik *et al.* 2000). Finally,

CCK-4 panic is not blocked by pretreatment with placebo or the nonantipanic GABA antagonist flumazenil (Bradwejn *et al.* 1994a).

Physiology

The behavioral effects of CCK agonists are accompanied by marked biological alterations, including robust increases in heart rate, blood pressure and minute ventilation (Bradwejn *et al.* 1990, 1991b, 1992a, 1998; Koszycki *et al.* 1998). CCK-4-induced dyspnea seems to be related to decreased vital capacity parameters without any apparent bronchoconstriction or change in respiratory resistance (Shlik *et al.* 1997b). As for neuroendocrine effects, CCK has been shown to increase plasma ACTH, cortisol, growth hormone and prolactin levels (Kellner *et al.* 1997; Shlik *et al.* 1997b; Dépôt *et al.* 1998; Koszycki *et al.* 1998).

Mechanisms

The neurotransmitter mechanism by which CCK-B receptor agonists provoke panic and concomitant biological changes has been the subject of considerable research activity. There is evidence that panic symptoms induced by CCK-4 is associated with selective stimulation of CCK-B receptors. Acute treatment with the selective CCK-B receptor antagonist L365-260 blocked CCK-4 induced panic in PD patients (Bradwejn *et al.* 1994b) and healthy volunteers (Lines *et al.* 1995). In addition, acute treatment with the CCK-B receptor agonist, CI-988, modestly attenuated the behavioral effects of CCK-4 in healthy subjects (Bradwejn *et al.* 1995), although it failed to antagonize CCK-4-induced panic in PD patients (van Megen *et al.* 1997). The results of CI-988 are difficult to interpret due to the poor bioavailability of this compound. While CCK-B receptors appear to be the principal mechanism by which CCK agonists induce symptoms of panic, there is growing recognition that CCK does not act in isolation and that it produces some of its effects by interacting with other neurotransmitter systems including serotonin (Koszycki *et al.* 1996; Shlik *et al.* 1997a; van Megen *et al.* 1997), norepinephrine (Le Mellédo *et al.* 1998) and the GABA-benzodiazepine complex (de Montigny 1989).

Imaging studies have shown that CCK-4 induced anxiety is associated with bilateral increases in extracerebral blood flow in the temporal artery region and CBF increases in the anterior cingulate gyrus, the claustrum-cortex-insular-amygdala region, and the cerebellar vermis (Benkelfat *et al.* 1995). This may reflect a change in brain tissue metabolic activity mediated by CCK which would demand more blood flow during panic. Regional CBF flow has also been measured at two time points as a function of CCK-4 injection (Javanmard *et al.* 1999). In this study, PET scans were conducted to capture brain activation during the 1st and 2nd minute after CCK-4 challenge. The earlier effects of CCK increased CBF in the hypothalamus, and the later effects of CCK increased CBF in the claustrum-insular region. In both early and late trials, CBF in the medial frontal cortex decreased. This work suggests a progression of brain activity with CCK stimulation starting with the hypothalamus and proceeding to the claustrum-insular cortex with an associated decrease in medial frontal brain activity. A recent investigation using brain stem auditory evoked potential (BSAEP) recordings found that CCK-4 exerts robust effects on the brain stem (Gunnarsson *et al.* 2000). These data are in keeping with current theories of CCK action whereby CCK leaks across the blood–brain barrier into circumventricular structures close to the nucleus tractus solitarius which contains ample CCK-A (for alimentary) and CCK-B receptors (Noble *et al.* 2000).

Evaluation of possible psychological mechanisms in CCK-4-induced panic indicate that cognitive appraisal processes, fear of anxiety sensations and baseline anxiety do not fully account for CCK-4's panicogenicity (Koszycki 1995). The influence of genetics on CCK-induced panic has not been evaluated. Recent work has shown that allelic variation of the CCK-B receptor gene may confer risk for PD (Kennedy *et al.* 1999), and it is conceivable that allelic variation of this gene influences panicogenic reactivity to CCK-B receptor stimulation with CCK agonists. Studies are currently underway to test this hypothesis.

In summary, CCK is a neurotransmitter which fulfills all of the proposed criteria for an ideal panicogenic agent. The mechanism by which CCK-4 provokes panic anxiety is complex, and involves stimulation of CCK-B receptors and other receptors systems with which it interacts.

Summary

Panicogens have been a useful tool to study the pathophysiology of panic attacks. Several panicogens have been reviewed in this chapter according to our

Table 15.2 Panicogens against Swain/Koszycki/Shlik/Bradwejn* criteria.

	Basic properties				Specificity		Clinical validation physiology			
	Safety	Affective and somatic	Naturalistic	Reliable	Specific	Elicit other anxiety	Blockable (antipanics)	Not placebo blockable	Cardiac and/or respiratory	HPA
Lactate	Yes	Yes	Yes	No	Yes	Yes	Yes	Yes	Yes	No
CO_2	Yes	Yes	Yes	Yes	Yes	N/K	Yes	Yes	Yes	No
Hypertonic saline	Yes	Yes	Yes	N/K	Yes	N/K	N/K	N/K	Yes	N/K
Caffeine	Yes	Yes	Dis.	No	Yes	Yes	N/K	N/K	Dis.	Yes
Doxepram	Yes	Yes	Dis.	N/K	Yes	N/K	N/K	N/K	Yes	No
Norepinephrine†	Yes	Yes	Yes	N/K	Yes	N/K	N/K	N/K	Yes	N/K
Yohimbine	Yes	Yes	Yes	N/K	Yes	Yes	Yes	Yes	Yes	N/K
Isoproterenol	Yes	Yes	Yes	N/K	Yes	N/K	Yes	Yes	Yes	No
Fenfluramine	No	Yes	Dis.	N/K	Yes	Dis.	N/K	N/K	N/K	Yes
mCPP	Dis.	Dis.	No	N/K	Yes	Dis.	Yes	N/K	Yes	Yes
Flumazenil	Yes	Dis.	Dis.	N/K	Yes	No	Yes	N/K	Yes	N/K
CCK	Yes	Yes	Yes	Yes	Yes	No	Yes	Yes	Yes	Yes

*Authors of this chapter. †Noradrenaline.

CCK, cholecystokinin; CO_2, carbon dioxide; Dis., disputed; mCPP, m-chlorophenylpiperazine; N/K, not known.

expanded criteria of an "ideal panicogen". The results of the review are summarized in Table 15.2. It is interesting that the metabolic/respiratory panicogens CO_2 and lactate activate the cardiorespiratory systems but are relatively ineffective in activating the HPA axis, while the noradrenergic, serotonergic and CCKergic panicogens activate both the cardio-respiratory and the HPA axis. Ultimately it appears that no panicogen meets all criteria of an "ideal" panicogen, but CCK-4 appears to most closely approximate such a compound.

In the future, challenge research may involve combinations of different panicogens in order to achieve a certain profile of physiological response, paired with more sophisticated experimental approaches including functional brain imaging. Further, more naturalistic behavioral challenges might be used such as public speaking testing and autobiographic scripts. This will lead to a better understanding of how the challenge agents work, how the brain works in health and illness, as well as leading to new nosological systems based on the underlying neurobiology which is just now beginning to be mapped out (Gorman *et al.* 2000). Consideration of brain development and gene activation in the development of the brain circuits that mediate panic will also likely figure prominently in panicogen research in order to improve early diagnosis and treatment of anxiety syndromes which include panic attacks.

References

Abelson, J.L., Glitz, D., Cameron, O.G. *et al.* (1992) Endocrine, cardiovascular and behavioral responses to clonidine in patients with panic disorder. *Biol Psychiatry* **32**, 18–25.

Abelson, J.L., Weg, J.G., Nesse, R.M. & Curtis, G.C. (1996) Neuroendocrine responses to laboratory panic: cognitive intervention in doxapram model. *Psychoneuroendocrinology* **21**, 375–90.

Albus, M., Zahn, P. & Breier, A. (1992) Anxiogenic properties of yohimbine. *Eur Arch Psychiatry Clin Neurosci* **241**, 337–44.

Antony, M.M., Brown, T.A. & Barlow, D.H. (1997) Response to hyperventilation and 5.5% CO_2 inhalation of subjects with types of specific phobia, panic disorder, or no mental disorder. *Am J Psychiatry* **154**, 1089–95.

Aronson, T.A., Carasiti, I., McBane, D. & Whitaker-Azmitia, P. (1989) Biological correlates of lactate sensitivity in panic disorder. *Biol Psychiatry* **26**, 463–77.

Asmundson, G.J. & Stein, M.B. (1994) Triggering the false suffocation alarm in panic disorder patients by using a voluntary breath-holding procedure. *Am J Psychiatry* **151**, 264–66.

Bailey, J.E., Argyropoulos, S., Kendrick, A., Nash, J., Lightman, S. & Nutt, D. (2001) Inhalation of 35% CO_2 results in subjective fear and activates the HPA axis in healthy volunteers. *J Psychopharmacol* **15**, A22.

Balon, R., Jordan, M., Pohl, R. & Yeragani, V.K. (1989) Family history of anxiety disorders in control subjects with lactate-induced panic attacks. *Am J Psychiatry* **14**, 1304–6.

Balon, R., Petty, F., Yeragani, V.K., Kramer, G.L. & Pohl, R. (1993) Intravenous sodium lactate decreases plasma GABA levels in man. *Psychopharmacology* **110**, 368–70.

Balon, R., Pohl, R., Yeragani, V.K., Rainey, J.M. Jr & Berchou, R. (1988) Follow-up study of control subjects with lactate- and isoproterenol-induced panic attacks. *Am J Psychiatry* **154**, 238–41.

Balon, R., Yeragani, V.K., Pohl, R., Muench, J. & Berchou, R. (1990) Somatic and psychological symptoms during isoproterenol-induced panic attacks. *Psychiatry Res* **32**, 103–12.

Bandelow, B., Wedekind, D., Pauls, J. *et al.* (2000) Salivary cortisol in panic attacks. *Am J Psychiatry* **157**, 454–6.

Barnes, N.M. & Sharp, T. (1999) A review of central 5-HT receptors and their function. *Neuropharmacology* **38**, 1083–1152.

Beck, J.G. & Berisford, M.A. (1992) The effects of caffeine on panic patients: response components of anxiety. *Behavior Therapy* **23**, 405–22.

Bell, C.J., Forshall, S., Adrover, M. *et al.* (2002) Does 5-HT restrain panic? A tryphophan depletion study in panic disorder patients recovered on paroxetine. *J Psychopharmacol* **16**, 5–14.

Bell, C.J. & Nutt, D.J. (1998) Serotonin and panic. *Br J Psychiatry* **172**, 465–71.

Bellodi, L., Perna, G., Caldirola, D., Arancio, C., Bertani, A. & Di Bella, D. (1998) CO_2-induced panic attacks: a twin study. *Am J Psychiatry* **155**, 1184–88.

Benkelfat, C., Bradwejn, J., Meyer, E. *et al.* (1995) Functional neuroanatomy of CCK-4-induced anxiety in normal healthy volunteers. *Am J Psychiatry* **152**, 1180–4.

Ben-Zion, I.Z., Meiri, G., Greenberg, B.D., Murphy, D.L. & Benjamin, J. (1999) Enhancement of CO_2-induced anxiety in healthy volunteers with the serotonin antagonist metergoline. *Am J Psychiatry* **156**, 1635–7.

Bertani, A., Perna, G., Arancio, C., Caldirola, D. & Bellodi, L. (1997) Pharmacologic effect of imipramine, paroxetine, and sertraline in 35% carbon dioxide sensitivity in panic patients: a double-blind, random, placebo-controlled study. *J Clin Psychopharmacol* **17**, 97–101.

Biber, B. & Alkin, T. (1999) Panic disorder subtypes: differential responses to CO_2 challenge. *Am J Psychiatry* **156**, 739–44.

Bond, A.J., Feizollah, S. & Lader, M.H. (1995) The effects of d-fenfluramine on mood and performance, and on neuro-endocrine indicators of 5-HT function. *J Psychopharmacol* **9**, 1–8.

Bonn, J.A., Harrison, J. & Rees, W.L. (1971) Lactate-induced anxiety, therapeutic application. *Br J Psychiatry* **119**, 468–71.

Boulenger, J.-P., Uhde, T.W., Wolff, A., III & Post, R.M. (1984) Increased sensitivity to caffeine in patients with panic disorders. *Arch Gen Psychiatry* **41**, 1067–71.

Bradwejn, J. & Koszycki, D. (1991) Comparison of CO_2-induced panic with cholecystokinin-induced panic in panic disorder. *Prog Neuro-psychopharmacol Biol Psychiatry* **15**, 237–9.

Bradwejn, J. & Koszycki, D. (1994) Imipramine antagonism of panicogenic effects of cholecystokinin tetrapeptide in panic disorder patients. *Am J Psychiatry* **151**, 261–3.

Bradwejn, J., Koszycki, D., Annable, L., Couëtoux du Tertre, A., Reines, S. & Karkanias, C. (1992a) A dose-ranging study of the behavioral and cardiovascular effects of CCK-tetrapeptide in panic disorder. *Biol Psychiatry* **32**, 903–12.

Bradwejn, J., Koszycki, D. & Bourin, M. (1991a) Dose ranging study of the effects of cholecystokinin in healthy volunteers. *J Psychiatr Neurosci* **16**, 91–5.

Bradwejn, J., Koszycki, D., Cöuetoux du Tertre, A. *et al.* (1994b) The panicogenic effects of cholecystokinin-tetrapeptide are antagonized by L-365 260, a central cholecystokinin receptor antagonist, in patients with panic disorder. *Arch Gen Psychiatry* **51**, 486–93.

Bradwejn, J., Koszycki, D., Cöuetoux du Tertre, A., Paradis, M. & Bourin, M. (1994a) Effects of flumazenil on cholecystokinin-tetrapeptide-induced panic symptoms in healthy volunteers. *Pychopharmacology* **114**, 257–61.

Bradwejn, J., Koszycki, D. & Meterissian, G. (1990) Cholecystokinin-tetrapeptide induces panic attacks in patients with panic disorder. *Can J Psychiatry* **35**, 83–5.

Bradwejn, J., Koszycki, D., Paradis, M., Reece, P., Hinton, J. & Sedman, A. (1995) Effect of CI-988 on cholecystokinin-tetrapeptide induced panic symptoms in healthy voluteers. *Biol Psychiatry* **38**, 742–6.

Bradwejn, J., Koszycki, D., Payeur, R., Bourin, M. & Borthwick, H. (1992b) Replication of action of cholecystokinin tetrapeptide in panic disorder: clinical and behavioral findings. *Am J Psychiatry* **149**, 962–4.

Bradwejn, J., Koszycki, D. & Shriqui, C. (1991b) Enhanced sensitivity to cholecystokinin-tetrapeptide in PD. *Arch Gen Psychiatry* **48**, 603–7.

Bradwejn, J., LeGrand, J.-M., Koszycki, D., Bates, J.H.T. & Bourin, M. (1998) Effects of cholecystokinin tetrapeptide on respiratory function in healthy volunteers. *Am J Psychiatry* **155**, 280–2.

Brawman-Mintzer, O., Lydiard, R.B., Bradwejn, J. *et al.* (1997) Effects of the cholecystokinin agonist pentagastrin in patients with generalized anxiety disorder. *Am J Psychiatry* **154**, 700–2.

Broocks, A., Bandelow, B., George, A. *et al.* (2000) Increased psychological responses and divergent neuroendocrine responses to m-CPP and ipsapirone in patients with panic disorder. *Int Clin Psychopharmacol* **15**, 153–61.

Bruce, M., Scott, N., Shine, P. & Lader, M. (1992) Anxiogenic effects of caffeine in patients with anxiety disorders. *Arch Gen Psychiatry* **49**, 867–9.

Buller, R., von Bardeleben, U., Maier, W. & Benkert, O. (1989) Specificity of lactate response in panic with concurrent depression and major depression. *J Affect Disord* **16**, 109–113.

Bystritsky, A., Craske, M., Maidenberg, E., Vapnik, T. & Shapiro, D. (2000) Autonomic reactivity of panic patients during a CO_2 inhalation procedure. *Depress Anxiety* **11**, 15–26.

Caldirola, D., Perna, G., Arancio, C., Bertani, A. & Bellodi, L. (1997) The 35% CO_2 challenge test in patients with social phobia. *Psychiatry Res* **71**, 41–8.

Calverley, P.M.A., Robson, R.H., Wraith, P.K. *et al.* (1983) The ventilatory effects of doxapram in normal man. *Clin Sci* **65**, 65–9.

Cameron, O.G., Lee, M.A., Curtis, G.C. & McCann, D.S. (1987) Endocrine and physiological changes during "spontaneous" panic attacks. *Psychoneuroendocrinology* **12**, 321–31.

Cameron, O.G., Model, J.G. & Hariharan, M. (1990) Caffeine and human cerebral blood flow: a positron emission tomography study. *Life Sciences* **47**, 1141–6.

Cameron, O.G., Zubieta, J.K., Grunhaus, L. & Minoshima, S. (2000) Effect of yohimbine on cerebral blood flow, symptoms, and physiological functions in humans. *Psychosom Med* **62**, 549–59.

Carr, D.B., Sheehan, D.V., Surman, O.S. *et al.* (1986) Neuroendocrine correlates of lactate-induced anxiety and their response to chronic alprazolam therapy. *Am J Psychiatry* **143**, 483–94.

Cavallini, M.C., Perna, G., Caldirola, D. & Bellodi, L. (1999) A segregation study of panic disorder in families of panic patients responsive to the 35% CO_2 challenge. *Biol Psychiatry* **46**, 815–20.

Charney, D.S., Breier, A., Jatlow, P.I. & Heninger, G.R. (1986) Behavioral, biochemical, and blood pressure responses to alprazolam in healthy subjects: interactions with yohimbine. *Psychopharmacology* **88**, 133–40.

Charney, D.S. & Bremner, J.D. (1999) The neurobiological basis of anxiety disorders. In: *The Neurobiology of Mental Illness* (D.S. Charney, E.J. Nestler & B.S. Bunney (eds), pp. 494–517). Oxford University Press, New York.

Charney, D.S., Galloway, M.P. & Heninger, G.R. (1984a) The effects of caffeine on plasma MHPG, subjective anxiety, autonomic symptoms and blood pressure in healthy humans. *Life Sciences* **35**, 135–44.

Charney, D.S., Goodman, W.K., Price, L.H., Woods, S.W., Rasmussen, S.A. & Heninger, G.R. (1988) Serotonin function in obsessive-compulsive disorder: a comparison of the effects of tryptophan and m-chlorophenylpiperazine in patients and healthy subjects. *Arch Gen Psychiatry* **45**, 177–85.

Charney, D.S. & Heninger, G.R. (1985a) Noradrenergic function and the mechanism of action of antianxiety treatment. II. The effect of long-term alprazolam treatment. *Arch Gen Psychiatry* **42**, 458–67.

Charney, D.S. & Heninger, G.R. (1985b) Noradrenergic function and the mechanism of action of antianxiety treatment. I. The effect of long-term imipramine treatment. *Arch Gen Psychiatry* **42**, 473–81.

Charney, D.S. & Heninger, G.R. (1986) Serotonin function in panic disorders. The effect of intravenous tryptophan in healthy subjects and patients with panic disorder before and during alprazolam treatment. *Arch Gen Psychiatry* **43**, 1059–65.

Charney, D.S., Heninger, G.R. & Breier, A. (1984b) Noradrenergic function in panic anxiety. *Arch Gen Psychiatry* **41**, 751–63.

Charney, D.S., Heninger, G.R. & Jatlow, P.I. (1985) Increased anxiogenic effects of caffeine in panic disorders. *Arch Gen Psychiatry* **42**, 233–43.

Charney, D.S., Heninger, G.R. & Redmond, D.E., Jr (1983) Yohimbine induced anxiety and increased noradrenergic function in humans: effects of diazepam and clonidine. *Life Sciences* **33**, 19–29.

Charney, D.S., Woods, S.W., Goodman, W.K. & Heninger, G.R. (1987a) Neurobiological mechanisms of panic anxiety: biochemical and behavioral correlates of yohimbine-induced panic attacks. *Am J Psychiatry* **144**, 1030–6.

Charney, D.S., Woods, S.W., Goodman, W.K. & Heninger, G.R. (1987b) Serotonin function in anxiety II. Effects of the serotonin agonist MCPP in panic disorder patients and healthy subjects. *Psychopharmacology* **92**, 14–24.

Charney, D.S., Woods, S.W. & Heninger, G.R. (1989) Noradrenergic function in generalized anxiety disorder: effects of yohimbine in healthy subjects and patients with generalized anxiety disorder. *Psychiatry Res* **27**, 173–82.

Charney, D.W., Woods, S.W., Keystal, J.H., Nagy, L.M. & Heninger, G.R. (1992) Noradrenergic neuronal dysregulation in panic disorder: the effects of intravenous yohimbine and clonidine in panic disorder patients. *Acta Psychiatr Scand* **86**, 273–82.

Charney, D.S., Woods, S.W., Nagy, L.M., Southwick, S.M., Krystal, J.H. & Heninger, G.R. (1990) Noradrenergic function in panic disorder. *J Clin Psychiatry* **51**(12) (Suppl. A), 5–11.

Cohen, M.E. & White, P.D. (1951) Life situations, emotions, and neurocirculatory asthenia (anxiety, neurosis, neurasthenia, effort syndrome). *Proc Assoc Res Nerv Ment Dis* **29**, 832–69.

Coplan, J.D., Goetz, G., Klein, D.F. *et al.* (1998) Plasma cortisol concentrations preceding lactate-induced panic. *Arch Gen Psychiatry* **55**, 130–6.

Coplan, J.D., Gorman, J.M. & Klein, D.F. (1992b) Serotonin related functions in panic anxiety: a critical overview. *Neuropsychopharmacology* **6**(3), 189–200.

Coplan, J.D. & Klein, D.F. (1996) Pharmacological probes in panic disorder. In: *Advances in the Neurobiology of Anxiety Disorders* (H.G. Westenberg, J.A. Den Boer & D.L. Murphy (eds), pp. 173–96). John Wiley & Sons, New York.

Coplan, J.D., Liebowitz, R., Gorman, J.M. *et al.* (1992a) Noradrenergic function in panic disorder effects of intravenous clonidine pretreatment on lactate induced panic. *Biol Psychiatry* **31**, 135–46.

Coryell, W. & Arndt, S. (1999) The 35% CO_2 inhalation procedure: test–retest reliability. *Biol Psychiatry* **45**, 923–7.

Coupland, N.J., Bell, C., Potokar, J., Dorkins, E. & Nutt, D.J. (2000) Flumazenil challenge in social phobia. *Depress Anxiety* **11**, 27–30.

Coupland, N.J., Lillywhite, A., Bell, C., Potokar, J. & Nutt, D.J. (1997) A pilot study of the effects of flumazenil in post-traumatic stress disorder. *Biol Psychiatry* **41**, 988–90.

Cowley, D.S. & Arana, G.W. (1990) The diagnostic utility of lactate sensitivity in panic disorder. *Arch Gen Psychiatry* **47**, 277–84.

Cowley, D.S., Dager, S.R. & Dunner, D.L. (1986) Lactate-induced panic in primary affective disorder. *Am J Psychiatry* **143**, 646–7.

Cowley, D.S., Dager, S.R. & Dunner, D.L. (1987) Lactate infusions in major depression without panic attacks. *J Psychiatric Res* **21**, 234–8.

Cowley, D.S., Dager, S.R., McClellan, J., Roy-Byrne, P.P. & Dunner, D.L. (1988) Response to lactate infusion in generalized anxiety disorder. *Biol Psychiatry* **24**, 409–14.

Cowley, D.S., Dager, S.R., Roy-Byrne, P.P., Avery, D.H. & Dunner, D.L. (1991) Lactate vulnerability after alprazolam versus placebo treatment of panic disorder. *Biol Psychiatry* **30**, 49–56.

Cowley, D.S. & Dunner, D.L. (1988) Response to sodium lactate in panic disorder: relationship to presenting clinical variables. *Psychiatry Res* **25**, 253–59.

Dager, S.R., Friedman, S.D., Heide, A. *et al.* (1999) Two-dimensional proton echo-planar spectroscopic imaging of brain metabolic changes during lactate-induced panic. *Arch Gen Psychiatry* **56**, 70–7.

Dager, S.R., Rainey, J.M., Kenny, M.A., Artru, A.A., Metzger, G.D. & Bowden, D.M. (1990) Central nervous system effects of lactate infusion in primates. *Biol Psychiatry* **27**, 193–204.

Davis, L.L., Clark, D.M., Kramer, G.L., Moeller, F.G. & Petty, F. (1999) D-fenfluramine challenge in post-traumatic stress disorder. *Biol Psychiatry* **45**, 928–30.

De Leeuw, A.S., den Boer, J.A., Slaap, B.R. *et al.* (1996) Pentagastrin has panic inducing properties in obsessive-compulsive disorder. *Psychopharmacology* **236**, 339–44.

De Montigny, C. (1989) Cholecystokinin induces panic like attacks in healthy volunteers. *Arch Gen Psychiatry* **465**, 511–17.

Deakin, J.F.W. & Graeff, F.G. (1991) t-HT and mechanisms of defence. *J Psychopharmacol* **5**, 305–15.

Den Boer, J.A. & Westenberg, H.G. (1988) Effect of a serotonin and noradrenaline uptake inhibitor in panic disorder, a double-blind comparative study with fluvoxamine and maprotiline. *Int Clin Psychopharmacol* **3**, 59–74.

Den Boer, J.A., Westenberg, H.G., Klompmakers, A.A. & van Lint, L.E.M. (1989) Behavioral biochemical and neuroendocrine concomitants of lactate-induced panic anxiety. *Biol Psychiatry* **26**, 612–22.

Dépôt. M., Caillé, G., Mukherjee, J., Katzman, M.A., Cadieux, A. & Bradwejn, J. (1998) Acute and chronic role of 5-HT3 neuronal system on behavioral and neuroendocrine changes induced by intravenous cholecystokinin tetrapeptide administration in humans. *Neuropsychopharmacology* **20**, 177–87.

Dorow, R., Horowski, R., Paschelke, G., Amin, M. & Baestrup, C. (1983) Severe anxiety induced by FG 7142, a α-carboline ligand for benzodiazepine receptors. *Lancet* **ii**, 98–9.

Drevets, W.C., Videen, T.Q., MacLeod, A.K., Haller, J.W. & Raichle, M.E. (1992) PET images of blood flow changes during anxiety: correction [letter]. *Science* **256** (5064), 1696.

Erzegovesi, S., Martucci, L., Henin, M. & Bellodi, L. (2001) Low versus standard dose mCPP challenge in obsessive-compulsive patients. *Neuropsychopharmacology* **24**, 31–6.

Facchinetti, F., Romano, G., Fava, M. & Genazzani, A.R. (1992) Lactate infusion induces panic attacks in patients with premenstrual syndrome. *Psychosom Med* **54**, 288–96.

George, D.T., Brewerton, T.D. & Jimerson, D.C. (1987) Comparison of lactate-induced anxiety in bulimic patients and healthy controls. *Psychiatry Res* **21** (3), 213–20.

George, D.T., Hibbeln, J.R., Ragan, P.W. *et al.* (2000) Lactate-induced rage and panic in a select group of subjects who perpetrate acts of domestic violence. *Biol Psychiatry* **47**, 804–12.

George, D.T., Lindquist, T., Nutt, D.J. *et al.* (1995) Effect of chloride or glucose on the incidence of lactate-induced panic attacks. *Am J Psychiatry* **152** (5), 692–7.

Germine, M., Goddard, A.W., Sholomskas, D.E. *et al.* (1994) Response to meta-chlorophenylpiperazine in panic disorder patients and healthy subjects: influence of reduction in intravenous dosage. *Psychiatry Res* **54**, 115–33.

Germine, M., Goddard, A.W., Woods, S.W., Charney, D.S. & Heninger, G.R. (1992) Anger and anxiety responses to m-chlorophenylpiperazine in generalized anxiety disorder. *Biol Psychiatry* **32**, 457–61.

Gijsman, H.J., van Greven, J.M.A., Tieleman, M.C. *et al.* (1998) Pharmacokinetic and pharmacodynamic profile of oral and intravenous metachlorophenylpiperazine in healthy volunteers. *J Clin Psychopharmacol* **18**, 289–95.

Goddard, A.W., Sholomskas, D.E., Walton, K.E. *et al.* (1994) Effects of tryptophan depletion in panic disorder. *Biol Psychiatry* **36**, 775–7.

Goddard, A.W., Woods, S.W., Sholomskas, D.E., Goodman, W.K., Charney, D.S. & Heninger, G.R. (1993) Effects of the serotonin reuptake inhibitor fluvoxamine on yohimbine-induced anxiety in panic disorder. *Psychiatry Res* **48**, 119–33.

Goetz, R.R., Klein, D.F. & Gorman, J.M. (1996) Symptoms essential to the experience of sodium lactate-induced panic. *Neuropsychopharmacology* **14**, 355–66.

Goetz, R.R., Klein, D.F., Gully, R. *et al.* (1993) Panic attacks during placebo procedures in the laboratory. Physiological and symptomatology. *Arch Gen Psychiatry* **50**, 280–85.

Goodman, W.K., McDougle, C.J., Price, L.H. *et al.* (1995) m-Chlorophenylpiperazine in patients obsessive-compulsive disorder: absence of symptom exacerbation. *Biol Psychiatry* **38**, 138–49.

Gorman, J.M., Askanazi, J., Liebowitz, M.R. *et al.* (1984) Response to hyperventilation in a group of patients with panic disorder. *Am J Psychiatry* **141**, 857–61.

Gorman, J.M., Battista, D., Goetz, R.R. *et al.* (1989) A comparison of sodium bicarbonate and sodium lactate infusion in the induction of panic attacks. *Arch Gen Psychiatry* **46**, 145–50.

Gorman, J.M., Charney, D.S., Fyer, M.R., Liebowitz, M.R. & Klein, D.F. (1987) Pharmacological provocation of panic attacks. In: *Psychopharmacology: The Third Generation of Progress* (H.Y. Meltzer (ed.), pp. 985–93). Raven Press, New York.

Gorman, J.M., Fyer, M.R., Goetz, R. *et al.* (1988b) Ventilatory physiology of patients with panic disorder. *Arch Gen Psychiatry* **45**, 31–9.

Gorman, J.M., Goetz, R.R., Dillon, D. *et al.* (1990a) Sodium D-lactate infusion in panic disorder patients. *Neuropsychopharmacology* **3**, 181–9.

Gorman, J.M., Goetz, R.R., Uy, J. *et al.* (1988a) Hyperventilation occurs during lactate-induced panic. *J Anxiety Disord* **2**, 193–202.

Gorman, J.M., Kent, J.M., Sullivan, G.M. & Coplan, J.D. (2000) Neuroanatomical hypothesis of panic disorder, revised. *Am J Psychiatry* **157**, 493–505.

Gorman, J.M., Levy, G.F., Liebowitz, M.R. *et al.* (1983) Effect of acute β-adrenergic blockade on lactate-induced panic. *Arch Gen Psychiatry* **40**, 1079–82.

Gorman, J.M., Liebowitz, M.R., Fyer, A.J. *et al.* (1985) Lactate infusions in obsessive-compulsive disorder. *Am J Psychiatry* **142**, 864–6.

Gorman, J.M., Papp, L.A., Martinez, J. *et al.* (1990b) High-dose carbon dioxide challenge test in anxiety disorder patients. *Biol Psychiatry* **28**, 743–57.

Griez, E. & van den Hout, M.A. (1986) CO_2 inhalation in the treatment of panic attacks. *Behav Res Ther* **24**, 145–50.

Gunnarsson, T., Mahoney, C., Shlik, J., Bradwejn, J. & Knott, V. (2000) Acute effects of cholecystokinin tetrapeptide on brain stem auditory evoked potentials in healthy volunteers. *Int J Psychopharmacol* **3** (Suppl. 1), S277.

Gurguis, G.N.M. & Uhde, T.W. (1990) Plasma 3-methoxy-4-hydroxyphenylethylene glycol (MHPG) and growth hormone responses to yohimbine in panic disorder patients and normal controls. *Psychoneuroendocrinology* **15**, 217–24.

Gurguis, G.N.M., Vitton, B.J. & Uhde, T.W. (1997) Behavioral, sympathetic and adrenocortical responses to yohimbine in panic disorder patients and normal controls. *Psychiatry Res* **71**, 27–39.

Guthrie, S.K., Grunhaus, L., Pande, A.C. & Hariharan, M. (1993) Noradrenergic response to intravenous yohimbine in patients with depression and comorbidity of depression and panic. *Biol Psychiatry* **34**, 558–61.

Guttmacher, L.B., Murphy, D.L. & Insel, T.R. (1983) Pharmacological models of anxiety. *Compr Psychiatry* **24**, 312–26.

Harrington, P.J., Schmidt, N.B. & Telch, M.J. (1996) Prospective evaluation of panic potentiation following 35% CO_2 challenge in nonclinical subjects. *Am J Psychiatry* **153**, 823–5.

Heninger, G.R., Charney, D.S. & Prince, L.H. (1988) α_2-Adrenergic receptor sensitivity in depression. *Arch Gen Psychiatry* **45**, 718–26.

Hetem, L.A.B., de Souza, C.J., Guimaraes, F.S., Zuardi, A.W. & Graeff, F.G. (1996) Effect of d-fenfluramine on human experimental anxiety. *Psychopharmacology* **127**, 276–82.

Hollander, E., DeCaria, C., Gully, R. *et al.* (1991) Effects of chronic fluoxetine treatment on behavioral and neuroendocrine responses to meta-chlorophenylpiperazine in obsessive-compulsive disorder. *Psychiatry Res* **36**, 1–17.

Hollander, E., Liebowitz, M.R., Cohen, B. *et al.* (1989) Prolactin and sodium lactate-induced panic. *Psychiatry Res* **28**, 181–91.

Hollander, E., Liebowitz, M.R., DeCaria, C. & Klein, D.F. (1990) Fenfluramine, cortisol, and anxiety. *Psychiatry Res* **31**, 211–13.

Hollander, E., Liebowitz, M.R., Gorman, J.M., Cohen, B., Fryer, A. & Klein, D.F. (1989) Cortisol and sodium lactate-induced panic. *Arch Gen Psychiatry* **46**, 135–140.

Javanmard, M., Shlik, J., Kennedy, S.H., Vaccarino, F.J., Houle, S. & Bradwejn, J. (1999) Neuroanatomic correlates of CCK-4 induced panic attacks in healthy humans: a comparison of two time points. *Biol Psychiatry* **45**, 872–82.

Jensen, C.F., Keller, T.W., Peskind, E.R. *et al.* (1997) Behavioral and neuroendocrine responses to sodium lactate infusion in subjects with post-traumatic stress disorder. *Am J Psychiatry* **152**, 266–8.

Jensen, C.F., Peskind, E.R., Veith, R.C. *et al.* (1991) Hypertonic saline infusion induces panic in patients with panic disorder. *Biol Psychiatry* **30**, 628–30.

Kahn, R.S., Asnis, G.M., Wetzler, S. & van Pragg, H.M. (1988) Neuroendocrine evidence for serotonin receptor hypersensitivity in panic disorder. *Psychopharmacology* **96**, 360–4.

Kahn, R.S. & Wetzler, S. (1991) m-Chlorophenylpiperazine as a probe of serotonin function. *Biol Psychiatry* **30**, 1139–66.

Keck, P.E., Jr, Taylor, V.E., Tugrul, K.C., McElroy, S.L. & Bennett, J.A. (1993) Valproate treatment of panic disorder and lactate-induced panic attacks. *Biol Psychiatry* **33**, 542–6.

Kellner, M., Herzog, L., Yassouridis, A., Holsboer, F. & Wiedermann, K. (1995) Possible role of atrial natriuretic hormone in pituitary-adrenocortical unresponsiveness in lactate-induced panic. *Am J Psychiatry* **152**, 1365–7.

Kellner, M., Knaudt, K., Jahn, H., Holsboer, F. & Wiedemann, K. (1998) Atrial natriuretic hormone in lactate-induced panic attacks: mode of release and endocrine and pathophysiological consequences. *J Psychiatric Res* **32**, 37–48.

Kellner, M., Wiedemann, K., Yassouridis, A. *et al.* (2000) Behavioral and endocrine response to cholecystokinin tetrapeptide in patients with post-traumatic stress disorder. *Biol Psychiatry* **41**, 107–11.

Kellner, M., Yassouridis, A. & Wiedemann, J.H. (1997) Influence of clonidine on psychopathological, endocrine and repiratory effects of cholecystokinin-tetrapeptide in patients with panic disorder. *Psychopharmacology* **133**, 55–61.

Kelly, D., Mitchell-Heggs, N. & Sherman, D. (1971) Anxiety and the effects of sodium lactate assessed clinically and physiologically. *Br J Psychiatry* **119**, 129–41.

Kennedy, J.L., Bradwejn, J., Koszycki, D. *et al.* (1999) Investigation of cholecystokinin system genes in panic disorder. *Mol Psychiatry* **4**, 284–5.

Kent, J.M., Papp, L.A., Martinez, J.M. *et al.* (2001) Specificity of panic response to CO_2 inhalation in panic disorder: a comparison with major depression and premenstrual dysphoric disorder. *Am J Psychiatry* **158**, 58–67.

Khanna, S., John, J.P. & Lakshmi Reddy, P. (2001) Neuroendocrine and behavioral responses to mCPP in obsessive-compulsive disorder. *Psychoneuroendocrinolgy* **26**, 209–23.

Klaassen, T., Ho Pian, K.L., Westenberg, H.G., den Boer, J.A. & van Praag, H.M. (1998) Serotonin syndrome after challenge with the 5-HT agonist metachlorophenylpiperazine. *Psychiatry Res* **79**, 207–12.

Klein, D. (1993) False suffocation alarms, spontaneous panics, and related conditions. *Arch Gen Psychiatry* **50**, 306–17.

Klein, E., Zohar, J., Geraci, M.F., Murphy, D.L. & Uhde, T.W. (1991) Anxiogenic effect of mCCP in patients with panic disorder: comparison to caffeine's anxiogenic effects. *Biol Psychiatry* **30**, 973–84.

Koszycki, D. (1995) Psychological factors and response to cholecystokinin. In: *Cholecystokinin and Anxiety: From Neuron to Behavior* (J. Bradwejn & E. Vasar (eds), pp. 87–99). R.G. Landes Co., Austin, TX.

Koszycki, D. & Bradwejn, J. (2002) Anxiety sensitivity does not predict fearful responding to 35% carbon dioxide in patients with panic disorder. *Psychiatry Res* **101**, 137–43.

Koszycki, D., Zacharko, R.M., Le Mellédo, J.-M. & Bradwejn, J. (1998) Behavioral, cardiovascular, and neuroendocrine profiles following CCK-4 challenge in healthy volunteers: a comparison of panickers and nonpanickers. *Depress Anxiety* **8**, 1–7.

Koszycki, D., Zarcharko, R.M., Le Mellédo, J.-M., Young, S.N. & Bradwejn, J. (1996) Effect of acute tryptophan depletion on behavioral, cardiovascular, and hormonal sensitivity to cholecystokinin-tetrapeptide challenge in healthy volunteers. *Biol Psychiatry* **40**, 648–55.

Kushner, M.G., Mackenzie, T.B., Fiszdon, J. *et al.* (1996) The effects of alcohol consumption on laboratory-induced panic and state anxiety. *Arch Gen Psychiatry* **53**, 264–70.

Le Mellédo, J.-M., Bradwejn, J., Koszycki, D., Bichet, D.G. & Bellavance, F. (1998) The role of the β-noradrenergic system in cholecystokinin-tetrapeptide-induced panic symptoms. *Biol Psychiatry* **44**, 364–6.

Le Mellédo, J.-M., Merani, S., Koszycki, D. *et al.* (1999) Sensitivity to CCK-4 in women with and without premenstrual dysphoric disorder (PMDD) during their follicular and luteal phases. *Neuropsychopharmacology* **20**(1), 81–91.

Le Mellédo, J.-M., Van Driel, M., Coupland, N.J. *et al.* (2000) Response to flumazenil in women with premenstrual dysphoric disorder. *Am J Psychiatry* **157**, 821–3.

Lee, Y.-J., Curtis, G.C., Weg, J.G. *et al.* (1993) Panic attacks induced by doxapram. *Biol Psychol* **33**, 295–7.

Lesch, K.P., Wiesmann, M., Hoh, A. *et al.* (1992) 5-HT1A receptor-effector system responsivity in panic disorder. *Psychopharmacology* **106**, 111–17.

Levin, A.P., Doran, A.R., Liebowitz, M.R. *et al.* (1987) Pituitary adrenocortical unresponsiveness in lactate-induced panic. *Psychiatry Res* **21** (1), 23–32.

Liebowitz, M.R., Copland, J.D., Martinez, J. *et al.* (1995) Effects of intravenous diazepam pretreatment of lactate-induced panic. *Psychiatry Res* **58**, 127–38.

Liebowitz, M.R., Fyer, A.J., Gorman, J.M. *et al.* (1984) Lactate provocation of panic attacks. I. Clinical and behavioral correlates. *Arch Gen Psychiatry* **41**, 764–70.

Liebowitz, M.R., Fyer, A.J., Gorman, J.M. *et al.* (1985a) Specificity of lactate infusions in social phobia versus panic disorder. *Am J Psychiatry* **142**, 947–50.

Liebowitz, M.R., Gorman, J.M., Fyer, A.J. *et al.* (1985b) Lactate provocation of panic attacks. II. Biochemical and physiological findings. *Arch Gen Psychiatry* **42**, 709–19.

Liebowitz, M.R., Gorman, J.M., Fyer, A.J., Dillon, D., Levitt, M. & Klein, D.F. (1986) Possible mechanisms for lactate's induction of panic. *Am J Psychiatry* **143**, 495–502.

Lindy, D.C., Walsh, B.T., Gorman, J.M. *et al.* (1988) Lactate infusions in patients with bulimia. *Psychiatry Res* **26**(3), 287–92.

Lines, C., Challenor, J. & Traub, M. (1995) Cholecystokinin and anxiety in normal volunteers: an investigation of the anxiogenic properties of pentagastrin and reversal by the cholecystokinin receptor subtype B antagonists L-3650260. *Brit J Clin Pharmacol* **39**, 235–42.

Lovallo, W.R., Al'absi, M., Blick, K. *et al.* (1996) Stress-like adrenocorticotropin responses to caffeine in young healthy men. *Pharmacol Biochem Behav* **55**, 365–9.

Lucas, P.B., Pickar, D., Kelsoe, J., Rapaport, M., Pato, C. & Hommer, D. (1990) Effects of acute administration of caffeine in patients with schizophrenia. *Biol Psychiatry* **28**, 35–40.

Lucey, J.V., O'Keane, V., Butcher, G., Clare, A.W. & Dinan, T.G. (1992) Cortisol and prolactin responses to d-fenfluramine in nondepressed patients with obsessive-compulsive disorder: a comparison with depressed and healthy controls. *Br J Psychiatry* **161**, 517–21.

Malizia, A.L., Cunningham, V.J., Bell, C.J., Liddle, P.F., Jones, T. & Nutt, D.J. (1998) Decreased brain GABA-A-benzodiazepine receptor binding in panic disorder: Preliminary results from a quantitative PET study. *Arch Gen Psychiatry* **55**, 715–20.

Mathew, R.J. & Wilson, W.H. (1988) Cerebral blood flow changes induced by CO_2 in anxiety. *Psychiatry Res* **23**, 285–94.

Matilla, M., Seppala, T. & Matilla, M.J. (1988) Anxiogenic effect of yohimbine in healthy subjects: comparison with caffeine and antagonism by clonidine and diazepam. *Int J Clin Psychopharmacol* **3** (3), 215–29.

McCann, U.D., Morgan, C.M., Geraci, M. *et al.* (1997) Effects of the 5-HT3 antagonist, ondansetron, on the behavioral and physiological effects of pentagastrin in patients with panic disorder and social phobia. *Neuropsychopharmacology* **17**, 360–9.

McCann. U.D., Eligulashvili, V. & Ricaurte, G.A. (1998) Adverse neuropsychiatric events associated with dexfenfluramine and fenfluramine. *Prog Neuropsychopharmacology Biol Psychiatry* **22**, 1087–102.

Miller, H.E.J., Deakin, J.F.W. & Anderson, I.M. (2000) Effect of acute tryptophan depletion on CO_2-induced

anxiety in patients with panic disorder and normal volunteers. *Br J Psychiatry* **176**, 182–8.

Mortimore, C. & Anderson, I.M. (2000) d-Fenfluramine in panic disorder: a dual role for 5-hydroxytryptamine. *Psychopharmacology* **149**, 251–8.

Murphy, D.L., Aulakh, C., Mazzola-Pomietto, P. & Briggs, N.C. (1996) Neuroendocrine responses to serotonergic agonists as indices of the functional status of central serotonin neurotransmission in humans: a preliminary comparative analysis of neuroendocrine endpoints versus other endpoint measures. *Behav Brain Res* **73**, 209–14.

Nardi, A.E., Valenca, A.M., Nascimento, I., Mezzasalma, M.A. & Zin, W.A. (2000) Double-blind acute clonazepam versus placebo in carbon dioxide-induced panic attacks. *Psychiatry Res* **94**(2), 179–84.

Nehlig, A., Daval, J.-L. & Debry, G. (1992) Caffeine and the central nervous system: mechanisms of action, biochemical, metabolic and psychostimulant effects. *Brain Research Reviews* **17**, 139–70.

Nesse, R.M., Cameron, O.G., Curtis, G.C., McCann, D.S. & Huber-Smith, M.J. (1984) Adrenergic function in patients with panic anxiety. *Arch Gen Psychiatry* **41**, 771–6.

Nickell, P.V. & Uhde, T.W. (1995) Dose-response of intravenous caffeine in normal volunteers. *Anxiety* **1**, 161–8.

Noble, F., Wank, S.A., Crawley, J.N. *et al.* (2000) International union of pharmacology. XXI. Structure, distribution, and functions of cholecystokinin receptors. *Pharmacological Reviews* **51**, 745–81.

Norman, T.R., Apostolopoulos, M., Burrows, G.D. & Judd, F.K. (1994) Neuroendocrine responses to single doses of buspirone in obsessive-compulsive disorder. *Int Clin Psychopharmacol* **9**, 89–94.

Nutt, D.J., Glue, P., Lawson, C. & Wilson, S. (1990) Flumazenil provocation of panic attacks: evidence for altered benzodiazepine receptor sensitivity in panic disorder. *Arch Gen Psychiatry* **47**, 917–25.

Nutt, D.J. & Lawson, C. (1992) Panic attacks. a neurochemical overview of the models and mechanisms. *Br J Psychiatry* **161**, 517–21.

Orlikov, A. & Ryzov, I. (1991) Caffeine-induced anxiety and increase of kynurenine concentration in plasma of healthy subjects: a pilot project. *Biol Psychiatry* **29**, 391–6.

Papp, L.A., Goetz, R., Cole, R. *et al.* (1989) Hypersensitivity to carbon dioxide in panic disorder. *Am J Psychiatry* **146**, 779–81.

Papp, L.A., Klein, D.F., Martinez, J. *et al.* (1993) Diagnostic and substance specificity of carbon-dioxide-induced panic. *Am J Psychiatry* **150**, 250–7.

Papp, L.A., Martinez, J.M., Klein, D.F. *et al.* (1997) Respiratory psychophysiology of panic disorder: three respiratory challenges in 98 subjects. *Am J Psychiatry* **154**, 1557–65.

Perna, G., Bertani, B., Arancio, C., Ronchi, P. & Bellodi, L. (1995b) Laboratory response of patients with panic obsessive-compulsive disorders to 35% CO_2 challenges. *Am J Psychiatry* **152**, 85–9.

Perna, G., Bertani, B., Cocchi, S., Bertani, A. & Gasperini, M. (1995c) 35% CO_2 challenge in panic and mood disorders. *J Affect Disord* **33**, 189–94.

Perna, G., Bertani, A., Gabriele, A. & Bellodi, L. (1997) Modification of 35% carbon dioxide hypersensitivity across 1 week of treatment with clomipramine and fluvoxamine: a double-blind, randomized, placebo-controlled study. *J Clin Psychopharmacol* **17**, 173–8.

Perna, G., Bussi, R., Allevi, L. & Bellodi, L. (1999a) Sensitivity to 35% carbon dioxide in patients with generalized anxiety disorder. *J Clin Psychiatry* **60**, 379–84.

Perna, G., Cocchi, S., Allevi, L., Bussi, R. & Bellodi, L. (1999b) A long-term prospective evaluation of first-degree relatives of panic patients who underwent 35% CO_2 challenge. *Biol Psychiatry* **45**, 365–7.

Perna, G., Cocchi, S., Bertani, A., Arancio, C. & Bellodi, L. (1994) Pharmacologic effect of toloxatone on reactivity to the 35% carbon dioxide challenge: a single-blind, random, placebo-controlled study. *J Clin Psychopharmacol* **14**, 414–18.

Perna, G., Cocchi, S., Bertani, A., Arancio, C. & Bellodi, L. (1995d) Sensitivity to 35% CO_2 in healthy first-degree relatives of patients with panic disorder. *Am J Psychiatry* **152**, 623–5.

Perna, G., Gabriele, A., Caldirola, D. & Bellodi, L. (1995a) Hypersensitivity to inhalation of carbon dioxide and panic attacks. *Psychiatry Res* **57**, 267–73.

Peskind, E.R., Jensen, C.F., Pascualy, M. *et al.* (1998) Sodium lactate and hypertonic sodium choloride induce equivalent panic incidence, panic symptoms, and hypernatremia in panic disorder. *Biol Psychiatry* **44**, 1007–16.

Pine, D.S., Coplan, J.D., Papp, L.A. *et al.* (1998) Ventilatory physiology of children and adolescents with anxiety disorders. *Arch Gen Psychiatry* **55**, 123–9.

Pine, D.S., Klein, R.G., Coplan, J.D. *et al.* (2000) Differential carbon dioxide sensitivity in childhood anxiety disorders and nonill comparison group. *Arch Gen Psychiatry* **57**, 960–7.

Pine, D.S., Weese-Mayer, D.E., Silvestri, J.M., Davies, M., Whitaker, A.H. & Klein, D.F. (1994) Anxiety and the congenital central hypoventilation syndrome. *Am J Psychiatry* **151**, 864–70.

Pitts, F.N. Jr & McClure, J.N. Jr (1967) Lactate metabolism in anxiety neurosis. *N Engl J Med* **277**, 1329–36.

Pohl, R., Balon, R. & Lycaki, H. (1994) Lactate-induced anxiety after imipramine and diazepam treatment. *Anxiety* **1**(2), 54–63.

Pohl, R., Pandey, G.N., Yeragani, V.K., Balon, R., Davis, J.M. & Berchou, R. (1993) β-Receptor responsiveness after desipramine treatment. *Psychopharmacology* **110**, 37–44.

Pohl, R., Yeragani, V.K. & Balon, R. (1990) Effects of isoproterenol in panic disorder patients after antidepressant treatment. *Biol Psychiatry* **28**, 203–14.

Pohl, R., Yeragani, V.K., Balon, R. *et al.* (1988a) Isoproterenol-induced panic attacks. *Biol Psychiatry* **24**, 891–902.

Pohl, R., Yeragani, V.K., Balon, R. & Lycaki, H. (1989) Lactate and isoproterenol infusions in bulimic patients. *Neuropsychobiology* **22**, 225–30.

Pohl, R., Yergani, V.K., Balon, R. & Lycaki, H. (1988b) The jitteriness syndrome in panic disorder patients treated with antidepressants. *J Clin Psychiatry* **49**, 100–4.

Pols, H.J., Hauzer, R.C., Meijer, J.A., Verburg, K. & Griez, E.J. (1996a) Fluvoxamine attenuates panic induced by 35% CO_2 challenge. *J Clin Psychiatry* **57**, 539–42.

Pols, H., Verburg, K., Hauzer, R., Meijer, J. & Griez, E. (1996b) Alprazolam premedication and 35% carbon dioxide vulnerability in panic patients. *Biol Psychiatry* **40**, 913–17.

Pols, H., Zandbergen, J., de Loof, C. *et al.* (1991) Attenuation of carbon dioxide-induced panic after clonazepman treatment. *Acta Psychiatr Scand* **84**, 885–6.

Pyke, R.E. & Greenberg, H.S. (1986) Norepinephrine challenges in panic patients. *J Clin Psychopharmacol* **6**, 279–85.

Rainey, J.M., Aleem, A., Ortiz, A., Yeragani, V., Pohl, R. & Berchou, R. (1987) A laboratory procedure for the induction of flashbacks. *Am J Psychiatry* **144**, 1317–19.

Rainey, J.M., Frohman, C.E., Freedman, R.R., Pohl, R.B., Ettedgui, E. & Williams, M. (1984a) Specificity of lactate infusion as a model of anxiety. *Psychopharmacol Bull* **20**, 45–57.

Rainey, J.M., Pohl, R.B., Williams, M., Knitter, E., Freedman, R.R. & Ettedgui, E. (1984c) A comparison of lactate and isoproterenol anxiety states. *Psychopathology* **17** (Suppl. 1), 74–82.

Rainey, M., Jr, Ettedgui, E., Pohl, B. *et al.* (1984b) The β-receptor: isoproterenol anxiety states. *Psychopathology* **17** (Suppl. 3), 40–51.

Rasmussen, S.A., Goodman, W.K., Woods, S.W., Henninger, G.R. & Charney, D.S. (1987) Effects of yohimbine in obsessive-compulsive disorder. *Psychopharmacology* **93**, 308–13.

Redmond, D.E. (1977) Alterations in the function of the nucleus locus ceruleus: a possible model for studies in anxiety. In: *Animal Models in Psychiatry and Neurology* (I. Hanin & E. Usdin (eds), 293–304). Pergamon Press, New York.

Reiman, E.M., Raichle, M.E., Robins, E. *et al.* (1986) The application of positron emission tomography to the study of panic disorder. *Am J Psychiatry* **143**, 469–77.

Reiman, E.M., Raichle, M.E., Robins, E. *et al.* (1989) Neuroanatomical correlates of a lactate-induced anxiety attack. *Arch Gen Psychiatry* **46**, 493–500.

Reschke, A.H., Mannuzza, S., Chapman, T.F. *et al.* (1995) Sodium lactate response and familial risk for panic disorder. *Am J Psychiatry* **152**, 277–9.

Rifkin, A., Klein, D., Dillon, D. & Levitt, M. (1981) Blockade by imipramine or desipramine of panic induced by sodium lactate. *Am J Psychiatry* **138**, 676–7.

Rowland, B.E. & Carlton, J. (1986) Neurobiology of an anorectic drug: fenfluramine. *Progress in Neurobiology* **27**, 13–62.

Roy-Byrne, P.P., Cowley, D.S., Greenblatt, D.J., Shader, R.I. & Hommer, D. (1990) Reduced benzodiazepine sensitivity in panic disorder. *Arch Gen Psychiatry* **47**, 534–8.

Salkovskis, P.M. & Clark, D.M. (1990) Affective responses to hyperventilation: a test of the cognitive model of panic. *Behav Res Ther* **28**, 51–61.

Sallee, F.R., Sethuraman, G., Sine, L. & Liu, H. (2000) Yohimbine challenge in children with anxiety disorders. *Am J Psychiatry* **157**, 1236–42.

Sandberg, D., Endicott, J., Harrison, W., Nee, J. & Gorman, J. (1993) Sodium lactate infusion in late luteal phase dysphoric disorder. *Psychiatry Res* **46**, 79–88.

Sanderson, W.C., Wetzler, S. & Asnis, G.M. (1994) Alprazolam blockade in CO_2-provoked panic in patients with panic disorder. *Am J Psychiatry* **151**, 1220–2.

Schmidt, N.B., Telch, M.J. & Jaimez, T.L. (1996) Biological challenge manipulation of $P{CO_2}$ levels: a test of Klein's (1993) suffocation alarm theory of panic. *J Abnorm Psychol* **105**, 446–54.

Schruers, K., Klaassen, T., Pols, H., Overbeek, T., Deutz, N.E.P. & Griez, E. (2000) Effects of tryptophan depletion on carbon dioxide provoked panic in panic disorder patients. *Psychiatry Res* **93**, 179–87.

Sevy, S., Brown, S.L., Wetzler, S. *et al.* (1994) Effects of alprazolam on increases in hormonal and anxiety levels induced by meta-chlorophenylpiperazine. *Psychiatry Res* **53**, 219–29.

Shear, M.K. (1986) Pathophysiology of panic: a review of pharmacologic provocation tests and naturalistic monitoring data. *J Clin Psychiatry* **4** (Suppl. 6), 18–26.

Shear, M.K., Fyer, A.J., Ball, G. *et al.* (1991) Vulnerability to sodium lactate in panic disorder patients given cognitive-behavioral therapy. *Am J Psychiatry* **148**, 795–97.

Shekhar, A. & Keim, S.R. (1997) The circumventricular organs form a potential neural pathway for lactate sensitivity: implications for panic disorder. *J Neurosci* **17**, 9726–35.

Shlik, J., Aluoja, A., Vasar, V., Vasar, E., Podar, T. & Bradwejn, J. (1997a) Effects of citalopram treatment on behavioral, cardiovascular and neuroendocrine response to cholecystokinin tetrapeptide challenge in patients with panic disorder. *Revue de psychiatrie et du neuroscience* **22**, 332–40.

Shlik, J., Vasar, V., Aluoja, A. *et al.* (1997b) The effect of cholecystokinin tetrapeptide on respiratory resistance in healthy volunteers. *Biol Psychiatry* **42**, 206–12.

Shlik, J., Vasar, E. & Vasar, V. (2000) Clonidine does not block CCK-4 induced panic in healthy volunteers. *Int J Neuropsychopharmacol* **3** (Suppl. 1), S290.

Sinha, S.S., Coplan, J.D., Martinez, J.A., Klein, D.F. & Gorman, J.M. (1999) Panic induced by carbon dioxide inhalation and lack of hypothalamic–pituitary–adrenal axis activation. *Psychiatry Res* **86**(2), 93–8.

Southwick, S.M., Krystal, J.H., Bremner, J.D. *et al.* (1997) Noradrenergic and serotonergic function in post-traumatic stress disorder. *Arch Gen Psychiatry* **54**, 749–58.

Southwick, S.M., Morgan, C.A., Charney, D.S. & High, J.R. (1999) Yohimbine use in a natural setting: effects on post-traumatic stress disorder. *Biol Psychiatry* **46**, 442–4.

Stein, M.B. *et al.* (1999) Single photon emission computed tomography of the brain with Tc-99m HMPAQ during sumatriptan challenge in obsessive-compulsive disorder: investigating the functional role of the serotonin auto-receptor. *Prog Neuropsychopharmacological Biol Psychiatry* **23**, 1079–99.

Stein, M.B. & Uhde, T.W. (1989) Depersonalization disorder: effects of caffeine and response to pharmacotherapy. *Biol Psychiatry* **26** (3), 315–20.

Ströhle, A., Kellner, M., Holsboer, F. & Wiederman, K. (1998) Effect of flumazenil in lactate-sensitive patients with panic disorder. *Am J Psychiatry* **155**, 610–12.

Ströhle, A., Kellner, M., Holsboer, F. & Wiederman, K. (2000) Behavioral, neuroendocrine, and cardiovascular response to flumazenil: no evidence for an altered benzodiazepine receptor sensitivity in panic disorder. *Biol Psychiatry* **45**, 321–6.

Sullivan, G.M., Coplan, J.D., Kent, J.M. & Gorman, J.M. (1999) The noradrenergic system in pathological anxiety: a focus on panic with relevance to generalized anxiety and phobias. *Biol Psychiatry* **46**, 1205–18.

Tancer, M.E., Black, B. & Brown, T.M. (1991) Phenomenology and neurobiology of social phobia: comparison with panic disorder. *J Clin Psychiatry* **52** (Suppl.), 31–40.

Tanum, L. & Malt, U.F. (1995) Sodium lactate infusion in fibromyalgia patients. *Biol Psychiatry* **38**, 559–61.

Targum, S.D. (1990) Differential responses to anxiogenic challenge studies in patients with major depressive disorder and panic disorder. *Biol Psychiatry* **28**, 21–34.

Targum, S.D. (1992) Cortisol response during different anxiogenic challenges in panic disorder patients. *Psychoneuroendocrinology* **17**(5), 453–8.

Targum, S.D. & Marshall, L.E. (1989) Fenfluramine provocation of anxiety in patients with panic disorder. *Psychiatry Res* **28**, 295–306.

Uhde, T.W. (1990) Caffeine provocation on panic: a focus on biological mechanisms. *Neurobiology of Panic Disorder.* Alan R. Liss, New York, pp. 219–42.

Uhde, T.W., Boulenger, J.-P., Jimerson, D.C. & Post, R.M. (1984) Caffeine: relationship to human anxiety, plasma MHPG, and cortisol. *Psychopharmacol Bull* 20, 426–30.

Uhde, T.W., Tancer, M.E., Rubinow, D.R. *et al.* (1992) Evidence for hypothalamo-growth hormone dysfunction in panic disorder: profile to growth hormone (GH) responses to clonidine, yohimbine, caffeine, glucose, GRF and TRH in panic disorder patients versus healthy volunteers. *Neuropsychopharmacology* 6(2), 101–18.

Van den Hout, M.A. & Griez, E. (1984) Panic symptoms after inhalation of carbon dioxide. *Br J Psychiatry* 144, 503–7.

Van der Wee, N., Fiselier, J., van Megen, H.G., Van Vliet, I. & Westenberg, H.G. (1999) Behavioral effects of rapid intravenous challenge with meta-chlorophenyl-piperazine (0.1 mg/kg) in patients with panic disorder and controls. *Eur Neuropsychopharmacol* 9 (Suppl. 5), S308.

Van Megen, H.G., Westenberg, H.G., den Boer, J.A., Haigh, J.R. & Traub, M. (1994) Pentagastrin induced panic attacks: enhanced sensitivity in panic disorder patients. *Psychopharmacology* 114, 449–55.

Van Megen, H.G., Westenberg, H.G., den Boer, J.A., Slaap, B. & Scheepmakers, A. (1997) Effect of the selective serotonin reuptake inhibitor fluvoxamiine on CCK-4-induced panic attacks. *Psychopharmacology* 129, 357–64.

Van Vliet, I.M., Slaap, B.R., Westenberg, H.G. & Den Boer, J.A. (1996) Behavioral, neuroendocrine, and biochemical effects of different doses of 5-HTP in panic disorder. *Eur Neuropsychopharmacol* 6, 103–110.

Veltman, D.J., van Zijderveld, G.A. & van Dyck, R. (1996) Epinephrine infusions in panic disorder: a double-blind placebo-controlled study. *J Affect Disord* 39, 133–40.

Veltman, D.J., van Zijderveld, G.A., van Dyck, R. & Bakker, A. (1998) Predictability, controllability, and fear of symptoms of anxiety in epinephrine-induced panic. *Biol Psychiatry* 44, 1017–26.

Verburg, C., Griez, E. & Meijer, A. (1994) A 35% carbon dioxide challenge in simple phobias. *Acta Psychiatr Scand* 90, 420–3.

Verburg, C., Griez, E., Meijer, J. & Pols, H. (1995) Discrimination between panic disorder and generalized anxiety disorder by 35% carbon dioxide challenge. *Am J Psychiatry* 152, 1081–3.

Verburg, C., Pols, H., de Leeuw, M. & Griez, E. (1998) Reliability of 35% carbon dioxide panic provocation challenge. *Psychiatry Res* 78, 207–14.

Westenberg, H.G. & den Boer, J.A. (1989) Serotonin function in panic disorder: effect of 1–5-hydroxytryptophan in patients and controls. *Psychopharmacology* 98, 283–5.

Wetzler, S., Asnis, G.M., DeLecuona, J.M. & Kalus, O. (1996) Serotonin function in panic disorder: intravenous administration of meta-chlorophenylpiperazine. *Psychiatry Res* 64, 77–82.

Woods, S.W., Charney, D.S., Delgado, P.L. & Heninger, G.R. (1990) The effect of long-term imipramine treatment on carbon dioxide-induced anxiety in panic disorder patients. *J Clin Psychiatry* 5, 505–7.

Woods, S.W., Charney, D.S., Goodman, W.K. & Heninger, G.R. (1988a) Carbon dioxide-induced anxiety. *Arch Gen Psychiatry* 45, 43–52.

Woods, S.W., Charney, D.S., Loke, J., Goodman, W.K., Redmond, D.E. Jr & Heninger, G.R. (1986) Carbon dioxide sensitivity in panic anxiety. *Arch Gen Psychiatry* 43, 900–9.

Woods, S.W., Charney, D.S., McPherson, C.A., Gradman, A.H. & Heninger, G.R. (1987) Situational panic attacks: behavioral, physiologic, and biochemical characterization. *Arch Gen Psychiatry* 44, 365–75.

Woods, S.W., Charney, D.S., Silver, J.M., Krystal, J.H. & Heninger, G.R. (1991) Behavioral, neuroendocrine, and cardiovascular response to the benzodiazepine receptor antagonist flumazenil in panic disorder. *Psychiatry Res* 36, 115–27.

Woods, S.W., Koster, K., Krystal, J.K. *et al.* (1988b) Yohimbine alters regional cerebral blood flow in panic disorder. *Lancet* 2, 678.

Woods, S.W., Krystal, J.H., D'Amico, C.L., Heninger, G.R. & Charney, D.S. (1988c) A review of behavioral and pharmacologic studies relevant to the application of CO_2 as a human subject model of anxiety. *Psychopharmacol Bull* 24, 149–53.

Woods, S.W., Krystal, J.H., Heninger, G.R. & Charney, D.S. (1989) Effects of alprazolam and clonidine on carbon dioxide-induced increases in anxiety ratings in healthy human subjects. *Life Sciences* 45, 233–42.

Yeragani, V.K., Pohl, R., Balon, R., Rainey, J.M., Berchou, R. & Ortiz, A. (1988) Sodium lactate infusions after treatment with tricyclic antidepressants: behavioral and physiological findings. *Biol Psychiatry* 24, 767–74.

Yeragani, V.K., Pohl, R., Srinivasan, K., Balon, R., Ramesh, C. & Berchou, R. (1995) Effects of isoproterenol infusions on heart rate variability in patients with panic disorder. *Psychiatry Res* 56, 289–93.

van Zijderveld, G.A., TenVoorde, B.J., Veltman, D.J. *et al.* (1997) Cardiovascular, respiratory, and panic reactions to epinephrine in panic disorder patients. *Biol Psychiatry* 41, 249–51.

van Zijderveld, G.A., van Doornen, L.J.P., van Faassen, I. *et al.* (1992) The psychophysiological effects of adrenaline infusions as a function of trait anxiety and aerobic fitness. *Anxiety Res* 4, 257–74.

van Zijderveld, G.A., Veltman, D.J., van Dyck, R. & van Doornen, L.J. (1999) Epinephrine-induced panic attacks and hyperventilation. *J Psychiatr Res* **33** (1), 73–8.

Zohar, J., Mueller, E.A., Insel, T.R., Zohar-Kadouch, R.C. & Murphy, D.L. (1987) Serotonergic responsivity in obsessive-compulsive disorder: comparison of patients and healthy controls. *Arch Gen Psychiatry* **44**, 946–51.

Zohar, J., Thomas, T.R., Zohar-Kadouch, R.C., Hill, J.R. & Murphy, D.L. (1988) Serotonergic responsivity in obsessive-compulsive disorder: effects of chronic clomipramine treatment. *Arch Gen Psychiatry* **45**, 167–72.

16 Panic Disorder and Medical Illness

T.S. Zaubler & W. Katon

Introduction

Panic disorder (PD) is a common, disabling psychiatric illness that is closely linked with several medical conditions and medically unexplained symptoms. Patients with PD will often select one of their most frightening symptoms and present to their physicians with cardiac, respiratory, gastrointestinal or neurologic complaints such as chest pain, palpitations, epigastric pain, lower abdominal pain, diarrhea, headache or dizziness (Zaubler & Katon 1998). Given the overlap between the symptoms associated with panic attacks and other medical illnesses, the vast majority of patients with PD present for treatment in the medical setting. It is often only after patients have gone to their primary care or emergency room physicians on multiple occasions that a correct diagnosis of PD is made and appropriate treatment is initiated. This chapter explores the association between PD and specific medical illnesses and medically unexplained symptoms.

Prevalence and utilization of medical services

The National Comorbidity Survey (NCS) Study found that the 12 month prevalence of PD in the community was 3.2% in women and 1.3% in men (Kessler *et al.* 1994; Table 16.1). Many people who do not meet full Diagnostic Statistical Manual, fourth edition (DSM-IV; American Psychiatric Association 1994) criteria for PD do experience occasional panic attacks with estimates for prevalence in the community ranging from 3.6% to 10% (Klerman *et al.* 1991). In the primary

care setting as many as 4–13% of patients meet criteria for PD and 16.5% experience panic attacks (Katon *et al.* 1986; Goodwin *et al.* 2001). Patients seen in the primary care setting who are particularly likely to have PD include (i) those with multiple, common medically unexplained symptoms; (ii) patients complaining of anxiety and tension (Schurman *et al.* 1985; Katon 1994); (iii) patients with hypochondriacal concerns about their medical symptoms (Simon & VonKorff 1991; Table 16.2); and (iv) patients with certain medical problems such as labile hypertension, mitral valve prolapse, asthma and chronic obstructive pulmonary disease and migraine headaches (Katon 1994; Zaubler & Katon 1998).

Utilization of primary care services by patients with PD is approximately three times greater than for most

Table 16.1 Prevalence of PD in community, primary care, and medically unexplained symptom samples.

Sample source	PD prevalence (%)
Community	1.3–3.2
Primary care	4–13
Primary care high utilizers	22
Chest pain/negative angiogram	43–61
Hypertensives screened for pheochromocytoma	28
Irritable bowel syndrome	29
Asthma	6.5–24
Unexplained dizziness	20
Headache	15

PD, panic disorder.

Table 16.2 Psychiatric disorder and increased probability of multiple unexplained physical symptoms. (From Simon & VonKorff 1991.)

Diagnosis	Odds ratio
PD	204
Schizophrenia	90
Mania	24
Major depression	17
Phobia	12

PD, panic disorder.

other primary care patients (Katon 1996). Data from the National Institute of Mental Health Epidemiologic Catchment Area (ECA) Program have shown that patients with PD are not only high utilizers of primary care services but also are more likely to seek treatment in emergency departments, inpatient medical settings and both inpatient and outpatient psychiatric settings (Markowitz et al. 1989; Klerman et al. 1991; Leon et al. 1995). Simpson et al. (1994) found that in the 10 years prior to a diagnosis of PD, patients with PD had significantly more visits to their primary care physicians, received more prescriptions for both psychotropic and nonpsychotropic medications, and had more hospital admissions, emergency room visits and diagnostic tests than a control group without psychiatric illness. Compared to patients with other psychiatric illnesses, patients with PD are significantly more likely to seek help from general medical and specialized mental health services, human service organizations and emergency departments (Markowitz et al. 1989; Leon et al. 1995).

The high rate of utilization of medical services by patients with PD may be due to several factors. Given the stigma attached to psychiatric illness, patients may be reluctant to accept a psychiatric explanation for their symptoms. Patients with PD also do characteristically experience their physical symptoms with great intensity and may be unaware that a psychiatric problem could cause such distressing physical symptoms. ECA program data have shown that patients with PD may be more likely to perceive their health as poor and in need of medical treatment than those with other psychiatric illnesses or those without any psychiatric illness (Klerman et al. 1991). Patients with PD may also catastrophize and misattribute their panic symptoms

as due to an acute medical illness such as myocardial infarction (Zaubler & Katon 1998).

Despite the high prevalence of PD in the medical setting and its association with increased utilization of medical services, it is often undiagnosed and untreated (Katon 1996). Fifer et al. (1994) found that anxiety symptoms in the medical setting are recognized and treated in only about 44% of anxious patients. In the emergency department, where patients with PD are likely to present with rapid heart beat or chest pain, physicians miss a diagnosis of PD 94% to 98% of the time (Yingling et al. 1993; Fleet et al. 1995). This under-recognition of PD in the medical setting leads to costly and unnecessary workups to investigate presumed medical etiologies for the somatic symptoms associated with PD (Simpson et al. 1994).

The consequences of PD

The low rates of detection of PD are of particular concern given the association between PD and significant functional disability and spiraling health care costs (Zaubler & Katon 1998). Patients with PD often develop financial problems. Up to 60% of patients with PD and 30% of patients with panic attacks are unemployed (Leon et al. 1995). Patients with PD are significantly more likely to receive public assistance or disability payments than patients with other psychiatric disorders (Klerman et al. 1991). They are at high risk for suicide and have high levels of family and social dysfunction (Markowitz et al. 1989; Katon et al. 1995). Their perception of their overall health and level of physical functioning is comparable to that of other patients with chronic medical illnesses such as diabetes and arthritis (Katon et al. 1995; Sherbourne et al. 1996). Patients who do not meet full criteria for PD but are experiencing panic attacks have been found to experience nearly comparably high rates of disability in vocational, familial and social functioning (Katon et al. 1995). Since panic attacks are more prevalent than PD, they may account for more functional disability within the community than PD.

While there is little information on the economic cost to society of PD, patients with PD undoubtedly often receive costly and unnecessary medical work ups. In a primary care practice, the likelihood of obtaining a positive diagnostic test for common symptoms such as chest pain and palpitations may range

Table 16.3 Costs of unrecognized PD (US$).

Chest pain	
Angiography	2000–3000
Echocardiography	350
Treadmill	150
Holter monitor	200
Irritable bowel syndrome	
Gastroscopy	300
Colonoscopy	500
Labile hypertension	
Pheochromocytoma	300
(Urinary catechol., VMA, met)	
Headache, dizziness	
MRI	1000
CAT scan	550
EEG	322

CAT, computed axial tomography; EEG, electroencephalograms; met, metanephrines; MRI, magnetic resonance angiography; PD, panic disorder; VMA, vanillylmandelic acid.

from 3% to 29% (Kroenke & Mangelsdorff 1989). Patients with PD are likely to present with many of these common symptoms and receive costly tests such as angiography, echocardiography, Holter monitoring and treadmill testing (Kroenke 1992; Katon 1996; Table 16.3). Salvador-Carulla *et al.* (1995) examined the costs associated with the treatment of PD (Fig. 16.1). They found that when comparing the costs pre- and post-treatment, treatment resulted in an increase in direct costs due to the increased use of mental health services. These costs were offset by a substantial decrease in indirect costs due to the increased productivity at, and decreased absenteeism from, work. Treatment of PD therefore may be associated with an overall decrease in costs to society.

Pathophysiology of panic

Patients with PD often report an interplay between stressful life events exacerbating or precipitating panic symptoms and ensuing physical symptoms which may also contribute to the experience of panic. Both stressful life events and changes in the internal homeostasis of organ systems can lead to changes in brain biochemistry that result in panic symptoms. There is strong evidence suggesting that a small cluster of noradrenergic neurones in the brain called the locus coerulus mediates the experience of panic symptoms (Redmond 1979).

The locus coerulus is activated in response to real or imagined external dangers in order to program the body to fight or flee. In patients with PD, the fight or

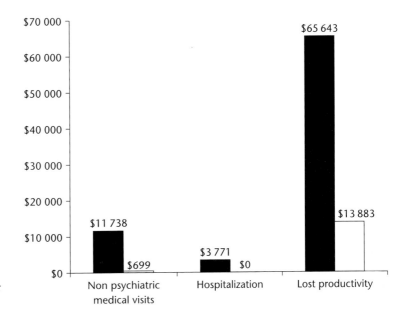

Fig. 16.1 Effect of diagnosis and treatment on cost of 61 patients with PD ■ 1 year before diagnosis; □ 1 year after diagnosis.

flight response is not appropriately calibrated so a panic response may occur in response to innocuous stimuli or even when there is an absence of any threatening stimulus. This miscalibration may result from stressful life circumstances which have been shown to cause a sustained alteration of synaptic transmission in the locus coerulus (Kandel 1983).

Changes in the body's internal homeostasis have also been shown to lead to altered synaptic transmission and increased firing of neurones in the locus coerulus (Kandel 1983; Svensson 1987; Katon & Roy-Byrne 1989). In animal studies, acute changes in blood pressure, arterial oxygen concentration and distension of the stomach, distal colon, rectum and urinary bladder have all been shown to lead to sustained activation of the locus coerulus (Svensson & Thoren 1979; Elam et al. 1984). The anxiety generated by these physiologic changes may be adaptive if it prompts the individual to seek help from the medical system for potentially harmful disease states that may be causing these changes in the body to occur. However, these internal homeostatic changes may also lead to locus coerulus activation in the absence of any disease state (Zaubler & Katon 1996).

An external stress may therefore lead to increased noradrenergic discharge, increased anxiety and a psychophysiologic illness such as irritable bowel syndrome or peptic ulcer disease. The changes in the body's internal homeostasis resulting from these illnesses may in turn lead to further locus coerulus activation and a vicious cycle of worsening anxiety. The emphasis that this pathophysiologic model of PD places on both external and internal stressors may help to explain why many patients with PD believe that their physical symptoms are causing their anxiety (Zaubler & Katon 1996).

PD and cardiac illness

There is considerable overlap between panic symptoms and the most common complaints of patients presenting for cardiologic evaluations. Of the 13 diagnostic symptoms of a panic attack (American Psychiatric Association 1994), five are typical for patients with cardiovascular diseases: chest pain, palpitations, shortness of breath, choking sensation, and sweating (Fleet et al. 2000). It can be exceedingly difficult to determine whether a patient's symptoms reflect a panic attack or true cardiac disease. Moreover, the two are not mutually exclusive. Many patients with substantiated cardiac illness also have comorbid panic attacks.

Chest pain

Chest pain is one of the most common symptoms associated with both panic attacks and heart disease. Between 25% and 57% of patients with PD experience chest pain (Jeejeebhoy et al. 2000). Conversely, Dammen et al. (1999) found that 38.2% of patients with chest pain seen in outpatient medical clinics have PD. Between 16% and 25% of patients presenting to an emergency room with a chief complaint of chest pain suffer from PD.

Medical work ups reveal no demonstrable cardiac basis for chest pain in over 50% of patients, and PD is 30–50 times more common in patients with noncardiac chest pain than in the general population (Fleet et al. 2000). In the outpatient setting, the prevalence of PD among patients with chest pain without coronary artery disease is 41.3% (Dammen et al. 1999). One study found that one-third of patients admitted to a cardiac care unit for a presumed myocardial infarction had PD, and 79% of patients with PD did not have conclusive evidence of cardiac disease (Carter et al. 1992).

The costs associated with medical evaluations for chest pain are enormous. In the primary care setting a workup for chest pain may cost several thousand dollars per patient, and more than 80% of these work ups are negative (Lavey & Winkle 1979; Kroenke & Mangelsdorff 1989; Zaubler & Katon 1996). Costs may spiral when patients are referred for angiography. Between 10% and 30% of patients referred for angiographic testing have minimal or no evidence of coronary artery disease (Lavey & Winkle 1979). One study found that in 1997 the cost for cardiac catheterizations in the US for patients without angiographic evidence of coronary artery disease was US$750 million (Carter et al. 1997).

While some patients with chest pain and normal angiograms are ultimately diagnosed with Prinzmetal's angina, costochondritis, mitral valve prolapse and esophageal motility disorders, between 43% and 61% of these patients were found to have PD (Bass et al. 1983; Beitman et al. 1987; Katon et al. 1988). Interestingly, among those patients with chest pain without angiographic findings, approximately 50% continue to experience significant vocational and social disabilities due to their chest pain 1 year after their angiograms (Ockene *et al.* 1980). Moreover, the presence of PD is one of the best predictors of persistent chest pain and disability in patients with normal angiograms (Beitman *et al.* 1991; Zaubler & Katon 1998).

Palpitations

Palpitations is another common symptom in patients both with PD and heart disease. Approximately 16% of patients seen in a medical setting complain of having palpitations, and 31% of these patients have been found to have PD, panic attacks or anxiety (Kroenke *et al.* 1990; Weber & Kapoor 1996). Among patients seen in outpatient cardiology practices, studies have found that over 20% of patients with palpitations have PD and approximately two-thirds of patients seen in this setting who have PD also report having palpitations (Morris *et al.* 1997). Compared to patients with palpitations without any psychiatric disorder, patients with palpitations and PD are typically more disabled, younger, and have more visits to the emergency room with somatic complaints (Jeejeebhoy *et al.* 2000). Many patients with palpitations undergo Holter monitoring as a workup for arrythmias. Studies have found that patients with normal Holter results are more hypochondriacal and have greater psychiatric morbidity and somatization than patients with documented arrhythmias (Barsky *et al.* 1994). Among patients undergoing Holter monitoring for palpitations, 18.6% have current PD and 27.6% have a lifetime prevalence of PD (Barsky *et al.* 1995). PD may therefore account for a significant percentage of the US$250 million spent annually in the US on Holter monitoring for palpitations (Katon 1996).

Panic-related cardiac symptoms in the absence of heart disease

There is an increasing body of research exploring possible perceptual, psychological and physiologic factors that may account for the link between PD and nonmedical cardiac symptoms. Patients with PD are often exquisitely sensitive to any homeostatic changes in their bodies. Clinicians frequently encounter patients who refuse to take medications due to the severity of side-effects they experience. There is considerable evidence that patients with PD have many somatic concerns and heightened bodily awareness. For example,

among patients undergoing Holter monitoring for palpitations, those that did not have any documented arrythmia had a much higher prevalence of PD, a greater fear of bodily sensations, increased hypochondriacal concerns and somatic complaints than those with arrhythmias (Barsky *et al.* 1994; Ehlers *et al.* 2000). Interestingly, PD patients are also more likely to misperceive their heartbeats than those with arrhythmias and no panic symptoms (Ehlers *et al.* 2000). Walker *et al.* (1990a) suggest that patients with PD may have distorted signal-to-noise ratios for internal body stimuli, thereby predisposing them to interpret background physiological activity and mild somatic symptoms as catastrophic events.

Some researchers have speculated that PD patients with cardiac symptoms may have a problem with cardiac nociception (Jeejeebhoy *et al.* 2000). Chest pain during cardiac catheterization can be elicited in patients with a history of medically unexplained cardiac symptoms by right ventricular pacing, contrast media injection into the left coronary artery or adenosine infusion (Cannon 1995). When performed on individuals with coronary artery disease, these procedures are typically painless.

Medically unexplained cardiac symptoms in patients with PD may reflect a syndrome of heightened sensitivity to visceral pain that occurs throughout the body. For example, patients with noncardiac chest pain have been found to have exaggerated pain sensitivity within the esophagus (Cannon 1995). These patients, similar to those with irritable bowel syndrome, have also been found to have abnormal sensitivity to inflation of balloon catheters in the upper and lower gastrointestinal tract (Moriarty & Dawson 1982). Heightened visceral pain sensitivity may therefore be attributed to increased anxiety and panic symptoms leading to hypervigilance toward internal body stimuli (Walker *et al.* 1995).

Microvascular angina

There is some research supporting the possibility of a physiologic explanation for noncardiac chest pain in patients with PD. A subset of angiographically normal patients with chest pain have been found to have dynamic blood flow abnormalities in the coronary microvasculature which are not detected by angiogram (Cannon 1988). The pain believed to be associated with this phenomenon is referred to as microvascular angina. Researchers have suggested that patients suffering from microvascular angina have a limited ability to increase blood flow in small cardiac vessels with increases in heart rate. Microvascular angina may account for chest pain in up to 75% of angiographically normal patients, and 40% of patients with microvascular angina have been found to have PD (Cannon 1988; Roy-Byrne *et al.* 1989). It remains unclear whether microvascular angina is due to a primary cardiac etiology with significant comorbidity with PD, or whether microvascular angina and PD have a common centrally mediated etiology (Roy-Byrne *et al.* 1989). Evidence supporting a central etiology comes from animal studies where central nervous system stimulation leads to spasm of small intramural coronary vessels (Wielgosz 1988), and positron emission tomography studies showing that patients experiencing chest pain with normal angiograms have been found to have characteristic patterns of cerebral activation (Rosen & Camici 2000). Patients with microvascular angina have also been found to have increased smooth muscle tone. Some researchers have speculated that patients with microvascular angina may have a "generalized abnormality of the smooth muscle" since the majority of them have been found to have bronchial hyper-reactivity to methacholine challenge tests, esophageal motility dysfunction, and abnormal resistance in large forearm arteries as measured by blood pressure cuff ischemia, in addition to increased vascular resistance in coronary arteries (Cannon 1988).

PD and coronary artery disease

While PD is common in patients with medically unexplained cardiac symptoms, it is also prevalent in patients with documented coronary artery disease (Zaubler & Katon 1996). Between 5% and 23% of patients with chest pain and angiographic evidence of significant coronary artery disease have PD (Bass *et al.* 1983). Among patients with chest pain seen in an emergency room and found to have acute cardiac ischemia, 19.4% have been diagnosed with PD. Sixty-two percent of patients referred for ambulatory electrocardiogram (ECG) recordings and found to have ECG abnormalities have been diagnosed with PD (Beitman *et al.* 1987; Katon *et al.* 1988; Chignon *et al.* 1993; Yingling *et al.* 1993). Between 9.2% and 12.4% of patients seen in cardiology practices have PD, and 40–62.5% of these patients with PD are found to have evidence of ischemic heart disease (Goldberg *et al.* 1990; Morris *et al.* 1997). PD is also a predictor of

persistent chest pain in 50% of patients with known coronary artery disease but no scintigraphic evidence of ischemia (Jeejeebhoy *et al.* 2000).

Because psychiatric and cardiac symptoms may be easily confused in patients with PD, patients with documented cardiac illness are especially likely to have PD misdiagnosed (Bridges & Goldberg 1985). These patients often present with crescendo angina, unresponsive to treatment with antianginal medications, yet potentially highly responsive to treatment with antipanic medication. Conversely, patients with potentially life threatening cardiac conditions such as paroxysmal supraventricular tachycardia, may be incorrectly labeled as having PD (Lessmeier *et al.* 1997). It is critical for clinicians to be cognizant of the overlapping cardiac symptoms shared by both PD and cardiac disease and minimize the risk of both false negative and false positive diagnoses of PD.

Establishing the diagnosis of PD in cardiac patients is especially important in light of research that has found that untreated panic symptoms may be associated with increased morbidity and mortality from heart disease (Coryell *et al.* 1982). Several large cohort studies, looking exclusively at male subjects, have found that high levels of anxiety increase the risk of fatal coronary heart disease by two to three times and the risk of sudden cardiac death by as much as six times that of patients with low anxiety levels, even when controlling for potential confounding variables such as family history of heart disease, cholesterol level or alcohol or cigarette use (Kawachi *et al.* 1994a,b).

Several pathophysiologic mechanisms have been postulated to account for this increased morbidity and mortality. The sympathetic autonomic effects of untreated PD such as tachycardia and hypertension may cause significant cardiac compromise in patients with coronary artery disease. (Katon 1990; Jeejeebhoy *et al.* 2000). Patients with PD are more likely to have increased blood pressure and dangerously high heart rates during treadmill stress testing than those without PD (Taylor *et al.* 1987). Hyperventilation, which is commonly associated with panic attacks, may lead to coronary spasm, ventricular arrhythmias and myocardial infarction (Kawachi *et al.* 1994a; Kaplan 1997).

There is evidence that PD may be associated with transient ischemic events, independent of the presence of hyperventilation. There is a growing body of research demonstrating that mental stress leads to myocardial ischemia in 50–70% of patients with coronary artery disease (Dakak *et al.* 1995). Mental stress is defined as the experience of a negative emotion such as depression or anxiety and may be elicited in a research setting by having a subject perform complicated arithmetic calculations or speaking publicly. Mental stress may therefore be a proxy for panic symptoms; although, further research, specifically on patients with PD, will need to confirm this. There is evidence that patients with coronary artery disease have endothelial dysfunction in diseased vessels resulting in impaired ability to dilate vessels during mental stress (Dakak *et al.* 1995; Fleet *et al.* 2000). This impaired ability to dilate vessels may be mediated by mental stress induced alterations in α-adrenoceptor activation and increased norepinephrine (noradrenaline) release resulting in smooth muscle contraction in diseased coronary vessels.

Alterations of the sympathovagal tone in the autonomic nervous system may help to establish a link between PD and sudden cardiac death (Kawachi *et al.* 1995). While increased sympathetic drive has traditionally been associated both with cardiac mortality and anxiety, researchers have recently shown that decreased parasympathetic (vagal) tone, as measured by the heart rate variability between inspiration and expiration, may play a critical role in the development of panic symptoms (George *et al.* 1989) and in mediating ventricular arrhythmias and cardiac death in patients with anxiety (Fleet *et al.* 2000; Gorman & Sloan 2000). Because of the lack of vagal excitation of the sinus node during inspiration the heart rate speeds up, while it slows down during expiration. Decreased

vagal tone leads to decreased heart rate variability, which has been shown to be associated with sudden cardiac death and may be so prevalent in patients with panic symptoms that it may be a "diagnostic marker" for PD (Yergani *et al.* 1993; Kawachi *et al.* 1995; Klein *et al.* 1995; Yergani *et al.* 1995). Patients with PD have also been found to have increased beat-to-beat QT variability. An increase in QT variability appears to be associated with symptomatic patients with dilated cardiomyopathy and also an increased risk of sudden death. (Yeragani *et al.* 2000). Further research is necessary to determine whether panic causes decreased heart rate and increased QT variability or vice versa, and whether these parameters can be restored to normal after patients have received effective treatment for their PD (Zaubler & Katon 1998). There is some preliminary evidence that treatment of PD with a selective serotonin reuptake inhibitor (SSRI) may normalize heart rate variability (Gorman & Sloan 2000).

Mitral valve prolapse and PD

Mitral valve prolapse (MVP), a condition which occurs when redundant mitral valve leaflets sag toward the left atrial chamber during ventricular systole, shares many symptoms with PD such as atypical chest pain, tachycardia, palpitations, dyspnea, lightheadedness, syncope, fatigue, and anxiety (Devereux *et al.* 1976; Zaubler & Katon 1996; Fig. 16.2). Given differences in the extent of mitral valve leaflet sagging

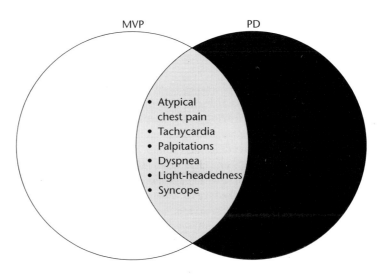

Fig. 16.2 Overlapping symptoms in patients with mitral valve prolapse (MVP) and panic disorder (PD).

necessary to make a diagnosis of MVP, the prevalence rates of this disorder have been estimated to range from 5% to 21%.

Because of the overlapping symptoms between MVP and PD, researchers have investigated the comorbidity between these two illnesses. While the prevalence of PD among individuals with MVP is not higher than it is for other cardiac illnesses, patients with both MVP and PD may be more likely to seek medical care for their cardiac symptoms than patients with MVP alone (Margraff et al. 1988; National Institute of Mental Health 1989). Studies investigating the rate of MVP among individuals with PD, on the other hand, have found a significant correlation. As many as 18% of patients with PD compared to 1% of control subjects without PD have been found to meet criteria for MVP. When a less stringent standard is used to make the diagnosis of MVP, up to 27% of patients with PD versus 12% of control subjects meet criteria for MVP (Margraff et al. 1988).

Given the high prevalence of MVP among patients with PD and the lack of any significantly increased comorbidity in the reverse direction, some researchers have speculated that PD may cause MVP (Zaubler & Katon 1996). The tachycardia, increased sympathetic discharge and high levels of catecholamines in the peripheral circulation associated with PD may cause desynchrony of ventricular contraction or anatomic abnormalities of the mitral valve leaflets resulting in MVP (Channick et al. 1981; Gorman et al. 1988). Moreover, researchers have found that MVP associated with PD may be clinically distinct from MVP occurring in the absence of PD (Weissman et al. 1987). Patients with MVP and PD have been found to have greater increases in mean blood pressure and heart rate during quiet standing and the early strain phase of the Valsalva maneuver than patients with MVP alone. On the other hand, patients with MVP alone have been found to have more syncope, increased orthostatic hypotension during quiet standing, a loss of normal age-dependent decrease of heart rate variability, and decreased 24-h epinephrine (adrenaline) excretion than patients with both MVP and PD (Zaubler & Katon 1996).

Given the comorbidity between PD and MVP it is important that PD not be overlooked in patients with MVP (National Institute of Mental Health 1989). Patients with MVP and panic symptoms are typically given beta-blockers with little improvement, leading to persistent and failed efforts to diagnose and treat the underlying psychopathology. Appropriate medication

for PD in patients with MVP is likely to provide the symptomatic relief that cardiac medication cannot achieve. Anti-panic medications have been shown to be equally effective in patients with PD and MVP as in patients with PD alone (Gorman et al. 1981; Grunhaus et al. 1984).

Idiopathic cardiomyopathy and PD

There is conflicting data regarding an association between PD and idiopathic cardiomyopathy, a disease characterized by progressive hypertrophy and dilatation of the myocardium (Zaubler & Katon 1996). Between 20% and 23% of patients with PD have been shown to have significant subclinical increases in left ventricular chamber size and mass. These changes may signify the early signs of a developing cardiomyopathy (Kahn et al. 1990). Researchers have speculated that the increased adrenergic tone, tachycardia and high peripheral catecholamine levels seen in patients with PD may lead to cardiomyopathy (Gillette et al. 1985; Kahn et al. 1987). Further evidence for this theory is suggested by studies where animals infused with catecholamines developed cardiomyopathic changes (Laks et al. 1973; Dargie & Goodwin 1982).

There is some evidence that as many as 51% of patients with idiopathic cardiomyopathy have PD, far greater than in patients with other severe cardiac conditions such as rheumatic or congenital heart disease (Kahn et al. 1987). A recent study by Griez et al. (2000), however, found that the prevalence of PD among patients with cardiomyopathy and cardiac failure was no higher than in patients with other cardiac diseases responsible for the cardiac failure.

Hypertension and PD

Researchers have found a significant association between PD and hypertension. Patients with PD have been found to have significantly higher rates of hypertension than controls without PD (Noyes et al. 1980; Katon 1984; Katon et al. 1986; White & Baker 1986; Balon et al. 1988). Davies et al. (1999) also found significantly higher rates of PD in hypertensive patients receiving treatment at primary care and hospital-based clinics compared to normotensive control subjects. Among hypertensive patients being screened for pheochromocytoma, an extremely rare chromaffin tissue tumor typically found in the adrenal gland, 35% met criteria for a lifetime diagnosis and 28% for a current diagnosis of PD. This is a strikingly high percentage given that only 0.1% of hypertensive patients actually do have a pheochromocytoma (Fogarty *et al.* 1994). Clearly all patients undergoing testing for pheochromocytoma should preliminarily be screened for PD (Zaubler & Katon 1998).

The association between PD and hypertension may in large part be mediated by the tendency of patients with PD to hyperventilate. Panic related hyperventilation, resulting in vascular contraction, has been shown to lead both to transient and sustained increases in blood pressure and tachycardia (Todd *et al.* 1995; Kaplan 1997). The increased adrenergic discharge seen in patients with PD may also eventually cause irreversible peripheral vasoconstriction resulting in chronic hypertension (National Institute of Mental Health 1989).

Gastrointestinal illness and PD

It is well recognized that functional gastrointestinal symptoms, characterized by the absence of any underlying structural or biochemical abnormality, are frequently comorbid with anxiety. The symptoms most commonly associated with PD are noncardiac chest pain of esophageal origin and irritable bowel syndrome.

PD is highly prevalent in patients with normal angiograms and chest pain (See PD and cardiac illness above). While there is little data regarding the prevalence of esophageal disorder in these patients, estimates suggesting an esophageal basis for the chest pain range between 20% and 60% (Maunder 1998).

Irritable bowel syndrome (IBS), characterized by intermittent diarrhea, constipation and abdominal pain, is a very common disorder accounting for 20–52% of new referrals to gastroenterologists (Drossman *et al.* 1988; Walker *et al.* 1990a). Between 8% and 17% of the general population experience significant disability due to IBS (Drossman *et al.* 1988; Lydiard *et al.* 1994). Given the high prevalence of IBS, it is extremely important that clinicians be aware of the well-established association between PD and irritable bowel syndrome (IBS) (Walker *et al.* 1990a; Lydiard *et al.* 1993; Walker *et al.* 1995). Walker *et al.* (1990b, 1995) found that the current and lifetime prevalence of PD among patients with IBS were 28% and 41%, respectively, compared

to a 3% current and 25% lifetime prevalence of PD among controls with inflammatory bowel diseases such as ulcerative colitis and Crohn's disease. Lydiard *et al.* (1993) found that 31% of patients with IBS met the criteria for PD. Conversely, among patients with PD, between 41% and 44% of patients have been diagnosed with IBS (Lydiard 1997). The association between PD and IBS is particularly noteworthy since there is substantial evidence that many patients with IBS, who are typically refractory to medical treatments, experience decreased gastrointestinal symptoms and pain with antidepressants and anxiolytics (Walker *et al.* 1990a; Lydiard 1997).

Several pathophysiologic models have been proposed to account for the association between IBS and PD. The enteric nervous system (ENS) is often referred to as the "little brain" because of the extensive neuronal interconnections in the gut and the elaborate communication between the ENS and central nervous system (CNS). The locus coerulus serves as an important link between the ENS and CNS. It is directly innervated by the medullary nucleus solitarius (the principal locus for afferent information from the gut) and receives afferent information from the viscera (Walker *et al.* 1990a). Locus coerulus activation may occur secondary to internal bowel events such as distension of the bowel or stomach. This activation may lead to increased anxiety and may affect gastrointestinal function through efferent connections to the gut. A vicious cycle may ensue with gastrointestinal activity eliciting locus coerulus discharge, leading to increased anxiety and gastrointestinal dysfunction (Zaubler & Katon 1996).

Some researchers have suggested that patients with IBS have an abnormality of central modulation of smooth muscle tone. In addition to experiencing hyperalgesia to colonic distension, patients with IBS often complain of extra-abdominal symptoms which may be due to smooth muscle dysfunction such as urinary frequency, urgency, retention, nocturia and hyper-reactive bronchi in response to methacholine challenge (White *et al.* 1991; Farthing 1995). Moreover, patients with noncardiac chest pain have abnormalities of smooth muscle tone in forearm arterioles, cardiac arterioles and extra-cardiac organ systems such as the esophagus, and increased sensitivity to cardiac as well as gastrointestinal pain (Cannon 1988; Cannon *et al.* 1994). Patients with panic symptoms as well as patients with functional gastrointestinal symptoms have also been found to have decreased vagal tone as measured by heart rate variability (Yeragani *et al.* 1993; Haug *et al.* 1994; Kawachi *et al.* 1995; Yergani *et al.* 1995). Decreased vagal tone may therefore be another possible CNS mechanism mediating the association between PD and functional gastrointestinal symptoms.

The neuropeptide cholecystokinin (CCK) may also account for the comorbidity between panic and functional gastrointestinal symptoms. CCK, commonly found in both the CNS and ENS, regulates gastrointestinal motility and induces panic-like attacks in the majority of patients with PD (De Montigny 1989; Maunder 1998).

Respiratory illness and PD

PD and respiratory illness share many symptoms such as hyperventilation-induced dyspnea, choking, suffocation, chest pain and increased anxiety. Because of these overlapping symptoms, researchers have established a clear association between PD and respiratory illness, with a particular focus on patients with asthma. Between 6.5% and 24% of asthmatic patients suffer from PD and as many as 42% of asthmatic patients experience panic attacks (Kinsman *et al.* 1973; Yellowlees *et al.* 1987; Yellowlees *et al.* 1988; Shavitt *et al.* 1992; Carr *et al.* 1994). Among patients referred for pulmonary function testing, 17% reported having panic attacks and 11% had PD (Pollack *et al.* 1996). Patients with PD are three times more likely to have asthma, bronchitis, emphysema, or allergy than patients without psychiatric illness and have a significantly higher prevalence of these illnesses compared to patients with other psychiatric disorders (Zandbergen *et al.* 1991; Spinhoven *et al.* 1994).

Panic symptoms lead to significantly increased disability and morbidity in patients with asthma. Patients with PD and asthma, independent of the magnitude of objective pulmonary dysfunction, have more frequent hospital admissions, longer hospital stays and more frequent steroid use than asthmatic patients without PD (Carr 1997). Patients with PD and asthma compared to asthmatic patients without PD are more likely to hyperventilate in response to stressful situations which, in part, may account for the increased morbidity seen in these patients. They tend to have bronchodilated airways and a decreased lower airway impedance to stressful stimuli (Carr *et al.* 1996).

Many pathophysiological mechanisms have been proposed to account for the association between respiratory illness and PD. Klein (1993) suggests that patients with PD have an abnormality in a "suffocation center" in the brain that prompts individuals to hyperventilate in response to a false perception of asphyxia due to subtle increases in arterial carbon dioxide (CO_2) levels. Patients with chronic obstructive pulmonary disease are likely to experience intermittent hypercapnia which may lead to increased locus coerulus activity, resulting in panic and hyperventilation (Zandbergen *et al.* 1991). This hypothesis is supported by the finding that exogenous CO_2 has been found to precipitate or worsen panic symptoms in most patients with PD. Autonomic nervous system abnormalities may lead to subclinical airway obstruction in patients with PD (Perna *et al.* 1994). A high prevalence of panic symptoms (35%) and disorder (10%) has also been found in patients with allergies, raising the possibility of immune system dysfunction mediating this association (Ramesh *et al.* 1991; Schmidt-Traub *et al.* 1995).

Distortions of cognitive processing may also account for the association between PD and respiratory illness. Patients with PD may catastrophize somatic sensations associated with respiratory illnesses. This, in turn, leads to excessive concern about respiratory symptoms regardless of their severity (Prozelius *et al.* 1992; Carr *et al.* 1994). Panic symptoms may also develop if a patient, having experienced frightening physical symptoms during a past respiratory illness, experiences similar but less severe symptoms that are reminiscent of the those from the past. This conditioning effect may account for the high prevalence of childhood respiratory illnesses (40%) and near death experiences due to asthma in patients with PD (Yellowlees *et al.* 1987, 1988; Zandbergen *et al.* 1991).

Neurologic illness and PD

There is an association between PD and several neurologic illnesses. Among patients presenting to their physician with complaints of headache nearly 15% have PD (Stewart *et al.* 1989, 1992). Patients with migraine headaches, compared to those without, are 3 times more likely to have PD and 12 times more likely to develop PD in the year following their migraine diagnosis (Merikangas *et al.* 1990; Breslau & Davis 1993). Dizziness is one of the most common panic symptoms reported in 50% to 90% of patients with PD (Asmundson *et al.* 1998). This has prompted researchers to explore an association between PD and vestibular dysfunction. The vast majority of studies exploring this association have found a very high prevalence of vestibular abnormalities in patients with PD (Asmundson *et al.* 1998). One carefully controlled study found that 93.1% of patients with PD and moderate agoraphobia have vestibular dysfunction compared to 41.7% of healthy control subjects (Jacob *et al.* 1996). Conversely, several studies have shown that approximately 20% of patients referred for audiologic and/or vestibular assessment have PD (Asmundson 1998). Given the increasingly well-established association between PD and dizziness, it is critical that clinicians routinely screen for PD in patients complaining of dizziness even when there is evidence of vestibular dysfunction.

Patients with a lifetime diagnosis of PD may have a two-fold increased risk of having a stroke compared to those with other psychiatric disorders or no psychiatric disorder (Weissman *et al.* 1990). The relatively high prevalence of left ventricular hypertrophy and hypertension in patients with PD may account for this association (Coryell *et al.* 1982). Studies investigating the association between seizure activity and PD have been less conclusive. Temporal lobe epilepsy and PD share many symptoms such as fear, terror, tachycardia, hyperventilation, flushing, diaphoresis, depersonalization and derealization. While there is little data supporting a clear association between these two illnesses, panic-like attacks have been reported in response to temperolimbic stimulation and are more likely to occur in individuals with right temporal lobe mass lesions or those who have had a right temporal lobectomy (Wall *et al.* 1985, 1986; Ghadirian *et al.* 1986; Lepola *et al.* 1990). Most patients with PD, however, have normal electroencephalograms (EEG) and computerized tomography (CT) findings (Lepola *et al.* 1990; Spitz 1991). Interestingly, in one study up to 70% of patients with psychogenic seizures were found to have PD (Snyder *et al.* 1994).

Conclusion

Patients with PD are very prevalent in the medical setting and account for significant overutilization of medical services, functional disability and increased morbidity. While it may be difficult to discern whether a patient's symptoms are due to an underlying medical problem or to PD, it is critical that clinicians be aware that PD and many different medical illnesses and medical symptoms are comorbid. Treatment of panic is equally efficacious whether or not there is comorbid medical illness. Moreover, without treatment the medical symptoms experienced by patients with PD will typically escalate leading to ever more costly and invasive medical investigations and growing distress in the patient who cannot find any relief from his or her panic symptoms. Further research is likely to provide greater understanding of the pathophysiologic links between PD and various medical illnesses, and the impact that treatment may have not only on ameliorating panic symptoms but also on decreasing morbidity in the medically ill with PD.

References

American Psychiatric Association (1994) *Diagnostic Statistical Manual of Mental Disorders*, 4th edn. American Psychiatric Association, Washington, D.C.

Asmundson, G., Larsen, D. & Stein, M. (1998) Panic disorder and vestibular disturbance: an overview of empirical findings and clinical evaluations. *J Psychosom Res* **44**, 107–20.

Balon, R., Ortiz, A., Pohl, R. & Yeragani, V.K. (1988) Heart rate and blood pressure during placebo-associated panic attacks. *Psychosom Med* **50**, 434–8.

Barsky, A.J., Cleary, P.D., Barnett, M.D., Christiansen, C.L. & Ruskin, J.N. (1994) The accuracy of symptom reporting by patients complaining of palpitations. *Am J Med* **97**, 214–21.

Barsky, A.J., Cleary, P.D., Coeytaux, R.R. & Ruskin, J.D. (1995) The clinical course of palpitations in medical outpatients. *Arch Intern Med* **155**, 1782–8.

Bass, C., Wade, C., Hand, D. & Jackson, G. (1983) Patients with angina with normal and near-normal coronary arteries: clinical and psychosocial state 12 months after angiography. *BMJ* **287**, 1505–8.

Beitman, B.D., Basha, I., Flaker, G. *et al.* (1987) Atypical or nonanginal chest pain: panic disorder or coronary artery disease? *Arch Intern Med* **147**, 1548–52.

Beitman, B.D., Kushner, M.G., Basha, I., Lamberti, J., Mukerji, V. & Bartels, K. (1991) Follow-up status of patients with angiographically normal coronary arteries and panic disorder. *JAMA* **265**, 1545–9.

Breslau, N. & Davis, G.C. (1993) Migraine, physical health and psychiatric disorder: a prospective epidemiologic study in young adults. *J Psychiatr Res* **27**, 211–21.

Bridges, K.W. & Goldberg, D.P. (1985) Somatic presentation of DSM-III psychiatric disorders in primary care. *J Psychosom Res* **29**, 563–9.

Cannon, R.O. 3rd, Quyyumi, A.A., Mincemoyer, R. *et al.* (1994) Imipramine in patients with chest pain despite normal coronary angiograms. *N Engl J Med* **330**, 1411–17.

Cannon, R.O., III (1988) Causes of chest pain in patients with normal coronary angiograms: the eye of the beholder. *Am J Cardiol* **62**, 306–8.

Cannon, R.O. 3rd (1995) The sensitive heart. A syndrome of abnormal cardiac pain. *Perception* **273**, 883–7.

Carr, R.E. (1997) Panic disorder and asthma: causes, effects and research implications. *J Psychosom Res* **44**, 43–52.

Carr, R.E., Lehrer, P.M. & Hochron, S.M. (1996) Effect of psychological stress on airway impedance in individuals with asthma and panic disorder. *J Abnorm Psychol* **105**, 137–41.

Carr, R.E., Lehrer, P.M., Rausch, L.L. & Hochron, S.M. (1994) Anxiety sensitivity and panic attacks in an asthmatic population. *Behav Res Ther* **32**, 411–18.

Carter, C., Maddock, R., Amsterdam, E., McCormick, S., Waters, C. & Billette, J. (1992) Panic disorder and chest pain in the coronary care unit. *Psychosomatics* **33**, 302–9.

Carter, C.S., Servan-Schreiber, D. & Perlstein, W.M. (1997) Anxiety disorders and the syndrome of chest pain with normal coronary arteries: prevalence and pathophysiology. *J Clin Psychiatry* **58**, 70–3.

Channick, B.J., Adlin, E.V., Marks, A.D. *et al.* (1981) Hyperthyroidism and mitral valve prolapse. *N Engl J Med* **305**, 497–500.

Chignon, J.M., Lepine, J.P. & Ades, J. (1993) Panic disorder in cardiac outpatients. *Am J Psychiatry* **150**, 780–5.

Coryell, W., Noyes, R. & Clancy, J. (1982) Excess mortality in panic disorder. *Arch Gen Psychiatry* **39**, 701–3.

Dakak, N., Quyyumi, A.A., Eisenhofer, G., Goldstein, D.S. & Cannon, R.O. (1995) Sympathetically mediated effects of mental stress on the cardiac microcirculation of patients with coronary artery disease. *Am J Cardiol* **76**, 125–30.

Dammen, T., Arnesen, H., Ekeberg, O., Husebye, T. & Friis, S. (1999) Panic disorder in chest pain patients referred for cardiological outpatient investigation. *J Intern Med* **245**, 497–507.

Dargie, H.J. & Goodwin, J.F. (1982) Catecholamines, cardiomyopathies and cardiac function. In: *Progress in Cardiology*, Vol. 11 (P.H. Yu & J.F. Goodwin (eds), pp. 93–106). Lea & Febiger, Philadelphia.

Davies, S.J., Ghahramani, P., Jackson, P.R. *et al.* (1999) Association of panic disorder and panic attacks with hypertension. *Am J Med* **107**, 310–16.

De Montigny, C. (1989) Cholecystokinin tetrapeptide induces panic-like attacks in healthy volunteers. *Arch Gen Psychiatry* **46**, 511–17.

Devereux, R.B., Perloff, J.K., Reiche, K. & Josephson, M.E. (1976) Mitral valve prolapse. *Circulation* **54**, 3–14.

Drossman, D.A., McKee, D.C., Sandler, R.S. *et al.* (1988) Psychosocial factors in the irritable bowel syndrome: a multivariate study of patients and nonpatients with irritable bowel syndrome. *Gastroenterology* **95**, 701–8.

Ehlers, A., Mayou, R.A., Sprigings, D.C. & Birkhead, J. (2000) Psychological and perceptual factors associated with arrhythmias and benign palpitations. *Psychosom Med* **62** (5), 693–702.

Elamm, Y., Svensson, T.H. & Thoren, P. (1984) Regulation of locus coerulus neurons and splanchnic sympathetic nerves by cardiovascular afferents. *Brain Res* **290**, 282–7.

Farthing, M.J. (1995) Irritable bowel, irritable body, or irritable brain? *BMJ* **310**, 171–5.

Fifer, S.K., Mathias, S.D., Patrick, D.L., Mazonson, P.D., Lubeck, D.P. & Buesching, D.P. (1994) Untreated anxiety among adult primary care patients in a health maintenance organization. *Arch Gen Psychiatry* **51**, 740–50.

Fleet, R.P., Dupais, G., Marchand, A., Burelle, D., Arsenault, A. & Beitman, B.D. (1996) Panic disorder in emergency department chest pain patients: prevalence, comorbidity, suicidal ideation and physician recognition. *Am J Med* **101**, 371–80.

Fleet, R.P., Lavoie, K. & Beitman, B.D. (2000) Is panic disorder associate with coronary artery disease? A critical review of the literature. *J Psychosom Res* **48**, 347–56.

Fogarty, J., Engle, C.C. Jr, Russo, J., Simon, G. & Katon, W. (1994) Hypertension and pheochromocytoma testing: the association with anxiety disorders. *Arch Fam Med* **3**, 55–60.

George, D.T., Nutt, D.J., Walker, W.V., Porges, S.W., Adinoff, B. & Linnoila, M. (1989) Lactate and hyperventilation substantially attenuate vagal tone in normal volunteers. *Arch Gen Psychiatry* **46**, 153–6.

Ghadirian, A.M., Gauthier, S. & Betrand, S. (1986) Anxiety attacks in a patient with a right temporal lobe meningioma. *J Clin Psychiatry* **47**, 270–1.

Gillette, P.C., Smith, R.T., Garson, A. *et al.* (1985) Chronic supraventricular tachycardia: a curable cause of congestive cardiomyopathy. *JAMA* **253**, 391–2.

Goldberg, R., Morris, P., Christian, F., Badger, J., Chapot, S. & Edlund, M. (1990) Panic disorder in cardiac outpatients. *Psychosomatics* **31**, 168–73.

Goodwin, R., Olfson, M., Feder, A., Fuenter, M., Pilowsky, D.J., Weissman, M.M. (2001) Panic and suicidal ideation in primary care. *Depress Anxiety* **14**(4), 244–6.

Gorman, J.M., Fyer, A.F., Glicklick, J., King, D.L. & Klein, D.F. (1981) Effect of imipramine on prolapsed mitral valves of patients with panic disorder. *Am J Psychiatry* **138**, 977–8.

Gorman, M., Goetz, R.R., Fyer, M. *et al.* (1988) The mitral valve prolapse–panic disorder connection. *Psychosom Med* **50**, 114–22.

Gorman, J.M. & Sloan, R.P. (2000) Heart rate variability in depressive and anxiety disorders. *Am Heart J* **140** (Suppl. 4), 77–83.

Griez, E.J., Mammar, N., Loirat, J., Djega, N., Trochut, J.N. & Bouhour, J.B. (2000) Panic disorder and idiopathic cardiomyopathy. *J Psychosom Res* **48**(6), 585–7.

Grunhaus, L., Gloger, S. & Birmacher, B. (1984) Clomipramine treatment for panic attacks in patients with mitral valve prolapse. *J Clin Psychiatry* **45**, 25–7.

Haug, T.T., Svebak, S., Haisken, T., Wilhelmsen, I., Berstad, A. & Ursin, H. (1994) Low vagal activity as mediating mechanism for the relationship between personality factors and gastric symptoms in functional dyspepsia. *Psychosom Med* **56**, 181–6.

Jacob, R.G., Furman, J.M., Durrant, J.D. & Turner, S.M. (1996) Panic, agoraphobia, and vestibular dysfunction. *Am J Psychiatry* **153**, 503–12.

Jeejeebhoy, F., Dorian, P. & Newman, D. (2000) Panic disorder and the heart: a cardiology perspective. *J Psychosom Res* **48**, 393–403.

Kahn, J.P., Drusin, R.E. & Klein, D.F. (1987) Idiopathic cardiomyopathy and panic disorder: clinical association in cardiac transplant candidates. *Am J Psychiatry* **144**, 1327–30.

Kahn, J.P., Gorman, J.M., King, D.L., Fyer, A.J., Liebowitz, M.R. & Klein, D.F. (1990) Cardiac left ventricular hypertrophy and chamber dilatation in panic disorder patients: implications for idiopathic dilated cardiomyopathy. *Psychiatry Res* **32**, 55–61.

Kandel, E.R. (1983) From metapsychology to molecular biology: explorations into the nature of anxiety. *Am J Psychiatry* 1277–93.

Kaplan, N.M. (1997) Anxiety induced hyperventilation: a common cause of symptoms in patients with hypertension. *Arch Intern Med* **157**, 945–8.

Katon, W. (1984) Panic disorder and somatization: a review of 55 cases. *Am J Med* **77**, 101–6.

Katon, W. (1993) Panic disorder in the medical setting. In: *National Institute of Mental Health*. 93 (3482). National Institute of Mental Health, Washington, D.C.

Katon, W. (1994) Primary care—psychiatry panic disorder module. In: *Treatment of Panic Disorder: a Consensus Development Conference* (B.E. Wolfe & J.D. Maser (eds), pp. 44–56). American Psychiatric Press, Washington, D.C.

Katon, W. (1996) Panic disorder: relationship to high medical utilization, unexplained physical symptoms, and medical costs. *J Clin Psychiatry* **57**(Suppl. 10), 11–18.

Katon, W. (1990) Chest pain, cardiac disease and panic disorder. *J Clin Psychiatry* **51**, 27–30.

Katon, W., Hall, M.L., Russo, J. *et al.* (1988) Chest pain: the relationship of psychiatric illness to coronary arteriography results. *Am J Med* **84**, 1–9.

Katon, W., Hollifield, M., Chapman, T., Mannuzza, S., Ballenger, J. & Fyer, A. (1995) Infrequent panic attacks: psychiatric comorbidity, personality characteristics, and functional disability. *J Psychiatr Res* **29**, 121–31.

Katon, W. & Roy-Byrne, P.P. (1989) Panic disorder in the medically ill. *J Clin Psychiatry* **50**, 299–302.

Katon, W., Vitiliano, P.P., Russo, J., Jones, M. & Anderson, K. (1986) Panic disorder: epidemiology in primary care. *J Fam Pract* **23**, 233–9.

Kawachi, I., Colditz, G.A., Ascherio, A. *et al.* (1994a) Prospective study of phobic anxiety and risk of coronary heart disease in men. *Circulation* **89**, 1992–7.

Kawachi, I., Sparrow, D., Vokonas, P.S. & Weiss, S.T. (1994b) Symptoms of anxiety and risk of coronary heart disease: the Normative Aging Study. *Circulation* **90**, 2225–9.

Kawachi, I., Sparrow, D., Vokonas, P.S. & Weiss, S.T. (1995) Decreased heart rate variability in men with phobic anxiety (data from the Normative Aging Study). *Am J Cardiol* **75**, 882–5.

Kessler, R.C., McGonagle, K.A. & Zhaos, S. (1994) Lifetime and 12-month prevalence of DSM III-R psychiatric disorders in the United States. *Arch Gen Psychiatry* **51**, 8–18.

Kinsman, R.A., Luparello, T., O'Banion, K. & Spector, S. (1973) Multidimensional analysis of the subjective symptomatology of asthma. *Psychosom Med* **35**, 250–67.

Klein, D.F. (1993) False suffocation alarms, spontaneous panics, and related conditions: an integrative hypothesis. *Arch Gen Psychiatry* **50**, 306–17.

Klein, E., Cnaani, E., Harel, T., Braun, S. & Ben-Haim, S.A. (1995) Altered heart rate variability in panic disorder patients. *Biol Psychiatry* **37**, 18–24.

Klerman, G.L., Weissman, M.M., Quellette, R., Johnson, J. & Greenwald, S. (1991) Panic attacks in the community: social morbidity and health care utilization. *JAMA* **265**, 742–6.

Kroenke, K. (1992) Symptoms in medical patients: an untended field. *Am J Med* **92** (Suppl. A), 3–6.

Kroenke, K., Arrington, M.E. & Mangelsdorff, A.D. (1990) The prevalence of symptoms in medical outpatients and the adequacy of therapy. *Arch Intern Med* **150**, 1685–9.

Kroenke, K. & Mangelsdorff, A.D. (1989) Common symptoms in ambulatory care: incidence, evaluation, therapy and outcome. *Am J Med* **86**, 262–6.

Laks, M.M., Morady, F. & Swan, H.J.C. (1973) Myocardial hypertrophy produced by chronic infusion of subhypertensive doses of norepinephrine in the dog. *Chest* **64**, 75–8.

Lavey, E.D. & Winkle, R.A. (1979) Continuing disability of patients with chest pain and normal coronary arteriograms. *Journal of Chronic Disease* **32**, 191–6.

Leon, A.C., Porter, A.L. & Weissman, M.M. (1995) The social costs of anxiety disorders. *Br J Psychiatry* **166** (Suppl. 27), 19–22.

Lepola, U., Nousiainen, U., Puranen, M., Reikkinen, P. & Rimon, R. (1990) EEG and CT findings in patients with panic disorder. *Biol Psychiatry* **28**, 721–7.

Lessmeier, T.J., Gamperling, D., Johnson-Liddon, V. *et al.* (1997) Unrecognized paroxysmal supraventricular tachycardia: potential for misdiagnosis as panic disorder. *Arch Intern Med* **157**, 537–43.

Lydiard, R.B. (1997) Anxiety and the irritable bowel syndrome: psychiatric, medical, or both? *J Clin Psychiatry* **58** (Suppl. 3), 51–8.

Lydiard, R.B., Fosser, M.D., Marsh, W. & Ballenger, J.C. (1993) Prevalence of psychiatric disorders in patients with irritable bowel syndrome. *Psychosomatics* **34**, 229–34.

Lydiard, R.B., Greenwald, S., Weissman, M.M., Johnson, J., Drossman, D.A. & Ballenger, J.C. (1994) Panic disorder and gastrointestinal symptoms: findings from the National Institute of Mental Health Epidemiologic Catchment Area project. *Am J Psychiatry* **151**, 64–70.

Margraff, J., Ehlers, A. & Roth, W.T. (1988) Mitral valve prolapse and panic disorder: a review of their relationship. *Psychosom Med* **50**, 93–113.

Markowitz, J.S., Weissman, M.M., Quellette, R., Lish, J.D. & Klerman, G.L. (1989) Quality of life in panic disorder. *Arch Gen Psychiatry* **46**, 984–92.

Maunder, R.G. (1998) Panic disorder associated with gastrointestinal disease: review and hypothesis. *J Psychosom Res* **44**, 91–105.

Merikangas, K.R., Angst, J. & Isler, H. (1990) Migraine and psychopathology: results of the Zurich cohort study of young adults. *Arch Gen Psychiatry* **47**, 849–53.

Moriarty, K.J. & Dawson, A.M. (1982) Functional abdominal pain: further evidence that the whole gut is affected. *BMJ* **284**, 1670–2.

Morris, A., Baker, B., Devins, G.M. & Shapiro, C.M. (1997) Prevalence of panic disorder in cardiac outpatients. *Can J Psychiatry* **42**, 185–90.

National Institute of Mental Health (1989) *Panic Disorder in the Medical Setting.* (ADM 89–1629, pp. 51–9.) US Govt. Print. Off., Washington, DC.

Noyes, R., Clancy, J., Hoenk, P.R. & Slymen, D.J. (1980) The prognosis of anxiety neurosis. *Arch Gen Psychiatry* **37**, 173–8.

Ockene, I.S., Shay, M.J., Alpert, J.S., Weiner, B.H. & Dolen, J.E. (1980) Unexplained chest pain in patients with normal coronary arteriograms. *N Engl J Med* **303**, 1249–52.

Perna, G., Marconi, C., Battaglia, M., Bertani, A., Panzacchi, A. & Bellodi, L. (1994) Subclinical impairment of lung airways in patients with panic disorder. *Biol Psychiatry* **36**, 601–5.

Pollack, M.H., Kradin, R., Otto, M.W. *et al.* (1996) Prevalence of panic in patients referred for pulmonary function testing at a major medical center. *Am J Psychiatry* **153**, 110–13.

Prozelius, J., Vest, M. & Nochomovitz, M. (1992) Respiratory function, cognitions, and panic in chronic pulmonary patients. *Behav Res Ther* **30**, 75–7.

Ramesh, C., Yeragani, V.K., Balon, R. & Pohl, R. (1991) A comparative study of immune status in panic disorder patients and controls. *Acta Pscyhiatr Scand* **84**, 396–7.

Redmond, D.E. (1979) New and old evidence for the involvement of a brain norepinephrine system in anxiety. In: *Phenomenology and Treatment of Anxiety* (W. Fann, J. Karacan, A.D. Pokoiny & R.L. Williams (eds), pp. 153–203). Spectrum, New York.

Rosen, S.D. & Camici, P.G. (2000) The brain–heart axis in the perception of cardiac pain: the elusive link between ischaemia and pain. *Ann Med* **32**, 350–64.

Roy-Byrne, P.P., Schmidt, P., Cannon, R.O., III, Diem, H. & Rubinow, D.R. (1989) Microvascular angina and panic disorder. *Int J Psychiatry Med* **19**, 315–25.

Salvador-Carulla, L., Segui, J., Fernandez-Cano, P. & Canet, J. (1995) Costs and offset effect in panic disorders. *Br J Psychiatry* **166** (Suppl. 27), 23–8.

Schmidt-Traub, S., Bamler, K.J. & Schaffrath-Rosario, A. (1995) More anxiety and other psychological disturbances in allergic patients? *Allergologie* **18**, 13–19.

Schurman, R.A., Kramer, P.D. & Mitchell, J.B. (1985) The hidden mental health network: treatment of mental illness by nonpsychiatrist physicians. *Arch Gen Psychiatry* **42**, 89–94.

Shavitt, R.G., Gentil, V. & Mandetta, R. (1992) The association of panic/agoraphobia and asthma: contributing factors and clinical implications. *Gen Hosp Psychiatry* **14**, 420–3.

Sherbourne, C.D., Wells, K.B. & Judd, L.L. (1996) Functioning and well-being of patients with panic disorder. *Am J Psychiatry* **153**, 213–18.

Simon, G.E. & VonKorff, M. (1991) Somatization and psychiatric disorder in the NIMH Epidemiologic Catchment Area Study. *Am J Psychiatry* **148**, 1494–500.

Simpson, R.J., Kazmierczak, Power, K.G. & Sharp, D.M. (1994) Controlled comparison of the characteristics of patients with panic disorder. *Br J Gen Pract* **44**, 352–6.

Snyder, S.L., Rosenbaum, D.H., Rowan, A.J. & Strain, J.J. (1994) SCID diagnosis of panic disorder in psychogenic seizure patients. *J Neuropsychiatry Clin Neurosci* **6**, 261–6.

Spinhoven, P., Ros, M., Westgeest, A. & Van Der Does, A.J. (1994) The prevalence of respiratory disorders in panic disorder, major depressive disorder and V-code patients. *Behav Res Ther* **32**, 647–9.

Spitz, M.C. (1991) Panic disorder in seizure patients: a diagnostic pitfall. *Epilepsia* **32**, 33–8.

Stewart, W.F., Linet, M.S. & Celentano, D.D. (1989) Migraine headaches and panic attacks. *Psychosom Med* **51**, 559–69.

Stewart, W.F., Shechter, A. & Liberman, J. (1992) Physician consultation for headache pain and history of panic: results from a population-based study. *Am J Med* **92** (Suppl. 1A), S35–S40.

Svensson, T.H. (1987) Peripheral, autonomic regulation of locus coerulus noradrenergic neurons in brain: putative implications for psychiatry and psychopharmacology. *Psychopharmacology* **92**, 1–7.

Svensson, T.H. & Thoren, P. (1979) Brain noradrenergic neurons in the locus coerulus: inhabitation by blood volume load through vagal afferents. *Brain Res* **172**, 174–8.

Taylor, C.B., King, R. & Ehlers, A. (1987) Treadmill exercise test and ambulatory measures in panic attacks. *Am J Cardiol* **60**, 48J–52J.

Todd, G.P., Chadwick, I.G., Yeo, W.W., Jackson, P.R. & Ramsay, L.E. (1995) Pressor effect of hyperventilation in healthy subjects. *J Hum Hypertens* **9**, 119–22.

Walker, E.A., Gelfand, A.N., Gelfand, M.D., Katon, W.J. (1995) Psychiatric diagnoses, sexual and physical victimization, and disability in patients with irritable bowel syndrome or inflammatory bowel disease. *Psychol Med* **25**, 1259–67.

Walker, E.A., Roy-Byrne, P.P. & Katon, W.J. (1990a) Irritable bowel syndrome and psychiatric illness. *Am J Psychiatry* **147**, 565–72.

Walker, E.A., Roy-Byrne, P.P., Katon, W., Li, L., Amos, D. & Jiranek, G. (1990b) Psychiatric illness and irritable bowel syndrome: a comparison with inflammatory bowel disease. *Am J Psychiatry* **147**, 1656–61.

Wall, M., Mielke, D. & Luther, J.S. (1986) Panic attacks and psychomotor seizures following right temporal lobectomy. *J Clin Psychiatry* **47**, 219.

Wall, M., Tuchman, M. & Mielke, D. (1985) Panic attacks and temporal lobe seizures associated with a right temporal lobe arteriovenous malformation: case report. *J Clin Psychiatry* **46**, 143–5.

Weber, B.E. & Kapoor, W.N. (1996) Evaluation and outcomes of patients with palpitations. *Am J Med* **100**, 138–48.

Weissman, M.M., Markowitz, J.S., Quellette, R., Greenwald, S. & Kahn, J.P. (1990) Panic disorder and cardiovascular/cerebrovascular problems: results from a community survey. *Am J Psychiatry* **147**, 1504–8.

Weissman, N.J., Shear, M.K., Kramer-Fox, R. & Devereux, R.B. (1987) Contrasting patterns of autonomic dysfunction in patients with mitral valve prolapse and panic attacks. *Am J Med* **82**, 880–8.

White, W.B. & Baker, C.H. (1986) Episodic hypertension secondary to panic disorder. *Arch Intern Med* **146**, 1129–30.

White, A.M., Stevens, W.H., Upton, A.R., O'Byrne, P.M. & Collins, S.M. (1991) Airway responsiveness to inhaled methacholine in patients with irritable bowel syndrome. *Gastroenterology* **100**, 68–74.

Wielgosz, A.T. (1988) Connecting the locus coerulus and the coronaries. *Am J Cardiol* **62**, 308–9.

Yellowlees, P.M., Alpers, J.H., Bowden, J.J., Bryant, G.D. & Ruffin, R.E. (1987) Psychiatric morbidity in patients with chronic airflow obstruction. *Med J Aust* **146**, 305–7.

Yellowlees, P.M., Hayner, S., Potts, N. & Ruffin, R.E. (1988) Psychiatric morbidity in patients with life-threatening asthma: initial report of a controlled study. *Med J Aust* **149**, 246–9.

Yeragani, V.K., Pohl, R., Jampala, V.C., Balon, R., Ramesh, C. & Srinivasan, K. (2000) Increased QT variability in patients with panic disorder and depression. *Psychiatry Res* **93** (3), 225–35.

Yeragani, V.K., Pohl, R., Berger, R. *et al.* (1993) Decreased heart rate variability in panic disorder patients: a study of power-spectral analysis of heart rate. *Psychiatry Res* **46**, 89–103.

Yeragani, V.K., Pohl, R., Srinivasan, K., Balon, R., Ramesh, C. & Berchou, R. (1995) Effects of isoproterenol infusions on heart rate variability in patients with panic disorder. *Psychiatry Res* **56**, 289–93.

Yingling, K.W., Lawson, R.W., Arnold, L.M. & Rouan, G.W. (1993) Estimated prevalences of panic disorder and depression among consecutive patients seen in an emergency department with acute chest pain. *J Gen Intern Med* **8**, 231–5.

Zandbergen, J., Bright, M., Pols, H., Fernandez, I., DeLoof, C. & Griez, E.J.L. (1991) Higher lifetime prevalence of respiratory diseases in panic disorder. *Am J Psychiatry* **148**, 1583–5.

Zaubler, T.S. & Katon, W. (1996) Panic disorder and medical comorbidity: a review of the medical and psychiatric literature. *Bull Menninger Clin* **60** (Suppl. A), 12–38.

Zaubler, T.S. & Katon, W. (1998) Panic disorder in the general medical setting. *J Psychosom Res* **44**, 25–42.

PART FOUR

Treatments

17 Benzodiazepines
C. Faravelli, S. Rosi & E. Truglia

Introduction

Following their introduction in the 1960s, the benzodiazepines rapidly displaced previous pharmacological treatments for anxiety disorders, such as the barbiturates and meprobamate, due to their effectiveness and safety. Benzodiazepines gained an enormous popularity and in the mid-1970s they had become the most widely prescribed class of psychotropic drugs in the world (Balter *et al.* 1974). Their widespread utilization, however, caused an increasing amount of concern, mostly because of the emerging evidence of their liability to cause abuse and dependence phenomena. This lead to a debate over the value of the benzodiazepines that often relied on emotive and ideological, rather than on scientific, issues.

Despite these concerns the benzodiazepines remain a widely prescribed, generally safe and effective treatment for many anxiety disorders because abuse and dependence do not seem to occur in the great majority of patients. However, it must be acknowledged that even in the absence of clear dependence phenomena, benzodiazepines are more difficult to discontinue than other antianxiety drugs. Moreover, benzodiazepines are not effective in treating depression, a condition that frequently coexists with anxiety (Nutt 2000). Given the present availability of other effective treatment options for anxiety, in the opinion of several expert groups the benzodiazepines are no longer a first-choice treatment for any anxiety disorder (with the possible exception of adjustment disorder with anxiety). On the other hand the use of benzodiazepines as adjunctive treatment in order to induce rapid control of specific symptoms (e.g., sleep or muscle tension), or in an emergency situation may be sensible.

Pharmacodynamics

The main effects of benzodiazepines are to decrease anxiety, produce sedation sleep, muscle relaxation, anterograde amnesia and to have anticonvulsant activity. These result from their action on the central nervous system (CNS). There are only two effects of these drugs that seem to derive from actions on peripheral tissues. One is coronary vasodilatation, occurring after intravenous administration of therapeutic doses and involving an inhibition of adenosine metabolism through the blocking of the nucleoside transporter (Seubert *et al.* 2000). The other is neuromuscular blockade that occurs only with very high doses possibly involving the motoneurones $GABA_A$ receptors (Rudolph *et al.* 1999; Crestani *et al.* 2001).

Benzodiazepines exert their actions on the CNS through the enhancement of the actions of γ-aminobutirric acid (GABA), the main inhibitory neurotransmitter in the mammalian brain. Two major subtypes of receptors ($GABA_A$ and $GABA_B$) mediate GABA action in the CNS. $GABA_B$ receptors are metabotropic receptors coupled to G proteins; $GABA_A$ receptors are responsible for most of the inhibitory neurotransmission in the CNS, are ionotropic receptors composed of five subunits assembled to form an integral chloride channel. Binding of two molecules of GABA increases the channel permeability to chloride ions which then hyperpolarizes the cell membrane and reduces the

Table 17.1 GABA$_A$ receptor ligands.

	GABA binding site	BDZ binding site	Barbiturate binding site	Steroid binding site	Other binding sites
Agonists	GABA,	BDZ muscimol	Barbiturates imidazopyridines, cyclopyrrolones	Allopregnanolone,	Anesthetics allotetrahydroethanol deoxycorticosterone
Antagonists	Bicuculline	Flumazenil	Picrotoxin	Pregnenolone	t-butylbicyclosulfate phosphorothionate
Inverse agonists		β-carbolines			

BDZ, benzodiazepine; GABA, γ-aminobutirric acid.

depolarizing effects of excitatory stimuli thus reducing neuronal excitability.

In the 1970s specific binding sites for the benzodiazepines, subsequently defined 'benzodiazepine receptors' were discovered in the CNS. The correlation between the GABA$_A$ receptor and the benzodiazepine receptor was subsequently shown, when it was observed that GABA potentiated benzodiazepine binding to this receptor. At the end of the 1980s the sequence and the functional expression of genes codifying for two GABA$_A$ receptor subunits were identified and it was shown that these subunits could form a functioning chloride channel (Mamalaki *et al.* 1987). Subsequently an additional component of the GABA$_A$ receptor that permitted formation of a chloride channel sensitive to benzodiazepines was identified, thus showing that GABA and benzodiazepine receptors were part of the same molecular complex (Pritchett *et al.* 1989). Benzodiazepines are positive allosteric modulators of the GABA$_A$ receptor; they do not directly open the chloride channel but binding to their receptor site, which is different from the GABA binding site, increases the opening frequency of the channel in the presence of GABA, without changing its opening time or conductance.

Each GABA$_A$ receptor is thought to consist of a pentamer made up of five subunits. Thus far, 16 different subunits have been identified and classified into seven families: six α (α_{1-6}), three β (β_{1-3}), three γ (γ_{1-3}) and single δ, ε, π and θ subunits. Additional complexity derives from ribonucleic acid (RNA) splice variants of some of these subunits (Charney *et al.* 2000). The exact subunit structures of native GABA$_A$ receptors remains unknown, but it is thought that most GABA receptors are composed of α, β and γ subunits that coassemble with a stochiometric ratio of 2: 2: 1.

The existence of several subunits and their coassembling determines the existence of various subtypes of GABA$_A$ receptors. These different subtypes of the benzodiazepine receptor have different distributions in the CNS and probably subserve different functions, through different sensitivity to benzodiazepines and other ligands. Although theoretically hundreds of thousands of different GABA$_A$ receptors could be assembled from the different subunits, there are constraints limiting their number (Sieghart *et al.* 1999).

Many compounds bind to GABA$_A$ receptors in different sites (Table 17.1). Benzodiazepine binding sites are on the α subunits, whereas the GABA binding sites are in the β subunits. Studies of cloned GABA$_A$ receptors have shown that the coassembly of two α and two β subunits produce a chloride channel receptor sensitive to GABA, barbiturates and their antagonists that binds benzodiazepines but is not sensitive to their effects (Valeyev *et al.* 1993). The coassembly of a γ subunit with α and β subunits is necessary to confer benzodiazepine sensitivity (Boileau *et al.* 1998). GABA, benzodiazepine and steroid binding sites are functionally interacting: the activation or the inhibition of one of these sites by its specific agonists or antagonists changes the other sites binding capacity resulting in positive or negative modulation of the channel activity. Benzodiazepines binding to their site facilitates GABA and barbiturate binding, and barbiturates binding to their site facilitate GABA and benzodiazepine binding.

The benzodiazepine binding site on the GABA$_A$ receptor is called the central benzodiazepine receptor. Three different binding sites have been identified and were initially called the BZ1, BZ2 and BZ3 binding sites. BZ1 and BZ2 sites are present only in the CNS neurones (central benzodiazepine receptors), while BZ3

Table 17.2 Different $GABA_A$ receptor subtypes, with different α subunits.

$GABA_A$ receptor (α_1–6 β_3 γ_2)	α subunit	Different affinity of different ligands for the binding site in the α subunit
A1	α_1	High affinity for zolpidem, CL 218 872, 2-oxoquazepam, β-carbolines
A2	α_2	Preferential affinity ligands do not exist for this site
A3	α_3	Low affinity for CL 218 872
A4	α_4	Insensitive to diazepam and imidazopyridines, sensitive to bretazenil
A5	α_5	Low affinity for imidazopyridines
A6	α_6	Insensitive to diazepam and imidazopyridines, cyclopyrrolones and CL 218 872

is expressed in the CNS by the glial cells and in the peripheral tissues, e.g., by steroidogenic cells in the adrenal cortex and in the testis and by other cells in the lungs, kidneys, liver, spleen, skin and blood (Beurdeley-Thomas *et al.* 2000; Marino *et al.* 2001); it is therefore called peripheral benzodiazepine receptor.

It is generally thought that BZ1 and BZ2 mediate the typical pharmacological effects of the benzodiazepines, while the physiological role of the peripheral receptor has not yet been defined, neither is there solid evidence that it is associated to the $GABA_A$ receptor. Recent studies suggest that BZ3 is located in the outer mitochondrial membrane, where it seems involved in the regulation of steroidogenesis, both in the peripheral tissues and in the CNS. Putative natural ligands of this receptor could be "endogenous" or "natural" benzodiazepines (or "endozepines") like the diazepam binding inhibitor and its two major processing products, the octaneuropeptide and the triakontatetraneuropeptide, also interacting with central-type benzodiazepine receptors and probably stimulating neurosteroid biosynthesis (Costa & Guidotti 1991; Papadoupolus *et al.* 1997; Do-Rego *et al.* 1998, 2001).

Recently a commission of the International Pharmacology Association has proposed to define benzodiazepine binding sites 'ω receptors', because these sites also interact with nonbenzodiazepinic ligands. Currently the BZ1 site, or ω_1 receptor, is associated to the combination of subunits α_1 β_3 γ_2, while the binding site BZ2, or ω_2 receptor, seems associated to the combination α_2 β_3 γ_2. Other binding sites, located on the subunits α_3, α_4, α_5 and α_6 have been recently identified and classified according to their affinity for different ligands (Table 17.2). Activities at different ω receptor subtypes may be associated with different pharmacological effects of benzodiazepine receptor ligands: ω_1

Table 17.3 Affinity of different ligands for the $GABA_A$ receptor benzodiazepine binding site.

Drug	IC50*
Triazolam	0.49
Imidazenil†	0.90
Clonazepam	0.95
Flunitrazepam	1.10
Lorazepam	2.47
Bretazenil†	2.60
Chlordesmethyldiazepam	2.75
Alprazolam	7.34
Diazepam	12.10
Flurazepam	12.50
Chlordiazepoxide	360.00

*IC50 = concentration (expressed in nMol/L) necessary to inhibit 50% of the flunitrazepam binding to rat cerebral cortex membranes.
†Nonbenzodiazepinic compounds.

receptors play an important role in the anxiolytic and sedative/hypnotic effects, whereas activity at ω_2 sites could be associated primarily with muscle relaxation (Griebel *et al.* 1999).

Receptor affinity or potency refers to the different affinity of various benzodiazepine receptor ligands for their binding site (Table 17.3). High potency benzodiazepines act at more minor doses than low potency ones because they have a higher affinity for the benzodiazepine receptor. Potency may influence not only the therapeutic dose, but also the possible specificity of action of certain benzodiazepines in certain clinical conditions; for instance, a higher efficacy on panic disorder has been suggested for high potency benzodiazepines (Gorman *et al.* 1989). Moreover, different

Table 17.4 Intrinsic activity of benzodiazepine receptor ligands.

Intrinsic activity	Compounds
Full agonists	Benzodiazepines
Partial agonists	Bretazenil, imidazenil, abecarnil
Antagonists	Flumazenil
Partial inverse agonists	RU 33965, sarmazenil, FG 7142
Full inverse agonists	β-carbolines

benzodiazepines may have different affinity for different receptor subtypes, with different clinical effects: for instance, it has been suggested that lormetazepam may be a potent hypnotic agent with less ataxic effect than other hypnotic benzodiazepines because it is more selective and acts potently on ω_1 receptors (Ozawa *et al.* 1991).

Benzodiazepine receptor ligands can act as agonists, antagonists or inverse agonists at the benzodiazepine receptor site (Table 17.4: Nutt & Malizia 2001). Agonists increase the amount of chloride current generated by the $GABA_A$ receptor activation and shift the GABA concentration-response curve to the left, while inverse agonists have opposite actions. Full inverse agonists, such as β-carbolines, produce effects that are opposite to those of full agonists: they are anxiogenic, proconvulsant, stimulating and memory activating. All of these effects can be blocked by antagonists at the benzodiazepine receptor site. Antagonists, for instance flumazenil, are molecules without intrinsic activity, in the absence of agonists or inverse agonists, an antagonist does not affect $GABA_A$ receptor function.

Partial agonists such as bretazenil, imidazenil and abecarnil are in an intermediary position; theoretically they offer the possibility to separate desired clinical effects (anxiolysis) from unwanted side-effects such as sedation, ataxia, memory disturbances or dependence. So far the data are not convincing, because a powerful partial agonist does not behave very differently from full agonists and a low potency partial agonist has not enough clinical activity (Haefely 1988; Griebel *et al.* 1999).

Partial inverse agonists, such as RU 33965, sarmazenil, FG 7142, are anxiogenic and memory activating and so may be useful in the treatment of age-associated memory impairment (Zhang *et al.* 1995), but they are not currently employed as therapeutic drugs. The benzodiazepines receptor response to compounds with different intrinsic activity is a dynamic property. For instance, after chronic benzodiazepine treatment, there is a change in the set-point of the receptor: agonist effects are attenuated, inverse agonist effects are enhanced, and antagonists become slightly inverse agonistic in their effects. An explanation for this finding is a receptor shift in the inverse-agonist direction. This change has been suggested to contribute to benzodiazepine withdrawal (Nutt & Malizia 2001). Changes in the efficacy of benzodiazepines, such as seen in tolerance, are associated with reduced expression of α_1 subunits during chronic administration and increased expression of α_4 subunits during withdrawal of benzodiazepines (Follesa *et al.* 2001). Differences in intrinsic activity and in receptor affinity may explain why different benzodiazepines, although producing similar pharmacological effects, exhibit differences in the specificity of the pharmacological effect and in the intensity of side-effects.

There is some recent evidence beginning to point out which $GABA_A$ receptor subunits are responsible for some specific *in vivo* effects of benzodiazepines. The mutation to arginine of a histidine residue at position 101 of the α_1 subunit renders receptors containing that subunit insensitive to the sedative, amnestic and, in part, the anticonvulsant effects of diazepam, while retaining sensitivity to anxiolytic, muscle-relaxant and ethanol enhancing effects (Rudolph *et al.* 1999; McKernan *et al.* 2000). Conversely, mice bearing the equivalent mutation in the α_2 subunit display insensitivity to anxiolytic effects of diazepam (Low *et al.* 2000). The attribution of specific behavioral effects of benzodiazepines to individual receptor subunits will help in the development of new compounds exhibiting fewer undesired side-effects. For example, the experimental compound L838 417 enhances the effects of GABA on receptors composed of α_2, α_3 or α_5 subunits but does not have efficacy on receptors containing the α_1 subunit; it is thus anxiolytic but not sedating (McKernan *et al.* 2000).

Pharmacokinetics

Table 17.5 summarizes the main pharmacokinetic parameters of the benzodiazepines that are most widely employed in the treatment of anxiety.

Table 17.5 Pharmacokinetic parameters of selected benzodiazepines.

	Peak plasma concentration after p.o. administration	Plasma protein binding (%)	Main metabolic pathway	Duration of action* (h)
Alprazolam	1.0–2.0	70	Oxidation (alprazolam-like)	Short-acting
Bromazepam	0.5–4.0	70	Oxidation (nordiazepam-like)	Short-acting
Brotizolam	0.5–2.0	90	Oxidation (alprazolam-like)	Short-acting
Chlordesmethyldiazepam	1.0–2.0	95	Oxidation (nordiazepam-like)	Long-acting
Chlordiazepoxide	1.0–2.0	95	Oxidation (pronordiazepam-like)	Long-acting
Clobazam	1.0–4.0	85	Oxidation (pronordiazepam-like)	Long-acting
Clonazepam	1.0–4.0	85	Nitroreduction	Intermediate-acting
Clorazepate	1.0–2.0	95	Oxidation (pronordiazepam-like)	Long-acting
Diazepam	0.5–1.5	95	Oxidation (pronordiazepam-like)	Long-acting
Etizolam	3.0	90	Oxidation (alprazolam-like)	Short-acting
Flunitrazepam	1.0	75	Nitroreduction	Short-acting
Flurazepam	0.5–1.0	95	Oxidation (pronordiazepam-like)	Long-acting
Halazepam	1.0–3.0	95	Oxidation (pronordiazepam-like)	Long-acting
Ketazolam	2.0–3.0	90	Oxidation (pronordiazepam-like)	Long-acting
Lorazepam	1.0–2.0	90	Direct conjugation	Short-acting
Lormetazepam	2.0		Direct conjugation	Short-acting
Midazolam	0.5–1.0	95	Oxidation (alprazolam-like)	Short-acting
Nitrazepam	0.5–7.0	85	Nitroreduction	Intermediate-acting
Nordiazepam	1.0–2.0	95	Oxidation (nordiazepam-like)	Long-acting
Oxazepam	2.0–3.0	95	Direct conjugation	Short-acting
Prazepam	2.5–6.0	95	Oxidation (pronordiazepam-like)	Long-acting
Quazepam	1.0–3.0	95	Oxidation (pronordiazepam-like)	Long-acting
Temazepam	2.5	95	Direct conjugation	Short-acting
Triazolam	1.0–2.0	90	Oxidation (alprazolam-like)	Short-acting

*Short-acting, drug or active metabolites with a half-life of less than 24 h; intermediate-acting, drug or active metabolites with a half-life of 24–48 h; long-acting, drug or active metabolites with a half-life of more than 48 h.

Absorption

The benzodiazepines are generally well absorbed following oral administration so their onset of action is limited by the absorption rate, rather than by the much more rapid passage from blood to brain (Greenblatt *et al.* 1983a,b). As benzodiazepines are generally highly lipophilic compounds they quickly cross the blood–brain barrier, as demonstrated by the rapid onset of action after intravenous administration, ranging from 15 s to 30 s to a few minutes (Arendt *et al.* 1983).

The absorption rate of benzodiazepines in the gut mostly depends on variations in their lipid solubility; as though all benzodiazepines have high lipophilicity, there are significant differences among the individual compounds. Therefore, the rate of absorption shows a broad variability, and peak plasma concentrations occur after an interval that ranges from 0.5 h to 1 h for those benzodiazepines with the highest lipophilicity to some hours for the less lipophilic agents (Shader *et al.* 1984). Rapidly absorbed benzodiazepines could be preferable whenever quick therapeutic effects are desirable; on the other hand, some patients may perceive a rapid onset of action as an unwelcome feeling of drowsiness or loss of control and therefore tolerate better slowly absorbed drugs (Greenblatt *et al.* 1983a). Given that speed of onset of drug action is considered as an important determinant of the reinforcing effects, it has been suggested that the speed of absorption may influence the relative potential for the abuse of a benzodiazepine (Busto *et al.* 1989; de Wit & Griffith

1991). Consequentially, although decisive evidence on this topic is still lacking, slowly absorbed drugs may offer some advantages when a high likelihood of abuse is suspected.

It must be remembered, however, that aside from the intrinsic characteristics of each compound, the absorption rate also depends on the pharmaceutical formulation. A good example is temazepam which is slowly absorbed from conventional tablet formulation but has a fast onset of action when prepared in a solution of propylene glycol. Such a liquid formulation was used in the early days to accelerate the speed of hypnotic onset but these gel-filled capsules became much sought after and abused as the liquid could be injected intravenously.

Benzodiazepine administration after a meal may result in delayed absorption because of the physiological slowing of gastric emptying (Greenblatt 1991). This has probably no clinical relevance unless a quick onset of action is absolutely necessary. Benzodiazepine absorption may be reduced in inflammatory gastrointestinal disease, although few data are available and the clinical significance of this observation is uncertain (Gubbins & Bertch 1991).

After oral administration benzodiazepines undergo a relevant first-pass hepatic inactivation which limits their bioavailability. Conversely, doses administered by sublingual route avoid first-pass metabolism and may therefore produce earlier and higher peak concentrations than do doses administered orally (Kroboth et al. 1995).

Following intramuscular injection, the absorption of benzodiazepines is generally erratic with the exception of lorazepam (Greenblatt et al. 1983a,b), which therefore should be considered as the drug of choice for intramuscular use. However, intramuscular injection seems to offer only marginal advantages in terms of speed of absorption when compared to oral or sublingual administration (Greenblatt et al. 1982) and should be reserved for noncollaborative patients.

Plasma protein binding

The binding of benzodiazepines to plasma proteins correlates with lipid solubility and ranges from about 70% for alprazolam to nearly 99% for diazepam. While there is currently no evidence of clinically significant effects due to competition with other protein-bound drugs, an increased incidence of side-effects from several benzodiazepines in patients with hypoalbuminemia has been reported (du Souich et al. 1993). In such patients lower doses should be used and careful clinical monitoring is therefore required. Again due to their high lipophilicity, benzodiazepines are quickly removed from plasma to brain and lungs. The distribution to this compartment is followed by a second-phase redistribution to less perfused areas, primarily the adipose tissue (Bailey et al. 1994).

Half-life and metabolism

Benzodiazepines are often classified according to their elimination half-life. It must be remembered, however, that the half-life of elimination should not be confused with duration of action (Task Force Report of the American Psychiatric Association 1990). In fact, for single dose or very short-term administration, such as in the short term or intermittent therapy of acute anxiety states or in the treatment of sleep disorders, the duration of action of benzodiazepines is strongly influenced by their lipid solubility, which in turn determines tissue distribution. Absorption and crossing of the blood–brain barrier are quicker for highly lipophilic compounds, but they are also have a higher brain clearance rate and are more rapidly redistributed from brain and blood to peripheral inactive compartments such as adipose tissue. This explains the fact that benzodiazepines with a long elimination half-life and a high lipophilicity, such as diazepam, may have a shorter duration of action than agents with a short elimination half-life but a lower lipophilicity, such as lorazepam (Greenblatt et al. 1983a,b).

With multiple dosing of benzodiazepines, however, half-life becomes a reliable index, since repeated administration leads to saturation of the adipose tissue, that serves as a depot for leaching out of the drug and its active metabolites (Bailey et al. 1994).

However, the benzodiazepines require metabolism by liver enzymatic systems to be biotransformed into more polar, water-soluble products which are readily eliminated through renal excretion (Shen 1997). They can therefore be classified according to their main metabolic pathway, which in turn is the main determinant of their actual duration of action on clinical grounds. The real clinical duration of their effect, is given by the sum of the parent compound plus all its active metabolites. 3-hydroxybenzodiazepines (lorazepam, lormetazepam, oxazepam and temazepam)

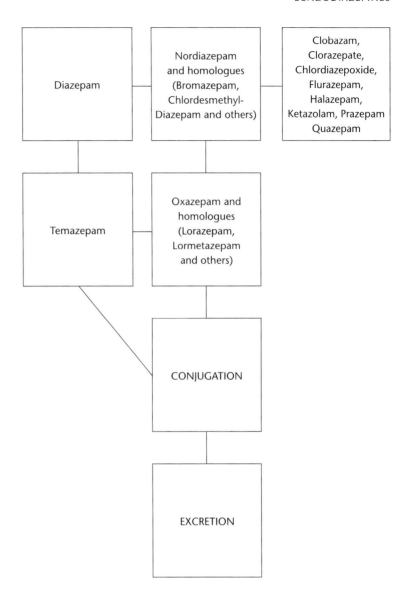

Fig. 17.1 Metabolism of pronordiazepam-like and of 3-hydroxybenzodiazepines.

do not require oxidative metabolism; they rapidly undergo glucuronide conjugation to inactive compounds which are quickly excreted by the kidney. Consequentially, they are short-acting drugs with no active metabolites and their elimination is not affected by inhibition or induction of the hepatic oxidative metabolism. Pronordiazepam-like benzodiazepines (Fig. 17.1), of which the prototype is diazepam, are long-acting compounds that require oxidation by cytochrome P450-dependent mono oxygenases (CYP 450) in the liver to nordiazepam or its homologues,

which are active compounds (in fact, they are often commercially available as prescription drugs) with a long elimination half-life, thus substantially contributing to the pharmacological activity of the parent drug. Nordiazepam and its homologues require further CYP 450-mediated oxidation to form oxazepam (or its halogenated homologues) which are rapidly conjugated and eliminated.

Other compounds (alprazolam-like benzodiazepines) also require CYP 450-mediated oxidation; the resulting metabolites have psychoactive properties, but they are rapidly inactivated through conjugation and thus do not contribute to the pharmacological activity of the parent drug. Compared with pronordiazepam-like benzodiazepines, these drugs have a short duration of action, but for both groups elimination can be influenced by conditions affecting the hepatic oxidative metabolism. 7-nitrobenzodiazepines, such as clonazepam, generally have an intermediate duration of action; they undergo reduction of the nitro group to form both active and inactive compounds. The combination of half-life and number of active metabolites is probably the main factor that may influence the choice of a specific benzodiazepine.

Drugs with a long clinical duration may offer the advantages of a sustained effect and of a lower likelihood of a discontinuation syndrome with rapid recurrence of anxiety symptoms if treatment is stopped abruptly. On the other hand with these agents drug accumulation is more frequent and therefore the risk of adverse events deriving from psychomotor impairment is considered as higher, especially in the elderly. Conversely, short-acting benzodiazepines are thought to be safer from this point of view, but they may result in more severe withdrawal phenomena with a consequentially higher risk of physiological dependence and they may more easily induce tolerance (Shader & Greenblatt 1993; Petursson 1994). However, it must be recognized that the existence of these relationships between half-life and unwanted effects of benzodiazepines has not always emerged, especially in pharmacoepidemiological studies. In fact, it has been suggested that dosage is a much more important determinant of whether a regimen is potentially hazardous than half-life (Cumming 1998; Salzman 1998).

The metabolism of benzodiazepines can be influenced by some conditions. Old age is associated with an impairment of the clearance of those benzodiazepines that are primarily metabolized by microsomal oxidation and consequentially an increase in their half-life may occur leading to an increased accumulation and subsequent adverse events during multiple dosage. Conversely, for those benzodiazepines metabolized mainly by glucuronide conjugation or nitroreduction there are minimal, if any, age-related decrements in clearance (Greenblatt et al. 1991; Hammerlein et al. 1998).

Liver disorders also lead to an impairment of the metabolism of benzodiazepines; although glucuronidation is not spared when liver disease is severe, the oxidative metabolism is much more affected (Rodighiero 1999). Consequentially, directly conjugated compounds should be preferred in the elderly or in patients with liver impairment. Several drugs affect the functions of the cytochrome P450 isoenzymes involved in the oxidative metabolism of benzodiazepines, leading to pharmacokinetic interactions some of which have clinical relevance (see Drug interactions); the likelihood of drug interactions is much reduced with directly conjugated compounds.

It is not clear whether renal impairment leads to clinically meaningful effects on the kinetics of benzodiazepines. A report has attributed the development of encephalopathy to the administration of benzodiazepines in patients on maintenance haemodialysis (Taclob & Needle 1976). Subsequent studies suggested that reduced plasma protein binding and secondary altered benzodiazepine distribution are possible and a reduction in the clearance of the unbound drugs has been proposed (Ochs et al. 1981; Greenblatt & Wright 1993). In the absence of more decisive evidence, careful monitoring of the emergence of unwanted effects is required and dosage reduction is advisable.

Benzodiazepines cross the placental barrier and are excreted into breast milk (Mortola 1989; Llewellyn & Stowe 1998). If the use of a benzodiazepine during breast-feeding is necessary, compounds with minimal distribution into breast milk and metabolites not significantly contributing to pharmacological activity, such as lorazepam, oxazepam or alprazolam are to be preferred (Chisholm & Kuller 1997).

Drug interactions

Although concurrent administration of benzodiazepines and tricyclic antidepressants (TCAs) is rather frequent; there is little evidence concerning the possibilities of relevant pharmacokinetic interactions (Silverman & Braithwaite 1973; Gram et al. 1974; Dugal et al. 1975; Deicken 1988) and the combination is generally considered as safe (General Practitioner Clinical Trials 1969; Wells et al. 1988). However, additive CNS depression is possible and may result in increased impairment of psychomotor performance (Moskowitz & Burns 1988). There are also a few reports of patients receiving amitriptyline and chlordiazepoxide who experienced manifestation of toxicity such as delusions, confusion, agitation or disorientation (Beresford et al. 1988).

Therefore, this combination requires some caution, especially when using TCAs with high sedation potential. A single study suggested that benzodiazepines coadministration may increase the risk of hepatitis induced by the TCA amineptine (Lefebure *et al.* 1984).

Combination therapy with a benzodiazepine and a selective serotonin reuptake inhibitor (SSRI) is also common. Some SSRIs are inhibitors of cytochrome P450 enzymes; therefore, there is a relevant potential for pharmacokinetic interactions with oxidatively metabolized benzodiazepines. Conversely, interactions with directly conjugated or nitroreduced benzodiazepines are less likely to occur. Both fluvoxamine and fluoxetine have been shown to determine relevant increases in the plasma levels of oxidatively metabolized benzodiazepines (Greenblatt *et al.* 1992; Fleishaker & Hulst 1994), while the potential for clinically relevant interactions with benzodiazepines is considered to be less for paroxetine, sertraline or citalopram (Sproule *et al.* 1997). Although there is a case report of delirium attributed to the interaction of fluoxetine and diazepam (Dent & Orrock 1997), the clinical relevance of the interactions between SSRIs and oxidatively metabolized benzodiazepines is still a debated issue. We hold the view that directly conjugated benzodiazepines should be preferred when such an association is planned.

The coadministration of monoamine oxidase inhibitors and benzodiazepines is generally safe (Suerinck & Suerinck 1966; Frommer 1967), although there are a few reports of adverse events such as massive oedema, excessive sweating and postural hypotension (Pathak 1977; Harris & McIntyre 1981) that have been attributed to this combination. Nefazodone is a potent inhibitor of cytochrome P450 enzymes; it can cause relevant increases of the plasma levels of oxidatively metabolized benzodiazepines leading to an increase in psychomotor impairment and sedation, and therefore this association is potentially hazardous. Conversely, directly conjugated benzodiazepines seem safe (Greene & Barbhaiya 1997; Rickels *et al.* 1998).

The combination of lithium carbonate and benzodiazepines is less frequently used, and there is very little evidence of adverse events with the exception of a single case of profound hypothermia in a patient taking lithium carbonate and diazepam (Naylor & McHarg 1977).

Various antiepileptic drugs, including carbamazepine, phenytoin and barbiturates, are inducers of hepatic enzymes involved in drug metabolism. Consequentially, chronic administration of these drugs may increase the metabolism of benzodiazepines thus possibly reducing their clinical effects (Lai *et al.* 1978; Khoo *et al.* 1980; Dhillon & Richens 1981; Scott *et al.* 1983). Conversely, benzodiazepines may increase phenytoin plasma levels (Vajda *et al.* 1971) and cases of phenytoin toxicity have been imputed to this interaction (Rogers *et al.* 1977) although other studies have not supported these findings (Saavedra *et al.* 1985).

Valproic acid may displace benzodiazepines from plasma protein binding sites and inhibit their metabolism thus increasing their plasma levels (Dhillon & Richens 1982; Samara *et al.* 1997), and adverse events, such as drowsiness and absence status in epileptic patients, have been attributed to this combination (Jeavons *et al.* 1977; Watson 1979). However, there is a lack of evidence concerning this association, despite both agents being not uncommonly used together in psychiatry and in other classes of patients.

There have been cases of cardiorespiratory collapse, including fatal ones, in patients who received coadministration of benzodiazepines and of the atypical antipsychotic clozapine (Sassim & Grohmann 1988; Friedman *et al.* 1991). Other adverse events reported in patients taking clozapine and benzodiazepines include hypersalivation, parotid swelling, sedation, ataxia and delirium (Cobb *et al.* 1991; Martin 1993; Jackson *et al.* 1995). Although a specific interaction between clozapine and benzodiazepines has not yet emerged, at the moment very careful monitoring of the patient is necessary with this combination (American Psychiatric Association 1997).

The therapeutic actions of levodopa can be antagonized by benzodiazepines in some patients (Brogden *et al.* 1971; Wodak *et al.* 1972). Although this interaction is probably very infrequent, it is advisable to monitor the patient in order to detect an eventual worsening of parkinsonian symptoms.

Several drugs commonly employed in the treatment of gastric and duodenal ulcers (and of related syndromes) have pharmacokinetic interactions with benzodiazepines. Antacids delay their rate of absorption, but the extent is unaffected and this interaction has probably little or no clinical relevance (Maton & Burton 1999). Prokinetic drugs such as metoclopramide or cisapride may occasion a slight increase in sedation, probably of little importance, when coadministered with benzodiazepines, possibly because they promote gastric emptying and thus accelerate their absorption from the small intestine (Negro 1998). Other drugs, namely the histamine H2-receptor antagonist cimetidine and the proton pump inhibitor omeprazole, impair the clearance of oxidatively metabolized benzodiazepines through inhibition of cytochrome P450 enzymes, while the metabolism of directly conjugated drugs seems unaffected (Negro 1998; Tanaka 1999). The occurrence and extent of effects on cognitive function with these combinations are not completely clear, although it has been reported that the interaction with omeprazole may involve some risk (Andre *et al.* 2000). Nevertheless, use of other H2-receptor antagonists should be preferred when coadministration is needed. These include famotidine, nizatidine and ranitidine, although for the latter there are some contrasting results, and proton pump inhibitors, such as lansoprazole and pantoprazole, seem not to interact with benzodiazepines (Negro 1998).

Some drugs employed in the treatment of infective diseases, such as the macrolide antibiotics erythromycin, triacetyloleandomycin and, to a lesser extent, roxithromycin (von Rosensteil & Adam 1995; Tanaka 1999) and the antifungals ketoconazole, itraconazole and fluconazole (Tanaka 1999; Venkatakrishnan *et al.* 2000), also significantly impair the clearance of oxidatively metabolized benzodiazepines. The resulting increase in duration and extent of effects seems relevant, so coadministration should best be avoided or the dosage of the benzodiazepines greatly reduced. Again, directly glucuronidated benzodiazepines seem safe.

A similar pharmacokinetic interaction has been described for isoniazid, although its clinical significance is not known (Self *et al.* 1999), and has been proposed for ciprofloxacin, but for the latter evidence is mixed and no significant effect on psychomotor performance has been demonstrated (Wijnands *et al.* 1990; Kamali *et al.* 1994). Recently, potentially dangerous interactions (again, probably related to inhibition of CYP enzymes) between the viral protease inhibitors saquinavir (Palkama *et al.* 1999), ritonavir (Greenblatt *et al.* 2000), and benzodiazepines have been described. Dosage reduction of benzodiazepines and careful monitoring are therefore suggested in patients taking these combinations.

Conversely, rifampicin is a potent inducer of the hepatic cytochrome P450 enzyme system in humans; a noteworthy increase of the clearance of oxidatively metabolized benzodiazepines (but not of directly conjugated drugs) has been shown and this can result in a reduction of their clinical effects (Borcherding *et al.* 1992).

Although not all studies are in accord, benzodiazepines may reduce digoxin clearance and increase its plasma concentrations. Especially in the elderly, a few cases of digoxin toxicity have been described, so patients receiving this combination should be closely monitored (Tollefson *et al.* 1984; Ochs *et al.* 1985; Guven *et al.* 1993). It has also been reported that β-blockers may reduce the clearance of some oxidatively metabolized benzodiazepines, but the results are mixed and directly conjugated benzodiazepines do not seem to be involved (Klotz & Reimann 1984; Ochs *et al.* 1987; Sonne *et al.* 1990; Scott *et al.* 1991). It has also been suggested that the association of β-blockers and benzodiazepines, including directly conjugated ones, may impair psychomotor performance (Betts *et al.* 1985; Sonne *et al.* 1990). The clinical relevance of these observations is uncertain; however, clinical monitoring in order to detect incipient signs of this potentially hazardous side-effect is recommended.

Diltiazem and verapamil can increase the plasma concentrations and the elimination half-life of benzodiazepines, and it has also been suggested that these associations should be avoided or the dose of the benzodiazepines reduced. (Kosuge *et al.* 1997). A case of benzodiazepine toxicity in which an interaction between amiodarone and clonazepam was suspected has been described (Witt *et al.* 1993) but there are no further data concerning this association.

Probenecid has been reported to impair the clearance of benzodiazepines by the kidney and their glucuronidation by the liver; the clinical relevance of this interaction is unknown but monitoring for increased drowsiness is suggested (Golden *et al.* 1994). Disulfiram inhibits the oxidative metabolism of benzodiazepines and the coadministration may result in increased drowsiness. The metabolism of directly conjugated benzodiazepines, but also of alprazolam, seems unaffected (Sellers *et al.* 1980; Diquet *et al.* 1990), although there is a case report of temazepam intoxication attributed to concomitant administration of disulfiram (Hardman *et al.* 1994). Diflunisal treatment can significantly decrease peak plasma concentration of benzodiazepines and therefore reduce their clinical action (van Hecken *et al.* 1985).

The coadministration of opioids and benzodiazepines is rather common in the treatment of pain and drug addiction. Although synergism has not been demonstrated, additive pharmacodynamic effects leading to enhanced CNS depression, especially of the respiratory center, are present (Pond *et al.* 1982; Tverskoy *et al.* 1989) and caution is therefore required. Similarly alcohol and benzodiazepines have well-established and dangerous additive CNS depressant actions (Ghodse 1994; Adams 1995). Pharmacokinetic interactions are also of interest; the acute effect of the ingestion of large amounts of alcohol is an impairment of the clearance of oxidatively metabolized benzodiazepines through competition for CYP enzymes, thus enhancing CNS toxicity. Conversely, the chronic consumption of large amounts of alcohol leads to the induction of CYP enzymes, which contributes to the well-known cross tolerance between alcohol and the benzodiazepines, although receptor based changes are probably also important (Lane *et al.* 1985; Fraser 1997). Patients taking benzodiazepines should always be warned against the potentially hazardous effects of the consumption of alcohol. While all benzodiazepines probably have similar pharmacodynamic interactions with alcohol, the likelihood of pharmacokinetic interactions is reduced with directly conjugated compounds, which therefore should be preferred in patients with alcohol abuse/dependence if benzodiazepine therapy is decided.

Cigarette smoking may reduce the effects of benzodiazepines, probably because of the stimulant actions of nicotine (Zevin & Benowitz 1999). Grapefruit juice has been shown to increase the bioavailability and the plasma conentrations of some benzodiazepines, but the clinical relevance of this interaction is unknown (Ameer & Weintraub 1997). Oral contraceptives have been reported to impair the liver oxidation of benzodiazepines and to increase their glucuronidation, although not all the studies are in agreement (Shenfield & Griffin 1991). The clinical relevance of these interactions is not clear, but selected patients may need a dosage increase of directly conjugated benzodiazepines or a reduction for oxidatively metabolized ones.

Side-effects

The most common side-effect of benzodiazepines is sedation deriving from their nonspecific depressive action on the CNS (Shader & Greenblatt 1993; Woods *et al.* 1995a). Sedation may be evidenced by a variety of symptoms including tiredness or drowsiness, light-headedness, difficulty concentrating, thinking or staying awake, apathy, confusion, muscle weakness, movement difficulties such as ataxia, difficulties with balance or dysarthria, blurring of vision, diplopia, vertigo and anterograde amnesia. These side-effects are generally dose-dependent and show significant interindividual variability. Because of the pharmacokinetic changes and of the reduction of baseline cognitive and motor skills that often accompany ageing, they are more evident in the elderly, in whom benzodiazepine therapy is a well-known risk factor for delirium (Meagher 2001). However, with doses within the therapeutic range benzodiazepines are very well tolerated by the great majority of patients; moreover, tolerance to their sedative side-effects (but not to their antianxiety action) generally develops after about 2 weeks of continuous use (Shader & Greenblatt 1993).

Nevertheless, even mild sedation may determine a potentially hazardous impairment of psychomotor performance. Although not all the studies are in agreement (Pierfitte *et al.* 2001), the literature mostly suggests that even at modest doses benzodiazepine therapy is a risk factor for falls and fractures in the elderly. Early studies suggested that long-acting benzodiazepines are more likely to increase the risk of falling, though subsequent evidence has been highly discordant (Cumming 1998; Leipzig *et al.* 1999; Wang *et al.* 2001). Benzodiazepine users also seem to be at increased risk of motor vehicle accidents (Barbone *et al.* 1998; Thomas 1998). On the other hand, it may be speculated that very anxious drivers may be accident prone because of their anxiety and the use of small doses of benzodiazepines could reduce the risk of car accidents.

Paradoxical CNS effects of benzodiazepines, such as increased feelings of anxiety, anger or hostility and behavioral disinhibition have been described but seem very rare (Rothschild *et al.* 2000).

Other possible side-effects of benzodiazepines (less common than sedation) include weight gain, skin rash, nausea, headache, sexual dysfunction and, in women, menstrual irregularities and anovulation; haematologic and hepatic reactions are rare (Charney *et al.* 2000). Benzodiazepines can lead to reduction in the upper airway muscle tone and respiratory depression through blunting of the arousal response to hypercapnia. In healthy adults with therapeutic doses this is not clinically relevant, but in patients suffering from chronic obstructive respiratory disease, or obstructive sleep apnea, caution is recommended (George 2000).

Dependence and withdrawal

The liability of benzodiazepines for abuse and dependence has been a matter of widespread concern and debate (Williams & McBride 1998; Lader 1999). In nonsubstance abusing populations benzodiazepine abuse is quite rare and the great majority of patients does not take higher doses than prescribed (Woods & Winger 1995b; Posternak & Mueller 2001). Benzodiazepine abuse mostly occurs in subjects with a history of previous or concurrent abuse of other drugs; in these patients consequentially benzodiazepine treatment should be avoided (Task Force Report of the American Psychiatric Association 1990).

The issue of benzodiazepine dependence is particularly controversial. It has been clearly demonstrated that chronic use at therapeutic dose can result in physiological dependence (Woods et al. 1995a). However, the majority of patients employ benzodiazepines for relatively short periods (Mellinger et al. 1984; Mant et al. 1988; Fiorio et al. 1990), thus suggesting that most subjects do not have particular difficulties in discontinuing these drugs. If strict criteria are employed, benzodiazepine dependence seems quite uncommon in psychiatric patients, possibly involving no more than 1% of them (Fleischhacker et al. 1986; Rifkin et al. 1989). However, in alcohol- or substance-abusing populations the prevalence is much higher (Ross 1993).

It must be remembered that experiencing some discomfort in discontinuing a medication does not necessarily imply dependence. In fact, the occurrence of clinical changes associated with the discontinuation of benzodiazepine therapy can reflect at least three different discontinuation syndromes, namely *recurrence*, *rebound* and *withdrawal* (Shader & Greenblatt 1993; Schweizer & Rickels 1998). These syndromes may frequently overlap and the distinction is often difficult in clinical practice; nevertheless, they have different theoretical implications, since only withdrawal clearly indicates the presence of physical dependence. Recurrence refers to the reappearance of essentially the same symptoms for which the drug was originally prescribed; it represents a manifestation of the persistence of the original disorder. Although recurrence can take place upon discontinuation of any antianxiety treatment, it is probably more common with benzodiazepines (Ballenger 2001).

Rebound is characterized by the return of anxiety symptoms which are similar or identical to those experienced by the subject before the start of treatment but to a higher level of intensity. Although this phenomenon is not limited to benzodiazepine therapy, it seems particularly frequent when discontinuing these drugs, possibly involving 15–30% of patients (Schweizer & Rickels 1998). Rebound anxiety has been observed after as little as 4 weeks of treatment at therapeutic doses; it is of mild or moderate severity and has generally a short duration but can be followed by recurrence. Risk factors for rebound anxiety when discontinuing benzodiazepine therapy include utilization of higher doses and of short-acting drugs and abrupt taper (Schweizer & Rickels 1998).

The benzodiazepine withdrawal syndrome generally includes, besides increased anxiety or irritability and insomnia, several other symptoms, largely autonomic in nature. Sweating, tachycardia, mild systolic hypertension, tremoulosness, dizziness, tinnitus, excessive sensitivity to light, sound or touch, altered taste, nausea, abdominal discomfort, depressed or dysphoric mood, fatigue, restlessness, agitation and, rarely, confusion, psychotic symptoms, and seizures may all be a part of the clinical picture. The syndrome generally appears in subjects treated for 6 months or longer, although it can be observed much earlier; it is generally of mild severity and rarely requires hospitalization. It tends to resolve in 3–6 weeks but again it can be followed by the recurrence of the original disorder (Shader & Greenblatt 1993; Schweizer & Rickels 1998). The existence of a persistent benzodiazepine discontinuation syndrome has been proposed (Ashton 1991), but there is little evidence to support this claim (Shader & Greenblatt 1993).

Utilization of higher doses and of short-acting benzodiazepines, longer duration of treatment, abrupt taper, female sex, higher levels of anxiety and depression before tapering, dysfunctional personality traits, previous or current alcohol or substance use disorders and a diagnosis of panic disorders may all increase the likelihood and the severity of the withdrawal syndrome (Schweizer & Rickels 1998).

In sum, although the issue of benzodiazepine dependence has been probably overemphasized, it must be acknowledged that a significant minority of patients, almost certainly larger than with other antianxiety therapies, will meet some difficulties in discontinuing these drugs.

Several strategies have been proposed for the discontinuation of chronic benzodiazepine use. Gradual tapering reduce the risk of discontinuation syndromes; reduction by 25% per week is a common regimen, but several clinicians tend to prefer slower tapering (Shader & Greenblatt 1993), especially in panic disorder where reduction by no more than 10% per week has been suggested (American Psychiatric Association 1998). Close monitoring of the patient's conditions, a high degree of flexibility and providing encouragement and emotional support are always advisable. Switching from short-acting to equivalent doses of longer acting benzodiazepines before starting taper also seems useful (Zitman & Couvee 2001). Besides these general measures various pharmacological approaches for benzodiazepine withdrawal have been suggested. Carbamazepine (Schweizer et al. 1991), valproate, trazodone (Rickels et al. 1999) and imipramine (Rickels et al. 2000b) seem effective in increasing taper success rates, although with little or no effect on withdrawal severity. The benefits of other drug therapies such as propranolol (Cantopher et al. 1990), clonidine (Goodman et al. 1986), alpidem (Lader et al. 1993), progesterone (Schweizer et al. 1995), dothiepin (Tyrer et al. 1996) and SSRIs (Zitman & Couvee 2001) seem limited or controversial. Cognitive-behavioral therapy also seems effective in facilitating benzodiazepine discontinuation (Spiegel 1999).

Effects on the fetus and baby

Although the literature is rather controversial, benzodiazepines do not seem to be major human teratogens but an increased risk for malformations, especially oral clefts, after first trimester exposition cannot be ruled out (Dolovich et al. 1998). In advanced pregnancy, benzodiazepine exposure can determine respiratory depression, lower Apgar scores, hypothermia, muscular hypotonicity, failure to feed and withdrawal symptoms in the newborn (Cohen & Rosenbaum 1998; American Academy of Pediatrics 2000). Utilization of benzodiazepines during the first trimester should be avoided; in later pregnancy, short-term administration of low doses is probably safe.

There are limited data regarding the safety of benzodiazepines in breast-feeding. However, CNS depression, weight loss and episodes of apnea have been described in the infant (Llewellyn & Stowe 1998); consequentially, the chronic use of benzodiazepines in breast-feeding women should be avoided (Mortola 1989). Utilization of small doses and for short courses, especially with short-acting drugs, is probably of low risk (Chisholm & Kuller 1997), but the infant should always be closely monitored for signs of sedation.

Overdose

Benzodiazepines are remarkably safe in overdose, except when combined with other CNS depressants, and pure benzodiazepine poisonings generally only induce a mild to moderate CNS depression (Gaudreault et al. 1991). However, fatal poisonings due to benzodiazepines taken alone or with alcohol only, although infrequent, do occur (Serfaty & Masterton 1993), mostly due to respiratory depression with aspiration of gastric contents (Hojer et al. 1989) and consequentially these drugs should not be assumed to be completely safe in patients at risk of suicide. Oxazepam has been suggested to be safer in overdose than other benzodiazepines, while flurazepam and temazepam seem to involve a higher risk of coma and fatal outcome (Serfaty & Masterton 1993; Buckley et al. 1995).

Clinical uses

A judgement on the efficacy of benzodiazepines in clinical practice depends on the choice of the therapeutic goals.

If the outcome is evaluated in terms of symptom reduction, as it is generally the case in clinical trials, then the efficacy of benzodiazepines in most anxiety disorders seems quite good and roughly comparable to that of other pharmacotherapies such as antidepressants. On the other hand, if the improvement of positive indicators of well being such as social or occupational functioning is taken into account, the impression on the efficacy of benzodiazepines is, in the opinion of many clinicians, less favorable.

Consequentially, some caution is required in the interpretation of the results of clinical trials, since the simple quantification of the reduction of anxiety symptoms may fail to capture some elements that are relevant for the patient's quality of life. For instance, it is a frequent observation that patients treated with SSRIs report much more often than those treated with benzodiazepines a reduction of their sensitivity to environmental stressors.

Moreover, while it is well known that comorbidity is a fundamental feature of anxiety disorders, in clinical trials patients suffering from comorbid conditions other than the disorder being investigated are generally excluded, thus making difficult to extend the findings to everyday clinical practice.

There is currently a growing consensus on the chronic nature of anxiety disorders and on the consequent need for long-term treatment in a substantial number of patients. The efficacy of benzodiazepine therapy is mantained during chronic administration. However, it must be remembered that the long-term use of a class of drugs that can potentially impair cognitive and psychomotor performance is less acceptable when there are alternative medications. This is true even if their overall tolerability may be not superior to that of the benzodiazepines but they have a lower impact on the patient's functioning.

On the other hand, it must be acknowledged that the careful use of benzodiazepines remains valuable in the clinical management of anxiety patients, for instance as a tool to increase compliance to the treatment with other drugs presenting a long latency of therapeutic action.

Panic disorder

Benzodiazepines are generally described as an effective and generally well-tolerated treatment option for panic disorder (PD: Kasper & Resinger 2001). Alprazolam (Ballenger et al. 1988; Cross-National Collaborative Panic Study et al. 1992; Noyes et al. 1996) and clonazepam (Tesar et al. 1991; Rosenbaum et al. 1997) have been studied most extensively. The efficacy of several other benzodiazepines, including adinazolam (Davidson et al. 1994), diazepam (Noyes et al. 1996), etizolam (Savoldi et al. 1990) and lorazepam (Schweizer et al. 1990) has also been demonstrated. Benzodiazepines are effective on several endpoint measures, including panic frequency, global anxiety and agoraphobic avoidance (den Boer 1998).

Regarding these symptom areas, meta-analyses comparing benzodiazepines with imipramine (Cox et al. 1992) or antidepressants in general (Clum et al. 1993; Gould et al. 1995; van Balkom et al. 1997) have suggested no significant difference in short-term efficacy. However, in a meta-analysis comparing SSRIs and benzodiazepines the former were found to be superior in alleviating panic attacks (Boyer 1995).

It is unclear whether the presence of comorbid depression affects negatively the response to benzodi-

azepine treatment (Lecrubier 1998). However, as consistently shown in meta-analyses, benzodiazepines are less effective than antidepressants in reducing depressive symptoms in PD patients (Cox et al. 1992; Clum et al. 1993; van Balkom et al. 1997).

It is now acknowledged that PD is a chronic condition and that long-term treatment is often necessary and offers significant benefits (Davidson 1998). The efficacy of benzodiazepines is maintained during long-term administration (Curtis et al. 1993; Schweizer et al. 1993); however, withdrawal symptoms are more likely to occur the longer a benzodiazepine is taken, especially at the high doses required for the treatment of PD. Moreover, there is evidence suggesting that benzodiazepine discontinuation may be especially difficult in PD when compared to other anxiety disorders (Schweizer & Rickels 1998).

The potential difficulties with withdrawal symptoms associated with the likelihood of abuse in subjects with drug or alcohol use disorders, the low efficacy on depressive symptoms and the potential for psychomotor impairment (a particular concern in PD patients given the relatively high doses of benzodiazepines required) are the main drawbacks of benzodiazepine treatment. For these reasons benzodiazepine monotherapy is not currently considered as a first-choice treatment for PD by the majority of experts (American Psychiatric Association 1998; Ballenger et al. 1998a).

The onset of therapeutic action of benzodiazepines is more rapid when compared to antidepressants (American Psychiatric Association 1998) and their short-term coadministration in the acute treatment of PD is a very common clinical practice. In fact, it has been shown (Woods et al. 1992; Goddard et al. 2001) that this combination facilitates a rapid clinical stabilization of panic symptoms, but findings on the maintenance of treatment gains and the occurrence of withdrawal symptoms when discontinuing benzodiazepines were contrasting, thus suggesting the need for further research.

Concurrent use of benzodiazepines and cognitive-behavioral therapy for PD is a highly controversial issue. Several cognitive-behavioral theorists have suggested that benzodiazepines may negatively interfere with psychological treatments (Jensen & Poulsen 1982; Sartory 1983; Gray et al. 1987), while other authors have proposed additive benefits (Lader & Mathews 1968; Wardle 1990) but evidence does not decisively support either claim (Spiegel & Bruce 1997).

Generalized anxiety disorder

The efficacy of benzodiazepines in the treatment of generalized anxiety disorder (GAD) is well established (Davidson 2001). There seems to be little difference between various benzodiazepines (Shader & Greenblatt 1993; Ballenger 1999). Diazepam (Rickels *et al.* 1993; Rickels *et al.* 2000a), alprazolam (Lydiard *et al.* 1997; Moller *et al.* 2001) and lorazepam (Cutler *et al.* 1993; Laakman *et al.* 1998) have been more extensively studied, but several other compounds, including adinazolam (Wilcox *et al.* 1994), bromazepam (Kragh-Sorensen *et al.* 1990), etizolam (Casacchia *et al.* 1990) and ketazolam (Bresolin *et al.* 1988), have been found to be superior to placebo. The efficacy of benzodiazepines seems to be maintained during long-term treatment (Shader & Greenblatt 1993).

Most studies agree that buspirone is as effective as benzodiazepines in reducing GAD symptoms; however, in a few investigations benzodiazepines were found to be superior (Laakman *et al.* 1998).

On the other hand, antidepressants have been consistently found to be equal or even superior in efficacy to benzodiazepines (Davidson 2001). Concerning specific symptom areas, studies are concordant in indicating that benzodiazepines are less effective than antidepressants or buspirone in reducing psychic symptoms of GAD. They may be more effective than these drugs in treating somatic symptoms, but not all this literature is in agreement (Rickels *et al.* 1982, 1993; Hohen-Saric *et al.* 1988; Rocca *et al.* 1997).

It has been shown that even in patients without comorbid major depression the presence of mild, subthreshold depressive symptoms may negatively affect the response of anxiety symptoms to benzodiazepines but not to antidepressants (Rickels *et al.* 1993). For this reason antidepressants should be favored over benzodiazepines as a first-line treatment for GAD (Ballenger *et al.* 2001) because of their efficacy against comorbid psychiatric disorders, such as depression, and of their safety in alcohol and substance abusers. Moreover, following discontinuation of pharmacotherapy the recurrence of anxiety symptoms in GAD patients occurs significantly more often with benzodiazepines in comparison to nonbenzodiazepine anxiolytics (Ballenger 2001). However, benzodiazepines are still a useful treatment option in patients who do not tolerate or fail to respond to antidepressants and as an adjunctive treatment for acute exacerbations of anxiety.

If benzodiazepine therapy is chosen, intermittent rather than continuous treatment should be considered. It has been shown (Rickels & Schweizer 1997) that even after a 4- to 6-week treatment period at least 50% of patients will remain symptom free for weeks or months, and about one-third will not experience the recurrence of anxiety after a 1-year follow-up. Consequentially, drug tapering and discontinuation after about 6 weeks of benzodiazepine treatment has been proposed as a useful strategy in order to distinguish patients who can receive intermittent therapy from those who will require chronic treatment (Ballenger 1999).

Social phobia

Clonazepam has been found to be an effective and generally well-tolerated treatment for social phobia (SP) both in open studies (Jefferson 2001) and in a double-blind, placebo-controlled study (Davidson *et al.* 1993). Open studies also suggest the efficacy of alprazolam (Jefferson 2001). In a controlled trial (Gelernter *et al.* 1991) that compared cognitive-behavioral therapy, alprazolam plus self-exposure, phenelzine plus self-exposure, and placebo plus self-exposure, all the four treatment conditions were associated with substantial improvements in severe and chronic social phobia with no treatment showing a clear superiority over the others, although a trend towards greater efficacy for phenelzine was suggested and the alprazolam-treated group showed a higher relapse rate on treatment discontinuation. Finally, bromazepam has been found to be superior to placebo in a double-blind study (Versiani *et al.* 1997).

In a recent meta-analysis, benzodiazepines resulted more effective than control conditions or psychological therapies, and as effective and tolerable as SSRIs (Fedoroff & Taylor 2001).

Duration of benzodiazepine treatment for SP is not well established. A 2-year follow-up study suggested that the gains acquired during a brief (10-week) treatment with clonazepam are substantially maintained (Sutherland *et al.* 1996); however, treatments received in the follow-up period might have accounted for that result and the persistence of social phobia symptoms despite the overall improvement suggested the need for

329

a longer treatment course. In a double-blind, placebo-controlled study of patients who responded well to 6 months treatment with clonazepam, continuation treatment for another 5 months produced a somewhat greater clinical benefit than a slow-taper discontinuation. Nevertheless, outcome was reasonably good in the discontinuation group with a relatively low relapse rate (Connor *et al.* 1998). In the same study, withdrawal difficulties were not found to represent a major problem.

In sum, although evidence is limited, benzodiazepines (especially clonazepam) seem a useful therapeutic tool for the treatment of SP. Nevertheless, they should probably be considered as a second choice when compared to SSRIs, for which a larger amount of efficacy data is available (Ballenger *et al.* 1998b).

Specific phobias

Benzodiazepines on an 'as needed' basis are frequently employed in order to reduce anxiety and to permit confrontation with the feared stimulus when exposure is sporadic and predictable, as is the case for flight phobia (Taylor & Arnow 1988). However, it has been suggested that their benefits are not maintained in subsequent confrontations; moreover, they may hinder the therapeutic effects of exposure (Wilhelm & Roth 1997). In any case, they only provide a symptomatic relief and do not cure the disorder. Behavioral therapies are currently considered as the treatment of choice for specific phobias; concurrent benzodiazepine use in patients undergoing behavior therapy has been a matter of debate and both positive (Lader & Mathews 1968; Wardle 1990) and negative (Jensen & Poulsen 1982; Sartory 1983; Gray 1987) effects on the outcome have been proposed. Overall, benzodiazepines should probably be reserved for those patients who are completely unable to endure exposure to the phobic stimulus (and consequentially to engage in exposure therapy) unless anxiety levels are reduced (Argyropoulos *et al.* 2000).

Post-traumatic stress disorder

Benzodiazepines do not seem to be an effective treatment for post-traumatic stress disorder (PTSD) and currently several experts tend to discourage their use in this disorder (Ballenger *et al.* 2000). Alprazolam has been shown to determine only a modest reduction in anxiety symptoms, while symptoms specific to PTSD were unimproved (Braun *et al.* 1990). Moreover, PTSD patients receiving long-term benzodiazepine therapy may have a very high potential for severe withdrawal reactions, even with gradual tapering (Risse *et al.* 1990). It must also be considered that PTSD has particularly high comorbidity rates with alcohol/substance use disorders (Jacobsen *et al.* 2001) and therefore PTSD patients could be at high risk for benzodiazepine abuse and dependence. Early benzodiazepine treatment has been evaluated in a controlled study as a preventive strategy in order to improve the psychiatric outcome in recent trauma survivors, but the results have been rather disappointing (Gelpin *et al.* 1996).

Obsessive-compulsive disorder

Some case reports and case series (Hewlett 1993) suggested that benzodiazepines may be of some utility in the treatment of obsessive-compulsive disorder (OCD), especially clonazepam, a benzodiazepine for which an action on serotoninergic neurotransmission has been proposed (Pranzatelli 1989). Clonazepam has been evaluated in a double-blind crossover study (Hewlett *et al.* 1992) in which over a 6-week period an efficacy comparable to that of clomipramine was found. Clonazepam improvement was unrelated to changes in anxiety and occurred early in treatment; a clinically significant response occurred in 40% of subjects failing clomipramine trials. Clonazepam augmentation to antidepressant therapy has also been reported to determine significant benefits (Leonard 1997). More research is needed; currently, given the scarcity of evidence, benzodiazepines should not be considered as a first-line treatment for OCD.

References

Adams, W.L. (1995) Interactions between alcohol and other drugs. *Int J Addict* 30, 1903–23.

Ameer, B. & Weintraub, R.A. (1997) Drug interactions with grapefruit juice. *Clin Pharmacokinet* 33, 103–21.

American Academy of Pediatrics (2000) Use of psychoactive medication during pregnancy and possible effects on the fetus and newborn. *Pediatrics* 105, 880–7.

American Psychiatric Association (1997) *Practice Guideline for the Treatment of Patients with Schizophrenia*. American Psychiatric Press, Washington, D.C.

American Psychiatric Association (1998) *Practice Guideline for the Treatment of Patients with Panic Disorder.* American Psychiatric Press, Washington, D.C.

Andre, M., Fialip, J., Zenut, M., Aumaitre, O. & Eschalier, A. (2000) Confusion mentale sous association inhibiteur de la pompe a protons-benzodiazepines: a propos de trois cas. *Therapie* **55**, 319–20.

Arendt, R.M., Greenblatt, D.J., deJong, R.H. *et al.* (1983) *In vitro* correlates of benzodiazepine cerebrospinal fluid uptake, pharmacodynamic action and peripheral distribution. *J Pharmacol Exp Ther* **227**, 98–106.

Argyropoulos, S.V., Sandford, J.J. & Nutt, D.J. (2000) The psychobiology of anxiolytic drug. Part 2: pharmacological treatments of anxiety. *Pharmacol Ther* **88**, 213–27.

Ashton, H. (1991) Protracted withdrawal syndromes from benzodiazepines. *J Subst Abuse Treat* **8**, 19–28.

Bailey, L., Ward, M. & Musa, M.N. (1994) Clinical pharmacokinetics of benzodiazepines. *J Clin Pharmacol* **34**, 804–11.

Ballenger, J.C. (1999) Current treatments of the anxiety disorders in adults. *Biol Psychiatry* **46**, 1579–94.

Ballenger, J.C. (2001) Overview of different pharmacotherapies for attaining remission in generalized anxiety disorder. *J Clin Psychiatry* **62** (Suppl. 19), 11–19.

Ballenger, J.C., Burrows, G.D., DuPont, R.L., Jr. *et al.* (1988) Alprazolam in panic disorder and agoraphobia: results from a multicenter trial. I. Efficacy in short-term treatment. *Arch Gen Psychiatry* **45**, 413–22.

Ballenger, J.C., Davidson, J.R.T., Lecrubier, Y. *et al.* (1998a) Consensus statement on panic disorder from the International Consensus Group on Depression and Anxiety. *J Clin Psychiatry* **59** (Suppl. 8), 47–54.

Ballenger, J.C., Davidson, J.R.T., Lecrubier, Y. *et al.* (1998b) Consensus statement on social anxiety disorder from the International Consensus Group on Depression and Anxiety. *J Clin Psychiatry* **59** (Suppl. 17), 54–60.

Ballenger, J.C., Davidson, J.R.T., Lecrubier, Y. *et al.* (2000) Consensus statement on post-traumatic stress disorder from the International Consensus Group on Depression and Anxiety. *J Clin Psychiatry* **61** (Suppl. 5), 60–6.

Ballenger, J.C., Davidson, J.R.T., Lecrubier, Y. *et al.* (2001) Consensus statement on generalized anxiety disorder from the International Consensus Group on Depression and Anxiety. *J Clin Psychiatry* **62** (Suppl. 11), 53–8.

Balter, M.B., Levine, J. & Manheimer, D. (1974) Cross-national study of the extent of anti-anxiety/sedative drug use. *N Engl J Med* **290**, 769–74.

Barbone, F., McMahon, A.D., Davey, P.G. *et al.* (1998) Association of road-traffic accidents with benzodiazepine use. *Lancet* **352**, 1331–6.

Beresford, T.P., Feinsilver, D.L. & Hall, R.C. (1988) Adverse reactions to a benzodiazepine-tricyclic antidepressant compound. *J Clin Psychopharmacol* **1**, 392–4.

Betts, T., Knight, R., Crowe, A., Blake, A., Harvey, P. & Mortiboy, D. (1985) Effects of β-blockers on the psychomotor performance in normal volunteers. *Eur J Clin Pharmacol* **28** (Suppl.), 39–49.

Beurdeley-Thomas, A., Miccoli, L., Oudard, S., Dutrillaux, B. & Poupon, M.F. (2000) The peripheral benzodiazepine receptors: a review. *J Neurooncol* **46**, 45–56.

Boileau, A.J., Kucken, A.M., Evers, A.R. & Czajkowski, C. (1998) Molecular dissection of benzodiazepine binding and allosteric coupling using chimeric γ-aminobutyric acid A receptor subunits. *Mol Pharmacol* **53**, 295–303.

Borcherding, S.M., Baciewicz, A.M. & Self, T.H. (1992) Update on rifampin drug interactions II. *Arch Intern Med* **152**, 711–16.

Boyer, W. (1995) Serotonin uptake inhibitors are superior to imipramine and alprazolam in alleviating panic attacks: a meta-analysis. *Int Clin Psychopharmacol* **10**, 45–9.

Braun, P., Greenberg, D., Dasberg, H. & Lerer, B. (1990) Core symptoms of post-traumatic stress disorder unimproved by alprazolam treatment. *J Clin Psychiatry* **51**, 236–8.

Bresolin, N., Monza, G., Scarpini, E. *et al.* (1988) Treatment of anxiety with ketazolam in elderly patients. *Clin Ther* **10**, 536–42.

Brogden, R.N., Speight, T.M. & Avery, G.S. (1971) Levodopa: a review of its pharmacological properties and therapeutic use with particular reference to parkinsonism. *Drugs* **2**, 262–400.

Buckley, N.A., Dawson, A.H., Whyte, I.M. & O'Connell, D.L. (1995) Relative toxicity of benzodiazepines in overdose. *BMJ* **310**, 219–21.

Busto, U., Bendayan, R. & Sellers, E.M. (1989) Clinical pharmacokinetics of nonopiate abused drugs. *Clin Pharmacokinet* **16**, 1–26.

Cantopher, T., Olivieri, S., Cleave, N. & Edwards, J.G. (1990) Chronic benzodiazepine dependence. A comparative study of abrupt withdrawal under propranolol cover versus gradual withdrawal. *Br J Psychiatry* **156**, 406–11.

Casacchia, M., Bolino, F. & Ecari, U. (1990) Etizolam in the treatment of generalized anxiety disorder: a double-blind study versus placebo. *Curr Med Res Opin* **12**, 215–23.

Charney, D.S., Mihic, S.J. & Harris, R.A. (2000) Hypnotics and sedatives. In: *Goodman & Gilman's. The Pharmacological Basis of Therapeutics*, 10th edn (J.G. Hardman & L.E. Limbird (eds), pp. 399–428. McGraw-Hill, New York.

Chisholm, C.A. & Kuller, J.A. (1997) A guide to the safety of CNS-active agents during breastfeeding. *Drug Saf* **17**, 127–42.

Clum, G.A., Clum, G.A. & Surls, R. (1993) A meta-analysis for panic disorder. *J Consult Clin Psychol* **61**, 317–26.

Cobb, C.D., Anderson, C.B. & Seidel, D.R. (1991) Possible interaction between clozapine and lorazepam. *Am J Psychiatry* **148**, 1606–7.

Cohen, L.S. & Rosenbaum, J.F. (1998) Psychotropic drug use during pregnancy: weighing the risks. *J Clin Psychiatry* **59** (Suppl. 2), 18–28.

Connor, K.M., Davidson, J.R., Potts, N.L. *et al.* (1998) Discontinuation of clonazepam in the treatment of social phobia. *J Clin Psychopharmacol* **18**, 373–8.

Costa, E. & Guidotti, A. (1991) Diazepam binding inhibitor (DBI): a peptide with multiple biological actions. *Life Sciences* **49**, 325–44.

Cox, B.J., Endler, N.S., Lee, P.S. & Swinson, R.P. (1992) A meta-analysis of treatments for panic disorder with agoraphobia: imipramine, alprazolam and *in vivo* exposure. *J Behav Ther Exp Psychiatry* **23**, 175–82.

Crestani, F., Low, K., Keist, R., Mandelli, M., Mohler, H. & Rudolph, U. (2001) Molecular targets for the myorelaxant action of diazepam. *Mol Pharmacol* **59**, 442–5.

Cross-National Collaborative Panic Study, Second Phase Investigators (1992) Drug treatment of panic disorder. Comparative efficacy of alprazolam, imipramine, and placebo. *Br J Psychiatry* **160**, 191–202.

Cumming, R.G. (1998) Epidemiology of medication-related falls and fractures in the elderly. *Drugs Aging* **12**, 45–53.

Curtis, G.C., Massana, J., Udina, C., Ayuso, J.L., Cassano, G.B. & Perugi, G. (1993) Maintenance drug therapy of panic disorder. *J Psychiatr Res* **27** (Suppl. 1), 127–42.

Cutler, N.R., Sramek, J.J., Keppel-Hesselink, J.M. *et al.* (1993) A double-blind, placebo-controlled study comparing the efficacy and safety of ipsapirone versus lorazepam in patients with generalized anxiety disorder: a prospective multicenter trial. *J Clin Psychopharmacol* **13**, 429–37.

Davidson, J.R.T. (1998) The long-term treatment of panic disorder. *J Clin Psychiatry* **59** (Suppl. 8), 17–21.

Davidson, J.R.T. (2001) Pharmacotherapy of generalized anxiety disorder. *J Clin Psychiatry* **62** (Suppl. 11), 46–50.

Davidson, J.R.T., Beitman, B., Greist, J.H. *et al.* (1994) Adinazolam sustained-release treatment of panic disorder: a double-blind study. *J Clin Psychopharmacol* **14**, 255–63.

Davidson, J.R.T., Potts, N., Richichi, E. *et al.* (1993) Treatment of social phobia with clonazepam and placebo. *J Clin Psychopharmacol* **13**, 423–8.

Deicken, R.F. (1988) Clonazepam-induced reduction in serum desipramine concentration. *J Clin Psychopharmacol* **8**, 71–3.

den Boer, J.A. (1998) Pharmacotherapy of panic disorder: differential efficacy from a clinical viewpoint. *J Clin Psychiatry* **59** (Suppl. 8), 30–6.

Dent, L.A. & Orrock, M.W. (1997) Warfarin–fluoxetine and diazepam–fluoxetine interaction. *Pharmacotherapy* **17**, 170–2.

de Wit, H. & Griffith, R.R. (1991) Testing the abuse liability of anxiolytic and hypnotic drugs in humans. *Drug Alcohol Depend* **28**, 83–111.

Dhillon, S. & Richens, A. (1981) Pharmacokinetics of diazepam in epileptic patients and normal volunteers following intravenous administration. *British J Clin Pharmacol* **12**, 841–4.

Dhillon, S. & Richens, A. (1982) Valproic acid and diazepam interaction *in vivo*. *British J Clin Pharmacol* **13**, 553–60.

Diquet, B., Gujadhur, L., Lamiable, D., Warot, D., Hayoun, H. & Choisy, H. (1990) Lack of interaction between disulfiram and alprazolam in alcoholic patients. *Eur J Clin Pharmacol* **38**, 157–60.

Dolovich, L.R., Addis, A., Vaillancourt, J.M.R., Power, J.D.B., Koren, G. & Einarson, T.R. (1998) Benzodiazepine use in pregnancy and major malformations or oral cleft: meta-analysis of cohort and case-control studies. *BMJ* **317**, 839–43.

Do-Rego, J.L., Mensah-Nyagan, A.G., Beaujean, D. *et al.* (2001) The octaneuropeptide ODN stimulates neurosteroid biosynthesis through activation of central-type benzodiazepine receptors. *J Neurochem* **76**, 128–38.

Do-Rego, J.L., Mensah-Nyagan, A.G., Feuilloley, M., Ferrara, P., Pelletier, G. & Vaudry, H. (1998) The endozepine triakontatetraneuropeptide diazepam-binding inhibitor [17–50] stimulates neurosteroid biosynthesis in the frog hypothalamus. *Neuroscience* **83**, 555–70.

Dugal, R., Caille, G., Albert, J.M. & Cooper, S.F. (1975) Apparent pharmacokinetic interaction of diazepam and amitriptyline in psychiatric patients: a pilot study. *Curr Ther Res Clin Exp* **18**, 679–86.

Fedoroff, I.C. & Taylor, S. (2001) Psychological and pharmacological treatments of social phobia: a meta-analysis. *J Clin Psychopharmacol* **21**, 311–24.

Fiorio, R., Bellantuono, C., Leoncini, M., Montemezzi, G., Micciolo, R. & Williams, P. (1990) The long-term use of psychotropic drugs: a follow-up in Italian general practice. *Human Psychopharmacology* **5**, 195–206.

Fleischhacker, W.W., Barnas, C. & Hackenberg, B. (1986) Epidemiology of benzodiazepine dependence. *Acta Psychiatr Scand* **74**, 80–3.

Fleishaker, J.C. & Hulst, L.K. (1994) A pharmacokinetic and pharmacodynamic evaluation of the combined administration of alprazolam and fluvoxamine. *Eur J Clin Pharmacol* **46**, 35–9.

Follesa, P., Cagetti, E., Mancuso, L. *et al.* (2001) Increase in expression of the $GABA_A$ receptor α_4 subunit gene induced by withdrawal of, but not long-term treatment with, benzodiazepine full or partial agonists. *Brain Res Mol Brain Res* **92**, 138–48.

Fraser, A.G. (1997) Pharmacokinetic interactions between alcohol and other drugs. *Clin Pharmacokinet* **33**, 79–90.

Friedman, L.J., Tabb, S.E., Worthington, J.J., Sanchez, C.J. & Sved, M. (1991) Clozapine—a novel antipsychotic agent. *N Engl J Med* **325**, 518–19.

Frommer, E.A. (1967) Treatment of childhood depression with antidepressant drugs. *BMJ* **1**, 729–32.

Gaudreault, P., Guay, J., Thivierge, R.L. & Verdy, I. (1991) Benzodiazepine poisoning. Clinical and pharmacological considerations and treatment. *Drug Saf* **6**, 247–65.

Gelernter, C.S., Uhde, T.W., Cimbolic, P. *et al.* (1991) Cognitive-behavioral and pharmacological treatments of social phobia. A controlled study. *Arch Gen Psychiatry* **48**, 938–45.

Gelpin, E., Bonne, O., Peri, T., Brandes, D. & Shalev, A.Y. (1996) Treatment of recent trauma survivors with benzodiazepines: a prospective study. *J Clin Psychiatry* **57**, 390–4.

General Practitioner Clinical Trials (1969) Chlordiazepoxide with amytriptiline in neurotic depression. *Practitioner* **202**, 437–40.

George, C.F. (2000) Perspectives on the management of insomnia in patients with chronic respiratory disorders. *Sleep* **23** (Suppl. 1), S31–5.

Ghodse, H. (1994) Combined use of drugs and alcohol. *Curr Opin Psychiatry* **7**, 249–51.

Goddard, A.W., Brouette, T., Almai, A., Jetty, P., Woods, S.W. & Charney, D. (2001) Early coadministration of clonazepam with sertraline for panic disorder. *Arch Gen Psychiatry* **58**, 681–6.

Golden, P.L., Warner, P.E., Fleishaker, J.C. *et al.* (1994) Effects of probenecid on the pharmacokinetics and pharmacodynamics of adinazolam in humans. *Clinical Pharmacol Ther* **56**, 133–41.

Goodman, W.K., Charney, D.S., Price, L.H., Woods, S.W. & Heninger, G.R. (1986) Ineffectiveness of clonidine in the treatment of the benzodiazepine withdrawal syndrome: report of three cases. *Am J Psychiatry* **143**, 900–3.

Gorman, J.M., Liebowitz, M.D., Fyer, A.J. & Stein, J. (1989) A neurochemical hypothesis for panic disorder. *Am J Psychiatry* **146**, 148–61.

Gould, R.A., Otto, M.W. & Pollack, M.H. (1995) A meta-analysis of treatment outcome for panic disorder. *Clin Psychol Rev* **15**, 819–44.

Gram, L.F. & Overo, K. & Kirk, L. (1974) Influence of neuroleptics and benzodiazepines on metabolism of tricyclic antidepressants in man. *Am J Psychiatry* **131**, 863–6.

Gray, J.A. (1987) Interactions between drugs and behavior therapy. In: *Theoretical Foundations of Behavior Therapy* (H.J. Eysenck & I. Martin (eds), pp. 433–47). Plenum, New York.

Greenblatt, D.J. (1991) Benzodiazepine hypnotics: sorting the pharmacokinetic facts. *J Clin Psychiatry* **52** (Suppl.), 4–10.

Greenblatt, D.J., Divoll, M., Harmatz, J.S. & Shader, R.I. (1982) Pharmacokinetic comparison of sublingual lorazepam with intravenous, intramuscular, and oral lorazepam. *J Pharm Sci* **71**, 248–52.

Greenblatt, D.J., Harmatz, J.S. & Shader, R.I. (1991) Clinical pharmacokinetics of anxiolytics and hypnotics in the elderly. Therapeutic considerations (Part I). *Clin Pharmacokinet* **21**, 165–77.

Greenblatt, D.J., Preskorn, S.H., Cotreau, M.M., Horst, W.D. & Harmatz, J.S. (1992) Fluoxetine impairs clearance of alprazolam but not of clonazepam. *Clin Pharmacol Ther* **55**, 479–86.

Greenblatt, D.J., Shader, R.I. & Abernethy, D.R. (1983a) Drug therapy. Current status of benzodiazepines, I. *N Engl J Med* **309**, 354–8.

Greenblatt, D.J., Shader, R.I. & Abernethy, D.R. (1983b) Drug therapy. Current status of benzodiazepines, II. *N Engl J Med* **309**, 410–16.

Greenblatt, D.J., von Moltke, L.L., Harmatz, J.S. *et al.* (2000) Alprazolam–ritonavir interaction: implications for product labeling. *Clin Pharmacol Ther* **67**, 335–41.

Greenblatt, D.J. & Wright, C.E. (1993) Clinical pharmacokinetics of alprazolam. Therapeutic implications. *Clin Pharmacokinet* **24**, 453–71.

Greene, D.S. & Barbhaiya, R.H. (1997) Clinical pharmacokinetics of nefazodone. *Clin Pharmacokinet* **33**, 260–75.

Griebel, G., Perrault, G., Letang, V. *et al.* (1999) New evidence that the pharmacological effects of benzodiazepine receptor ligands can be associated with activities at different BZ θ receptor subtypes. *Psychopharmacology (Berl)* **146**, 205–13.

Gubbins, P.O. & Bertch, K.E. (1991) Drug absorption in gastrointestinal disease. Clinical pharmacokinetic and therapeutic implications. *Clin Pharmacokinet* **21**, 431–47.

Guven, H., Tuncok, Y., Guneri, S., Cavdar, C. & Fowler, J. (1993) Age-related digoxin–alprazolam interaction. *Clin Pharmacol Ther* **54**, 42–4.

Haefely, W. (1988) Partial agonists of the benzodiazepine receptor: from animal data to results in patients. *Adv Biochem Psychopharmacol* **45**, 275–92.

Hammerlein, A., Derendorf, H. & Lowenthal, D.T. (1998) Pharmacokinetic and pharmacodynamic changes in the elderly. Clinical implications. *Clin Pharmacokinet* **35**, 49–64.

Hardman, M., Biniwale, A. & Clarke, C.E. (1994) Temazepam toxicity precipitated by disulfiram.

Harris, A.L. & McIntyre, N. (1981) Interaction of phenelzine and nitrazepam in a slow acetylator. *Br J Clin Pharmacol* **12**, 254–5.

van Hecken, A.M., Tjandramaga, T.B., Verbesselt, R. & de Schepper, P.J. (1985) The influence of diflunisal on the pharmacokinetics of oxazepam. *Br J Clin Pharmacol* **20**, 225–34.

Hewlett, W.A. (1993) The use of benzodiazepines in obsessive-compulsive disorder and Tourette's syndrome. *Psychiatr Ann* **23**, 309–16.

Hewlett, W.A., Vinogradov, S. & Agras, W.S. (1992) Clomipramine, clonazepam, and clonidine treatment of obsessive-compulsive disorder. *J Clin Psychopharmacol* **12**, 420–30.

Hohen-Saric, R., McLeod, D.R. & Zimmerli, W.D. (1988) Differential effects of alprazolam and imipramine in generalized anxiety disorder: somatic versus psychic symptoms. *J Clin Psychiatry* **49**, 293–301.

Hojer, J., Baehrendtz, S. & Gustafsson, L. (1989) Benzodiazepine poisoning: experience of 702 admissions to an intensive care unit during a 14-year period. *J Intern Med* **226**, 117–22.

Jackson, C.W., Markowitz, J.S. & Brewerton, T.D. (1995) Delirium associated with clozapine and benzodiazepine combinations. *Ann Clin Psychiatry* **7**, 139–41.

Jacobsen, L.K., Southwick, S.M. & Kosten, T.R. (2001) Substance use disorders in patients with post-traumatic stress disorder: a review of the literature. *Am J Psychiatry* **158**, 1184–90.

Jeavons, P.M., Clark, J.E. & Maheshwari, M.C. (1977) Treatment of generalized epilepsies of childhood and adolescence with sodium valproate ("epilim"). *Dev Med Child Neurol* **19**, 9–25.

Jefferson, J.W. (2001) Benzodiazepines and anticonvulsants for social phobia (social anxiety disorder). *J Clin Psychiatry* **62** (Suppl. 1), 50–3.

Jensen, H.H. & Poulsen, J.C. (1982) Amnesic effects of diazepam: "drug dependence" explored by state-dependent learning. *Scand J Psychol* **23**, 107–11.

Kamali, F., Herd, B., Edwards, C., Nicholson, E. & Wynne, H. (1994) The influence of ciprofloxacin on the pharmacokinetics and pharmacodynamics of a single dose of temazepam in the young and elderly. *J Clin Pharm Ther* **19**, 105–9.

Kasper, S. & Resinger, E. (2001) Panic disorder: the place of benzodiazepines and selective serotonin reuptake inhibitors. *Eur Neuropsychopharmacol* **11**, 307–21.

Khoo, K.C., Mendels, J., Rothbart, M. *et al.* (1980) Influence of phenytoin and phenobarbital on the disposition of a single oral dose of clonazepam. *Clin Pharmacol Ther* **28**, 368–75.

Klotz, U. & Reimann, J.W. (1984) Pharmacokinetic and pharmacodynamic interaction study of diazepam and metoprolol. *Eur J Clin Pharmacol* **26**, 223–6.

Kosuge, K., Nishimoto, M., Kimura, M., Umemura, K., Nakashima, M. & Ohashi, K. (1997) Enhanced effect of triazolam with diltiazem. *Br J Clin Pharmacol* **43**, 367–72.

Kragh-Sorensen, P., Holm, P., Fynboe, C. *et al.* (1990) Bromazepam in generalized anxiety. Randomized, multipractice comparisons with both chlorprothixene and placebo. *Psychopharmacology (Berl)* **100**, 383–6.

Kroboth, P.D., McAuley, J.W., Kroboth, F.J., Bertz, R.J. & Smith, R.B. (1995) Triazolam pharmacokinetics after intravenous, oral, and sublingual administration. *J Clin Psychopharmacol* **15**, 259–62.

Laakmann, G., Schule, C., Lorkowski, G., Baghai, T., Kuhn, K. & Ehrentraut, S. (1998) Buspirone and lorazepam in the treatment of generalized anxiety disorder in outpatients. *Psychopharmacology (Berl)* **136**, 357–66.

Lader, M.H. (1999) Limitations on the use of benzodiazepines in anxiety and insomnia: are they justified? *Eur Neuropsychopharmacol* **9** (Suppl. 6), S399–405.

Lader, M.H., Farr, I. & Morton, S. (1993) A comparison of alpidem and placebo in relieving benzodiazepine withdrawal symptoms. *Int Clin Psychopharmacol* **8**, 31–6.

Lader, M.H. & Mathews, A.M. (1968) A psychological model of phobic anxiety and desensitization. *Behav Res Ther* **6**, 411–21.

Lai, A.A., Levy, R.H. & Cutler, R.E. (1978) Time-course of interaction between carbamazepine and clonazepam in normal man. *Clin Pharmacol Ther* **24**, 316–23.

Lane, E.A., Guthrie, S. & Linnoila, M. (1985) Effect of ethanol on drug and metabolite pharmacokinetic. *Clin Pharmacokinet* **10**, 228–47.

Lecrubier, Y. (1998) The impact of comorbidity on the treatment of panic disorder. *J Clin Psychiatry* **59** (Suppl. 8), 11–14.

Lefebure, B., Castot, A., Danan, G., Elmalem, J., Jean-Pastor, M.J. & Efthymiou, M.L. (1984) Hepatites aux antidepresseurs. *Therapie* **39**, 509–16.

Leipzig, R.M., Cumming, R.G. & Tinetti, M.E. (1999) Drugs and falls in older people: a systematic review and meta-analysis. I. Psychotropic drugs. *J Am Geriatr Soc* **47**, 30–9.

Leonard, H.L. (1997) New developments in the treatment of obsessive-compulsive disorder. *J Clin Psychiatry* **58** (Suppl. 14), 39–45.

Llewellyn, A. & Stowe, Z.N. (1998) Psychotropic medications in lactation. *J Clin Psychiatry* **59** (Suppl. 2), 41–52.

Low, K., Crestani, F., Keist, R. *et al.* (2000) Molecular and neuronal substrate for the selective attenuation of anxiety. *Science* **290**, 131–4.

Lydiard, R.B., Ballenger, J.C. & Rickels, K. (1997) A double-blind evaluation of the safety and efficacy of abecarnil, alprazolam, and placebo in outpatients with generalized anxiety disorder. *J Clin Psychiatry* **58** (Suppl. 11), 11–18.

Mamalaki, C., Stephenson, F.A. & Barnard, E.A. (1987) The GABA$_A$/benzodiazepine receptor is a heterotetramer of homologous α and β subunits. *EMBO J* **6**, 561–5.

Mant, A., Duncan-Jones, P., Saltman, D. *et al.* (1988) Development of long-term use of psychotropic drugs by general practice patients. *BMJ* **296**, 251–4.

Marino, F., Cattaneo, S., Cosentino, M. *et al.* (2001) Diazepam stimulates migration and phagocytosis of human neutrophils: possible contribution of peripheral-type benzodiazepine receptors and intracellular calcium. *Pharmacology* **63**, 42–9.

Martin, S.D. (1993) Drug-induced parotid swelling. *Br J Hosp Med* **50**, 426.

Maton, P.N. & Burton, M.E. (1999) Antacids revisited: a review of their clinical pharmacology and recommended therapeutic use. *Drugs* **57**, 855–70.

McKernan, R.M., Rosahl, T.W., Reynolds, D.S. *et al.* (2000) Sedative but not anxiolytic properties of benzodiazepines are mediated by the GABA$_A$ receptor α_1 subtype. *Nat Neurosci* **3**, 587–92.

Meagher, D.J. (2001) Delirium: optimizing management. *BMJ* **322**, 144–9.

Mellinger, G.D., Balter, M.B. & Uhlenhuth, E.H. (1984) Prevalence and correlates of the long-term regular use of anxyolitics. *JAMA* **251**, 375–9.

Moller, H.J., Volz, H.P., Reimann, I.W. & Stoll, K.D. (2001) Opipramol for the treatment of generalized anxiety disorder: a placebo-controlled trial including an alprazolam-treated group. *J Clin Psychopharmacol* **21**, 59–65.

Mortola, J.F. (1989) The use of psychotropic agents in pregnancy and lactation. *Psychiatr Clin North Am* **12**, 69–87.

Moskowitz, H. & Burns, M. (1988) The effects on performance of two antidepressants, alone and in combination with diazepam. *Prog Neuropsychopharmacol Biol Psychiatry* **12**, 783–92.

Naylor, G.J. & McHarg, A. (1977) Profound hypothermia on combined lithium carbonate and diazepam treatment. *BMJ* **2**, 22.

Negro, R.D. (1998) Pharmacokinetic drug interactions with anti-ulcer drugs. *Clin Pharmacokinet* **35**, 135–50.

Noyes, R. Jr, Burrows, G.D., Reich, J.H. *et al.* (1996) Diazepam versus alprazolam for the treatment of panic disorder. *J Clin Psychiatry* **57**, 349–55.

Nutt, D.J. (2000) Treatment of depression and concomitant anxiety. *Eur Neuropsychopharmacol* **10** (Suppl. 4), S433–7.

Nutt, D.J. & Malizia, A.L. (2001) New insights into the role of the GABA$_A$ benzodiazepine receptor. *Br J Psychiatry* **179**, 390–6.

Ochs, H.R., Greenblatt, D.J., Friedman, H. *et al.* (1987) Bromazepam pharmacokinetics: influence of age, gender, oral contraceptives, cimetidine, and propranolol. *Clin Pharmacol Ther* **41**, 562–70.

Ochs, H.R., Greenblatt, D.J., Kaschell, H.J., Klehr, U., Divoll, M. & Abernethy, D.R. (1981) Diazepam kinetics in patients with renal insufficiency or hyperthyroidism. *Br J Clin Pharmacol* **12**, 829–32.

Ochs, H.R., Greenblatt, D.J. & Verburg-Ochs, B. (1985) Effect of alprazolam on digoxin kinetics and creatinine clearance. *Clin Pharmacol Ther* **38**, 595–8.

Ozawa, M., Nakada, Y., Sugimachi, K., Akai, T. & Yamaguchi, M. (1991) Interaction of the hypnotic lormetazepam with central benzodiazepine receptor subtypes θ_1, θ_2 and θ_3. *Nippon Yakurigaku Zasshi* **98**, 399–408.

Palkama, V.J., Ahonen, J., Neuvonen, P.J. & Olkkola, K.T. (1999) Effect of saquinavir on the pharmacokinetics and pharmacodynamics of oral and intravenous midazolam. *Clin Pharmacol Ther* **66**, 33–9.

Papadoupolus, V., Amri, H., Bouirad, N. *et al.* (1997) Peripheral benzodiazepine receptor in cholesterol transport and steroidogenesis. *Steroids* **62**, 21–8.

Pathak, S.K. (1977) Gross oedema during treatment for depression. *BMJ* **1**, 1220.

Petursson, H. (1994) The benzodiazepine withdrawal syndrome. *Addiction* **89**, 1455–9.

Pierfitte, C., Macouillard, G., Thicoipe, M. *et al.* (2001) Benzodiazepines and hip fractures in elderly people: case-control study. *BMJ* **322**, 704–8.

Pond, S.M., Tong, T.G., Benowitz, N.L., Jacob, P. & Rigod, J. (1982) Lack of effect of diazepam on methadone metabolism in methadone-maintained addicts. *Clin Pharmacol Ther* **31**, 139–43.

Posternak, M.A. & Mueller, T.I. (2001) Assessing the risks and benefits of benzodiazepines for anxiety disorders in patients with a history of substance abuse or dependence. *Am J Addict* **10**, 48–68.

Pranzatelli, M.R. (1989) Benzodiazepine-induced shaking behavior in the rat: structure-activity and relation to serotonin and benzodiazepine receptors. *Exp Neurol* **104**, 241–50.

Pritchett, D.B., Sontheimer, H., Shivers, B.D. *et al.* (1989) Importance of a novel GABA$_A$ receptor subunit for benzodiazepine pharmacology. *Nature* **338**, 582–5.

Rickels, K., DeMartinis, N. & Aufdembrinke, B. (2000a) A double-blind, placebo-controlled trial of abecarnil and diazepam in the treatment of patients with generalized anxiety disorder. *J Clin Psychopharmacol* **20**, 12–18.

Rickels, K., DeMartinis, N., Garcia-Espana, F., Greenblatt, D.J., Mandos, L.A. & Rynn, M. (2000b) Imipramine and buspirone in treatment of patients with generalized anxiety disorder who are discontinuing long-term benzodiazepine therapy. *Am J Psychiatry* **157**, 1973–9.

Rickels, K., Downing, R., Schweizer, E. & Hassman, H. (1993) Antidepressants for the treatment of generalized anxiety disorder. A placebo-controlled comparison of imipramine, trazodone, and diazepam. *Arch Gen Psychiatry* **50**, 884–95.

Rickels, K. & Schweizer, E. (1997) The clinical presentation of generalized anxiety in primary-care settings: practical concepts of classification and management. *J Clin Psychiatry* **58** (Suppl. 11), 4–10.

Rickels, K., Schweizer, E., Case, W.G. *et al.* (1998) Nefazodone in major depression: adjunctive benzodiazepine therapy and tolerability. *J Clin Psychopharmacol* **18**, 145–53.

Rickels, K., Schweizer, E., Garcia Espana, F., Case, G., DeMartinis, N. & Greenblatt, D. (1999) Trazodone and valproate in patients discontinuing long-term benzodiazepine therapy: effects on withdrawal symptoms and taper outcome. *Psychopharmacology (Berl)* **141**, 1–5.

335

Rickels, K., Wiseman, K., Norstad, N. *et al.* (1982) Buspirone and diazepam in anxiety: a controlled study. *J Clin Psychiatry* **43**, 81–6.

Rifkin, A., Doddi, S., Karajgi, B., Hasan, N. & Alvares, L. (1989) Benzodiazepine use and abuse by patients at outpatients clinics. *Am J Psychiatry* **146**, 1331–2.

Risse, S.C., Whitters, A., Burke, J., Chen, S., Scurfield, R.M. & Raskind, M.A. (1990) Severe withdrawal symptoms after discontinuation of alprazolam in eight patients with combat-induced post-traumatic stress disorder. *J Clin Psychiatry* **51**, 206–9.

Rocca, P., Fonzo, V., Scotta, M., Zanalda, E. & Ravizza, L. (1997) Paroxetine efficacy in the treatment of generalized anxiety disorder. *Acta Psychiatr Scand* **95**, 444–50.

Rodighiero, V. (1999) Effects of liver disease on pharmacokinetics. An update. *Clin Pharmacokinet* **37**, 399–431.

Rogers, H.J., Haslam, R.A., Longstreth, J. & Lietman, P.S. (1977) Phenytoin intoxication during concurrent diazepam therapy. *J Neurol Neurosurg Psychiatry* **40**, 890–5.

Rosenbaum, J.F., Moroz, G. & Bowden, C.L. (1997) Clonazepam in the treatment of panic disorder with or without agoraphobia: a dose–response study of efficacy, safety, and discontinuance. *J Clin Psychopharmacol* **17**, 390–400.

Ross, H.E. (1993) Benzodiazepine use and anxiolytic abuse and dependence in treated alcoholics. *Addiction* **88**, 209–18.

Rothschild, A.J., Shindul-Rothschild, J., Viguera, A., Murray, M. & Brewster, S. (2000) Comparison of the frequency of behavioral disinhibition on alprazolam, clonazepam, or no benzodiazepine in hospitalized psychiatric patients. *J Clin Psychopharmacol* **20**, 7–11.

Rudolph, U., Crestani, F., Benke, D. *et al.* (1999) Benzodiazepine actions mediated by specific γ-aminobutirric acid$_A$ receptor subtypes. *Nature* **401**, 796–800.

Saavedra, I.N., Aguilera, L.I., Faure, E. & Galdames, D.G. (1985) Phenytoin/clonazepam interaction. *Ther Drug Monit* **7**, 481–4.

Salzman, C. (1998) Addiction to benzodiazepines. *Psychiatr Q* **69**, 251–61.

Samara, E.E., Granneman, R.G., Witt, G.F. & Cavanaugh, J.H. (1997) Effect of valproate on the pharmacokinetics and pharmacodynamics of lorazepam. *J Clin Pharmacol* **37**, 442–50.

Sartory, G. (1983) Benzodiazepines and behavioral treatment of phobic anxiety. *Behav Psychother* **11**, 204–17.

Sassim, N. & Grohmann, R. (1988) Adverse drug reactions with clozapine and simultaneous application of benzodiazepines. *Pharmacopsychiatry* **21**, 306–7.

Savoldi, F., Somenzini, G. & Ecari, U. (1990) Etizolam versus placebo in the treatment of panic disorder with agoraphobia: a double-blind study. *Curr Med Res Opin* **12**, 185–90.

Schweizer, E., Case, W.G., Garcia-Espana, F., Greenblatt, D.J. & Rickels, K. (1995) Progesterone coadministration in patients discontinuing long-term benzodiazepine therapy: effects on withdrawal severity and taper outcome. *Psychopharmacology (Berl)* **117**, 424–9.

Schweizer, E., Pohl, R., Balon, R., Fox, I., Rickels, K. & Yeragani, V.K. (1990) Lorazepam versus alprazolam in the treatment of panic disorder. *Pharmacopsychiatry* **23**, 90–3.

Schweizer, E. & Rickels, K. (1998) Benzodiazepine dependence and withdrawal: a review of the syndrome and its clinical management. *Acta Psychiatr Scand* **98** (Suppl. 393), 95–101.

Schweizer, E., Rickels, K., Case, W.G. & Greenblatt, D.J. (1991) Carbamazepine treatment in patients discontinuing long-term benzodiazepine therapy. Effects on withdrawal severity and outcome. *Arch Gen Psychiatry* **48**, 448–52.

Schweizer, E., Rickels, K., Weiss, S. & Zavodnick, S. (1993) Maintenance drug treatment of panic disorder. I. Results of a prospective, placebo-controlled comparison of alprazolam and imipramine. *Arch Gen Psychiatry* **50**, 51–60.

Scott, A.K., Cameron, G.A. & Hawksworth, G.M. (1991) Interaction of metoprolol with lorazepam and bromazepam. *Eur J Clin Pharmacol* **40**, 105–9.

Scott, A.K., Khir, A.S., Steele, W.H., Hawksworth, G.M. & Petrie, J.C. (1983) Oxazepam pharmacokinetics in patients with epilepsy treated long-term with phenytoin alone or in combination with phenobarbitone. *Br J Clin Pharmacol* **16**, 441–4.

Self, T.H., Chrisman, C.R., Baciewicz, A.M. & Bronze, M.S. (1999) Isoniazid drug and food interactions. *Am J Med Sci* **317**, 304–11.

Sellers, E.M., Giles, H.G., Greenblatt, D.J. & Naranjo, C.A. (1980) Differential effects of benzodiazepine disposition by disulfiram and ethanol. *Arzneimittelforschung* **30**, 882–6.

Serfaty, M. & Masterton, G. (1993) Fatal poisonings attributed to benzodiazepines in Britain during the 1980s. *Br J Psychiatry* **163**, 386–93.

Seubert, C.N., Morey, T.E., Martynyuc, A.E., Cucchiara, R.F. & Dennis, D.M. (2000) Midazolam selectively potentiates the A$_{A2}$—but not A1—receptor-mediated effects of adenosine: role of nucleoside transport inhibition and clinical implications. *Anesthesiology* **92**, 567–77.

Shader, R.I. & Greenblatt, D.J. (1993) Use of benzodiazepines in anxiety disorders. *N Engl J Med* **328**, 1398–405.

Shader, R.I., Pary, R.J., Harmatz, J.S., Allison, S., Locniskar, A. & Greenblatt, D.J. (1984) Plasma concentrations and clinical effects after single oral doses of prazepam, clorazepate, and diazepam. *J Clin Psychiatry* **45**, 411–13.

Shen, W.W. (1997) The metabolism of psychoactive drugs: a review of enzymatic biotransformation and inhibition. *Biol Psychiatry* **41**, 814–26.

Shenfield, G.M. & Griffin, J.M. (1991) Clinical pharmacokinetics of contraceptive steroids. An update. *Clin Pharmacokinet* **20**, 15–37.

Sieghart, W., Fuchs, K., Tretter, V. *et al.* (1999) Structure and subunit composition of GABA_A receptors. *Neurochem In* **34**, 379–85.

Silverman, G. & Braithwaite, R.A. (1973) Benzodiazepines and tricyclic antidepressant plasma levels. *BMJ* **3**, 18–20.

Sonne, J., Dossing, M., Loft, S. *et al.* (1990) Single dose pharmacokinetics and pharmacodynamics of oral oxazepam during concomitant administration of propranolol and labetalol. *Br J Clin Pharmacol* **29**, 33–7.

du Souich, P., Verges, J. & Erill, S. (1993) Plasma protein binding and pharmacological response. *Clin Pharmacokinet* **24**, 435–40.

Spiegel, D.A. (1999) Psychological strategies for discontinuing benzodiazepine treatment. *J Clin Psychopharmacol* **19** (Suppl. 2), S17–22.

Spiegel, D.A. & Bruce, T.J. (1997) Benzodiazepines and exposure-based cognitive behavior therapies for panic disorder: conclusions from combined treatment trials. *Am J Psychiatry* **154**, 773–81.

Sproule, B.A., Naranjo, C.A., Brenmer, K.E. & Hassan, P.C. (1997) Selective serotonin reuptake inhibitors and CNS drug interactions. A critical review of the evidence. *Clin Pharmacokinet* **33**, 454–71.

Suerinck, A. & Suerinck, E. (1966) Etats depressifs en milieu sanatorial et inhibiteurs de la mono-amine oxydase. (Resultats therapeutiques par l'association d'iproclozide et de chlordiazepoxide.) A propos de 146 observations. *Journal de Medecine de Lyon* **47**, 573–9.

Sutherland, S.M., Tupler, L.A., Colket, J.T. & Davidson, J.R. (1996) A 2-year follow-up of social phobia. Status after a brief medication trial. *J Nerv Ment Dis* **184**, 731–8.

Taclob, L. & Needle, M. (1976) Drug-induced encephalopathy in patients on maintenance haemodialysis. *Lancet* **2**, 704–5.

Tanaka, E. (1999) Clinically significant pharmacokinetic drug interactions with benzodiazepines. *J Clin Pharm Ther* **24**, 347–55.

Task Force Report of the American Psychiatric Association (1990) *Benzodiazepine Dependence, Toxicity, and Abuse.* American Psychiatric Association, Washington, D.C.

Taylor, C.B. & Arnow, B.A. (1988) *The Nature and Treatment of Anxiety Disorders.* Free Press, New York.

Tesar, G.E., Rosenbaum, J.F., Pollack, M.H. *et al.* (1991) Double-blind, placebo-controlled comparison of clonazepam and alprazolam for panic disorder. *J Clin Psychiatry* **52**, 69–76.

Thomas, R.E. (1998) Benzodiazepine use and motor vehicle accidents. Systematic review of reported association. *Can Fam Physician* **44**, 799–808.

Tollefson, G., Lesar, T., Grothe, D. & Garvey, M. (1984) Alprazolam-related digoxin toxicity. *Am J Psychiatry* **141**, 1612–14.

Tverskoy, M., Fleyshman, G., Ezry, J., Bradley, E.L. & Kissin, I. (1989) Midazolam–morphine sedative interaction in patients. *Anesth Analg* **68**, 282–5.

Tyrer, P., Ferguson, B., Hallstrom, C. *et al.* (1996) A controlled trial of dothiepin and placebo in treating benzodiazepine withdrawal symptoms. *Br J Psychiatry* **168**, 457–61.

Vajda, F.J., Prineas, R.J. & Lovell, R.R. (1971) Interaction between phenytoin and the benzodiazepines. *BMJ* **1**, 346.

Valeyev, A.Y., Barker, J.L., Cruciani, R.A., Lange, G.D., Smallwood, V.V. & Mahan, L.C. (1993) Characterization of the γ-aminobutyric acid A receptor-channel complex composed of α1 β2 and α1 β3 subunits from rat brain. *J Pharmacol Exp Ther* **265**, 985–91.

van Balkom, A.J.L.M., Bakker, A., Spinhoven, P., Blaauw, B.M.J.W., Smeenk, S. & Ruesink, B. (1997) A meta-analysis of the treatment of panic disorder with or without agoraphobia: a comparison of psychopharmacological, cognitive-behavioral and combination treatments. *J Nerv Ment Dis* **185**, 510–16.

Venkatakrishnan, K., von Moltke, L.L. & Greenblatt, D.J. (2000) Effects of the antifungal agents on oxidative drug metabolism: clinical relevance. *Clin Pharmacokinet* **38**, 111–80.

Versiani, M., Nardi, A.E., Figueira, I., Mendlowicz, M. & Marques, C. (1997) Double-blind placebo controlled trial with bromazepam in social phobia. *Jornal Brasileiro de Psiquiatria* **46**, 167–71.

von Rosensteil, N.A. & Adam, D. (1995) Macrolide antibacterials. Drug interactions of clinical significance. *Drug Saf* **13**, 105–22.

Wang, P.S., Bohn, R.L., Glynn, R.J., Mogun, H. & Avorn, J. (2001) Hazardous benzodiazepine regimens in the elderly: effects of half-life, dosage and duration on risk of hip fracture. *Am J Psychiatry* **158**, 892–8.

Wardle, J. (1990) Behavior therapy and benzodiazepines: allies or antagonists? *Br J Psychiatry* **156**, 163–8.

Watson, W.A. (1979) Interaction between clonazepam and sodium valproate. *N Engl J Med* **300**, 678–9.

Wells, B.G., Evans, R.L., Ereshefsky, L. *et al.* (1988) Clinical outcome and adverse effect profile associated with concurrent administration of alprazolam and imipramine. *J Clin Psychiatry* **49**, 394–9.

Wijnands, W.J., Trooster, J.F., Teunissen, P.C., Cats, H.A. & Vree, T.B. (1990) Ciprofloxacin does not impair the elimination of diazepam in humans. *Drug Metab Dispos* **18**, 954–7.

Wilcox, C.S., Ryan, P.J., Morrissey, J.L. *et al.* (1994) A fixed-dose study of adinazolam-SR tablets in generalized anxiety disorder. *Prog Neuropsychopharmacol Biol Psychiatry* **18**, 979–93.

Wilhelm, F.H. & Roth, W.T. (1997) Acute and delayed effects of alprazolam on flight phobics during exposure. *Behav Res Ther* **35**, 831–41.

Williams, D.D.R. & McBride, A. (1998) Benzodiazepines: time for reassessment. *Br J Psychiatry* **173**, 361–2.

Witt, D.M., Ellsworth, A.J. & Leversee, J.H. (1993) Amiodarone–clonazepam interaction. *Ann Pharmacother* **27**, 1463–4.

Wodak, J., Gilligan, B.S., Veale, J.L. & Dowty, B.J. (1972) Review of 12 months' treatment with L-dopa in Parkinson's disease, with remarks on unusual side effects. *Med J Aust* **2**, 1277–82.

Woods, J.H., Katz, J.L. & Winger, G. (1995a) Abuse and therapeutic use of benzodiazepines and benzodiazepine-like drugs. In: *Psychopharmacology: the Fourth Generation of Progress* (F.E. Bloom & D.J. Kupfer (eds), pp. 1777–91). Raven Press, New York.

Woods, J.H. & Winger, G. (1995b) Current benzodiazepine issues. *Psychopharmacology (Berl)* **118**, 107–15.

Woods, S.W., Nagy, L.M., Kolesar, A.S., Krystal, J.H., Heninger, G.R. & Charney, D.S. (1992) Controlled trial of alprazolam supplementation during imipramine treatment of panic disorder. *J Clin Psychopharmacol* **12**, 32–8.

Zevin, S. & Benowitz, N.L. (1999) Drug interactions with tobacco smoking. An update. *Clin Pharmacokinet* **36**, 425–38.

Zhang, W., Koelher, K.F., Zhang, P. & Cook, J.M. (1995) Development of a comprehensive pharmacophore model for the benzodiazepine receptor. *Drug Des Discov* **12**, 193–248.

Zitman, F.G. & Couvee, J.E. (2001) Chronic benzodiazepine use in general practice patients with depression: an evaluation of controlled treatment and taper-off. *Br J Psychiatry* **178**, 317–24.

18

Selective Serotonin Reuptake Inhibitors in the Treatment of the Anxiety Disorders

J.C. Ballenger

Introduction

A review of the selective serotonin reuptake inhibitors (SSRIs) in the treatment of the anxiety disorders (ADs) is particularly appropriate at this point in time. Over the last several years the SSRIs have become the treatment of choice in each of the ADs, in the opinion of many experts (Ballenger *et al*. 1998a–c, 1999b, 2000, 2001). That one class of agents would become the preferred treatment across all five ADs is surprising, but it is a conclusion now supported by numerous rigorously designed and conducted double-blind trials of the SSRIs in all of these disorders. The evidence supportive of this conclusion will be reviewed in this chapter for each of the five ADs —obsessive-compulsive disorder, panic disorder, social anxiety disorder, generalized anxiety disorder, and post-traumatic stress disorder. The clear efficacy demonstrated for one or more of the SSRIs in all five ADs, and the increased tolerability of the SSRIs over previous treatments has led to the widespread conclusion of their being the first-line choice in all these disorders.

This chapter will review these studies, beginning with the historically first area of investigation—obsessive-compulsive disorder—and then panic disorder, social anxiety disorder, generalized anxiety disorder, and post-traumatic stress disorder. Attempts will be made to present most, if not all, of the trials of all five of the SSRIs (fluoxetine, paroxetine, sertraline, fluvoxamine, and citalopram) when data are available. Although this review will mostly be concerned with studies of efficacy, issues of dose, side-effects, clinical use, relapse, and length of treatment, comparisons between the SSRIs and previous medications, etc., will be included when there are empirically derived data leading to clinical suggestions.

Obsessive-compulsive disorder

The use of the SSRIs in obsessive-compulsive disorder (OCD) may be unique because it appears that only drugs which have potent serotonin-enhancing effects are effective in OCD. Although the tricyclic antidepressants (TCAs) and other nonspecific antidepressants are effective in depression and other anxiety syndromes, they are not effective in the treatment of OCD. This has included imipramine and nortriptyline (Volavka *et al*. 1985), and desipramine.

The first agent shown to be effective in OCD was clomipramine, which was observed in the 1960s (Fernandex & Lopez-Ibor 1967) and in large, well-controlled, placebo trials in the 1980s. Although technically a TCA, clomipramine's effects are primarily on serotonin with lesser effects on norepinephrine (noradrenaline), dopamine, acetylcholine (Hall & Ogren 1984). The earliest studies of clomipramine were small but consistently demonstrated efficacy which was later confirmed in larger trials (Thoren *et al*. 1980; Ananth *et al*. 1981; Insel *et al*. 1983).

In many ways, the large database with clomipramine sets the standard for a pharmacological treatment of OCD. In the large initial multicenter flexible-dose trials (Deveaugh-Geiss *et al*. 1989), the average dose was 249 mg/day, and most patients are treated within the range of 150–250 mg/day (Pigott *et al*. 1990). There were only 10–15% of patients who responded to placebo, with ~70% of clomipramine patients attaining at least some clinically significant improvement. However, most responders experienced a reduction in symptoms of only ~40% and complete resolution was rare (~10%) (Clomipramine Collaborative Study 1991).

Despite its efficacy, the principal issue with the use of clomipramine is its significant side-effects. The principal side-effects are of an anticholinergic nature and typically include dry mouth, blurred vision, but also sexual difficulties and seizures at higher doses (Deveaugh-Geiss *et al.* 1989).

Because clomipramine was the treatment of choice before the advent of the SSRIs, comparisons between the two will be made where available. In general, clomipramine and the SSRIs have comparable efficacy in most trials in the modern era, but it is the increased side-effects with clomipramine that significantly differentiate clomipramine from the SSRIs.

Fluoxetine

Fluoxetine was the first SSRI suggested to be effective in OCD in a number of open trials. In perhaps the first trial, Turner treated 10 OCD patients and reported that it was effective (Turner *et al.* 1985). This was followed by a trial in 1986 by Fontaine and colleagues in nine OCD patients. In a subsequent larger trial with 50 patients, fully 86% of these responded to fluoxetine, often at high doses (as high as 100 mg/day). Jenike reported a similar experience with over 250 patients treated with a mean dose of 75.1 ± 11.3 mg/day in an open trial (Jenike 1990). They were among the first to suggest that high doses would be necessary.

In the first long-term fluoxetine treatment of OCD, Levine *et al.* (1988) treated 75 OCD patients in an open setting over a 5-month period. At the end of the trial, all but two were receiving 80 mg/day. They observed significant reduction in OCD symptomatology after the first few weeks, and these substantial improvements continued over several months.

The first placebo controlled multicenter trial (Tollefson *et al.* 1994b) was a 13-week, fixed-dose (20, 40, or 60 mg/day) trial demonstrating that all three doses were significantly more effective than placebo. There was a trend suggesting greater efficacy at the highest dose (60 mg). The two American trials (Tollefson *et al.* 1994a) had a sample size of 355 and observed significant differences between fluoxetine and placebo from week 5 on. The European trial involved 217 patients and again compared 20, 40, and 60 mg to placebo (Montgomery *et al.* 1993). There were similar findings but less statistical significance, probably because of the smaller sample size and because the European trial was

8 weeks versus 13 weeks in the two American trials (Montgomery *et al.* 1993).

Paroxetine

The first results from paroxetine were from a fixed-dose study of 348 patients in a 12-week trial comparing placebo to 20, 40, or 60 mg/day of paroxetine (Wheadon *et al.* 1993). On the Yale–Brown Obsessive Compulsive Scale (Y-BOCS) and the National Institutes of Mental Health-Obsessive Compulsive (NIMH-OC) Scale a significant difference was observed between placebo, 20, 40 and 60 mg/day. Interestingly, more severely ill patients (Y-BOCS > 26) demonstrated greater response to 60 mg/day than 40 mg. This study would suggest that the target dose in OCD with paroxetine is 40 mg/day, although 60 mg/day may be necessary in the more severely ill patients.

In a second large study, paroxetine in flexible doses (10–60 mg/day) was compared to clomipramine (25–250 mg/day) and placebo. The mean dose for paroxetine in this trial was 37.5 mg/day and clomipramine 113.1 mg/day (Zohar & Judge 1996). This was a 12-week trial and involved 406 subjects, again using the Y-BOCS and NIMH-OC as primary outcome measures. Significant differences from placebo were observed at week 6, and paroxetine and clomipramine were both significantly better than placebo by week 12 on both the obsession and compulsion subscales of the Y-BOCS. Baseline scores on the Y-BOCS were in the moderate to severe range (25–27). A reduction of at least 25% in the Y-BOCS was observed in 55% in both the paroxetine and clomipramine groups. Not, surprisingly, paroxetine was significantly better tolerated than clomipramine with adverse effects in 16% of the paroxetine group and 28% of the clomipramine and leading to withdrawal in 9% of the paroxetine group and 17% with clomipramine.

The findings of Rosenberg *et al.* (1999) of an open-label study treatment of OCD in children is important because of the early onset of this disorder in many patients. They treated 20 patients, ages 8–17. Doses ranged from 10 to 60 mg/day with outcome as measured by the Children's Yale–Brown Obsessive Compulsive Scale (CY-BOCS), which decreased significantly from 30.6 ± 3.5 to 21.6 ± 3.8 ($P = 0.00005$). Side-effects included hyperactivity in three younger patients, which required dosage reduction, as well as insomnia, anxiety, and headache, but no patients were discontinued because of side-effects.

There are almost no reports of long-term treatment of OCD with SSRIs. However, there was an extension trial following one of the paroxetine studies providing some long-term safety, tolerability, and efficacy data (Dunbar *et al.* 1995). A total of 263 patients were treated with paroxetine (20–60 mg/day) in a 12-week open-label trial. Those who responded in the first phase were re-randomized in a double-blind fashion to either paroxetine or placebo to assess the prevention of relapse. This multicenter, 12-month extension study was divided into two 6-month phases. In the first 12 weeks, patients improved an average of 5.70 points from a mean baseline of 25.45 points on the Y-BOCS. In the remainder of the first 6 months, they improved an additional 5.11 points. After re-randomization, fewer patients in the paroxetine cell relapsed (59% vs. 38%) when compared to placebo (*P* = 0.05), reaching significance 2 weeks after randomization. There was a 2.7 times greater chance of relapse on placebo versus paroxetine. Also pertinent to note is that in this second 6 months, patients continued to improve on paroxetine. Paroxetine was well-tolerated even to 60 mg/day over the 1-year trial. Most common side-effects in the first 6 months were abnormal ejaculation (22.6%), somnolence (22.4%), and headache (19.8%). In the second 6 months in those patients continued on paroxetine, 9.7% had abnormal dreams and 6.7% increased appetite.

Fluvoxamine

Fluvoxamine was actually the earliest SSRI to be studied in OCD in the 1980s in small studies (Price *et al.* 1987; Goodman *et al.* 1989b). In these early trials, responses were seen in the first couple of weeks, but they became significant after 6–8 weeks (Price *et al.* 1987; Goodman *et al.* 1989b). In the Goodman trial, nine of 21 were rated as responders compared to no responders on placebo. Jenike and colleagues reported a 10-week trial with the maximum dose of 294 mg/day. Side-effects were generally mild and of the SSRI class (fatigue, insomnia, headache). Fluvoxamine was an effective treatment of OCD compared to placebo in this trial (Greist *et al.* 1995d; Goodman *et al.* 1996).

Recent multicenter, placebo-controlled trials of fluvoxamine have been completed. Two trials each including 160 patients studied fluvoxamine for 10 weeks, finding significant advantages over placebo from 6 weeks through the remainder of the trial. On the NIMH-OC Scale in one study and the Clinical Global Improvement

(CGI) Scale on the other, significant advantage over placebo was observed as early as 4 weeks at ~250 mg/day. Mean reductions in Y-BOCS were ~20% with 5% reductions in the placebo group. Most common side-effects were again the typical SSRI side-effects of nausea, asthenia, somnolence, insomnia, and sexual side-effects.

In a smaller trial comparing fluvoxamine to clomipramine in a double-blind, 10-week comparison, there was no significant difference in average reduction on the Y-BOCS. Reductions of 33% were seen in fluvoxamine and 31% in the clomipramine group, although some measures actually favored fluvoxamine (e.g. obsessive-free interval: Freeman *et al.* 1994).

Sertraline

In a small (*N* = 87) flexible-dose, 8-week trial, sertraline was studied in doses ranging 50–200 mg/day and a significant effect when compared to placebo was observed (*P* < 0.05: Chouinard *et al.* 1990). A larger flexible-dose trial (*N* = 167) of 12-week duration found similar efficacy (*P* < 0.05: Kronig *et al.* 1999). In a 12-week fixed-dose trial, approximately 80 patients each were compared on 50, 100, and 200 mg/day to placebo (Greist *et al.* 1995c). Efficacy was significantly greater in the 50 and 200 mg/day dose groups; however, this was marginal in the 100 mg/day group, where statistical significance was reached only on the NIMH-OC Scale. It is unclear whether the small but nonsignificant differences in 100 mg cell would have been positive had the study been larger. Side-effects were the expected diarrhea, insomnia, nausea, anorexia, sexual side-effects, tremor, and weight gain.

Citalopram

A 24-week open trial suggested that 20–60 mg/day of citalopram was effective in treating OCD with a 50% Y-BOCS reduction in 20 of 29 patients (Koponen 1997) and a recent double-blind, placebo-controlled trial has demonstrated its effectiveness in a controlled fashion. In a 12-week, fixed-dose study comparing 20, 40, and 60 mg/day, all three doses were found to be effective and equally tolerable (Montgomery 2000). There was a suggestion that the highest dose was associated with the earliest and most significant response. Mundo *et al.* (1997) have recently completed a small 10-week trial (*N* = 30) comparing citalopram to fluvoxamine and paroxetine in a single-blind trial. Doses were of fluvoxamine 290 ± 31 mg, paroxetine 53.3 ± 10 mg, and citalopram 50.9 ± 10.4 mg. All three drugs were effective with no discernable difference in this small trial with 40% of citalopram patients having a 35% Y-BOCS reduction.

In a small open trial in children and adolescents, 18 of 23 experienced a moderate or marked response, usually at 50 mg/day (Thomsen 1997).

SSRIs compared to clomipramine

The question of whether SSRIs are comparable in terms of efficacy with the well-established clomipramine is a critical question given their increased tolerability and clear efficacy. The issue of the relative efficacy between the two has been the object of considerable research and analysis. Two of the meta-analyses (Greist *et al.* 1995b; Stein *et al.* 1995) suggest that there were greater effects seen with clomipramine than with the SSRIs. However, subsequent analyses (Cox & Swinson 1993; Piccanelli *et al.* 1995) fail to find such a difference. Also, there are considerable methodological problems with relying on these studies which span a large number of studies that were different in design and quality and, in particular, which stretch over an extended period of time. The early trials of clomipramine had low placebo responses rates and seem to be treating a different patient population than current trials, which appear to involve patients with a more intermittent and perhaps milder disorder. Certainly a more reliable method is a direct head-to-head comparison between clomipramine and the SSRIs, and there are several recent ones. There have now been comparison studies with fluoxetine (two), fluvoxamine (five), paroxetine (one), sertraline (one), and citalopram (one). There were almost no differences comparing these SSRIs to clomipramine, although in the sertraline trial (Biserbe *et al.* 1997) sertraline was observed to be better than clomipramine. In the paroxetine trial, paroxetine was significantly better than clomipramine in treating comorbid depression (Zohar & Judge 1996).

Another measure of comparability is the "cross-over response." Piggott *et al.* (1990) utilized a sequential treatment design and found that 65% of patients who had responded to clomipramine, subsequently also responded to fluoxetine. Conversely, if a patient had responded to fluoxetine, 80% of these patients also subsequently responded to clomipramine; however, if

a patient failed to respond to clomipramine, only 20% ultimately responded to fluoxetine.

Predictors of response

Other research suggests that patients with schizotypal personalities respond less well to pharmacotherapy (Baer & Jenike 1992), and subsequent studies find essentially the same thing with comorbid social anxiety disorder (Carrasco *et al.* 1992). Probably the most well-documented and accepted predictor is the negative predictor of a concomitant tic disorder (Baer 1994; McDougle *et al.* 1994). The presence of a tic also predicts a better response to SSRIs combined with neuroleptics (McDougle 1994).

However, there appears to be no relationship between OCD symptoms or symptom types and response to treatment (Baer 1994).

Dose of SSRI

For some time the clinical opinion has been that higher doses of SSRIs are needed to treat OCD than to treat depression or the other ADs. These clinical opinions have found empirical support in recent large fixed-dose studies. This was clear in the large fluoxetine trials in which 40 and 60 mg were effective, whereas 20 mg failed to be more effective than placebo (Montgomery *et al.* 1993). This was again seen in the paroxetine trials (Wheadon *et al.* 1993) in that 40 and 60 mg were effective, whereas 20 mg was not. As mentioned, the higher doses were also more efficacious in the more severely ill.

Augmentation strategies

A series of medications have been suggested and studied, primarily in open trials, to try to augment the frequently limited clinical response to antidepressants. These have included lithium, clonazepam, buspirone, haloperidol, trazodone, methylphenidate, and others (Jenike 1988, 1990a). Most have been disappointing, with some suggestion that clonazepam (Jenike 1998) might be effective, and also pimozide (Goodman *et al.* 1989a) in patients with a concomitant tic disorder.

Side-effects

The principal advantage of the SSRIs in the treatment of OCD has been the increased tolerability because of fewer side-effects than with clomipramine. Since most patients need to be treated for longer periods of time, tolerability can be a major issue. For instance, in a comparison trial of clomipramine versus sertraline (Biserbe *et al.* 1997) there was significantly more withdrawal from clomipramine (26%) than sertraline (11%).

This is certainly also true in terms of more serious side-effects. Overdose from SSRIs have generally been benign, but "5-days" dosage of clomipramine is potentially fatal, frequently from cardiotoxicity. Although rare, convulsions are significantly higher with clomipramine (1.5–2.0%) compared to SSRIs (0.1–0.5%).

Length of treatment

Clinical experience in open trials suggests that patients with OCD continue to improve for quite some time, certainly the first several months. As previously mentioned, Zohar and Judge (1996) reported that patients continued to improve for the first 6 months of treatment and further still in the second 6 months of treatment, providing the best evidence of a long-term response. It was also observed in 118 patients treated with sertraline (Greist *et al.* 1995a) that not only was the initial 12-week response maintained, further small gains occurred over the follow-up period. In one smaller study, patients continued to respond and improve on sertraline for a 2nd year as well (Rasmussen *et al.* 1997).

Relapse

It appears clear that most OCD patients will maintain their improvement and perhaps improve as long as they continue SSRI treatment. However, there are two placebo-controlled trials that document a high relapse rate if clomipramine is discontinued (Pato *et al.* 1988; Leonard *et al.* 1991). Most patients relapsed within the first 2 months (Steiner *et al.* 1995).

Therefore, it seems clear that most patients who maintain their SSRI treatment of OCD will maintain their clinical response and most will lose that response if medication is discontinued. However, most patients do subsequently regain their clinical response if restarted on medication.

It is of interest that contrary to the treatment of depression, doses needed for improvement may be safely reduced during the maintenance phase (Pato *et al.* 1990).

Panic disorder

Like OCD, the treatment of panic disorder (PD) with antidepressants began in the 1960s with the TCA imipramine and monoamine oxidase inhibitor (MAOI) phenelzine. Both were demonstrated to be effective treatments (Sheehan *et al.* 1980). In the late 1980s the high-potency benzodiazepines (BZs), particularly alprazolam and clonazepam, were shown to be also effective (Ballenger *et al.* 1988), although their beneficial effects were much more rapid, occurring in the 1st week or two.

However, the use of clomipramine and fluvoxamine in Europe, and then paroxetine and fluoxetine in the US, documented that the SSRIs were equally effective and better tolerated than available TCAs or BZs (Boyer 1995). In fact, in 1995 the NIMH in the US convened an expert panel that concluded that SSRIs should be the treatment of first choice in the pharmacological treatment of PD (Jobson & Potter 1995). This was at a time when there were, in fact, few trials published with SSRIs; however, since that time, multiple trials have been published which will be outlined below. Subsequent expert panels convened by the American Psychiatric Association (APA) and the International Consensus Group for Anxiety and Depression (Ballenger *et al.* 1998b) have reached the same conclusion.

Although the study of PD has focused on the alleviation of the prominent panic attacks, the studies reviewed below will refer to efficacy of SSRIs and their ability to treat the entire PD syndrome. This includes reducing panic attacks but also anticipatory anxiety, avoidance behavior, depression, and improving function. Although the reduction in panic attacks and the percentage of patients free of panic attacks will be reported, the better, more recent multidomain outcome measures will be reported when available (Shear *et al.* 1994).

Clomipramine

As is the case in OCD, clomipramine's experience needs to be reviewed because of its similarly prominent place in the evolution in the psychopharmacology of PD. Clomipramine was one of the first serotonergic agents studied in Europe, where it became the treatment of choice.

The first studies (Gloger *et al.* 1981) suggested that 75% of patients benefited from treatment. The first large scientifically rigorous trial was performed by Johnston and colleagues with a sample of 108 women studied in an 8-week, placebo-controlled, double-blind trial (Johnston *et al.* 1988). This trial provided the first definitive evidence of clomipramine's effectiveness against the full range of panic symptoms.

Several further trials documented impressive results with clomipramine. Fahy and colleagues (1992) studied 79 patients comparing clomipramine to lofepramine and placebo, finding that 93% of the clomipramine patients were panic-free at 24 weeks. In a small trial ($N = 18$), Hoffart and colleagues (1993) demonstrated that 17 of 18 previous nonresponders had a significant reduction in symptoms in a 12-week, placebo-controlled, double-blind study.

Two studies led to the acceptance of clomipramine as the treatment of choice in Europe. Cassano and colleagues compared clomipramine to what was thought to be the best treatment for PD at that time, imipramine (Cassano *et al.* 1988). Although both medications were effective, clomipramine was actually more effective on several outcome measures and had a more rapid onset of action in the 2nd week. Modigh and colleagues also compared imipramine to clomipramine in a 12-week trial (Modigh *et al.* 1992). Clomipramine led to greater improvement on almost all of the principal outcome measures. Again, improvement on clomipramine was noted significantly earlier (week 4 vs. week 8) than with imipramine. This was replicated more recently in an 8-week trial comparing low dose (50 mg/day) clomipramine to imipramine (114 mg/day) (Gentil *et al.* 1993).

Comparisons to the SSRIs and clomipramine will be included in the review of each SSRI when available. However, in almost every trial the SSRI and clomipramine have been observed to have comparable positive effects, but the SSRI is better tolerated, leading to fewer dropouts.

Fluvoxamine

Clinical use of fluvoxamine in PD in Europe has a long history, but controlled trials began to appear in the late 1980s and early 1990s. In a 6-week trial ($N = 58$), den Boer and colleagues compared clomipramine and fluvoxamine (den Boer *et al.* 1987). The two drugs appeared relatively equal in efficacy, with two-thirds of the patient groups having an excellent response. In a larger trial of 188 patients, Asnis (1992) also reported

significant effects of fluvoxamine over placebo with a 64% versus 42% responding ($P < 0.002$) with an early onset (end of week 1) on some measures. Hoehn-Saric and colleagues demonstrated the effectiveness of fluvoxamine in 50 panic patients with a mean dose of 206.8 mg/day, again with two-thirds of patients becoming panic-free versus 22% on placebo (Hoehn-Saric *et al.* 1993).

In larger ($N = 117$) 8-week multicenter trials, Hoehn-Saric *et al.* (1994) again reported excellent results against the symptoms of PD. Similarly, Woods *et al.* (1994) in a study of 189 PD patients again found almost two-thirds (64%) of fluvoxamine patients became panic-free versus 40% of placebo patients, again with improvement beginning in the 1st or 2nd week. In the only negative trial, Nair and colleagues compared fluvoxamine, imipramine, and placebo in 148 patients (Nair *et al.* 1996). There was a very high dropout in the fluvoxamine cell (62%), probably explaining the failure to observe a positive response.

In a recent multicenter, 12-week trial involving 229 patients, Dewolf *et al.* (1995) demonstrated clear effectiveness of fluvoxamine in outpatients.

In one of the earliest long-term trials of an SSRI in panic, Holland *et al.* (1994) demonstrated that fluvoxamine's initial gains were maintained for a full year. Fluvoxamine was well-tolerated, and improvement was excellent in over 80% of the patients.

Fluvoxamine has been compared to cognitive-behavioral therapy in several studies. Black and colleagues (1993) studied 55 patients in an 8-week trial with a mean dose of 230 mg/day of fluvoxamine. In this particular trial, fluvoxamine was shown to be superior to both cognitive-behavioral therapy and placebo. There was a very high response (90%) of moderate or marked improvement versus only 50% with cognitive therapy and 39% with placebo. Sharpe and colleagues (1996) followed up this trial in 190 patients but found fluvoxamine and cognitive-behavioral therapy to be comparable. However, doses of fluvoxamine were only 150 mg in this trial. In another trial (de Beurs *et al.* 1995) fluvoxamine's efficacy was doubled by an effective psychotherapy.

As mentioned, trials have begun to compare these agents to each other and to clomipramine. J. den Boer and colleagues have compared fluvoxamine to clomipramine (den Boer *et al.* 1987) and essentially reported equal efficacy with both medications, with two-thirds of patients having excellent responses. There was some evidence that clomipramine's onset of action was earlier than fluvoxamine, but there were higher doses utilized for clomipramine (150 mg/day vs. 100 mg/day of fluvoxamine). Fluvoxamine was compared to the reversible MAOI brofaromine by van Vliet (1996), who demonstrated comparable efficacy.

Citalopram

Citalopram has been utilized in Europe for quite some time, although introduced to the US only relatively recently. There have been relatively few studies in PD. In the first publication of an open trial, Humble and colleagues reported results with 20 PD patients (Humble et al. 1989). Thirteen of 17 patients experienced significant symptomatic relief with doses averaging 40 mg/day. These patients were subsequently followed in a 15-month maintenance trial (Humble & Wistedt 1992). During this time they maintained their initial response and extended it in certain areas.

In the first, and to-date only, multicenter, well-controlled trial, Wade et al. (1997) compared clomipramine to citalopram in 479 PD patients. They were studied in an 8-week, double-blind, placebo-controlled trial and then followed for a year. Although citalopram was clearly effective, its positive effects were not observed until week 12. The follow-up trial was for a year and 279 of the initial patients participated in this long-term trial (Lepola et al. 1998). Over the 12-month period, patients in the citalopram and clomipramine groups both maintained their responses and generally gradually improved. At the end of 12 months, patients in the 20–30 mg citalopram group had the greatest response, closely followed by the 40–60 mg range. Almost all patients remaining in the trial at 1 year were free of panic attacks.

Fluoxetine

Although fluoxetine was the first true SSRI released in the US, its use in PD was limited to clinical situations and open trials until recently. The first report was by Gorman et al. (1987) with 16 patients in an open trial. It was observed that most patients had a positive response beginning around week 6, and they labeled 7 of 16 subjects responders. However, half of the patients dropped out of the trial because of side-effects, principally the hyperactivity–jitteriness syndrome. This group subsequently studied 25 patients beginning

with only 5 mg/day of fluoxetine (vs. 10 mg) and gradually increasing the dose as tolerated. In this group, 76% of the patients had a moderate or better response and marked reduction in the initial hyperactivity side-effects with only 16% dropping out (Schneier et al. 1991). Pecknold reported results in an 8-week open trial in 28 patients with 33% of patients being panic-free by the end of week 3, and half by week 8 with a mean dose of 20 mg/day. Again in an open trial, Copland reported 10 of 12 panic patients having at least moderate improvement.

In the first large, multicenter, fixed-dose (10 mg and 20 mg), placebo-controlled trial, Michelson et al. (1998) reported positive results for 20 mg of fluoxetine, but not 10 mg or placebo, in overall responses to treatment. Panic attack reductions were more complex, with significant reductions with 10 mg but not 20 mg in the intent-to-treat sample but significant differences in the completer analysis for both doses. This trial is a good example of the limited value of using panic attacks as an outcome measure. In fact, there were no differences between either dose of fluoxetine and placebo on the number of patients who were completely panic-free. On the other hand, improvements in anxiety, avoidance, functional impairment, and in the CGI Scale scores did show efficacy for fluoxetine over placebo. Although it is possible that these results suggest a lower potency for fluoxetine in treating PD, it is more likely that this trial represents the vagaries of utilizing simple panic attack outcome measures.

Eighty-eight patients who responded to fluoxetine and 32 placebo responders from the initial treatment trial were randomized to fluoxetine and placebo in a continuation trial and demonstrated continued improvement (Michelson et al. 1999).

In a large (N = 366) international, multicenter trial comparison with moclobemide, both drugs were about equally effective with 70% being panic free on fluoxetine at week 8 (Tiller et al. 1999). In a year extension, almost all patients were much or very much improved on the CGI Scale.

Paroxetine

The first publications of well-controlled placebo trials with a true SSRI other than fluvoxamine were studies published in Europe by Oehrberg et al. (1995) and in the US by Ballenger et al. (1998c). The study of paroxetine's effects in PD is the most extensive of all the SSRIs.

The Oehrberg study was a large ($N = 120$) trial performed in seven Danish centers. All patients received cognitive-behavioral therapy and either 40 or 60 mg of paroxetine or placebo. Paroxetine was demonstrated to be effective by week 6 across the parameters measuring panic attacks, as well as other measures (e.g. anxiety, global response and dysfunction). Significant responses were observed at weeks 3 and 6 and for the remainder of the trial.

In a large 12-week multicenter trial ($N = 367$), LeCrubier and colleagues (1997a) reported a comparison of paroxetine, clomipramine, and placebo. By week 12, 50.9% of paroxetine patients versus 36.7% of clomipramine and 31.6% of placebo patients were free of panic attacks. The number of panic attacks in the paroxetine group fell from 21.2/week to 5.2/week versus 26.4/week to 16.6/week on placebo. The majority of these patients (80%) had agoraphobia and there was significant improvement for both paroxetine and clomipramine in agoraphobia, anxiety, and functional disability (work, social and family). The effects of both clomipramine and paroxetine were comparable, although in this trial paroxetine's effects were observed earlier, and it was clearly better tolerated than clomipramine.

This same large multicenter trial followed 176 patients for 1 year in 32 centers in 11 European countries. Of the original sample, 116 (66%) completed the study and 60 patients (34%) withdrew. The largest percentage of patients withdrew from the placebo-treated cell (42%), then clomipramine (35%), and then paroxetine (25%). The percentage of patients withdrawing because of side-effects was the highest in the clomipramine group (19%), with the paroxetine group (7.4%) not significantly different from the placebo group (6.7%). Although side-effects tended to improve in both active agents, there was a higher percentage of patients with sweating and dry mouth on clomipramine than paroxetine.

The patients continued to improve throughout the long-term trial with almost 85% of the paroxetine group being panic free versus 72.4% of clomipramine and 59% of placebo patients at the end of the long-term extension. Secondary measures of anxiety and agoraphobia also continued to improve over that time period. The Sheehan Disability Scale (SDS) demonstrated continued improvement with paroxetine and clomipramine over the entire follow-up period. This study provides perhaps the best evidence of continued long-term improvement in PD over at least the 1st year of treatment.

The first controlled trial of an SSRI published in the US was of a double-blind, fixed-dose, placebo-controlled trial carried out in 20 centers in the US and Canada (Ballenger et al. 1998c). Ballenger and colleagues studied 278 patients over a 10-week trial comparing placebo to paroxetine doses of 10, 20, or 40 mg/day. This trial documented that 40 mg (but not 20 or 10 mg) of paroxetine was significantly better than placebo or most outcome measures, including panic attacks, and global severity. At week 1, patients free of panic attacks on 40 mg (86%) were significantly greater than those at 20 mg (65.2%), 10 mg (67.4%), and placebo (50.0%). CGI Scale scores also favored 40 mg of paroxetine. Avoidance declined, although not significantly, while agoraphobic fears were significantly lower, again favoring the 40 mg dose of paroxetine. The significant improvements in anxiety and depression ratings also favored the 40 mg dose, definitively illustrating that the target dose for paroxetine in PD is 40 mg.

In the first trial in panic disorder in Japan, a carefully performed placebo controlled trial reported that 82% on paroxetine had a moderate or better improvement versus 43.5% on placebo ($P < 0.0001$) (Kamijim, presented at Panic Meeting, Tokyo, 2/4/01).

In an unpublished study, Ballenger and colleagues (Ballenger et al. 2001) followed 138 responders from the dose–response study described above in a 6-month extension trial. After 3-months treatment on current medication, responders were re-randomized in a double-blind fashion to either same-dose paroxetine or placebo. In patients crossing from paroxetine to placebo, 30% (11/37) relapsed while only 5% (2/43) of patients continuing on paroxetine relapsed ($P = 0.002$). The relapse rate seen in the group switching from paroxetine 40 mg/day to placebo was highest, with 54% meeting criteria versus 17% relapsing from the lower dosage groups (10 and 20 mg/day). Relapse was generally within 14 days crossing over to placebo and in the two patients remaining on paroxetine it was at 14 and 28 days. Given the abrupt medication withdrawal in this trial, it was difficult to distinguish early relapse and withdrawal symptoms in some patients; however, that there is a higher relapse rate coming off paroxetine after 6 months of treatment is quite clear.

Sertraline

Experience with sertraline is relatively recent and consists of two large, flexible-dose, multicenter trials (Londberg *et al.* 1998; Pohl *et al.* 1998; Pollack *et al.* 1998). In the trial reported by Pohl *et al.* (1998), a sample of 168 patients were studied for 10 weeks. The drop in panic attacks (77%) on sertraline was significantly greater than placebo (51%) and significantly more patients (62%) were panic free (46% placebo). Reductions in time spent worrying, the Multicenter Panic Anxiety Scale, and the Hamilton Anxiety Rating Scale (HAM-A) failed to reach statistical significance, but improvements on the CGI and Quality of Life Scales did. Two almost identical trials with a total of 352 patients from 20 US and Canadian centers were reported by Londberg *et al.* (1998) and Pollack (1998). Patients were treated with flexible dosing to 200 mg/day. Panic attacks were reduced significantly more in the sertraline group beginning at week 2. Sertraline patients also had a significant reduction in global CGI Scale scores by week 4.

In the trial reported by Pollack (1998), reduction in panic attacks were significantly greater by week 2 (*P* = 0.04), and in CGI Scale scores by week 4, although endpoint differences in panic-free status was not significantly different (57% sertraline, 47% placebo). However, there were highly significant differences in high end state functioning with 35% of the sertraline patients meeting criteria versus 17% of placebo (*P* = 0.03), and this is certainly a better outcome measure than panic-free status.

There were also significant advantages for sertraline on the CGI Scale, global evaluation ratings, and the multidomain Panic Disorder Severity Scale (PDSS) (*P* = 0.03), perhaps the best available outcome measure in PD. This study also provided for the first time outcome measures of quality of life which highly favored sertraline (*P* = 0.003). There were improvements in mood, work, and family, as well as leisure activities. Sertraline patients also had significantly higher scores on measures of satisfaction with life and the medication.

In the fixed-dose study reported by Lundberg (1998), patients experienced a 65% decrease in the number of panic attacks (39% placebo). There were significant reductions in other measures and also in anticipatory anxiety measured by the HAM-A. There were no differences between the doses (50, 100, 200 mg/day).

Sertraline was well tolerated in these trials with an 8.3% discontinuation rate for adverse events (versus 2.3% placebo). Principal side-effects were nausea, dry mouth, diarrhea and ejaculation failure. There was very little hyperactivity or jitteriness at the beginning with only a 6% dropout rate in the 1st week, perhaps because of the low starting dose (25 mg/day). Although the higher rate for discontinuation very early in treatment for sertraline (10.5% vs. 0% for placebo) does suggest that even lower initial doses might be helpful.

Recommended doses

Probably the only definitive target dose supported by empirical data is with paroxetine. In one trial, 40 mg was clearly significantly better than both placebo and 10 and 20 mg doses (Ballenger 1998c). Although some patients respond to lower doses and some patients might require higher doses, the average patient should be increased to 40 mg if tolerated.

Some early studies suggested that clomipramine might be effective as low as 25 mg/day (Gloger *et al.* 1981, 1989), and this was recently confirmed in a large (*N* = 180) double-blind placebo-controlled trial (Caillard *et al.* 1999) finding that 60 mg was as effective as 150 mg/day and better tolerated. However most recent studies have treated patients between 150 and 250 mg/day.

The sertraline studies found it to be effective in the range of 50–200 mg/day in flexible-dose trials (Pollack 1998), and the fixed-dose trial found no difference in efficacy in the 50, 100, and 200 mg groups. Therefore, no definitive statement can be made about a target dose and most experts recommend that patients be treated between 100 and 150 mg/day.

In the citalopram studies comparing 20–30 mg and 60–90 mg, both ranges were better than placebo in the reduction of panic symptomatology. However, the 20–30 mg range appeared to be more effective than the higher dose (Lepola 1998). Although the results with 10 mg of fluoxetine were significant, results with 20 mg were across a broader range of outcome measures and suggest 20 mg should be the target dose for fluoxetine in PD (Michelson *et al.* 1998). Although clinical use has suggested that some patients will respond better at higher doses, this has not been formally studied. Interestingly, one recent trial reported that stabilized patients could maintain their initial improvement with once a week dosing, presumably because of the 4–5 week half-life of fluoxetine (Emmanuel *et al.* 1999).

Probably the most important issue with dosing is the clear experience that panic patients should begin treatment with as low a dose as possible. This is perhaps particularly true with fluoxetine which clinical experience would suggest is best started with a dosage range of 2.5–5.0 mg/day with slow increases. Roy-Byrne and Wingerson (1992) reported that actually beginning with 2 mg/day of fluoxetine enabled a group of patients who had previously been unable to successfully begin treatment with fluoxetine to do so. Routine practice is to begin paroxetine at 10 mg, and fluvoxamine and sertraline at no more than 25 mg/day and lower if possible.

Comparison between the SSRIs in panic disorder

Not surprisingly, there are relatively few studies comparing the SSRIs in the treatment of PD. As previously described, paroxetine and clomipramine have been directly compared in short-term and long-term treatment (LeCrubier *et al.* 1997a,b). In that trial, efficacy was largely comparable, although on some measures paroxetine's effects appeared to be more rapid and there were greater reductions in secondary symptoms of anxiety, disability and depression. The principal difference between the two was the better tolerability of paroxetine.

Also as mentioned, den Boer and colleagues have compared fluvoxamine to clomipramine, again finding them to be roughly comparable with some suggestion that clomipramine was more effective in reducing anxiety and depression (den Boer 1987). In a comparison between citalopram and clomipramine, both drugs were effective with little differences (Wade 1997).

Generalized anxiety disorder

Controlled trials of antidepressants in generalized anxiety disorder (GAD) are much more limited and quite recent. The only SSRI studied in placebo-controlled trials or even open trials has been paroxetine. However, the SNRI venlafaxine, has been studied in a series of short-term studies, and in one 6-month study and has been demonstrated to be effective (Davidson *et al.* 1999; Gelenberg *et al.* 2000; Hackett *et al.* 2000).

Paroxetine

The first formal study of an SSRI (paroxetine) was a comparison with imipramine and a BZ (2′-chlor-

desmethyldiazepam) in an 8-week trial (Rocca *et al.* 1997). This trial involved 81 patients and compared 20 mg of paroxetine to 50–100 mg of imipramine and 3–6 mg/day of 2′-chlordesmethyldiazepam. Overall paroxetine was more effective than the BZ and approximately equal to imipramine, although efficacy of paroxetine over 2′-chlordesmethyl diazepam was apparent from week 4, whereas imipramine's superiority was only from week 8. The improvement in the HAM-A score for paroxetine of 15.6 versus 11.8 for 2′-chlordesmethyl diazepam was significant ($P > 0.01$) at week 4, while the improvement of imipramine (13.9) was significant at week 8 ($P > 0.05$). As seen in previous studies, both antidepressants tended to improve the psychological symptoms whereas the BZ led to greater improvements in physical symptoms. Generally, differences in side-effects were as expected with greater anticholinergic side-effects in the imipramine group (dry mouth 56% vs. 8% paroxetine, and constipation 39% vs. 8% paroxetine), more than with the BZ (10% and 5%, respectively). Drowsiness was also more common with BZs and nausea more common with paroxetine. Dropout was lowest with paroxetine (17% vs. 20% BZ and 31% imipramine).

A large, multicenter, fixed-dose, placebo-controlled trial compared efficacy of 20 and 40 mg of paroxetine versus placebo over an 8-week period in 566 patients (Bellew *et al.* 2000a). The primary efficacy outcome measure was the HAM-A with the secondary outcome measure the CGI Scale. Both doses of paroxetine led to significant reductions in the HAM-A total score versus placebo ($P > 0.001$). There were also significant differences between the doses of paroxetine versus placebo in the percentage of CGI Scale responders (1 or 2) with 62% of the 20 mg and 68% of the 40 mg paroxetine versus 46% of placebo patients having a 1 or 2 on the CGI Scale ($P > 0.001$) (Bellew 2000a). In this fixed-dose trial, quality of life questionnaires (EuroQol-5D) and visual analogue scales demonstrated a significant change on both measures in the paroxetine treatment groups demonstrating a significant improvement in quality of life even over this 8-week trial (Bellew *et al.* 2000b). Although there was no significant difference between response in the 20 and 40 mg groups in the HAM-A, more patients were rated as responders at 40 mg than at 20 mg, suggestive of a difference. Significant effects for both doses of paroxetine were seen in the first two items of the HAM-A (anxiety and tension items), as well as the psychic and somatic anxiety subscales. The SDS functional disability scores were significantly reduced in both dosage groups.

There was also a significant improvement over placebo in disability in the paroxetine patients. Changes on the SDS from baseline to week 8 were reductions of 6.1 for 20 mg paroxetine, 6.6 for 40 mg. and 3.0 for placebo, significant differences for both doses ($P > 0.001$).

There were also two large, multicenter, double-blind, placebo-controlled 8-week flexible-dose trials reported by Pollack and colleagues (2001) in the US and by McCafferty and colleagues (2000) in Europe. These two studies utilized flexible dosing after an initial dose of 10 mg/day and increases to 20–50 mg/day. A total of 324 patients were treated in the two studies. Significant reductions in these flexible-dose trials were observed in eight of 10 efficacy measures including the HAM-A total, the anxiety and tension items (items 1 and 2), the psychic anxiety item, the CGI Scale, and the SDS. Interestingly, the Somatic Anxiety Scale was reduced but only at a trend level.

On the HAM-A item 1 (anxiety and worry), which is perhaps the item most representative of core GAD symptomatology, the paroxetine group had significantly greater improvement compared to placebo, beginning at week 1 and lasting throughout the trial. On what many consider to be the other characteristic item, the HAM-A item 2 (tension), significant differences for paroxetine began in week 3 and were present at week 8. Significantly more paroxetine patients ($P < 0.007$) had a CGI Scale improvement score of 1 (very much improved) or 2 (much improved) (62% vs. 47% with placebo). Similarly, if responders were defined as a HAM-A total score of <10, significantly more patients in the paroxetine (55%) were responders than placebo (37%). Paroxetine was well-tolerated over the dose range of 20–50 mg/day.

In a similarly designed, multicenter, double-blind, placebo flexible-dose trial, Baldwin (Baldwin *et al.* 1999; Baldwin 2000b) studied 372 patients with either paroxetine or placebo. Results were very similar to previous trials in that the paroxetine group showed significant improvements in the HAM-A total score compared to placebo ($P > 0.05$). Again, there was a higher proportion of paroxetine patients considered to be responders on the CGI Scale (73% vs. 55%).

In a recent trial by Stocchi and colleagues (2001), a large sample of 652 GAD patients were treated with paroxetine (20–50 mg/day) for 8 weeks. Responders were defined as those whose CGI Scale severity of illness score decreased by at least 2 points (and ≤ 3). Responders were randomized to double-blind treatment with either the same dose of paroxetine ($N = 278$) or placebo ($N = 288$), and they were treated for an additional 6 months. The primary outcome measure of this study was the number of patients relapsing during double-blind therapy. There was a significant difference between paroxetine and placebo with only 10.9% of patients continued on paroxetine relapsing, versus 39.9% on placebo ($P > 0.001$). There was also a significant difference in favor of paroxetine in time to relapse as well. Secondary measures of efficacy also significantly favored paroxetine. This study demonstrated an almost five-fold increase in relapse if paroxetine is not continued after the initial acute trial (8 weeks).

This is the only longer term treatment trial of GAD with an SSRI and it clearly showed significant continued improvement over the 6-month extension in the cell treated with paroxetine. Remission was defined by reduction of the HAM-A to = 7 (Ballenger 1999a). At the end of the initial single blind phase, 42.5% of patients had achieved remission. At the end of the double-blind continuation, fully 72% were in remission, compared to 34% on placebo ($P > 0.001$).

Equally important, the number of patients converting from either nonresponders or partial responders to full remission almost doubled over a 6-month period. These data suggest a significant difference in the way of treating GAD. It would appear that patients with a partial response should be continued on paroxetine with the expectation that many partial responders would convert to complete responders over the additional 6 months of treatment. A similar result has been found in the venlafaxine trials and suggests that treatment of GAD with antidepressants should be at least 6–8 months and probably at least a year or more at least if some initial response is observed.

Dose

As mentioned, the trials with paroxetine found no significant difference between 20 and 40 mg in the fixed-dose trials. However there was a suggestion that there was a higher percentage of responders with the 40 mg/day group. At this point, most clinicians would begin treatment with paroxetine at 10 or 20 mg and increase to at least to 20 mg. If there is a poor response, then treatment to 40 mg would be recommended.

Length of treatment

As mentioned, the only long-term data suggest that response continues to improve over at least 8 months of treatment. This led to recent recommendations that treatment, if successful, should continue for at least a year before consideration of tapering and discontinuation (Ballenger 2001).

Other effects

In a fascinating, uncontrolled study with 29 GAD patients, treatment with paroxetine for 4–6 months was associated with significant improvement in problematic personality traits (Allgulander et al. 1998). Improvements on the Temperament and Character Inventory (Cloninger et al. 1994) included a decrease in harm avoidance ($P = 0.0001$) and novelty seeking ($P = 0.006$), as well as a positive increase in self-directedness ($P = 0.0004$). This is an interesting result extending the medication response beyond symptom reduction and bears further study.

Post-traumatic stress disorder

Although post-traumatic stress disorder (PTSD) has been a recognized condition and diagnosis for over 20 years, there are relatively few trials of modern medications in this disorder. In fact, the earliest reports of open trials with SSRIs in this condition are <10 years old, and the double-blind controlled trials have been completed only in the last few years and will be reviewed below.

Fluvoxamine

As SSRIs began to be utilized in PTSD, among the first reports was a report by den Boer et al. (1991). J. den Boer and colleagues studied 24 World War II resistance fighters given 300 mg/day for 12 weeks. Eleven subjects (46%) completed the trial, while nine discontinued because of gastrointestinal side-effects, sleep problems, and unspecified physical complaints. There were statistically significant improvements on a PTSD Scale they developed for this trial and other, more standard measures. Five of the study patients asked to continue on fluvoxamine at the end of the trial. It is unclear what the appropriate interpretation of this study is; whether there is low response to fluvoxamine in PTSD, or poor tolerance to the drug.

In another open trial, Marmar et al. (1996) observed improvement in 11 combat veterans with chronic PTSD. Only one subject dropped out and, in general, side-effects were mild and of the type expected for an SSRI (headache, nausea, insomnia, sedation). In this trial fluvoxamine was associated with significant improvement on the hyperarousal, avoidance, and intrusion symptom clusters on both patient- and clinician-rated scales. Additional secondary positive effects were seen in anxiety, hostility, depression, and the global SCL-90.

There are no as-yet double-blind placebo-controlled trials with fluvoxamine.

Fluoxetine

McDougle et al. (1991) treated 20 Vietnam veterans with doses of fluoxetine ranging from 20 to 40 mg in a long trial (mean 26 weeks). Twenty of the 23 patients completed at least 4 weeks, with the principal side-effects being gastrointestinal. Mean doses were 35 mg/day. Approximately two-thirds of patients were deemed responders on the CGI Scale and longer duration of treatment seemed to be a predictor of those who would respond.

Davidson et al. (1991) treated five patients with civilian trauma with doses again ranging from 20 to 80 mg for 8–32 weeks. Fluoxetine was seen to have very significant improvement on both the intrusive and avoidance symptom clusters.

Shay (1992) treated 18 depressed Vietnam veterans. They noted decreased explosiveness, and impulsivity in 13 of the 18, with responses as early as week 1. The average response, however, occurred between weeks 3 and 6 in this retrospective study. Reductions in depression ratings were also observed. Side-effects were significant in this patient sample, with insomnia often requiring the addition of trazodone, as well as diarrhea, nausea, and reductions in libido.

Nagy and colleagues (1993) studied 27 PTSD combat veterans, again with doses 20–80 mg for 10 weeks. They utilized the modern Clinician Administered PTSD Scale (CAPS-II) and observed decreases from a mean of 64 down to 42, which, although statistically significant, was a relatively small reduction. They observed improvement in the numbing and avoidance, hyperarousal, and re-experiencing symptom clusters. Improvement generally took 6 weeks or longer, again suggesting longer-term therapy and perhaps higher doses were necessary to produce improvement. Disappointingly, functional outcome measures demonstrated only minimal improvement.

The first double-blind trial of an SSRI in PTSD was that by van der Kolk et al. (1994). Fluoxetine was given up to a maximum of 60 mg/day (mean 40 mg/day) to 31 military PTSD victims and 13 civilian PTSD victims in a 5-week trial. They did observe an overall positive effect for fluoxetine despite a very high dropout rate, with side-effects typical of an SSRI, diarrhea, sweating, and headaches. This was the first trial to note a difference in response between male and female and in civilian versus military groups. In the predominantly female civilian group, fluoxetine lead to significantly greater improvement in the re-experiencing and numbing domains, as well as in depression and lability. However, combat veterans failed to respond in terms of PTSD symptoms, although depression did improve. However, neither hyperarousal nor hostility improved.

In two matched trials, Connor et al. (1999) and Hertzberg et al. (2000) utilized fluoxetine up to 60 mg/day over a 12-week period. The Conner trial demonstrated that fluoxetine was superior to placebo in the civilian group in terms of the severity of PTSD symptoms, stress reactivity, functional disability, and high end-state function. They observed specific improvements on the intrusion and avoidance domains, as well as improvement in foreshortened future but little benefit for nightmares (Meltzer-Brody et al. 2000). Interestingly, Hertzberg and colleagues failed to observe any drug-placebo differences. With the identical study design, the principal difference was that the patients studied in this trial were PTSD combat veterans. Consistent with suggestions from earlier TCA and MAOI trials, this trial provided additional evidence with SSRIs that civilian PTSD trauma patients would respond better than combat PTSD victims.

Sertraline

Kline et al. (1994) studied sertraline in 10 Vietnam PTSD veterans with comorbid depression. They were treated over 12 months with a mean dose of 98.5 mg/day (range 5–150 mg/day). Interestingly, in this combat veteran population, 63% of the participants appeared to respond despite the fact that they had all been poor responders to other treatments or poorly tolerated previous treatments. They raised the issue that drug treatment improved PTSD victims' resiliency or ability to deal with stressful life events.

Rothbaum et al. (1996) studied five women who had been raped. Doses varied between patients, some treated as low as 50 mg and others at 150 mg. Four of the five were felt to be responders, and sertraline was well-tolerated, despite typical SSRI side-effects.

In the first double-blind placebo-controlled trial, Brady and colleagues reported results from treatment with flexible doses between 15 and 200 mg/day in 94 patients compared to 93 on placebo (Brady et al. 2000). Sertraline was associated with significantly greater improvement on 3 of 4 of the primary outcome measures (CGI-S, CGI-I, CAPS-II total severity score). There was a trend level improvement for the Impact of Event Scale (IES). They defined responders as those who had a reduction of >30% on the CAPS-II total severity score and a CGI Scale score of 1 (very much improved) or 2 (much improved). Using this definition, 53% of the sertraline cell and 32% of the placebo cell were classified as responders by week 12. Improvement was noted in the symptom domains of avoidance, numbing, and increased arousal but were not observed on the re-experiencing-intrusion measures. There was also no significant drug-placebo difference in males, perhaps a reflection of poor response in the subsample of veteran PTSDD subjects, mostly males. Response was observed as early as week 2 in this trial. In a trial with a matching design, Davidson and colleagues found very similar results, demonstrating a significant response to sertraline across many of the same outcome measures (Davidson et al. 2001).

Paroxetine

In the first trial of paroxetine, Marshall et al. (1998) studied 17 patients with chronic PTSD from civilian trauma with doses from 10 to 60 mg for 12 weeks. Mean reduction of PTSD symptoms on the Davidson Trauma Scale (DTS) was 48% and 11 of the 17 (65%) patients were rated as responders (1 or 2) on the CGI Scale. Improvement was noted in all three symptom clusters of re-experiencing, numbing, and hyperarousal. Interestingly, various components of PTSD symptom clusters responded at different times in this 12-week trial. Outcome measures included patient ratings, the treating physician, as well as independent evaluators using the modern PTSD Scale, the DTS and the IES. Mean reduction in PTSD scores by the independent evaluator was 48%.

Paroxetine has been subsequently studied in three large multicenter placebo-controlled trials (Stein *et al.* 1999; Beebe *et al.* 2000; Stein 2000): one fixed-dose and two flexible-dose trials. Beebe and colleagues studied 551 patients in a fixed-dose study comparing 20 or 40 mg/day to placebo in a 12-week, double-blind, placebo-controlled trial in 59 centers in the US (Beebe *et al.* 2000). Principal outcome measures were the CAPS-II and the percentage of responders on the CGI Scale. Secondary measures included changes in all three symptom clusters (re-experiencing, avoidance, hyperarousal) of the CAPS-II, the DTS, the Treatment Outcome PTSD Scale (TOPS), and the SDS. Patient improvement in the paroxetine cell on the CAPS-II was significantly greater for both 20 mg ($P < 0.001$) and 40 mg ($P < 0.001$). On the CGI-I, patients on paroxetine, both 20 and 40 mg, were significantly more likely to reach a 1 or 2 on the CGI Scale by endpoint ($P < 0.001$). On the secondary measures, both doses of paroxetine significantly improved the TOPS ($P < 0.001$). On the CGI Scale, 63% of the 20 mg group were rated as responders, 57% of the 40 mg group versus 37% of placebo. There were also significantly greater responses for paroxetine on the DTS, functional impairment on the SDS, as well as comorbid depression as measured by the MADRS. Side-effects were again of the expected SSRI class, i.e. nausea, asthenia, diarrhea, sexual, and sedation. There were no significant differences between doses in any of the outcome measures.

Perhaps most importantly, response was significant in all three of the PTSD symptom clusters, re-experiencing ($P < 0.001$), avoidance ($P < 0.001$), and hyperarousal ($P < 0.001$), and in both men and women.

Results from the first large multicenter double-blind placebo-controlled 12-week flexible-dose trial, with 307 patients treated with between 20 and 50 mg (mean 32.5 mg/day) were presented by Stein (2000). Again, on the principal outcome measure of the CAPS-II, there was significantly greater improvement compared to placebo ($P < 0.001$). Again, there was significantly greater improvement in all three PTSD symptom clusters (re-experiencing, avoidance, hyperarousal). There were significantly more responders (CGI Scale score 1 or 2) in the paroxetine cell beginning at week 1 and at the end of the trial (59% vs. 39%). The TOPS total scores were reduced significantly greater in the

paroxetine group ($P < 0.001$) and on the DTS total scores. Paroxetine was well-tolerated with the typical SSRI side-effects.

In the second flexible-dose (20–50 mg) multicenter double-blind placebo-controlled 12-week trial (Stein *et al.* 1999), the same design was utilized with 322 patients treated with a mean dose of 31.3 mg/day. Significant improvement was observed on the CAPS-II and TOPS total scores on paroxetine versus placebo ($P < 0.05$). Statistically greater improvement with paroxetine was observed in the re-experiencing symptom domain and, although numerical improvements were observed for the other two clusters, these did not reach statistical significance. Significantly more responders were seen on the CGI Scale in the paroxetine cell (50%) than in the placebo cell (43.5%). Improvements in disability in social and family life were significantly greater in the paroxetine cell, and although there were numerical differences in favor of paroxetine in the work item on the SDS, this was not statistically significant, probably because of the small numbers of patients. Side-effects were again minimal.

All three of these trials were quite similar in methodology, length, patient recruitment, outcome measures, etc., and therefore can be pooled. In the combined sample, there were a total of 1180 patients with 676 on paroxetine and 504 on placebo. Demographics of the patients were well-balanced within each study and within each treatment group. All three trials used the CAPS-II total score as their primary outcome measure and observed statistically greater improvement on paroxetine ($P < 0.001$). The proportion of patients deemed rated as responders on paroxetine (57%) was significantly greater than those on placebo (39%: $P < 0.001$). In the pooled dataset on the CAPS-II, there was a statistically significant improvement in the re-experiencing symptom domain ($P < 0.001$), the avoidance-numbing cluster ($P < 0.001$), and the hyperarousal cluster ($P < 0.001$), which were significantly greater than placebo from week 4.

Importantly, reductions on the CAPS-II were significant in both men and women and in all trauma types (Marshall 1998; Stein 2000). Unlike other trials, outcome was not affected by gender, whether PTSD trauma was military or civilian, or even by the time since the trauma itself, the severity of PTSD, or depressive symptoms at baseline. Interestingly, unlike the fluoxetine and sertraline studies, response to paroxetine was across all symptom clusters, genders, and trauma type. It is unclear whether this broader and more extensive treatment response is related to differences with paroxetine or methodological differences between the trials. Since re-experiencing symptoms are the most critical symptoms in PTSD patients, and developing successful treatments for military PTSD is critical, these potentially important differences need to be followed up.

Social anxiety disorder (social phobia)

Research in social anxiety disorder (social phobia) has generally lagged behind the other ADs, and this is certainly true of psychopharmacological treatments. There are preliminary studies with fluvoxamine, sertraline, and fluoxetine, but the only SSRI that has been studied extensively in well-controlled trials is paroxetine. These data will be reviewed below.

Fluvoxamine

The earliest trials (van Vliet *et al.* 1994) studied 30 outpatients in a double-blind, placebo-controlled, 12-week trial. They treated patients with 150 mg/day of fluvoxamine, and 28 patients completed the trial, 15 on fluvoxamine and 13 on placebo. Fluvoxamine's efficacy was demonstrated across the full range of the outcome measures with significant differences between fluvoxamine and placebo on most. Using the definition of a reduction of 50% or more on the Liebowitz Social Phobia Scale (Liebowitz 1987), 46% of the subjects on fluvoxamine and 7% on placebo were rated as responders. All of the symptom factors of the SCL-90 showed a statistically significant advantage for fluvoxamine.

If the patients felt they were sufficiently improved, they could continue for another 12 weeks. All 15 patients in the fluvoxamine cell elected to continue, but none in the placebo group, certainly an early indication of fluvoxamine's effectiveness. In the 12-week follow-up of responders on fluvoxamine, patients continued to improve, and their social anxiety and avoidance continued to decrease.

Stein *et al.* (1999) recently completed a 12-week multicenter placebo controlled trial of fluvoxamine with a larger sample ($N = 92$). Patients were treated with an average fluvoxamine dose of 202 mg/day. Statistically significant differences favoring fluvoxamine

over placebo were found on most outcome measures. The CGI Scale response rate on fluvoxamine was 43% versus 23% in the placebo group.

Sertraline

In the first trial studying sertraline in social anxiety disorder in a small patient sample of 12 patients, patients were treated with a mean dose of sertraline of 133 mg/day in a cross-over flexible-dose design with doses ranging from 50 to 200 mg/day. Despite the small sample, they were able to demonstrate a 50% response rate for sertraline versus only 9% for placebo after 10 weeks. There were also statistically significant changes favoring sertraline on the LSAS (Katzelnick *et al.* 1994).

Van Ameringen *et al.* (1999) have presented preliminary results from a large controlled study of sertraline. The CGI-I responder rate of 53% for sertraline was significantly greater than the 29% for placebo. This study had a large sample of 203 patients, 134 on sertraline and 69 on placebo.

Although these studies differ greatly in design and quality, they provide a preliminary estimate that ~50% of patients with social anxiety disorder will have a good response to sertraline.

Fluoxetine

Sternbach (1990) reported two responders to fluoxetine and Schneier *et al.* (1992) reported that seven of 12 responded. Similarly, Black *et al.* (1992) reported that 10 of 14 had moderate or marked improvement and Van Ameringen *et al.* (1993) 10 of 13. Perugi *et al.* (1995) reported 13 of 19 responded and Fairbanks *et al.* (1997) eight of 10 children and adolescents responded. In one double-blind trial comparing 20–60 mg of fluoxetine to placebo, Kobak *et al.* (2002) failed to observe a drug placebo difference. In this trial, placebo responses were higher than most recent trials and fluoxetine's lower (drop in LSAS of 22.6 points vs. 23.4 on placebo), which the authors suggested may related to lower doses or study design.

Further double-blind trials with fluoxetine are warranted.

Citalopram

There has been a single case report describing citalopram's efficacy in social anxiety disorder. In this case report, three patients treated with citalopram were reported to have good responses (Lepola *et al.* 1994). In a 12-week open trial with 22 patients, 86% were rated as responders (CGI Scale score 1 or 2) on 40 mg/day (Bouwer & Stein 1998). Again, controlled trials are needed to compare citalopram's efficacy to the other, better-studied agents.

Paroxetine

The only SSRI adequately studied and reported in social anxiety disorder is paroxetine with a series of well-controlled, acute, and for the first time, long-term maintenance-relapse prevention trials.

The first report of the use of paroxetine in social anxiety disorder was by Mancini and Van Ameringen (1996) who studied 18 patients in a 12-week open trial with doses that began at 10 mg/day of paroxetine and which were increased based on tolerability and response. Responders were patients who attained a CGI = 1 (markedly improved) or CGI = 2 (moderately improved) and 15 of 18 (83.3%) of the paroxetine patients met that criteria, with nine of the 15 responders actually having a marked improvement. There were statistically significant improvements in paroxetine on most measures with CGI Scale severity of illness scores being reduced from 5.3 at baseline to 3.7 at the end of the study ($P < 0.001$).

In a similar report appearing the same year, Stein *et al.* (1996) reported the results of a 12-week double-blind comparison of paroxetine and placebo in 36 patients. Patients were treated with 10–50 mg/day. At the end of 12 weeks, responders were continued on paroxetine or tapered and discontinued with placebo substitution. At the end of the acute phase trial, 77% of the paroxetine patients (22/30) were defined as responders (CGI = 1 or 2). The LSAS was reduced from 75.1 ± 25.4 (moderately severe) to 37.2 ± 32.5 (normal or mildly ill) ($P < 0.0005$). Sixteen of the responders were randomized in the 12-week continuation phase with eight remaining on the same dose of paroxetine and eight slowly tapered and put then on placebo. Of the patients randomized to placebo, five of the eight (63%) relapsed versus only one of the eight (13%) continued on paroxetine.

In the first of the large multicenter placebo-controlled trials (Stein *et al.* 1998), 187 patients were treated for 12 weeks with flexible doses (20–50 mg) of paroxetine or placebo. The effects of paroxetine were significantly

greater than placebo on almost all outcome measures at all points. On the principal outcome measure of the CGI Scale improvement responder categorization (1 or 2), 50 of the 91 (55%) were rated as responders versus 22 of the 92 (23.9%) of the placebo group at week 12. Also, the LSAS Scale total scores decreased from a baseline score of 78 by a mean of 30.5 (39.1%) in the paroxetine group versus falling from 83.5 by mean of 14.5 (17.4%) on placebo. Sixty-six percent of the paroxetine group finished the trial with the most common reasons for dropout being adverse effects (15%). Seventy-seven percent of the placebo cell completed the trial with the most common reason for discontinuation being lack of efficacy (11%).

Efficacy was initially observed at week 4 and continued throughout each week of the trial. Paroxetine was also significantly greater on five of the six secondary efficacy measures including the SDS (work and social life). Most side-effects were mild to moderate and were the expected SSRI class side-effects of headache, sexual difficulties, somnolence, and nausea.

In a second multicenter, flexible-dose trial using similar methodology, Baldwin and colleagues (1999) also reported that paroxetine was quite effective and well-tolerated. This was also a 12-week randomized, double-blind, placebo-controlled trial conducted in 39 centers in Europe and South Africa. The sample included 290 patients assigned to paroxetine doses between 20 and 50 mg/day or placebo. The primary outcome measure was the LSAS, and paroxetine produced significantly greater improvement on LSAS total score from baseline with a drop of 29.4 versus 15.6 on placebo ($P < 0.001$). Similar efficacy of paroxetine versus placebo was seen in the CGI Scale responders (1 or 2) with 65.7% versus 32.4% ($P < 0.001$) at week 12. Efficacy was observed from week 4 throughout the remainder of the trial.

Of the paroxetine group, 47% received 20–30 mg/day with remainder receiving 40–50 mg/day with a mean daily dose for paroxetine at week 12 being 34.4 mg/day. The reduction in LSAS scores were from baseline moderate-severe levels down to the moderate-mild levels of secondary impairment.

In the secondary measures significantly greater efficacy for paroxetine was again observed in the Social Avoidance and Distress Scale (SADS) ($P = 0.032$). Patients on paroxetine fell from a moderate/marked level of disability at baseline to levels of mild disability with reductions of ~30%. Improvement in levels of function were in all three areas of work, social, and family life.

Although the common adverse events of nausea, asthenia, and insomnia were observed, there was actually little difference in the adverse experience reported by the paroxetine and placebo groups with 74.1% and 68.2% reporting adverse effects. Of the patients reporting serious side-effects, there were slightly more in the paroxetine group (4.3% vs. 1.3%) with none considered to be actually secondary to paroxetine.

Although paroxetine did reduce the baseline HAM-D ratings significantly more than the placebo group, covariate analysis demonstrated that the changes in the primary social anxiety disorder variables were independent of effects on depression as measured by the HAM-D.

In a connected follow-up trial by Allgulander (1999), a total of 99 patients were treated with flexible doses of paroxetine (50–20 mg) or placebo for 3 months. Improvement in the paroxetine cell was seen from week 4 on the principal outcome measure of the LSAS which significantly favored paroxetine. The proportion of responders (much or very much improved) on the CGI Scale was greater on paroxetine (70.4%) than placebo (8.3%) ($P = 0.0001$). The reduction in LSAS in the paroxetine group was 33.4% compared to 8.6% on placebo ($P = 0.0001$). Paroxetine was also significantly superior to placebo in the secondary outcome measures of the Brief Social Phobia Scale (BSPS), the SDS, and the Fear of Negative Evaluation Scale (FNES).

As mentioned, there are some long-term data as patients from several of these trials were followed in long-term placebo-controlled extensions. Patients from the large study reported by Stein *et al.* (1998) were followed for an additional 28-week extension to the acute 12-week study. Patients receiving paroxetine for the entire 36 weeks ($N = 40$) not only maintained their improvement but improved further with the number of responders rising from 27/40 to 29/31 at follow-up. In his trial, Allgulander followed up patients by interviewing them again after a total treatment period of 32 months. They were able to interview 36 of 92 patients at 32 months and observed that efficacy of paroxetine was maintained and significantly augmented during the extended treatment period.

A recent long-term multicenter trial was presented by Hiar *et al.* (2000). Four hundred and thirty-seven patients were treated in an initial 12-week single-blind paroxetine treatment, and 323 of those were continued

in a long-term 24-week treatment study with 257 completing. Significantly more patients on placebo (39%) relapsed than those on paroxetine (14%). Similarly, the LSAS was reduced significantly more in the paroxetine group ($P < 0.0001$).

Conclusions

With the publication in the last few years of large, well-controlled, multicenter trials comparing SSRIs to placebo in all of the five principal ADs, it is now clear that the SSRIs are quite effective and well-tolerated in each of those disorders. As reviewed, paroxetine has now been demonstrated in well-controlled trials to be significantly more effective than placebo in all five ADs. Fluoxetine, sertraline, and fluvoxamine have also been studied in well-controlled trials in some of these disorders, demonstrating similar efficacy and tolerability. Citalopram has been less well-studied, but appears to also be effective in probably most of these conditions. As has been reviewed in this chapter, the SSRIs are now recommended by most expert and consensus groups as the treatment of choice in each of the five ADs.

This is itself fairly remarkable and represents the clear evolution of the treatment of choice from clomipramine in OCD and BZs in GAD and PD. The change to recommending SSRIs in GAD is perhaps the biggest change. Previously, the mainstay of treatment had been the BZs, and, to a lesser extent, buspirone. This change also recognizes that GAD is a long-term condition and that the SSRIs are more appropriate as long-term agents. Also given the high rate of depression and other ADs in GAD, the recommendation of the use of SSRIs makes all the more sense.

The demonstration of efficacy of several SSRIs in the treatment of PTSD also represents a major therapeutic advance. In this often difficult-to-treat and chronic condition, finding a well-tolerated and nonabuseable treatment is important.

Most of the SSRIs in the treatment of these five primary ADs are now being recommended for at least 1–2 years treatment which is yet another change, and recognizes the chronic nature of all five conditions in most patients. Although this is a somewhat understudied area, the studies that are available demonstrate that acute response is maintained with the SSRIs as long as the medication is continued. Also when patients are studied for longer periods, improvement continues and a larger group of patients become responders or even enter the remission group. Although this does need further study, there are now sufficient data to document the value of maintenance treatment, at least 6–12 months in each condition, and generally 12–24 months in most. Given the high rate of comorbidity, both acutely and especially over the long-term with these disorders, the case for utilizing SSRIs to treat each of the five disorders for at least 1–2 years is now unequivocal. It is less well-studied how treatment with the SSRIs for these conditions compares with psychotherapy, and there is need for well-controlled trials comparing these two treatments utilized alone and in combination. Although combination treatment may offer the ideal treatment as suggested by some trials, this is not supported by all trials and needs further study.

References

Allgulander, C. (1999) Paroxetine in social anxiety disorder: a randomized placebo-controlled study. *Acta Psychiatr Scand* 100, 193–8.

Allgulander, C., Cloninger, C.R. Przybeck T.R. & Brandt, L. (1998) Changes on the temperament and character inventory after paroxetine treatment in volunteers with generalized anxiety disorder. *Psychopharmacol Bull* 34, 165–6.

Ananth, J., Pecknold, J., Van Den Steen, N. & Engelsman, F. (1981) Double-blind study of clomipramine and amitriptyline in obsessive neurosis. *Prog Neuropsychopharmacol* 5, 257–62.

Asnis, G.M. (1992) Effects of fluvoxamine on the treatment of panic disorder: a placebo-controlled trial. *An Psiquiatric (Madrid)* 8 (Suppl. 1), 78.

Baer, L. (1994) Factor analysis of symptom subtypes of obsessive-compulsive disorder and their relation to personality and tic disorders. *J Clin Psychiatry* 55, 18–23.

Baer, L. & Jenike, M. (1992) Personality disorders in OCD. *Psychiatr Clin North Am* 15, 803–12.

Baldwin, D.S. (2000a) Clinical experience with paroxetine in social anxiety disorder. *Int Clin Psychopharmacol* 15 (Suppl. 1), S19–S24.

Baldwin, D.S. (2000b) SSRIs in the treatment of generalised anxiety disorder SB satellite symposium during European College of Neuropsychophmaracology, Munich, September 10.

Baldwin, D., Bobes, J., Stein, D.J. *et al.* (1999) Paroxetine in social phobia/social anxiety disorder. Randomized, double-blind, placebo-controlled study. *Br J Psychiatry* 175, 120–6.

Ballenger, J.C. (1999a) Clinical guidelines for establishing remission in patients with depression and anxiety. *J Clin Psychiatry* 60S(22), 29–34.

Ballenger, J.C. (1999b) Current treatments of the anxiety disorders in adults. *Biol Psychiatry* 46, 1579–94.

Ballenger, J.C. (1999c) Selective serotonin reuptake inhibitors (SSRIs) in panic disorder. In: *Panic Disorder: Clinical Diagnosis and Management* (D. Nutt, J.C. Ballenger & J. Lepine (eds), 159–78). Martin Dunitz, London.

Ballenger, J.C., Burrows, G.D., DuPont, R.L. *et al.* (1988) Alprazolam in panic disorder and agoraphobia: results of a multicenter trial. 1. Efficacy in short-term treatment. *Arch Gen Psychiatry* 45, 413–22.

Ballenger, J.C., Davidson, J.R. *et al.* (1998a) Consensus statement on social anxiety disorder from the International Consensus Group on Depression and Anxiety. *J Clin Psychiatry* 59 (Suppl. 17), 54–60.

Ballenger, J.C., Davidson, J.R., Lecrubier, Y. *et al.* (2000) Consensus statement on post-traumatic stress disorder from the International Consensus Group on Depression and Anxiety. *J Clin Psychiatry* 61 (Suppl. 5), 60–6.

Ballenger, J.C., Davidson, J.R., Lecrubier, Y., Nutt, D.J., Baldwin, D.S. & den Boer, J.A. (1998b) Consensus statement on panic disorder from the International Consensus Group on Depression and Anxiety. *J Clin Psychiatry* 59 (Suppl. 8), 7–54.

Ballenger, J.C., Davidson, J.R.T., Lecrubier, Y. *et al.* (2001) Consensus statement on generalized anxiety disorder from the International Consensus Group on Depression and Anxiety. *J Clin Psychiatry* 62 (Suppl. 11), 53–8.

Ballenger, J.C., Steiner, M., Bushness, W. & Gergel, I. (1998c) Double-blind, fixed-dose, placebo-controlled study of paroxetine in the treatment of panic disorder. *Am J Psychiatry* 155, 36–42.

Bellew, K.M., McCafferty, J.P., Lyengar, M. *et al.* (2000a) Short-term efficacy of paroxetine in generalized anxiety disorder: a double-blind placebo controlled trial. Presented at the 153rd Annual Meeting of the American Psychiatric Association, Chicago, May 13–18 (NR253).

Bellew, K.M., McCafferty, J.P. & Zaninelli, R. (2000b) Paroxetine improves quality of life in patients with generalized anxiety disorder. *Int J Neuropsychopharmacol* 3 (Suppl. 1), S226–S7.

de Beurs, E., van Balkom, A., Lange, A., Koele, P. & van Dyck, R. (1995) Treatment of panic disorder with agoraphobia: comparison of fluvoxamine, placebo, and psychological panic management combined with exposure and of exposure *in vivo* alone. *Am J Psychiatry* 152(5), 683–91.

Biserbe, J.C., Lane, R.M. & Flament, M.F. (1997) A double-blind comparison of sertraline and clomipramine in outpatients with obsessive-compulsive disorder. *Eur Psychiatry* 12, 82–93.

Black, B., Uhde, T.W. & Tancer, M.E. (1992) Fluoxetine for the treatment of social phobia [letter]. *J Clin Psychopharmacol* **12**, 293–5.

Black, D.W., Wesner, R., Bowers, W. & Gabel, J. (1993) A comparison of fluvoxamine, cognitive therapy, and placebo in the treatment of panic disorder. *Arch Gen Psychiatry* **50**, 44–50.

den Boer, M., Op der Belde, W., Falger, R.J.R., Hoveas, J.E., deGroen, J.H.M. & van Duijn, H. (1991) Fluvoxamine treatment for chronic PTSD. *Psychother Psychosomat* **57**, 158–63.

den Boer, J.A., Westenberg, H.G.M. & Kamerbeek, W.D.J. (1987) Effect of serotonin uptake inhibitors in anxiety disorders: a double-blind comparison of clorimipramine and fluvoxamine. *Int Clin Psychopharmacol* **2**, 21–32.

Bouwer, C. & Stein, D.J. (1998) Use of the selective serotonin reuptake inhibitor citalopram in the treatment of generalized social phobia. *J Affect Disord* **49**, 79–82.

Boyer, W. (1995) Serotonin uptake inhibitors are superior to imipramine and alprazolam in alleviating panic attacks: a meta-analysis. *Int Clin Psychopharmacol* **10**, 45–9.

Brady, K., Pearlstein, T., Asnis, G.M. *et al.* (2000) Efficacy and safety of sertraline treatment of post-traumatic stress disorder: a randomized controlled trial. *JAMA* **283**, 1837–44.

Caillard, V., Rouillion, F., Viel, J.F. & Markabi, S. & The French University Antidepressant Group (1999) Comparative effects of low and high doeses of clomipramine and placebo in panic disorder: a double-blind controlled study. *Acta Psychiatr Scand* **99**, 51–8.

Carrasco, J., Hollander, E., Schneier, F. & Liebowitz, M. (1992) Treatment outcome of OCD with comorbid social phobia. *J Clin Psychiatry* **53**, 387–91.

Cassano, G.B., Petracca, A. & Perugi, G. (1988) Clomipramine for panic disorder. I. The first 10 weeks of a long-term comparison with imipramine. *J Affect Disord* **14**, 123–7.

Chouinard, G., Goodman, W.K., Greist, J.H., Jenike, M.A., Rasmussen, S.A. & White, K. (1990) Results of a double-blind serotonin uptake inhibitor sertraline in the treatment of obsessive-compulsive disorder. *Psychopharmacol Bull* **26** (3), 279–84.

Clomipramine Collaborative Study Group (1991) Clomipramine in the treatment of patients with OCD. *Arch Gen Psychiatry* **48**, 730–8.

Cloninger, C.R., Przybeck, T.R., Syrakic, D.M. *et al.* (1994) The Temperament and Character Inventory (TCI): a guide to its development and use. Center for Psychobiology of Personality, Washington University, St. Louis, MO.

Connor, K.M., Sutherland, S.M., Tupler, L.A. *et al.* (1999) Fluoxetine in post-traumatic stress disorder. Randomised, double-blind study. *Br J Psychiatry* **175**, 17–22.

Cox, B.J. & Swinson, R.P. (1993) Clomipramine, fluoxetine, and behavior therapy in the treatment of obsessive-compulsive disorder: a meta-analysis. *J Behav Therap Exp Psychiat* **24**, 149–53.

Davidson, J.R.T., DuPont, R.L., Hedges, D. *et al.* (1999) Efficacy, safety, and tolerability of venlafaxine extended release and buspirone in outpatients with generalized anxiety disorder. *J Clin Psychiatry* **60**, 528–30.

Davidson, J., Roth, S. & Newman, E. (1991) Fluoxetine in post-traumatic stress disorder. *J Trauma Stress* **4**, 419–23.

Davidson, J.R.T., Rothbaum, B.O., van der Kolk, B.A., Sikes, C.R. & Farfel, G.M. (2001) Multicenter, double-blind comparison of sertraline and placebo in the treatment of post-traumatic stress disorder. *Arch Gen Psychiatry* **58**(5), 485–92.

DeVeaugh-Geiss, J., Katz, R.J., Landau, P. *et al.* (1991) Clomipramine in the treatment of patients with obsessive-compulsive disorder. *Arch Gen Psychiatry* **31**, 45–9.

DeVeaugh-Geiss, J., Katz, R., Landau, P., Goodman, W. & Rasmussen, S. (1990) Clinical predictors of treatment response in OCD: exploratory analyses from multicenter trials of clomipramine. *Psychopharmacol Bull* **26**, 54–9.

DeVeaugh-Geiss, J., Landau, P. & Katz, R. (1989) Treatment of obsessive-compulsive disorder with clomipramine. *Psychology Annals* **19**, 97–101.

Dewulf, L., Hendericx, B. & Lesaffre, E. (1995) Epidemiological data of patients with fluvoxamine: results from a 12-week non-comparative multicentre study. *Int Clin Psychopharmacol* **9** (Suppl. 4), 67–72.

Dunbar, G.C., Steiner, M. & Bushnell, W.D. (1995) Long-term treatment and prevention of relapse of obsessive compulsive disorder with paroxetine [abstract]. *Eur Neuro Psychopharmacol* **5**, 372.

Emmanuel, N.T., Ware, M. & Brawman-Mintzer, O. (1999) Once weekly dosing of fluoxetine in the maintenance of remission in panic disorder. *J Clin Psychiatry* **69**, 299–301.

Fahy, T.J., O'Rourke, D.O., Bropky, J. *et al.* (1992) The Galway study of panic disorder. I. Clomipramine and lofepramine in DSM-III-R panic disorder: a placebo-controlled trial. *J Affect Disord* **25**, 63–76.

Fairbanks, J.M., Pine, D.S., Tancer, N.K. *et al.* (1997) Open fluoxetine treatment of mixed anxiety disorders in children and adolescents. *J Child Adolesc Psychopharmacol* **7**, 17–29.

Fernandex, C.E. & Lopez-Ibor, J.J. (1967) Monochlorimipramine in the treatment of psychiatric patients resistant to other therapies. *Actas Luso Esp Neurological Psiquiatrics Cienc* **26**, 119–47.

Fontaine, R. & Choiinard, G. (1986) An open clinical trial of fluoxetine in the treatment of obsessive-compulsive disorder. *J Clin Psychopharmacol* **6**, 98–101.

Freeman, C.P.L., Trimble, M.R., Deakin, J.F.W. *et al.* (1994) Fluvoxamine versus clomipramine in the treatment of obsessive-compulsive disorder: a multicenter, randomized, double-blind, parallel group comparison. *J Clin Psychiatry* **55**(7), 301–5.

Gelenberg, A.J., Lydiard, R.B., Rudolph, R.L. *et al.* (2000) Efficacy of venlafaxine extended-release capsules in non-depressed outpatients with generalized anxiety disorder. *JAMA* **283**, 3082–8.

Gentil, V., Lotufoo-Neto, F., Andrade, L. *et al.* (1993) Clomipramine, a better reference drug for panic/agoraphobia. I. Effectiveness comparison with imipramine. *J Psychopharmacol* **7**(4), 316–24.

Gloger, S., Grunhaus, L., Birmacher, B. & Troudarf, T. (1981) Treatment of spontaneous panic attacks with clomipramine. *Am J Psychiatry* **138**, 1215–17.

Gloger, S., Grunhaus, L., Gladic, D. *et al.* (1989) Panic attacks and agoraphobia: low-dose clomipramine treatment. *J Clin Psychopharmacol* **9**, 28–32.

Goodman, W.K., Kozak, M.J., Liebowitz, M. & White, K.L. (1996) Treatment of obsessive-compulsive disorder with fluvoxamine: a multicenter, double-blind, placebo-controlled trial. *Int Clin Psychopharmacol* **11**, 21–30.

Goodman, W.K., Price, L.P., Anderson, G.M. *et al.* (1989a) Drug response and obsessive-compulsive disorder subtypes. APA Symposium, May 8, 1989. American Psychiatric Association Meetings, San Francisco, CA.

Goodman, W.K., Price, L.H., Rasmussen, S.A., Delgado, P.I., Henninger, G.R. & Charney, D.S. (1989b) Efficacy of fluvoxamine in obsessive-compulsive disorder. *Arch Gen Psychiatry* **46**, 35–44.

Gorman, J.M., Liebowitz, M.R. & Fyer, A.J. (1987) An open trial of fluoxetine in the treatment of panic attacks. *J Clin Psychopharmacol* **7**, 329–32.

Greist, J., Chouinard, G. & Duboff, E. (1995a) Double-blind parallel comparison of three dosages of sertraline and placebo in outpatients with OCD. *Arch Gen Psychiatry* **51**, 559–67.

Greist, J.H., Chouinard, G., DuBoff, E. *et al.* (1995c) Double-blind parallel comparison of three dosages of sertraline and placebo in outpatients with obsessive-compulsive disorder. *Arch Gen Psychiatry* **52**, 289–95.

Greist, J., Jefferson, J., Koback, K., Katzelnick, D. & Serlin, R. (1995b) Efficacy and tolerability of serotonin inhibitors in obsessive-compulsive disorder: a meta-analysis. *Arch Gen Psychiatry* **52**, 53–60.

Greist, J.H., Jenike, M.A., Robinson, D.S. & Rasmussen, S.A. (1995d) Efficacy of fluvoxamine in obsessive-compulsive disorder: results of a multicenter, double-blind, placebo-controlled trial. *Eur J Clin Res* **7**, 195–204.

Hackett, D., Meoni, P., White, C. & Rasmussen, J. (2000) Efficacy of short and long-term venlafaxine ER treatment as somatic and psychic symptoms of GAD. *Eur Neuropsychopharmacol* **10** (Suppl. 10), 337.

Hall, H. & Ogren, S. (1984) Effects of antidepressant drugs on histamine H_1-receptors in the brain. *Life Sci* **34**, 597–605.

Hertzberg, M.A., Feldman, M.E., Beckham, J.C., Hudler, H.A. & Davidson, J.R.T. (2000) Lack of efficacy for fluoxetine in PTSD: a placebo-controlled trial in combat veterans. *Ann Clin Psychiatry* **59**, 460–4.

Hiar, T., Castrogiovanni, P., Domenech, J., Stocchi, F. & Van Ameringen, M. (2000) CINP, Brussels.

Hoehn-Saric, R., Fawcett, J., Munjack, D.J. & Roy-Byrne, P.P. (1994) A multicenter, double-blind, placebo-controlled study of fluvoxamine in the treatment of panic disorder. In: *Neuropsychopharmacology. Part 2. Oral Communications and Poster Abstracts of the XIXth Collegium International Neuropsychopharmacologicum Congress.* Abstract P-58-33, Washington, D.C.

Hoehn-Saric, R., McLeod, D.R. & Hipsley, P.A. (1993) Effect of fluvoxamine on panic disorder. *J Clin Psychopharmacol* **13**, 321–6.

Hoffart, A., Due-Madsen, J., Lande, B. *et al.* (1993) Clomipramine in the treatment of agrophobic inpatients resistant to behavioral therapy. *J Clin Psychiatry* **54**, 481–7.

Holland, R.I., Fawcett, J., Hoehn-Saric, R. *et al.* (1994) Long-term treatment of panic disorder with fluvoxamine in outpatients who had completed double-blind studies. *Neuropsychopharmacology* **10**(35) (Part 2), 1025.

Humble, M., Koczkas, C. & Wistedt, B. (1989) Serotonin and anxiety: an open study of citalopram in panic disorder. In: *Psychiatry Today VIII World Congress of Psychiatry Abstracts* (C.N. Stefanis, C.R. Soldatos & A.D. Rabavilas (eds), p. 151). Elsevier, New York.

Humble, M. & Wistedt, B. (1992) Serotonin, panic disorder and agorphobia: short-term and long-term efficacy of citalopram in panic disorder. *Int Clin Psychopharmacol* **6** (Suppl. 5), 21–39.

Insel, T.R., Murphy, D.L., Cohen, R.M., Alterman, I., Kilts, C. & Linnoila, M. (1983) Obsessive-compulsive disorder—a double-blind trial of clomipramine and clorgyline. *Arch Gen Psychiatry* **40**, 605–12.

Jenike, M.A. (1990a) The pharmacological treatment of obsessive-compulsive disorders. *Int Rev Psychiatry* **2**, 411–25.

Jenike, M.A. (1998) Drug treatment of obsessive-compulsive disorder. In: *Obsessive-compulsive Disorders: Practical Management*, 3rd edn (M.A. Jenike, L. Baer & W.E. Minichiello (eds), pp. 469–532). Mosby, St Louis, MO.

Jenike, M.A. & Baer, L. (1988) An open trial of buspirone in obsessive-compulsive disorder. *Am J Psychiatry* **145**, 1285–6.

Jenike, M.A., Hyman, S., Baer, L. *et al.* (1990b) A controlled trial of fluvoxamine in obsessive-compulsive disorder: implications for a serotonergic theory. *Am J Psychiatry* **147**(9), 1209–15.

Jobson, K.O. & Potter, W.Z. (1995) International psychopharmcology algorithm project report. *Psychopharmacol Bull* **31**, 457–507.

Johnston, D.G., Troyer, I.E. & Whitsett, S.F. (1988) Clomipramine treatment of agoraphobic women: an 8-week controlled trial. *Arch Gen Psychiatry* **45**, 453–9.

Katzelnick, D., Jefferson, J. et al. (1994) Sertraline in social phobia: a double-blind, placebo-controlled cross-over pilot study. Presented at the 34th Annual Meeting of NCDEU, May 31–June 3, 1994. Marco Island, FL.

Kline, N.A., Dow, B.M., Brown, S.A. & Matloff, J.A. (1994) Sertraline efficacy in depressed combat veterans with post-traumatic stress disorder. *Am J Psychiatry* **151**, 621.

Kobak, K.A., Greist, J.H., Jefferson, J.W. & Katzelnick, D.J. (2002) Fluoxetine in social phobia: a double-blind, placebo-controlled pilot study. *J Clin Psychopharmacol* **22**(3), 257–62.

van der Kolk, B.A., Dreyfuss, D., Michaels, M. et al. (1994) Fluoxetine in post-traumatic stress disorder. *J Clin Psychiatry* **55**, 517–22.

Koponen, H., Lepola, U., Leinonen, E., Jokinen, R., Penttinen, J. & Turtonen, J. (1997) Citalopram in the treatment of obsessive-compulsive disorder: a single-blind study. *J Clin Psychopharmacol* **17**, 267–71.

Kronig, M.H., Apter, J., Asnis, G. et al. (1999) Placebo-controlled, multicenter study of sertraline treatment for obsessive-compulsive disorder. *J Clin Psychopharmacol* **19**, 172–6.

LeCrubier, I., Bakker, A. & Judge, R. (1997) A comparison of paroxetine, clomipramine, and placebo in the treatment of panic disorder. *Acta Psychiatr Scand* **95**, 145–52.

LeCrubier, Y., Judget, R. & The Collaborative Paroxetine Study Investigators (1997) Long-term evaluation of paroxetine, clomipramine, and placebo in panic disorder. *Acta Psychiatr Scand* **95**, 153–60.

Leonard, H.L., Swedo, S.E., Lenane, M.C. et al. (1991) A double-blind desipramine substitution during long-term clomipramine treatment in children and adolescents with obsessive-compulsive disorder. *Arch Gen Psychiatry* **48**, 922–7.

Lepola, U., Koponen, H. & Leinonen, E. et al. (1994) Citalopram in the treatment of social phobia: a report of three cases. *Pharmacopsychiatry* **27**, 186–8.

Lepola, U., Wade, A.G. & Leinonen, E.V. (1998) A controlled prospective, 1-year study of citalopram in the treatment of panic disorder. *J Clin Psychiatry* **59**, 528–32.

Levine, R., Hoffman, J.S., Knepple, E.D. & Kenin, M. (1988) Long-term fluoxetine treatment of a large number of obsessive-compulsive patients. *J Clin Psychopharmacol* **9**, 281–3.

Liebowitz, M.R. (1987) Social phobia. *Mod Probl Pharmacopsychiatry* **22**, 141–73.

Londborg, P.D., Wolkow, R. & Smith, W.T. (1998) Sertraline in the treatment of panic disorder. *Br J Psychiatry* **173**, 54–60.

Mancini, C. & van Ameringen, M. (1996) Paroxetine in social phobia. *J Clin Psychiatry* **57**(11), 519–22.

Marmar, C.R., Schoenfeld, F., Weiss, D.S. et al. (1996) Open trial of fluvoxamine treatment for combat-rated post-traumatic stress disorder. *J Clin Psychiatry* **57** (Suppl. 8), 66–72.

Marshall, R.D., Schneier, F.R., Fallon, B.A. et al. (1998) An open trial of paroxetine in patients with noncombat-related, chronic post-traumatic stress disorder. *J Clin Psychopharmacol* **11**, 325–7.

McCafferty, J. et al. (2000) Paroxetine is effective in the treatment of generalised anxiety disorder: Results from a randomized placebo-controlled flexible-dose study. *Eur Neuropsychopharmacol* **10** (Suppl. 3), S348.

McDougle, C., Goodman, W., Leckman, J., Lee, N., Heninger, G. & Price, L. (1994) Halperidol addition in fluvoxamine-refractory obsessive-compulsive disorder: a double-blind, placebo-controlled study in patients with and without tics. *Arch Gen Psychiatry* **51**, 302–8.

McDougle, C.J., Southwick, S.M., Charney, D.S. et al. (1991) An open trial of fluoxetine in the treatment of post-traumatic stress disorder. *J Clin Psychopharmaco* **11**, 325–7.

Meltzer-Brody, S., Connon, K.M., Churchill, E. et al. (2000) Symptom-specific effects of fluoxetine in post-traumatic stress disorder. *Int Clin Psychopharmacol* **15**(4), 227–31.

Michelson, D., Lydiard, R.B., Pollack, M.H., Tamura, R.N., Hoog, S.L. & Tepner, R. (1998) Outcome assessment and clinical improvement in panic disorder: evidence from a randomized assessment and clinical improvement in panic disorder: evidence from a randomized controlled trial of fluoxetine and placebo. *Am J Psychiatry* **155**, 1570–7.

Michelson, D., Pollack, M. & Lydiard, R. (1999) Continuing treatment of panic disorder after acute response: randomised, placebo-controlled trial with fluoxetine. *Br J Psychiatry* **172**, 213–18.

Modigh, K., Westberg, P. & Eriksson, E. (1992) Superiority of clomipramine over imipramine in the treatment of panic disorder: a placebo-controlled trial. *J Clin Psychopharmacol* **51**(45), 53–8.

Montgomery, S.A. (2000) Long-term treatment of GAD. First International Forum on Mood and Anxiety Disorders, December 2, 2000, Monte Carlo.

Montgomery, S.A., Kasper, S., Stein, D. et al. (2001) Citalopram 20, 40 and 60 mg are all effective and well-tolerated compared with placebo in obsessive-compulsive disorder. *Int Clin Psychopharmacol* **16**(2), 75–86.

Montgomery, S.A., McIntyre, A., Osterheider, M. et al. (1993) A double-blind, placebo-controlled study of fluoxetine in patients with DSM-III-R obsessive-compulsive disorder. *Eur Neuropsychopharmacol* **3**, 143–52.

Mundo, E., Bianchi, L. & Bellodi, L. (1997) Efficacy of fluvoxamine, paroxetine, and citalopram in the treatment of obsessive-compulsive disorder: a single-blind study. *J Clin Psychopharmacol* **17**, 267–71.

Nagy, L.M., Morgan, C.A., Southwick, S.M. & Charney, D.S. (1993) Open prospective trial of fluoxetine for post-traumatic stress disorder. *J Clin Psychopharmacol* **13**, 107–14.

Nair, N.P., Bakish, D. & Saxena, B. (1996) Comparison of fluvoxamine, imipramine, and placebo in the treatment of outpatients with panic disorder. *Anxiety* **2**, 192–8.

Oehrberg, S., Christiansen, P.E. & Behnek, K. (1995) Paroxetine in the treatment of panic disorder, a randomized double-blind placebo controlled study. *Br J Psychiatry* **167**, 374–9.

Pato, M., Hill, J. & Murphy, D.L. (1990) A clomipramine dosage reduction study in the course of long-term treatment of OCD patients. *Psychopharmacol Bull* **26**, 211–14.

Pato, M.T., Zohar-Kodouch, R., Zohar, J. *et al.* (1988) Return of symptoms after discontinuation of clomipramine in patients with obsessive-compulsive disorder. *Am J Psychiatry* **145**, 1521–5.

Perse, T.L., Greist, J.H., Jefferson, J.W., Rosenfeld, J.W. & Dar, R. (1987) Fluvoxamine treatment of obsessive-compulsive disorder. *Am J Psychiatry* **144**, 1543–8.

Perugi, G., Nassini, S., Lenzi, M., Simonini, E., Cassano, G.B. & McNair, D.M. (1995) Treatment of social phobia with fluoxetine. *Anxiety* **1**, 282–6.

Piccinelli, M., Pini, S., Bellantuono, C., Wilkinson, G. (1995) Efficacy of drug treatment in obsessive compulsive disorder. *Br J Psychiat* **166**, 421–43.

Piggott, T.A., Pato, M.T., Bernstein, S.E. *et al.* (1990) Controlled comparisons of clomipramine and fluoxetine in the treatment of obsessive-compulsive disorder. *Arch Gen Psychiatry* **47**, 1543–50.

Pohl, R.B., Wolkow, R.M. & Clary, C.M. (1998) Sertraline in the treatment of panic disorder: a double-blind multi-center trial. *Am J Psychiatry* **155**(9), 1189–95.

Pollack, M.H., Otto, M.W. & Worthington, J.J. (1998) Sertraline in the treatment of panic disorder: a flexible-dose multicenter trial. *Arch Gen Psychiatry* **55**, 1010–16.

Pollack, M.H., Zaninelli, R., Goddard, A. *et al.* (2001) Paroxetine in the treatment of generalized anxiety disorder: results of a placebo-controlled, flexible dosage trial. *J Clin Psychiatry* **62**(5), 350–7.

Price, L.H., Goodman, W.K., Charney, D.S. *et al.* (1987) Treatment of severe obsessive-compulsive disorder with fluovoxamine. *Am J Psychiatry* **144**, 1059–61.

Rasmussen, S., Hacket, E., DuBoff, E. *et al.* (1997) A 2-year study of sertraline in the treatment of obsessive-compulsive disorder. *Int Clin Psychopharmacol* **12**, 309–16.

Rocca, P., Fonzo, V., Scotta, M., Zanalda, E. & Ravizza, L. (1997) Paroxetine efficacy in the treatment of generalized anxiety disorder. *Acta Psychiatr Scand* **95**, 444–50.

Rosenberg, D.R., Steward, C.M., Fitzgerald, K.D. *et al.* (1999) Paroxetine open-label treatment of pediatric outpatients with obsessive-compulsive disorder. *J Am Acad Child Adolesc Psychiat* **38**, 1180–5.

Rothbaum, B.O., Ninan, P.T. & Thomas, L. (1996) Sertraline in the treatment of rape victims with post-traumatic stress disorder. *J Trauma Stress* **9**, 865–71.

Roy-Byrne, P.P. & Wingerson, D. (1992) Pharmacotherapy of anxiety disorders. In: *Review of Psychiatry*, Vol. II (A. Tasman & M.B. Riba (eds), pp. 260–84). American Psychiatric Press, Washington, D.C.

Schneier, F.R., Chin, S.J., Hollander, E. & Liebowitz, M.R. (1992) Fluoxetine in social phobia [letter]. *J Clin Psychopharmacol* **12**, 62–4.

Schneier, F.R., Liebowitz, M.R. & Davies, S.O. (1991) Fluoxetine in panic disorder. *J Clin Psychopharmacol* **10**, 119–21.

Sharpe, D.M., Power, K.G., Simpson, R.J. *et al.* (1996) Fluvoxamine, placebo and cognitive behavior therapy used alone and in combination in the treatment of panic disorder and agoraphobia. *J Anxiety Disord* **30**, 233–41.

Shay, J. (1992) Fluoxetine reduces explosiveness and elevates mood of Vietnam combat veterans with PTSD. *J Trauma Stress* **5**, 97–101.

Shear, M.K., Brown, T.A. & Barlow, D.H. (1997) Multicenter collaborative Panic Disorder Severity Scale. *Am J Psychiatry* **154**, 1571–5.

Shear, M.K. & Maser, J.D. (1994) Standardized assessment for panic disorder research. *Arch Gen Psychiatry* **147**, 507–9.

Sheehan, D., Ballenger, J.C. & Jacobson, G. (1980) Treatment of endogenous anxiety with phobic hysterical and hypochondriacal symptoms. *Arch Gen Psychiatry* **37**, 51–9.

Stein, D.J. (2000) Improving treatment options—new clinical data on paroxetine. CINP 2000.

Stein, M.B., Chartier, M.J., Hazen, A.L. *et al.* (1996) Paroxetine in the treatment of generalized social phobia: open-label treatment and double-blind placebo-controlled discontinuation. *J Clin Psychopharmacol* **16**, 218–22.

Stein, M.B., Fyer, A.J., Davidson, J.R.T., Pollack, M.H. & Wiita, B. (1999) Fluvoxamine treatment of social phobia (social anxiety disorder): a double-blind, placebo-controlled study. *Am J Psychiatry* **156**(5), 746–60.

Stein, M.G., Liebowitz, M.R. *et al.* (1998) Paroxetine treatment of generalized social phobia (social anxiety disorder): a double-blind, placebo-controlled study. *Am J Psychiatry* **156**, 756–60.

Steiner, M., Bushnell, W., Gergel, I. & Wheadon, D. (1995) Long-term treatment with paroxetine in outpatients with OCD: an extension of the fixed-dose study. American Psychiatric Association Annual Meeting, New Research Abstracts, May 9–12, 1995. Miami, FL.

Sternbach, H. (1990) Fluoxetine treatment of social phobia [letter]. *J Clin Psychopharmacol* **10**, 230–1.

Stocchi, F., Nordera, G., Jokinen, R. *et al.* (2001) Maintained efficacy of paroxetine in GAD. Presented at the 7th World Congress of Biological Psychiatry, July 1–6, 2001. Berlin, Germany.

Thomsen, P.H. (1997) Child and adolescent obsessive-compulsive disorder treated with citalopram: findings from an open trial of 23 cases. *J Child Adolesc Psychopharmacol* **7**, 157–66.

Thoren, P., Asberg, M., Cronholm, B., Jornestedt, L. & Traskman, L. (1980) Clomipramine treatment in obsessive-compulsive disorder. I. A controlled clinical trial. *Arch Gen Psychiatry* **37**, 1281–5.

Tiller, J.W.G., Bouwer, C. & Behnke, K. (1999) Moclobemide and fluoxetine for panic disorder. *Eur Arch Psychiatry Clin Neurosci* **249** (Suppl. 1S), 7–10.

Tollefson, G., Birkett, M., Koran, L. & Genduso, L. (1994a) Continuation treatment of OCD: double-blind and open-label experience with fluoxetine. *J Clin Psychiatry* **55**, 69–78.

Tollefson, G.D., Rampey, A.H., Potvin, J.H. *et al.* (1994b) A multicenter investigation of fixed-dose fluoxetine in the treatment of obsessive-compulsive disorder. *Arch Gen Psychiatry* **51**, 559–67.

Turner, S.M., Jacob, R.G., Beidel, D.C. *et al.* (1985) Fluoxetine treatment of obsessive-compulsive disorder. *J Clin Psychopharmacol* **5**, 207–12.

Van Amerigen, M.A., Lane, R.M., Walker, J.R. *et al.* (1999a) Sertraline treatment of social phobia: a 20-week, double-blind, placebo-controlled study. Presented at XI. World Congress of Psychiatry; August 7, Hamburg, Germany.

Van Ameringen, M., Mancini, C. & Streiner, D.L. (1993) Fluoxetine efficacy in social phobia. *J Clin Psychiatry* **54**, 27–32.

Van Ameringen, M.A., Swinson, R.P. *et al.* (1999b) *A Placebo-Controlled Study of Sertraline in Generalized Social Phobia NR330.* American Psychiatric Association, Washington, D.C.

van Vliet, I.M., den Boer, J.A. & Westenberg, H.G. (1994) Psychopharmacological treatment of social phobia: a double-blind placebo controlled study of fluvoxamine. *Psychopharmacology* **115**, 128–34.

van Vliet, I.M., den Boer, J.A., Westenberg, H.G. *et al.* (1996) A double-blind comparative study of brofaramine and fluoxetine in outpatients with panic disorder. *J Clin Psychopharmacol* **16**, 299–306.

Volavka, J., Neziroglu, F. & Yaryura-Tobias, J.A. (1985) Clomipramine and imipramine in obsessive-compulsive disorders. *Psychiatr Res* **14**, 85–93.

Wade, A.G., Lepola, U. & Koponen, H.J. (1997) The effect of citalopram in panic disorder. *Br J Psychiatry* **170**, 549–53.

Wheadon, D., Bushnell, W.D. & Steiner, M. (1993) A fixed-dose comparison of 20, 40 or 60 mg of paroxetine to placebo in the treatment of obsessive-compulsive disorder. Presented at the American College of Neuropsychopharmacology Annual Meeting, December. Puerto Rico.

Woods, S., Black, D., Brown, S. *et al.* (1994) Fluvoxamine in the treatment of panic disorder in outpatients: A double-blind, placebo-controlled study. In: *Neuropsychopharmacology. Part 2. Oral Communications and Poster Abstracts of the XIXth Collegium International Neuropsychopharmacologicum Congress.* Abstract P-58-37. Washington, D.C.

Zohar, J. & Judge, R. (1996) Paroxetine versus clomipramine in the treatment of obsessive-compulsive disorder. *Br J Psychiatry* **169**, 468–74.

19 Treatment of Anxiety Disorders with Tricyclic Antidepressants

R. Rosenberg

Introduction

During the last two decades extensive research has widened the indications of antidepressant drugs to include most, if not all, anxiety disorders including obsessive-compulsive disorder. Randomized controlled trials have demonstrated the efficacy of antidepressants on major anxiety components (Ballenger 1999; Zohar *et al*. 2000) and basic neurobiological research has given important insights into the pathophysiology of anxiety disorders (Goddard & Charney 1997; Coplan & Lydiard 1998) and the pharmacodynamics of antidepressants (Sanchez & Hyttel 1999).

Panic disorder and obsessive-compulsive disorder have been the most extensively studied of the anxiety disorders, and results from controlled drug trials have influenced the development of neurobiological models of these disorders (Charney *et al*. 1993; Coplan & Lydiard 1998; Sanchez & Hyttel 1999). Disturbances in serotonergic neurotransmission have been suggested to be essential components in the pathophysiology of several anxiety disorders (Zohar *et al*. 2000).

In this chapter evidence from controlled trials with the classical tricyclic antidepressants (TCAs) will be shortly reviewed. A major issue to be addressed in this chapter is whether the appearance of the specific serotonin reuptake inhibitors (SSRIs) and other new antidepressant compounds means an end to the use of the TCAs in the treatment of anxiety disorders.

Panic disorder

The benefit of imipramine treatment of panic attacks was already demonstrated by Klein in 1964 (Klein 1964). According to his influential theory (Klein *et al*. 1981) the core symptom of panic disorder (PD) is recurrent panic attacks, some of which are spontaneous while others are precipitated by phobic stimuli. Anticipatory anxiety and agoraphobia are suggested to be sequela to recurrent panic attacks which eventually are followed by depression as a demoralization phenomenon (Rosenberg *et al*. 1991). Hence, standardized assessments should include measures of panic attacks, anticipatory anxiety, phobic symptoms, comorbidity (especially agoraphobia and depression) and global improvement (Shear & Maser 1994). Most studies from the 1990s present data on such measures.

The heuristic validity of PD has generally been accepted. However, with respect to the validity of the putative nosological entity, important issues still need clarification, especially comorbidity issues with affective disorders. The high comorbidity between PD and affective disorders (Rosenberg & Jensen 1994) suggests that antipanic effects of antidepressants might be secondary to their efficacy on depressive symptoms. Multicenter studies enrolling large samples of patients allow analyses of subgroups to elucidate this important problem.

The affinities to serotonergic and noradrenergic transporters vary across TCAs (Sanchez & Hyttel 1999). In this connection, it is theoretically interesting that amongst the two most frequently studied TCAs clomipramine has a higher affinity for the serotonin transporter than imipramine.

Imipramine and clomipramine

Studies from the 1980s

In a series of studies published in the 1980s, the antipanic efficacy of imipramine (IMI) and (clomipramine) CMI was suggested from several double-blind placebo controlled trials of 6–12 weeks duration (Rosenberg et al. 1999). However, sample sizes were modest, i.e., less than 25 in each treatment cell and some studies allowed concomitant psychotherapy. Methodological restrictions called for larger multicenter studies, which fulfilled modern requirements of standardized diagnostic assessment and of clinical phenomenology of PD.

The early literature of panic studies has been traditionally reviewed, for instance, by Liebowitz et al. (1988), Balestrieri et al. (1989), and Matuzas and Jack (1991),

and subjected to several meta-analyses (Wilkinson et al. 1991; Boyer 1995; Gould et al. 1995; van Balkom et al. 1997: Table 19.1). Most reviewers agree upon the efficacy of the TCAs, especially IMI, on various clinical components of PD.

In Wilkinson et al.'s (1991) meta-analysis the median effect sizes for several important clinical parameters based on 13 studies on antidepressants (12 with IMI) and six on benzodiazepines were calculated. The treatment median effect size for TCAs was 0.55 indicating moderate improvement. The effect size for panic attacks was fairly low [0.27], but panic attacks were not systematically registered in all studies. It was also registered that the effect sizes varied widely (from 0.002 to 0.76) on panic attacks in individual studies. The effects sizes for IMI and benzodiazepines were quite similar.

Boyer (1995) calculated an *improvement ratio* defined as improvement on active drug divided by that on placebo based on nine studies with IMI and three with CMI. For IMI the mean improvement ratio for the nine studies was 1.90 (range 1.00–2.97) and for CMI (the three studies) 2.43 (range 1.66–5.41). However, Boyer evaluated only efficacy for completers

Table 19.1 Panic disorder. Meta-analysis of short-term TCA treatment trials.

Study	N	Years	Double-blind placebo control only	Outcome TCA > placebo/control	Comments
Wilkinson et al. (1991)	13	1964–1986	Yes	Yes	Comprehensive study, effect sizes calculated for major outcome measure
Boyer (1995)	15	1980–1992	Yes	Yes	Panic free was main outcome measure (four studies other anxiety measure); only completer analysis; clomipramine and SSRIs combined
Gould et al. (1995)	43 (9)*	1980–1994	No	Yes	Comprehensive analyses of efficacy of drugs and psychotherapy. Special analyses on antidepressants vs. placebo, statistical testing of effect sizes
van Balkom et al. (1997)	106	1964–1995	No	Yes (antidepressants)	Antidepressants evaluated as a group including some SSRIs. The combination of antidepressants with exposure *in vivo* is the most potent short-term treatment for agoraphobia

*Antidepressants vs placebo.

TCA, tricyclic antidepressants; SSRIs, specific serotonin reuptake inhibitors.

in the trials and only considered one major outcome (i.e. panic attacks). Boyer also analysed results from trials with SSRIs. Boyer subsumed CMI under the concept of *serotonin reuptake inhibitors*. Interestingly, the meta-analysis demonstrated that serotonin reuptake inhibitors were significantly superior to both IMI and the benzodiazepine alprazolam.

Multicenter studies in the 1990s

Flaws in evaluating the literature by meta-analysis have recently been underlined by Klein (2000), and Klerman (1988) was an early advocate for giving high priority to quality aspects of controlled trials in evaluating drug efficacy. Many of such requirements (i.e., randomized placebo controlled double-blind design, standardized assessment, absence of concomitant psychotherapy and statistical analysis of intent to treat, and completer samples) have been fulfilled in multicenter studies (Cross-National Collaborative Panic Study 1992: Table 19.2) although even such large studies may be subject to methodological criticism.

Imipramine

Cross-National Collaborative Panic Study

In phase II of the Cross-National Collaborative Panic Study (1992) IMI, alprazolam and placebo were compared in an 8-week trial. IMI was efficacious on a wide range of panic phenomenology including panic attacks, anticipatory anxiety and phobic avoidance behavior. However, for completers of the trial no differences were seen on the primary outcome measure panic attack.

An important finding was that the efficacy of IMI was not restricted to the amelioration of panic attacks, but comprised a spectrum of clinically relevant symptoms including phobic avoidance behavior, even in the absence of concomitant psychotherapy. Furthermore, it was found that improvement as in the treatment of depression with TCAs was gradual over weeks. In contrast, the benzodiazepine alprazolam had a faster mode of action. After 8 weeks both drugs had similar profiles of efficacy.

Affective symptoms A substantial proportion of the patients had affective symptoms. Among panic patients, 16% fulfilled the criteria for current major depressive episode, 16% for past major depressive episode, and 12% for dysthymia.

Deltito *et al.* (1991) analysed a subgroup of patients (*N* = 312) from the CNCPS applying strict criteria to

rule out affective symptoms, i.e., current or previous affective episode as well as dysphoria. They found that the clinical response to IMI or alprazolam was *independent* of the presence of current or past affective symptoms. Analyses relying on general linear models on the importance of current major depressive episodes are in accordance with this conclusion (Maier *et al.* 1991). Detailed analysis of panic patients with *dysthymia* did not suggest this syndrome to be of major clinical relevance for the outcome of drug treatment of PD (Rosenberg & Jensen 1994).

Although patients with affective symptoms did improve significantly, patients with current major depressive episode improved less, probably due to higher scores at baseline on most anxiety and affective scales (Rosenberg & Jensen 1994). No significant differences were observed between IMI and alprazolam considering subgroups defined by affective symptoms.

These results strongly indicate that IMI has specific efficacy on core symptoms of PD independent on the presence of affective symptoms.

Avoidance behavior Twenty-two percent of the patients had uncomplicated PD, 40% limited phobic avoidance, while 36% had agoraphobia.

The role of avoidance behavior has been further analysed applying analysis of variance within the framework of a linear model to test the efficacy of active drugs in different subgroups of patients (Maier *et al.* 1991a,b). Patients with extensive avoidance behavior (agoraphobia) profited the most from treatment with active drugs but, surprisingly, specific drug effects were most pronounced in avoidance behavior. PD uncomplicated by avoidance behavior responded nearly equally well to alprazolam, IMI, and placebo, while phobic avoidance was significantly improved by both drugs.

In summary On a spectrum of symptoms PD patients improve on short-term IMI treatment independent of comorbid affective or phobic symptoms. The improvement is gradual over several weeks. However, patients with agoraphobia may have a better response to drugs than patients with uncomplicated PD.

Other multicenter studies

The efficacy of IMI in PD has been substantiated by later multicenter studies (Nair *et al.* 1996; Barlow *et al.* 2000). Barlow *et al.* (2000) included 312 patients in a study where drugs and psychosocial therapies were

Table 19.2 Panic disorder. Some placebo-controlled studies of TCAs.

Study	Year	Diagnosis	TCA (N/drop out)	Placebo (N/drop out)	Dose (/24 h)	Duration (weeks)	Other therapy	Efficacy	Comments
Taylor et al.	1990	PD	IMI 26 ALP 27	26	IMI 147 mg ALZ 3.7 mg	8	Not given	I = ALZ > P	Drugs not efficacious on panic attacks ALZ > IMI at some measures
Andersch et al.	1991	PD +/− AG	IMI 41 (27%) ALP 41 (5%)	41 (54%)	IMI 170 mg ALZ 4.6 mg	8	Not given	IMI = ALZ > P	Scandinavian sample of the CNCPS
Fahy et al.	1992	PD +/− AG	CMI 27 (33%) LOF 26 (8%)	26 (8%)	CMI 100 mg LOF 140 mg	6	Behavioral counseling 1 h every 1–2 wks	CMI = LOF > P	Short period; concommitant psychotherapy; follow-up protocol 12–24 wk
Modigh et al.	1992	PD +/− AG	CMI 29 (%) IMI 22 (18%)	17 (41%)	CMI 100 mg IMI 124 mg	12	Diazepam max. 15 mg/day	CMI > IMI = P	IMI not better than placebo; reduction of diazeam for CMI
CNCPS	1992	PD +/− AG	IMI 391 (30%) ALZ 386 (17%)	391 (44%)	IMI 155 mg ALP 5.7 mg	8	Not given	IMI = ALZ > P	High proportion of placebo responders
Gentil et al.	1993	PD +/− AG	CMI 20 (12%) IMI 20 (10%)	20 (33%)	CMI 50 mg IMI 141 mg	8	—	CMI > IMI > P	Active placebo, PA not assessed
Nair et al.	1996	PD +/− AG	IMI 42 (31%) FLU 43 (31%)	47 (57%)	IMI (x: 165 mg) FLU (x: 171 mg)	8	Oxazepam chloralhydrate	IMI > FLU = P	By chance fewer PA at baseline
Lecrubier et al.	1997	PD +/− AG	CMI 121 (36%) PAR 33 (27%)	123 (36%)	CMI (range 10–150 mg) PAR (range 10–60 mg)	12	Chloralhydrate p.n.	CMI = PAR > P	High proportion of placebo responders
Wade et al.	1997	PD +/− AG	CMI 98 (26%) CIT 281 (17%)	96 (26%)	CMI (60–90 mg) CIT (10–15/20–30/40–60 mg)	8	Not given	CMI = CIT > P	Phobias not assessed
Caillard et al.	1999	PD	CMI 30–60 mg, 61 (25%) CMI 75–100 mg, 62 (37%)	57 (45%)	CMI 30–60 mg CMI 75–100 mg	8	Not given	CMI > P (both dosages)	Plasma level of active drug was not measured
Barlow et al.	2000	PD	IMI 83* (39%)	24 (58%)	IMI <300 mg (12 wk): 214–349 mg)	12	Benzodiazepines limited use	IMI > P	Panic Disorder Severity Scale, but not for CGI

*Experimental design included more treatment groups.

AG, agoraphobia; ALZ, alprazolam; BUS, busirone; CGI, Clinical Global Improvement; CMI, clomipramine; CIT, citalopram; CNCPS, Cross-National Collaborative Panic Study; FLU, fluvoxamine; IMI, imipramine; LOF, lofepramine; P, placebo; PA, panic attacks; PAR, paroxetine; PD, panic disorder; TCAs, tricyclic antidepressants; ZIM, zimelidine.

compared in an acute treatment phase with a 12-weeks duration and after 6 months of maintenance therapy in responders. The groups were followed up for 6 months after treatment discontinuation. Data from the IMI and the placebo group are shown in Table 19.2. Interestingly, IMI treated patients improved on the Panic Disorder Severity Scale after 3 months, but not on the Clinical Global Scale (CGI) as compared with placebo. However, after 6 months of maintenance, IMI was also significantly better on the CGI suggesting that maximum improvement may require a time period longer than generally studied in controlled trials.

Clomipramine

CMI-paroxetine and citalopram multicenter studies

The SSRIs have been studied extensively in PD (see Chapter 18), but in two large multicenter studies CMI has been included as a reference drug.

Lecrubier *et al.* (1997) compared CMI with paroxetine in a double-blind placebo controlled study and a multicenter study with PD, while Wade *et al.* (1997) studied the effects of the TCA as measured against citalopram. The design, methods and main results are presented in Table 19.3. Studies included a long-term

Table 19.3 Panic disorder. Multicenter studies comparing CMI and SSRIs (paroxetine and citalopram).

	CMI vs. paroxetine: Lecrubier *et al.* (1997)	CMI vs. citalopram: Wade *et al.* (1997)

Design and methodology	DB-pla N : 367
	Flexible dose
	PAR: 20–60 mg
	    10–20 mg: 31%
	    20–40 mg: 37%
	    40–60 mg: 31%
	CMI: 50–150 mg 12 wk
		DB-pla N : 475
		Fixed dose
		CIT: 10–60 mg
		    10–15 mg: 35%
		    20–30 mg: 34%
		    40–60 mg: 32%
		CMI: 60–90 mg 8 wk

Patients	PD 20% PD + AG 75% Female 60% Age 35 yrs	PD 25% PD + AG 75% Female 70% Age 38 yrs

Results	Panic free
	    CMI 37%
	    PAR 51%
	    PLA 32%
	Anxiety symptoms: significant decrease
	Global improvement
	    PAR 46%
	    CMI 36%
	    PLA 24%
	Phobias: significant decrease
		Panic free
		    CMI 50%
		    CIT 57%
		    PLA 30%
		Anxiety symptoms: significant decrease
		Global improvement
		    PAR 41%
		    CMI 39%
		    PLA 21%
		Phobias: not studied

Drop-outs (due to side-effects)	Drop-outs:
	    CMI 27 (15%)
	    PAR 29 (7%)
	    PLA 36 (11%)
		Drop-outs:
		    CMI 26(10%)
		    CIT 18 (7%)
		    PLA 26 (7%)

Long-term study	36 weeks (*N* = 176/367 = 48%); drop-outs 34% Efficacy sustained or increased*	52 weeks (*N* = 279/475 = 59%); drop outs 36% Efficacy sustained or increased†

*Lecrubier *et al.* (1997). †Lepola *et al.* (1997).

AG, agoraphobia; CIT, citalopram; CMI, clomipramine; DB-pla, double-blind placebo-controlled study; PAR, paroxetine; PD, panic disorder; PLA, placebo; SSRIs, specific serotonin reuptake inhibitors.

extension treatment phase. There were some minor differences in methodology, but essentially the same results were obtained in both studies; however, phobic symptoms were not addressed in Wade *et al.* (1997).

In the study of Lecrubier *et al.* (1997), CMI patients improved slowly with respect to panic attacks and the drug was not significantly better than placebo before week 12. Paroxetine had a faster mode of action. When other outcome measures were considered (anxiety, phobia, disability, and others) the active drugs gave better improvement compared to placebo from week 9. There were no significant differences between the active components throughout the trial.

In Wade *et al.* (1997) which compared CMI with citalopram, dosage for CMI was 60–90 mg/day and for citalopram 10–15, 20–30 or 40–60 mg/day. There was an increasing number of panic-free patients in all groups, but the improvement was significantly higher for CMI and citalopram (20–30 and 40–60 mg/day) treated patients. Similar improvements were observed for measures of depressive symptoms.

Number of dropouts and side-effects reported were fairly similar in the two studies (Table 19.3).

It may be argued that relatively low dosages of CMI were applied, especially in the Wade *et al.* (1997) study, but problems concerning adequate CMI-dosages have recently been addressed in a multicenter study.

Clomipramine low/high-dose multicenter study
Caillard *et al.* (1999) studied the efficacy of two doses of CMI (30–60 and 75–100 mg/day) in an 8-week placebo controlled multicenter study (Table 19.2). Several outcome measures were applied. CMI was significantly superior to placebo chiefly but not for all measures. It was concluded that both CMI dose schedules were more efficacious than placebo especially with respect to global improvement, and that the low dose was at least as effective as the high dose, sometimes more so. CMI was well-tolerated, the low dose being better tolerated. It was discussed whether more improvement on phobic symptoms would have been obtained by a longer trial period and higher doses of CMI. The plasma level of active drug was not measured.

Lotufo-Neto *et al.* (2001) treated 81 PD patients with or without agoraphobia with flexible doses of CMI under single-blind conditions. Seventy percent reached full remission in 16.2 ± 6.5 weeks, with a mean dose of 89 ± 8 mg/day. After a maintenance phase (4–6 months) the medication was tappered and discontinued with placebo substitution under double-blind conditions. Sixty-three percent of the patients were followed-up for up to 3 years. Twenty percent remained asymptomatic, 37% experienced a relapse 5.2 ± 4.9 weeks, while 43% experienced recurrence 42.9 ± 35 weeks after discontinuation.

Table 19.2 summarized some major drug trials from the 1990s (Taylor *et al.* 1990; Andersch *et al.* 1991; CNCPS 1992; Fahy *et al.* 1992; Modigh *et al.* 1992; Gentil *et al.* 1993; Nair *et al.* 1996; Lecrubier *et al.* 1997; Wade *et al.* 1997; Caillard *et al.* 1999; Barlow *et al.* 2000).

In summary Although the SSRIs studies focused on the new antidepressants, CMI was included as a reference drug and further support for the efficacy of CMI was obtained in both large studies. It may be argued that the studies were somewhat biased against CMI by fairly low-dose prescription of CMI, but the Caillard *et al.* (1999) study justifies such approach.

Other TCAs

Compared with IMI and CMI much less evidence is available for the clinical efficacy of other TCAs in PD.

Fahy *et al.* (1992) compared CMI with lofepramine in a placebo-controlled trial where some behavioral counseling were also given (Table 19.2). By the end of the acute phase at week 6 a pronounced placebo effect was seen. Forty-two percent had zero panic attacks compared with 67% in the active drug groups. However, on several other outcome measures both drugs were superior to placebo.

Interestingly, no tendency for relapse was noted in the 3 months following taper-off of medication from week 12 to week 24. This is in contrast to a similar study of Clark *et al.* (1994).

Studies applying a much less rigorous design suggest desimipramine (Kalus *et al.* 1991) and nortriptyline (Munjack *et al.* 1988) as efficacious. A double-blind study by Den Boer & Westenberg (1988) is theoretically interesting, as they compared fluvoxamine, a SSRI, and maprotilin, a specific noradrenergic uptake inhibitor. The former drug appears to be potent antipanic agent, while the latter had slight effect on depressive symptoms (cf. Boyer 1995).

Sasson *et al.* (1999) applied a double-blind cross-over comparison of CMI and desimipramine in a

16-week double-blind study including 17 patients with PD. Both drugs led to a significant reduction of panic attacks, but CMI was superior to desimipramine on several ratings of anxiety.

Tolerability and side-effects

The well-known spectrum of side-effects of TCAs (anticholinergic, cardiovascular, and others) may be a major hindrance for their wider applicability in panic patients, who are assumed to be very sensitive to any symptoms imitating anxiety attacks, such as palpitations and tremor. An initial exacerbation of anxiety symptoms has frequently been noticed, and experts advise more gradual dose increase when treating panic patients than is used with depressed patients (Klerman *et al.* 1993). High dropout rates have often been noticed in controlled trials of TCAs. In the CNPCS significantly more patients dropped out in the IMI group (30%) compared with the benzodiazepin alprazolam group (17%), but not in comparison with the placebo group (40%). Low-dose CMI may be sufficient for some patients and is better tolerated than high doses.

Compared with the SSRIs, CMI is also less well-tolerated, but an advocate for CMI could claim that the difference between CMI and the SSRIs are of minor clinical relevance with respect to side-effects.

Discontinuation symptoms have also been described for antidepressants, but have not been observed as a major problem in controlled studies.

Long-term treatment

PD is generally conceived as a chronic and recurrent disabling syndrome. The optimal time to discontinue treatment has not been determined (Lecrubier *et al.* 1997). In a comprehensive review of the course and outcome of panic patients by Roy-Burne and Cowley (1994) it is concluded that while most patients improve by modern treatment, few are cured. The presence of agoraphobia, depression and personality disorders indicated a poorer prognosis. Thus, a majority of patients may require long-term treatment. In a review by Burrows *et al.* (1993) from 1993 it was concluded that long-term treatment with TCA did not lead to loss of efficacy. On drug withdrawal, high rates of relapse were observed. A recent study (Mavissakalian & Perel 1999) reports similar findings.

Katschnig *et al.* (1995) followed up 423 patients from the CNCPS. The mean duration and follow-up was 47 months (range 27–73 months). The course of PD was not uniform. Long duration of illness and severe phobic avoidance at baseline were predictors for an unfavorable course.

It is reassuring that long-term efficacy for CMI and SSRIs was found in the extension phase of the studies by two reviewed SSRI-CMI studies (Lecrubier & Judge 1997; Lepola *et al.* 1998). The therapeutic gain by drug treatment was present during the long-term treatment period and even tended to increase.

In a study by Barlow *et al.* (2000), IMI was compared with cognitive therapy and placebo. Responders of the acute phase were then seen monthly for 6 months (maintenance phase) and then followed up for 6 months after treatment continuation. Six months after discontinuation, response rates decreased for IMI from 60% to 20% indicating that for some patients, continuous drug treatment is required.

In summary Tolerance to TCAs in PD has not been a major problem. In contrast, greater improvement may be expected by a longer treatment period. However, continuous treatment may be required for patients with long duration of illness and phobic avoidance.

Optimizing TCA treatment

A dose of 150–200 mg of IMI is assumed to be the most appropriate initial target dose, but as in the treatment of depression plasma, monitoring antidepressants should have a more prominent role in the future considering the genetic polymorphism for cytochrome P450 isozymes (Meyer *et al.* 1996).

There is evidence that some patients may improve on low dose (10–50 mg) CMI treatment (Gloger *et al.* 1989; Modigh 1989; Caillard *et al.* 1999). The presence of agoraphobia may require higher dosages (Gloger *et al.* 1989). Plasma levels of CMI have seldom been applied. Modigh *et al.* (1992) compared IMI and CMI, but found no significant relations between plasma concentrations of IMI or CMI or their metabolites in relation to clinical response. Marcourakis *et al.* (1999) have reported relationships between improvement and ratios of CMI/dose and desmethylclomipramine. Thus, further studies are needed.

Mavissakalian and Perel (1995) have published an 8-week, double-blind placebo controlled dose-ranging trial in 80 panic patients with agoraphobia. They used weight-adjusted doses of IMI: (low) 0.5 mg/kg/day, (medium) 1.5 mg/kg/day, or (high) 3.0 mg/kg/day. Plasma levels of IMI and N-methylimipramine and response to treatment were ascertained after 4 and 8 weeks. There was a significant positive dose–response relationship. For phobias, the best total drug plasma levels were in the range of 110–140 mg/mL. Higher doses had a detrimental effect. For PD, improvement was observed by increasing dose, but rendered no improvement beyond 140 mg/mL.

A predictor analysis (Mavissakalian & Perel 1996) of the data for the plasma concentrations of IMI, desmethylimipramine and total drug concentration demonstrated that IMI and total drug concentration were better predictors of most outcome measures considered than desmethylimipramine. As this major metabolite has higher noradrenergic affinity than IMI, the author suggests that the antipanic and antiphobic activities are predominantly mediated by serotonergic mechanisms (cf. Den Boer & Westenberg 1988; Boyer 1995).

An important clinical implication is that drug efficacy may decrease by increasing total plasma concentration indicating the existence of a "therapeutic window." If replicated in future studies, this finding is further support for using therapeutic drug monitoring in optimizing TCA treatment of PD.

Conclusion

Among the TCAs, IMI and CMI have been most extensively studied. Both drugs are efficacious in the treatment of PD, and patients benefit across most important clinical aspects, including panic attacks, anticipatory anxiety and phobic avoidance behavior. This improvement is not dependent on the treatment of concurrent affective symptoms.

CMI is suggested to be more efficacious than IMI indicating that drugs with predominantly serotonergic affinity may be clinically more efficacious in the treatment of PD. Panic patients may be especially sensitive to the well-known spectrum of side-effects of the drugs, which may limit their role in the long-term treatment of a chronic disorder. Low-dose efficacy has been demonstrated for clomipramine with better tolerance.

In studies comparing CMI with SSRIs some differences in efficacy and side-effects in favor of the SSRIs (paroxetine and citalopram) have been found, but the clinical relevance hereof might be questioned.

Obsessive-compulsive disorder

Introduction

Obsessive-compulsive disorder (OCD) has been considered a rare and chronically disabling illness. Recent epidemiological research applying modern diagnostic criteria has found that the prevalence of the disorder is higher than previously estimated (Pélissolo *et al.* 1998: see also Chapter 6). The strikingly low placebo response established in early studies (e.g., The Clomipraine Collaborative Study Group 1991) has not subsequently been consistently corroborated (Zohar & Judge 1996), which indicates that OCD may follow courses of varying severity. Nevertheless, in the treatment of OCD antidepressant drug treatment is considered a major breakthrough. The pharmacological outcome literature of OCD can be divided into four phases: (i) open studies in the 1970s, (ii) smaller controlled studies published in the 1980s, (iii) two major multicenter studies of the efficacy of CMI, the most serotonergic TCA, at the beginning of the 1990s, and, (iv) several recent SSRI-studies which have questioned the claim of CMI as a drug of first choice in OCD treatment.

Studies from the 1980s

According to Liebowitz *et al.* (1988) and Montgomery *et al.* (1998) the benefit of CMI in OCD was initially demonstrated in the late 1960s and affirmed in several open studies in the 1970s. According to the seminal review of Liebowitz *et al.* (1988) at least 10 controlled studies published in the 1980s started the use of TCA in Diagnostic Statistical Manual, 3rd edition (DSM III: American Psychiatric Association 1980) anxiety disorders. This is supported by a more recent meta-analysis of the efficacy of drug treatment by Piccinelli *et al.* (1995). CMI has been compared with nortriptyline, desimipramine, amitriptyline and IMI in studies of small sample size ($N = 19–24$), and typical short duration (i.e., 4–6 weeks) (Piccinelli *et al.* 1995). Placebo control was not used consistently. Nevertheless, evidence of the efficacy of CMI was obtained on obsessional and compulsory symptoms, as well as on concomitant anxiety and depression.

Furthermore, it was suggested early on that CMI was more efficacious than other TCAs involving less affinity for serotonergic reuptake proteins, although such a difference was not demonstrated in all studies (Liebowitz *et al.* 1988). Based on a meta-analysis of eight trials testing CMI against TCAs with no selective serotonergic activity, including the monoamine oxidase inhibitors (MAOIs) clorgyline and phenelzine, Picinelli *et al.* (1995) concluded that CMI was superior to other antidepressants on obsessive-compulsive symptoms considered together with anxiety, depression and global clinical improvement. In psychosocial adjustment no difference was obtained.

In the 1980s it was often debated whether the efficacy of the TCAs was attributable to their antidepressant activity or to a specific effect on obsessional and compulsory symptoms (The Clomipramine Collaborative Study Group 1991).

Multicenter studies in the 1990s

The Clomipramine Collaborative Study Group published an important paper on two double-blind studies at 21 centers evaluating the therapeutic efficacy, safety, and tolerance of up to 300 mg/day of CMI in 520 patients with OCD diagnosed according to DSM-III (The Clomipramine Collaborative Study Group 1991). It was a placebo-controlled study applying standardized outcome measures of obsessions and compulsions (Yale-Brown Obsessive Compulsive Scale [Y-BOCS], National Institutes of Mental Health [NIMH] Global Scale, and the Hamilton Rating Scale for Depression [HAM-D]) to control for concomitant depressive symptoms. After a 2- to 4-week washout period patients entered a 2-week single-blind placebo period. During the following 10 weeks, patients with qualifying scores on these scales were randomly assigned to either CMI or placebo. Qualifying score was >15 on Y-BOCS at three weekly assessments (maximum score 15), >6 on the NIMH Global Scale (range of clinical OCD 7–15), and <17 on the 17-item HAM-D.

Two-hundred and thirty-nine patients with a duration of OCD for at least 2 years entered Study I, while 281, who had been ill for at least 1 year, were included in Study II. The patients had all had OCD for a long time (mean 14–16 years). Mean scores on the HAM-D were 6–7 in the two studies reassuring that concomitant depressive symptoms were not prevalent.

The two studies gave almost identical results for the major outcome scales demonstrating a pronounced effect of CMI and weak placebo response. The mean response was thus a reduction in Y-BOCS scores of 38% and 44% in Studies I and II, respectively, in comparison with 3% and 5% for placebo treated patients. Statistically significant differences were obtained

from week 1–2 through week 10. The efficacy of CMI increased almost linearly through the trial. The time course of improvement was similar for scores on the NIMH Global Scale, but shortly after statistically significant differences were obtained (week 2 Study I, week 5 Study II). At the visits later on in the trial, when compared with 10% in the placebo group, 55% of patients treated with CMI considered themselves as much or very much improved and the physicians gave similar ratings. Half of the CMI-treated patients had NIMH global scores in the normal or subclinical range.

Because of a forced titration schedule the studies did not permit determination of the optimum daily dosage, but for the majority of patients maximum dosage ranged from 150 to 250 mg/day. Well-known anticholinergic side-effects were seen more often in the CMI group, but it was concluded that CMI was well-tolerated. Temporary elevation of some hepatic enzymes was observed in 18 patients taking CMI compared to only one in the placebo group. Seizures were seen in one CMI-treated patient and in three other patients during the 1 year continuation study. Among the CMI-treated patients, 9% discontinued prematurely as compared with 2% in the placebo group.

The study was followed up by a 1-year double-blind extension phase. The number of CMI patients fulfilling the 1-year period was sufficient to suggest that the efficacy was maintained or even increased (Katz *et al.* 1990).

The importance of this study is evident for several reasons. It included (i) substantially larger samples of patients than previous studies, (ii) only nondepressed patients were included, and, (iii) standardized assessment on target symptoms was applied.

In summary In OCD treatment CMI is efficacious in a clinically meaningful sense. High dosages, up to 300 mg/day administered over 10 weeks or more, may be required to optimize drug efficacy. Efficacy is maintained through continued treatment for at least 1 year. Based on such firm evidence, CMI has for a long time been considered a reference drug for OCD. The multicenter studies indicated that OCD is a disorder with no response to placebo. Furthermore, serotonergic theories on OCD were strongly supported.

The SSRI era

Treatment of OCD with SSRIs is thoroughly reviewed in Chapter 18, but part of the literature will be addressed in the following in order to clarify the future role of CMI in the SSRI era.

Meta-analyses

With the documentation of the efficacy of SSRIs in OCD, several meta-analyses have addressed the clinically important question regarding the relative efficacy and tolerance of serotonergic reuptake inhibitors (SRIs). Greist *et al.* (1995) compared the results from four large multicenter placebo controlled trials which used similar, although not identical designs including Y-BOCS and CGI as outcome measures. The above-mentioned multicenter CMI study ($N = 520$) was compared with studies on fluoxetine ($N = 355$), fluvoxamine ($N = 320$) and sertraline ($N = 325$). All four drugs were decisively better than placebo with CMI being significantly more effective than the remaining three from which no difference in effect size was found.

Surprisingly, the total dropout rate (side-effect plus lack of efficacy) was significantly lower for CMI than for each of the other compounds. There were no significant differences in dropouts caused by side-effects

(CMI, 8%; fluoxetine 12%; fluvoxamine, 15%; and sertraline, 10%).

Summarizing six meta-analyses of pharmacological and psychological treatment (Greist *et al.* 1995; Piccinelli *et al.* 1995; Stein *et al.* 1995; Abramowitz 1997; Kobak *et al.* 1998; van Balkom *et al.* 1998), Kobak *et al.* (1998) were stricken by the relative consistency in the order of effect sizes for the SRI. Their analysis was thus consistent with previous meta-analyses suggesting that CMI stood out from the rest of the SRIs in terms of clinical efficacy (Table 19.4). Similar advantages for CMI have been suggested for depressed in-patients (Vestergaard *et al.* 1993).

It has been suggested that patients with OCD are less sensitive to TCA side-effects as they suffer from an incapacitating disorder (The Clomipramine Collaborative Study Group 1991). Based on meta-analytical evidence CMI was suggested to be more efficacious than SSRIs. If so, it may still be a reference drug in the SSRI era. However, when reading meta-analyses caution must be taken (Fallon *et al.* 1998) and to decide on the relative efficacy of drugs treatment a head-to-head

Table 19.4 OCD. Some meta-analysis of serotonergic drugs. (Modified after Kobak *et al.* 1998.)

Study	Kobak *et al.* (1998)	Abramowitz (1997)	Greist *et al.* (1995)	Stein *et al.* (1995)	Piccinelli *et al.* (1995)	van Balkom (1994)
No. of studies	77	32	4	30	36	56
Year (range)	1973–1997	1975–1995	1986–1991	1988–1994	1975–1994	1970–1993
Drug						
CMI	1.11	1.31	1.48	1.71	1.41	1.46
FLX	0.86	0.68	0.83	1.39	0.57	1.39
FLU	0.79	1.28	0.50	1.14	0.57	1.18
SER	0.52	0.37	0.45	0.77	0.52	0.45
PAR	0.56	N/a	N/a	N/a	N/a	N/a
SSRIs (mean)	0.68	0.78	0.59	1.10	0.55	1.01
Comments	Studies not excluded due to poor methodology; drugs also compared to behavior therapy	Only randomized studies with multiple treatment or control groups	Four large multicenter placebo controlled studies	Studies with single medication of >6 wk duration and no concomitant psychotherapy	Randomized double-blind drug trials in peer-reviewed journals	Studies with antidepressants and/or psychotherapy

CMI, clomipramine; FLU, fluvoxamine; FLX, fluoxetine; OCD, obsessive-compulsive disorder; PAR, paroxetine; SER, sertraline; SSRIs, specific serotonin reuptake inhibitors.

comparison in the same study is needed (Montgomery *et al.* 1998).

Direct comparison of CMI and SSRIs

Between 1990 and 1997, several studies comparing CMI and fluoxetine, fluvoxamine and sertraline were published (Freeman *et al.* 1994; Koran *et al.* 1996; Lopez-Ibor *et al.* 1996; Zohar & Judge 1996; Bisserbe *et al.* 1997). Some studies including a substantial number of patients are presented in Table 19.5. Similar efficacy was found for all drugs studied. A placebo group was included in the study of Zohar and Judge (1996). Interestingly, a much larger placebo response was observed in comparison with the classical 1991 study of CMI (The Clomipramine Collaborative Study Group 1991). Thus, a reduction of 25% or more in total Y-BOCS scores by CMI, paroxetine and placebo were obtained by 55%, 55% and 35%, respectively.

Table 19.5 also shows dropout rates, reported adverse effects and the percentage of patients who dropped out due to side-effects. Marked differences were not observed between the drugs. In general, CMI-treated patients made complaints of anticholinergic or hypotensive symptoms, while patients on SSRIs reported higher frequencies of insomnia and nervousness. In a meta-analysis of 62 randomized controlled trials, including 6029 patients with major depression (Anderson & Tomenson 1995), SSRIs were reported to be somewhat better tolerated as is also evidenced by dropout rates caused by side-effects. However, the clinical relevance of the overall fairly small difference was questioned.

Affective comorbidity

In order to address the important question of drug efficacy in patients with significant comorbidity, Hoehn-Saric *et al.* (2000) have studied the efficacy in patients selected to have concurrent OCD and major depressive disorder (MDD). Sertraline (up to 200 mg/day) was compared with desimipramine (up to 300 mg/day) over 12 weeks. The SSRI was more effective in reducing both OCD and MDD symptoms than desimipramine (a primarily noradrenergic reuptake inhibitor). Sertraline had a milder spectrum of side-effects. This study demonstrates that sertraline is efficacious in patients with OCD and MDD, i.e., in two highly comorbid disorders. Interestingly, the noradrenergic drug was less potent even with respect to depressive symptoms.

Route of administration

CMI is the only SRI available for intravenous injection. Clinically significant improvement in drug treatment of OCD usually takes about 6 weeks, and one cannot predict which patient will respond to treatment. Koran *et al.* (1998) have used an intravenous pulse loading of CMI in a small study of 15 patients in a randomized double-blind placebo controlled trial. Interestingly, evidence was obtained that intravenous pulse loadings led to a faster rate of improvement, and the authors suggest that this route of administration may be valuable, especially for patients who have failed oral treatment trials. Salle *et al.* (1998) have reported growth hormone after the intravenous CMI challenge predicted response to treatment after 8 weeks. These interesting studies need replications.

Plasma concentrations

Mavissakalien *et al.* (1990) have reported that OCD responders had significantly higher CMI plasma levels and a trend toward lower desmethylclomipramine/CMI ratios.

Conclusion

Due to its marked effects on core symptoms, CMI from the early 1990s has been considered a reference drug for OCD treatment. The improvement is not a consequence of its antidepressive efficacy. As in PD, CMI is considered more efficacious than other TCAs. However, its role is questioned by the appearance of the SSRIs as evidence of greater therapeutic efficacy of CMI demonstrated in meta-analyses has not been confirmed in a head-to-head comparison studies. Furthermore, SSRIs have a better profile with respect to side-effects and safety.

Generalized anxiety disorder

The efficacy of TCAs in generalized anxiety disorder (GAD) has been less frequently studied than has been the case with PD and OCD. In evaluation of the literature it should be emphasized that diagnostic criteria for GAD have changed from DSM-III to DSM-IV (American Psychiatric Association 1994), so that worry (apprehensive expectation) now has a prominent role

Table 19.5 OCD. Comparison of clomipramine with other SSRIs.

Study	Year	Diagnosis	Drug (N/drop-out)	Placebo (N/drop-out)	Dose (/24 h)	Duration (weeks)	Adverse effect	Efficacy
Freeman et al.	1994	OCD No depression	CMI 30 (37%) FLU 32 (19%)	No	CMI (100–250 mg) FLU (100–250 mg)	10	Reported CMI 80% FLU 88% Withdrawn CMI 13% FLU 16%	CMI = FLU
López-Ibor et al.	1996	OCD No depression	CMI 25 (16%) FLX 30 (16%)	No	CMI 150 mg FLX 40 mg	8	Reported CMI > 10% FLX > 10% Withdrawn CMI 4% FLX 3.3%	CMI > FLX (response rate) CMI = FLX (rating scales)
Koran et al.	1996	OCD No depression	CMI 42 (36%) FLU 37 (23%)	No	CMI (100–250 mg) FLU (100–300 mg)	12	Reported CMI > 10% FLU > 10% Withdrawn CMI 17% FLU 14%	CMI = FLU
Zohar & Judge	1996	OCD No depression	CMI 99 (34%) PAR 201 (24%)	PLA 99 (39%)	CMI (50–250 mg) PAR (20–60 mg)	12	Reported CMI: 81% PAR: 86% PLA: 79% Withdrawn CMI: 17% PAR: 9% PLA: 6%	CMI = PAR > P
Bisserbe et al.	1997	OCD <18 HAM-D	CMI 82 (43%) SER 86 (27%)	No	CMI (105 mg) SER (135 mg)	16	Reported CMI: 70% SER: 65% Withdrawn CMI: 26% SER: 11%	SER = CMI SER > CMI (16 wk)

ALP, alprazolam; BUS, buspirone; CMI, clomipramine; FLU, fluvoxamine; FLX, fluoxetine; HAM-D, Hamilton Rating Scale for Depression; IMI, imipramine; OCD, obsessive-compulsive disorder; P, placebo; PAR, paroxetine; SER, sertraline; SSRIs, specific serotonin reuptake inhibitors; ZIM, zimelidine.

among diagnostic criteria. In recent years, the validity of GAD as a diagnostic entity has been thoroughly discussed (Brown 1997; Barlow & Wincze 1998; Judd *et al.* 1998).

Among early studies from 1974 to 1986 reviewed by Liebowitz *et al.* (1988) and Johnstone *et al.* (1980) demonstrated a significant effect of amitriptyline on anxiety and depressive symptoms in a large group of neurotic patients. The efficacy of the antidepressant was not different from that of diazepam. In a large placebo-controlled comparison of IMI and chlordiazepoxide antianxiety effects of IMI was by the 2nd week increasingly better as compared with those of benzodiazepine (Kahn *et al.* 1986). Even when excluding patients with panic-phobic symptoms, this still demonstrated superior antianxiety effects of IMI.

Hoehn-Saric *et al.* (1988) studied a group of patients with a DSM-III diagnosis GAD (N = 60). Alprazolam was compared with IMI in 6 weeks applying a flexible dosage schedule. The benzodiazepine was more effective during early treatment, but after 2 weeks both drugs were equally effective. However, the benzodiazepine was suggested to be more effective in attenuating somatic symptoms, while IMI in comparison had an enhanced effect on psychic symptoms, such as dysphoria and negative anticipatory thinking. It was concluded that patients with chronic worries obtain better results on antidepressants than on benzodiazepine. This study is of special interest in view of the criteria for GAD in DSM-IV.

Similar findings were reported in an 8-week placebo controlled study of Rickels *et al.* (1993) who compared IMI (mean 143 mg/day), trazodone (255 mg/day) and diazepam (25 mg/day) in 230 patients with a DSM-III diagnosis of GAD. Psychic symptoms such as tensions, apprehension and worry were more responsive to the antidepressants. Surprisingly, no difference in attrition was observed, but with the exception of drowsiness, both antidepressants caused more side-effects than diazepam. Significant improvements were not notable for the antidepressants until the 3rd week of treatment.

Rocca *et al.* (1997) compared IMI with chlordesmethyldiazepam and paroxetine in 81 patients with a DSM-IV diagnosis of GAD. A similar picture appeared. The benzodiazepine led to fast improvement, but after the 4th week more improvements were seen among patients treated with the antidepressants. These drugs administered later on predominantly affected psychic symptoms and, as the benzodiazepine had more effect on somatic symptoms, Hoehn-Saric *et al.* (1988) have

suggested that somatic symptoms and hyperarousal respond to drugs acting on the γ-aminobutyric acid (GABA) system, whereas psychic symptoms respond to treatment affecting the noradrenergic or serotonergic symptom.

In summary In spite of the few controlled trials in GAD, a consistent picture has emerged demonstrating antianxiety efficacy of the TCAs studied, especially on those psychic symptoms that in DSM-IV are mandatory for the diagnosis of GAD. As for most other anxiety disorders, improvement is gradual with significant effect after about 3 weeks.

Post-traumatic stress disorder

There has been growing interest in drug treatment of post-traumatic stress disorder (PTSD) as the course is often chronic and leads to disability (Ballenger *et al.* 2000; Kessler 2000). Theories on the neurobiology of the disorder (Charney *et al.* 1993; Nutt 2000) suggest various mechanisms by which drugs may benefit PTSD patients.

In the 1980s it was suggested that antidepressants might benefit patients with PTSD, but there have been few placebo-controlled studies of PTSD. Frank *et al.* (1988) published a double-blind randomized trial on the effect of IMI (N = 12) and phenelzine (N = 11) in 34 male veterans with PTSD. Both drugs significantly improved PTSD symptoms, especially the more specific anxiety symptoms assessed by the Impact of Event Scale, a scale focusing on symptoms specific to PTSD, and particularly for phenelzine.

In 1990, Davidson *et al.* (1990) published an 8-week trial where amitriptyline (50–300 mg/day) was compared with placebo in 46 veterans with chronic PTSD. Efficacy was measured both by observer and self-rated scales. Patients who completed 4 weeks (N = 40) improved more with amitriptyline on the HAM-D. In the group completing 8 weeks of treatment (n = 33), the drug was superior to placebo on HAM-D, HAM-A, CGI Severity, and Impact of Event Scales. However, at the end of treatment, 64% of the amitriptyline and 72% of the placebo samples still met the diagnostic criteria for PTSD. Drug-placebo differences were greater in the presence of comorbidity in general, although recovery rates were uniformly low in the presence of major depression, PD, and alcoholism.

An extension of this study was published in 1993 (Davidson *et al.* 1993). At this point, 62 patients had entered the trial, and, as expected, drug improvement on the above mentioned scales was substantiated. Better response to amitriptyline was observed on several items from the scales, including depressed mood, insomnia, anorexia, loss of libido and hypochondriases. From the self-rated Impact of Event Scale the symptom "pictures about it keep popping into my mind" also responded better to the drug. Overall 14 patients responded to amitriptyline, whereas 15 failed. Drug response was related to lower baseline levels of depression, neuroticism, combat intensity, anxious mood, impaired concentration, somatic symptoms, feeling of guilt, and one intrusion and four avoidance symptoms of PTSD. Similar relationships were not observed in the placebo group indicating a specific drug effect.

Kosten *et al.* (1991) compared IMI (50–300 mg/day, $N = 23$), phenelzine (15–75 mg/day, $N = 19$) and placebo ($N = 18$) in an 8-week trial of male veterans. By week 5, both drugs significantly reduced PTSD symptoms as assessed by the Impact of Event Scale, but IMI gave less improvement (25%) than phenelzine (44%), and only on the intrusion subscale, not the avoidance subscale. Anxiety measured by the Covi Scale did not improve. Overall IMI appeared to be less effective than the MAOI. Neither depressive symptoms nor simple antidepressive effect were suggested to be accountable for treatment results. The role of noradrenergic-specific drugs is questionable (Ballenger *et al.* 2000).

Davidson *et al.* (1997) have reviewed seven placebo-controlled trials including different antidepressants in the treatment of both combat and noncombat patients with PTSD. Interestingly, drug response rates in both groups appeared similar, but placebo response rated was suggested low in combat veterans, but high among civilians.

In summary Although some efficacy for TCAs has been shown in PTSD, controlled studies are few, and recent studies have focused on the SSRIs (see Chapter 18). The future role of the TCAs will depend on results from future trials comparing TCAs and more recent antidepressants.

Social phobia

Surprisingly, no placebo-controlled study with TCAs has been performed on patients with social phobia (Ballenger *et al.* 1998) in contrast to studies with other antidepressants, such as MAOI (Versiani 2000) and, recently, SSRIs (Stein *et al.* 1998; Allgulander 1999). Among the reasons for this, may be that trials in the 1980s and the 1990s focused on PD and OCD, and that the growing evidence for the diagnostic validity of social phobia has coincided with the appearance of the SSRIs and other new antidepressants.

However, social phobia is a disorder that is highly comorbid with other anxiety disorders, for instance PD. As TCA treatment typically lead to improvement of most symptoms, it would be reasonable to assume that TCAs may benefit social phobic symptoms, as well as worry and other affective symptoms which often incapacitate patients with social phobia. As for PTSD, the future role of the TCAs will depend on results from future trials comparing TCAs and more recent antidepressants.

Conclusion

The group of classical TCAs has had an important position in the psychopharmacological treatment and for the pathophysiological conceptions of anxiety disorders. An extensive body of evidence testifies to their efficacy in the treatment of PD and OCD, but support for therapeutic efficacy is available for other anxiety disorders except for social phobia. The effect on anxiety symptoms is not secondary to amelioration of depressive symptoms.

Evidence suggests that CMI is more efficacious than other TCAs and it is tempting to attribute this to CMI's higher affinity for the serotonin transport. In the 1990s CMI obtained the status of a drug of reference in OCD. Interestingly, evidence from a meta-analysis has suggested that CMI is more efficacious than the SSRIs. However, direct comparison of the serotonergic drug has not substantiated this finding.

The disadvantages of the TCAs are their well-known side-effects (especially anticholinergic) and toxicity in overdose. However, although the lower tolerance of the TCAs is often stated to be a major disadvantage in comparison with new antidepressants, especially the SSRIs, the latter compounds are far from free from side-effects. In terms of empirical evidence, such as reported side-effects and dropout rates, the differences are in favor of the SSRIs, but many studies do not report striking differences between TCAs and more recent antidepressants. Nevertheless, there is general consensus that the SSRIs have a more favorable safety (Thoren *et al.* 1980; Montgomery *et al.* 1998) profile. Furthermore, during treatment depressed patients on SSRIs are more likely to complete a course of adequate dose and duration than patients who initiate therapy on a TCA (Donoghue 2000).

However, it would be premature to conclude that the role of the TCAs, such as that of the CMI, has been completely defined. In a world with comprehensive biological variations among human beings it may be wise to have drugs with broader pharmacodynamic profiles than the new antidepressants, such as the SSRIs.

References

Abramowitz, J.S. (1997) Effectiveness of psychological and pharmacological treatments for obsessive-compulsive disorder: a quantitative review. *J Consult Clin Psychol* **65**(1), 44–52.

Allgulander, C. (1999) Paroxetine in social anxiety disorder: a randomized placebo-controlled study. *Acta Psychiatr Scand* **100**(3), 193–8.

American Psychiatric Association (1980) *Diagnostic Statistical Manual of Mental Disorders*, 3rd edn. American Psychiatric Association, Washington, D.C.

American Psychiatric Association (1994) *Diagnostic Statistical Manual of Mental Disorders*, 4th edn. American Psychiatric Association, Washington, D.C.

Andersch, S., Ottosson, J.-O., Bech, P. *et al.* (1991) Efficacy and safety of alprazolam, imipramine, and placebo in the treatment of panic disorder. *Acta Psychiatr Scand* **83** (Suppl. 365), 18–27.

Anderson, I.M. & Tomenson, B.M. (1995) Treatment discontinuation with selective serotonin reuptake inhibitors compared with tricyclic antidepressants: a meta-analysis. *BMJ* **310**, 1433–8.

Balestrieri, M., Ruggeri, M. & Bellantuono, C. (1989) Drug treatment of panic disorder—a critical review of controlled clinical trials. *Psychiatr Dev* **4**, 337–50.

Ballenger, J.C. (1999) Current treatments of the anxiety disorders in adults. *Biol Psychiatry* **46**(11), 1579–94.

Ballenger, J.C., Davidson, J.R., Lecrubier, Y. *et al.* (1998) Consensus statement on social anxiety disorder from the International Consensus Group on Depression and Anxiety. *J Clin Psychiatry* **59** (Suppl. 17), 54–60.

Ballenger, J.C., Davidson, J.R., Lecrubier, Y. *et al.* (2000) Consensus statement on post-traumatic stress disorder from the International Consensus Group on Depression and Anxiety. *J Clin Psychiatry* **61** (Suppl. 5), 60–6.

Barlow, D.H., Gorman, J.M., Shear, M.K. & Woods, S.W. (2000) Cognitive-behavioral therapy, imipramine, or their combination for panic disorder: a randomized controlled trial. *JAMA* **283**(19), 2529–36.

Barlow, D.H. & Wincze, J. (1998) DSM-IV and beyond: what is generalized anxiety disorder? *Acta Psychiatr Scand Suppl* **393**, 23–9.

Bisserbe, J.C., Lane, R.M., Flament, M.F. & Franco–Belgian OCD Study Group (1997) A double-blind comparison of sertraline and clompramine in outpatients with obsessive-compulsive disorder. *Eur Psychiatry* **12**, 82–93.

Boyer, W. (1995) Serotonin uptake inhibitors are superior to imipramine and alprazolam in alleviating panic attacks: a meta-analysis. *Int Clin Psychopharmacol* **10**(1), 45–9.

Brown, T.A. (1997) The nature of generalized anxiety disorder and pathological worry: current evidence and conceptual models. *Can J Psychiatry* **42**, 817–25.

Burrows, G.D., Judd, F.K. & Norman, T.R. (1993) Long-term drug treatment of panic disorder. *J Psychiatr Res* **27** (Suppl. 1), 111–25.

Caillard, V., Rouillon, F., Viel, J.F. & Markabi, S. (1999) Comparative effects of low and high doses of clomipramine and placebo in panic disorder: a double-blind controlled study. *Acta Psychiatr Scand* **99**(1), 51–8.

Charney, D.S., Deutch, A.Y., Krystal, J.H., Southwick, S.M. & Davis, M. (1993) Psychobiologic mechanisms of post-traumatic stress disorder. *Arch Gen Psychiatry* **50**, 295–305.

Clark, D.M., Salkovskis, P.M., Hackmann, A., Middleton, H., Anastasiades, P. & Gelder, M. (1994) A comparison of cognitive therapy, applied relaxation and imipramine in the treatment of panic disorder. *Br J Psychiatry* **164**, 759–69.

Clomipramine Collaborative Study Group (The) (1991) Clomipramine in the treatment of patients with obsessive-compulsive disorder. The Clomipramine Collaborative Study Group [see comments]. *Arch Gen Psychiatry* **48**, 730–8.

Coplan, J.D. & Lydiard, R.B. (1998) Brain circuits in panic disorder. *Biol Psychiatry* **44**, 1264–76.

Cross-National Collaborative Panic Study (CNCPS) (1992) Drug treatment of panic disorder. Comparative efficacy of alprazolam, imipramine, and placebo. *Br J Psychiatry* **160**, 191–202.

Davidson, J.R., Kudler, H.S., Saunders, W.B. *et al.* (1993) Predicting response to amitriptyline in post-traumatic stress disorder. *Am J Psychiatry* **150**(7), 1024–9.

Davidson, J., Kudler, H., Smith, R. *et al.* (1990) Treatment of post-traumatic stress disorder with amitriptyline and placebo. *Arch Gen Psychiatry* **47**, 259–66.

Davidson, J.R., Malik, M.L. & Sutherland, S.N. (1997) Response characteristics to antidepressants and placebo in post-traumatic stress disorder. *Int Clin Psychopharmacol* **12**(6), 291–6.

Deltito, J.A., Argyle, N. & Klerman, G.L. (1991) Patients with panic disorder unaccompanied by depression improve with alprazolam and imipramine treatment. *J Clin Psychiatry* 52, 121–7.

Den Boer, J.A. & Westenberg, H.G. (1988) Effect of a serotonin and noradrenaline uptake inhibitor in panic disorder: a double-blind comparative study with fluvoxamine and maprotiline. *Int Clin Psychopharmacol* 3(1), 59–74.

Donoghue, J. (2000) Antidepressant use patterns in clinical practices: comparisons among tricyclic antidepressants and selective serotonin reuptake inhibitors. *Acta Psychiatr Scand Suppl* 403, 57–61.

Fahy, T.J., O'Rourke, D., Brophy, J., Schazmann, W., Sciascia, S. (1992) The Galway Study of Panic Disorder. I. Clomipramine and lofepramine in DSM-III-R panic disorder: a placebo-controlled trial. *Journal of Affect Disord* 25, 63–75.

Fallon, B.A., Liebowitz, M.R., Campeas, R. *et al.* (1998) Intravenous clomipramine for obsessive-compulsive disorder refractory to oral clomipramine: a placebo-controlled study. *Arch Gen Psychiatry* 55(10), 918–24.

Frank, J.B., Kosten, T.R., Giller, E.L. & Dan, E. (1988) A randomized clinical trial of phenelzine and imipramine for post-traumatic stress disorder. *Am J Psychiatry* 145, 1289–91.

Freeman, C.P., Trimble, M.R., Deakin, J.F., Stokes, T.M. & Ashford, J.J. (1994) Fluvoxamine versus clomipramine in the treatment of obsessive-compulsive disorder: a multicenter, randomized, double-blind, parallel group comparison. *J Clin Psychiatry* 55(7), 301–5.

Gentil, V., Lotufo-Neto, F., Andrade, L. *et al.* (1993) Clomipramine, a better reference drug for panic/agoraphobia. I. Effectiveness comparison with imipramine. *J Psychopharmacol* 7, 316–24.

Gloger, S., Grunhaus, L., Gladic, D., O'Ryan, F., Cohen, L. & Codner, S. (1989) Panic attacks and agoraphobia: low-dose clomipramine treatment. *J Clin Psychopharmacol* 9(1), 28–32.

Goddard, A.W. & Charney, D.S. (1997) Toward an integrated neurobiology of panic disorder. *J Clin Psychiatry* 58 (Suppl. 2), 4–11.

Gould, R.A., Otto, M.W. & Pollack, M.H. (1995) A meta-analysis of treatment outcome for panic disorder. *Clin Psychol Rev* 15, 819–44.

Greist, J.H., Jefferson, J.W., Kobak, K.A., Katzelnick, D.J. & Serlin, R.C. (1995) Efficacy and tolerability of serotonin transport inhibitors in obsessive-compulsive disorder. A meta-analysis. *Arch Gen Psychiatry* 52(1), 53–60.

Hoehn-Saric, R., McLeod, D.R. & Zimmerli, W.D. (1988) Differential effects of alprazolam and imipramine in generalized anxiety disorder: somatic versus psychic symptoms. *J Clin Psychiatry* 49(8), 293–301.

Hoehn-Saric, R., Ninan, P., Black, D.W. *et al.* (2000) Multicenter double-blind comparison of sertraline and desipramine for concurrent obsessive-compulsive and major depressive disorders. *Arch Gen Psychiatry* 57(1), 76–82.

Johnstone, E.C., Owens, D.G., Frith, C.D. *et al.* (1980) Neurotic illness and its response to anxiolytic and antidepressant treatment. *Psychol Med* 10(2), 321–8.

Judd, L.L., Kessler, R.C., Paulus, M.P., Zeller, P.V., Wittchen, H.U. & Kunovac, J.L. (1998) Comorbidity as a fundamental feature of generalized anxiety disorders: results from the National Comorbidity Study (NCS). *Acta Psychiatr Scand Suppl* 393, 6–11.

Kahn, R.J., McNair, D.M., Lipman, R.S. *et al.* (1986) Imipramine and chlordiazepoxide in depressive and anxiety disorders. II. Efficacy in anxious outpatients. *Arch Gen Psychiatry* 43(1), 79–85.

Kalus, O., Asnis, G.M., Rubinson, E. *et al.* (1991) Desipramine treatment in panic disorder. *J Affect Disord* 21, 239–44.

Katschnig, H., Amering, M., Stolk, J.M. *et al.* (1995) Long-term follow-up after a drug trial for panic disorder. *Br J Psychiatry* 167(4), 487–94.

Katz, R.J., DeVeaugh-Geiss, J. & Landau, P. (1990) Clomipramine in obsessive-compulsive disorder. *Biol Psychiatry* 28(5), 401–14.

Kessler, R.C. (2000) Post-traumatic stress disorder: the burden to the individual and to society. *J Clin Psychiatry* 61 (Suppl. 5), 4–12.

Klein, D.F. (1964) Delineation of two drug-responsive anxiety syndromes. *Psychopharmacologia* 5, 397–408.

Klein, D.F. (1981) Anxiety reconceptualized. In: *Anxiety: New Research and Changing Concepts* (D.F. Klein & J. Rabkin (eds), pp. 235–63). Raven Press, New York.

Klein, D.F. (2000) Flawed meta-analyses comparing psychotherapy with pharmacotherapy. *Am J Psychiatry* 157(8), 1204–11.

Klerman, G.L. (1988) Overview of the Cross-National Collaborative Panic Study. *Arch Gen Psychiatry* 45, 407–12.

Klerman, G.L., Hirschfeld, R.M.A., Weissman, M.M. *et al.* (eds) (1993) *Panic Anxiety and its Treatments*. American Psychiatric Press, Washington, D.C.

Kobak, K.A., Greist, J.H., Jefferson, J.W., Katzelnick, D.J. & Henk, H.J. (1998) Behavioral versus pharmacological treatments of obsessive-compulsive disorder: a meta-analysis. *Psychopharmacology* 136(3), 205–16.

Koran, L.M., McElroy, S.L., Davidson, J.R., Rasmussen, S.A., Hollander, E. & Jenike, M.A. (1996) Fluvoxamine versus clomipramine for obsessive-compulsive disorder: a double-blind comparison. *J Clin Psychopharmacol* 16(2), 121–9.

Koran, L.M., Pallanti, S., Paiva, R.S. & Quercioli, L. (1998) Pulse loading versus gradual dosing of intravenous clomipramine in obsessive-compulsive disorder. *Eur Neuropsychopharmacol* 8(2), 121–6.

Kosten, T.R., Frank, J.B., Dan, E., McDougle, C.J. & Giller, E.L.J. (1991) Pharmacotherapy for post-traumatic stress disorder using phenelzine or imipramine. *J Nerv Ment Dis* **179**, 366–70.

Lecrubier, Y., Bakker, A., Dunbar, G. & Judge, R. (1997) A comparison of paroxetine, clomipramine and placebo in the treatment of panic disorder. Collaborative Paroxetine Panic Study Investigators. *Acta Psychiatr Scand* **95**(2), 145–52.

Lecrubier, Y. & Judge, R. (1997) Long-term evaluation of paroxetine, clomipramine and placebo in panic disorder. Collaborative Paroxetine Panic Study Investigators. *Acta Psychiatr Scand* **95**(2), 153–60.

Lepola, U.M., Wade, A.G., Leinonen, E.V. *et al.* (1998) A controlled, prospective, 1-year trial of citalopram in the treatment of panic disorder. *J Clin Psychiatry* **59**(10), 528–34.

Liebowitz, M.R., Fyer, A.J., Gorman, J.M. *et al.* (1988) Tricyclic therapy of the DSM-III anxiety disorders: a review with implications for further research. *J Psychiatr Res* **22** (Suppl. 1), 7–32.

Lopez-Ibor, J.J., Jr, Saiz, J., Cottraux, J. *et al.* (1996) Double-blind comparison of fluoxetine versus clomipramine in the treatment of obsessive-compulsive disorder. *Eur Neuropsychopharmacol* **6**(2), 111–18.

Lotufo-Neto, F., Bernik, M., Ramos, R.T. *et al.* (2001) A dose-finding and discontinuation study of clomipramine in panic disorder. *J Psychopharmacol* **15**(1), 13–17.

Maier, W., Rosenberg, R., Argyle, N. *et al.* (1991a) Subtyping panic disorder by major depression and avoidance behavior and the response to active treatment. *Eur Arch Psychiatry Clin Neurosci* **241**, 22–30.

Maier, W., Roth, S.M., Argyle, N. *et al.* (1991b) Avoidance behavior: a predictor of the efficacy of pharmacotherapy in panic disorder? *Eur Arch Psychiatry Clin Neurosci* **241**, 151–8.

Marcourakis, T., Gorenstein, C., Ramos, R.T. & Da Motto, S.J. (1999) Serum levels of clomipramine and desmethyl-clomipramine and clinical improvement in panic disorder. *J Psychopharmacol* **13**(1), 40–4.

Matuzas, W. & Jack, E. (1991) The drug treatment of panic disorder. *Psychiatr Med* **9**, 215–43.

Mavissakalian, M.R., Jones, B., Olson, S. & Perel, J.M. (1990) Clomipramine in obsessive-compulsive disorder: clinical response and plasma levels. *J Clin Psychopharmacol* **10**(4), 261–8.

Mavissakalian, M.R. & Perel, J.M. (1995) Imipramine treatment of panic disorder with agoraphobia: dose ranging and plasma level-response relationships. *Am J Psychiatry* **152**(5), 673–82.

Mavissakalian, M.R. & Perel, J.M. (1996) The relationship of plasma imipramine and N-desmethylimipramine to response in panic disorder. *Psychopharmacol Bull* **32**(1), 143–7.

Mavissakalian, M.R. & Perel, J.M. (1999) Long-term maintenance and discontinuation of imipramine therapy in panic disorder with agoraphobia. *Arch Gen Psychiatry* **56**(9), 821–7.

Meyer, U.A., Amrein, R., Balant, L.P. *et al.* (1996) Antidepressants and drug-metabolizing enzymes—Expert Group Report. *Acta Psychiatr Scand* **93**(2), 71–9.

Modigh, K. (1989) Antidepressant drugs in anxiety disorders. *Acta Psychiatr Scand* **76** (Suppl. 335), 57–71.

Modigh, K., Westberg, P. & Eriksson, E. (1992) Superiority of clomipramine over imipramine in the treatment of panic disorder: a placebo-controlled trial. *J Clin Psychopharmacol* **12**, 251–61.

Montgomery, S.A. (1998) SSRIs in obsessive-compulsive disorder. In: *SSRIs in Depression and Anxiety* (S.A. Montgomery & J.A. Den Boer (eds), pp. 149–72). John Wiley & Sons, Chichester.

Munjack, D.J., Usigli, R., Zulueta, A. *et al.* (1988) Nortriptyline in the treatment of panic disorder and agoraphobia with panic attacks. *J Clin Psychopharmacol* **8**, 204–7.

Nair, N.P., Bakish, D., Saxena, B., Amin, M., Schwartz, G. & West, T.E. (1996) Comparison of fluvoxamine, imipramine, and placebo in the treatment of outpatients with panic disorder. *Anxiety* **2**(4), 192–8.

Nutt, D.J. (2000) The psychobiology of post-traumatic stress disorder. *J Clin Psychiatry* **61** (Suppl. 5), 24–9.

Pélissolo, A. & Lépine, J.-P. (1998) Epidemiology of depression and anxiety disorders. In: *SSRIs in Depression and Anxiety* (S.A. Montgomery & J.A. Den Boer (eds), pp. 1–21). John Wiley & Sons, Chichester.

Piccinelli, M., Pini, S., Bellantuono, C. & Wilkinson, G. (1995) Efficacy of drug treatment in obsessive-compulsive disorder. A meta-analytic review. *Br J Psychiatry* **166**(4), 424–43.

Rickels, K., Downing, R., Schweizer, E. & Hassman, H. (1993) Antidepressants for the treatment of generalized anxiety disorder. A placebo-controlled comparison of imipramine, trazodone, and diazepam. *Arch Gen Psychiatry* **50**(11), 884–95.

Rocca, P., Fonzo, V., Scotta, M., Zanalda, E. & Ravizza, L. (1997) Paroxetine efficacy in the treatment of generalized anxiety disorder. *Acta Psychiatr Scand* **95**(5), 444–50.

Rosenberg, R. (1999) Treatment of panic disorder with tricyclics and MAOIs. In: *Panic Disorder: Clinical Diagnosis, Management and Mechanisms* (D. Nutt, J.C. Ballenger & J.-P. Lépine (eds), pp. 125–44). Martin Dunitz Ltd, London.

Rosenberg, R. & Jensen, P.N. (1994) Treatment of panic disorder with alprazolam and imipramine: clinical relevance of DSM-III dysthymia. *Eur Psychiatry* **9**, 27–32.

Rosenberg, R., Ottosson, J.O., Bech, P., Mellergard, M. & Rosenberg, N.K. (1991) Validation criteria for panic disorder as a nosological entity. *Acta Psychiatr Scand* **83** (Suppl. 365), 7–17.

Roy-Byrne, P.P. & Cowley, D.S. (1994) Course and outcome in panic disorder: a review of recent follow-up studies. *Anxiety* **1**(4), 151–60.

Sallee, F.R., Koran, L.M., Pallanti, S., Carson, S.W. & Sethuraman, G. (1998) Intravenous clomipramine challenge in obsessive-compulsive disorder: predicting response to oral therapy at 8 weeks. *Biol Psychiatry* **44**(3), 220–27.

Sanchez, C. & Hyttel, J. (1999) Comparison of the effects of antidepressants and their metabolites on reuptake of biogenic amines and on receptor binding. *Cell Molecular Neurobiology* **19**(4), 467–89.

Sasson, Y., Iancu, I., Fux, M., Taub, M., Dannon, P.N. & Zohar, J. (1999) A double-blind cross-over comparison of clomipramine and desipramine in the treatment of panic disorder. *Eur Neuropsychopharmacol* **9**(3), 191–6.

Shear, M.K. & Maser, J.D. (1994) Standardized assessment for panic disorder research. A conference report. *Arch Gen Psychiatry* **51**(5), 346–54.

Stein, M.B., Liebowitz, M.R., Lydiard, R.B., Pitts, C.D., Bushnell, W. & Gergel, I. (1998) Paroxetine treatment of generalized social phobia (social anxiety disorder): a randomized controlled trial. *JAMA* **280**(8), 708–13.

Stein, D.J., Spadaccini, E. & Hollander, E. (1995) Meta-analysis of pharmacotherapy trials for obsessive-compulsive disorder. *Int Clin Psychopharmacol* **10**(1), 11–18.

Taylor, C.B., Hayward, C., King, R. *et al.* (1990) Cardiovascular and symptomatic reduction effects of alprazolam and imipramine in patients with panic disorder: results of a double-blind, placebo-controlled trial. *J Clin Psychopharmacol* **10**, 112–18.

Thoren, P., Asberg, M., Cronholm, B., Jornestedt, L. & Traskman, L. (1980) Clomipramine treatment of obsessive-compulsive disorder. I. A controlled clinical trial. *Arch Gen Psychiatry* **37**(11), 1281–5.

van Balkom, A.J., Bakker, A., Spinhoven, P., Blaauw, B.M., Smeenk, S. & Ruesink, B. (1997) A meta-analysis of the treatment of panic disorder with or without agoraphobia: a comparison of psychopharmacological, cognitive-behavioral, and combination treatments. *J Nerv Ment Dis* **185**(8), 510–16.

van Balkom, A.J., De Haan, E., van Oppen, P., Spinhoven, P., Hoogduin, K.A. & Van Dyck, R. (1998) Cognitive and behavioral therapies alone versus in combination with fluvoxamine in the treatment of obsessive-compulsive disorder. *J Nerv Ment Dis* **186**(8), 492–9.

Versiani, M. (2000) A review of 19 double-blind placebo-controlled studies in social anxiety disorder (social phobia). *World J Biol Psychiatry* **1**, 27–33.

Vestergaard, P., Gram, L.F., Kragh-Sorensen, P., Bech, P., Reisby, N. & Bolwig, T.G. (1993) Therapeutic potentials of recently introduced antidepressants. *Danish University Antidepressant Group Psychopharmacological Series* **10**, 190–8.

Wade, A.G., Lepola, U., Koponen, H.J., Pedersen, V. & Pedersen, T. (1997) The effect of citalopram in panic disorder. *Br J Psychiatry* **170**, 549–53.

Wilkinson, G., Balestrieri, M., Ruggeri, M. & Bellantuono, C. (1991) Meta-analysis of double-blind placebo-controlled trials of antidepressants and benzodiazepines for patients with panic disorders. *Psychol Med* **21**, 991–8.

Zohar, J. & Judge, R. (1996) Paroxetine versus clomipramine in the treatment of obsessive-compulsive disorder. OCD Paroxetine Study Investigators. *Br J Psychiatry* **169**(4), 468–74.

Zohar, J. & Westenberg, H.G. (2000) Anxiety disorders: a review of tricyclic antidepressants and selective serotonin reuptake inhibitors. *Acta Psychiatr Scand Suppl* **403**, 39–49.

20 Buspirone in the Treatment of Anxiety Disorders

K. Rickels, S. Khalid-Khan & M. Rynn

Introduction

This paper focuses on efficacy and safety of the aza-pirone buspirone for the treatment of anxiety disorders (Eison 1990). Buspirone is the only serotonergic medication that is not a selective serotonin reuptake inhibitor (SSRI) presently approved for the treatment of generalized anxiety disorders in many countries. Buspirone acts as a partial agonist at the 5-HT1A serotonin receptor subtype. Its primary mechanism of action is not serotonin reuptake inhibition. Other 5-HT1A partial agonists, such as ipsapirone, gepirone, tandospirone, flesinoxan, all do possess some anxiolytic and some mild antidepressant properties, but the daily doses needed to produce such effects also produce an unacceptable number of adverse events (Cutler *et al.* 1993; Rickels *et al.* 1997; Stahl *et al.* 1998). Antagonists of the 5-HT2 serotonin receptor (e.g. ritanserin) and the 5-HT3 receptor (e.g., ondansetron, zacopride, zatosetron) have also been studied as possible anxiolytics but with little success (Cutler *et al.* 1993; Schweizer & Rickels 1995; Olivier *et al.* 2000). Thus buspirone is the only azapirone 5-HT1A partial agonist with a favorable adverse event profile and demonstrated anxiolytic efficacy.

Mechanism of action/pharmacokinetic properties

5-HT1A drugs such as buspirone, gepirone and others appear to act as partial agonists at the postsynaptic 5-HT1A population of serotonin receptors located at the hippocampus, but as full agonists at the presynaptic 5-HT1A serotonergic autoreceptors, located in the dorsal raphe nucleus (De Montigny & Blier 1992). Binding to these receptors enables these drugs to influence the activity of serotonergic neurones through receptor down-regulation. In addition buspirone also has a moderate affinity for presynaptic dopamine D2 receptors. It is not known, however, whether this affinity for dopamine receptors contributes to the anxiolytic properties of buspirone (Tunnicliff 1991; Pecknold 1994).

Acute application of buspirone and of other aza-pirones to presynaptic dorsal raphe autoreceptors results in inhibition of serotonergic neurones firing, while increasing noradrenergic firing in the locus ceruleus (Eison & Temple 1986). Serotonergic functioning generally recovers following continued administration, presumably due to down-regulation of the 5-HT1A autoreceptors. In contrast, postsynaptic hippocampal 5-HT1A receptors do not appear to down-regulate, although they show reduction in serotonergic functions after acute treatment. Chronic administration of the azapirones, as with traditional antidepressants, causes a down-regulation of 5-HT2 receptors, possibly explaining their moderate antidepressant properties.

Buspirone has a short elimination half-life of 2–3 h with a weakly active 1-(2-pyrimidinyl)-piperazine (1-PP) metabolite that does not itself bind to 5-HT1A receptors and has α_2-adrenergic antagonistic properties. There is no interaction between the binding of benzodiazepines and buspirone. Buspirone does not bind to the γ-aminobutyric acid (GABA) benzodiazepine complex nor is buspirone blocked by the benzodiazepine receptor antagonist flumazenil (Goa & Ward 1986).

Buspirone is 100% absorbed after oral administration (Jajoo *et al.* 1989). The oral bioavailability is approximately 5% after extensive first-pass metabolism, and a linear relationship between acute oral dose and area under the plasma concentration-time curve (AUC) was demonstrated. A mean maximum plasma concentration (C max) of 1.7 μg/L was reported after a single 20 mg dose; however, there was considerable interindividual variation (Gammans *et al.* 1985). Buspirone and food taken together approximately doubled the AUC of unchanged buspirone compared with values obtained fasting. The first-pass metabolism of buspirone (Mayol *et al.* 1983) is decreased by taking food with buspirone but the clinical significance of these findings is not known. Buspirone is >95% bound to plasma proteins, with about 70% of the bound fraction binding to albumin and 30% to α_1-acid glycoprotein (Gammans *et al.* 1986).

Buspirone undergoes extensive metabolism so that less than 1% of an administered dose is excreted unchanged in the urine. There are seven major and five minor metabolites that have been identified, and the major metabolic pathways are hydroxylation and dealkylation. The N-dealkylated metabolite 1-PP also appears to have weak anxiolytic activity (approximately 20% of the level of activity of buspirone) in animal studies. The elimination half-life (t ^{1}/2) of buspirone in healthy subjects ranges from 2 to 11 h.

Compared to patients with normal hepatic function, in patients with cirrhosis the mean values for AUC, C max, and t ^{1}/2 of buspirone were significantly greater (Dalhoff *et al.* 1987; Barbhaiya *et al.* 1994). In patients with marked renal impairment, decreased clearance (up to 50%) and increased C max and AUC values (Barbhaiya *et al.* 1994) have been reported for buspirone and its metabolite 1-PP. However, the pharmacokinetic values of buspirone were unchanged in patients with only acute mild to moderate renal impairment (Caccia *et al.* 1988). In elderly healthy subjects (aged >65) compared with young healthy subjects, no significant differences in the pharmacokinetic values of buspirone or 1-PP were found (Gammans *et al.* 1989).

Sedation and psychomotor function

Buspirone has a low potential for sedation. When single or multiple doses of 5 mg buspirone were given,

much less daytime sedation was seen with buspirone than with alprazolam 0.5 mg, diazepam 5 mg or lorazepam 1 mg (Dement *et al.* 1991). Comparing buspirone with diazepam, sedation in subjects with a single 10 mg dose of buspirone was less marked than with the same dose of diazepam (Boulenger *et al.* 1989). In a placebo-controlled study in patients with generalized anxiety disorder (GAD), buspirone 10–20 mg/day given for 3 weeks produced no sedation when compared with baseline assessment or placebo response neither during treatment nor after sudden discontinuation (De Roeck *et al.* 1989). Interestingly, in one study buspirone was reported to be in fact slightly stimulatory when compared to placebo in patients with insomnia (Manfredi *et al.* 1991).

Several psychomotor and cognitive studies with healthy subjects demonstrated that buspirone did not have the same impairing psychomotor effects as the benzodiazepines. Performance ability was evaluated by various measures such as the digit symbol substitution test, signal identification tasks, finger-tapping, peg board, and reaction time. Comparing single or multiple doses of buspirone with several benzodiazepines and placebo, no significant differences in performance ability was found in healthy volunteers between buspirone and placebo; however, significantly more impairment was observed with the benzodiazepines (Boulenger *et al.* 1989; Schaffler & Klausnitzer 1989; Greenblatt *et al.* 1994).

Driving skills, using a driving simulator (Moskowitz & Smiley 1982) did not show significant buspirone-placebo differences. Driving-related skills were assessed between buspirone 20 mg/day and diazepam 15 mg/day given for 4 weeks in 24 outpatients with GAD (van Laar *et al.* 1992), again demonstrating the lack of sedation and of driving impairment when compared to diazepam.

In tests of memory function, assessed as immediate and delayed recall, buspirone appears to have minimal effects when compared to the benzodiazepines. Buspirone given in 5–30 mg single doses to young healthy subjects had no effect on immediate or delayed recall (Schaffler & Klausnitzer 1989). In anxious subjects, Lucki *et al.* (1987) confirmed that the benzodiazepine, diazepam, but not buspirone caused significant impairment of delayed recall when compared to placebo (Fig. 20.1). When elderly patients were tested for the same measures, buspirone in 20 mg single-dose or multiple-doses (15 mg/day) also had significantly

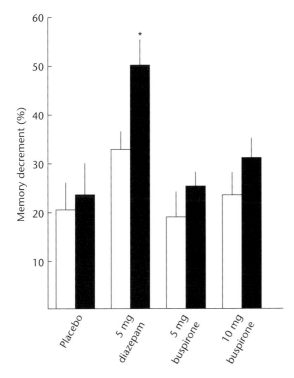

Fig. 20.1 The effect of antianxiety drugs on percentage memory decrement, expressed as the percentage of words that were remembered immediately after the list was read that could no longer be recalled after the 20 min delay. (*) indicates that diazepam (■) increased the memory decrement when compared with the corresponding value at baseline (□) ($P < 0.01$). (Taken from Lucki *et al.*, 1987, with permission.)

less effect on memory function as compared to the benzodiazepine alprazolam (Hart *et al.* 1991).

Abuse potential and dependence liability

The data that are available on buspirone show that it has little potential for abuse or dependence (Troisi *et al.* 1993). For example, in individuals with a history of drug abuse (Sellers *et al.* 1992), buspirone and lorazepam were compared on whether or not they liked their medication. Buspirone (15, 30, 60 and 120 mg/70 kg) was rated by subjects as significantly "less liked" than lorazepam (1, 2, 4 and 8 mg/70 kg). In fact, buspirone produced a dose-dependent increase in subjects "disliking" the drug whereas lorazepam produced a dose-dependent increase in drug "liking."

Compared to the benzodiazepines, no discontinuation (withdrawal) symptoms were ever demonstrated for buspirone. Rickels *et al.* (1988) were the first group to search for possible evidence of physical dependence by treating chronically anxious patients for 6 months with either buspirone or the benzodiazepine, clorazepate, substituting drug with placebo abruptly at the end of the treatment and maintaining patients on placebo for 4 weeks. Significantly more withdrawal symptoms were produced by the long half-life benzodiazepine clorazepate than by buspirone (Fig. 20.2).

Fig. 20.2 Mean symptoms scores before and during withdrawal on the Physician Checklist of Withdrawal Symptoms ($N = 61$). *Indicates significant differences between both clorazepate dipotassium and buspirone hydrochloride groups. BU, buspirone; CL, clorazepate. (Taken from Rickels *et al.*, 1998, with permission.)

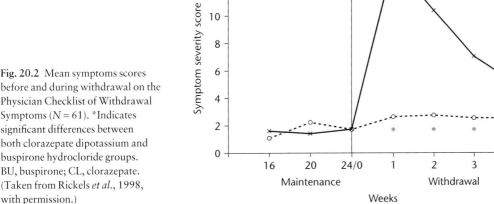

Toxicity and adverse events

Newton *et al.* (1986), using data from 17 clinical trials, reported on frequency of adverse events for buspirone ($N = 477$) and placebo ($N = 464$). The most commonly reported adverse events were dizziness (12%), drowsiness (10%), nausea (8%), headache (6%), nervousness (5%), fatigue (4%), insomnia (3%), lightheadedness (3%), dry mouth (3%), and excitement (2%). However, patients receiving placebo also reported drowsiness, insomnia, fatigue and dry mouth at similar frequency.

The relative frequencies of adverse effects associated with buspirone and diazepam are illustrated in Fig. 20.3. While diazepam caused significantly more drowsiness, fatigue, weakness, and depression than buspirone, buspirone produced significantly more nausea and nervousness.

The ability of patients to tolerate buspirone appears to depend little on their age. A meta-analysis of over 6000 patients demonstrated that no difference existed in the incidence of adverse events reported between patients aged ≥65 years and patients <65 years, with the exception of a slightly higher incidence of dizziness in elderly patients (7.8% vs. 6.2%) (Robinson *et al.* 1988).

A multicenter, unblinded trial was conducted to test the tolerability of buspirone, prescribed in the daily dosage of 15–30 mg/day during chronic use. Of 852 patients enrolled, 424 patients received buspirone for 6 months and 264 for 12 months (Rakel 1990). Over the total study period only 12% of patients ended therapy because of adverse events. It was of particular interest that the frequency of adverse events was the same after 1 month and after 12 months of treatment. No withdrawal syndrome occurred when treatment was abruptly discontinued.

Sexual dysfunction was studied in noncomparative trials in a large number of patients. It appears that not only does buspirone not cause any sexual dysfunction but it may improve sexual dysfunction caused by persistent anxiety (Othmer & Othmer 1987). Buspirone also has been reported to reverse sexual dysfunction caused by SSRIs (Norden 1994).

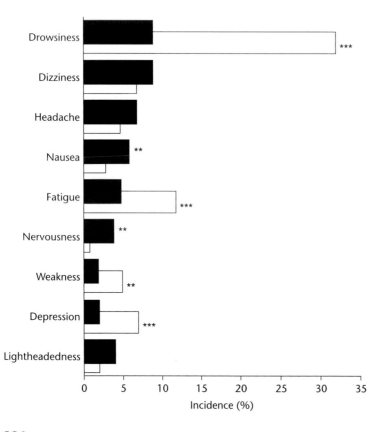

Fig. 20.3 Comparative incidence of adverse effects of buspirone ($N = 984$) (■) and diazepam ($N = 427$) (□) from clinical trials ** $P < 0.01$, *** $P < 0.001$. (Taken from Fulton & Brogden 1997, with permission.)

There is very little published data on buspirone overdose, and the data that are available suggest that buspirone is not toxic in overdose (Langlois & Paquette 1994). In clinical pharmacology trials, dosages of up to 375 mg/day were used in healthy subjects. As subjects were titrated up to this high daily dose, the following symptoms were observed: nausea, vomiting, gastric distress, drowsiness, miosis, and dizziness (Newton *et al.* 1986). In another study, 25 cases of buspirone overdose were studied. Out of these 25 cases, 10 subjects had taken only buspirone. Drowsiness was the most commonly reported symptom. Forty-eight percent of patients had no symptoms, 40% had minor symptoms, 8% had moderate symptoms and one patient died. The patient who died was on a tricyclic antidepressant which was the most likely cause of death. Taken by itself no deaths have been associated with an overdose of buspirone alone (Newton *et al.* 1986).

Interactions between buspirone and tricyclic antidepressants have not been reported. For example, the addition of 30 mg/day of buspirone in 18 patients taking imipramine 75–150 mg/day (Pollicino *et al.* 1992) for treatment of depression, had no significant effect on steady-state plasma concentrations of imipramine or its active metabolite desipramine. In another study, 184 patients on 15 mg of buspirone, and an antidepressant, retrospectively compared to a matched group receiving buspirone alone, reported identical adverse events frequencies (25.7% vs. 26.1%: Napoliello 1986). Nevertheless, when combining serotonergic medications one must look out for the possibility of the development of a serotonergic syndrome.

No interactions were observed in healthy subjects when buspirone was combined with triazolam (Boulenger *et al.* 1993) or alprazolam (Buch *et al.* 1999). Alcohol being added to single or multiple dose administration of buspirone also had little effect on performance tasks (Erwin *et al.* 1986), and in schizophrenic patients who were taking haloperidol, concomitant treatment with buspirone did not alter haloperidol steady-state plasma concentrations (Jann *et al.* 1996). The addition of grapefruit juice (Lilja *et al.* 1998), diltiazem and verapamil (Lamberg *et al.* 1998) significantly increased buspirone plasma concentrations, probably via inhibition of the cytochrome P-450, 3A$_4$ isoenzyme.

Other clinical reports demonstrated the safety of combining buspirone with cimetidine (Gammans *et al.*

1987), bronchodilators (mostly theophylline and terbutaline: Kiev & Domantay 1988), and nonsteroidal anti-inflammatory agents (Kiev & Domantay 1989).

While benzodiazepines can be problematic in their use in respiratory diseases because of their propensity to cause respiratory depression, buspirone does not cause respiratory depression (Craven & Sutherland 1991). For example, in healthy subjects, 10 mg diazepam depressed the ventilatory response to CO_2 rebreathing, whereas buspirone did not. Buspirone also produced less depression of load compensation than diazepam. Two placebo-controlled trials conducted in patients with chronic obstructive pulmonary disease indicated no negative effect on respiratory drive when taking buspirone 20–60 mg/day (Rapaport *et al.* 1991; Argyropoulou *et al.* 1993). In one study (Rapaport *et al.* 1991), an improvement in exercise tolerance was shown by buspirone, and a reduction in the sensation of dyspnea was shown by both studies. While a few single dose studies in healthy volunteers reported an increase of plasma prolactin (Gregory *et al.* 1990; Anderson & Cowen 1992) with buspirone, Tollefson *et al.* (1989), prescribing buspirone 10–30 mg/day for 4 weeks to patients with GAD, found no significant effect of buspirone on plasma prolactin or growth hormone levels.

Therapeutic efficacy in GAD

GAD is often a chronic condition which interferes with the daily functioning of patients. It has a waxing and waning course interspersed with long intervals where the patient is relatively free of anxiety. Anxiety has been treated with various psychotherapeutic approaches and medications. The acute phase of anxiety in chronically anxious patients is clearly managed best by anxiolytic medications like the benzodiazepines. However, it is very difficult for most of the chronically anxious patients to sustain remission of their anxiety symptoms. Less than 50% of chronically anxious patients will have sustained remission of symptoms after stopping acute medication treatment (Rickels & Schweizer 1990). Some percentage of chronically anxious patients may need to be treated for years. Benzodiazepines have been used for a long time for the treatment of anxiety; however, they are sedating and with prolonged use do cause physical dependence. Consequently, research for nonbenzodiazepine anxiolytics has been actively

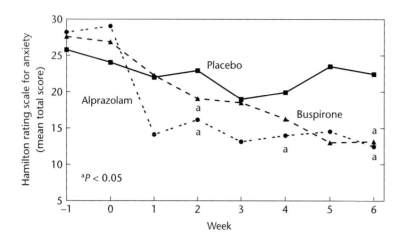

Fig. 20.4 Alprazolam vs. buspirone in the treatment of outpatients with generalized anxiety disorder (From Enkelmann, 1991, with permission.)

pursued by the pharmaceutical industry which eventually produced the anxiolytic buspirone.

In the past 20 years a number of double-blind studies, some of them placebo-controlled, others only active drug controlled, have been conducted and proven buspirone's efficacy in the alleviation of anxious symptoms in patients suffering from GAD. Most of these were placebo lead in, randomized, double-blind studies designed to minimize any placebo effect. The primary measure of efficacy was the Hamilton Anxiety Rating Scale (HAM-A) (Hamilton 1959). Patients were generally required to have a HAM-A score of at least 18 when admitted to the trial.

After treatment periods of 4–6 weeks, buspirone produced similar reduction in total HAM-A scores as compared to such benzodiazepines as alprazolam, bromazepam, clobazam, diazepam, lorazepam, oxazepam, and clorazepate. In studies including placebo control, buspirone-treated patients usually had statistically significantly greater reduction in HAM-A total scores at end-point than those receiving placebo. Results reported by Enkelmann (1991) are given in Fig. 20.4 as being representative of results obtained in most studies.

All published placebo controlled, double-blind trials that also included a benzodiazepine showed equal efficacy to a standard benzodiazepine and significantly better response than placebo (Goldberg & Finnerty 1979; Rickels et al. 1982; Pecknold et al. 1989; Bohm et al. 1990a; Enkelmann 1991; Laakman et al. 1998; Lader & Scotto 1998). Additional nonplacebo controlled, double-blind studies compared buspirone against

several benzodiazepines and demonstrated equal efficacy for both treatments (Goldberg & Finnerty 1982; Wheatley 1982; Cohn et al. 1986a; Cohn & Rickels 1989; Feighner & Cohen 1989; Murphy et al. 1989; Strand et al. 1990; Dimitriou et al. 1992; Sacchetti et al. 1994). One of the most salient clinical features of buspirone, compared with the benzodiazepines, is its *gradual, relatively slow onset of action*, with many patients taking 2–4 weeks to respond (Rickels et al. 1988; Pecknold et al. 1989; Enkelmann 1991: see also Fig. 20.4). This slow onset of action makes buspirone less useful for the treatment of transient, situational, or acute anxiety. A similar gradual onset of action has been reported for the treatment of anxiety symptoms with antidepressants (Rickels et al. 1993). Buspirone's slow onset of action appears to be derived from its lack of sedative and muscle relaxing properties, as well as its lack of action at the GABA receptor complex. Psychic symptoms of anxiety, which are diagnostically considered core features of GAD in the Diagnostic Statistical Manual, fourth edition (DSM-IV: American Psychiatric Association 1994), respond faster to buspirone when compared to the benzodiazepines while the reverse is true for somatic symptoms (Rickels et al. 1982). Similar observations were made for antidepressants (Rickels et al. 1993; Davidson et al. 1999).

Because of the more gradual onset of efficacy as compared to benzodiazepine-treated patients, patients considered for buspirone therapy should be prepared differently for such therapy than patients being placed on a benzodiazepine. Patients should be informed that buspirone is less sedating and has a more gradual onset of action than the benzodiazepines. Patients should be encouraged to give buspirone more time to work. Patients can be further assured that if they are in need of prolonged therapy, buspirone does not cause physical dependence and withdrawal symptoms upon discontinuation, and thus represents a safer drug than the benzodiazepines for long-term treatment. Finally, patients can be informed that there is preliminary evidence that long-term treatment with buspirone, in contrast to long-term treatment with benzodiazepines does not decrease the ability to learn new coping skills. Preliminary data to support such assumptions have been provided by Rickels and Schweizer who conducted follow-up evaluations after patients completed a 6-month maintenance trial with buspirone and clorazepate (Rickels & Schweizer 1990). At 6-month follow-up ($N = 45$), it was observed that of 34% of patients treated with clorazepate, but only 13% of those treated with buspirone, had returned to regular antianxiety drug use (benzodiazepines); in addition, several clorazepate treated patients were using a benzodiazepine on an as-needed basis. At 40-month follow-up ($N = 34$), it was observed that none of the available patients formerly treated with buspirone were taking either regular or as-needed anxiolytic medication, whereas of those patients treated with clorazepate, 30% were taking a benzodiazepine regularly and 25% on an as-needed basis. Thus, >50% of patients treated for 6 months with clorazepate, and none of the patients treated for 6 months with buspirone were still receiving medication at the 40-month follow-up (Rickels & Schweizer 1990). Scheibe (1996) reported a similar observation.

Schweizer et al. (1986) were the first authors to observe that prior benzodiazepine use affected treatment outcome in that patients treated with buspirone who had received prior benzodiazepines responded less well than those previously untreated with a benzodiazepine. At that time the authors speculated that this effect may have been related to the treatment expectations of patients based on earlier experience with benzodiazepines, which may prejudice clinical outcome. Particularly, benzodiazepine-treated patients may have expected sedation and/or euphoria, side-effects they hardly experienced with buspirone. More recently, DeMartinis et al. (2000) reviewed a large data set and examined the response to buspirone treatment as a function of patients who were never treated with ben-

zodiazepines, were remotely treated (>1 month ago), or were recently treated with benzodiazepines (<1 month ago). Results clearly indicated that treatment response to buspirone in patients who had recently terminated benzodiazepine treatment was significantly impaired when compared to patients who had either never been treated or had been treated several months ago with a benzodiazepine (Fig. 20.5). Therefore, the recommendation is made that initiation of buspirone therapy in such patients should be undertaken cautiously and be combined with appropriate patient education.

Elderly patients

Buspirone also has demonstrated anxiolytic effectiveness and safety in the elderly. The advantages of using buspirone in the elderly is that it is nonsedating, spares cognitive and memory functions. In addition it does not produce respiratory depression, impair psychomotor performance, nor potentiate the effects of alcohol or other central nervous system (CNS) depressants. There is also the apparent absence of new or unexpected adverse reactions when buspirone is added to the existing treatment regimen, which may include gastrointestinal, cardiac, and antihypertensive agents (Goldberg 1994).

Buspirone has been assessed for its efficacy in geriatric patients with anxiety in a number of trials (Robinson et al. 1988; Bohm et al. 1990b; Ritchie & Cox 1993). In a meta-analyses of 6574 patients who were treated with at least 15 mg of buspirone daily, 605 patients were at least 65 years of age. The total HAM-A scores were decreased by 54% in elderly and 65% in the younger patients after 4-weeks of treatment (Robinson et al. 1988). In another multicenter, noncomparative trial, 175 anxious patients aged 65 years or older were treated with buspirone 15–45 mg daily for 6 weeks (Ritchie & Cox 1993). The mean reduction in total HAM-A scores was 61% after treatment and 81% of patients had marked or moderate improvement on the Clinical Global Impressions (CGI) Scale. Finally, Boehm et al. (1990) reported results of a double-blind, placebo-controlled trial of buspirone in 20 anxious patients over 65 years old. After 4 weeks of random assignment to buspirone 5–30 mg/day or placebo, buspirone-treated patients showed a statistically significant decrease in HAM-A and CGI on scores compared with placebo. The medication was well tolerated.

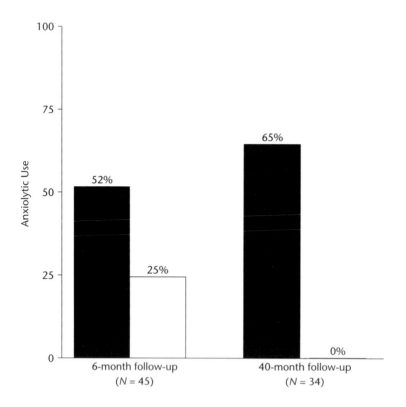

Fig. 20.5 Anxiolytic use at 6-month and 40-month follow-up after 6-month treatment with clorazepate (■) or buspirone (□). (Modified from Rickels & Schweizer, 1990, with permission.)

Children

Only two open studies report on the use of buspirone in children, one in young children at a daily dose of 5–15 mg (Kutcher *et al.* 1992), and one in adolescents at a daily dose of 15–30 mg (Simeon *et al.* 1994). Some beneficial effects were noticed by 6 weeks of treatment.

Replacement of benzodiazepines by buspirone

Since buspirone does not exhibit cross-tolerance to the benzodiazepines, and thus does not block benzodiazepine withdrawal symptoms, patients should never be abruptly switched from a benzodiazepine to a buspirone. When switching benzodiazepine-treated patients to buspirone, it is beneficial to initiate buspirone therapy concurrently for 2–4 weeks before tapering the benzodiazepine gradually. While some studies, in which the benzodiazepine was abruptly replaced with buspirone, have shown no benefit for buspirone facilitating benzodiazepine withdrawal (Schweizer & Rickels 1986), other studies have shown

some beneficial results when buspirone was started several weeks before the benzodiazepine taper process was started (Udelman & Udelman 1990; Chiaie *et al.* 1995; Rickels *et al.* 2000).

Dosage and administration

The recommended initial dosage of buspirone is 15 mg/day administered in 2–3 divided doses. The dosage should be increased to 30 mg daily (5–10 mg/day increments at intervals of 3 days) to achieve the optimal therapeutic response. The recommended maximum daily dosage is 45 mg in the UK and 60 mg in the US.

There are no firm recommendations regarding dosage adjustments in patients with hepatic or renal insufficiency. Although there appears to be some reduction in the elimination of buspirone or the active *N*-dealkylated metabolite (1-PP) in such patients, interpatient variation in pharmacokinetic parameters is substantial. Dosage adjustments may be necessary in patients with severe renal or hepatic impairment. No age-related dosage adjustments are necessary in elderly patients.

Therapeutic efficacy for unapproved indications

Mixed anxiety-depression

It was observed that patients with GAD with subsyndromal depressive symptoms reported improvement in their depressive symptoms during treatment with buspirone (Feighner *et al.* 1982). This sparked an interest in buspirone as an antidepressant as there is a high (about 25–35%) reported comorbidity for major depression and GAD (Brown & Barlow 1992). This has led some researchers (Tyrer *et al.* 1992) to suggest that the two disorders might be seen as different manifestations of one underlying diathesis. Genetic analyses done on women having major depression and GAD (Kendler *et al.* 1992) suggest that the genetic vulnerability for both disorders is largely shared. Thus, it was no surprise when the first open-label study (Schweizer *et al.* 1986) carried out in depression found buspirone to have antidepressant properties.

Since then, several large placebo-controlled studies have demonstrated the antidepressant efficacy of buspirone in patients who also exhibited symptoms of anxiety. In one study with 155 outpatients with major depression and at least moderate amounts of anxiety (with HAM-A scores ≥15), 70% of patients reported moderate to marked improvement on buspirone, compared with 35% on placebo (Rickels *et al.* 1991). The mean daily dose of buspirone in this study was 56 mg. Two other double-blind studies, one involving 140 outpatients with major depression and concomitant anxiety (scores ≥18 on both the Hamilton Anxiety and Depression scales: Fabre 1990), and the other involving 80 outpatients with GAD and secondary symptoms of depression (Sramek *et al.* 1996), confirmed the findings by Rickels *et al.* (1991).

In a trial by Schweizer *et al.* (1998) 177 geriatric outpatients, with a minimum age of 65 years and suffering from major depression, were treated under double-blind conditions with buspirone, imipramine, or placebo. Compared with placebo, there was a statistically significant (and comparable) antidepressant effect observed for both buspirone (mean daily dose = 38 mg) and imipramine (mean daily dose = 89 mg). Global moderate/marked improvement was observed in 80% of buspirone, 86% of imipramine, but only 49% of placebo patients.

When buspirone was added to fluoxetine, paroxetine, citalopram or fluvoxamine in small noncomparative

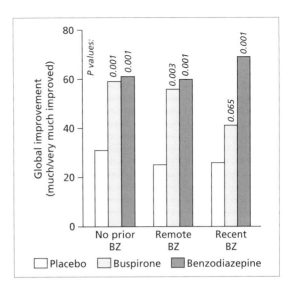

Fig. 20.6 Global improvement after 4 weeks of treatment (LOCF data set) as a function of treatment and prior benzodiazepine use. (Modified from DeMartinis *et al.*, 2000, with permission.)

studies of depressed patients not or only partially responding to SSRI antidepressants, additional improvements beyond that produced by the antidepressants were seen (Dimitriou & Dimitriou 1998; Landen *et al.* 1998; Gonul *et al.* 1999). In summary, evidence is accumulating that buspirone is useful as an augmentation agent in the treatment of treatment-resistant patients with major depression, but also as a single agent in the treatment of depressed patients with significant symptoms of anxiety.

Panic disorder

Since buspirone has been found efficacious for treating GAD, it was also studied in panic disorder (PD). Two double-blind, placebo-controlled trials have been performed (Pohl *et al.* 1989; Sheehan *et al.* 1993). Buspirone appears to have no efficacy compared with placebo and it is significantly less efficacious than both alprazolam and imipramine. This is not surprising since in preclinical trials it has been seen that buspirone increases the firing rate in the locus ceruleus (Eison & Temple 1986) and PD is associated with noradrenergic hyperactivity (Charney & Heninger 1985). In light of this information buspirone should not be prescribed for the treatment of PD.

389

Post-traumatic stress disorder

Post-traumatic stress disorder (PTSD) as a diagnosis has been increasingly recognized. Currently, promising treatment results have come from the SSRI antidepressants. In animals, 5-HT1A medications have shown benefit in reducing the behavioral effects of inescapable shock, which may serve as an experimental model for PTSD (De Montigny & Blier 1992). The use of buspirone to treat PTSD has been reported only in open-label case reports and case series. The cases reported include patients with highly chronic combat-related PTSD, sometimes complicated by a history of alcoholism, and civilian PTSD of more recent origin. The doses used were in the range of 30–60 mg/day, with time to response ranging from approximately 1–4 weeks. The results suggest that daily doses of 30–60 mg may have some benefit, not only for associated depressive and anxious symptomatology, but also for the core symptoms of flashbacks, nightmares, and intrusive thoughts (Duffy & Molloy 1994). The small number of cases reported, the lack of formal diagnostic evaluations and outcome measures, and the frequent use of concomitant psychotherapy suggest that the reported results be interpreted with caution. A controlled trial may be worthwhile undertaking.

Social phobia

Social phobia has recently received increased clinical attention. It is a common disorder, with a lifetime prevalence estimated at 2%. Only several open-label studies have been reported on (Schweizer & Rickels 1994). For example, in one pilot study of 21 patients (Munjack et al. 1991) the mean daily buspirone dose for responders was 57 mg compared with a dose of 38 mg for nonresponders. This suggests the effective dose in social phobia of buspirone may be more in the range for that used to treat depression (Rickels et al. 1991). More recently, a double-blind, placebo controlled trial conducted with a small number of patients ($N = 30$) could not confirm buspirone's efficacy in this disorder (Vliet et al. 1997). The small sample size may explain these negative findings. A controlled clinical trial would be of clinical interest.

Obsessive-compulsive disorder

Buspirone's efficacy as a primary treatment for obsessive-compulsive disorder (OCD) has been assessed with only one small double-blind, placebo-controlled, cross-over study. Eighteen patients were treated by Pato et al. (1991) with both 6 weeks of clomipramine (mean dose = 225 mg) and 6 weeks of buspirone (mean dose = 60 mg), interrupted by 3–4 weeks on placebo. Improvement achieved with buspirone was comparable to that with clomipramine, with 56% of patients reporting more than a 20% improvement in the Yale-Brown Obsessive Compulsive Scale (Y-BOCS), and 78% reporting more than 20% improvement on the National Institute of Mental Health OCD scale. The efficacy and safety of buspirone when used to augment SSRIs for the treatment of OCD has been examined in several small sample-size studies. These studies were reviewed by Schweizer and Rickels (1994). For example, Jenike et al. (1991) studied 20 treatment-resistant patients. All patients received 80 mg/day of fluoxetine for 12 weeks. About 10 of the 20 patients received adjunctive treatment with 45–60 mg/day of buspirone for 8 weeks and 10 patients remained for all 20 weeks on fluoxetine. Augmentation with buspirone showed a significant improvement in the Y-BOCS with a mean five point between-group difference score. Since these initial results are promising, especially when used as augmentation, further studies are indicated.

Premenstrual syndrome

The fact that premenstrual syndrome (PMS) patients have prominent mixed symptoms of anxiety, depression, and irritability makes buspirone a potentially promising treatment for PMS. There is preliminary evidence that the alteration in 5-HT1A receptor functions in the late lutel phase may contribute to the pathogenesis of PMS. Some preliminary evidence has been provided by two placebo-controlled, small sample-size studies for the efficacy of buspirone in treating the symptoms of PMS. The first study (Rickels et al. 1989) showed modest efficacy. This may have been due to the fact that the treatment with buspirone was not continuous, but was intermittent, and was limited to the last 2 weeks of the menstrual cycle. Brown et al. (1990) used daily doses of buspirone in the range of 30–60 mg throughout the cycle, with modest results. Considering this evidence, buspirone might be of interest as an alternative in the treatment of PMS since it is well-tolerated and does not cause either sedation or physical dependence.

Smoking cessation

A few studies have looked at the effects of treatment with buspirone on the withdrawal symptoms associated with smoking cessation. A randomized, placebo-controlled, double-blind study by West *et al.* (1991) used a low daily dose of 15 mg of buspirone in 61 smokers. In this study there was no difference in the severity of withdrawal, but 47% of patients (vs. 16% for placebo), were able to remain abstinent for the 4-week follow-up period. Buspirone was found by Hilleman *et al.* (1992) to significantly decrease irritability, craving, restlessness, and sad mood when compared with double-blind placebo. The very short 7-day follow-up period showed buspirone to increase the rate at which subjects were able to stay successfully abstinent. In a third double-blind study (Cinciripini *et al.* 1995), which enrolled 101 smokers receiving buspirone ≤60 mg daily or placebo in addition to a smoking cessation program, it was shown that buspirone's efficacy was only apparent in smokers who also had a high level of initial anxiety.

Alcohol and substance dependence

The medication treatment of drug dependence has been the subject of extensive research. There are three reasons for this approach: to decrease psychiatric comorbidity (e.g., anxiety and depression) that commonly occurs in persons with drug dependence, to decrease withdrawal syndromes that occur when the drug of abuse is stopped, and to reduce craving for the drug of abuse that occurs after successful withdrawal symptoms are over (Kushner *et al.* 1990). Buspirone has no abuse potential and it has a minimal additive effect on psychomotor and cognitive function when coadministered with alcohol (Mattila *et al.* 1982). This makes it a promising alternative to the benzodiazepines in the pharmacologic management of dependence and withdrawal. It has been suggested that anxiety and alcoholism may share a common pathophysiological abnormality that is mediated via serotonergic neurotransmission.

Buspirone has been assessed in a few double-blind, placebo-controlled trials, most of which involved anxious outpatients with coexisting alcohol-use disorders. In most of these studies (Tollefson *et al.* 1992; Kranzler *et al.* 1994) it was seen that patients who were on buspirone were significantly more likely to continue with treatment than patients who were on placebo. Anxiety and alcohol consumption were decreased in these trials after treatment with buspirone. Malcolm *et al.* (1992) found no beneficial effect of buspirone over placebo in anxious inpatient alcoholics.

Agitation and aggressive behavior

Buspirone has been studied for its potential in the treatment of agitation in a few small trials. For example, in 26 patients with Alzheimer's disease, a double-blind trial compared haloperidol to buspirone (Cantillon *et al.* 1996). Buspirone reduced tension (rated on objective physical signs and motor behavior) and anxiety scores to a significantly greater extent. Patients with organic disorders, including patients with dementia and traumatic brain injury, also frequently display aggressive, irritable and hostile behaviors, which can be difficult to treat and manage effectively. Several open-label case reports have found buspirone, in the daily dosage range of 15–45 mg per day, to be modestly effective in reducing hostile, aggressive, and irritable behavior, as well as restlessness and agitation (Gualtieri 1991; Ratey *et al.* 1992). Buspirone has also been found to be effective against aggressive behaviors in mentally retarded and autistic patients, in whom the self-injurious behaviors are also reduced (Realmuto *et al.* 1989). In addition, in an open-label study with 15–60 mg daily of buspirone, it was found that 11 male patients with a history of coronary artery disease and Type A personalities had reduced anxiety, impatience, irritability, and perceived levels of stress (Littman *et al.* 1993). Given the well-established link between serotonergic function and aggression, the role of buspirone in organically based aggression and agitation deserves further clinical research.

Children with pervasive developmental disorders

Many children with pervasive developmental disorders (PDD) have particular characteristics of increased anxiety and dysregulation of affect (Cohen *et al.* 1986). When symptoms are troublesome or disruptive (i.e., hyperactivity, aggression, impulsivity, anxiety, irritability, temper tantrums, and stereotyped or self-injurious behaviors) medications are frequently prescribed (Buitelaar *et al.* 1995). In children with PDD, the following symptoms are also frequently seen: intense generalized anxiety, extreme phobias (e.g., fear of annihilation or fear of bodily disintegration), recurrent panic episodes, and inappropriate affect.

Neuroleptics, such as haloperidol and pimozide, have been shown to improve hyperactivity, aggression, and stereotypes in children with autism (Campbell *et al.* 1978) and pervasive developmental disorders, not otherwise specified (PDD-NOS) (Joshi *et al.* 1988). In children with PDD, the use of neuroleptics on a long-term basis is limited due to the side-effects of drug-related dyskinesias, excessive sedation, impaired cognition and fatigue. In addition, neuroleptic drugs have not been found to be very effective in these children (Campbell *et al.* 1988).

Buitelaar *et al.* (1998) evaluated the efficacy and safety of buspirone in the management of anxiety and irritability in children with PDD. The twenty-two subjects, 6–17 years old, included DSM-III-R (American Psychiatric Association 1987) diagnosed PDD-NOS (N = 20) and autistic disorder (N = 2) subjects. Buspirone was used to treat these subjects in dosages ranging from 15 to 45 mg/day in an open-label trial lasting 6–8 weeks. Those who responded continued treatment with buspirone and were followed for up to 12 months. Marked therapeutic response was seen in nine subjects and a moderate response in seven subjects after 6–8 weeks of treatment. Minimal side-effects were reported and one patient developed abnormal involuntary movements. It can be extrapolated from these results that buspirone may be useful for treating symptoms of anxiety and irritability in children with PDD; however, double-blind placebo-controlled trials are clearly needed.

Body dysmorphic disorder

Although preliminary data suggest that serotonin reuptake inhibitors may be effective in treating body dysmorphic disorder (BDD), a substantial percentage of patients have no response or respond only partially to SSRIs. The efficacy of buspirone augmentation of SSRIs in BDD was therefore evaluated in an open study (Phillips 1996). Thirteen patients with DSM-IV BDD who had not responded, or had responded only partially to an SSRI had buspirone added to the SSRI. Six of these subjects (46%) improved. Three patients who decreased or discontinued buspirone experienced an increase in symptom severity. BDD symptoms again

improved in the one subject who resumed treatment. Side-effects were minimal and well-tolerated in all but one subject. These data, while preliminary, suggest that buspirone augmentation of SSRIs may be useful for BDD and warrant further investigation in a controlled trial.

Migraine headaches

In an open-label, 10-week study (Pascual & Berciano 1991), 33 migraine headache patients used daily doses of 15–20 mg of buspirone. Seventy-six percent of patients reported moderate to marked improvement on buspirone. Since no placebo controlled studies are available, these data are hard to interpret.

Tardive dyskinesia

In a 12-week, open-label study with independent, blinded assessment, buspirone in doses up to 180 mg/day was found to yield moderate improvements in the symptoms of tardive dyskinesia in eight patients (Moss *et al.* 1993). This confirms previous case reports (Neppe 1989). It should be noted that all but one of these patients were on concomitant neuroleptics, and it is possible that such high doses of buspirone may have increased neuroleptic plasma level (Goff *et al.* 1991). Again, controlled studies are indicated.

Conclusion

Buspirone, the first nonbenzodiazepine anxiolytic introduced into psychiatry, is a safe anxiolytic compound with relatively few side-effects. It causes little sedation and consequently has no negative effects on psychomotor and cognitive functions, including memory and driving skills. It is well tolerated and safe in overdose. Patients do not suffer discontinuation or withdrawal symptoms when buspirone is abruptly stopped, even after many months of treatment. Reassessment of continued need for buspirone therapy is therefore simple without the risk of rebound anxiety, a phenomenon that makes temporary discontinuation of benzodiazepines frequently a challenge. Since buspirone does not interact with alcohol, it is a safer alternative to the benzodiazepines for those anxious patients who request the ability to have occasional alcohol intake.

Many controlled clinical trials have demonstrated buspirone's anxiolytic efficacy to be equal to that of the benzodiazepines and significantly better than that of placebo. The perception among some clinicians that buspirone has slightly lower anxiolytic efficacy than the benzodiazepines may well be related to its relatively slow onset of efficacy and its lack of sedative effects, effects which might be particularly missed by patients recently treated with a benzodiazepine. Consequently, patients switched from a benzodiazepine to buspirone should be well prepared and informed about what to expect from buspirone therapy and in which way buspirone differs from the benzodiazepines. Some clinicians prefer buspirone to the benzodiazepines in the long term (more than 4 weeks) treatment of anxious patients for two main reasons. One reason is the lack of withdrawal symptoms to occur on treatment discontinuation and the other its moderate antidepressant properties that allow treatment of the many anxious patients who also suffer from depressive symptoms at a diagnostic subthreshhold level. Since buspirone does not have the fast onset of action of the benzodiazepines, it is not indicated for the short-term (i.e., 1–14 days) treatment of situational or temporary anxiety conditions. However, it should be considered one of the treatments of choice for the more chronically anxious patients in need of more than 4–6 weeks of treatment, many of whom are suffering from GAD.

As with any marketed medication, over the years buspirone, approved for the treatment of generalized anxiety, has been tried by clinicians for a variety of unapproved indications, sometimes with success, but more often with inconsistent or negative results. Frequently, such uses are based primarily on uncontrolled studies or case reports. Nevertheless, there exists some evidence based on placebo-controlled trials, that buspirone possesses moderate antidepressant properties in depressed patients with secondary symptoms of anxiety. In addition, buspirone seems to augment the effects of antidepressants in those patients who either did not or only partially responded to antidepressants alone. A number of potential additional indications for the use of buspirone are discussed, not to suggest efficacy but to encourage physicians to explore the potential usefulness of buspirone in patients who are not responding to other treatments.

References

American Psychiatric Association (1987) *Diagnostic Statistical Manual of Mental Disorders*, 3rd edn revised. American Psychiatric Association, Washington, D.C.

American Psychiatric Association (1994) *Diagnostic Statistical Manual of Mental Disorders*, 4th edn. American Psychiatric Association, Washington, D.C.

Anderson, I.M. & Cowen, P.J. (1992) Effect of pindolol on endocrine and temperature responses to buspirone in healthy volunteers. *Psychopharmacology* 106, 428–30.

Argyropoulou, P., Patakas, D., Koukou, A. et al. (1993) Buspirone effect on breathlessness and exercise performance in patients with chronic obstructive pulmonary disease. *Respiration* 60, 216–20.

Barbhaiya, R.H., Shukla, J.A., Pfeffer, M. et al. (1994) Disposition kinetics of buspirone in patients with renal or hepatic impairment after administration of single and multiple doses. *Eur J Clin Pharmacol* 46, 41–7.

Bohm, C., Placchi, M., Stallone, F. et al. (1990a) A double-blind comparison of buspirone, clobazepam, and placebo in patients with anxiety treated in a general practice setting. *J Clin Psychopharmacol* 10, 385–425.

Bohm, C., Robinson, D.S., Gammans, R.E. et al. (1990b) Buspirone therapy in anxious elderly patients: a controlled clinical trial. *J Clin Psychopharmacol* 10 (Suppl.), 47–51.

Boulenger, J.-P., Gram, L.F., Jolicoeur, F.B. et al. (1993) Repeated administration of buspirone: absence of pharmacodynamic or pharmacokinetic interaction with triazolam. *Hum Psychopharmacol* 8, 117–24.

Boulenger, J.P., Squillace, K., Simon, P. et al. (1989) Buspirone and diazepam: comparison of subjective, psychomotor and biological effects. *Neuropsychobiology* 22, 83–9.

Brown, T.A. & Barlow, D. (1992) Comorbidity among anxiety disorders: implications for treatment and DSM-IV. *J Consult Clin Psychol* 60, 835–44.

Brown, C.S., Ling, F.W., Farmer, R.G. et al. (1990) Buspirone in the treatment of premenstrual syndrome. *Drug Ther Bull* 8 (Suppl.), 112–16.

Buch, A.B., Van Harken, D.R., Seidehamel, R.J. et al. (1999) A study of pharmacokinetic interaction between buspirone and alprazolam at steady state. *J Clin Pharmacol* 33, 1104–9.

Buitelaar, J.K. (1995) Psychopharmacological approaches to childhood psychotic disorders. In: *Advances in the Neurobiology of Schizophrenia.* (J.A. Den Boer, H.G.M. Westenberg & H.M. Van Praag (eds), pp. 429–57). John Wiley & Sons, New York.

Buitelaar, J.K., Rutger, J., van der Gaag & van der Hoeven, J. (1998) Buspirone in the management of anxiety and irritability in children with pervasive developmental disorders: results of an open-label study. *J Clin Psychiatry* 59, 56–9.

Caccia, S., Vigano, G.L., Mingardi, G. *et al.* (1988) Clinical pharmacokinetics of oral buspirone in patients with impaired renal function. *Clin Pharmacokinet* **14**, 171–7.

Campbell, M., Adams, P., Perry, R. *et al.* (1988) Tardive and withdrawal dyskinesia in autistic children: a prospective study. *Psychopharmacol Bull* **24**, 251–5.

Campbell, M., Anderson, L.T., Meier, M. *et al.* (1978) A comparison of haloperidol and behavior therapy and their interaction in autistic children. *J Am Acad Child Psychiatry* **17**, 640–55.

Cantillon, M., Brunswick, R., Molina, D. *et al.* (1996) Buspirone versus haloperidol. A double-blind trial for agitation in a nursing home population with Alzheimer's disease. *Am J Geriatr Psychiatry* **4**, 236–67.

Charney, D.S. & Heninger, G.R. (1985) Noradrenergic function and the mechanism of action of antianxiety treatment. I. The effect of long-term alprazolam treatment. *Arch Gen Psychiatry* **42**, 458–67.

Chiaie, R., Pancheri, P., Cassacchia, M. *et al.* (1995) Assessment of the efficacy of buspirone in patients affected by generalized anxiety disorder, shifting to buspirone from prior treatment with lorazepam: a placebo-controlled, double-blind study. *J Clin Psychopharmacol* **15**, 12–19.

Cinciripini, P.M., Lapitsky, L., Seay, S. *et al.* (1995) A placebo-controlled evaluation of the effects of buspirone on smoking cessation: differences between high- and low-anxiety smokers. *J Clin Psychopharmacol* **15**, 182–91.

Cohen, D.J., Paul, R. & Volkmar, F.R. (1986) Issues in the classification of pervasive and other developmental disorders: toward DSM-IV. *J Am Acad Child Psychiatry* **25**, 213–20.

Cohn, J.B., Bowden, C.L., Fisher, J.G. & Rodos, J. (1986a) Double-blind comparison of buspirone and clorazepate in anxious outpatients. *Am J Med* **80**, 10–16.

Cohn, J.B. & Rickels, K. (1989) A pooled, double-blind comparison of the effects of buspirone, diazepam and placebo in women with chronic anxiety. *Curr Med Res Opin* **11**, 304–20.

Craven, J. & Sutherland, A. (1991) Buspirone for anxiety disorders in patients with severe lung disease [letter]. *Lancet* **338**, 249.

Cutler, N., Sramek, J., Hesselink, J.M.K. *et al.* (1993) A double-blind, placebo-controlled study comparing the efficacy and safety of ipsapirone versus lorazepam in patients with generalized anxiety disorder: a prospective multicenter trial. *J Clin Psychopharmacol* **13**, 429–37.

Dalhoff, K., Poulsen, H.E., Garred, P. *et al.* (1987) Buspirone pharmacokinetics in patients with cirrhosis. *Br J Clin Pharmacol* **24**, 547–50.

Davidson, J.R., Dupont, R.L., Hedges, D. & Haskins, J.T. (1999) Efficacy, safety, and tolerability of venlafaxine extended release and buspirone in outpatients with generalized anxiety disorder. *J Clin Psychiatry* **60**, 528–35.

De Montigny, C. & Blier, P. (1992) Potentiation of 5-HT neurotransmission by short-term lithium: *in vivo* electrophysiological studies. *Clin Neuropsychopharmacol* **15**, 610A–11A.

De Roeck, J., Dluydts, R., Schotte, C. *et al.* (1989) Explorative single-blind study on the sedative and hypnotic effects of buspirone in anxiety patients. *Acta Psychiatr Scand* **79**, 129–35.

Demartinis, N., Rynn, M., Rickels, K. & Mandos, L. (2000) Prior benzodiazepine use and buspirone response in the treatment of generalized anxiety disorder. *J Clin Psychiatry* **61**, 91–4.

Dement, W.C., Seidel, W.F., Cohen, S.A. *et al.* (1991) Effects of alprazolam, buspirone and diazepam on daytime sedation and performance. *Drug Invest* **3**, 148–56.

Dimitriou, E.C. & Dimitriou, C.E. (1998) Buspirone augmentation of antidepressant therapy. *J Clin Psychopharmacol* **18**, 465–9.

Dimitriou, E.C., Parashos, A.J. & Giouzepas, J.S. (1992) Buspirone versus alprazolam. A double-blind comparative study of their efficacy, adverse effects and withdrawal symptoms. *Drug Invest* **4**, 316–21.

Duffy, J.D. & Molloy, P.F. (1994) Efficacy of buspirone in the treatment of post-traumatic stress disorder: an open trial. *Ann Clin Psychiatry* **6**, 33–7.

Eison, A.S. & Temple D.L., Jr (1986) Buspirone. Review of its pharmacology and current perspectives on its mechanism of action. *Am J Med* **80**, 1–9.

Eison, A.S. (1990) Azapirones. mechanism of action in anxiety and depression. *Drug Ther* **20** (Suppl.), 3–8.

Enkelmann, R. (1991) Alprazolam versus buspirone in the treatment of outpatients with generalized anxiety disorder. *Psychopharmacology* **105**, 428–32.

Erwin, C.W., Linnoila, M., Hartwell, J. *et al.* (1986) Effects of buspirone and diazepam, alone and in combination with alcohol, on skilled performance and evoked potentials. *J Clin Psychopharmacol* **6**, 199–209.

Fabre, L.F. (1990) Buspirone in the management of major depression: a placebo-controlled comparison. *J Clin Psychiatry* **51** (Suppl.), 55–61.

Feighner, J.P. & Cohen, J.B. (1989) Analysis of individual symptoms in generalized anxiety—a pooled, multistudy, double-blind evaluation of buspirone. *Neuropsychobiology* **21**, 124–30.

Feighner, J.P., Merideth, C.H. & Hendrickson, G.A. (1982) A double-blind comparison of buspirone and diazepam in outpatients with generalized anxiety disorder. *J Clin Psychiatry* **43**, 103–7.

Fulton, B. & Brogden, R.N. (1997) Buspirone. An updated review of its clinical pharmacology and therapeutic applications. *CNS Drugs* **7**, 68–88.

Gammans, R.E., Kerns, E.H. & Bullen, W.W. (1985) Capillary gas chromatographic-mass spectrometric determination of buspirone in plasma. *J Chromatogr* **345**, 285–97.

Gammans, R.E., Mayol, R.F. & Labudde, J.A. (1986) Metabolism and disposition of buspirone. *Am J Med* **80** (Suppl. 3B), 41–51.

Gammans, R.E., Pfeffer, M., Westrick, M.L. *et al.* (1987) Lack of interaction between cimetidine and buspirone. *Pharmacotherapy* **7**, 72–9.

Gammans, R.E., Westrick, M.L., Shea, J.P. *et al.* (1989) Pharmacokinetics of buspirone in elderly subjects. *J Clin Pharmacol* **29**, 72–8.

Goa, K.L., Ward, A. & Buspirone, A. (1986) Preliminary review of its pharmacological properties and therapeutic efficacy as an anxiolytic. *Drugs* **32**, 114–29.

Goff, D.C., Midha, K.K., Brotman, A.W. *et al.* (1991) An open trial of buspirone added to neuroleptics in schizophrenic patients. *J Clin Psychopharmacol* **11**, 193–7.

Goldberg, H.L. & Finnerty, R.J. (1979) The comparative efficacy of buspirone and diazepam in the treatment of anxiety. *Am J Psychiatry* **136**, 1184–7.

Goldberg, H.L. & Finnerty, R. (1982) Comparison of buspirone in two separate studies. *J Clin Psychiatry* **43**, 87–91.

Goldberg, R.J. (1994) The use of buspirone in geriatric patients. *J Clin Psychiatry* **12**, 31–2.

Gonul, A.S., Oguz, A., Yabanoglu, I., Aslan, S.S. & Turan, T. (1999) Buspirone and pindolol in augmentation therapy of treatment-resistant depression. *Eur Neuropsychopharmacol* **9** (Suppl. 5), S215.

Greenblatt, D.J., Harmatz, J.S., Gouthro, T.A. *et al.* (1994) Distinguishing a benzodiazepine agonist (triazolam) from a nonagonist anxiolytic (buspirone) by electroencephalography: kinetic-dynamic studies. *Clin Pharmacol Ther* **56**, 100–11.

Gregory, C.A., Anderson, I.M. & Cowen, P.J. (1990) Metergoline abolishes the prolactin response to buspirone. *Psychopharmacology Berl* **100**, 283–4.

Gualtieri, C.T. (1991) Buspirone for the behavior problems of patients with organic brain disorders [letter]. *J Clin Psychopharmacol* **11**, 280–1.

Hamilton, M.A. (1959) The assessment of anxiety states by rating. *Br J Med Psychol* **32**, 50–5.

Hart, R.P., Colenda, C. & Hamer, R.M. (1991) Effects of buspirone and alprazolam on the cognitive performance of normal elderly subjects. *Am J Psychiatry* **148**, 73–7.

Hilleman, D.E., Mohiuddin, S.M., Del Core, M.G. *et al.* (1992) Effect of buspirone on withdrawal symptoms associated with smoking cessation. *Arch Intern Med* **152**, 350–2.

Jajoo, H.K., Mayol, R.F., LaBudde, J.A. *et al.* (1989) Metabolism of the antianxiety drug buspirone in human subjects. *Drug Metab Dispos* **17**, 634–40.

Jann, M.W., Huang, H.F., Chang, T.P. *et al.* (1996) Lack of pharmacokinetic interactions between buspirone and haloperidol in schizophrenic patients [abstract no. P-2–1]. *Eur Neuropsychopharmacol* **6** (Suppl. 3), 37.

Jenike, M.A., Baer, L. & Buttolph, L. (1991) Buspirone augmentation of fluoxetine in patients with obsessive-compulsive disorder. *J Clin Psychiatry* **52**, 13–14.

Joshi, P.T., Capozzoli, J.A. & Coyle, J.T. (1988) Low-dose neuroleptic therapy for children with childhood-onset pervasive developmental disorder. *Am J Psychiatry* **145**, 335–8.

Kendler, K.S., Neale, M.C., Kessler, R.C. *et al.* (1992) Major depression and generalized anxiety disorder: same genes, (partly) different environments? *Arch Gen Psychiatry* **49**, 716–22.

Kiev, A. & Domantay, A.G. (1988) A study of buspirone coprescribed with bronchodilators in 82 anxious ambulatory patients. *J Asthma* **25**, 281–4.

Kiev, A. & Domantay, A.G. (1989) A study of buspirone coprescribed with nonsteroidal antiinflammatory drugs in 150 anxious ambulatory patients. *Curr Ther Res* **46**, 1086–90.

Kranzler, H.R., Burleson, J.A. & Del, B.F.K. *et al.* (1994) Buspirone treatment of anxious alcoholics: a placebo-controlled trial. *Arch Gen Psychiatry* **51**, 702–31.

Kushner, M.G., Sher, K.J. & Beitman B.D. (1990) The relation between alcohol problems and the anxiety disorders. *Am J Psychiatry* **147**, 685–95.

Kutcher, S.P., Reiter, S., Gardener, D.M. *et al.* (1992) The pharmacotherapy of anxiety disorders in children and adolescents. *Psychiatr Clin North Am* **15**, 41–66.

Laakman, G., Schule, C., Lorkowski, G., Baghai, T., Kuhn, K. & Ehrentraut, S. (1998) Buspirone and lorazepam in the treatment of generalized anxiety disorder in outpatients. *Psychopharmacology* **136**, 357–66.

van Laar, M.W., Volkerts, E.R. & van Willigenburg, A.P. (1992) Therapeutic effects and effects on actual driving performance of chronically administered buspirone and diazepam in anxious outpatients. *J Clin Psychopharmacol* **12**, 86–95.

Lader, M. & Scotto, J.C. (1998) A multicenter double-blind comparison of hydroxyzine, buspirone and placebo in patients with generalized anxiety disorder. *Psychopharmacology* **139**, 402–6.

Lamberg, T.S., Kivisto, K.T. & Neuvonen, P.J. (1998) Effects of verapamil and diltiazem on the pharmacokinetics and pharmacodynamics of buspirone. *Clin Pharmacol Ther* **63**, 640–5.

Landen, M., Bjorling, G., Agren, H. & Fahlen, T. (1998) A randomized, double-blind, placebo-controlled trial of buspirone in combination with an SSRI in patients with treatment-refractory depression. *J Clin Psychiatry* **59**, 664–8.

Langlois, R.P. & Paquette, D. (1994) Sustained bradycardia during fluvoxamine and buspirone intoxication. *Can J Psychiatry* **39**, 126–7.

Lilja, J.J., Kivisto, K.T., Backman, J.T., Lamberg, T.S. & Neuvonen, P.J. (1998) Grapefruit juice substantially increases plasma concentrations of buspirone. *Clin Pharmacol Ther* **64**, 655–60.

Littman, A.B., Fava, M., McKool, K. *et al.* (1993) Buspirone therapy for Type A behavior, hostility, and perceived stress in cardiac patients. *Psychother Psychosom* **59**, 107–10.

Lucki, I., Rickels, K., Giesecke, A. & Geller, A. (1987) Differential effects of the anxiolytic drugs, diazepam and buspirone on memory function. *Br J Clin Pharmacol* **23**, 207–11.

Malcolm, R., Anton, R.F., Randall, C.L. *et al.* (1992) A placebo-controlled trial of buspirone in anxious inpatient alcoholics. *Alcohol Clin Exp Res* **16**, 1007–13.

Manfredi, R.L., Kales, A., Vgontzas A. *et al.* (1991) Buspirone: sedative or stimulant effect? *Am J Psychiatry* **148**, 1213–17.

Mattila, M.J., Aranko, K. & Seppala, T. (1982) Acute effects of buspirone and alcohol on psychomotor skills. *J Clin Psychiatry* **43**, 56–60.

Mayol, R.F., Gammans, R.E., Mackenthun, A.V. *et al.* (1983) The effect of food on the bioavailability of buspirone HCl [abstract]. *Clin Res* **31**, 631a.

Moskowitz, H. & Smiley, A. (1982) Effects of chronically administered buspirone and diazepam on driving-related skills performance. *J Clin Psychiatry* **43**, 45–55.

Moss, L.E. & Neppe, V.M. & Drevets, W.C. (1993) Buspirone in the treatment of tardive dyskinesia. *J Clin Psychopharmacol* **13**, 204–9.

Munjack, D.J., Bruns, J., Baltazar, P.L. *et al.* (1991) A pilot study of buspirone in the treatment of social phobia. *J Anxiety Disord* **5**, 87–98.

Murphy, S.M., Owen, R. & Tyrer, P. (1989) Comparative assessment of efficacy and withdrawal symptoms after 6 and 12 weeks' treatment with diazepam or buspirone. *Br J Psychiatry* **154**, 529–34.

Napoliello, M.J. (1986) A study of buspirone coprescribed with antidepressants in 184 anxious ambulatory patients. *Curr Ther Res* **40**, 917–23.

Neppe, V.M. (1989) High-dose buspirone in a case of tardive dyskinesia [letter]. *Lancet* **2**, 8677.

Newton, R.E., Marunycz, J.D., Alderdice, M.T. *et al.* (1986) Review of the side-effect profile of buspirone. *Am J Med* **80** (Suppl. 3B), 17–21.

Norden, M.J. (1994) Buspirone treatment of sexual dysfunction associated with selective serotonin reuptake inhibitors. *Depression* **2**, 109–12.

Olivier, B., van Wijngaarden, I. & Soudijn, W. (2000) 5-HT3 receptor antagonists and anxiety; a preclinical and clinical review. *Eur Neuropsychopharmacol* **10**, 77–95.

Othmer, E. & Othmer, S.C. (1987) Effect of buspirone on sexual dysfunction in patients with generalized anxiety disorder. *J Clin Psychiatry* **48**, 201–3.

Pascual, J. & Berciano, J. (1991) An open trial of buspirone in migraine prophylaxis: preliminary report. *Clin Neuropharmacol* **14**, 245–50.

Pato, M.T., Pigott, T.A., Hill, J.L. *et al.* (1991) Controlled comparison of buspirone and clomipramine in obsessive-compulsive disorder. *Am J Psychiatry* **148**, 127–9.

Pecknold, J.C. (1994) Serotonin 5-HT1A agonists. a comparative review. *CNS Drugs* **2**, 234–51.

Pecknold, J.C., Matas, M., Howarth, B.G. *et al.* (1989) Evaluation of buspirone as an antianxiety agent: buspirone and diazepam versus placebo. *Am J Psychiatryry* **34**, 766–71.

Phillips, K.A. (1996) An open study of buspirone augmentation of serotonin-reuptake inhibitors in body dysmorphic disorder. *Psychopharmacol Bull* **32**(1), 175–80.

Pohl, R., Balon, R., Yeragani, V.K. *et al.* (1989) Serotonergic anxiolytics in the treatment of panic disorder: a controlled study with buspirone. *Psychopathology* **22** (Suppl. 1), 60–7.

Pollicino, A.M., Spina, E., Campo, G.M. *et al.* (1992) Pharmacokinetics interactions between tricyclic antidepressants and other psychotropic drugs in depressed patients. *Pharmacol Res* **25** (Suppl. 2), 210–11.

Rakel, R.E. (1990) Long-term buspirone therapy for chronic anxiety: a multicenter international study to determine safety. *South Med J* **83**, 194–8.

Rapaport, D.M., Greenberg, H.E. & Goldring, R.M. (1991) Differing effects of the anxiolytic agents buspirone and diazepam on control of breathing. *Clin Pharmacol Ther* **49**, 394–401.

Ratey, J.J., Leveroni, C.L., Miller, A.C. *et al.* (1992) Low-dose buspirone to treat agitation and maladaptive behavior in brain-injured patients: two case reports [letter]. *J Clin Psychopharmacol* **12**, 362–4.

Realmuto, G.M., August, G.J. & Garfinkel, B.D. (1989) Clinical effect of buspirone in autistic children. *J Clin Psychopharmacol* **9**, 122–5.

Rickels, K. & Schweizer, E. (1990) The clinical course and long-term management of generalized anxiety disoder: *J Clin Psychopharmacol* **10**, 101S–10S.

Rickels, K., Amsterdam, J.D., Clary, C. *et al.* (1991) Buspirone in major depression: a controlled study. *J Clin Psychiatry* **52**, 34–8.

Rickels, K., DeMartinis, N., Garcia-Espana, F., Greenblat, D., Mandos, L. & Rynn, M. (2000) Imipramine and buspirone in treatment of patients with generalized anxiety disorder who are discontinuing long-term benzodiazepine therapy. *Am J Psychiatry* **157**, 1973–9.

Rickels, K., Downing, R., Scheweizer, E. & Hassman, H. (1993) Antidepressants for the treatment of generalized anxiety disorder: a placebo-controlled comparison of imipramine, trazodone, and diazepam. *Arch Gen Psychiatry* **50**, 884–95.

Rickels, K., Freeman, E. & Sondheimer, S. (1989) Buspirone in treatment of premenstrual syndrome. *Lancet* **1**, 777.

Rickels, K., Schweizer, E., Csanalosi, I. *et al.* (1988) Long-term treatment of anxiety and risk of withdrawal: prospective comparison of clorazepate and buspirone. *Arch Gen Psychiatry* **45**, 444–50.

Rickels, K., Schweizer, E., DeMaritinis, N., Mandos, L. & Mercer, C. (1997) Gepirone and diazepam in generalized anxiety disorder: a placebo-controlled trial. *J Clin Psychopharmacol* **17**, 272–7.

Rickels, K., Wiseman, K., Norstad, N. *et al.* (1982) Buspirone and diazepam in anxiety: a controlled study. *J Clin Psychiatry* **43**, 81–6.

Ritchie, L.D. & Cox, J. (1993) A multicenter study of buspirone in the treatment of anxiety disorders in the elderly. *Br J Clin Res* **4**, 131–9.

Robinson, D., Napoliello, M.J. & Schenk, J. (1988) The safety and usefulness of buspirone as an anxiolytic drug in the elderly versus young patients. *Clin Ther* **10**, 740–6.

Sacchetti, E., Zerbini, O., Banfi, F. *et al.* (1994) Overlap of buspirone with lorazepam, diazepam and bromazepam in patients with generalized anxiety disorder: findings from a controlled, multicenter, double-blind study. *Hum Psychopharmacol* **9**, 409–22.

Schaffler, K. & Klausnitzer, W. (1989) Placebo-controlled study on acute and subchronic effects of buspirone versus bromazepam utilizing psychomotor and cognitive assessments in healthy volunteers. *Pharmacopsychiatry* **22**, 26–33.

Scheibe, G. (1996) Four-year follow-up in 40 outpatients with anxiety disorders: buspirone versus lorazepam. *Eur J Pscyhiat* **10**, 25–34.

Schweizer, E., Amsterdam, J., Rickels, K. *et al.* (1986) Open trial of buspirone in the treatment of major depressive disorder. *Psychopharmacol Bull* **22**, 183–5.

Schweizer, E. & Rickels, K. (1986) Failure of buspirone to manage benzodiazepine withdrawal. *Am J Psychiatry* **143**, 1590–2.

Schweizer, E. & Rickels, R. (1994) New and emerging clinical uses for buspirone. *J Clin Psychiatry Monograph* **12**, 1.

Schweizer, E. & Rickels, K. (1995) Buspirone and related 5-HT compounds as anxiolytics. In: *Hypnotics and Anxiolytics* (D.J. Nutt & W.B. Mendelson (eds), pp. 447–66). Bailliere Tindall, London.

Schweizer, E., Rickels, K. & Lucki, I. (1986) Resistance to the anti-anxiety effect of buspirone in patients with a history of benzodiazepine use. *N Engl J Med* **314**, 719–20.

Schweizer, E., Rickels, K., Hassman, H. & Garcia-Espana, F. (1998) Buspirone and imipramine for the treatment of major depression in the elderly. *J Clin Psychiatry* **59**, 175–83.

Sellers, E.M., Schneiderman, J.F., Romacch, M.K. *et al.* (1992) Comparative drug effects and abuse liability of lorazepam, buspirone, and secobarbital in nondependent subjects. *J Clin Psychopharmacol* **12**, 79–85.

Sheehan, D.V., Raj, A.B., Harnett-Sheehan, K. *et al.* (1993) The relative efficacy of high-dose buspirone and alprazolam in the treatment of panic disorder: a double-blind placebo-controlled study. *Acta Psychiatr Scand* **88**, 1–11.

Simeon, J.G., Knott, V.J., Dubois, C. *et al.* (1994) Buspirone therapy of mixed anxiety disorders in childhood and adolescence: a pilot study. *J Child Adolesc Psychophamacol* **4**, 159–70.

Sramek, J.J., Tansman, M., Suri, A. *et al.* (1996) Efficacy of buspirone in generalized anxiety disorder with coexisting mild depressive symptoms. *J Clin Psychiatry* **57**, 287–91.

Stahl, S.M., Kaiser, L., Roeschen, J., Kepper-Hesselink, J.M. & Orazem, J. (1998) Effectiveness of ipsapirone, a 5-HT1A partial agonist, in major depressive disorder. Support for the role of 5-HT1A receptors in the mechanism of action of serotonergic antidepressants. *Int J Neuropsychopharmacol* **1**, 11–18.

Strand, M., Hetta, J., Rosen, A. *et al.* (1990) A double-blind, controlled trial in primary care patients with generalized anxiety: a comparison between buspirone and oxazepam. *J Clin Psychiatry* **51** (Suppl.), 40–5.

Tollefson, G.D., Godes, M., Montague-Clouse, J. *et al.* (1989) Buspirone: effects on prolactin and growth hormone as a function of drug level in generalized anxiety. *J Clin Psychopharmacol* **9**, 132–6.

Tollefson, G.D., Montague-Clouse, J. & Tollefson, S.L. (1992) Treatment of comorbid generalized anxiety in a recently detoxified alcoholic population with a selective serotonergic drug (buspirone). *J Clin Psychopharmacol* **12**, 19–26.

Troisi, I.I.J.R., Critchfield, T.S. & Griffiths, R.R. (1993) Buspirone and lorazepam abuse liability in humans. Behavioral effects, subjective effects and choice. *Behav Pharmacol* **4**, 217–30.

Tunnicliff, G. (1991) Molecular basis of buspirone's anxiolytic action. *Pharmacol Toxicol* **69**, 149–56.

Tyrer, P., Seivewright, N., Ferguson, B. *et al.* (1992) The general neurotic syndrome: a coaxial diagnosis of anxiety, depression and personality disorder. *Acta Psychiatr Scand* **85**, 201–6.

Udelman, H.D. & Udelman, D.L. (1990) Concurrent use of buspirone in anxious patients during withdrawal from alprazolam therapy. *J Clin Psychiatry* **51**(9) (Suppl.), 46–50.

Vliet, I.M., den Boer, J.A.D., Westenberg, H.G.M. & Ho Pian, K.L. (1997) Clinical effects of buspirone in social phobia: a double-blind placebo-controlled study. *J Clin Psychiatry* **58**, 164–8.

West, R., Hajek, P. & McNeill, A. (1991) Effect of buspirone on cigarette withdrawal symptoms and short-term abstinence rates in a smokers' clinic. *Psychopharmacology* **104**, 91–6.

Wheatley, D. (1982) Buspirone. Multicenter efficacy study. *J Clin Psychiatry* **43**, 92–4.

21 Antihistamines in the Treatment of Psychic and Somatic Anxiety States

M.M.M.P. Van Moffaert

Introduction

The global prevalence of anxiety disorder lies between 2% and 5% (Angst & Wicki 1992) and both generalized anxiety and panic disorder are among the psychiatric conditions that have to be dealt with most frequently in general practice. Anxiety states are frequently found to express themselves in somatization: general practitioners as well as somatic specialists find that between 10% and 30% of their patients suffer from somatized anxiety through unexplained somatic symptoms. Not only masked depression but also anxiety may underlie unexplained symptoms of a cardiac or gastrointestinal nature (Van Moffaert & Jannes 1987).

The skin, however, as the most visible, expressive and accessible organ, proves to be the target of choice for somatization, which ranges from subjective symptoms such as pruritus—as a sign of tension—to self-provoked lesions as a result of scratching and skin picking—as the psychomotoric and behavioral exteriorization of tension and anxious stress (Van Moffaert 1982).

Although this somatization of anxiety, particularly in a dermatological context, has been extensively researched in its clinical, neurobiological and psychodynamic aspects, its treatment remains very much under discussion. The choice of drug treatment of psychic and somatic types of anxiety requires special attention, mainly because anxiety disorders tend to become chronic, especially in women, and because some of the most widely used anxiolytic drugs, benzodiazepines in particular, have major drawbacks, including diminishing effects in the long term, the possibility of dependence and of memory impairment and, particularly in the elderly, an increased risk of falls with fractures as a result of myorelaxant activity.

The use of antihistamines, hydroxyzine in particular, may offer an alternative or an addition to the current armamentarium for the treatment of anxiety. As the antihistaminic and antipruritus effects of hydroxyzine are an asset in dermatology, its efficacy has been investigated in psychodermatological conditions such as psychogenic pruritus and anxiety with dermatological somatization.

Somatization of anxiety in general liaison-psychiatry settings

Clinical experience shows that somatized anxiety is frequently encountered in different fields of somatic medicine, and that its clinical picture differs from that routinely seen in general psychiatric practice. Cardiologists are faced with "cardiac neurosis." Gastroenterologists have to deal with irritable bowel syndrome, which is often a particular mixture of somatized anxiety and depression. In dentistry preintervention anxiety is common, specially in children. In dermatology many aesthetically disabling diseases such as eczema, psoriasis, alopecia, urticaria, and rosacea, engender anxiety, often in the form of a social fear of being found ugly and repugnant. In emergency medicine a prompt differential diagnosis is often hard to make because of anxiety-related clinical situations. A typical anxious patient presents him or herself as a medical emergency case with cardiac pain and dyspnea. In one single year more than 100 patients were admitted to the Emergency Department of the University Hospital of

Ghent, Belgium, with a demand for immediate medical help, while in fact they suffered from an anxiety state (Van Moffaert *et al.* 1988).

Anxiety is characterized by autonomic arousal symptoms and unexplained physical symptoms. A hypochondriacal fixation on these autonomic concomitant symptoms of anxiety often creates a vicious circle of anxious and psychosomatic symptoms, thus creating hybrid syndromes of anxio-depressive states, panic disorder with reactive depression, or adjustment disorders with anxiety and depressive mood (Widlocher *et al.* 1983). In women there is a 2–4 times higher overall prevalence of anxiety, phobia and panic than in men, and anxiety may typically connect with the procreative cycle of the female. Furthermore, premenstrual tension syndrome, postnatal depression and climacteric depression are syndromes in which agitation and anxiety coexist with a range of physical symptoms. Indeed, comorbidity and somatization are altogether more prevalent in women. (Van Moffaert 1987).

It is a fallacy to regard anxiety disorder as a mild condition which may be left to its natural course. Recent research has clearly indicated that anxiety has an unfavorable prognosis with chronicity, comorbidity with depression, as well as higher cardiovascular morbidity, perhaps even mortality. Also a higher suicide risk has been mentioned, as anxiety symptoms are found to constitute a specific marker in the 2 weeks prior to a suicide attempt (Van Moffaert 1987). Anxiety must alert the physician to vigilance and an interventionist approach. Not only the psychological compounds of generalized anxiety must be dealt with, but its psychosomatic and psychomotoric components are often pivotal. Further empirical research is required into the treatment of different subtypes of anxiety in liaison settings, e.g., concentration difficulties, insomnia, fatigue, irritability and worry, hypervigilance, and anticipatory anxiety.

Anxiety and psychodermatological disorders

Both dermatologists and general practitioners should be particularly aware of the interaction between anxiety and psychosomatic dermatological symptoms. Indeed, anxiety and psychodermatological symptoms are intricately intertwined, both on the emotional and behavioral level and in a causative and a reactive way

(Wittkower & Lester 1960). Anxiety states may be contributive, concomitant or secondary to a skin disorder. They may be accompanied by skin arousal phenomena, they may result in skin-damaging behavior, they can trigger a relapse of a pre-existing dermatosis, while in turn dermatosis may cause anxiety (Van Moffaert 1992).

Anxiety states may be accompanied by an arousal of physical perceptions and by psychophysiological signs such as flushing, whitening of the skin, or pilo-erection. The psychosomatic clinical picture is complicated by the fact that because of their visibility, and hence their negative impact on self-image, these dermatological symptoms add to the detriment of the patient's psychological well-being. The dermatological symptoms may eventually lead to psychiatric comorbidity in the form of social phobia or obsessive-compulsive behavior.

On the other hand, anxiety states contain a behavioral component to the extent that they tend to increase and intensify displacement activities, i.e., gestures that mimic washing or grooming rituals and that are performed by primates and humans in stressful situations. The self-touching, scratching, even picking displacement behavior naturally focuses on the skin and may lead to full-blown psychodermatological disorders. Thus anxiety can result in excoriations and facial lesions that are aggravated and perpetuated in a neurotic pattern that can further lead to depression and social phobia (Van Moffaert 1982). Also psychic anxiety that is accompanied by pruritus is sometimes relieved by scratching (without itching as a trigger) as a kind of displacement behavior (Fjellner *et al.* 1985).

Anxiety is both causative and reactive in general tension-provoking itch, a condition that leads to scratching as a tension reducing habit (Van Moffaert 1989). Many skin disorders, acne and alopecia in particular, are complicated by social phobia. Dermatoses of the genital area generally cause deterioration of the patient's sex life (Panconesi 1984). This connection is often overlooked, and it is strongly recommended to inquire explicitly about the patient's sexual activity and feelings of sexual (un)attractiveness (Koblenzer 1987).

Anxious patients tend to express their tensions in obsessive-compulsive behavior such as nail biting (onychophagy), hair pulling (trichotillomania, trichophagy), or excoriations. The essential feature of trichotillomania is the recurrent pulling out of one's hair with noticeable hair loss as a result. Like nail-biting, lip-biting and excoriations, trichotillomnia is a behavior that is in origin part of normal human self-grooming but that in anxious patients may escalate to an obsessive–compulsive syndrome. The patient with trichotillomania selects an area of the scalp to be pulled and ritualistically twists, then scrutinizes and possibly even eats (trichophagy) the hair after it has been extracted (Koo & Strauss 1987).

Anxiety has an even stronger negative impact on pre-existing dermatological conditions. It is not only a causative factor in all kinds of somatization on the skin, but it is also a major determinant in the onset and the severity of many dermatological disorders. Eczema, alopecia areata, psoriasis and urticaria are strongly affected by the anxiety that accompanies both non-specific stress factors and specific stressful life events such as the threat of loss through separation. This anxious component can also trigger a relapse and affect the duration of the disorder as well as the patient's drug compliance. Although the primary cause of atopic dermatitis (also known as neurodermatitis) is clearly immunological, anxiety factors play a part in precipitating and maintaining the lesions, and have a strong impact on the itch-scratch cycle. In infantile eczema the role of anxiety factors is beyond question (Beveridge 1974).

Attacks or relapses of alopecia areata may be induced by anxiety factors, neurotic personality features and psycho-immunological disturbances. Similarly, neuro-endocrinological investigations suggest that patients with psoriasis suffer not only from biological vulnerability, but also from personality features that make them perceive and interpret challenging situations as more anxiogenic than normal. Furthermore, experimental work has confirmed that patients with psychogenic pruritus have distinctive character features that are anxiety-related, such as "semipermeability of their emotional balance" (that is extreme vulnerability to social stress), an inability to manage aggressive tendencies, character armoring (resistance to other people's emotions), and exaggerated cleanliness. Also chronic hyperhidrosis (excessive sweating) is generally accepted to be related to anxiety and stress factors. Clinical improvement in the condition has been achieved through biofeedback therapies that reduce the symptoms and the underlying anxiety associated with the condition (Whitlock 1970).

An additional problem characteristic for skin conditions is that they often lead to reactive psychological problems and psychiatric disorders such as depression and social anxiety, because the direct visibility of the skin lesions can easily lead to undeserved professional and social stigmatization. Dermatological patients tend to experience a "leper complex," as their appearance inevitably lowers their self-esteem. In addition they have to cope with the practical inconvenience caused by the dermatosis and its treatment, which often includes occlusive dressings and the need to wear a bath cap or to apply smelly ointments.

Body dysmorphic disorder (BDD) is another anxiety-related psychosomatic skin problem. It is the obsessive fear of a major skin defect or of minor conditions such as blemishes and red spots, or wrinkling and changing of the skin with ageing (Hay 1990). The imagined or exaggerated defects, the perception of which lies on a continuum from over-valued ideas to outright psychosis, become the focus of obsessive thought or phobic avoidance. BDD on the skin can lead to urgent requests for incisive dermatological treatment (laser therapy or transplant) and/or cosmetic surgery.

Finally, the treatment of anxiety in a psychopharmacological context should always be part of an approach that combines medical and psychobiobehavioral management. The temporary use of an anxiolytic compound is justified to reduce the psychological stress, tension, anxiety, hostility or irritation underlying a dermatosis. If the anxiety is reduced, the intensity of the scratching or the general interfering with the skin is lowered, and the skin will have the opportunity to heal.

Antihistamines: hydroxyzine (Atarax®, Vistaril®)

Antihistaminic drugs are not widely used in psychiatry, with the exception of diphenhydramine i.v. for the treatment of acute dystonic reaction and of hydroxyzine as a sedative, antiemetic and antipruritus agent. Centrally acting antihistamines are of limited use as anxiolytics, but hydroxyzine, an antihistamine that was synthetized in Belgium, was developed as a minor tranquilizer with antihistaminergic properties (Natens 1992). The substance is chemically unrelated to the phenothiazines, the benzodiazepines or meprobamate. It is a piperazine derivative whose core action is the suppression of activity in certain key regions of the subcortical area of the central nervous system. However, hydroxyzine is not a direct corticodepressant. The anxiolytic effect of hydroxyzine is probably through a modulating role of the H1 receptor (Leonard 1999). For the treatment of pruritus the sedative effect is significant since the nonsedative H1 antagonists are less effective. The anti-allergic effect of hydroxyzine is partially based on its active metabolite cetirizine.

Hydroxyzine has been tried in many clinical situations for the relief of anxiety and tension, with or without the association of neurotic anxiety. Since the early 1960s it has been used to treat both psychic and somatic anxiety in its many syndromes: predentistry or preoperative anxiety, stress related syndromes, etc.

The histamine receptors antagonist properties of hydroxyzine have made its use in dermatological disorders widespread. In particular in the management of pruritus, certainly of histamine-mediated pruritus, chronic urticaria, and atopic dermatoses, hydroxyzine has proved useful.

As the use of benzodiazepines is limited in view of the risks of dependency, overcompliance and withdrawal effects such as rebound anxiety, antihistamines and hydroxyzine, in particular, have been used as tranquilizers in patients with psychic and somatic anxiety.

Hydroxyzine trials in diverse anxiety states

Open studies

Most open trials with hydroxyzine have failed to meet the selection criteria of the current Diagnostic Statistical Manual, fourth edition (DSM-IV: American Psychiatric Association [APA] 1994) inclusion criteria of generalized anxiety disorder (GAD). However, all patients in the trials discussed here were suffering from some sort of anxiety syndrome, either anxiety as a psychiatric illness ("anxiety neurosis"), trait anxiety as part of a personality disorder, or state anxiety related to stress, e.g., preoperative anxiety, in particular preceding dental surgery.

In 54 elderly patients suffering from anxiety and various cardiac disorders, Shalowitz (1956) found good (76%) to partial (19%) efficacy after treatment with 30–100 mg/day hydroxyzine during 1–6 months. Neither significant side-effects nor adverse effects on biological parameters were observed. Settel (1957) obtained good results in 76% of 83 patients suffering from neurotic anxiety by treating them with hydroxyzine 2–3 × 10–25 mg/day during 2–10 weeks. Garber (1958) treated 143 anxious neurotics with hydroxyzine

10–50 mg b.i.d. or t.i.d. during up to 18 months with more than 80% efficacy.

In a trial by Smigel et al. (1959) 101 elderly patients suffering from anxiety and confusion were treated with hydroxyzine 3 × 25 mg/day during 3–9 months with excellent anxiolytic results in 54% of patients, good results in 36% and partial results in 10%. Also the associated symptoms of confusion were found to have improved.

Of 2025 adults and children given hydroxyzine to relieve the tension of fear of an impending dental intervention, 91.6%, experienced good to excellent symptomatic control (Alexander 1960). As a result, diverse dental procedures were greatly expedited and undue strain upon the patient and dentist was effectively averted. No evidence of toxicity was observed. Patients were able to leave the office unaccompanied. The high degree of therapeutic efficacy of hydroxyzine was judged in its absence of injurious effects, its ease of administration, and its patient acceptability. In 93% of the 41 neurotic children treated by Litchfield (1960) hydroxyzine 10–30 mg/day during 2–36 weeks had a good effect on anxiety and emotional tension.

In Lipton's study (1961) 51 neurotic or psychotic patients were treated with hydroxyzine 50 mg to 200 mg t.i.d. for up to 16 months, with good efficacy in 70% for anxious symptoms and little efficacy for psychotic symptoms. Shalowitz (1961) treated 450 patients with anxiety neurosis with hydroxyzine 30–400 mg/day during several months to up to 4.5 years of follow-up, with good to excellent efficacy in 89% of patients. In patients with psychosis, severe agitation and depression with psychomotoric retardation, there were no good results.

In a study in which 26 children aged between 4 and 15 with anxiety expressed in hyperactivity, insomnia, tics, and enuresis, were treated with 3 × 10 mg hydroxyzine/day during 17 months, a good efficacy in 39% of all patients, and partial remission in 19% was found (Piuck 1963).

These open studies dealt with anxiety in different clinical contexts. They did not meet our current diagnostic specificity. As they relied on clinical evaluation as the main instrument of measurement they fall short of the current methodological requirements for objective quantification of psychopathology. However, their wide clinical range covering various states of anxiety demonstrated the anxiolytic action of hydroxyzine. Hydroxyzine is believed to merit the consideration of the dental profession as a possible adjunct to conventional techniques, to be used routinely whenever patients express or exhibit anxious tensions regarding dental visits. Hydroxyzine has also been widely used to treat anxiety in conjunction with bodily symptoms in the context of psychosomatic syndromes, because of its beneficial effect on somatized anxiety, in particular cardiac anxiety.

Hydroxyzine is more effective in treating anxiety of a neurotic nature than in relieving psychotic anxiety. The lack of habituation to the anxiolytic effects of the substance make it useful for chronic and intermittent administration. It has few, if any side-effects. The initial drowsiness that has been observed, disappears with the continuation of the treatment. It is well tolerated and no long-term abnormalities in biological parameters have been found.

Double-blind versus placebo studies

In 51 women with postpartum anxiety Reisner (1967) compared hydroxyzine 300 mg/day (25 patients) with placebo (16 patients). Improvement was found on parameters such as activity, communication, aggressivity, sleep, and tension, in the hydroxyzine group: an average of 7.25 versus 3.23 in the placebo group. In 56 prisoners diagnosed with anxiety the efficacy of hydroxyzine 4×100 mg/day was compared with placebo with sequential periods of 4 weeks (Breslow 1968). Anxiety and agitation were reduced in 96.4% of prisoners treated with hydroxyzine, while the placebo response was not more than 38.3%.

A double-blind, cross-over study was conducted with 100 children with behavioral disorders (Manchanda *et al.* 1969). Each group was given either hydroxyzine (2×25–50 mg/day) or placebo for 6 weeks, and the reverse during the next 6 weeks. After the first 6-week period a global reduction of 82.5% in the symptoms was seen in the hydroxyzine group and 24.3% in the placebo group. This significant improvement was sustained in 77.6% of cases during the last 6-week period (on placebo) and attained 88% (on hydroxyzine). Symptoms that improved most significantly included behavioral dysfunction, sleep pattern, appetite, sexual and emotional problems, and psychosomatic and hysterical symptoms. The improvement was less noticeable for speech and motor disturbances and social behavior.

In a trial with 51 anxious neurotic adults, Goldberg and Finnerty (1973) compared hydroxyzine with placebo. After a 4-week period the results showed a global improvement—hydroxyzine better than placebo, and on subitems such as tension and anxiety (hydroxyzine better than placebo), depression (no difference from placebo), and insomnia (hydroxyzine better than placebo).

A population of 26 anxious insomniacs were treated with hydroxyzine (2×12.5 mg $+ 1 \times 25$ mg daily) versus placebo. In the hydroxyzine group a significant and immediate relief of anxiety and insomnia was observed. After 1 week the difference with placebo grew smaller (Laffont & Cathala 1987).

In a multicenter, double-blind, randomized study, with a sounder methodology and an adequate patient selection, Ferreri *et al.* (1995) demonstrated the efficacy and tolerance of hydroxyzine and its beneficial effect on sleep, as well as stress and anxiety associated with coronary disease in 110 anxious adults. Of 110 patients with GAD, 56 patients were treated with hydroxyzine (at a fixed dose of 50 mg) against 54 with placebo. After 1 week of treatment, the anxiety was significantly more reduced in the hydroxyzine group. This beneficial effect was maintained throughout the trial period, and lasted till 1 week after discontinuation. Hantouche and Ferreri (1995) commented on methodological improvements in comparison with earlier studies. The patients were selected in accordance with the DSM-III-R (APA 1987) inclusion criteria, and the measurement was performed with the Hamilton Anxiety Rating Scale, the Tyrer Brief Anxiety Scale and the Ferreri Anxiety Rating Diagram (FARD).

Most recently, the efficacy and safety of hydroxyzine was studied in 55 patients with generalized anxiety and somatoform disorders (cardioneurosis as well as maladaptation) (Smulevich *et al.* 1999). The patients in the hydroxyzine group were given a daily dose of 50 mg for 28 days. Overall the score value of the Hamilton Anxiety Scale dropped by 10, the reduction being more obvious in patients with somatic anxiety.

These trials show some superiority of hydroxyzine versus placebo in treating GAD and related disorders. They confirm the main findings of the open label previous studies. Furthermore, they intimate the long-term maintenance of efficacy. The fast onset of action of hydroxyzine, especially on irritability, concentration difficulties, apprehension, and contact difficulties, its large spectrum of efficacy, and its maintenance of action after discontinuation make it an asset in the treatment of a number of anxiety states. Moreover, these trials confirm the absence of dependency and hydroxyzine's lack of organ toxicity. However, even in the more recent studies some methodological shortcomings remain, e.g., blurred patient selection, diverse populations (prisoners, children), diagnostic overlaps, and insufficiently defined inclusion criteria.

Comparative studies

Early studies

A population of 143 patients with withdrawal symptoms of severe alcohol addiction were tested with hydroxyzine (4×25 mg/day i.m.) versus chlorpromazine (4×25 mg/day i.m.) and reserpine (4×0.25 mg/day i.m.). The withdrawal symptoms were substantially reduced in 86% of the patients in the hydroxyzine group, in 84% in the chlorpromazine group, and in 78% in the reserpine group. Also in a population of 60 alcohol-addicted patients with diverse psychiatric comorbidity the efficacy of hydroxyzine (4×100 mg/day during 21 days) was compared to that of chlordiazepoxide (4×25 mg/day during 21 days) and placebo (Knott & Beard 1967). Hydroxyzine significantly improved the anxiety, agitation and hostility. Chlordiazepoxide did not differ significantly from placebo for the anxious symptoms but seemed to alleviate depression significantly.

In 98 patients divided into two groups of severity of anxiety, the efficacy of hydroxyzine 3×100 mg/day was compared to meprobamate 3×400 mg/day (Clyne et al. 1968). In 40 patients with mild anxiety, eight of the 14 patients (57%) in the hydroxyzine group improved versus 12 of the 26 (46%) in the meprobamate group. Among the 58 patients with severe anxiety, improvement occurred in 25 of the 27 (92%) patients treated with hydroxyzine, and in 24 of the 31 (77%) patients treated with meprobamate. In a double-blind and cross-over study including 24 patients Kellner et al. (1968) compared the efficacy of hydroxyzine (3×50 mg/day), with that of diazepam (3×5 mg/day) and placebo, and found a superior result for diazepam versus hydroxyzine and placebo. Williams (1968) compared hydroxyzine (2×100 mg/day), during 14 days with chlorpromazine (2×50 mg/day) in 32 anxious patients. Global anxiety scores were reduced 40% and 37%, respectively, with hydroxyzine and chlorpromazine, phobic symptoms with 29% and 44%, inactivity with 36% and 40%, and insomnia with 71% and 53%.

In 70 mixed anxiety-depressive patients Silver et al. (1969) compared the efficacy of hydroxyzine (25–200 mg/day), with amitriptyline (25–200 mg/day), and the association of both drugs during 8 weeks. The Brief Psychiatric Rating Scale (BPRS), the Verdun Target Symptom Rating Scale (VTSRS) and the Wittenborn Psychiatric Rating Scale (WPRS) showed significant positive results for hydroxyzine on the items of anxiety, tension and hostility.

Rickels et al. (1970) compared in 130 patients with anxiety neurosis the efficacy of hydroxyzine (55 patients, 4×100 mg/day) during 4 weeks with chlordiazepoxide (51 patients, 4×10 mg/day) and placebo (24 patients). Drop-out for adverse events was registered in 31% of patients in the hydroxyzine group, in 25% of patients in the chlordiazepoxide group, and in 12% of patients in the placebo group, leaving 97 patients for end analysis. Hydroxyzine was found to have a comparable efficacy to chlordiazepoxide and to be significantly better than placebo for the anxiety neurotic symptoms.

In 400 patients with alcohol addiction the efficacy of hydroxyzine (4×100 mg/day) was compared with that of chlordiazepoxide (4×50 mg/day), chlorpromazine (4×100 mg/day) and thiamine (4×100 mg/day). No significant improvement was found, except for thiamine and chlorpromazine (Klett et al. 1971).

A study of 210 patients indicated the anxiolytic and sedating activity 30 min and 60 min after administration of hydroxyzine (50, 100, or 150 mg i.m.) versus diazepam (5, 10 or 15 mg i.m.) and placebo (in association with pentobarbitone) (Forrest & Brown 1973, proceedings 27th AMA). The results were more favorable for hydroxyzine, while diazepam did not improve anxiety any more than placebo. A study in 76 patients with anxiety neurosis compared hydroxyzine (10 patients, 225 mg/day) with meprobamate (8 patients, 1800 mg/day), phenobarbital (9 patients, 30 mg/day), doxepin (40 patients, 225 mg/day), and chlordiazepoxide (9 patients, 90 mg/day), with a duration of 28 days. All treatments resulted in a significant symptom reduction (Saint Laurent et al. 1977). Tornetta (1977) compared the efficacy of hydroxyzine (50 mg), diazepam (5 mg), and placebo (in association with pethidine) in 280 patients. Compared to pretreatment the number of emotionally calm patients increased in the hydroxyzine group from 17% to 54%, in the diazepam group from 21% to 46%, and in the placebo group from 10% to 34%. There was no significant difference between the groups as far as sedation was concerned.

The efficacy of hydroxyzine (50 mg), was compared to physostigmine (2 mg), haloperidol (5 mg), and meperidine (50 mg), in two administrations with an interval of 20 min All three compounds yielded comparative results for anxiety and tension (Castellani *et al.* 1982).

Recent studies

Samuelian *et al.* (1995) treated 30 patients suffering from GAD (DSM-III criteria: APA 1980) with hydroxyzine 100 mg/day compared blindly to lorazepam 4 mg/day. The anxiety was measured with the Hamilton Anxiety Rating Scale and the Covi Scale for Anxiety (CAS). Although both treatments showed a comparable antianxiety effect, the hydroxyzine group showed a higher improvement on cognitive functions as measured by the BEC 86 rating scale.

Lemoine *et al.* (1997) studied 154 outpatients with GAD (DSM III-R criteria: APA 1987), followed up by general practitioners during 2 months. The patients were long-term consumers (at least 3 months) of 2 mg/day of lorazepam and were withdrawn using transiently hydroxyzine or placebo. Clinical evaluations for anxiety (Hamilton Anxiety Rating Scale [HARS], Zung), sleep (Spiegel), benzodiazepine withdrawal syndrome (Tyrer), adverse reactions and clinical global effects, show that with abrupt or progressive discontinuation, with or without hydroxyzine support, with half or with full dosage, lorazepam withdrawal proved to be feasible even after a long-term benzodiazepine treatment. Despite a high initial level of anxiety under lorazepam (HARS = 21 ± 10 at D0), after a 1-month period of withdrawal (under placebo or hydroxyzine) followed by a 2-month period without any treatment, 75% patients were totally free of any drug and their level of anxiety was significantly reduced. The transient prescription of hydroxyzine 25 mg t.i.d. for markedly anxious patients and of hydroxyzine 50 mg t.i.d. for patients presenting a withdrawal symptomatology is regarded as a satisfactory treatment option.

Lader and Scotto (1998) reported the efficacy of hydroxyzine and of buspirone, controlled by placebo, in a double-blind, parallel group, multicenter study conducted with a total of 244 patients, 70% female, with GAD in primary care. The patients were allocated randomly to treatments with hydroxyzine (12.5 mg morning and mid-day, 25 mg evening), buspirone (5 mg morning and mid-day, 10 mg evening) or placebo (three capsules/day) for 4 weeks. The Clinical Global Im-

provement (CGI) and self-rating (Hospital Anxiety and Depression [HAD]) scales showed both hydroxyzine and buspirone to be more efficacious than placebo. The somnolence associated with hydroxyzine was transient, and both active treatments were very well tolerated. In a review comparing his study with Ferreri *et al.*'s (1995) study, Lader (1999) concluded that hydroxyzine was a useful treatment for GAD.

The possible cognitive impairment as a result of anxiolytic medication in general has received special attention (Hindmarch *et al.* 1990). De Brabander and Deberdt (1990) investigated the effects of hydroxyzine on attention and memory. In a double-blind, crossover study with hydroxyzine 50 mg, lorazepam 2 mg, and placebo, it was found that hydroxyzine resulted in neither short-term nor long-term memory and concentration impairment. Although the sedative effect of hydroxyzine 50 mg and lorazepam 2 mg were comparable, hydroxyzine had no effect on memory, concentration and psychomotoric performance. In a second trial, with the same study design, De Brabander *et al.* (1992) focused on memory impairment in elderly volunteers. They found that hydroxyzine had no negative effect on memory and concentration, while lorazepam significantly caused memory impairment.

Wesnes *et al.* (1996) conducted a double-blind, placebo controlled, four-way cross-over study to assess the effects of a benzodiazepine (lorazepam 1 mg), a tricyclic antidepressant (amitriptyline 75 mg), and hydroxyzine (25 mg) on cognitive functioning, resting electroencephalogram (EEG), and the evoked potential in healthy male and female volunteers. Cognitive performance was assessed with a selection of tests from the Cognitive Drug Research Computerized Assessment System. Of all the drugs compared, amitriptyline showed the greatest magnitude of attention impairment and the longest duration of effect. Working memory was impaired by all compounds, most markedly by amitriptyline, while hydroxyzine had the smallest effect on secondary memory.

Shamsi *et al.* (1999) investigated whether hydroxyzine had any disruptive effects on cognitive functioning and sleep in comparison to lorazepam. In their study, 81 patients with a clinical diagnosis of GAD were randomized into a double-blind, parallel group design for 28 days, to receive either hydroxyzine (50 mg/day) ($N = 42$) or lorazepam (3 mg/day) ($N = 39$). The clinical questionnaire, the Milford Memory Test, and the Leeds Sleep Evaluation Questionnaire showed that patients reported a clinical improvement of their cognitive functioning and awakening from sleep following both treatments. It was concluded that hydroxyzine offered the possibility of effective relief of generalized anxiety, without causing significant impairment of cognitive functioning.

Early insomnia is often a concomitant problem in anxious patients, especially in those diagnosed with mixed anxiety depression (Van Moffaert 1994a). Hindmarch *et al.* (1990) performed a polysomnographic, double-blind, placebo-controlled study with 12 volunteers and found positive effects of hydroxyzine on sleep induction and sleep quality, without behavioral toxicity, that is day-time somnolence, the following day. In a similar study neither hangover effects nor disturbances in short-term memory were recorded (Alford *et al.* 1992).

In an early study Shalowitz (1956) observed that habituation or addiction to hydroxyzine was not noted during the entire period of the trial. More recently Barranco and Bridger (1976) stated that hydroxyzine is of interest because in its extensive clinical history there have been no documented cases of significant abuse, habituation, or physical dependence. Unlike most other anxiolytic agents, hydroxyzine is not listed under the Controlled Substances Act of 1970.

Most comparative studies of the efficacy and tolerance of hydroxyzine used a benzodiazepine as a comparator, as the current treatment of GAD mostly relies on benzodiazepines. However, the drawbacks of benzodiazepines have recently been investigated more thoroughly. Indeed, the anxiolytic effects of a benzodiazepine treatment sometimes lessen in the long term (Lader 1999). Furthermore, the use of benzodiazepines may imply cognitive impairment (Hindmarch *et al.* 1990). Finally, there is concern about the dependence potential of benzodiazepines and the emergence of rebound anxiety on discontinuation (Lader 1999).

Although hydroxyzine is associated with transient somnolence, particularly in high dosages, the comparative studies show hydroxyzine to be generally well tolerated and clinically efficacious in GAD and in various anxiety-related conditions. Indeed, equivalent results in anxiolytic efficacy were found comparing hydroxyzine with benzodiazepines. No addictive properties or withdrawal reactions have been reported, even after abrupt discontinuation. In all the decades of use there have been no reports on hydroxyzine causing cognitive impairment, nor dependence.

Special indications: psychodermatology

In psychodermatology hydroxyzine has established itself as a symptom relieving agent for pruritus related dermatoses. Robinson *et al.* (1957) reported on the use of hydroxyzine in the treatment of 479 patients with various dermatoses in which emotional stress was thought to be a factor. Subjective evaluation, based on the patients' statements lead to the conclusions that the ataractic effect was satisfactory in 378 patients who experienced some degree of relief from tension. The authors concluded that hydroxyzine is valuable as an adjunctive therapy in the treatment of patients with dermatoses in which emotional tension is a determinant.

In a study with 1987 patients, Robinson and Robinson (1958) found that hydroxyzine and meprobamate were useful to lessen or control emotional tension in patients with various dermatoses. In a double-blind, cross-over study with 20 patients with a history of pruritus resulting from urticaria, atopic dermatitis, or contact dermatitis (Baraf 1976), the patients received hydroxyzine 25 mg t.i.d. and cyproheptadine 4 mg t.i.d. alternatively for 7 days each. Although the degree of pruritus was reduced by both drugs, hydroxyzine was significantly more effective than cyproheptadine in relieving the itching as assessed both subjectively by the patients and objectively by the dermatologist.

Cotterill *et al.* (1981), a dermatologist with a special interest in psychiatry, mentioned a case of prurigo pigmentosa that was treated with hydroxyzine orally (dosage unknown) and cortisone topically. The itching and the papular eruption, along with the pigmentation, had nearly completely disappeared after 6 months of therapy.

Clinical experience with various dermatological conditions (Van Moffaert 1994b) shows that the inclusion of hydroxyzine in the treatment may positively change the course of a psychodermatological condition because of its simultaneous actions on the anxiety component and on the sensory symptoms (pain or itching).

General conclusions

Especially in primary care, GAD and anxious personality traits are among the most frequent and chronic psychiatric problems the social impairment of which is regularly underestimated. There is a tendency to trivialize GAD as "minor psychiatry," but pathological anxiety states are genuinely disabling and distressing conditions. The comorbidity (simultaneous or sequential) of anxiety disorders with mood disorders (major depression, dysthymia) or with other anxiety subtypes, e.g., panic disorder, complicates the picture (Van Moffaert *et al.* 1983). Anxiety states are accompanied by arousal of the autonomous nervous system causing physiological dysregulations. The anxious patients, above all Mediterranean migrant patients (Van Moffaert 1998), perceive these bodily changes in a hypochondriacal way, which exacerbates the anxiety even more. In addition, many anxious patients suffer from some form of sleep disturbance, especially early insomnia.

Since the 1960s the pharmacological treatment of anxiety has been dominated by the use of various benzodiazepines. However, the growing awareness on the possible drawbacks of benzodiazepine use may review the possibilities of a relatively "ancient" drug like hydroxyzine. Most open trials with hydroxyzine in the 1960s and 1970s are not up to present-day standards of comparative drug investigation. They employed imprecise selection criteria, they included special populations, such as children and prisoners, and they used different dosages of hydroxyzine and comparators. The mode of anxiolytic action of hydroxyzine remained speculative. The early data, some of which have subsequently been confirmed by methodologically sounder double-blind placebo-controlled studies, indicate that hydroxyzine provides effective relief of anxiety in GAD as well as in a broad spectrum of pathological anxiety states such as situational anxiety, preoperative anxiety, somatized anxiety with pruritus as a specific target (Ferreri & Hantouche 1998).

Hydroxyzine is claimed to be effective in acute anxiety and as a maintenance treatment, both on the psychic and on the somatic component (pruritus in particular) of anxiety. Indeed, hydroxyzine proves to be useful where rapid relaxation is needed, as in pre-dentistry anxiety, and where the anxiety-reducing effect continues, as in psychosomatic conditions, which are long-term by nature. However, the transient drowsiness and sedation of hydroxyzine has been stressed to the extent that for some researchers and clinicians hydroxyzine is no anxiolytic but merely a sedative. The scientific data available warrant the conclusion that hydroxyzine gives rapid relief of acute anxiety. Symptoms of psychic and somatic anxiety, the apprehension and the cognitive symptoms of anxiety are relieved without obvious cognitive impairment. More recent data indicate a lack of habituation to its anxiolytic effect. Therefore hydroxyzine can be easily discontinued without rebound phenomena. Hydroxyzine does not induce dependence. This may be emphasized in view of recent reports on benzodiazepine withdrawal. Although benzodiazepines may not be called addictive in the proper sense, their use does require caution. Hydroxyzine may offer an even safer alternative. A further, somewhat speculative advantage of hydroxyzine over benzodiazepines is the suggestion that anxiolytics augment resistance to psychotherapy (Hantouche & Vahia 1999). Clinical experience with hydroxyzine appears to indicate its lessening effect on impulsivity and its lack both of behavioral toxicity and of any negative effects on cognitive functioning. In combination with psychotherapy, hydroxyzine might therefore facilitate the patient's acceptance of psychotherapy and enhance its efficacy.

Anecdotally sedating antihistamines have been useful for early insomnia by virtue of their soporific effect, and it should be emphasized that their bedtime use is warranted, but there is as yet no sufficient evidence to support the effectiveness of sedating antihistamines in the treatment of sleep disturbances (Van Moffaert 1994a).

The latter comment also applies to the use of hydroxyzine in dermatology and psychodermatology. The majority of trials on the use of hydroxyzine in dermatology are flawed in terms of the sample size or the study design. Empirically hydroxyzine is found to be useful in a variety of psychophysiological skin symptoms. Its specific efficacy, if any, requires further investigation in controlled trials. It must be emphasized that the objective assessment of the efficacy of psychotropic drugs in psychodermatological disorders is particularly difficult. On the one hand, psychotropic agents may reduce the psychiatric symptoms of psychodermatological disorders initially and subsequently (and often only indirectly) have an effect on the somatic symptoms. On the other hand, this distinct patient population is particularly sensitive to placebo response.

On the basis of further research hydroxyzine might be assigned a more appropriate place, however peripheral, in the current psychopharmacological arsenal of anxiety treatments.

References

Alexander, A. (1960) Evaluation of an ataract (hydroxyzine) in 2025 patients as an adjunct in oral surgery. *West Virgina Dental Journal* **34**, 56–9.

Alford, C., Rombout, N., Jones, J., Foley, S., Idzikowski, C. & Hindmarch, I. (1992) Acute effects of hydroxyzine on nocturnal sleep and sleep tendency the following day: a C-EEG study. *Human Psychopharmacology* **7**, 25–35.

American Psychiatric Association (APA) (1980) *Diagnostic Statistical Manual of Mental Disorders*, 3rd edn. American Psychiatric Association, Washington, D.C.

American Psychiatric Association (APA) (1987) *Diagnostic Statistical Manual of Mental Disorders*, 3rd edn revised. American Psychiatric Association, Washington, D.C.

American Psychiatric Association (APA) (1994) *Diagnostic Statistical Manual of Mental Disorders*, 4th edn. American Psychiatric Association, Washington, D.C.

Angst, J. & Wicki, W. (1992) The Zurich Study: recurrent brief anxiety. *Eur Arch Psychiatry Clin Neurosci* **241**, 196–300.

Baraf, C.S. (1976) Treatment of pruritus in allergic dermatoses: an evaluation of the relative efficacy of cyproheptadine and hydroxyzine. *Curr Ther Res Clin Exp* **19**(1), 32–8.

Barranco, S.F. & Bridger, W. (1976) Treatment of anxiety with oral hydroxyzine: an overview. *Curr Ther Res Clin Exp* **22**(1–2), 217–27.

Beveridge, G.W. (1974) Diseases of the skin: infantile eczema. *BMJ* I, 154–5.

Breslow, I.H. (1968) Evaluation of hydroxyzine palmoate concentrate as an ataractic: Double-blind cross-over study in a neurotic male prison group. *Curr Ther Res Clin Exp* **10**, 421–7.

Castellani, S., Giannini, A.J., Boeringa, J.A. & Adams, P.M. (1982) Phencylidine intoxication: assessment of possible antidotes. *Clin Toxicol* **19**, 313–19.

Clyne, M.B., Freeling, P. & Ginsborg, S. (1968) A comparative trial between two tranquilizers. *Practitioner* **201**, 496–8.

Cotterill, J.A., Ryatt, K.S. & Greenwood, R. (1981) Prurigo pigmentosa. *Br J Dermatol* **105**(6), 707–10.

Covi, L. & Lipman, R.S. (1984) Primary depression or primary anxiety? A possible psychometric approach to diagnostic dilemma. *Clin Neuropharmacol* **7** (Suppl.), 501.

De Brabander, A. & Deberdt, W. (1990) Effects of hydroxyzine on attention and memory. *Human Psychopharmacology* **5**, 357–62.

De Brabander, A. & Deberdt, W. (1992) Effets de l'hydroxyzine sur l'attention et al mémoire chez le sujet âgè. *Acto Psychiat Belg* **92**, 370–82.

Ferreri, M., Darcis, T., Natens, J. *et al.* (1995) A multicenter, double-blind, placebo-controlled study investigating the anxiolytic efficacy of hydroxyzine in patients with generalized anxiety. *Hum Psychopharmacol* **10**, 181–7.

Ferreri, M. & Hantouche, E.G. (1998) Recent clinical trials of hydroxyzine in generalized anxiety disorder. *Acta Psychiatr Scand* **98** (Suppl. 393), 102–8.

Fjellner, B., Arnetz, B., Eneroth, P. *et al.* (1985) Pruritus during standardized mental stress. *Acta Derm Venereol* **65**, 199–205.

Garber, R.C. Jr (1958) Management of tension and anxiety states with hydroxyzine hydrochloride. *J Fla Med Assoc* **45**, 549–52.

Goldberg, H.L. & Finnerty, R.J. (1973) The use of hydroxyzine (Vistaril®) in the treatment of anxiety neurosis. *Psychosomatics* **14**, 39–41.

Hantouche, E. & Ferreri, M. (1995) Trouble anxiété généralisée. apperçu sur l'évolution des concepts cliniques et thérapeutiques. Exemple de l'hydroxyzine avec analyse détaillée de ses effets sur l'échelle FARD. *Nervure* **8**, 9–15.

Hantouche, E. & Vahia, V.N. (1999) Interactions between psychotherapy and drug therapy in generalized anxiety disorder. *Hum Psychopharmacol* **14**, 87–93.

Hay, G.G. (1990) Dysmorphophobia. *Br J Psychiatry* **116**, 399–406.

Hindmarch, I., Rombaut, N. & Alford, C. (1990) Psychopharmacological effects of hydroxyzine on sleep and daytime functions. *TW Neurologie Psychiatrie*, **4**, 16–17.

Kellner, R., Kelly, A. & Sheffield, B.F. (1968) The assessment of changes in anxiety in a drug trial: a comparison of methods. *Br J Psychiatry* **114**, 863–9.

Klett, C.J., Hollister, L.E., Caffey, E.M. & Kaim, S.C. (1971) Evaluating changes in symptoms during acute alcohol withdrawal. *Arch Gen Psychiatry* **24**, 174–8.

Knott, D.H. & Beard, J.D. (1967) A study of drugs in the management of chronic alcoholism. *Am Fam Physician* **13**, 80–5.

Koblenzer, C.S. (1987) *Psychocutaneous Disease*. Grune & Stratton Inc., Orlando.

Koo, J.M. & Strauss, G.D. (1987) Psychopharmacologic treatment of psychocutaneous disorders: a practical guide. *Semin Dermatol* **6**, 83–93.

Lader, M. (1999) Anxiolytic effect of hydroxyzine: a double-blind trial versus placebo and buspirone. *Hum Psychopharmacol* **14**, 94–103.

Lader, M. & Scotto, J.C. (1998) A multicenter double-blind comparison of hydroxyzine, buspirone and placebo in patients with generalized anxiety disorder. *Psychopharmacology* **139**, 402–6.

Laffont, F. & Cathala, H.P. (1987) Effet de l'hydroxyzine (Atarax) sur le sommeil chez les insomniaques non déprimés et anxieux. *Revue de Médecine et de L'internat* **25**, 21–4.

Lemoine, P., Touchon, J. & Billardon, M. (1997) Comparaison de six différentes modalités de sevrage du Lorazepam: une étude controlée, hydroxyzine versus placebo. *Encéphale* **23**(4), 290–9.

Leonard, B.E. (1999) New developments in the pharmacological treatment of anxiety. *Hum Psychopharmacol* **14**, 52–9.

Lipton, M.I. (1961) High dosages of hydroxyzine in outpatient treatment of severe neuroses and psychoses. *Pa Med J* **64**, 60–2.

Litchfield, H. (1960) Clinical pediatric experience with ataractic agent in less severe emotional states. *N Y State J Med* **60**(14), 518–23.

Manchanda, S.S., Kishore, B., Jain, C.K. *et al.* (1969) Hydroxyzine hydrochloride in the management of children with behavior problems. *Indian Pediatr* **6**(8), 538–49.

Natens, J. (1992) Present position of hydroxyzine and related ataractic drugs in the treatment of anxiety. Molecular pharmacology. *Int. Acad. Biomed. Drug. Res. Basel, Karger* **3**, 78–84.

Panconesi, E. (1984) *Stress and Skin Diseases: Psychosomatic Dermatology.* Lippincott, Philadelphia.

Piuck, C.L. (1963) Clinical impressions of hydroxyzine and other tranquilizers in a child guidance clinic. *Dis Nerv Syst* **24**, 483–8.

Reisner, J.G. (1967) Hydroxyzine for controlling postpartum anxiety: a double-blind study. *Nebr State Med J* **52**, 498–9.

Rickels, K., Gordon, P.E., Zamostien, B.R., Case, W., Hutchison, J. & Chung, H. (1970) Hydroxyzine and chlordiazepoxide in anxious neurotic outpatients: a collaborative controlled study. *Compr Psychiatry* **11**, 457–74.

Robinson, R.C.V. & Robinson, H.M. (1958) Control of emotional tension in dermatoses. *South Med J* **51**, 509–13.

Robinson, H.M., Robinson, R.C.V. & Strahan, J.F. (1957) Hydroxyzine hydrochlozide (Atarax®). A new tranquillizer. *South Med J* **50**, 1282–7.

Saint Laurent, J., Ban, T.A. & Carle, R. (1977) Doxepin in the treatment of neuroses: a comparative clinical study of doxepin, chlordiazepoxide, hydroxyzine, meprobamate and phenobarbital. *Curr Ther Res Clin Exp* **22**, 316–20.

Samuelian, J.C., Billardon, M. & Guillou, N. (1995) Retentissement sur les fonctions cognitives de deux traitements axiolytiques chez des patients souffrant d'anxiété généralisée. *Encephale* **21**, 147–53.

Settel, E. (1957) Clinical observation on the use of hydroxyzine in anxiety-tension states and senile agitation. *American Practitioner and Digest of Treatment* **8**, 1584–8.

Shalowitz, M. (1956) Hydroxyzine: a new therapeutic agent for senile anxiety states. *Geriatrics* **11**, 312–15.

Shalowitz, M. (1961) Evaluation of Ataraxic® (hydroxyzine) in long-term therapy. *International Record of Medicine* **174**, 357–61.

Silver, D., Beaubien, J., Ban, T.A., Saxena, B.M. & Bennett, J. (1969) Hydroxyzine, amitriptyline and their combination in the treatment of psychoneurotic patients. *Curr Ther Res Clin Exp* **11**(11), 663–9.

Smigel, J.O., Lowe, K.J. & Green, M. (1959) Emotional and psychic problems of institutionalized geriatric patients: evaluation of hydroxyzine. *J Am Geriatr Soc* **7**, 61–6.

Smulevich, A.B., Syrkin, A.L., Drobizhev, M., Ivanov, S.V., Lebedeva, O.I. & Andreev, A.M. (1999) Therapy of cardioneurotic diseases in general practice: clinical experience with Atarax®. *Klin. Medical (Mosk.)* **4**(77/1), 43–6. [in Russian].

Tornetta, F. (1977) A comparison of droperidol, diazepam and hydroxyzine hydrochloride as premedication. *Anesth Analg* **56**(4), 496–500.

Van Moffaert, M. (1982) Psychosomatics for the practising dermatologist. *Dermatologica* **165**, 73–84.

Van Moffaert, M. (1987) The borderline of depression. *Acta Psychiatrica Belgica* **87**, 257–9.

Van Moffaert, M. (1989) Management of self-mutilation. Confrontation and the integration of psychotherapy and psychotropic drug treatment. *Psychother Psychosom* **51**, 180–6.

Van Moffaert, M. (1992) Psychodermatology. An overview. *Psychother Psychosom* **58**, 125–36.

Van Moffaert, M. (1994a) Sleep disorders and depression. The "chicken and egg" situation. *J Psychosom Res* **38**, 9–13.

Van Moffaert, M. (1994b) Clinical features and drug treatment of psychodermatological disorders. *CNS Drugs* **1**(3), 193–200.

Van Moffaert, M. (1998) Transcultural psychiatry in Mediterranean migrants in Belgium. In: *Clinical Methods in Transcultural Psychiatry* (S. Okpaku (ed.), pp. 301–20). American Psychiatric Association Press, New York.

Van Moffaert, M., Dierick, M., De Meulemeester, F. & Vereecken, A. (1983) The treatment of depressive anxiety states associated with psychosomatic symptoms. *Acta Psychiatrica Belgica* **83**(5), 525–39.

Van Moffaert, M. & Jannes, C. (1987) An update of panic disorders, somatization, biological markers and outcome. *Acta Psychiatrica Belgica* **87**(3), 332–45.

Van Moffaert, M., Spiers, R., Buylaert, W. & Van Brantegem, J. (1988) Panic as a medical emergency. *Tijdschrift Voor Psychiatrie* **10**, 644–65. [in Dutch].

Wesnes, K.A., Meulenberg, O., Vermeij, B. *et al.* (1996) The acute cognitive effect of amitriptyline, hydroxyzine and lorazepam in volunteers. *J Psychopharmacol* **10**(3) (Suppl.), A51, abstract 204.

Whitlock, F.A. (1970) *Psychophysiological Aspects of Skin Diseases*. W.B. Saunders, London.

Widlocher, D., Lecrubier, Y. & Le Goc, Y. (1983) The place of anxiety in depressive symptomatology. *Br J Clin Pharmacol* 15(2), 171–9.

Williams, N. (1968) Chlorpromazine and hydroxyzine in treatment of situational anxiety. *Clin Med* 45, 48–50.

Wittkower, E.D. & Lester, E. (1960) Hautkrankheiten in psychosomatischer Sicht. *Acta Psychosomatica. Documenta Geigy* 6, 1–39.

Anxiety Disorders: New Antidepressants

R.B. Hidalgo & J.R.T. Davidson

Introduction

In this chapter we will review the antidepressants nefazodone, mirtazapine and venlafaxine regarding their chemical structure, mechanism of action, pharmacokinetics, side-effects and toxicity, drug interactions and, finally, their clinical use, specifically in the treatment of anxiety disorders.

This group of antidepressants resembles some tricyclic antidepressants, in that they have a dual action on serotonergic and noradrenergic reuptake. Nevertheless these newer antidepressants have a much better profile regarding side-effects, mainly due to the lack of anticholinergic and cardiovascular adverse effects.

Nefazodone

Nefazodone is a phenylpiperazine antidepressant with predominantly, although not exclusively, serotonergic actions. Its mechanism of action, pharmacokinetics, side-effects, toxicity, drug interactions and clinical efficacy will be reviewed.

Mode of action

Nefazodone is an antidepressant with two pharmacologic actions on the serotonin (5-HT) system, namely a potent blockade of the postsynaptic 5-HT2 receptor and moderate inhibition of synaptosomal 5-HT reuptake. In addition, nefazodone moderately blocks norepinephrine reuptake and shows weak α_1-adrenergic antagonism, but has no significant anticholinergic, antidopaminergic and antihistaminic activity (Taylor *et al.*

1995). This dual action on serotonin distinguishes nefazodone from selective serotonin reuptake inhibitors (SSRIs). Its mechanism of action is thought to be the result of its enhancement of serotonin-mediated neurotransmission, *presumably through 5-HT1A receptor stimulation.*

Nefazodone is structurally related to trazodone, which has stronger α_1-adrenergic antagonist action. As a result, nefazodone is less likely to cause the characteristic postural hypotension, sedation, and priapism that may occur with the use of trazodone. Another advantage of its pharmacodynamic profile is the absence of common side-effects seen with SSRIs, like gastrointestinal symptomatology (i.e., nausea, vomiting), sexual dysfunction and tremor. Nefazodone and trazodone are the antidepressants with the highest affinity for the 5-HT1A receptor. The nature of this affinity *remains* unclear since, on the one hand, Frazer (1997) espoused antagonist properties, whereas Nutt (1996) described this action on the 5-HT1A receptor as agonist and as a possible way for nefazodone to treat depression and anxiety.

Because of nefazodone's blockade of the 5-HT2 receptor, it was thought that it may have a preferred action as antidepressant and a more benign side-effect profile.

Another differentiating pharmacologic feature of nefazodone is its favorable effect on sleep, as evidenced by sleep laboratory studies, which show that it decreases arousal and increases stage 2 sleep without suppressing rapid-eye movement (REM) sleep (Cohn *et al.* 1996). In addition, nefazodone has been shown to increase sleep efficiency, decrease natural awakening and stage 1 sleep in comparative studies versus fluoxetine, to a greater extent than with fluoxetine and, in contrast to most antidepressants, does not suppress REM sleep (Armitage *et al.* 1997; Gillin *et al.* 1997; Rush *et al.* 1998). Of clinical importance, nefazodone is unlikely to induce activation, anxiety or insomnia. Such side-effects have proved troublesome with many other antidepressants, especially during the first weeks of treatment. Early onset activation associated with SSRIs may require concomitant anxiolytic or hypnotic/sedative treatment (Rascati 1995). Moreover, nefazodone is not associated with significant changes in body weight, as may be present with antidepressants like tricyclic antidepressants (TCAs), some SSRIs, and mirtazapine (Caplik *et al.* 1994; Davis *et al.* 1997; Feighner *et al.* 1998; Sussman & Ginsberg 1998). This pharmacologic profile, differing from other antidepressants offers a number of potential advantages for nefazodone compared with existing agents.

Pharmacokinetics

Nefazodone is rapidly and completely absorbed after oral administration and peak plasma level is reached after 1–3 h. Its bioavailability is 15–23%, due to an extensive first pass metabolism. Plasma steady-states are reached within 3–4 days from treatment initiation or from dosage changing.

Nefazodone has three metabolites: hydroxynefazodone and triazoledione are the two major metabolites, and m-chlorophenylpiperizine (mCPP) is a minor metabolite. Hydroxynefazodone and, in a lower range, mCPP, are both active on the serotonergic system.

Due to its nonlinear kinetics, mean plasma concentrations of nefazodone and its metabolites, are greater than expected with higher doses. Greater area-under-the-curve, higher peak plasma concentrations, and prolonged elimination half-life are seen in patients of extreme ages (i.e. very young and very elderly patients), especially among females.

Nefazodone's binding to plasma proteins is greater than 99% and its elimination is by liver metabolism. Nefazodone is a strong inhibitor of cytochrome P450 III_{A4} isoenzyme, something that leads to potentiating interactions with certain benzodiazepines (e.g., alprazolam and triazolam *and some antihistamines* [see p. 413]). mCPP is metabolized by the cytochrome P450 isoenzyme IID_6.

Due to its pharmacokinetic profile, the dosage of nefazodone has to be reduced in patients with liver disease and patients who are very elderly. On the other hand, patients with renal dysfunction do not show need for dosing adjustment.

Adverse events, toxicity and safety

The most frequent adverse events observed with nefazodone in placebo-controlled trials were somnolence, dry mouth, nausea, dizziness, constipation, asthenia, light-headedness, blurred vision, confusion and abnormal vision (Markus 1996). These effects were reported in treatments using up to 600 mg of nefazodone. Most of the common side-effects decreased in severity and many of them disappeared with time. Nevertheless, dry mouth persisted in 44% of patients after 6 weeks of treatment.

Several adverse events showed a higher incidence as the dosage increased (i.e., doses up to 500 or 600 mg/day vs. ≤300 mg/day). These adverse events were visual disturbances (e.g., visual tracings), confusion, blurred vision, tinnitus, dizziness, nausea, somnolence, and constipation.

Five side-effects were more likely to lead to discontinuation of treatment: nausea, dizziness, insomnia, asthenia and agitation.

Regarding laboratory testing, nefazodone was only associated with higher incidence of decreased hematocrit (1.6%) compared to placebo (0.6%). This finding was considered to be nonclinically significant. The investigators did not find differences in the incidence of liver function tests between nefazodone and placebo.

A 3.6% incidence of serious adverse events was reported among depressed patients treated with nefazodone in short or long-term clinical trials ($N = 3496$). These serious adverse events were mostly due to hospitalizations (psychiatric or for treatment of a pre-existing condition) and the investigators described them as unlikely to be related with nefazodone therapy. Likewise the 10 deaths that occurred during or shortly after nefazodone treatment were not attributed to the use of nefazodone. Among the 3496 patients, nine patients committed suicide. In five of them the suicide occurred within 1 month of discontinuing treatment. *Moreover*, suicides among patients suffering from depression are always difficult to interpret as a straightforward effect of a medication, since suicide is one of the most feared consequences of depression itself. In addition, in some of these patients other antidepressants were being used.

Apparently there was no serious cardiovascular toxicity reported with nefazodone in the elderly and nonelderly populations. However, nefazodone was not used in patients who had unstable heart conditions or who had had a recent myocardial infarction.

Nefazodone appears to be safe in overdose, the most common symptoms in this situation being drowsiness and vomiting. All cases of overdose recovered completely without sequelae.

Patients with liver impairment should be started on a lower dose and increases should occur slowly aiming for an overall lower dosage. Apparently patients with renal impairment did not show alterations in nefazodone's pharmacokinetics. Thus, no dose adjustment is required for these patients. However, accumulation of nefazodone and its metabolites may occur with chronic administration in those with severe renal impairment. Hence, in such patients care is advised in dosing and evaluating clinical response. Regarding serious adverse events in elderly populations, no significant differences were found among the 488 elders treated with nefazodone when compared with younger patients. However, as was described before, lower doses are needed at the beginning of treatment in this group, especially among females.

There are no data to our knowledge on the safety of nefazodone in children, adolescents, and during pregnancy.

Drug interactions

As described before, the liver metabolizes nefazodone. Therefore, it is likely to result in some drug-drug interreactions with other medications, since most drugs are metabolized via liver. There are specific enzymes responsible for this metabolism; namely, cytochrome P450 isoenzymes. Nefazodone is a substrate of, and a potent inhibitor of, the III_{A4} isoenzyme *in vitro* and *in vivo* (Davis *et al.* 1997). Consequently, drug–drug interactions are to be expected with any medication metabolized by the same coenzyme and coadministration of these drugs must be cautiously considered, especially for medications with which increased plasma concentrations are associated with higher risk of cardiotoxicity. Examples of these medications are cisapride, terfenadine, astemizole and pimozide; all of which are contraindicated in combination with nefazodone for that reason. Drug–drug interactions were also found in the area under the curve at steady state for alprazolam

(two-fold increase) and triazolam (four-fold increase). Nevertheless the pharmacokinetics of nefazodone remained unaltered (Markus 1996). Contrarily, lorazepam, which is not metabolized by III_{A4} isoenzyme, is not affected when coadministered with nefazodone (Green *et al.* 1995).

Unlike some SSRIs (i.e., fluoxetine and paroxetine) which are potent inhibitors of the IID_6 isoenzyme, nefazodone was found to be a very weak inhibitor of such isoenzyme (*in vitro*). Consequently, nefazodone has either minimal or no interactions with drugs like cimetidine, desipramine, haloperidol, phenytoin and propranolol. Nefazodone does not inhibit the IA_2 isoenzyme (*in vitro*) and no pharmacokinetic interaction was observed with theophylline (Markus 1996).

Monoamine oxidase inhibitors (MAOIs) are contraindicated in case of a patient taking nefazodone and vice versa. Nefazodone should not be used unless at least 2 weeks have passed after discontinuation of a MAOI and, contrarily, when switching from nefazodone to a MAOI the minimum time of wash-out should not be less than 1 week.

Clinical use

Regrettably, only few single-blind studies have been conducted with nefazodone in the treatment of anxiety disorders. To our best knowledge there is no data available from double-blind placebo controlled investigations of this drug for the treatment of specific anxiety disorders However, there is some useful available information from double-blind research studies of the efficacy of nefazodone in treating depressed patients with comorbid anxiety. These studies will be presented here.

Panic disorder

DeMartinis *et al.* (1996) conducted an open-label trial in 14 adults (mean age 34 ± 15 years) with panic disorder (PD) which was often comorbid with other psychiatric disorders. Fifty-seven percent (N = 8) had comorbid major depression, and 21% had depression not otherwise specified (NOS) or minor depressive symptoms. Thirty-six percent had comorbid generalized anxiety disorder (GAD), three of whom had both major depression and GAD. Only three patients in the sample (21%) had noncomorbid panic disorder. Subjects were treated for 8 weeks with nefazodone up to 600 mg/day (mean maximal daily dose 407 mg) in a flexible dosage regimen. Eighty-six percent of the patients completed the 8 weeks. Counting the drop outs as nonrespondents, 71% of the sample ($N = 10$) had a Clinical Global Impressions (CGI) Scale score of much or very much improved by the endpoint visit. The number of panic attacks decreased from 5.4 at baseline to 2.1 at week 8 ($P < 0.05$), phobic anxiety decreased as well. Five of the eight patients with comorbid major depression were considered respondents, as well as 3/5 patients showing comorbid GAD. Nefazodone was well-tolerated by patients and none of the participants withdrew from the study because of side-effects.

Berigan *et al.* (1998) also presented a case report of a patient who had PD with agoraphobia and a history of poor tolerance for SSRI medications. The authors treated the patient with nefazodone (up to 400 mg/day) after a trial with paroxetine in which the subject showed improvement in his PD and functioning, but also had a sexual dysfunction that was interfering in his marriage. Nefazodone was well tolerated, with side-effects (visual disturbances) fading after 1 week of treatment, *and sexual function returned*. Nefazodone showed to have good efficacy in treating PD, as the patient remained free of symptoms after 6 months of continued treatment with nefazodone and self-relaxation techniques when under stress.

Bystritsky *et al.* (1999) reported a small 12-week open-label trial in which 10 patients meeting Diagnostic Statistical Manual, fourth edition (DSM-IV: American Psychiatric Association 1994) criteria for noncomorbid PD or PD with agoraphobia were treated with a flexible dose of nefazodone (50–400 mg/day). At the end of the study nine patients were rated as much improved with seven patients being panic free and in full remission.

Generalized anxiety disorder

One small open-label trial has presented the effects of nefazodone in patients with GAD (Hedges *et al.* 1996). Twenty-one subjects (12 female; nine male) were treated with nefazodone up to 600 mg/day for 8 weeks. All subjects met criteria for DSM-IV GAD and did not carry comorbid diagnosis, other than two patients with comorbid social phobia. The effect of nefazodone was monitored by the Hamilton Rating Scale for Anxiety (HAM-A) and the CGI Scale. Fifteen of the 21 subjects completed the study. Three subjects dropped because of adverse events and three withdrew for personal reasons. Eighty percent of participants who completed the trial ($N = 12$) were rated as either very much or much improved, 7% ($N = 1$) as minimally improved, and 13% ($N = 2$) as unchanged. No subjects were rated as worse. Both patients with comorbid social phobia also showed improvement in the HAM-A and were rated as responders in the CGI. Regarding adverse events, those affecting primarily central nervous system (CNS) were the most common with 37% of the patients reporting drowsiness or fatigue, 21% reporting headache, and 21% reporting insomnia.

Post-traumatic stress disorder

Hidalgo *et al.* (1999) reported the results from six open-label trials in the treatment of post-traumatic stress disorder (PTSD) with nefazodone. One hundred and five patients with chronic PTSD were treated acutely (6–12 weeks) with nefazodone with doses up to 600 mg/day, and 92 of them were entered in their intent-to-treat analysis. The authors evaluated outcome and predictors of response. Using different response criteria (e.g., drop in scores between baseline and endpoint of at least 30%, 40% and 50%) they found response rates of 46%, 36% and 26%, respectively. Nefazodone showed a broad spectrum of action in all cluster symptoms to a significant extent. Predictors of response included age, sex and trauma type; with younger patients, women, noncombat trauma survivors showed the highest response to treatment. However, these results should be interpreted cautiously since, among post-traumatic patients, combat trauma, which usually presents in men, often shows poor response to treatment and represents a clinical challenge. It should be noted that in this particular sample combat veterans represented 71.4% of the total ($N = 81$).

Two major *placebo-controlled* studies of nefazodone have been completed, but results have not been presented yet.

Social anxiety disorder

Van Ameringen *et al.* (1999) conducted an open-label trial in which nefazodone was administered to 23 patients with a primary diagnosis of DSM-IV social phobia, generalized type. Social phobics (men aged 34.8 ± 9.8 years: mean duration of illness 21 ± 9.9 years) were treated with nefazodone 200–600 mg/day (mean dose at endpoint 435.9 ± 116 mg/day) for 12 weeks. Twenty-one of the 23 patients who participated in the trial completed the 12 weeks of treatment. The two patients who dropped out from the study withdrew because of lack of efficacy. Interestingly, 13 patients had at least one comorbid psychiatric condition (dysthymia, $N = 5$; major depression, obsessive-compulsive disorder (OCD) and specific phobia, $N = 3$ each; PD with agoraphobia, $N = 2$; alcohol abuse and dependence, $N = 1$). Seventy percent were considered respondents ($N = 16$), meaning a CGI Scale improvement score of "markedly improved" ($N = 6$) or "moderately improved" ($N = 10$). Seven patients were nonresponders (30%), including the two who dropped out of the study. Interestingly, many patients with comorbid psychiatric disorders showed reduction in their symptomatology, and the one patient with alcohol dependence showed a substantial decrease in alcohol consumption. However, patients with comorbid specific phobia did not show a change in their specific phobic avoidance. Seventy-four percent of patients showed nefazodone-related side-effects, but none of these side-effects led to withdrawal of subjects from the trial. The most common side-effects were fatigue/sedation, nausea, poor memory and visual disturbances. The authors concluded that nefazodone may have a role in the treatment of generalized social phobia.

Anxiety associated with depression

As mentioned above, some double-blind, placebo-controlled trials have been conducted with depressed patients with comorbid anxiety.

Fontaine *et al.* (1994) reported that nefazodone showed a very significant reduction of symptoms at the 6-week endpoint compared with placebo, as did imipramine in patients with depression and comorbid anxiety symptoms. The HAM-A was included as one of the outcome measurements. Nefazodone produced a greater reduction in anxiety compared with placebo (–10.5 on HAM-A: $P < 0.01$) by the end of treatment. The group treated with imipramine as the active control also showed reduced anxiety compared with placebo, but to a lesser extent (–9 on HAM-A: $P < 0.05$). Another interesting finding of this trial is that neither placebo nor imipramine showed a significant anxiolytic effect over 6 weeks of treatment on the patient rated Symptom Checklist-90. However, nefazodone produced a progressive improvement in this scale up to 6 weeks that was statistically significant by the end of the 1st week of treatment.

Fawcett *et al.* (1995) reported a meta-analysis of six major randomized clinical trials of the efficacy of nefazodone in treating anxiety and agitation associated with depression. The data included 817 depressed patients. Nefazodone produced a significant reduction in somatic anxiety (Hamilton Rating Scale for Depression [HAM-D], item 11) by week 4 of treatment, compared with imipramine and placebo ($P < 0.01$). This reduction persisted up to the termination of the study. Nefazodone was described as having an excellent safety profile with only 5% of patients discontinuing because of adverse experiences, compared with 17% for imipramine and 5% for placebo. Moreover the authors pointed out that nefazodone did not provoke unwanted activating side-effects during early treatment as may happen with tricyclics and SSRIs.

In another report, Nelson (1994) presented the result of an open-label trial of nefazodone in the treatment of depression with and without comorbid OCD. Eighteen depressed patients entered in the study and were treated with nefazodone for 8 weeks. Nine of the 15 individuals who completed the study also met criteria for OCD. Nefazodone was found to be effective as antidepressant as well as anxiolytic among participants with major depression alone or associated with OCD. A trend toward antiobsessional efficacy was seen among those with OCD. The degree of its anxiolytic effect was found to be significantly correlated with the degree of antidepressant effect. Nefazodone was generally well-tolerated and the most commonly reported side-effects were dizziness, joint pain, dry mouth and sedation.

These studies are suggestive for efficacy of nefazodone in anxiety disorders. Moreover, since anxiety often presents with comorbid depression, and vice-versa, an agent that works for both symptom groups may represent a useful tool for clinical practice, allowing treatment with only one drug, which may increase compliance and reduce the possibility of drug inter-reactions.

Mirtazapine

Mirtazapine is a new antidepressant with a novel and unique pharmacologic profile that differs from the other antidepressants (i.e. tricyclics, SSRIs, serotonin noradrenergic reuptake inhibitors [SNRIs]). Mirtazapine is the first noradrenergic and specific serotonergic antidepressant (NaSSA).

Table 22.1 Mechanism of action of mirtazapine.

Blockade of α_2-auto and heteroreceptors	Increases noradrenergic and serotonergic transmission. Antidepressant effect
Weak affinity for α_1-receptors	Allows noradrenergic action provoking firing of serotonergic neurones and serotonin release, further increasing serotonergic transmission. Antidepressant effect
Blockade of 5-HT2	Lack of anxiety and insomnia. No sexual dysfunction. Can cause weight gain
Blockade of 5-HT3	Lack of gastrointestinal problems. No nausea
No action on 5-HT1	Allows serotonin to act on these receptors. Anxiolytic and antidepressant effects
Blockade of H1	Anxiolytic effect but can cause drowsiness and weight gain

Mode of action

Mirtazapine enhances noradrenergic and 5-HT neurotransmission by a blockade of the presynaptic α_2-adrenoreceptors located presynaptically on noradrenergic terminals and α_2-heteroreceptors, which are located on serotonergic nerve terminals. These two types of receptors have inhibitory functions on the release of norepinephrine (noradrenaline) and serotonin, respectively. By blocking them, mirtazapine increases both noradrenergic and serotonergic neurotransmission. Norepinephrine released in this form stimulates α_1-adrenoceptors on the serotonergic cell body, further potentiating serotonin release by increasing the firing rate of serotonergic neurones. This is possible because mirtazapine has a weak affinity for α_1-adrenoreceptors.

The overall effect of mirtazapine is increase of noradrenergic and serotonergic neurotransmission. Moreover, mirtazapine specifically enhances the 5-HT1-mediated neurotransmission, because it blocks 5-HT2 and 5-HT3 receptors which accounts for its benign profile regarding therapeutic actions and side-effects (blockade of 5-HT2 and 5-HT3 may contribute to mirtazapine's anxiolytic and sleep improving effects and lack of side-effects such as anxiety, sexual dysfunction, and nausea).

Even though mirtazapine has a strong affinity for histamine receptors and can be sedative at lower doses, this is often less of a problem at higher doses, possibly because of noradrenergic mediated activation provoked by mirtazapine, increases to offset the sedative effect.

Furthermore, mirtazapine shows low or very low affinity for α_1-adrenergic, cholinergic and dopaminergic receptors, which permits this drug to have a low incidence of adrenergic (tachycardia, orthostatic hypotension), cholinergic (dry mouth, constipation, etc.) and dopaminergic side-effects, which have proven to be quite frequent with older antidepressants (Table 22.1).

Pharmacokinetics

Within the normal dose range (15–45 mg/day), mirtazapine follows linear pharmacokinetics. It is rapidly and well absorbed after oral administration and shows a bioavailability of 50% after single or multiple doses. Its absorption is not affected by the presence of food in the stomach. The half-life elimination is 20–40 h and steady state is reached in 3–5 days.

Mirtazapine's binding to plasma proteins is around 85%, is nonspecific and reversible. Its biotransformation occurs in the liver. Cytochrome P450 isoenzymes 2D6 and 1A2 are involved in the production of the hydroxy metabolite, and the 3A4 isoenzyme is involved in the formation of the demethyl and N-oxide metabolites. Besides the primary active compound, mirtazapine, the only other active metabolite is demethylmirtazapine, which in animal studies has shown an activity ten-fold lower than the parent compound.

Mirtazapine and its metabolites are eliminated in urine and feces within a few days after oral administration. Approximately 100% of the dose is excreted within 4 days in the urine (up to 85%) and faeces (up to 15%). Because of this pharmacokinetic pathway, the dose of mirtazapine should be lowered in the presence of hepatic or renal impairment. Hepatic impairment may diminish metabolism and increase half-life up to 40%, resulting in higher plasma levels. Renal impairment causes decreased clearance of mirtazapine and significantly increased plasma concentration. Thus, whenever a patient with renal and/or hepatic impairment is treated with mirtazapine, cautious dose escalation and monitoring is recommended.

Adverse events, toxicity and safety

Overall mirtazapine seems to have a benign side-effect profile. Montgomery (1995) reviewed the accumulated data on the safety of this dual antidepressant and concluded that participants taking mirtazapine had fewer side-effects than patients taking placebo and amitriptyline (65%, 76% and 87%, respectively). Only dry mouth, drowsiness, sedation, increased appetite, and weight gain were more frequent with mirtazapine than placebo. Mirtazapine was found to have significantly lower side-effects when compared with amitriptyline. Patients taking mirtazapine complained significantly less often of anticholinergic symptoms (i.e. dry mouth, constipation, abnormal accommodation and abnormal vision), cardiac symptoms (palpitations and tachycardia) and neurological symptoms (tremor and vertigo) than amitriptyline treated patients. Moreover, the majority of all other side-effects were noted more frequently in the amitriptyline-treated sample. Interestingly, sexual dysfunction, a common adverse event, among patients taking antidepressants, was either similar or lower in recipients taking mirtazapine than in patients under placebo treatment. When compared with amitriptyline, sexual dysfunction was also less frequent with mirtazapine, although the difference did not reach a statistically significant level.

Mirtazapine also showed a more favorable tolerability than other antidepressants like clomipramine (Richou et al. 1995), doxepin (Mattila et al. 1995), and trazodone (Van Moffaert et al. 1995).

Regarding SSRI antidepressants, several studies have been conducted to compare them with mirtazapine. In a study that included 133 patients with major depression, the tolerability of mirtazapine was compared with fluoxetine (Wheatley et al. 1998). Mirtazapine was associated with more reports of dry mouth, blurred vision and somnolence than fluoxetine, while fluoxetine presented with more frequent incidences of headache, nausea and dizziness. A similar study was reported by Leinonen et al. (1999) comparing mirtazapine with citalopram. The authors concluded that mirtazapine was associated with a significantly higher incidence of increased appetite and weight gain, and significantly lower incidence of nausea and sweating. Another study compared mirtazapine with paroxetine (Benkert et al. 2000). In this trial the authors reported that mirtazapine had significantly lower incidences of nausea, vomiting, sweating, and tremor; and significantly higher incidence of weight increase and flu-like symptoms.

Blockade of H1 receptors has a sedative effect and also causes drowsiness. Such blockade may also be related with weight increase. Mirtazapine, given its high affinity for H1 receptors, shows sedation and drowsiness (Montgomery 1995). However, tolerance develops to these side-effects with time.

The weight gain observed with mirtazapine may be one potential drawback for patients presented with overeating and/or with other concerns about this issue. However, in patients with weight loss this may be an advantage, an issue that might be of particular importance among the elderly.

Regarding toxicity, mirtazapine seems to have less serious sequelae associated with overdose when compared with other antidepressants, especially with tricyclics. In reported cases of overdose, transient somnolence was the most important symptom, without any clinically relevant changes in vital signs or the electrocardiogram (Montgomery 1995). Another case report described an 81-year-old-woman who took 900 mg of mirtazapine and 210 mg of midazolam. The patient presented in the admission to the hospital with a comatose state that resolved spontaneously within 1 h. The subsequent somnolence disappeared completely after 3 days. Neither respiratory nor cardiovascular functions were compromised and no seizures were observed (Hoes & Zijpveld 1996).

Drug interactions

Even though different P450 isoenzymes metabolize mirtazapine, this drug does not seem to be a potent inhibitor, so it is unlikely to have clinically important interactions with other medications. Furthermore, mirtazapine's binding to plasma proteins is relatively low. However, results from investigations conducted with a wide range of other drugs regarding potential interactions are still unavailable.

Psychomotor performance may be impaired when combining mirtazapine and diazepam or ethanol (Mattila et al. 1989; Kuitunen 1994; Sisten & Zikov 1995).

Mirtazapine should be avoided in patients taking MAOIs, although, to our knowledge, no case reports of toxic interactions exist.

Clinical use

Unfortunately, mirtazapine has not been extensively evaluated as a treatment for anxiety disorders in the research arena. However, three small open-label trials have been conducted to study the efficacy of mirtazapine in GAD, PD and PTSD. These result along with preliminary information from another unpublished study will be presented here.

Generalized anxiety disorder

Goodnick *et al.* (1999) conducted a small open-label study with 10 patients suffering from depression with comorbid GAD. Patients received mirtazapine (15–45 mg/day) for 8 weeks. The authors reported significant improvements on the HAM-A, the HAM-D, and the Beck Depression Inventory (BDI) noticeable since the 1st week and persisting throughout the study.

Panic disorder

Carpenter *et al.* (1999) reported the results of a small open-label study in which 10 adult outpatients with a primary diagnosis of PD where treated with mirtazapine for 16 weeks. Based on all available data, 70% of the sample showed an acute response (defined as Clinical Global Impression-Improvement (CGI-1) = 2 or 3) by weeks 5–7, and six continued to have a positive long-term response (defined as response at the 16-week endpoint, except for one patient who formally concluded the study at week 12 because of moving to another state). Regrettably, concomitant medications were allowed in this trial (i.e., low doses of benzodiazepines, if they were used previously for at least 2 months; and in two patients SSRIs to which there had not been an adequate response).

Falkai (1999) referred to unpublished data in a recent article regarding a study conducted to evaluate the efficacy of mirtazapine in the treatment of PD. Apparently, mirtazapine reduced panic attacks in number and intensity.

Post-traumatic stress disorder

Connor *et al.* (1999) reported the results of a small pilot study of six outpatients with severe, chronic PTSD and substantial comorbidity who were treated with mirtazapine, up to 45 mg/day for 8 weeks. Fifty percent of the sample showed improvement of 50% or more from baseline using a global rating. Moreover, improvements were noted on both interviewer-administered and self-rated scales of PTSD, and of depression. The

authors acknowledged the limitations of the study, mainly related with high psychiatric comorbidity and the size of the sample.

Venlafaxine

Venlafaxine is the first medication in a new class of antidepressants known as serotonin noradrenergic reuptake inhibitors (SNRIs). This medication is available in two different formulations: immediate release (IR) and extended release (XR).

Mode of action

Venlafaxine and its active metabolite, O-desmethylvenlafaxine (ODV), are potent inhibitors of reuptake of both norepinephrine and serotonin and, more weakly, of dopamine. Venlafaxine has a very similar action to the serotonin reuptake inhibitors at lower doses but, at higher doses, norepinephrine reuptake inhibition predominates. Unlike TCAs that also have this dual action, venlafaxine and its metabolite lack anticholinergic actions and effects on cardiac conduction. Moreover, they have little affinity for muscarinic, H1-histaminic, or α-adrenergic receptors *in vitro*. They do not show monoamine oxidase A or B inhibitory activity.

Pharmacokinetics

Venlafaxine is well-absorbed and extensively metabolized in the liver after oral administration, with a bioavailability of 45%. ODV is the only major active metabolite.

XR formulation has a lower rate of absorption but to the same extent when compared with the IR tablets.

Recommended starting dose for the IR formulation is generally 75 mg/day, divided in two or three doses. *The maximum dose studied in controlled trials is 375 mg/day, but higher doses have been recommended in unresponsive patients by many clinicians and investigators.* The XR formulation simplifies dosing, with a once-daily dose. *Food does not affect the bioavailability of venlafaxine or its active metabolite.*

After absorption, venlafaxine undergoes extensive presystemic metabolism in the liver. *In-vitro* studies had shown that the formation of ODV is catalysed by CYP2D6; and this was confirmed clinically, showing that patients with low CYP2D6 levels had increased levels of venlafaxine and lower levels of ODV, compared with subjects with normal levels of CYP2D6. Renal elimination of venlafaxine and its metabolites is the principal route for excretion.

Venlafaxine and its metabolites have diminished clearance in patients with hepatic cirrhosis and severe renal impairment; in these patients the dose of venlafaxine has to be reduced. However, in healthy elderly patients there is no need for dosage adjustment.

Adverse events, toxicity and safety

Venlafaxine has *low* affinity for muscarinic cholinergic, histaminic, or α-adrenergic receptors; hence it has low incidence of side-effects related with them (i.e. sedation, orthostatic hypotension, etc.).

Venlafaxine can cause a dose-related increase in blood pressure in some patients. This effect becomes apparent with doses higher than 101 mg/day (i.e. sustained elevation of blood pressure was 3–4% higher in patients receiving 101–300 mg/day of venlafaxine than in patients taking placebo) (Rudolph & Derivan 1996).

Venlafaxine presents a side-effect profile similar to that of SSRIs; however, it does not seem to have the stimulant action that may occur with fluoxetine. The adverse event most frequently reported with the XR formulation is nausea. Other common adverse events include insomnia, dizziness, somnolence, headaches, asthenia, nervousness, anorexia, sweating and dry mouth. Abnormalities of sexual function were also described (abnormal ejaculation and impotence in men, and decreased libido (package insert, Wyeth Laboratories, Inc., revised December 30, 1999).

There have been three reports on possible venlafaxine withdrawal syndrome (Farah & Lauer 1996; Louie *et al.* 1996; Dallal & Chouinard 1998). These reports complete a total of 10 patients who presented withdrawal symptoms after discontinuation of venlafaxine. The symptoms described involved mainly the gastrointestinal system (i.e., nausea, abdominal distention, gastrointestinal distress) and CNS (i.e., headaches, anxiety, agitation, tinnitus, tremors, vertigo, akathisia, dizziness, bizarre dreams, and auditory hallucinations). Other reported withdrawal symptoms were fatigue, congested sinus and tachycardia. Noteworthy is that this symptomatology resolved when venlafaxine was restarted. The authors acknowledge

the importance of gradual tapering when discontinuing venlafaxine, which in some cases may take more than 4 weeks.

Regarding overdose, in the premarketing evaluation of venlafaxine there were 14 reports of acute overdose, either alone or in combination with other drugs and/or alcohol. All 14 patients recovered without untoward effects. Among patients included in the premarketing evaluation of venlafaxine XR, there were two overdoses in depression trials, either alone or in combination with other drugs. In trials for the treatment of GAD, two patients had acute overdose. In all these cases patients recovered without sequelae. In postmarketing experience, overdose with venlafaxine has occurred predominantly in combination with alcohol and/or other drugs. The findings in these cases were ECG changes (i.e., prolongation of QT interval, bundle branch block, QRS prolongation), sinus and ventricular tachycardia, bradycardia, hypotension, altered level of consciousness (ranging from somnolence to coma), seizures, vertigo and death (package insert, Wyeth Laboratories, Inc., revised December 30, 1999).

Drug interactions

Venlafaxine is extensively metabolized by the hepatic cytochrome P450 enzyme system, mainly by CYP2D6 isoenzyme. This isoenzyme is subject to genetic polymorphism, hence venlafaxine's metabolism varies from patient to patient. Nevertheless, the total amount of venlafaxine and ODV was similar in CYP2D6-poor and CYP2D6-extensive metabolizers; this suggests that no dose adjustment is necessary when venlafaxine is coadministered with a CYP2D6 inhibitor.

Venlafaxine hydrochloride showed neither *in vivo* nor *in vitro* significant inhibition or effect on isoenzymes CYP1A2, CYP2C9, CYP2D6, and CYP3A4 (Ereshefsky 1996). These findings point out that venlafaxine as favorable drug interaction profile.

Clinical use

Venlafaxine is the nonSSRI antidepressant most extensively evaluated in a double-blind fashion for the treatment of both depression and anxiety. Moreover, in 1999 venlafaxine XR became the only antidepressant approved by the US Food and Drug Administration for the treatment of GAD.

Here we will present data available to date for the use of venlafaxine and venlafaxine XR in the treatment of anxiety disorders.

Generalized anxiety disorder

Johnson *et al.* (1998) presented the results of an small open-label prospective study with 11 patients, in which venlafaxine was highly effective in mitigating symptoms of GAD in 73% of the population ($N = 8$). Positive responses were detected early in treatment and with relatively low doses of venlafaxine (12.5–187.5 mg/day).

Venlafaxine XR has also been found effective in the treatment of GAD. Aguiar *et al.* (1998) reported the results of a double-blind placebo controlled study in 377 patients with GAD without comorbid major depression. In this study venlafaxine XR (225 mg/day) appeared to be significantly more effective than placebo, as measured on the Clinical Global Impression-Severity (CGI-S) and HAM-A. Additionally, venlafaxine XR in doses of 75 mg/day and 150 mg/day was found to be significantly better than placebo and buspirone on the Hospital Anxiety and Depression (HAD) Scale, a patient-rated scale (Davidson *et al.* 1999).

Davidson *et al.* (1999) published the results of a randomized, double-blind study comparing the efficacy and safety of venlafaxine XR and buspirone in outpatients with GAD without comorbid major depression. The efficacy analysis included 365 patients who were treated with venlafaxine 75 or 150 mg/day, buspirone 30 mg/day, or placebo. Patients taking venlafaxine XR had significantly lower adjusted mean HAM-A psychic anxiety factor, CGI-I, and CGI-S scores than placebo-treated patients, although no effect was found on the HAM-A total scores. The HAD anxiety subscale scores for both doses of venlafaxine XR were also significantly better than those for buspirone from week 2 and continuing through the study. The authors acknowledged that higher doses of buspirone might have been more effective. The investigators concluded that once-daily administration of venlafaxine XR, 75 or 150 mg, is an effective, safe, and well-tolerated treatment for patients with GAD without comorbid major depression. Venlafaxine was significantly superior to placebo and comparable to, or slightly better than, buspirone.

Another randomized, double-blind, parallel-group, placebo controlled study with patients with GAD without depression was reported by Rickels *et al.* (2000). In this trial, patients were randomly assigned to receive either placebo or venlafaxine XR at one of three dose levels (75, 150 or 225 mg/day) for up to 8 weeks. Three-hundred and forty-nine patients were entered for the efficacy analysis which showed that venlafaxine demonstrated superiority in all three dosages, beginning as early as week 1 and maintained throughout the entire 8 weeks of the study. Venlafaxine XR had statistically significantly lower adjusted mean scores on the HAM-A total score and psychic anxiety factor, on the CGI-S item, and on the CGI-I item at endpoint when compared with placebo. Moreover, the three venlafaxine XR treatment groups showed important anxiolytic effect on the Hospital Anxiety and Depression Scale's anxiety subscale. The authors also noted that even though all three groups treated with venlafaxine showed some efficacy, further inspection of the data showed most positive results in the group receiving 225 mg/day.

Positive results were also presented by Gelenberg *et al.* (2000) from a long-term study with nondepressed outpatients with GAD. In this study 251 participants were randomly assigned to receive either placebo or venlafaxine XR (75, 150 or 225 mg/day) for 28 weeks. The efficacy analysis was conducted on data from 238 patients (123 in the placebo group and 115 in the venlafaxine XR group). Response to treatment was defined as either a reduction in HAM-A total score of 40% or more from baseline or a CGI-I score of 1 or 2. Patients treated with venlafaxine XR showed response rates in the HAM-A total score significantly better than those of patients receiving placebo. Similar results were observed for CGI-I, with significantly more patients receiving venlafaxine XR responding than patients in the placebo group.

Panic disorder

Four cases of PD treated with venlafaxine were reported by Geracioti (1995). All the patients responded to very modest doses of venlafaxine (12.5–18.75 mg twice daily). Papp *et al.* (1998) conducted a small open-label trial in which 13 patients with PD were treated with venlafaxine for up to 10 weeks (mean daily dose at the end of the trial was 93.4 mg). All 10 patients who completed the study were *responders*.

Effects of venlafaxine were reported in *25 patients from one site from a multicenter double-blind placebo controlled trial of PD*. Patients taking venlafaxine showed statistically significant changes on the CGI-I items at endpoint compared with patients in the placebo group (effect size 0.89) (Pollack *et al.* 1996).

Social anxiety disorder

Kelsey (1995) reported a case series of 9 patients with a history of failure to respond or unable to tolerate SSRIs who were treated with venlafaxine for 4–12 weeks (mean final dose 146.5 mg/day). Patients showed a significant improvement in the social phobia subscale of the Fear Questionnaire ($P < 0.02$) and in the social/leisure subscales of the Sheehan Disability Scale ($P < 0.02$). Overall, 8 of the 9 patients were respondents to venlafaxine.

In a more recent study conducted in Italy by Altamura *et al.* (1999) 12 patients with social phobia (with or without concomitant avoidant personality disorder) who were nonresponders to SSRIs responded to a 15-weeks trial with venlafaxine (doses from 112.5 mg/day to 187.5 mg/day). Venlafaxine improved social phobia and/or avoidant personality disorder symptomatology, as measured by a decrease in Liebowitz Social Anxiety Scale total scores ($P < 0.05$).

Larger, placebo-controlled, multicenter trials are now ongoing.

Obsessive-compulsive disorder

Ananth *et al.* (1995) presented two cases of patients with OCD who responded to venlafaxine treatment. In both cases patients had a history of failure to respond or tolerate SSRI medications. These patients showed a dramatic response to 150 mg/day of venlafaxine.

Rauch *et al.* (1996) conducted a 12-week open-label trial of venlafaxine in 10 outpatients with OCD (mean daily dose 308.3 mg/day). Overall improvement attributed to venlafaxine was observed in 30% of these patients. The investigators concluded that venlafaxine has potential antiobsessional efficacy.

A small, 8 week, double-blind, placebo-controlled trial of venlafaxine in 30 outpatients with OCD was reported by Yaryura-Tobias and Neziroglu (1996). Venlafaxine showed to be beneficial in 6 *patients*, while in three patients the condition remained unchanged and in five patients the condition became worse. In contrast, none of the patients in the placebo group ($N = 14$) showed improvement and their drop out rate was higher. The authors acknowledged that the number of patients who might have benefited from venlafaxine would have been higher if the study had been carried out for a longer duration (and if higher

dosages of venlafaxine than that used [225 mg/day] had been employed).

Post-traumatic stress disorder

To our knowledge, only one case of PTSD (with co-morbid major depression) treated with venlafaxine was reported (Hamner & Frueh 1998). The authors presented a male Vietnam combat veteran with history of resistance to several serotonergic agents who successfully responded to a trial with venlafaxine. This patient showed substantial improvement with venlafaxine 150 mg/day and further improvement was observed after an increase of the dose up to 225 mg/day.

Anxiety associated with depression

Rudolph *et al.* (1998) reported a meta-analysis of the efficacy of venlafaxine in the treatment of anxiety associated with depression. The authors performed a pooled analysis of six short-term trials of venlafaxine, retrospectively measuring anxiety in patients with depression and anxiety. Three of these trials were placebo-controlled of three fixed-dosage range groups and the remaining were placebo- and active-drug-controlled studies (the active comparators were imipramine in two of them and trazodone in the third). Overall, venlafaxine was given 2–3 times daily (dose range 50–375 mg/day). All studies had a duration of 6 weeks, with the exception of one that lasted 12 weeks. Anxious-depressed participants taking venlafaxine showed greater improvement than those under placebo beginning at week 3, according to the HAM-D anxiety/somatization factor score, and beginning at week 1, according to the anxiety psychic item score. These effects were maintained at endpoint. Moreover, venlafaxine treatment caused highly significant ($P <$ or $= 0.001$) improvement in depression scores in patients who were anxious at baseline when compared with participants taking placebo. In *one* trial using imipramine as the active comparator, an advantage for venlafaxine over imipramine was observed by week 3 for both anxiety variables in this study and maintained *for* the anxiety/somatization factor. In the other two (one using trazodone and one imipramine as the active controls), no consistent differences were detected between venlafaxine and the active comparator. The authors of this meta-analysis concluded that venlafaxine is effective in relieving anxiety in patients who have anxiety associated with depression, and think of venlafaxine as an adequate single drug option for first-line treatment of patients with comorbid anxiety and depression.

Venlafaxine XR was also studied in the treatment of outpatients with depression and anxiety ($N = 359$). Silverstone and Ravindran (1999) conducted a randomized double-blind, placebo-controlled study of the efficacy and safety of once daily venlafaxine XR (dose range 75–225 mg/day) and fluoxetine (dose range 20–60 mg/day). Patients were randomly assigned to once daily venlafaxine XR, fluoxetine, or placebo for 12 weeks. Venlafaxine XR and fluoxetine were significantly superior ($P < 0.05$) to placebo on the HAM-D total score beginning at week 2 and continuing through the study. At endpoint, the HAM-D response (reduction of 50% or more from baseline) was 43% for placebo, 62% for fluoxetine, and 67% for venlafaxine ($P < 0.05$). The HAM-A response (also defined as 50% decrease in score from baseline) was significantly higher with venlafaxine XR than with fluoxetine at week 12. The authors concluded that venlafaxine XR is an effective and well-tolerated option for the treatment of major depression associated with anxiety and appears to be superior to fluoxetine.

A case report of a patient with coexisting major depression and OCD treated with venlafaxine was reported by Zajecka et al. (1990). The authors present a female patient who failed to respond to several other conventional antidepressants but who, in her obsessive-compulsive symptoms, responded to venlafaxine.

Conclusions

The possible common neurobiochemical roots of anxiety disorders and depression may partially explain why antidepressants can be used for the treatment of anxiety disorder with clinical success. Even though further double-blind research needs to be done, it is clear that nefazodone, mirtazapine and venlafaxine may represent useful tools in that area. Moreover, as previously stated, venlafaxine XR has already been approved by the US Food and Drug Administration for the treatment of GAD. Additionally, it is very common for different anxiety disorders to present concomitantly with depression, which makes nefazodone, mirtazapine, and venlafaxine a valuable option as a single drug treatment, which may increase not only the treatment efficacy but also its compliance and reduce the possible drug interactions.

References

Altamura, A.C., Pioli, R., Vitto, M. & Mannu, P. (1999) Venlafaxine in social phobia: a study in selective serotonin reuptake inhibitor nonresponders. Int Clin Psychopharmacol 14(4), 239–45.

Ananth, J., Burgoyne, K., Smith, M. & Swartz, R. (1995) Venlafaxine for treatment of obsessive-compulsive disorder. Am J Psychiatryry 152(12), 1832.

American Psychiatric Association (1994) Diagnostic Statistical Manual of Mental Disorders, 4th edn. American Psychiatric Association, Washington, D.C.

Armitage, R., Yonkers, K., Cole, D. & Rush, J. (1997) A multicenter, double-blind comparison of the effects of nefazodone and fluoxetine on sleep architecture and quality of sleep in depressed outpatients. J Clin Psychopharmacol 17, 161–8.

Benkert, O., Szegedi, A. & Kohnen, R. (2000) Mirtazapine compared with paroxetine in major depression. J Clin Psychiatry 61(9), 656–63.

Berigan, T.R., Casas, A. & Harazin, J. (1998) Nefazodone and the treatment of panic. J Clin Psychiatry 59(5), 256–7.

Bystritsky, A., Rosen, R., Suri, R. & Vapnik, T. (1999) Pilot open-label study of nefazodone in panic disorder. Depress Anxiety 10(3), 137–9.

Caplik, J., Talukder, E., Roberts, D. et al. (1994) Nefazodone and body-weight change: a comparison of nefazodone and imipramine in placebo-controlled trials of treatment for major depression. Neuropsychopharmacology 10 (Suppl. 3, Part 2), S220.

Carpenter, L.L., Leon, Z., Yasmin, S. & Price, L.H. (1999) Clinical experience with mirtazapine in the treatment of panic disorder. Ann Clin Psychiatry 11(2), 81–6.

Cohn, C.K., Robinson, D.S., Roberts, D.L. et al. (1996) Responders to anti-depressant drug treatment: a study comparing nefazodone, imipramine, and placebo inpatients with major depression. J Clin Psychiatry 57 (Suppl. 2), 15–18.

Connor, K.M., Davidson, J.R.T., Weisler, R.H. & Ahearn, E. (1999) A pilot study of mirtazapine in post-traumatic stress disorder. Int Clin Psychopharmacol 14, 29–31.

Dallal, A. & Chouinard, G. (1998) Withdrawal and rebound symptoms associated with abrupt discontinuation of venlafaxine. J Clin Psychiatry 18(4), 343–4.

Davidson, J.R.T., DuPont, R.L., Hedges, D. & Haskins, J.T. (1999) Efficacy, safety, and tolerability of venlafaxine extended release in outpatients with generalized anxiety disorder. J Clin Psychiatry 60(8), 528–35.

Davis, R., Whittington, R. & Bryson, H.M. (1997) Nefazodone. A review of its pharmacology and clinical efficacy in the management of major depression. Drugs 53(4), 608–36.

DeMartinis, N.A., Schweizer, E. & Rickels, K. (1996) An open-label trial of nefazodone in high comorbidity panic disorder. J Clin Psychiatry 57, 245–8.

Ereshefsky, L. (1996) Drug–drug interactions involving antidepressants: focus on venlafaxine. *J Clin Psychopharmacol* **16**(3) (Suppl. 2), S37–S50.

Falkai, P. (1999) Mirtazapine: other indications. *J Clin Psychiatry* **60**, 36–40.

Farah, A. & Lauer, T. (1996) Possible venlafaxine withdrawal syndrome. *Am J Psychiatry* **153**(4), 576.

Fawcett, J., Marcus, R., Anton, S., O'Brien, K. & Schwiderski, U. (1995) Response of anxiety and agitation symptoms during nefazodone treatment of major depression. *J Clin Psychiatry* **56** (Suppl. 6), 37–42.

Feighner, J., Targum, S.D., Bennett, M.E. *et al.* (1998) A double-blind, placebo-controlled trial of nefazodone in the treatment of patients hospitalized for major depression. *J Clin Psychiatry* **59**(5), 246–53.

Fontaine, R., Ontiveros, A., Elie, R. *et al.* (1994) A double-blind comparison of nefazodone, imipramine, and placebo in major depression. *J Clin Psychiatry* **55**, 234–41.

Frazer, A. (1997) Antidepressants. *J Clin Psychiatry* **58** (Suppl. 6), 9–25.

Gelenberg, A.J., Lydiard, R.B., Rudolph, R.L., Aguiar, L., Haskins, J.T. & Salinas, E. (2000) Efficacy of venlafaxine extended release capsules in nondepressed outpatients with generalized anxiety disorder. A 6-month randomized controlled trial. *JAMA* **283**(23), 3082–8.

Geracioti, T.D. Jr (1995) Venlafaxine treatment of panic disorder: a case series. *J Clin Psychiatry* **56**, 408–10.

Gillin, J.C., Rapaport, M., Erman, M., Winokur, A. & Albala, B. (1997) A comparison of nefazodone and fluoxetine on mood and on objective, subjective, and clinician-rated measures of sleep in depressed patients: a double-blind, 8-week clinical trial. *J Clin Psychiatry* **58**, 185–92.

Goodnick, P.J., Puig, A., DeVane, C.L. & Freund, B.V. (1999) Mirtazapine in major depression with comorbid generalized anxiety disorder. *J Clin Psychiatry* **60**(7), 446–8.

Green, D.S., Salazar, D.E., Dockens, R.C. *et al.* (1995) Coadministration of nefazodone and benzodiazepines. IV. A pharmacokinetic interaction study with lorazepam. *J Clin Psychopharmacol* **15**, 409–16.

Hamner, M.B. & Frueh, B.C. (1998) Response to venlafaxine in a previously antidepressant treatment-resistant combat veteran with post-traumatic disorder. *Int Clin Psychopharmacol* **13**, 233–4.

Hedges, D.W., Reimherr, F.W., Strong, R.E., Halls, C.H. & Rust, C. (1996) An open trial of nefazodone in adult patients with generalized anxiety disorder. *Psychopharmacol Bull* **32**, 671–6.

Hidalgo, R., Hertzberg, M.A., Mellman, T. *et al.* (1999) Nefazodone in post-traumatic stress disorder: results from six open-label trials. *Int Clin Psychopharmacol* **14**(2), 61–8.

Hoes, M.J.A.J.M. & Zijpveld, J.H.B. (1996) First report of mirtazapine overdose. *Int Clin Psychopharmacol* **11**, 147.

Johnson, M.R., Emanuel, N., Crawford, M., Lydiard, R.B. & Villareal, G. (1998) Treatment of generalized anxiety disorder with venlafaxine: a series of 11 cases. *J Clin Psychopharmacol* **18**, 418–19.

Kelsey, J.E. (1995) Venlafaxine in social phobia. *Psychopharmacol Bull* **31**, 767–71.

Kuitunen, T. (1994) Drug and ethanol effects on the clinical test for drunkenness: single dose of ethanol, hypnotic drugs and antidepressant drugs. *Pharmacol Toxicol* **75**, 91–8.

Leinonen, E., Skarstein, J., Behnke, K. & Agren Hans, Helsdingen, J.T. (1999) Efficacy and tolerability of mirtazapine versus citalopram: a double-blind, randomized study in patients with major depressive disorder. *Int Clin Psychopharmacol* **14**(6), 329–37.

Louie, A.K., Lannon, R.A., Kiesh, M.A. & Lewis, T.B. (1996) Venlafaxine withdrawal reaction. *Am J Psychiatry* **153**, 1652.

Markus, R.N. (1996) Safety and tolerability profile of nefazodone. *J Psychopharmacol* **10** (Suppl. 1), 11–17.

Mattila, M., Jaaskelainen, J., Jarvi, R. *et al.* (1995) A double-blind study comparing the efficacy and tolerability of Org 3770 and doxepin in patients with major depression. *Eur Neuropsychopharmacol* **5**, 441–6.

Mattila, M., Mattila, M.J., Vrijmoed-de-Vries, M. & Kuitunen, T. (1989) Actions and interactions of psychotropic drugs on human performance and mood: single doses of Org 3770, amitriptyline and diazepam. *Pharmacol Toxicol* **65**, 81–8.

Montgomery, S.A. (1995) Safety of mirtazapine: a review. *Int Clin Psychopharmacol* **10** (Suppl. 4), 37–45.

Nelson, E.C. (1994) An open-label study of nefazodone in the treatment of depression with and without comorbid obsessive-compulsive disorder. *Ann Clin Psychiatry* **6**(4), 249–53.

Nutt, D. (1996) Early action of nefazodone in anxiety associated with depression. *J Psychopharmacol* **10** (Suppl. 1), 18–21.

Papp, L.A., Sinha, S.S., Martinez, J.M. *et al.* (1998) Low-dose venlafaxine treatment in panic disorder. *Psychopharmacol Bull* **34**, 207–9.

Pollack, M.H., Worthington, J.J., III, Otto, M.W. *et al.* (1996) Venlafaxine for panic disorder: results from a double-blind, placebo-controlled study. *Psychopharmacol Bull* **32**, 667–70.

Rascati, K. (1995) Drug utilization review of concomitant use of specific serotonin reuptake inhibitors or clomipramine with antianxiety/sleep medications. *Clin Ther* **17**(4), 786–90.

Rauch, S.L., O'Sullivan, R.L. & Jenike, M.A. (1996) Open treatment of obsessive-compulsive disorder with venlafaxine. a series of 10 cases. *J Clin Psychopharmacol* **16**, 81–4.

Richou, H., Ruimy, P., Charbaut, J. *et al.* (1995) A multi-center, double-blind, clomipramine-controlled efficacy and safety study of Org 3770. *Hum Psychopharmacol* **10**, 263–71.

Rickels, K., Pollack, M.H., Sheehan, D.V. & Haskins, J.T. (2000) Efficacy of extended-release venlafaxine in non-depressed outpatients with generalized anxiety disorder. *Am J Psychiatry* **157**(6), 968–74.

Rudolph, R.L. & Derivan, A. (1996) The safety and tolerability of venlafaxine hydrochloride: analysis of the clinical trials database. *J Clin Psychopharmacol* **16**(2), S54–S61.

Rudolph, R., Entsuah, R. & Chitra, R. (1998) A meta-analysis of the effects of venlafaxine on anxiety associated with depression. *J Clin Psychopharmacol* **18**(2), 136–44.

Rush, J.A., Armitage, R., Gillin, J.C. *et al.* (1998) Comparative effects of nefazodone and fluoxetine on sleep in outpatients with major depressive disorder. *Biol Psychiatry* **44**, 3–14.

Silverstone, P.H. & Ravindran, A. (1999) Once-daily venlafaxine extended release (XR) compared with fluoxetine in outpatients with depression and anxiety. *J Clin Psychiatry* **60**(1), 22–8.

Sisten, J.M.A. & Zikov, M. (1995) Mirtazapine: clinical profile. *CNS Drugs* **4** (Suppl. 1), 39–48.

Sussman, N. & Ginsberg, D. (1998) Rethinking side effects of the selective reuptake inhibitors: sexual dysfunction and weight gain. *Psychiatr Ann* **28**(2), 89–97.

Taylor, D.P., Carter, R.B., Eison, A.S. *et al.* (1995) Pharmacology and neurochemistry of nefazodone, a novel antidepressant drug. *J Clin Psychiatry* **56** (Suppl. 6), 3–11.

Van Ameringen, M., Mancini, C. & Oakman, J.M. (1999) Nefazodone in social phobia. *J Clin Psychiatry* **60**(2), 96–100.

Van Moffaert, M., de Wilde, J., Vereecken, A. *et al.* (1995) Mirtazapine is more effective than trazodone: a double-blind controlled study of hospitalized patients with major depression. *Int Clin Psychopharmacol* **10**, 3–9.

Wheatley, D.P., van Moffaert, M., Timmerman, L. & Kremer, C.M.E. (1998) Mirtazapine: efficacy and tolerability in comparison with fluoxetine in patients with moderate to severe major depressive disorder. *J Clin Psychiatry* **59**(6), 306–12.

Yaryura-Tobias, J.A. & Neziroglu, F.A. (1996) Venlafaxine in obsessive-compulsive disorder. *Arch Gen Psychiatry* **53**, 653–4.

Zajecka, J.M., Fawcett, J. & Guy, C. (1990) Coexisting major depression and obsessive-compulsive disorder treated with venlafaxine. *J Clin Psychopharmacol* **10**(2), 152–3.

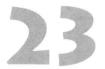

23

Cognitive Behavioral Treatment of Anxiety Disorders

S.A. Falsetti, A. Combs-Lane & J.L. Davis

Introduction

There are now many cognitive behavioral interventions available for the treatment of anxiety disorders. In this chapter we will review cognitive behavioral therapy (CBT) for the treatment of post-traumatic stress disorder, generalized anxiety disorder, social phobia, panic disorder, and obsessive-compulsive disorder. For each disorder, we provide descriptions of treatment, as well as review the literature on the efficacy of these treatments. Overall, the research suggests that CBT is an effective treatment option for those suffering from anxiety disorders.

Common elements of CBTs across anxiety disorders

CBTs for anxiety disorders are based on similar principles, namely that anxiety affects physiological, cognitive, and behavioral domains of functioning. In other words, the anxiety disorders generally include symptoms across these domains and the CBTs are aimed at these areas. Thus, most comprehensive CBT protocols include components that target the physiological symptoms of anxiety, such as progressive muscle relaxation or diaphragmatic breathing, a cognitive restructuring component that targets anxiety provoking thoughts, and a behavioral component that targets avoidance behaviors via imaginal or *in vivo* exposure. In addition, for some disorders, such as generalized anxiety disorder and obsessive-compulsive disorder, there may also be a response prevention component in which patients are instructed to refrain from engaging in certain behaviors.

Empirical studies for CBTs for anxiety disorders

CBT treatment alternatives for post-traumatic stress disorder

CBT is widely used and highly effective in the treatment of post-traumatic stress disorder (PTSD). Cognitive processing therapy (CPT: Resick & Schnicke 1993), developed for the treatment of PTSD in rape victims, employs mainly a cognitive approach. This treatment focuses on changes in cognition that result from trauma. Stress inoculation training (SIT: Kilpatrick *et al.* 1982) and multiple channel exposure therapy (MCET: Falsetti 1997; Falsetti & Resnick 2000a,b) are also CBTs. Prolonged exposure, developed by Foa and colleagues, is discussed in Chapter 24, and thus, will not be further addressed in this chapter. We will review the components of the above mentioned treatments, and then present the research on efficacy. For full descriptions of SIT, CPT, and MCET, readers are referred to the following resources: (i) SIT: Kilpatrick *et al.* (1982), Veronen and Kilpatrick (1983), Resick *et al.* (1988), Resnick *et al.* (1992), Foa *et al.* (1993); (ii) CPT: Resick and Schnicke (1990), Resick (1992), Resick and Schnicke (1992, 1993), Calhoun *et al.* (1993); and (iii) MCET: Falsetti (1997); Falsetti and Resnick (2000a,b); Falsetti *et al.* (2001).

Stress inoculation training
SIT, based on learning theory, was originally developed from Meichenbaum (1974) stress inoculation and was adapted by Kilpatrick *et al.* (1982) and Veronen and Kilpatrick (1983) to treat the fear and anxiety

experienced by rape victims. SIT consists of three treatment phases: education, skill building, and application (Resick & Jordan 1988). Generally treatment requires eight to 14 sessions, depending upon the individual needs of the patient and the specific approach.

The first two sessions are psychoeducational in nature and include an overview of treatment, a presentation about how the fear response develops based on learning theory, information about sympathetic nervous system arousal, and instruction in progressive muscle relaxation. Patients are asked to practice progressive relaxation and to identify cues that trigger fear reactions. Practice of relaxation training, identification of fear cues, and identification of safety factors are practised outside of sessions as homework.

The second phase of treatment focuses on skills building and emphasizes the development of coping skills. Most descriptions of SIT include diaphragmatic breathing, thought stopping, covert rehearsal, guided self-dialogue, and role playing (Kilpatrick et al. 1982; Resick & Jordan 1988; Resnick & Newton 1992). In addition, Resick and Jordan (1988) include the "quieting reflex," a brief relaxation technique developed by Stroebel (1983), and problem-solving techniques. These techniques are described in the references provided above, thus will not be described again here.

The final phase of treatment is the application phase of treatment. The goal is to have patients integrate and apply the skills they have learned and to use the following steps of stress inoculation: (i) assess the probability of feared event; (ii) manage escape and avoidance behavior with thought stopping and the quieting reflex; (iii) control self-criticism with guided self-dialogue; (iv) engage in the feared behavior; and (v) use self-reinforcement. Patients are asked to develop fear hierarchies in order to continue exposure work after therapy has ended. The final session consists of a review of the training program.

Cognitive processing therapy

CPT was developed by Resick and Schnicke (1990, 1992, 1993) for rape victims suffering from PTSD and depression. Resick and Schnicke proposed that PTSD consists of more than a fear network. Victims may also suffer from other strong feelings such as disgust, shame, and anger. As a framework for understanding how other intense emotions might develop, they have highlighted the work of Hollon et al. (1988) who have

suggested that when a person is exposed to information that is schema discrepant, assimilation or accommodation takes place. Put simply, this means that when something unusual happens that we cannot fit into a category (schema), or is not consistent with what we expect (i.e., rapes only happen to bad people who walk in dark alleys at night), then we must either alter the information (assimilation), or alter our schemas (accommodation). Examples of assimilation include self-blaming statements ("It must be my fault because I was wearing a short skirt," or "Maybe it wasn't really rape because I didn't fight"), whereas accommodation often results in extreme cognitive distortions (such as, "I never feel safe," "I trust no one," and "I have to be in control at all times"). The goals of CPT are to integrate the event, process emotions, and accommodate schema, while maintaining or achieving a healthy outlook and balanced perception of the world. Furthermore, the following beliefs, which McCann and colleagues (McCann et al. 1988; McCann & Pearlman 1990) have identified as being affected by victimization, are also a focus of CPT: safety, trust, power, esteem, and intimacy.

CPT provides exposure to the traumatic memory and training in challenging maladaptive cognitions. This treatment may be better than exposure alone because it also provides corrective information regarding misattributions or other maladaptive beliefs (Resick & Schnicke 1993). CPT is focused on identifying and modifying "stuckpoints," which are inadequately processed conflicts between prior schema and new information (i.e. the traumatic event). Stuckpoints are also proposed to arise from (i) negative, conflicting schemata imposed by others (victim blame); (ii) an avoidant coping style, or (iii) no relevant schema in which to store the information.

CPT, as described by Resick and Schnicke (1993), can be conducted in either group or individual sessions, and can be completed in 12 weekly sessions. The content of treatment includes a cognitive information processing explanation of traumatic event reactions, and writing assignments about the meaning of the event. This is followed by education regarding basic feelings and how changes in self-statements can affect emotions. Patients are also taught how to identify the connections between actions, beliefs, and consequences, and are asked to write accounts of the traumatic event and read it repeatedly. The accounts also expose stuckpoints.

In addition, several of the sessions focus on developing skills to analyse and confront stuckpoints and other maladaptive self-statements regarding the traumatic event. This is followed by a series of sessions that cover the five belief areas proposed by McCann *et al.* (1988). The final session is devoted to review and planning for the future.

Multiple channel exposure therapy

MCET was adapted from CPT (Resick & Schnicke 1993), SIT (Kilpatrick *et al.* 1982) and "mastery of your anxiety and panic" (Barlow & Craske 1989) treatments. The utility of this treatment approach is based on the high prevalence of PTSD and panic attacks. Generally, cognitive-behavioral treatments for PTSD are hypothesized to work by exposure to the feared memory of the traumatic event or by exposure to cues (i.e., places, situations, smell, sounds) that are not in and of themselves dangerous, but which became associated with fear at the time of a traumatic event. During the course of these treatments the patient initially experiences high levels of physiological arousal which, with successful treatment, decreases over the course of repeated sessions until extinction occurs. However, for patients who have panic attacks, and who are fearful of the attacks this may be very overwhelming, and thus not feasible. MCET is unique in that it provides exposure to physiological arousal symptoms prior to cognitive and behavioral exposure. This is hypothesized to decrease fear of physiological arousal symptoms experienced in PTSD and panic attacks, thus when exposure to traumatic memories and cues is conducted, patients will be less fearful of physiological reactions (Resnick & Newton 1992).

MCET is a 12-week treatment that has been conducted in groups and individually, and is applicable for individuals who have experienced many different types of traumatic events. Exposure to the physiological channel is conducted through interoceptive exposure to physiological reactions. Exposure to the cognitive channel is conducted through writing assignments about the traumatic event. Finally, exposure to the behavioral channel is conducted through *in vivo* exposure to conditioned cues to the traumatic event. Exposure to panic symptoms then serves not only to decrease fear of the symptoms themselves, but also provides exposure to the physiological component of fear associated with trauma, and thereby weakens the association of physiological arousal and the traumatic memory.

In addition to the exposure components, MCET also provides education about PTSD and panic symptoms, and includes several cognitive components to address distorted cognitions about trauma. Cognitive skills are employed to assist participants in challenging distorted thinking and to fully process traumatic memories. Worksheets addressing disruptions in beliefs about safety, trust, esteem, and power/competency have been adapted from CPT.

Efficacy of SIT, CPT and MCET

Studies that have investigated SIT, CPT, and MCET have supported the efficacy of these treatments. Veronen and Kilpatrick (1983) reported that SIT was effective in treating fear, anxiety, tension, and depression in 15 female rape victims treated with 20 h of SIT. Veronen and Kilpatrick (1983) also conducted a comparison study; utilizing SIT, peer counseling, and systematic desensitization. They reported that the patients who completed SIT had improved from pre- to post-treatment, but unfortunately no comparisons among treatments could be conducted.

Foa *et al.* (1991) compared SIT, exposure treatment, supportive counseling, and a no treatment control group. The SIT approach in this study differed from that described by Kilpatrick *et al.* (1982) in that it did not include instructions for *in vivo* exposure to feared situations. Foa *et al.* reported that all of the treatments led to some improvement in anxiety, depression, and PTSD. SIT was indicated to be the most effective treatment for PTSD at immediate follow-up, whereas at a 3.5-month follow-up patients who had participated in the exposure treatment had less PTSD symptoms.

More recently, Foa *et al.* (1999) conducted another study comparing prolonged exposure (PE), SIT and their combination in female assault victims. As in the 1991 study, SIT was modified by excluding the *in vivo* exposure component, so as not to be confounded with PE. Participants were 79 women who had experienced a physical or sexual assault and met the criteria for PTSD. Treatment was conducted individually and consisted of nine sessions, two times per week. Results from the intent to treatment sample indicated that PE was superior to SIT and PE-SIT on post-treatment anxiety and global social adjustment at follow-up, and had larger effect sizes on PTSD severity, depression, and anxiety, whereas SIT and PE-SIT did not differ significantly from each other on any outcome measure. Results using only treatment completers indicated that all three active treatments reduced PTSD and depression compared to women randomly assigned to a wait-list control group and that these gains were maintained at 3-, 6- and 12-month follow-ups. There are several alternative explanations for the superiority of PE compared to the other treatments. First, there was a trend towards significance for more women who did not work in the PE-SIT (43%) and SIT (30%) groups compared to the PE (19%) and control groups (8%). It is possible that the women who did not work may have been more functionally impaired in ways that were not assessed and that this interfered with their ability to participate in treatment. Indeed, more women also dropped out from these groups. Alternatively, it is also possible that more women actually got better and dropped out for this reason, thus reducing the success rates of the these treatments compared to SIT in the intent-to-treat analyses. It is also possible that the added load of doing both treatments in the same amount of time did not allow for enough time to develop the coping skills in SIT. Finally, an important component of SIT, *in vivo* exposure was left out, which may have decreased the effectiveness of SIT.

Resick *et al.* (1988) compared SIT, assertion training, and supportive psychotherapy plus information, and a wait-list control group. They reported that all three treatments were effective in reducing symptoms, with no significant differences between treatments. The patients on the wait-list control did not improve. At a 6-month follow-up, improvement was maintained in relation to rape-related fears, but not on depression, self-esteem, and social fears.

Results of CPT have been promising. Resick and Schnicke (1992) reported significant improvements with CPT on depression, and PTSD measures pretreatment to 6-months post-treatment for 19 sexual assault survivors who were at least 3 months postrape at the start of treatment. Therapy was conducted in group format over 12 weeks and a wait-list control group was also employed. Rates of PTSD went from a pretreatment rate of 90% to a post-treatment rate of 0%. Rates of major depression decreased from 62% to 42%. Further evaluation of the treatment indicates usefulness of both group and individual formats, with somewhat higher efficacy for treatment administered

in individual sessions (Resick & Schnicke 1993). A large controlled study has recently been completed to further test this treatment.

Falsetti and Resnick completed a controlled study of MCET. Falsetti *et al.* (2001) reported on preliminary data from the study. Data analyses were conducted on the pretreatment variables of the randomly assigned treatment group ($N = 7$), randomly assigned control only group ($N = 10$) and the controls then treatment ($N = 5$), to determine if there were any differences among these groups. Results of these analyses indicated there were no differences, thus the treatment data of the "controls, then treatment" were combined with data from treatment group. At post-treatment, only 8.3% of subjects in the MCET treatment condition met criteria for PTSD compared to 66.7% of subjects in the minimal attention control group. Panic attacks and related symptoms also decreased significantly. All subjects were experiencing panic attacks at the initial evaluation. At the post-evaluation, 93.3% of the minimal attention control group subjects had experienced at least one panic attack in the past month, compared to only 50% of the treatment group. Interference of the panic attacks in the past month was assessed on a 0–4 point scale. Pretreatment both groups reported moderate to severe interference. Post-treatment the control group did not change, whereas the treatment group mean dropped significantly to below mild. Finally, both groups experienced a decrease in depressive symptoms as measured by the Beck Depression Inventory (BDI).

Marks *et al.* (1998) completed a controlled study with 87 patients comparing PE alone, cognitive restructuring alone, combined PE and cognitive restructuring, and relaxation without prolonged exposure or cognitive restructuring. They found that exposure alone, cognitive restructuring alone, and exposure plus cognitive restructuring, all produced marked improvement and were generally superior to relaxation training alone. Therapists conducting the treatment in the study reported that doing the combination treatment was more difficult than doing either alone. Interestingly, combining these two treatments did not appear to enhance treatment effect. However, similar to Foa *et al.* (1999) study, the combination treatment was given in the same amount of time as the other treatment alone, thus patients may not have had enough time to thoroughly integrate all they had learned. Other studies that have compared CBT with exposure therapy include a study with refugees (Paunovic & Öst 2001), and a study by Tarrier *et al.* (1999a,b). These studies suggest that CBT and exposure are equally effective in reducing the symptoms of PTSD. However, given that many of these treatments are reporting good end-state functioning in only a proportion of patients (Marks *et al.* 1998: 53% exposure, 32% cognitive restructuring, 32% exposure + cognitive restructuring; Foa *et al.* 1999: 57% exposure, 42% SIT, 36% PE-SIT; Tarrier *et al.* 1999a: 59% exposure, 42% cognitive therapy [CT]), it would seem a worthwhile endeavor to conduct treatment outcome studies with combinations of cognitive and behavioral techniques over a longer period of time to determine if this would improve outcome for a larger number of PTSD sufferers.

Generalized anxiety disorder

There is a growing literature regarding the efficacy of cognitive behavioral treatments for generalized anxiety disorder (GAD). These generally include components of treatments that are directed at reducing physiological symptoms, but are also more comprehensive in that they are directed at other prominent aspects of GAD including attentional biases, worry and worry behaviors. In reviewing the treatment outcome literature for CBT of GAD, we identified 13 controlled clinical trials.

The CBT approaches developed for the treatment of GAD generally include teaching coping skills such as relaxation training for the somatic symptoms, teaching cognitive restructuring skills for the catastrophic thoughts associated with GAD, and providing exposure and response prevention to worry behaviors. Brown *et al.* (1993), for instance, have developed a 12–15 session manualized treatment that begins with psychoeducation about anxiety, teaches progressive muscle relaxation and uses cognitive restructuring to challenge worrying thoughts. In addition, worry exposure is conducted which requires the patient to use imagery to expose themselves to the worst feared outcome of their worry and to generate alternative outcomes. This procedure is designed to habituate the patient to their worries and worst possible outcomes as well to enable them to consider alternative outcomes. Finally, patients are taught to decrease worry behaviors, such as repeated safety checking behaviors, and to better manage their time and problem solving.

Similarly, Borkovec & Roemer (1996) describe a comprehensive treatment package that includes relaxation training, cognitive restructuring and behavioral components. Unique to this treatment are the use of self-monitoring and early cue detection in various arenas (i.e., images, thoughts, physiological reactions, emotions, and behaviors), and self-control desensitization to elicit affect and to counter avoidance. Further, given the inflexible nature of GAD, the authors emphasize the instruction of numerous skills for each component of treatment and encourage patients to utilize different methods to increase their coping repertoire.

Evidence for the efficacy of these types of therapies has been found in several studies. Overall, the findings indicate that CBT is an efficacious option for the treatment of GAD. All of the CBT treatments were found to be significantly better than no treatment, reporting rates of 40–60% improvement (Butler *et al.* 1987; Durham & Turvey 1987; Barlow *et al.* 1992; Borkovec & Costello 1993; Durham *et al.* 1999).

Butler *et al.* (1991) randomly assigned 57 participants to one of three conditions: CBT, behavior therapy (BT) alone, or a wait-list control group. Of these, CBT was found to be the most effective and long lasting. The CBT conditions was based on the work of Beck *et al.* (1985), and the BT condition consisted of anxiety management training, which focused on progressive muscle relaxation, breathing retraining, and exposure, but did not include cognitive components. Results indicated that at post-treatment, the CBT group showed significant improvement compared to the wait-list control group on 15/16 measures, and 6/16 compared to the BT group; whereas the BT group was significantly improved on 4/16 measures, compared to the wait-list control group. Results were maintained at the 6-month follow-up with the CBT group doing better on 3/6 measures of anxiety, 1/4 measures of depression, and 5/6 measures of cognition. Based on a score for clinically significant change, they found that 32% of CBT and 16% of BT groups met the criteria at post-treatment, and 42% of CBT and 5% of BT met the criteria at the 6-month follow-up. Finally, while 47% of the sample was taking medications at the beginning of treatment, only three patients (5%) in the overall remained on medications at the end of the study.

Barlow *et al.* (1992) in a comparison study of relaxation, CT, relaxation plus CT, and wait-list control conditions, found all treatments to be about equally effective compared to no treatment. Relaxation consisted of applied progressive muscle relaxation, and CT was based on the work of Beck *et al.* (1985).

Results indicated that all treatment groups showed significant improvements relative to the wait-list control and these gains were maintained at the 2-year follow-up. No differences were found among treatment groups in terms of the assessment measures, treatment responders, or high end-state functioning. Further, for those individuals taking anxiolytic medication, their use decreased significantly across treatment and follow-up. Of interest, patients in the applied relaxation group did as well as the other groups with respect to end-state functioning, indicating that perhaps other components of treatment were not necessary. However, upon further examination, it was noted that the drop out rates for this group were much higher (38%) than for the other active treatments (24% CT; 8% CBT). Limitations of this study include high attrition rates, which restrict the conclusions that can be drawn from the results, and there was somewhat high residual anxiety in many patients.

In a similar study, Borkovec and Costello (1993) compared applied relaxation (AR), CBT (using the treatment package described above by Borkovec & Roemer (1996), and nondirective (ND) treatment. Sessions were held twice a week for 12 sessions. Results indicated that AR and CBT were superior to the ND treatment at the post-treatment assessment, and were not different from each other. At the 12-month follow-up, treatments gains were noted for both the AR and CBT groups, with the latter showing more significant improvements. The ND group showed losses in previous gains at follow-up. Although it appears that the ND group did not fare as well as the other treatments, a full 25% still met criteria for high end-state functioning at 1 year, suggesting that more research needs to determine if ND treatment may be adequate for a segment of GAD patients (1996). Indeed, other studies have also found positive results using ND treatments with this population (Blowers et al. 1987; Borkovec et al. 1987; Borkovec & Mathews 1988).

Durham et al. (1994) compared CT, analytic psychotherapy, and anxiety management in 110 patients (32% male, 67% female) referred by a psychiatrist or a general practitioner. Patients were randomly assigned to one of three treatments, CT, analytic-based psychotherapy (AP), or anxiety management (AM). Additionally, participants in the CT and AP were randomly assigned to either "high contact" (16–20 sessions over 6 months) or "low contact" (8–10 sessions over 6 months), whereas patients in the AM treatment were all assigned to the low contact condition. Eighty of the original 110 patients completed the treatment and there were no significant group differences in drop-out rates. No effects were found for contact or treatment by contact. At post-treatment and follow-up, CT was superior to AP with 60% and 20%, respectively, scoring in the normative range of functioning. The low contact conditions were compared across all three groups and results indicated that at post-treatment, CT was superior to AP, but there were no significant differences between AM and CT. At follow-up, CT and AM were superior to AP, and CT showed the broadest improvement in functioning overall. Durham et al. (1999) later conducted a 1-year follow-up to this study, and reported that CT remained superior to AP.

In addition to these studies, findings of treatment outcome studies of Durham and Turvey (1987), Borkovec and Mathews (1988), White et al. (1992), and Bowman et al. (1997) also lend support to the efficacy of CBT for GAD. White et al. (1992) reported that CT, behavioral therapy and cognitive behavioral treatment (all group therapies) were all equally effective and more effective than a placebo condition or wait-list control. Durham and Turvey (1987) compared CT and BT and found them to be about equally effective; reporting improvement rates of 50–60%. Borkovec et al. (1987) compared CT with ND therapy and, later, in another study (Borkovec & Costello 1993) with self-control desensitization and ND therapy, and found that all groups improved. Bowman et al. (1997) compared self-examination therapy with a wait-list and found it to be better; however, the percentage of subjects with clinically significant change was somewhat low, suggesting that perhaps CT and CBTs may continue to be more efficacious treatment choices. Although cognitive behavioral techniques have been shown to be effective in the treatment of GAD, a recent report suggests that other treatments, which lack the same level of empirical support, are nonetheless being used more consistently than are cognitive behavioral treatments (Goisman et al. 1999).

Controlled comparisons of pharmacological and non-pharmacological treatments are still relatively sparse in the area of GAD treatment. We were able to find three such studies and review these here. Lindsay et al. (1987) compared CBT, anxiety management training (AMT), benzodiazepine treatment, and a wait-list control group. There were 40 participants who were randomly assigned to treatment, with treatment lasting

4 weeks in duration. In the drug condition, lorazepam was administered, starting with 1 mg three times a day for 10 days, 1 mg twice a day for 10 days, and 1 mg as needed for the last 10 days. Results indicated that the drug treatment was associated with the greatest initial improvement; however, the benefits for this group decreased over time. In contrast, the CBT and AMT groups made significant and consistent improvements throughout treatment, and were not different from each other. At a 3-month follow-up, comparisons between the CBT and AMT groups revealed the groups had maintained their treatment gains.

Power *et al.* (1989) randomly assigned 31 patients to either CBT, diazepam, or placebo. In the drug conditions, patients received placebo for 1 week and then 5 mg of either diazepam or placebo three times per day for 6 weeks, followed by 2 weeks of placebo. CBT was based on Beck & Emery's work (A.T. Beck & G. Emery (1979) Cognitive therapy of anxiety and phobic disorders. Unpublished Treatment Manual of the Center for Cognitive Therapy, Philadelphia) and included progressive muscle relaxation. In addition, graded exposure was utilized to decrease anxiety. Results indicated that CBT was superior to diazepam and placebo at the post-treatment assessment. With respect to rates of treatment seeking in the 12-months following the study, 30% of the CBT group, 70% of the diazepam group, and 55% of the placebo group sought either pharmacological or nonpharmacological treatment.

Power *et al.* (1990) extended their previous study by comparing CBT, diazepam, placebo, the combination of CBT plus diazepam, and the combination of CBT plus placebo. Patients included 19 men and 72 women who were randomly assigned to groups. Participants in the drug conditions (diazepam or placebo) were given a placebo three times per day for the 1st week, followed by 6 weeks of either diazepam or placebo. In the diazepam condition, participants received graded withdrawal for the remaining 3 weeks. The CBT group had a maximum of seven sessions over a 9-week period. Results at post-treatment and 6-month follow-up revealed that CBT, including CBT alone and the combination of CBT and diazepam, was superior to other treatments. Further, compared to other treatments, CBT was associated with fewer participants seeking treatment in the follow-up period.

In summary, CBT appears to be an effective treatment for GAD. Because GAD has a strong cognitive component, the inclusion of cognitive techniques to challenge worry thoughts seems particularly salient. It is not known how much imaginal exposure adds to the cognitive components. In the future, dismantling studies that address this would be helpful. It is also unclear how effective a CBT treatment protocol would be compared to a protocol focusing only on *in vivo* exposure and response prevention. Additional comparative studies of this nature would assist in developing the most effective and efficient treatments for GAD.

CBT for social phobia

It has only been in recent years, as social phobia (SP) has become recognized as a significant mental health problem, that cognitive behavioral researchers have begun investigating the effectiveness of CBT for this disorder. Despite the relative "newness" of this area, however, considerable research has been conducted. Several types of behavioral and cognitive behavioral techniques and treatments have been investigated, including systematic desensitization, imaginal flooding, applied muscle relaxation, graduated exposure, social skills training, cognitive approaches, and combined cognitive restructuring and graduated exposure (Schneier 1991). It is beyond the scope of this paper to review every study conducted in this area, and, thus, we refer the reader to more comprehensive reviews of this literature (Turner *et al.* 1992; Heimberg *et al.* 1993; Shear & Beidel 1998) and to the chapter on behavioral therapy of anxiety disorders. Our purpose will be to highlight some of the CBT studies that have been conducted, to demonstrate the breadth of CBT protocols that have been investigated, and to provide the reader with a representative overview of the effectiveness of these treatments both in comparison to other cognitive behavioral treatments and to pharmacotherapy.

Social skills training is probably one of the earliest interventions for SP (Turner *et al.* 1992). Social skills training is based on the underlying theory that social phobics have inadequate or inappropriate social skills that contribute to their social anxiety. However, research in this area suggests that this is only true for a subset of social phobics (Emmelkamp *et al.* 1985). Despite this apparent limiting factor of social skills training, Turner *et al.* (1992) point out that, regardless if social skills are actually a problem, training provides counterconditioning through behavioral rehearsal, and thus, may be beneficial to all social phobics, regardless of level of social skills.

Social skills training typically includes instruction, modeling, role rehearsal, self-monitoring, and home-work practice. Investigations of social skills training have generally yielded mixed results. Falloon *et al.* (1981) investigated the efficacy of social skills training with 16 social phobics and found significant improvement on self-report instruments, but no change on *in vivo* performance from pre- to post-treatment.

Stravynski *et al.* (1982) added a cognitive restructuring component to social skills training and compared this to social skills training in 22 social phobics who also had a diagnosis of avoidant personality disorder. They found no group differences post-treatment in the two groups, suggesting that the cognitive restructuring component did not add significantly to treatment effects. When treated and untreated behaviors were compared, results indicated that frequency of performance and associated anxiety improved in both groups. Lucock & Salkovskis (1988) investigated the efficacy of a cognitive social skills training with eight subjects and found marked improvement.

Butler *et al.* (1984) compared exposure therapy alone with exposure therapy plus AM and a wait-list control. Both treatment groups demonstrated significant improvements compared to the wait-list control group. Comparisons of the two treatment groups indicated that the exposure plus AM groups showed more improvement on the Fear of Negative Evaluation Scale and the Social Avoidance and Distress Scale. Follow-up at 6 months indicated that the exposure plus AM group had significantly more improvement on these same scales and several other self-rating subscales. Differences were not found on clinical ratings, the Beck Depression Inventory, or several subscales of the Fear Questionnaire.

Emmelkamp *et al.* (1985) conducted a study comparing the effectiveness of exposure, rational-emotive therapy, and self-instructional training in 34 socially phobic subjects. Results indicated no significant differences in self-report measures between groups at post-treatment. However, rational-emotive subjects had lower scores on the Phobic Anxiety Scale than self-instructional subjects. Exposure subjects did not differ from these two treatments combined. A 1-month follow-up indicated that the exposure group scored significantly lower on the Phobic Anxiety Scale compared to the other two groups combined.

In addition to social skills training and therapies that largely consist of exposure, some treatments also include cognitive components. Heimberg and colleagues have developed a cognitive-behavioral group therapy (CBGT) for SP that has received considerable investigation. Heimberg *et al.* (1990) compared CBGT to a placebo treatment group. The treatment consisted of 12 group sessions for 49 subjects. CBGT included education about anxiety, as well as cognitive restructuring and exposure components. The placebo condition included presentations about anxiety, and discussion of coping methods for difficult situations. The CBGT group demonstrated significantly better improvement than the placebo group on ratings of phobic severity at post-treatment and 6-month follow-up. Differences were not found on maximum anxiety ratings or the ratio of positive to negative thoughts or on self-report instruments at post-treatment. However, at 6-month follow-up the CBGT group was significantly better than the placebo group on maximum anxiety ratings and ratio of positive to negative thoughts compared to the placebo group. A subset of these subjects ($N = 19$) were later recontacted and agreed to participate in a long-term follow-up study (Heimberg *et al.* 1993). Patients were assessed an average of 5.5 years after they had finished treatment. The patients who had received the CBGT had higher functioning on several measures compared to those who underwent the placebo condition. Overall, 89% of the CBGT and 44% of the placebo patients were judged to be clinically improved by independent raters.

CBGT has also been compared to exposure alone and a wait-list control (Hope *et al.* 1990, paper presented at the annual meeting of the Phobia Society of America, Washington, D.C.). Both of the active treatments were found to be more effective than no treatment, and CBGT was found to be more effective than exposure alone in reducing anxiety in a behavioral test. However, the exposure alone treatment was found to be more effective than CBGT on several other measures at post-test. At follow-up, there were no differences in the two active treatments. The investigators noted that the patients receiving CBGT in this study had improved substantially less than in their other studies, and they were unsure how to interpret this or the above finding. Overall, however, the findings of Heimberg and colleagues have been impressive and warrant further investigation. In addition to the studies described here, other researchers have also investigated CBTs that include exposure and cognitive restructuring components (Mattick *et al.* 1989) and report favorable results.

Studies comparing cognitive behavioral treatments to pharmocotherapy have also been conducted with social phobics, although more research in this area is needed before any firm conclusions can be drawn. Clark and Agras (1991) conducted a comparison study of buspirone alone, buspirone plus CBT, CBT with placebo, and placebo alone. These researchers reported that the CBT groups improved significantly more than the drug only groups. The buspirone group did not appear to be significantly different than the placebo group. In fact, the CBT plus placebo group did better than the CBT plus buspirone group. These findings could be interpreted to indicate that buspirone may decrease the effectiveness of CBT for SP.

Gerlenter *et al.* (1991) compared cognitive behavioral group treatment with phenelzine, alprazolam, and placebo in a sample of 65 patients. In the medication groups, patients were also instructed to do self-exposure to phobic situations. All treatments, including the placebo plus self-instruction exposure resulted in improvements on self-report measures. The results indicated that phenelzine was superior on a measure of trait anxiety; however, other results for between-group comparisons indicated that treatment effects were very similar at follow-up. At a 2-month follow-up, patients who received CBGT or phenelzine had maintained their gains and those who received alprazolam or placebo had deteriorated.

Overall, the investigations of cognitive behavioral treatments for SP have indicated that these procedures are superior to no treatment, to placebo, and to some medications. In comparison to phenelzine these treatments appear to be at least equally effective. However, replications and further study of these treatments are needed.

CBT for panic disorder

CBT for panic disorder (PD) consists of a variety of techniques, and treatment typically includes relaxation training, cognitive restructuring, and exposure therapy. CBT is provided in a structured format and generally consists of 12–16 sessions. Patients are instructed to complete homework assignments between therapy sessions, such as reading educational materials, monitoring and recording thoughts and behaviors, and engaging in practice exercises.

CBT for PD routinely involves the introduction of relaxation training in the initial stages of therapy to target physiological arousal symptoms. In addition to decreasing arousal levels, relaxation training has been posited to decrease anticipatory anxiety and avoidance behaviors, improve habituation to anxiety during exposure, and enhance information processing (Rachman 1980; Michelson & Marchione 1991). Two forms of relaxation training have been employed in CBT for PD: breathing retraining and progressive muscle relaxation.

Research indicates that hyperventilation is involved in the occurrence of panic attacks for approximately 50–80% of panic attack sufferers (Garssen *et al.* 1983). Breathing retraining addresses symptoms of hyperventilation by promoting abdominal breathing in a slow, rhythmic pattern. Patients are first provided with an explanation of the physiological basis of hyperventilation, followed by an in-session demonstration of the effects of over-breathing. Then, patients are taught to breathe comfortably at the rate of 8–10 breaths/min, and to apply this technique during stressful situations.

Chronic anxiety, also referred to as anticipatory anxiety, and tension are also commonly experienced by individuals with PD. Progressive muscle relaxation (PMR) is a relaxation technique that is designed to target persistent anxiety symptoms. PMR involves a systematic procedure of tensing and relaxing specific muscle groups, focusing on one muscle group a time. PMR was originally developed by Jacobson (1938), modified by Wolpe (1958), and standardized in its current form by Bernstein and Borkovec (1973). More recently, Öst (1987) introduced a version of AR that teaches patients to utilize cue-controlled relaxation in various settings, including stressful situations in which panic attacks are likely to occur.

In addition to targeting physiological symptoms of anxiety, CBT addresses cognitive processes that are believed to maintain both the recurrence of acute panic episodes and persistence of anticipatory anxiety and avoidance. Cognitive restructuring is a key component of CBT for PD and is designed to address maladaptive beliefs and cognitions. The patient is taught to identify core cognitions associated with anxious responding, such as overestimating the probability of dangerous events or imagining the worst possible outcome. In addition, cognitive restructuring for PD targets cognitive misappraisals that normal bodily sensations are frightening, dangerous, or potentially lethal (Beck & Emery 1985; Clark *et al.* 1985; Clark 1986). Patients are taught to identify dysfunctional thoughts, schemas, and beliefs, and to modify beliefs related to anxiety, avoidance behaviors, and panic attacks. With respect to somatic sensations, individuals are taught to recognize and modify distorted beliefs about the potential consequences of bodily sensations.

Exposure-based techniques are utilized in both CBT and behavioral therapies for treating the spectrum of anxiety disorders. In the case of CBT for PD, both *in vivo* and interoceptive exposure are used to extinguish anxiety and avoidance behaviors. *In vivo* exposure involves exposure to activities and situations that were previously avoided and is therefore, particularly useful for agoraphobic avoidance behaviors (see Chapter 24). Interoceptive exposure is designed to extinguish anxiety associated with physical sensations that are misinterpreted as frightening or dangerous. Patients engage in exercises that induce physical sensations that are similar to those experienced during a panic attack. For instance, cardiac-related symptoms are produced by having patients run up a flight of stairs, while hyperventilation symptoms are created by having patients breathe through a narrow straw. The patient is encouraged to use cognitive restructuring to correct misappraisals that may arise during the exposure exercise. Through repeated exposure to the feared sensations, anxiety and avoidance behaviors are eliminated.

Several manualized treatments have been developed to target the symptoms of PD with and without agoraphobia. Although these treatments generally employ similar techniques, they differ with respect to the target population for which they were developed. Panic control treatment (PCT), developed by Barlow and Craske (1989), was created for use in an individual therapy context and includes interoceptive exposure, cognitive restructuring, and breathing retraining components. The manual, *Mastery of Your Anxiety and Panic* (MAP: Barlow & Craske 1989), is presented in a workbook format and includes reading materials and monitoring forms. PCT has subsequently been modified and incorporated into treatment designed to assist individuals with discontinuation of anxiety medication (Hegel *et al.* 1994; Spiegel *et al.* 1994; Bruce *et al.* 1995, 1999; Otto *et al.* 1996), and has also been implemented in both group (Otto *et al.* 1999) and self-directed formats (Hecker *et al.* 1996).

Several other CBT protocols have been introduced that have been shown to be effective at reducing panic symptoms. Clum (1990) published *Coping with Panic*, a resource that was designed to be used as a self-help

guide or with the assistance of a therapist. The book provides psychoeducation about the etiology and nature of PD, covers relaxation, breathing retraining, cognitive restructuring, and exposure, and instructs the reader in how to implement these techniques. In controlled studies, findings indicate that this self-help treatment was superior to wait-list control conditions, and as effective as therapist-directed treatments using the same protocol in both individual and group formats (Gould *et al.* 1993; Lidren *et al.* 1994; Gould & Clum 1995). This line of research provides additional support for the efficacy of CBT for PD, and suggests that effective treatment may be possible for individuals who do not have access to, or cannot afford, treatment provided by a mental health professional.

The efficacy of CBT for PD has been studied in a number of controlled research trials. Comparative studies and reviews have consistently found CBT for PD to be as effective or superior to alternative treatments (Clum 1989; Michelson & Marchione 1991; Gould *et al.* 1995). In a meta-analysis, Gould *et al.* (1995) found cognitive-behavioral treatments for PD to be associated with the highest mean effect size (ES: $ES = 0.68$), followed by the combination of CBT and pharmacological treatments ($ES = 0.56$) and pharmacological treatments alone ($ES = 0.47$).

Oei *et al.* (1999) reviewed 35 empirical studies evaluating treatments for PD with agoraphobia, including 20 studies that compared CBT to other treatments or compared components of CBT. Across the studies, cognitive restructuring, paradoxical interventions, breathing and relaxation training, various exposure-based treatments, and pharmacological treatments were used. Although the studies differed with respect to the outcome measures that were administered, CBT was generally effective in reducing the frequency and severity of panic attacks and fear and avoidance behaviors. A number of studies also found indirect benefits associated with CBT, including reductions in general anxiety and depression, as well as improvements in behavioral and cognitive measures.

Focusing solely on studies evaluating CBT for PD, it is difficult to draw conclusions about the "best" CBT treatment. For one, a large number of treatment combinations exist, and there are relatively few studies examining specific combinations. Second, each study tends to employ a slightly different treatment protocol, varying with respect to the information that is presented and the duration of treatment. The one exception is with panic control treatment (PCT). A series of studies have been conducted examining the effectiveness of PCT, and treatment has been conducted similarly across studies. The initial data indicated that PCT alone and PCT combined with relaxation had substantial benefits, with 85% and 87% of respective group participants reporting no panic attacks at the post-test, compared to 36% of the wait-list control group and 60% of the relaxation group (Barlow *et al.* 1989). A 2-year follow-up of this study revealed that the greatest long-term benefits were associated with PCT alone, with 81% of participants remaining panic free, compared to only 43% of participants in the combined PCT and relaxation condition and 36% of the participants in the relaxation alone condition (Craske *et al.* 1991). Thus, PCT was effective over both the short- and long-term, while PMR produced initial benefits that were not maintained at follow-up.

Subsequent studies have examined the efficacy of PCT relative to pharmacological treatments. Klosko *et al.* (1990) evaluated the efficacy of PCT compared to alprazolam, drug placebo, and wait-list control conditions. Findings at post-treatment showed PCT to be superior to all other conditions based on the proportion of participants who were panic-free (87% in the PCT condition, 50% in the alprazolam condition, 36% in the drug placebo condition, and 33% in the wait-list condition). In addition, Barlow *et al.* (2000) compared PCT to imipramine, the combination of PCT and imipramine, drug placebo, and the combination of PCT and placebo. Findings indicated that both imipramine and PCT were superior to placebo. However, imipramine demonstrated greater short-term benefits with respect to panic severity ratings, whereas PCT was associated with fewer adverse reactions and greater long-term benefits.

The efficacy of various CBT combinations has been examined across multiple studies, with mixed results. Studies have demonstrated that paradoxical intervention is more effective than the combination of exposure and paradoxical intervention (Ascher 1981), that exposure-based therapies are more effective than cognitive restructuring (Emmelkamp *et al.* 1978), and that cognitive restructuring is more effective than guided mastery (Hoffart 1995). However, studies have also been inconclusive, particularly in comparing the effectiveness of CBT vs. exposure therapy.

Overall, research supports the use of both CBT and exposure therapy. However, it is still unclear whether CBT, which includes both cognitive and exposure components, is advantageous compared to exposure therapy alone. Numerous studies have found that cognitive restructuring and exposure therapy are equally effective in treating PD (Emmelkamp & Mersch 1982; Marchione *et al.* 1987; Michelson *et al.* 1988; Öst 1987, 1988; Öst *et al.* 1993; Beck *et al.* 1994; Bouchard *et al.* 1996; Burke *et al.* 1997). Research also indicates that the combination of cognitive restructuring or relaxation training with exposure therapy is equally as effective as exposure therapy alone (Murphy *et al.* 1998). Therefore, it has been argued that the logical choice is the treatment containing fewer components (i.e., exposure), which theoretically requires less time to implement. However, this remains an empirical question, and additional research is needed to determine the effectiveness of specific techniques through dismantling studies.

A number of dismantling studies have been conducted, including comparisons of different relaxation techniques and comparisons of CT versus exposure-based techniques. As previously noted, one challenge in evaluating the effectiveness of CBT treatments for PD is the inclusion of multiple treatment components in a single treatment. Furthermore, the rationale for treatment often proposes that each component is essential and that various components are interdependent, making it difficult to isolate and test the effectiveness of specific components. For instance, in the case of breathing retraining, protocols typically include both cognitive restructuring and interoceptive exposure. Similarly, cognitive restructuring is routinely conducted in conjunction with behavioral techniques, including exposure-based components. Although cognitive therapists argue that it is through alterations in cognitive processing that individuals achieve a reduction in panic symptoms and a change in behavior, behavior therapists propose the opposite, that behavior change brings about alterations in cognition.

Relaxation training has received considerable attention in dismantling studies. Research by Clark and colleagues (Clark *et al.* 1985; Salkovskis *et al.* 1986) supports the use of breathing retraining for correcting anxiety-producing misinterpretations of hyperventilatory symptoms during panic attacks. However, only a few comparative studies have examined the efficacy of breathing retraining relative to other CBT techniques, and findings have been inconclusive. One study found breathing retraining to be equally effective to *in vivo* exposure in the short term, and more effective at 6-month follow-up (Bonn *et al.* 1984). In contrast, other studies have found breathing retraining to produce inferior results compared to *in vivo* exposure and interoceptive exposure (de Ruite *et al.* 1989; Craske *et al.* 1997). Based on their review of the literature, Garssen *et al.* (1992) suggested that breathing retraining may only be effective to the extent that it provides individuals with a method of distraction and a sense of control. In contrast, Ley (1993) responded to Garssen *et al.*'s review, arguing that breathing retraining is an effective treatment for reducing PD symptoms.

In contrast to Craske *et al.*'s (1991) finding that PMR did not have long-term benefits for reducing panic symptoms, other studies have found AR to be an effective treatment (Öst 1988). After receiving AR training, Öst (1988) reported that 100% of participants were panic-free at follow-up. Subsequent controlled studies have found AR to be equally effective compared to CT and *in vivo* exposure (Michelson *et al.* 1988; Michelson & Marchione 1991; Öst *et al.* 1993; Öst & Westling 1995; Michelson *et al.* 1996). However, across studies, treatments that employ a combination of techniques have reported better outcomes compared to relaxation training alone (Barlow *et al.* 1989; Craske *et al.* 1991).

Although all CBT treatments include a CT component, only a few controlled outcome studies have examined the effectiveness of CT alone compared to other CBT techniques for PD. Michelson *et al.* (1988) evaluated the effectiveness of graduated exposure, paradoxical intention, and progressive deep muscle relaxation. The paradoxical intention condition addressed the cognitive dimension in that patients were taught to recognize their fears and to try and "reverse" their ideas and thoughts. Findings indicated that the different techniques were equivalent in their effectiveness, producing significant improvements in the dependent measures at post-treatment and at a 3-month follow-up. However, across all conditions, patients were told to apply their respective strategy to phobic situations, which introduced an element of exposure therapy to treatment. This complicates the interpretation of these findings to the extent that each treatment condition did not provide a valid measure of a single technique.

A similar complication existed in the study conducted by Öst *et al.* (1993), comparing AR, *in vivo* exposure, and cognitive treatment. Cognitive treatment was based on Beck and Emery (1985) rationale,

and included self-instruction training (Meichenbaum 1977). Participants were taught to record their negative thoughts, to develop positive self-instructions, and to recognize alternative explanations for negative emotions. All three conditions were equally effective in reducing anxiety and fears, and decreasing measures of behavioral avoidance. However, all conditions included instructions to engage in self-exposure. As Öst *et al.* acknowledged, this limits the conclusions that can be drawn about the findings in that self-exposure itself has been shown to be an effective treatment for PD.

Clearly, there is a need for additional dismantling studies examining the relative effectiveness of CBT techniques. Because of the manner in which many CBT techniques are interdependent, it is quite challenging to isolate specific components in the context of treatment. Despite these limitations, there is a growing body of literature that supports the efficacy of various CBT techniques and their combination in the treatment of PD.

CBT for obsessive-compulsive disorder

Cognitive behavioral treatments for obsessive-compulsive disorder (OCD) include both exposure-based techniques and CT. Similar to other CBT protocols, treatment for OCD is implemented in a time-limited format, consisting of 12–16 sessions. Because of factors that may interfere with the patient's motivation for treatment, such as high levels of distress and depressed mood, sessions may be scheduled twice per week in the initial stages of treatment. In addition, CBT therapists emphasize the importance of regular attendance, especially once exposure with response prevention is initiated (Steketee 1993). Since there is great variety among patients with respect to the content of their obsessions and compulsions, CBT is typically conducted in the context of individual therapy. However, the effectiveness of group treatment for OCD has recently been investigated (McLean *et al.* 2001).

Exposure-based techniques, such as systematic desensitization, *in vivo* and imaginal exposure, and exposure combined with response prevention (i.e., prevention of performing rituals), have been employed in the treatment of OCD. Exposure is designed to promote habituation of anxiety associated with obsessions and eliminate engagement in compulsive behaviors. *In vivo* exposure involves exposure to real-life situations (e.g. touching a surface that may be contaminated with germs), while imaginal exposure targets obsessive fears and the imagined consequences of the fears (e.g. imagining oneself or a loved one becoming ill as a result of being exposed to germs). The most common behavioral technique is exposure with response prevention, which consists of exposure to fear-provoking thoughts and situations, combined with the strict prevention of ritualistic behaviors (see Chapter 24).

CT has also been incorporated into treatment for OCD, and is designed to target and modify irrational thoughts and beliefs associated with the development and maintenance of obsessions and compulsions. Several types of irrational beliefs have been identified in association with OCD, including: (i) the overestimation of threat, risk, and harm; (ii) the over-importance of thoughts; (iii) the importance of controlling one's thoughts; (iv) doubt and uncertainty; (v) perfectionism; (vi) guilt, inflated responsibility, and shame; and (vii) rigidity and morality (Steketee 1993; Obsessive Compulsive Cognitions Working Group 1997). In CBT, patients are taught to identify and challenge their irrational thoughts and beliefs. Therapists teach patients to estimate the realistic probability of an event occurring, and to anticipate the seriousness of the event if it occurred. Initially, patients require considerable direction and feedback from the therapist in order to effectively challenge beliefs. Over time, with successful treatment, individuals adopt a new cognitive approach that allows them to disregard intrusive thoughts and to resist engaging in compulsive behaviors. CT is often used in conjunction with exposure-based techniques, which provides an opportunity to use cognitive restructuring in confronting anxiety-provoking situations.

Salkovskis and colleagues (Salkovskis 1996, Salkovskis 1998) has developed a cognitive treatment for OCD, based on cognitive theory, that incorporates elements of exposure with response prevention and CT using Beck's techniques (Salkovskis 1985, 1989). Salkovskis (1996) has suggested that the goal of treatment is to modify dysfunctional beliefs about excessive responsibility through cognitive restructuring and behavioral exposure. Freeston and colleagues have subsequently modified and elaborated upon Salkovskis' CBT treatment to create a structured CBT program (Freeston et al. 1996, 1997). This treatment protocol includes cognitive restructuring, a focus on neutralizing strategies in conjunction with exposure, in vivo exposure practices, followed by additional cognitive restructuring and relapse prevention.

A second manualized treatment for OCD has been developed that includes in vivo exposure, imaginal exposure, and ritual prevention (Kozak & Foa 1997; Steketee 1993), as well as formalized cognitive components (van Oppen & Arntz 1994). Erroneous beliefs are thought to be disconfirmed during the course of exposure therapy. Thus, therapists assist patients in challenging their beliefs to the degree that this enables the patient to engage in exposure exercises. For instance, in conducting exposure to fears of contracting an illness through contact with a medical setting, the therapist and patient may discuss the probability of the feared outcome and assess the level of risk.

There are numerous studies that have evaluated the efficacy of various exposure-based therapies (see Chapter 24). Comparatively fewer studies have examined treatments containing a distinct cognitive intervention component. Cognitive-based techniques may be particularly important for patients who do not engage in overt compulsive rituals (Freeston et al. 1997), or who refuse to participate in exposure-based treatments (Clark 2000). In one of the first reviews of CBT for OCD, James and Blackburn (1995) concluded that there was not enough data by which to judge the effectiveness of CT for OCD. Compared to the available literature on CT, a large number of studies have been conducted evaluating exposure with response prevention, and researchers have acknowledged that cognitive restructuring is routinely employed in conjunction with exposure-based techniques (Abramowitz 1996; Foa et al. 1998). Therefore, while more recent reviews of CBT for OCD have not focused on the contribution of CT per se, in many studies, CT components have been included in exposure-based treatments (Abramowitz 1996, 1998). In the absence of dismantling studies, it is difficult to determine the degree to which each component contributes to the favorable outcomes observed with exposure therapy.

There are a several studies that have examined the efficacy of CT in the treatment of OCD. Accumulating data from case study reports support the use of cognitive restructuring combined with exposure therapy (Salkovskis & Warwick 1985; Kearny & Silverman 1990; Ladouceur et al. 1993, 1995; O'Kearney 1993; Clark 2000; Wilhelm 2000). In all cases, the combination of exposure and CT produced clinically significant improvements in OCD symptoms. Freeston et al. (1997) evaluated the efficacy of CBT in a sample of patients who reported obsessions but engaged in no overt compulsions. Patients were randomly assigned to treatment or a wait-list condition. Treatment consisted of cognitive restructuring related to four types of obsessional thinking (Salkovkis & Westbrook 1989), coupled with exposure to obsessional thoughts or situations related to the thoughts. Freeston *et al.* (1997) found that CBT was associated with clinically significant improvement at post-treatment for 77% of treatment completers, with gains maintained by 59% at a 6-month follow-up.

Controlled studies have also been conducted to examine the efficacy of CT versus other CBT techniques. In one of the first randomized group studies, patients were assigned to either self-instructional training plus exposure with response prevention or exposure with response prevention alone (Emmelkamp *et al.* 1980). Both groups received instruction in PMR at the beginning of treatment, and treatment consisted of 12 sessions. Findings indicated that both groups improved, however, the exposure with response prevention group exhibited less avoidance compared to the group that had received self-instructional training, suggesting that exposure with response prevention was superior to self-instructional training.

In subsequent studies, Emmelkamp and colleagues (Emmelkamp *et al.* 1988; Emmelkamp & Beens 1991) examined the efficacy of rational emotive therapy (RET) as a cognitive treatment for OCD. Emmelkamp *et al.* (1988) randomly assigned patients to RET or exposure with response prevention. The results indicated that exposure with response prevention was associated with roughly comparable rates of improvement (51%) at post-treatment compared to RET (40%) in terms of reductions in anxiety and distress ratings. In a second study, Emmelkamp and Beens (1991) compared a combination of RET and exposure with response prevention to exposure with response prevention alone. The exposure component was implemented in a self-directed format. After six sessions, the authors reported that CT was associated with a 25% mean reduction in anxiety, while exposure with response prevention resulted in a 23% reduction. With the completion of all 12 treatment sessions, results indicated that both groups improved on the majority of measures and there were no significant between group differences. Thus, research by Emmelkamp and colleagues suggests that RET may be an effective treatment for OCD when combined with exposure therapy, but that exposure

with response prevention alone may be sufficient to reduce OCD symptoms.

A more contemporary version of CT was evaluated by van Oppen *et al.* (1995). They employed Beck's model of CT combined with the work of Salkovskis (1985) in the area of OCD. Patients in the CT condition were taught to identify maladaptive beliefs, to appraise the degree to which they were overestimating threat and inflating personal responsibility, and to challenge these beliefs. Individuals were randomly assigned to exposure therapy with response prevention or CT, with both treatments consisting of 16 sessions. At post-treatment, both groups demonstrated significant improvement in OCD symptoms on the majority of measures, with the CT condition reporting slightly better rates of improvement compared to the exposure condition.

To evaluate the degree to which CBT is associated with cognitive changes following treatment, McLean *et al.* (2001) conducted a controlled study comparing CBT, exposure with response prevention, and wait-list conditions. Treatment was provided in a group format, and consisted of 12 weekly sessions that lasted 2.5 h per week. The CBT condition was based on the work of Freeston *et al.* (1996), Salkovskis (1996), and van Oppen and Arntz (1994), and included cognitive restructuring, with a focus on specific types of faulty appraisals that are common to OCD, and behavioral experiments to test appraisals. Exposure was facilitated by a therapist in session, and home-based exposure assignments were given. At post-treatment, both groups demonstrated statistically significant improvement compared to the wait-list condition. However, exposure was mildly to moderately superior to CBT on many of the outcome measures. The authors suggest this finding may have pertained to the group format, which may have made cognitive restructuring difficult because cognitions tend to be complex and idiosyncratic in nature. In contrast to expectations, OCD-related beliefs did not change following treatment on the majority of measures, with the exception of one scale pertaining to perceptions of responsibility. Specifically, both treatment groups scored significantly lower than the wait-list group.

In addition to evaluating the relative efficacy of CBT techniques, research has also examined the effectiveness of CBT treatments compared to pharmacological treatments (van Balkom *et al.* 1994; Abramowitz 1997). van Balkom *et al.* (1994) conducted a meta-analysis and found that serotonergic antidepressants, BT, and the combination of the two, resulted in significant rates of improvement compared to placebo. Across the treatment conditions, van Balkom *et al.* concluded that BT was superior to serotonergic antidepresants, and that the combination of BT and antidepressants was more effective than medication alone. More recently, Abramowitz (1997) conducted a meta-analysis and included both psychosocial and pharmacological treatments for OCD. Results indicated that exposure was more effective than PMR, that cognitive interventions were as effective as exposure procedures, and that serotonergic medication was effective, whereas non-serotonergic medication was not. Of all pharmacological treatments reviewed by van Balkom *et al.*, clomipramine was the most effective.

Overall, research supports the effectiveness of CBT for OCD. Exposure-based procedures have received widespread empirical support. Because CBT includes both exposure and cognitive techniques, dismantling studies comparing the effectiveness of exposure versus CT may be impractical. Rather, research is needed to determine if there are certain conditions under which one treatment, or combination of treatments, produces a more favorable therapeutic outcome. For example, it may be possible to identify subtypes of OCD and compare different treatment combinations across the different subtypes. Ideally, this would improve the effectiveness of treatments, as well as achieve a higher level of sophistication in treatment planning.

Discussion and future directions

Across the various anxiety disorders, CBT has been shown to be an effective treatment. The time-limited, relatively structured format of CBT is often appealing to both therapist and patient. CBT has gained increasing support because it offers a cost-effective treatment alternative, and is amenable to research evaluating its efficacy. Furthermore, a real strength of CBT is its reliance on theory, assessment, and measurable outcomes.

Based on the current state of knowledge, there are several areas where information is lacking and will need to be addressed in future research. First, the majority of studies evaluating the effectiveness of CBT have employed relatively select samples and been conducted in research settings. Thus, the extent to which CBT for anxiety disorders is generalizable to other

populations, elderly patients, and nonresearch settings is unclear (Sanderson *et al.* 1998). Research is needed to examine the efficacy of CBT in "real world" settings, including factors such as the ability of less-well trained clinicians to implement CBT with a diverse sample of patients.

Second, on a related note, the degree to which cognitive behavioral interventions for anxiety disorders effectively address issues of comorbidity needs to be addressed. Affective disorders and substance abuse are highly prevalent among anxiety disordered individuals (Kessler *et al.* 1994). Furthermore, a large proportion of individuals meet criteria for more than one anxiety disorder diagnosis (Kessler *et al.* 1994). Researchers have begun to consider the potential for comorbid diagnoses to affect treatment outcomes and to design treatments that target comorbid symptoms (e.g., Falsetti & Resnick 1998). However, more research is needed in this area so that we can gain a better understanding of what treatments are effective for particular presenting problems.

Finally, we need to address how to make treatment more accessible to patients in need of services. In controlled clinical trials, a certain proportion of patients fail to complete treatment. Now that we have identified efficacious treatments, it is necessary for patients to be willing to complete treatment in order for it to be beneficial. Thus, researchers need to attend to adverse reactions associated with treatments, as well as attrition. Efforts to determine methods of making CBT more accessible to patients should greatly contribute to our knowledge.

References

Abramowitz, J.S. (1996) Variants of exposure and response prevention in the treatment of obsessive-compulsive disorder: a meta-analysis. *Behav Ther* **27**, 583–600.

Abramowitz, J.S. (1997) Effectiveness of psychological and pharmacological treatments for obsessive-compulsive disorder: a quantitative review. *J Consult Clin Psychol* **65**, 44–52.

Abramowitz, J.S. (1998) Does cognitive-behavioral therapy cure obsessive-compulsive disorder? A meta-analytic evaluation of clinical significance. *Behav Ther* **29**, 339–55.

Ascher, L.M. (1981) Employing paradoxical intention in the treatment of agoraphobia. *Behav Res Ther* **19**, 533–42.

van Balkom, A.J.L.M., van Oppen, P., Vermeulen, A.W.A. *et al.* (1994) A meta-analysis on the treatment of obsessive-compulsive disorder: a comparison of antidepressants, behavior, and cognitive therapy. *Clin Psychol Rev* **14**, 359–81.

Barlow, D.H. & Craske, M.G. (1989) *Mastery of Your Anxiety and Panic.* Graywind Publications, Albany, NY.

Barlow, D.H., Craske, M.G., Cerny, J.A. & Klosko, J.S. (1989) Behavioral treatment of panic disorder. *Behav Ther* **20**, 261–82.

Barlow, D.H., Gorman, J.M., Shear, M.K. & Woods, S.W. (2000) Cognitive-behavioral therapy, imipramine, or their combination for panic disorder: a randomized controlled trial. *JAMA* **283**, 2529–36.

Barlow, D.H., Rapee, R.M. & Brown, T.A. (1992) Behavioral treatment of generalized anxiety disorder. *Behav Ther* **23**, 551–70.

Beck, A.T., Emery, G. & Greenburg, R.L. (1985) *Anxiety Disorders and Phobias: a Cognitive Perspective.* Basic Books, New York.

Beck, G.J., Stanley, M.A., Baldwin, L.E., Deagle, E.A. & Averill, P.M. (1994) Comparison of cognitive therapy and relaxation training for panic disorder. *J Consult Clin Psychol* **62**, 818–26.

Bernstein, D.A. & Borkovec, T.D. (1973) *Progressive Relaxation Training: a Manual for the Helping Professions.* Research Press, Champagne, IL.

Blowers, C., Cobb, J. & Mathews, A. (1987) Generalized anxiety: a controlled treatment study. *Behav Res Ther* **25**, 493–502.

Bonn, J.A., Readhead, C.P.A. & Timmons, B.H. (1984) Enhanced adaptive behavioral response in agoraphobic patients pretreated with breathing retraining. *Lancet* **2**, 665–9.

Borkovec, T.D. & Roemer, L. (1996) Generalized anxiety disorder. In: *Handbook of the Treatment of the Anxiety Disorders* (C.G. Lindemann (ed.), pp. 81–118). Jason Aronson, Inc, Northvale, NJ.

Borkovec, T.D. & Costello, E. (1993) Efficacy of applied relaxation and cognitive behavioral therapy in the treatment of generalized anxiety disorder. *J Consult Clin Psychol* **61**, 611–19.

Borkovec, T.D. & Mathews, A.M. (1988) Treatment of nonphobic anxiety disorders: a comparison of nondirective, cognitive, and coping desensitization therapy. *J Consult Clin Psychol* **56**, 877–84.

Borkovec, T.D., Mathews, A.M., Chambers, A. *et al.* (1987) The effects of relaxation training with cognitive or nondirective therapy and the role of relaxation-induced anxiety in the treatment of generalized anxiety. *J Consult Clin Psychol* **55**, 883–8.

Bouchard, S., Gauthier, J., Laberge, B., French, D., Pelletier, M. & Godbout, C. (1996) Exposure versus cognitive restructuring in the treatment of panic disorder with agoraphobia. *Behav Res Ther* **34**, 213–24.

Bowman, D., Scogin, F., Floyd, M., Patton, E. & Gist, L. (1997) Efficacy of self-examination therapy in the treatment of generalized anxiety disorder. *J Couns Psychol* **44**, 267–73.

Brown, T.A., O'Leary, T.A. & Barlow, D.H. (1993) Generalized anxiety disorder. In: *Clinical Handbook of Psychological Disorders*, 2nd edn (D.H. Barlow (ed.), pp. 137–88). The Guilford Press, New York.

Bruce, T.J., Spiegel, D.A., Gregg, S.F. & Nuzzarello, A. (1995) Predictors of aprazolam discontinuation with and without cognitive behavior therapy in panic disorder. *Am J Psychiatry* **152**, 1156–60.

Bruce, T.J., Spiegel, D.A. & Hegel, M.T. (1999) Cognitive behavioral therapy helps prevent relapse and recurrence of panic disorder following aprazolam discontinuation: a long-term follow-up of the Peoria and Dartmouth studies. *J Consult Clin Psychol* **67**, 151–6.

Burke, M., Drummond, L.M. & Johnston, D.W. (1997) Treatment choice for agoraphobic women: exposure or cognitive-behaviour therapy? *Br J Clin Psychol* **36**, 409–20.

Butler, G., Cullington, A., Hibbert, G. *et al.* (1987) Anxiety management for persistent generalized anxiety. *Br J Psychiatry* **151**, 535–42.

Butler, G., Cullington, A., Munby, M., Amies, P. & Gelder, M. (1984) Exposure and anxiety management in the treatment of social phobia. *J Consult Clin Psychol* **52**, 642–50.

Butler, G., Fennell, M., Robson, P *et al.* (1991) Comparison of behavior therapy and cognitive behavior therapy in the treatment of generalized anxiety disorder. *J Consult Clin Psychol* **59**, 167–75.

Calhoun, K.S., Resick, P.A. (1993) Treatment of PTSD in rape victims. In: *Clinical Handbook of Psychological Disorders*, 2nd edn (D.H. Barlow (ed.), pp. 48–98). The Guilford Press, New York.

Clark, D.A. (2000) Cognitive behavior therapy for obsessions and compulsions: New applications and emerging trends. *J Contemp Psychother* **30**, 129–47.

Clark, D.B. & Agras, S. (1991) The assessment and treatment of performance anxiety in musicians. *Am J Psychiatry* **148**, 598–605.

Clark, D.M. (1986) A cognitive approach to panic. *Behav Res Ther* **24**, 461–70.

Clark, D.M., Salkovskis, P.M. & Chalkley, A.J. (1985) Respiratory control as a treatment for panic attacks. *J Behav Ther Exp Psychiatry* **16**, 23–30.

Clum, G.A. (1989) Psychological interventions versus drugs in the treatment of panic. *Behav Ther* **20**, 429–57.

Clum, G.A. (1990) *Coping with Panic.* Brooks/Cole Publishing, Pacific Grove, CA.

Craske, M.G., Brown, T.A. & Barlow, D.H. (1991) Behavioral treatment of panic disorder: a 2-year follow-up. *Behav Ther* **22**, 289–304.

Craske, M.G., Rowe, M., Lewin, M. & Noriega-Dimitri, R. (1997) Interoceptive exposure versus breathing retraining within cognitive-behavioral therapy for panic disorder with agoraphobia. *Br J Clin Psychol* **36**, 85–99.

Durham, R.C., Murphy, R., Allan, T. *et al.* (1994) Cognitive therapy, analytic psychotherapy and anxiety management training for generalized anxiety disorder. *Br J Psychiatry* **165**, 315–23.

Durham, R.C. & Turvey, A.A. (1987) Cognitive therapy versus behavior therapy in the treatment of chronic general anxiety. *Behav Res Ther* **25**, 229–34.

Emmelkamp, P.M.G. & Beens, H. (1991) Cognitive therapy with obsessive-compulsive disorder: a comparative evaluation. *Behav Res Ther* **29**, 292–300.

Emmelkamp, P.M.G., Kuipers, A.C. & Eggeraat, J.B. (1978) Cognitive modification versus prolonged exposure *in vivo*: a comparison of agoraphobics as subjects. *Behav Res Ther* **16**, 33–41.

Emmelkamp, P.M.G. & Mersch, P.P. (1982) Cognitive and exposure *in vivo* in the treatment of agoraphobia: Short-term and delayed effects. *Cog Ther Res* **6**, 77–88.

Emmelkamp, P.M.G., Mersch, P.P., Vissia, F. & van der Helm, M. (1985) Social phobia: a comparative evaluation of cognitive and behavioral interventions. *Behav Res Ther* **23**, 365–9.

Emmelkamp, P.M.G., van der Helm, M., van Zanten, B.L. & Plochg, I. (1980) Treatment of obsessive-compulsive patients: The contribution of self-instructional training to the effectiveness of exposure. *Behav Res Ther* **18**, 61–6.

Emmelkamp, P.M.G., Visser, S. & Hoekstra, R.J. (1988) Cognitive therapy versus exposure *in vivo* in the treatment of obsessive-compulsives. *Cog Ther Res* **12**, 103–14.

Falloon, I.R.H., Lloyd, G.G. & Harpin, R.E. (1981) The treatment of social phobia: real-life rehearsal with non-professional therapist. *J Nerv Ment Dis* **169**, 180–4.

Falsetti, S.A. (1997) Treatment of PTSD with comorbid panic attacks. *PTSD Clinical Quarterly* **7**, 46–8.

Falsetti, S.A. & Resnick, H.S. (2000a) Cognitive-behavioral treatment of PTSD with comorbid panic attacks. *J Contemp Psychol* **30**, 163–79.

Falsetti, S.A. & Resnick, H.S. (2000b) Treatment of PTSD using cognitive and cognitive behavioral therapies. *J Cognit Psychother* **14**, 97–122.

Falsetti, S.A., Resnick, H.S., Davis, J. & Gallagher, N.A. (in press) Treatment of PTSD with panic attacks: combining cognitive processing therapy with panic control treatment techniques. *Group Dynamics: Theory, Research and Practice* **5**, 252–60.

Foa, E.B., Dancu, C.V., Hembree, E.A., Jaycox, L.H., Meadows, E.A. & Street, G.P. (1999) A comparison of exposure therapy, stress inoculation training, and their combination for reducing post-traumatic stress disorder in female assault victims. *J Consult Clin Psychol* **67**, 194–200.

Foa, E.B., Franklin, M.E. & Kozak, M.J. (1998) Psychosocial treatments for obsessive-compulsive disorder: literature review. In: *Obsessive-Compulsive Disorder: Theory, Research, and Treatment.* (R.P. Swinson, M.M. Antony, S. Rachman & M.A. Richter (eds), pp. 258–76). Guilford Press, New York.

Foa, E.B., Rothbaum, B.O., Riggs, D.S. & Murdock, T.B. (1991) Treatment of post-traumatic stress disorder in rape victims: a comparison between cognitive-behavioral procedures and counseling. *J Consult Clin Psychol* **59**, 715–23.

Foa, E.B., Rothbaum, B.O. & Steketee, G.S. (1993) Treatment of rape victims. *J Interpers Viol* **8**, 256–76.

Freeston, M.H., Ladouceur, R., Gagnon, F. *et al.* (1997) Cognitive-behavioral treatment of obsessive thoughts: a controlled study. *J Consult Clin Psychol* **65**, 405–13.

Freeston, M.H., Rhéaum, J. & Ladouceur, R. (1996) Correcting faulty appraisals of obsessional thoughts. *Behav Res Ther* **34**, 433–46.

Garssen, B., de Ruiter, C. & van Dyck, R. (1992) Breathing retraining. A rational placebo. *Clin Psychol Rev* **12**, 141–54.

Garssen, B., van Veenendaal, W. & Bloemink, R. (1983) Agoraphobia and the hyperventilation syndrome. *Behav Res Ther* **21**, 643–9.

Gerlenter, C.S., Uhde, T.W., Cimbolic, P. *et al.* (1991) Cognitive behavioral and pharmacological treatments for social phobia: a controlled study. *Arch Gen Psychiatry* **48**, 938–45.

Goisman, R.M. & Warshaw, M.G. & Keller, M.B. (1999) Psychosocial treatment prescriptions for generalized anxiety disorder, panic disorder, social phobia 1991–96. *Am J Psychiatry* **156**, 1819–21.

Gould, R.A. & Clum, G.A. (1995) Self-help plus minimal therapist contact in the treatment of panic disorder: a replication and extension. *Beh Ther* **26**, 533–46.

Gould, R.A., Clum, G.A. & Shapiro, D. (1993) The use of bibliotherapy in the treatment of panic: a preliminary investigation. *Beh Ther* **24**, 241–52.

Gould, R.A., Otto, M.W. & Pollack, M.H. (1995) A meta-analysis of treatment outcome for panic disorder. *Clin Psychol Rev* **15**, 819–44.

Hecker, J.E., Losee, M.C., Fritzler, B.K. & Fink, C.M. (1996) Self-directed versus therapist-directed cognitive behavioral treatment for panic disorder. *J Anxiety Disord* **10**, 253–65.

Hegel, M.T., Ravaris, C.I. & Ahles, T.A. (1994) Combined cognitive-behavioral and time-limited alprazolam treatment of panic disorder. *Beh Ther* **25**, 183–95.

Heimberg, R.G., Dodge, C.S., Hope, D.A. *et al.* (1990) Cognitive behavioral treatment of social phobia: comparison to a credible placebo control. *Cognit Res Ther* **14**, 1–23.

Heimberg, R.G., Salzman, D.G., Holt, C.S. *et al.* (1993) Cognitive behavioral group treatment for social phobia:

effectiveness at 5-year follow-up. *Cognit Res Ther* **17**, 325–39.

Hoffart, A. (1995) A comparison of cognitive and guided mastery therapy of agoraphobia. *Behav Res Ther* **33**, 423–34.

Hollon, S.D. & Garber, J. (1988) *Cognitive Therapy*. In: *Social Cognition and Clinical Psychology: a Synthesis* (L.Y. Abramson (ed.), pp. 204–53). Guilford, New York.

Jacobson, E. (1938) *Progressive Relaxation*. University of Chicago Press, Chicago.

James, I.A. & Blackburn, I.M. (1995) Cognitive therapy with obsessive-compulsive disorder. *Br J Psychiatry* **166**, 444–50.

Kearny, C.A. & Silverman, W.K. (1990) Treatment of an adolescent with obsessive-compulsive disorder by alternating response prevention and cognitive therapy: an empirical analysis. *J Behav Ther Exp Psychiatry* **21**, 39–47.

Kessler, R.C., McGonagle, K.A., Zhao, S. *et al.* (1994) Lifetime and 12-month prevalence of DSM-III-R psychiatric disorders in the United States: results from the National Comorbidity Survey. *Archives of General Psychiatry* **51**, 8–19.

Kilpatrick, D.G., Veronen, L.J. & Resick, P.A. (1982) Psychological sequelae to rape. In: *Behavioral Medicine: Assessment and Treatment Strategies* (D.M. Doleys, R.L. Meredith & A.R. Ciminero (eds), pp. 473–97). Plenum, New York.

Klosko, J.S., Barlow, D.H., Tassinari, R. & Cerny, J.A. (1990) A comparison of alprazolam and behavior therapy in treatment of panic disorder. *J Consult Clin Psychol* **58**, 77–84.

Kozak, M.J. & Foa, E.B. (1997) *Mastery of Obsessive-Compulsive Disorder: a Cognitive-Behavioral Approach* The Psychological Corporation, San Antonio, TX.

Ladouceur, R., Freeston, M.H., Gagnon, F., Thibodeau, N. & Dumont, J. (1993) Idiographic considerations in the behavioral treatment of obsessional thoughts. *J Behav Ther Exp Psychiatry* **24**, 301–10.

Ladouceur, R., Freeston, M.H., Gagnon, F., Thibodeau, N. & Dumont, J. (1995) Cognitive-behavioral treatment of obsessions. *Behav Mod* **19**, 247–57.

Ley, R. (1993) Breathing retraining in the treatment of hyperventilatory complaints and panic disorder: a reply to Garssen, de Ruiter, and van Dyck. *Clin Psychol Rev* **13**, 393–408.

Lidren, D.M., Watkins, P.L., Gould, R.A., Clum, G.A., Asterino, M. & Tulloch, H.L. (1994) A comparison of bibliotherapy and group therapy in the treatment of panic disorder. *J Consult Clin Psychol* **62**, 865–9.

Lindsay, W.R., Gamsu, C.V., McLaughlin, E. *et al.* (1987) A controlled trial of treatments for generalized anxiety. *Br J Clin Psychol* **26**, 3–15.

Lucock, M.P. & Salkovskis, P.M. (1988) Cognitive factors in social anxiety and its treatment. *Behav Res Ther* **26**, 297–302.

Marchione, K.E., Michelson, L., Greenwald, M. & Dancu, C. (1987) Cognitive behavioral treatment of agoraphobia. *Behav Res Ther* **25**, 319–28.

Marks, I., Lovell, K., Noshirvani, H., Livanou, M. & Thrasher, S. (1998) Treatment of post-traumatic stress disorder by exposure and/or cognitive restructuring. *Arch Gen Psychiatry* **55**, 317–25.

Mattick, R.P., Peters, L. & Clarke, J.C. (1989) Exposure and cognitive restructuring for severe social phobia. *Beh Ther* **20**, 3–23.

McCann, L. & Pearlman, L.A. (1990) *Psychological Trauma and the Adult Survivor: Theory, Therapy and Transformation*. Brunner/Mazel, Inc., New York.

McCann, L., Sakheim, D.K. & Pearlman, L.A. (1988) Trauma and victimization: a model of psychological adaptation. *Couns Psychol* **16**, 531–94.

McLean, P.D., Whittal, M.L., Thordarson, D.S. *et al.* (2001) Cognitive versus behavior therapy in the group treatment of obsessive-compulsive disorder. *J Consult Clin Psychol* **69**, 205–14.

Meichenbaum, D. (1974) *Cognitive Behavior Modification*. General Learning Press, Morristown, NJ.

Meichenbaum, D. (1977) *Cognitive Behavior Modification: an Integrative Approach*. Plenum Press, New York.

Michelson, L. & Marchione, K. (1991) Behavioral, cognitive and pharmacologic treatments of panic disorder with agoraphobia: critique and synthesis. *J Consult Clin Psychol* **59**, 100–14.

Michelson, L.K., Marchione, K.E., Greenwald, M., Testa, S. & Marchione, N.J. (1996) A comparative outcome and follow-up investigation of panic disorder with agoraphobia: The relative and combined efficacy of cognitive therapy, relaxation training, and therapist-assisted exposure. *J Anxiety Disord* **10**, 297–330.

Michelson, L., Mavissakalian, M. & Marchione, K. (1988) Cognitive-behavioral and psychophysiological treatments of agoraphobia. Clinical, behavioral, and psychophysiological outcomes. *J Consult Clin Psychol* **53**, 913–25.

Murphy, M.T., Michelson, L.K., Marchione, K., Marchione, N. & Testa, S. (1998) The role of self-directed *in vivo* exposure in combination with cognitive therapy, relaxation training, or therapist-assisted exposure in the treatment of panic disorder with agoraphobia. *J Anxiety Disord* **12**, 117–38.

O'Kearney, R. (1993) Additional considerations in the cognitive-behavioral treatment of obsession ruminations—a case study. *J Behav Ther Exp Psychiatry* **24**, 357–65.

Obsessive Compulsive Cognitions Working Group. (1997) Cognitive assessment of obsessive-compulsive disorder. *Behav Res Ther* **35**, 667–81.

Oei, T.P.S., Llamas, M. & Devilly, G.J. (1999) The efficacy of cognitive processes of cognitive behavior therapy in the treatment of panic disorder with agoraphobia. *Behav Cognit Psychother* 27, 63–88.

van Oppen, P. & Arntz, A. (1994) Cognitive therapy for obsessive-compulsive disorder. *Behav Res Ther* 32, 79–87.

van Oppen, P., de Haan, E., van Balkom, A.J.L.M. *et al.* (1995) Cognitive therapy and exposure *in vivo* in the treatment of obsessive-compulsive disorder. *Behav Res Ther* 33, 379–90.

Öst, L.G. (1987) Applied relaxation: description of a coping-technique and review of controlled studies. *Behav Res Ther* 25, 379–409.

Öst, L.G. (1988) Applied relaxation versus progressive relaxation in the treatment of panic disorder. *Behav Res Ther* 26, 13–22.

Öst, L.G. & Westling, B.E. (1995) Applied relaxation versus cognitive behavior therapy in the treatment of panic disorder. *Behav Res Ther* 32, 145–58.

Öst, L., Westling, B.E. & Hellström, K. (1993) Applied relaxation, exposure *in vivo*, and cognitive methods in the treatment of panic disorder with agoraphobia. *Behav Res Ther* 31, 383–94.

Otto, M.W., Jones, J.C., Craske, M.G. & Barlow, D.H. (1996) *Stopping Anxiety Medication: Panic Control Therapy for Benzodiazepine Discontinuation (Therapist Guide)*. Psychological Corporation, New York.

Otto, M.W., Pollack, M.H., Penava, S.J. & Zucker, B.G. (1999) Group cognitive behavior therapy for patients failing to respond to pharmacotherapy for panic disorder: a clinical case series. *Behav Res Ther* 37, 763–70.

Paunovic, N. & Öst, L.G. (2001) Cognitive behavioral therapy versus exposure therapy in the treatment of PTSD in refugees. *Behav Res Ther* 39, 1183–97.

Power, K.G., Jerrom, D.W.A., Simpson, R.J. *et al.* (1989) A controlled comparison of cognitive behavior therapy, diazepam, and placebo in the management of generalized anxiety. *Behav Psychother* 17, 1–14.

Power, K.G., Simpson, R.J., Swanson, V. *et al.* (1990) A controlled comparison of cognitive-behavior therapy, diazepam, and placebo, alone and in combination, for the treatment of generalized anxiety disorder. *J Anxiety Disord* 4, 267–92.

Rachman, S.J. (1980) Emotional processing. *Behav Res Ther* 7, 237–45.

Resick, P.A. (1992) Cognitive treatment of crime-related post-traumatic stress disorder. In: *Aggression and Violence Throughout the Life Span* (R.D. Peters, R.J. McMahon & V.L. Quinsey (eds), pp. 171–91. Sage, Newbury Park, CA.

Resick, P.A., Jordan, C.G., Girelli, S.A., Hutter, C.H. & Marhoefer-Dvorak, S. (1988) A comparative outcome study of behavioral group therapy for sexual assault victims. *Behav Ther* 19, 385–401.

Resick, P.A. & Schnicke, M.K. (1990) Treating symptoms in adult victims of sexual assault. *J Interpers Viol* 5, 488–506.

Resick, P.A. & Schnicke, M.K. (1992) Cognitive processing therapy for sexual assault victims. *J Consult Clin Psychol* 60, 748–56.

Resick, P.A. & Schnicke, M.K. (1993) *Cognitive Processing Therapy for Rape Victims: a Treatment Manual*. Sage, Newbury Park, CA.

Resnick, H.S. & Newton, T. (1992) *Assessment and Treatment of Post-Traumatic Stress Disorder in Adult Survivors of Sexual Assault*. In: *Treating PTSD* (D. Foy (ed.), pp. 99–126). Guilford, New York.

de Ruite, C., Rijken, H., Garssen, B. & Kraaimaat, F. (1989) Breathing retraining, exposure and a combination of both in the treatment of panic disorder with agoraphobia. *Behav Res Ther* 27, 647–56.

Salkovkis, P.M. & Westbrook, D. (1989) Behavior therapy and obsessional ruminations: can failure be turned into success? *Behav Res Ther* 27, 149–60.

Salkovskis, P.M. (1985) Obsessional-compulsive problems: a cognitive-behavioral analysis. *Behav Res Ther* 23, 571–83.

Salkovskis, P.M. (1989) Cognitive-behavioral factors and the persistence of intrusive thoughts in obsessional problems. *Behav Res Ther* 27, 677–82.

Salkovskis, P.M. (1996) Cognitive-behavioral approaches to the understanding of obsessional problems. In: *Current Controversies in Anxiety Disorders* (R.M. Rapee (eds), 103–33). Guilford, New York.

Salkovskis, P.M. (1998) Psychological approaches to the understanding of obsessional problems. In: *Obsessive-Compulsive Disorder: Theory, Research, and Treatment* (R.P. Swinson, M.M. Antony, S. Rachman & M.A. Richter (eds), pp. 33–50). Guilford, New York.

Salkovskis, P.M., Jones, D.R.O. & Clark, D.M. (1986) Respiratory control in the treatment of panic attacks. Replication and extension with concurrent measures of behavior and P_{CO_2}. *Br J Psychiatry* 148, 526–32.

Salkovskis, P.M. & Warwick, H.M.C. (1985) Cognitive therapy of obsessive-compulsive disorder: treating treatment failures. *Behav Psychother* 13, 243–55.

Sanderson, W.C., Raue, P.J. & Wetzler, S. (1998) The generalizability of cognitive behavior therapy for panic disorder. *J Cognit Psychother* 12(4), 323–30.

Schneier, F.R. (1991) Social phobia. *Psychiatr Ann* 21, 349–53.

Shear, M.K. & Beidel, D.C. (1998) Psychotherapy in the overall management strategy for social anxiety disorder. *J Clin Psychiatry* 59 (Suppl. 17), 39–44.

Spiegel, D.A., Bruce, T.J., Gregg, S.F. & Nuzzarello, A. (1994) Does cognitive behavior therapy assist slow-taper aprazolam discontinuation in panic disorder? *Am J Psychiatry* 151, 876–81.

Steketee, G.S. (1993) *Treatment of Obsessive-Compulsive Disorder*. Guilford, New York.

Stravynski, A., Marks, I. & Yule, W. (1982) Social skills problems in neurotic outpatients: Social skills training with and without cognitive modification. *Arch Gen Psychiatry* **39**, 1378–85.

Stroebel, C.F. (1983) *Quieting Reflex Training for Adults: Personal Workbook (or Practitioners guide)*. DMA. Audio Cassette Publications, New York.

Tarrier, N., Pilgrim, H., Sommerfield, C. *et al.* (1999b) A randomized trial of cognitive therapy and imaginal exposure in the treatment of chronic post-traumatic stress disorder. *J Consult Clin Psychol* **67**, 13–18.

Tarrier, N., Sommerfield, C., Pilgrim, H. & Humpreys, L. (1999a) Cognitive therapy or imaginal exposure in the treatment of post-traumatic stress disorder. *Br J Psychiatry* **175**, 571–5.

Turner, S.M., Beidel, D.C. & Townsley, R.M. (1992) Behavioral treatment of social phobia. In: *Handbook of Clinical Behavior Therapy*, 2nd edn (S.M. Turner, K.S. Calhoun & H.E. Adams (eds), pp. 326–31). John Wiley & Sons, New York.

Veronen, L.J. & Kilpatrick, D.G. (1983) Stress management for rape victims. In: *Stress Reduction and Prevention* (D. Meichenbaum & M.E. Jaremko (eds), pp. 341–74). Plenum, New York.

White, J., Keenan, M. & Brooks, N., (1992) Stress control. A controlled comparative investigation of large group therapy for generalized anxiety disorder. *Behav Psychol* **20**, 97–114.

Wilhelm, S. (2000) Cognitive therapy for obsessive-compulsive disorder. *Journal of Cognitive Psychotherapy: an International Quarterly* **14**, 245–59.

Wolpe, J. (1958) *Psychotherapy by Reciprocal Inhibition*. Stanford University Press, Stanford, CA.

24 Exposure Therapy in the Treatment of Anxiety Disorders

S.P. Cahill & E.B. Foa

Introduction

The term *exposure therapy* refers to a group of psychological interventions that have in common the intentional confrontation with feared, but otherwise safe objects, situations, and thoughts or memories for the purpose of reducing fear reactions to the same or similar stimuli in the future. Examples of distinct exposure therapy techniques that have been developed include systematic desensitization and other variations based on Wolpe's (e.g. 1958) concept of reciprocal inhibition; imaginal and *in vivo* flooding (Boulougouris & Marks 1969); and implosive therapy (Stampfl & Levis 1967). Other terms for therapeutic techniques based on exposure to feared stimuli include exposure and ritual prevention (e.g. Meyer 1966; used primarily in the literature on obsessive-compulsive disorder), prolonged exposure (e.g. Foa *et al.* 1991; used primarily in the literature on post-traumatic stress disorder), and direct therapeutic exposure (Boudewyns & Shipley 1983).

In this chapter, we provide a historical overview of the development of exposure therapy and illustrate its efficacy in the treatment of various anxiety conditions. It may be noted in advance that effective treatments incorporating exposure techniques have been developed for all of the primary anxiety disorders currently recognized in the Diagnostic Statistical Manual, fourth edition (DSM-IV: American Psychiatric Association [APA] 1994) nomenclature. However, the unique contribution of exposure therapy to outcome has been best established in the treatment of specific phobias, agoraphobia, obsessive-compulsive disorder (OCD), post-traumatic stress disorder (PTSD), and acute stress disorder (ASD). Indeed, the American Psychological Association's Division 12 Task Force on the Promotion and Dissemination of Psychological Interventions (Chambless *et al.* 1998) has designated variations of exposure therapy as "Well-Established Treatments" for agoraphobia, specific phobia, and OCD. In addition, The Task Force has designated exposure therapy as "Probably Efficacious Treatments" for PTSD and social phobia, while systematic desensitization received the same designation for animal phobias, public speaking anxiety, and social anxiety. Variations of exposure therapy are also incorporated into cognitive-behavioral treatment packages for panic disorder (PD) and generalized anxiety disorder (GAD), although less systematic work has been done isolating the role of exposure in these treatment packages in comparison to treatments for phobias, OCD, and PTSD.

Historical survey of the development of exposure therapy and evidence for its efficacy

The history of exposure therapy has its roots in the early behaviorist tradition in psychology beginning with work by John Watson and his students. In 1920 Watson and Rayner published their now infamous case of little Albert in which they putatively instilled a fear of white rats in a 9-month-old child through the process of Pavlovian conditioning. In the first phase of their case study, they demonstrated that Albert was not afraid of a range of stimuli, including a white rat, a white rabbit, masks with and without hair, a dog, a monkey, and a piece of burning newspaper. They also demonstrated that he showed a significant startle reaction and emotional distress in response to a loud noise produced by striking a hammer on a steel bar. In the second phase of their study, the rat was placed in front of Albert and then the hammer was struck on the bar. After seven separate pairings of the rat with the loud noise, Albert was observed to cry in response to the rat alone. In addition, the fear of rats generalized to a variety of white fuzzy objects such as cotton, a white rabbit, and a Santa Claus mask.

In a second famous case study, Watson's student, Mary Cover Jones (1924), treated Peter, a 34-month-old-boy who was afraid of white fuzzy objects including a white rabbit, fur coats, and cotton wool. Peter was treated by arranging for him to play with three other nonfearful children while the rabbit was present in the room. In addition, Peter was fed favorite foods as the rabbit was gradually brought closer to him. At first, the rabbit's presence anywhere in the room was distressing to Peter but, as his fear declined, he was able tolerate the rabbit being brought progressively closer to him until he was able to hold the rabbit on his lap and allow the rabbit to nibble at his fingers.

Taken together, the case studies of little Albert and Peter illustrate what were to become the two foundational assumptions of early behavioral models of the acquisition and treatment of anxiety problems: that fears and phobias were acquired through Pavlovian conditioning which could in turn be unlearned. Unfortunately, little was done initially with these observations towards the systematic development and evaluation of procedures to be used for treating anxiety. In part this may be attributed to failures to replicate the apparent ease of conditioning fear reactions in humans (e.g. English 1929; Bregman 1934). It remained for a South African psychiatrist who received some training in Hull's behavioral theory named Joseph Wolpe to systematically develop a system of psychotherapy for neurotic disorders based on principles of conditioning.

Systematic desensitization

Prior demonstrations of "experimental neurosis" in cats indicated that exposing them to uncontrollable electrical shock (Masserman 1943) resulted in, among other responses, a suppression of feeding when the cats were returned to the cage in which they had been shocked. Wolpe devised a treatment plan for such cats that was similar to Mary Cover Jones' procedure. Specifically, Wolpe took advantage of an observation that the cats' feeding behavior was less disrupted in rooms other than the one in which the shock had been administered. In fact, he had a series of four rooms that were increasingly less similar to the experimental room which appeared to produce a generalization gradient, such that the disruption in feeding was progressively less as the rooms became less similar. He began treatment of the cats in the least similar room. When feeding was no longer disrupted, he moved the cats to the next room where feeding continued and so on until, over a series of sessions, the cats were willing to eat even when placed in the cage where the shock had been administered.

To explain his observations, Wolpe invoked Sherrington's (1961 [originally published 1906]) concept of reciprocal inhibition, the notion that eliciting one response can inhibit the elicitation of another response. Specifically, the appetitive behavior elicited by food was inhibited by the defensive behavior originally elicited by the shock and subsequently conditioned to features of the experimental room and the training cage. However, because the defensive behavior was weaker in nonexperimental rooms, it was inhibited by the appetitive behavior elicited by food. This permitted counter-conditioning of the fear by the appetitive responses to features of the room. The conditioned appetitive appetite responses then generalized to the next room thereby allowing training to continue, and this process of counter-conditioning and stimulus generalization continued until the conditioned appetitive behavior was strong enough to inhibit the fear elicited by the experimental room and the training cage itself.

Although eating in the presence of fear eliciting stimuli may, as in the case of Peter, be appropriate in the treatment of children, Wolpe realized it was not practical for the routine treatment of adults. One solution to the problem of devising a practical application of this principle of *Psychotherapy Through Reciprocal Inhibition* (Wolpe 1958) is systematic desensitization, which involves the pairing of muscle relaxation induced through the procedures described by Jacobson (1938) with mental images of fear evoking situations. Because the relaxation induced by the Jacobsonian "tense and relax" procedure is weak relative to a strong fear response, a hierarchy of fear situations was designed so that patients could begin treatment with stimuli that elicited a weak fear reaction relative to the relaxation response. The patients then progressively work their way up the hierarchy until they are able to imagine the highest scene on the hierarchy without significant distress.

Systematic desensitization quickly became the focus of numerous clinical reports and controlled research during the mid-to-late 1960s. The first controlled study of systematic desensitization was conducted by Lang and Lazovik (1963), who compared systematic desensitization with a waitlist control condition in the treatment of students with a fear of snakes. Results indicated that neither group showed any change over a training period during which subjects in the systematic desensitization group separately practiced the relaxation procedures and constructed the hierarchy. However, after implementing pairings of the imagined snake scenes with relaxation, subjects in the desensitization group improved while the control group did not. In a follow-up study (Lang et al. 1965) found desensitization to be superior to a pseudotherapy that, like desensitization, included training in relaxation and hierarchy construction. However, after this initial preparation, subjects in the pseudotherapy condition engaged in relaxation and positive imagery. Davison (1968) replicated the efficacy of systematic desensitization in treating students with a fear of snakes, while other researches demonstrated its efficacy in treating students with a fear of rats (e.g. Cook 1966) and test anxiety (e.g. Emory & Krumboltz 1967).

In a landmark study, Gordon Paul (1966) investigated the efficacy of systematic desensitization in the treatment of highly distressed students with a fear of public speaking or other forms of social anxiety. Comparison groups in the study included (a) insight-orientated psychotherapy, which was congruent with the orientation of the therapists in the study (b) an attention-placebo condition in which subjects were given a pill placebo they were told was a drug that reduced anxiety in stressful situations and then were exposed to a task that was supposed to be stressful but in fact induced drowsiness, and (c) waitlist. Results revealed that both treatments were superior to waitlist. In addition, systematic desensitization was superior to insight-orientated psychotherapy and attention-placebo treatments, while the latter two did not differ from one another. This pattern of outcome was maintained up to 2 years after the completion of

treatment, which had consisted of five sessions over a period of 6 weeks.

In 1969, Paul (1969) surveyed the literature and identified 75 papers "on the application of systematic desensitization therapy by more than 90 different therapists with nearly 1000 different clients" (Paul 1969, p. 145). Although 55 of these papers consisted of case reports and single group studies, 20 of the papers reported controlled group design studies. In summarizing the results of his review, Paul wrote:

> The findings were overwhelmingly positive, and for the first time in the history of psychological treatments, a specific therapeutic package reliably produced measurable benefits for clients across a broad range of distressing problems in which anxiety was of fundamental importance. "Relapse" and "symptom substitution" were notably lacking, although the majority of authors were attuned to these problems. Investigations of equal quality and scope have not been carried out with other treatment techniques considered appropriate for similar problems, and cross-study comparisons where control is absent have little meaning. (p. 159)

Despite solid evidence for its efficacy, the use of systematic desensitization has fallen out of favor. This has been for both theoretical and practical reasons. Research into two key procedural features of systematic desensitization (use of a hierarchy and relaxation to inhibit anxiety) have not consistently yielded results in line with predictions that would be derived from Wolpe's theory of reciprocal inhibition. For example, Krapfl (1967, cited in Bandura 1969) found that implementing the fear hierarchy in descending order (from the most to the least fearful), rather than in the conventional ascending order, did not reduce the efficacy of treatment. Even more problematic for reciprocal inhibition theory are results from studies investigating the role of relaxation in systematic desensitization. It is true that some studies that have compared brief scene presentations of fear related images with and without concurrent relaxation have found better results for the traditional desensitization procedure (e.g. Davison 1968). However, pairing feared images with relaxation is by no means necessary for fear reduction to occur, and several studies have found that relaxation during imagery does not always enhance outcome (e.g. McGlynn 1973). Indeed, a critical review of select studies addressing this issue (McGlynn *et al.* 1981) concluded that, although there apparently are some conditions under which "graduated aversive imaging must be paired with relaxation in order to be clinically therapeutic," there are other conditions under which "graduated aversive imaging is clinically therapeutic in its own right" (p. 168). In particular, relaxation appears to be more critical to outcome when stimulus duration times were kept very short. For example, Sue (1975) compared desensitization procedures with and without relaxation utilizing either 5 s or 30 s imaginal presentations. When relaxation was omitted, longer presentation times were associated with better outcome, while duration had no effect on outcome when relaxation was included.

Further evidence suggests a very different role for effects of relaxation in systematic desensitization than as a counter-conditioning agent. Lang *et al.* (1970) found the individuals who benefited most from systematic desensitization displayed greater heart-rate reactivity in response to aversive imagery on early trials, followed by a decline in heart-rate reactivity with repetition. Based on these and other data, Mathews (1971) suggested the role of relaxation in systematic desensitization may actually be to enhance the vividness of imagery and thereby enhance the effects of imagery on autonomic reactivity. Borkovec and Sides (1979) directly tested this hypothesis and found that, indeed, standard systematic desensitization was associated with greater image vividness, greater heart-rate reactivity, and better outcome than control conditions that provided equivalent exposure in which relaxation was either not provided, or was provided but kept separate from the exposure. Such results are clearly contrary to the hypothesis that the efficacy of systematic desensitization is brought about by relaxation inhibiting anxiety.

In addition to the lack of support for the theory of reciprocal inhibition, systematic desensitization faced three related practical limitations. First, while systematic desensitization appeared to produce good results with specific phobias and social anxiety, little success was achieved when participants suffered severe agoraphobia (e.g. Gelder & Marks 1966) or OCD (Cooper *et al.* 1965). Second, systematic desensitization assumes that fear reduction to an image of an object or situation will transfer to the actual object or situation, and indeed this is sometimes the case. However, this is not inevitably the case, and progress up the imaginal hierarchy during therapy is often greater than the progress obtained on a behavioral test (e.g. Lang *et al.* 1965; Davison 1968; Barlow *et al.* 1969). This has been referred to as "the transfer gap" in systematic desensitization (Barlow *et al.* 1969). Third, alternative procedures involving prolonged *in vivo* exposure that violated the theoretical boundary conditions of reciprocal inhibition theory (e.g. high-intensity exposure in the absence of any explicit counter-conditioning agent) were being found effective in the treatment of agoraphobia (e.g. Agras *et al.* 1968; Leitenberg *et al.* 1970) and OCD (Meyer 1966; Meyer & Levy 1973), and more effective than systematic desensitization in the treatment of specific phobias (Bandura *et al.* 1969).

Implosive therapy, imaginal flooding, *in vivo* exposure and participant modeling

In contrast to Wolpe's graduated approach to exposure in which the duration of individual exposures were quite short and it was thought important to minimize the level of anxiety during exposures, implosive therapy (Stampfl & Levis 1967) and imaginal flooding (Boulougouris & Marks 1969) emphasized prolonged exposure to high-intensity stimuli in order to achieve fear reduction. This treatment approach to exposure therapy has been closely associated with Mowrer's (1947) two-factor theory of avoidance. The two factors in Mowrer's theory of avoidance are Pavlovian fear conditioning through the pairing of conditioned stimulus (CS) with an aversive unconditioned stimulus (US), and instrumental conditioning of an escape response through negative reinforcement. In a typical avoidance conditioning paradigm, rats are placed in a shuttle box and provided a series of learning trials. On each trial, a CS is first presented (e.g. a tone). If the subject responds by crossing over to the other side of the shuttle box, the CS is terminated and nothing else happens until the next trial. If the subject does not respond during the CS, then an aversive US (e.g. electric shock) is applied and remains on until the subject shuttles to the other side of the box or a maximum duration is met. During early trials, this arrangement results in a series of pairings between the CS and US that result in fear conditioning to the CS. In addition, the escape-from-shock trials result in negative reinforcement of the shuttle response. As trials continue, the subject begins to make the shuttle response during the CS.

While responses during the CS permit the subject to avoid the US, theoretically Mowrer proposed that responding continues to be reinforced through fear reduction and such responses are therefore better understood as "escape-from-fear" trials, rather than "avoidance-of-shock" trials. At the same time, however, the escape-from-fear trials operationally constitute Pavlovian extinction trials in which the CS occurs in the absence of the US. Hence, as the CS undergoes extinction, the magnitude of reinforcement on these trials should decrease resulting in a lagged decline in the escape response. If by this point the experimenter has removed the shock contingency, then both the Pavlovian fear response and the instrumental escape responses will eventually undergo extinction. An illustration of the interplay between Pavlovian and instrumental contingencies was illustrated by McAllister *et al.* (1986). Rats in this study were first provided with a series of Pavlovian fear conditioning trials in which they received pairings of a light with shocks. After this initial conditioning, subjects were given a series of trials in which they could escape from the light by jumping over a hurdle. Importantly, no additional shocks were presented during these escape-from-fear trials. Trials were continued until subjects stopped responding and the dependent variable was the subjects' latency to respond. Results indicated that latency to respond rapidly decreased over the first 25 trials. This reduction in latency to respond implies the strengthening effect of reinforcement via fear reduction. Acquisition of the escape response was followed by another period of 25 trials in which the latency to respond was relatively stable, and latencies to response gradually increased over a series of 250 additional trials reflecting extinction of both fear and escape responding.

Levis, Stampfl, and their colleagues (Levis & Stampfl 1972; Boyd & Levis 1976; Levis & Boyd 1979) further investigated procedural parameters that promote rapid acquisition and prolonged resistance to extinction of avoidance responding and offered the serial-CS hypothesis as an extension of two-factor theory. It has been demonstrated that having a chain of CSs (e.g. a tone followed by a light) prior to the US (e.g. CS1 → CS2 → US) results in rapid acquisition of an avoidance response and extreme resistance to extinction, compared to a standard single-CS condition. Theoretically, the increased resistance to extinction in the serial-CS condition is due to periodic second-order

Pavlovian conditioning trials of CS1 by CS2. Specifically, the serial presentation of stimuli permits both CS1 and CS2 to become associated with the US. However, CS2 will condition faster and stronger than CS1 due to its closer proximity to the US. As shuttle responses are strengthened, they begin to occur first during CS2 and then during CS1. Responding during CS1 has two important consequences. First, fear responses to CS1 gradually undergo extinction. Second, however, responses during CS1 prevent exposure to CS2 and thereby protect CS2 from undergoing extinction (the conservation of anxiety hypothesis). Only when there is sufficient exposure to CS1 to result in a failure to respond to CS1 does exposure to CS2 occur. Failure to respond to CS1 results in CS2 occurring which, because it has not yet undergone extinction, continues to elicit a strong fear response. The fear response elicited by CS2 motivates the shuttle response, while termination of CS2 following by the shuttle response provides further negative reinforcement and thereby strengthens the shuttle response. In addition, the sequence of CS1 being followed by CS2 serves as a second order Pavlovian conditioning trial and thereby temporarily reconditions fear to CS1. This process of oscillating between CS1 and CS2 continues until both stimuli have undergone adequate extinction trials for shuttle responding to cease altogether (assuming the US no longer occurs).

Stampfl (1987) has further extended this hypothesis by considering the effects of having different response requirements depending on where in the serial-CS chain the response occurs. Specifically, he has proposed that even greater resistance to extinction can occur when the response that terminates the equivalent of CS1 is substantially less effortful than the response required to terminate CS2 because the more effortful response requires greater reinforcement to be maintained than does the less effortful response. Taken together, these extensions of two-factor theory (the serial-CS hypothesis, the conservation of anxiety hypothesis, and the effects of differential response requirements) have been proposed to account for the highly persistent nature of avoidance behavior seen in anxiety disorders and some experimental situations (Levis 1989, 1991; Stampfl 1991).

The general therapeutic recommendations to come from this line of theorizing and basic research are two-fold: Treatment should involve: (i) exposure to all of the relevant feared CSs; and (ii) prevention or blocking of the avoidance (i.e. escape-from-fear) responses. Furthermore, unlike Wolpe and his theory of reciprical inhibition, the view of Pavlovian extinction endorsed by theorists such as Stampfl and Levis was not wed any specific hypothesized underlying mechanism. Rather, it was based on experimental observations that extinction, even to strongly conditioned CSs, occurs given adequate exposure in the absence of the US. This approach naturally favored massed exposure. Furthermore, from the serial-CS perspective, exposure to CS2 would be expected to have a greater effect of reducing responding to CS1 than the reverse. Therefore, the CS extinction/two-factor approach also tended to target stimuli higher up in the fear hierarchy early in treatment, as compared to the gradual approach of systematic desensitization.

Three related approaches to exposure, to a greater or lesser extent, derive from the theoretical aspects of two-factor theory and share the common procedural elements of prolonged and repeated exposure to relatively high intensity feared, but otherwise safe, stimuli: prolonged *in vivo* exposure (*in vivo* flooding), prolonged imaginal exposure (imaginal flooding), implosive therapy, and participant modeling/guided mastery. *In vivo* exposure is distinguished from imaginal exposure and implosive therapy in that it involves direct exposure to actual feared objects or situations, whereas imaginal exposure and implosive therapy rely on imagery.

Imaginal flooding and implosive therapy both share reliance on imagery as the modality for stimulus exposure, but differ in the content included in the imagery. The content for imaginal flooding includes imagery of feared situations or activities along with feared thoughts, images, or memories identified as problems by the patient. Implosive therapy includes such content but also includes cues hypothesized by the therapist to be relevant to the particular case, the basis of which includes hypotheses derived from pychodynamic theory. Thus, implosive imagery may include themes related to aggressive and sexual impulses and Oedipal conflicts.

A variation of *in vivo* exposure therapy, called participant modeling (Blanchard 1970) or guided mastery (Williams 1990), initially had its roots in two-factor theory (Bandura *et al.* 1969) but is now closely associated with Bandura's social learning theory and specifically with the concept of self-efficacy (Bandura 1977). Self-efficacy refers to an individual's belief that he or she is able to perform some particular task. According to the theory of self-efficacy, phobic avoidance is not due to being afraid of the phobic stimulus. Rather, fear and avoidance are both due to low self-efficacy, the belief that one cannot cope effectively with the phobic stimulus. From this perspective, treatments are not effective because they reduce, but because they promote mastery experiences and increase self-efficacy. Procedurally, participant modeling is said to differ from more traditional approaches to *in vivo* exposure in that the therapist is actively involved in demonstrating and guiding the patient to successful experiences with the feared object. In many cases, the therapist may use "response induction aides" to assist patients in gaining success experiences. For example, in treating snake phobics, the therapist may first demonstrate to the patient how to safely touch, handle and control a harmless snake and then coach the patient in performing the same behaviors, but first while wearing protective gloves and then repeating the exercise without gloves only when the patient feels a sense of self-efficacy in handling the snake. By contrast, more traditional approaches to *in vivo* exposure are often less active. Patients, for example, may be asked to simply sit and look at a snake in a cage, with instructions to attempt greater contact with the snake (reaching into the cage, touching the snake, picking it up, etc.) when their fear at the earlier step has decreased but without the therapist serving as an active model and the use of response induction aides.

What does the research literature say about the efficacy of these different forms of exposure therapy for reducing fear and avoidance? Extensive research beginning in the mid 1960s has consistently shown variations of prolonged imaginal and *in vivo* exposure to be highly effective in reducing fear and avoidance among a variety of populations.

Agoraphobia and specific phobias

There is no question about the efficacy of prolonged exposure in the treatment of agoraphobia and of a variety of simple phobias, such as fears of insects, small animals, heights and enclosed spaces, flying, and dental treatment. As noted earlier, several early studies demonstrating the efficacy of systematic desensitization utilized snake phobics as subjects (e.g. Lang & Lazovik 1963; Lang *et al.* 1965; Davidson 1968). How well do other approaches to exposure compare with systematic desensitization and with one another? Marks *et al.* (1971) utilized a crossover design to compare the efficacy of imaginal flooding with that of systematic desensitization using a mixed group of specific phobics and agoraphobics. Results revealed the two treatments were equally effective in the treatment of specific phobias but imaginal flooding was more effective than systematic desensitization in the treatment of agoraphobia. Gelder *et al.* (1973) found systematic desensitization and imaginal flooding were both more effective than a nonspecific treatment control condition among a mixed sample of specific phobics and agoraphobics, but did not find imaginal flooding to be any more effective than systematic desensitization even among the agoraphobics.

Conflicting results about comparative efficacy of imaginal and *in vivo* flooding in the treatment of agoraphobia were reported by a UK research group (Johnston *et al.* 1976; Mathews *et al.* 1976) relative to studies by Emmelkamp and colleagues in the Netherlands. For example, the UK group found that 8-weekly sessions of imaginal exposure followed by 8-weekly sessions of *in vivo* exposure produced comparable results as 16-weekly sessions of *in vivo* exposure alone or 16-weekly sessions of imaginal and *in vivo* exposure. By contrast, Emmelkamp and Wessels (1975) found four sessions of *in vivo* exposure with or without additional imaginal exposure to be superior to four sessions of imaginal exposure alone.

A series of studies comparing participant modeling with other forms of exposure therapy by Albert Bandura, Lloyd Williams, and their colleagues conducted over a period of 20 years has produced consistent support for the superiority of participant modeling in the treatment of specific phobias and agoraphobia. For example, Bandura *et al.* (1969) compared a systematic desensitization and two variations of modeling, symbolic modeling and participant modeling, with a waitlist control group in the treatment of snake phobia. Symbolic modeling consisted of watching a movie of several different individuals interacting with snakes, starting with the models handling toy snakes and gradually working up to allowing a large snake to be draped over the models' bodies and allowing the snake to crawl freely on the models. Results revealed that, compared to the waitlist condition, all three treatments resulted in significant increases in the behavioral approach test (BAT), accompanied by significant decreases in anxiety. Among the active treatments, participant modeling was more effective at increasing performance on the BAT than either symbolic modeling or systematic desensitization; both

symbolic and participant modeling were more effective than systematic desensitization in reducing fear during the BAT, but the two modeling methods did not differ from one another.

In a series of three similarly designed studies, Williams and colleagues compared participant modeling with a more passive form of *in vivo* exposure in which the therapist did not model successful performance or actively assist subjects in completing the therapeutic activities. Rather, the therapist served primarily as a monitor to record the subjects' performance and their self-reported levels of distress during the task. Williams *et al.* (1984) studied a mixed group of driving phobics and acrophobics, while Williams *et al.* (1985) studied acrophobics only, and Williams and Zane (1989) studied agoraphobics. In all three studies, the active treatments were found to be superior to waitlist, while participant modeling was found to be superior to passive exposure. Ost *et al.* (1997) have recently reported the superiority of participant modeling conducted in groups over other forms of group exposure therapy in the treatment of spider phobia.

Obsessive-compulsive disorder

Previously thought to be a disorder that was particularly resistant to treatment, Meyer (1966) reported successful outcome in two cases of OCD with a combination of prolonged exposure to obsession-related cues combined with the prevention of compulsive rituals. Meyer & Levy (1973) subsequently reported success in 10 out of 15 cases treated with exposure and ritual prevention, and that only two cases of relapse occurred during a 5–6 years follow-up period (Meyer *et al.* 1974). Since then, similar positive outcomes have been reported by a number of different research groups. Foa and Kozak (1996) reviewed 13 studies that reported short-term outcome for exposure and ritual prevention in the treatment of OCD in which the original authors reported responder rates on 330 subjects. After an average of 15 sessions (range 10–25), 83% of subjects were classified as responders. Foa and Kozak (1996) also reviewed 16 studies that reported long-term outcome in which responder rates were reported for a total 376 subjects. After an average follow-up interval of 29 months, 76% of subjects were classified as responders. In addition, exposure and ritual prevention has been found to be superior to a variety of comparison conditions including placebo medication (Marks *et al.* 1980), relaxation (Fals-Stewart *et al.*

1993), and anxiety management training (Lindsay *et al.* 1997).

Treatment for OCD typically involves a combination of imaginal exposure to obsessional thoughts/feared consequences and *in vivo* exposure to specifically feared objects, situations, activities, etc., plus ritual prevention, in which subjects are explicitly instructed to not perform their compulsive rituals. To what extent do the different treatment components contribute to treatment outcome? Available evidence suggests that exposure and ritual prevention each contribute to outcome and that there are differential effects of exposure and ritual prevention on the severity of obsessional distress and frequency of compulsive rituals. Foa *et al.* (1980a) utilized a crossover design to investigate this question among a group of compulsive washers. Half of the subjects received 2 weeks of treatment with 2 h of daily exposure plus additional exposure homework, but without any instructions to refrain from washing, followed by 2 weeks of treatment with strict response prevention, but without any instructions to explicity confront feared stimuli. The remaining half of subjects received the same treatment components in the opposite order. Results revealed greater reduction in the levels of distress reported *in vivo* exposure test when exposure procedures were implemented, but a greater reduction in the amount of time spent washing when ritual prevention was implemented. In a subsequent study, Foa *et al.* (1984) randomly assigned subjects to receive *in vivo* exposure alone, response prevention alone, or their combination. Consistent with the prior results, exposure alone was more effective in reducing fear during an *in vivo* test while response prevention alone was more effective in decreasing the amount of time spent engaging in their rituals. In addition, the combined treatment was more effective than either of the individual treatment components on both outcomes (time spent washing, distress experienced during an *in vivo* test).

Two studies have compared imaginal with *in vivo* exposure in the treatment of OCD (Rabavilas *et al.* 1976; Foa *et al.* 1985). Contrary to what has been found for specific phobias and agoraphobia, the two treatment modalities yielded comparable results. Foa *et al.* (1980b) took up the question as to whether the combination of imaginal and *in vivo* exposure plus ritual prevention would be more effective than *in vivo* exposure plus ritual prevention (no imaginal exposure). Both groups showed significant improve-

ment following acute treatment, with no differences between conditions. At follow-up, however, there was a tendency for subjects who received *in vivo* exposure alone to show relapse on measures of obsessional distress and urges to engage in rituals, while subjects in the combined groups tended to show further improvement. A more recent study, however, failed to replicate this finding (De Araujo *et al.* 1995).

Post-traumatic stress disorder

Exposure therapy for the treatment of PTSD typically combines imaginal exposure to the memory of the trauma, sometimes called "reliving," and *in vivo* exposure to safe, but otherwise avoided people, places, things, and activities that remind the survivor of the trauma and trigger intense negative emotional reactions. The efficacy of exposure therapy in the treatment of PTSD has been demonstrated in several specific trauma populations, including male combat veterans (Cooper & Clum 1989; Keane *et al.* 1989; Boudewyns & Hyer 1990; Boudewyns *et al.* 1990; Glynn *et al.* 1999), female victims of sexual or nonsexual assaults (Foa *et al.* 1991, 1999; Echeburua *et al.* 1997; Resick & Nishith 2001 presented at the 35th Annual Convention of the Association for Advancement of Behavior Therapy; Rothbaum & Astin 2001 presented at the 35th Annual Convention of the Association for Advancement of Behavior Therapy) and motor vehicle accidents (Fecteau & Nikki 1999), as well mixed-gender samples following a variety of traumatic events (Marks *et al.* 1998; Devilly & Spence 1999; Tarrier *et al.* 1999) and mixed-gender refugees (Paunovic & Ost 2001). Furthermore, exposure therapy has been studied more extensively than other treatments for PTSD and the efficacy of exposure therapy compares favorably with all other forms of therapy to which it has been compared, including relaxation (Echeburua *et al.* 1997; Marks *et al.* 1998); supportive counseling (Foa *et al.* 1991); stress inoculation training (Foa *et al.* 1991, 1999); cognitive therapy (Marks *et al.* 1998; Tarrier *et al.* 1999) and cognitive processing therapy (Resick & Nishith 2001 presented at the 35th Annual Convention of the Association for Advancement of Behavior Therapy); and eye movement desensitization and reprocessing (EMDR) (Devilley & Spence 1999; Rothbaum & Astin 2001 presented at the 35th Annual Convention of the Association for Advancement of Behavior Therapy). Contrary to expectations, combination treatments comprised by adding elements of stress inoculation training (Foa *et al.* 1999), cognitive therapy (Marks *et al.* 1998; Foa *et al.* 2001 presented at the 35th Annual Convention of the Association for Advancement of Behavior Therapy; Paunovic & Ost 2001), or couples therapy (Glynn *et al.* 1999) have consistently failed to increase the efficacy of exposure therapy, and in some cases may even slightly hamper the efficacy of exposure therapy.

A similar pattern of results appears from three studies of a brief (four to five sessions) cognitive behavioral treatment combining breathing and relaxation training, imaginal and *in vivo* exposure, and cognitive restructuring in treatment of ASD/prevention of PTSD. Treatment in this program typically begins about 2 weeks after the traumatic event. Foa *et al.* (1995) investigated the efficacy of this brief CBT intervention relative to a matched untreated comparison group. Immediately after the intervention, fewer women in the treatment condition (10%) met the criteria for PTSD than in a matched assessment-only control group (70%). However, this group difference disappeared at a follow-up assessment occurring 5.5 months after the assault. Thus, the brief prevention program appeared to accelerate the women's rate of recovery. Bryant *et al.* (1998) utilized this same intervention with male and female survivors of either motor vehicle or industrial accidents who met DSM-IV (APA 1994) criteria for ASD. Left untreated, the development of ASD shortly after a traumatic event is associated with an elevated risk of subsequently developing PTSD (Harvey & Bryant 1998). Results revealed that fewer participants receiving the brief prevention program met criteria for PTSD at both the post-treatment (8%) and the 6-month follow-up (17%) assessments compared to supportive counseling (83% and 67% for the post-treatment and follow-up assessments, respectively). In a follow-up study, Bryant *et al.* (1999) again compared brief CBT with supportive counseling, and this time added a third group that received the exposure therapy elements of the brief CBT program without relaxation training or cognitive restructuring. Following the brief intervention, 14% of subjects who received exposure therapy and 20% of subjects who received the full CBT program met the criteria for PTSD, in comparison to 56% of subjects who received supportive counseling.

Social phobia

Perhaps more so than any of the preceding disorders, both the rationale and empirical data strongly support

the importance of adding one or more elements to exposure therapy in the treatment of social anxiety. The two additional components that have received the most attention have been training in specific social skills thought to be lacking in the repertoire of social phobics and cognitive restructuring of beliefs related to the fear of negative evaluation. According to the socials skills deficit model, individuals with social anxiety lack certain skills to interact effectively with others. As a result they experience fewer interpersonal rewards and experience more interpersonal punishments. This leads them to avoid social interactions when possible, thereby further limiting their ability to acquire more effective social skills. Alternatively, the cognitive model argues that social anxiety is not the result of lacking in social skills, but rather is the result of acquiring a range of negative beliefs about themselves and others. Specifically, social phobics view others as being critical of them (Leary *et al.* 1988) and that others hold expectations they are not likely to be able to meet (Wallace & Alden 1991).

There is research evidence supporting both hypotheses that socially anxious individuals (i) may perform less skilfully in social situations and (ii) that socially anxious individuals view themselves more negatively than do others (Clark & Wells 1995). Furthermore, there is evidence that interventions directed at these components may be effective in reducing social anxiety. In a recent meta-analysis, Taylor (1996) summarized the outcome of 25 studies of treatments for social phobia that yielded a total of 42 within-group effect sizes for two control conditions (waitlist and pill placebo) and four active treatments (exposure, cognitive therapy, exposure plus cognitive therapy, and social skills training). Results of the meta-analysis revealed that all active treatments resulted in significantly better outcome than waitlist. However, only the combination of exposure therapy plus cognitive restructuring resulted in significantly better outcome than pill placebo. The additive effects of each component of treatment was clearly demonstrated in a pair of studies conducted by Mattick and colleagues. In the first study, Mattick and Peters (1988) compared exposure alone with exposure plus cognitive restructuring. Although both groups improved, there was somewhat better outcome for the combined treatment, particularly at the 3 month follow-up assessment. In the second study, Mattick *et al.* (1989) compared the efficacy of each component alone as well as their combination against a waitlist control group. Compared to the waitlist control group, all three treatments were found to be effective in reducing social anxiety. Again, however, outcome was best among subjects who received the combined treatment.

One particularly well-studied treatment package has been Heimberg's cognitive behavioral group therapy (CBGT) for social anxiety (Heimberg *et al.* 1995). The program consists of 12 weekly group sessions consisting of education about their underlying cognitive behavioral model of social anxiety, in-session role playing of social interactions, homework *in vivo* exposure exercises, and cognitive restructuring implemented before, during, and after each exposure (role plays and *in vivo* homework assignments). Two studies (Heimberg *et al.* 1990; Lucas & Telch, 1993, presented at the 27th Annual Convention of the Association for Advancement of Behavior Therapy) found CBGT to be more effective than an attention control group that received education about social anxiety and nondirective group therapy. The latter study also compared CBGT with the same treatment administered individually, finding treatment outcome was similar whether it was provided individually or in a group format. Hope *et al.* (1995) dismantled CBGT by comparing the full program with just the exposure component. Contrary to expectations, the exposure alone condition was actually somewhat superior to CBGT immediately after treatment, although the difference disappeared by the 6 month follow-up. The authors question these results on the basis that the results for CBGT were not as strong as observed in the previous studies, which they attributed to subject attrition in some of the therapy groups. Heimberg *et al.* (1998) compared CBGT with the previously described attention control, phenelzine, and placebo. Immediately after treatment, both active treatments were more effective than their respective control groups and there were no differences between the active treatments. Responders to each treatment subsequently entered a 6 month follow-up phase, during which it was found that 50% of the medication responders relapsed compared to only 17% of group therapy responders.

Generalized anxiety disorder

Considerably less research has been conducted on use of exposure therapy in the treatment of GAD compared to any of the other anxiety disorders. Rather treatment packages have tended to focus on the use of relaxation strategies and cognitive restructuring. Given

the generalized nature of the concerns in GAD, ergo the name "generalized anxiety disorder," the limited use of exposure therapy may reflect difficulties in specifying clear targets for imaginal and *in vivo* exposure. A notable exception is a pair of studies by Borkovec and colleagues. Borkovec and Costello (1993) compared applied relaxation training to a cognitive behavioral package that included applied relaxation, self-control desensitization, and brief cognitive therapy. Self-control desensitization is similar to standard systematic desensitization in that it uses a hierarchical presentation of imaginally presented fear-relevant cues. It differs from standard systematic desensitization, however, in that relaxation is only one of several possible coping strategies the patient may employ to reduce their anxiety during the imaginal practices. Coping self-statements and cognitive challenges are also used to help reduce anxiety during imaginal exposure. Both applied relaxation alone and the CBT package were more effective than supportive listening. Although there were no differences between the treatments immediately after treatment, the CBT group maintained their gains better at the 12 month follow-up than the applied relaxation group. In a recently completed dismantling study, Borkovec *et al.* (2002) compared three treatment conditions: (i) applied relaxation plus self-control desensitization; (ii) cognitive therapy; and (iii) their combination. All three groups displayed significant improvements on measures of anxiety and depression that were well-maintained, with only 17% of subjects meeting diagnostic criteria for GAD at a 2-year follow-up assessment. No significant differences were observed among the treatments.

Interoceptive exposure

A relatively recent addition to the exposure therapy armamentarium is interoceptive exposure, which has been added to cognitive-behavioral treatment packages for PD (Barlow 1988). Interoceptive exposure involves intentionally provoking internal cues associated with fear and anxiety, such as heavy breathing and its consequences (hyperventilation, chest pain, dizzyness), tachycardia, sweating, trembling, etc., for the purpose of reducing distress and anxiety associated with them. These sensations may by induced through physiological challenge procedures such as lactate infusions (e.g. Pitts & McClure 1967) and inhalation of carbon dioxide (CO_2) (van den Hout & Griez 1982; Woods *et al.* 1987), as well as a variety of behavioral exercises such as intentional over-breathing, spinning in a chair, rapid stair-stepping, and breathing through a thin straw, among others.

At least three factors appear to be important in the historical development of interoceptive exposure techniques. One factor was previously discussed dissatisfaction with the efficacy of *in vivo* exposure in the treatment of agoraphobia: despite clearly being superior to imaginal forms of exposure, *in vivo* exposure alone still left many patients with significant residual impairment (Jansson & Ost 1982). This lead researchers to look for adjunctive strategies to add to *in vivo* exposure. A second factor was Goldstein and Chambless's (1978) influential reanalysis of agoraphobia in which they proposed that agoraphobic avoidance was motivated by a "fear of fear" that was acquired through a form of Pavlovian interoceptive conditioning.

Having suffered one or more panic attacks, these people become hyperalert to their sensations and interpret feelings of mild to moderate anxiety as signs of oncoming panic attacks and react with such anxiety that the dreaded episode is almost invariably induced. This is analogous to the phenomenon described by Razran (1961) as interoceptive conditioning in which the conditioned stimuli are internal bodily sensations. In the case of fear of anxiety, a client's own physiological arousal becomes the conditioned stimuli for the powerful conditioned response of a panic attack. (Razran 1961, p. 55).

A third factor was a convergence of observations from several apparently unrelated procedures that all resulted in symptom reduction, including: (a) repeated exposure to panic provocation procedures, such as repeated administration of lactate (e.g. Bonn *et al.* 1971) or repeated inhalation of CO_2 (e.g. Haslam 1974); (b) other procedures that provoked physical sensations similar to panic, such as running (Orwin 1973); and (c) imaginal exposure to fears not obviously related to the target complaint (i.e. imagining being eaten by tigers when the target complaint is agoraphobia; Watson & Marks 1971). Such disparate findings did not make much sense under the then prevailing notion of agoraphobia being a fear of public places. However, they do make sense under the twin assumptions that the relevant cues in each case are the stimulus consequences of physiological arousal induced by the various procedures and that the emotional reactions to such cues are subject to reduction with repeated exposure.

The efficacy of cognitive-behavioral programs for PD incorporating interoceptive exposure techniques has since been demonstrated in a number of controlled studies. Barlow *et al.* (1989) compared a comprehensive cognitive behavioral program that combined psychoeducation, breathing retraining, applied relaxation, interceptive exposure, and cognitive restructure to several control conditions, including a similar CBT program without the applied relaxation component, applied relaxation only, and waitlist. At the post-treatment assessment, more than 70% of participants in the two treatment conditions that incorporated interoceptive exposure were panic free in comparison to 40% of patients in the relaxation condition, and 33% in the waitlist condition. In a second study, Klosko *et al.* (1990) compared the full CBT program to alprazolam, placebo, and waitlist control. After treatment, 87% of participants in the CBT were panic free compared to 50% in the alprazolam condition, 36% in the placebo condition, and 33% in the waitlist condition. Craske *et al.* (1995) compared a condensed version of the full CBT package (four 60–90 min sessions, compared to 15 60 min sessions in the previous studies) with nondirective supportive therapy. At the post-treatment assessment, 53% of participants who experienced at least one panic attack during the week preceding the pretreatment assessment were panic free in the week after treatment compared to 8% of participants in the supportive therapy condition. In the most recent study by this group of researchers, Barlow *et al.* (2000) compared their comprehensive CBT program, to which *in vivo* exposure along with interoceptive exposure, cognitive restructuring, breathing retraining, and applied relaxation, to imipramine alone, imipramine plus CBT, placebo alone, and placebo plus CBT. After treatment, significantly more participants were classified as treatment responders in the CBT (49%) imipramine (46%) conditions, compared to placebo (22%). The two combined treatment conditions (CBT plus imipramine and CBT plus placebo) were numerically superior to the individual treatment conditions (60% and 57% treatment responders, respectively).

Other research groups have demonstrated the efficacy of CBT interventions incorporating interoceptive exposure exercises. Telch *et al.* (1993) compared a CBT program that combined psychoeducation, cognitive therapy, breathing retraining, and interoceptive exposure to waitlist. After treatment, 85% of patients undergoing CBT were panic free in comparison to only 30%

of those in the waitlist condition. Clark *et al.* (1994) compared CBT to applied relaxation and imipramine. Fully 90% of participants in the CBT condition were panic free at the end of treatment, compared to 50% of participants in the applied relaxation condition, 55% in the imipramine condition, and only 7% in the waitlist condition. In a second study by this group (Clark *et al.* 1999), the full (12 sessions) CBT program was compared with a briefer version (five sessions) of the same treatment that utilized home-study materials to supplement the therapy sessions. At the post-treatment assessment, significantly more participants who received CBT (79% in the full treatment program and 71% in the brief treatment program) were panic free in comparison to waitlist (8%).

The studies discussed above, and others (e.g. Beck *et al.* 1992; Gould *et al.* 1993; Gould & Clum 1995), clearly indicate that CBT programs incorporating interoceptive exposure are consistently better than waitlist or placebo control conditions, more effective than relaxation, and as or more effective than some medications. However, these CBT packages include other active treatment components as well, most notably cognitive therapy. Mavissakalian *et al.* (1983) and Marchione *et al.* (1987) both found that adding cognitive restructuring to *in vivo* exposure substantially improved outcome, although Williams and Rappaport (1983) found that adding cognitive restructuring decreased the efficacy of *in vivo* exposure based on the guided mastery model.

Evidence that interoceptive exposure contributes to the efficacy of CBT programs comes from three additional sources. First, there are controlled studies demonstrating that repeated interoceptive exposure alone, through repeated physiological challenge procedures or strenuous exercise, can result in symptom reduction. For example, Griez and van den Hout (1986) utilized a crossover design to compare the efficacy of the β-blocker propranolol and repeated inhalations of CO_2. Each phase of the study lasted 2 weeks, separated by a 2-week no-intervention period. Although the frequency of panic attacks declined during both treatments, only CO_2 inhalation was associated with decreased scores on a questionnaire measure of fear of bodily sensations. More recently, Broocks *et al.* (1998) compared the efficacy of 10 weeks of aerobic exercise (running 4 miles, three times per week), clomipramine, and pill placebo. Relative to placebo, both treatments were effective in reducing symptoms of anxiety and depression. However, compared to aerobic exercise, clomipramine

was associated with fewer dropouts and it worked more rapidly and more thoroughly on symptom reduction.

Second, a meta-analysis conducted by Gould *et al.* (1995) obtained a mean post-treatment effect size of .88 from seven studies comparing CBT with waitlist control. This may be contrasted with an effect size of .53 from four studies comparing cognitive restructuring plus *in vivo* exposure with *in vivo* exposure alone, raising the possibility that interoceptive exposure is a more powerful adjunct to therapy than is cognitive restructuring. However, as the authors note, it would be premature to draw a firm conclusion about the relative efficacy of interoceptive exposure and cognitive therapy as add-on therapies to cognitive restructuring. The comparison condition used in the computation of effect sizes for the *in vivo* exposure plus cognitive restructuring combination (i.e. *in vivo* exposure alone) is a more powerful control group than the one used to compute effect sizes for the CBT interventions that included interoceptive exposure (i.e. the waitlist).

Third, relevant dismantling studies/component analyses designed to evaluate the contribution of interoceptive exposure to the larger treatment package are beginning to appear. In the first such study, Craske *et al.* (1997) compared two CBT groups, both of which incorporated cognitive restructuring and *in vivo* exposure. In addition, one group also included interoceptive exposure, while the other group included breathing retraining instead. The two treatments were equally effective on most outcome measures. However, the group that received interoceptive exposure had better outcome on panic frequency both immediately after treatment and at 6-month follow-up. Hecker *et al.* (1998) utilized a crossover design to compare the efficacy of cognitive therapy and interoceptive exposure. Each group received four sessions of each treatment, but in reverse order. Although the authors expected cognitive therapy to be superior, improvement in both conditions was comparable and the order of treatments did not affect outcome. On average, subjects improved during the first phase of treatment and maintained their gains. In the most recent study, Ito *et al.* (2001) compared three variations of self-conducted exposure therapy (meetings with therapist generally lasted 30 min and focused on developing homework assignments) with one another and a waitlist control. The three active treatments were *in vivo* exposure alone, interoceptive exposure alone, and combined *in vivo* and interoceptive exposure. All three treatments were superior to the waitlist condition, and no significant differences were observed among the three exposure conditions. Post-treatment effect sizes comparing each treatment to waitlist on a measure of phobic avoidance were 2.5, 3.0, and 1.6 for *in vivo*, interoceptive, and combined exposure conditions, respectively.

Virtual reality

Recent advances in computer technology may make conducting exposure therapy easier through the use of virtual technology. The potential for using virtual technology in the conduct of exposure therapy has been hinted at through a growing number of case studies (see Glanz *et al.* 1996 for a review). Published case studies in which virtual technology has appeared effective include cases of acrophobia (Rothbaum *et al.* 1995b), claustrophobia (Botella *et al.* 1998), flight phobia (Rothbaum *et al.* 1996; Wiederhold *et al.* 1998), and spider phobia (Carlin *et al.* 1997).

Two published randomized controlled trials utilizing virtual technology have also been reported. Rothbaum *et al.* (1995a) compared virtual reality exposure therapy with a waitlist control condition in treating 20 college students with a fear of heights. Results revealed significantly greater improvement for subjects receiving virtual reality exposure, although seven of the 10 subjects in this condition also practised *in vivo* exposure although they had not been instructed to do so. Thus, the outcome results probably reflect the effects of both virtual and real exposure. However, it is likely that engaging in virtual exposure made it easier for these subjects to subsequently practice real life exposures. Rothbaum *et al.* (2000) compared virtual reality exposure with standard *in vivo* exposure in the treatment of the fear of flying. This study also included a waitlist control group. After completing treatment, subjects took a commercial flight to evaluate their willingness to fly and their anxiety during the flight. Compared to waitlist, both treatments were effective, no differences were observed between the two active treatment conditions, and treatment gains were maintained at 6-month follow-up.

Summary

The above review indicates that exposure therapy is a highly effective intervention in its own right for most anxiety disorders, and is an important element of most effective CBT packages for anxiety problems, regardless of which diagnosis. That said, not all forms of exposure therapy are equally effective, and this may be further qualified that how exposure therapy is best applied may be moderated by some extent to the anxiety disorder under consideration. We offer the following more specific conclusions and recommendations.

1 *In vivo* exposure appears to be more effective than imaginal exposure. This is most clearly seen in the treatment of specific phobias and agoraphobia, and should be used in these instances whenever possible. Furthermore, the participant modeling approach to *in vivo* exposure, where the therapist is actively involved in helping the patient to master the exposure tasks appears especially effective. A potential disadvantage of *in vivo* exposure are the added burdens on the therapist involved in conducting therapy sessions outside the convenience of the office and the need to be creative in obtaining appropriate stimuli for *in vivo* exposures (e.g. obtaining several examples of bugs or insects).

2 Imaginal exposure is especially useful when the feared stimuli are intrusive thoughts, images, or memories as in the cases of OCD and PTSD. Imaginal exposure may also be useful when the feared stimuli are difficult to obtain for use in *in vivo* exposure. Imaginal exposure may also be useful as a stepping stone toward a particular *in vivo* exercise if the *in vivo* exercise cannot itself be broken down into smaller achievable steps.

3 In the future, virtual reality technology may become more widely available as a third exposure medium. Although the number of studies on virtual technology is still limited, the results appear as though it may be as effective as *in vivo* exposure. Once the technology becomes more widely available, this may become a convenient and possibly cost-efficient way to conduct exposure.

4 Interoceptive exposure exercises have significantly helped to advance the treatment of PD.

References

Agras, W.S., Leitenberg, H. & Barlow, D.H. (1968) Social reinforcement in the modification of agoraphobia. *Arch Gen Psychiatry* **19**, 423–7.

American Psychiatric Association (APA) (1994) *Diagnostic Statistical Manual of Mental Disorders*, 4th edn. American Psychiatric Association, Washington, D.C.

Bandura, A. (1969) *Principles of Behavior Modification*. Holt, Rinehart & Winston, New York.

Bandura, A. (1977) Self-efficacy: toward a unifying theory of behavioral change. *Psychol Rev* **84**, 191–215.

Bandura, A., Blanchard, E.B. & Ritter, B. (1969) The relative efficacy of desensitization and modeling approaches for inducing behavioral, affective, and attitudinal changes. *J Pers Soc Psychol* **13**, 173–99.

Barlow, D.H. (1988) *Anxiety and its Disorders: the Nature and Treatment of Anxiety and Panic*. Guilford, New York.

Barlow, D.H., Craske, M.G., Cerny, J.A. & Klosko, J.S. (1989) Behavioral treatment of panic disorder. *Behav Ther* **20**, 261–82.

Barlow, D.H., Gorman, J.M., Shear, M.K. & Woods, S.W. (2000) Cognitive-behavioral therapy, imipramine, or their combination for panic disorder: a randomized controlled trial. *JAMA* **283**, 2529–36.

Barlow, D.H., Leitenberg, H., Agras, W.S. & Winczel, J.P. (1969) The transfer gap in systematic desensitization: an analog study. *Behav Res Ther* **7**, 191–6.

Beck, A.T., Sokol, L., Clark, D.M., Berchick, R. & Wright, F. (1992) A crossover study of focussed cognitive therapy for panic disorder. *Am J Psychiatry* **149**, 778–83.

Blanchard, E.B. (1970) Relative contributions of modeling, informational influences, and physical contact in extinction of phobic behavior. *J Abnorm Psychol* **76**, 55–61.

Bonn, J.A., Harrison, J. & Rees, W.L. (1971) Lactate-induced anxiety: therapeutic implications. *Br J Psychiatry* **119**, 468–70.

Borkovec, T.D. & Costello, E. (1993) Efficacy of applied relaxation and cognitive-behavioral therapy in the treatment of generalized anxiety disorder. *J Consult Clin Psychol* **61**, 611–19.

Borkovec, T.D., Newman, M.G., Pincus, A.L. & Lytle, R. (2002) A Component analysis of cognitive-behavioral therapy for generalized anxiety disorder and the role of interpersonal problems. *J Consult Clin Psychol* **70**, 288–98.

Borkovec, T.D. & Sides, J.K. (1979) The contribution of relaxation and expectancy to fear reduction via graded, imaginal exposure to feared stimuli. *Behav Res Ther* **17**, 529–40.

Botella, C., Banos, R.M., Perpina, C., Villa, H., Alcaniz, M. & Rey, A. (1998) Virtual reality treatment of claustrophobia: a case report. *Behav Res Ther* **36**, 239–46.

Boudewyns, P.A. & Hyer, L. (1990) Physiological response to combat memories and preliminary treatment outcome in Vietnam veterans: PTSD patients treated with direct therapeutic exposure. *Behav Ther* **21**, 63–87.

Boudewyns, P.A., Hyer, L., Woods, M.G., Harrison, W.R. & McCranie, E. (1990) PTSD among Vietnam veterans: an early look at treatment outcome using direct therapeutic exposure. *J Traumatic Stress* **3**, 359–68.

Boudewyns, P.A. & Shipley, R.H. (1983) *Flooding and Implosive Therapy: Direct Therapeutic Exposure in Clinical Practice*. Plenum Publishing Co., New York.

Boulougouris, J.C. & Marks, I.M. (1969) Implosion (flooding): a new treatment for phobias. *BMJ* **2**, 721–3.

Boyd, T.L. & Levis, D.J. (1976) The effects of single-component extinction of a three-component serial CS on resistance to extinction of the conditioned avoidance response. *Learning and Motivation* **7**, 517–31.

Bregman, E.O. (1934) An attempt to modify the emotional attitudes of infants by the conditioned response technique. *J Genet Psychol* **45**, 169–98.

Broocks, A., Bandelow, B., Pekrun, G. *et al.* (1998) Comparison of aerobic exercise, clomipramine, and placebo in the treatment of panic disorder. *Am J Psychiatry* **155**, 603–9.

Bryant, R.A., Harvey, A.G., Dang, S.T., Sackville, T. & Basten, C. (1998) Treatment of acute stress disorder: a comparison of cognitive-behavior therapy and supportive counseling. *J Consult Clin Psychol* **66**, 862–6.

Bryant, R.A., Sackville, T., Dangh, S.T., Moulds, M. & Guthrie, R. (1999) Treating acute stress disorder: an evaluation of cognitive behavior therapy and supportive counseling techniques. *Am J Psychiatry* **156**, 1780–6.

Carlin, A.S., Hoffman, H.G. & Weghorst, S. (1997) Virtual reality and tactile augmentation in the treatment of spider phobia: a case report. *Behav Res Ther* **35**, 153–8.

Chambless, D.L., Baker, M.J., Baucom, D.H. *et al.* (1998) Update on empirically validated therapies II. *The Clinical Psychologist* **51**, 3–16.

Clark, D.M., Salkovoskis, P.M., Hackmann, A. *et al.* (1994) A comparison of cognitive therapy, applied relaxation and imipramine in the treatment of panic disorder. *Br J Psychiatry* **164**, 759–69.

Clark, D.M., Salkovskis, P.M., Hackmann, A. *et al.* (1999) Brief therapy for panic disorder: a randomized controlled trial. *J Consult Clin Psychol* **67**, 583–9.

Clark, D.M. & Wells, A. (1995) A cognitive model of social phobia. In: *Social Phobia: Diagnosis Assessment and Treatment* (R.G. Heimberg, M.R. Liebowitz, D.A. Hope & F.R. Schneier (eds), pp. 69–93). Guilford Press, New York.

Cook, G. (1966) The efficacy of two desensitization procedures: an analogue study. *Behav Res Ther* **4**, 17–24.

Cooper, N.A. & Clum, G.A. (1989) Imaginal flooding as a supplementary treatment for PTSD in combat veterans: a controlled study. *Behav Ther* **20**, 381–91.

Cooper, J.E., Gelder, M.G. & Marks, I.M. (1965) Results of behavior therapy in 77 psychiatric patients. *BMJ* **1**, 1222–5.

Craske, M.G., Maidenberg, E. & Bystritsky, A. (1995) Brief cognitive-behavioral versus nondirective therapy for panic disorder. *J Behav Ther Exp Psychiatry* **26**, 113–20.

Craske, M.G., Rowe, M., Lewin, M. & Noriega-Dimitri, R. (1997) Interoceptive exposure versus breathing retraining within cognitive-behavioral therapy for panic disorder with agoraphobia. *Br J Clin Psychol* **36**, 85–99.

Davidson, G.C. (1968) Systematic desensitization as a counterconditioning process. *J Abnorm Psychol* **73**, 91–9.

De Araujo, L.A., Ito, L.M., Marks, I.M. & Deale, A. (1995) Does imaginal exposure to the consequences of not ritualising enhance live exposure for OCD? A controlled study: I. main outcome. *Br J Psychiatry* **167**, 65–70.

Devilly, G.J. & Spence, S.H. (1999) The relative efficacy and treatment distress of EMDR and a cognitive-behavior trauma treatment protocol in the amelioration of post-traumatic stress disorder. *J Anxiety Disord* **13**, 131–57.

Echeburua, E., Corral, P.D., Zubizarreta, I. & Sarasua, B. (1997) Psychological treatment of chronic post-traumatic stress disorder in victims of sexual aggression. *Behav Mod* **21**, 433–56.

Emery, J.R. & Krumboltz, J.D. (1967) Standard versus individualized hierarchies in desensitization to reduce test anxiety. *J Counsel Psychol* **14**, 204–9.

Emmelkamp, P.M.G. & Wessels, H. (1975) Flooding in imagination vs. flooding *in vivo*: a comparison with agoraphobics. *Behav Res Ther* **13**, 7–15.

English, H.B. (1929) Three cases of the conditioned fear response. *J Abnorm Soc Psychol* **24**, 221–5.

Fals-Stewart, W., Marks, A.P. & Schafer, J. (1993) A comparison of behavioral group therapy and individual behavior therapy in treating obsessive compulsive disorder. *J Nerv Ment Dis* **181**, 189–93.

Fecteau, G. & Nikki, R. (1999) Cognitive behavioral treatment of post-traumatic stress disorder after motor vehicle accident. *Behav Cog Psychother* **27**, 201–14.

Foa, E.B., Dancu, C.V., Hembree, E.A., Jaycox, L.H., Meadows, E.A. & Street, G.P. (1999) A comparison of exposure therapy, stress inoculation training, and their combination for reducing post-traumatic stress disorder in female assault victims. *J Consult Clin Psychol* **67**, 194–200.

Foa, E.B., Hearst-Ikeda, D. & Perry, K.J. (1995) Evaluation of a brief cognitive-behavior program for the prevention of chronic PTSD in recent assault victims. *J Consult Clin Psychol* **63**, 948–55.

Foa, E.B. & Kozak, M.J. (1996) Psychological treatment for obsessive compulsive disorder. In: *Long-term Treatments of Anxiety Disorders* (M.R. Mavissakalian & R.P. Prien (eds), pp. 285–309. American Psychiatric Press, Washington, D.C.

Foa, E.B., Rothbaum, R.O., Riggs, D.S. & Murdock, T.B. (1991) Treatment of post-traumatic stress disorder in rape victims: a comparison between cognitive-behavioral procedures and counseling. *J Consult Clin Psychol* **59**, 715–23.

Foa, E.B., Steketee, G. & Grayson, J.B. (1985) Imaginal and *in vivo* exposure: a comparison with obsessive-compulsive checkers. *Behav Ther* **16**, 292–302.

Foa, E.B., Steketee, G., Grayson, J.B., Turner, R.M. & Latimer, P. (1984) Deliberate exposure and blocking of obsessive-compulsive rituals: immediate and long-term effects. *Behav Ther* **15**, 450–72.

Foa, E.B., Steketee, G. & Milby, J.B. (1980a) Differential effects of exposure and response prevention in obsessive-compulsive washers. *J Consult Clin Psychol* **48**, 71–9.

Foa, E.B., Steketee, G., Turner, R.M. & Fischer, S.C. (1980b) Effects of imaginal exposure to feared disasters in obsessive-compulsive checkers. *Behav Res Ther* **18**, 449–55.

Gelder, M.G., Banchroft, J.H.J., Gath, D.H., Johnston, D.W., Mathews, A.M. & Shaw, P.M. (1973) Specific and non-specific factors in behaviour therapy. *Br J Psychiatry* **123**, 309–19.

Gelder, M.G. & Marks, I.M. (1966) Severe agoraphobia: a controlled prospective trial of behavior therapy. *Br J Psychiatry* **112**, 309–19.

Glanz, K., Durlach, N.I., Barnett, R.C. & Aviles, W.A. (1996) Virtual reality (VR) for psychotherapy: from the physical to the social environment. *Psychotherapy* **33**, 464–73.

Glynn, S.M., Eth, S., Randolph, E.T. *et al.* (1999) A test of behavioral family therapy to augment exposure for combat-related post-traumatic stress disorder. *J Consult Clin Psychol* **67**, 243–51.

Goldstein, A.J. & Chambless, D.L. (1978) A reanalysis of agoraphobia. *Behav Ther* **9**, 47–59.

Gould, R.A. & Clum, G.A. (1995) Self-help treatment for panic disorder: a replication and extension. *Behav Ther* **26**, 533–46.

Gould, R.A., Clum, G.A. & Shapiro, D. (1993) The use of bibliotherapy in the treatment of panic: a preliminary investigation. *Behav Ther* **24**, 241–52.

Gould, R.A., Otto, M.W. & Pollack, M.H. (1995) A meta-analysis of treatment outcome for panic disorder. *Clin Psychol Rev* **15**, 819–44.

Griez, E. & van den Hout, M.A. (1986) CO_2 inhalation in the treatment of panic attacks. *Behav Res Ther* **24**, 145–50.

Harvey, A.G. & Bryant, R.A. (1998) The relationship between acute stress disorder and post-traumatic stress disorder: a prospective evaluation of motor vehicle accident survivors. *J Consult Clin Psychol* **66**, 507–12.

Haslam, M.T. (1974) The relationship between the effect of lactate infusion on anxiety states, and their amelioration by carbon dioxide inhalation. *Br J Psychiatry* **125**, 88–90.

Hecker, J.E., Fink, C.M., Vogeltanz, N.D., Thorpe, G.L. & Sigmon, S.T. (1998) Cognitive restructuring and interoceptive exposure in the treatment of panic disorder: a crossover study. *Behav Cognit Psychother* **26**, 115–31.

Heimberg, R.G., Dodge, C.S., Hope, D.A., Kennedy, C.R., Zollo, L.J. & Becker, R.E. (1990) Cognitive behavioral group treatment for social phobia: comparison with a credible placebo control. *Cognit Ther Res* **14**, 1–23.

Heimberg, R.G., Juster, H.R., Hope, D.A. & Mattia, J.I. (1995) Cognitive behavioral group treatment for social phobia: description, case presentation and empirical support. In: *Social Phobia: Clinical and Research Perspectives* (M.B. Stein (ed.), pp. 293–321). American Psychiatric Press, Washington, D.C.

Heimberg, R.G., Liebowitz, M.R., Hope, D.A. *et al.* (1998) Cognitive-behavioral group therapy versus phenelzine in social phobia: 12-week outcome. *Arch Gen Psychiatry* **55**, 1133–41.

Hope, D.A., Heimberg, R.G. & Bruch, M.A. (1995) Dismantling cognitive-behavioral group therapy for social phobia. *Behav Res Ther* **33**, 637–50.

van den Hout, M.A. & Griez, E. (1982) Cardovascular and subjective responses to inhalation of carbon dioxide. *Psychother Psychosom* **37**, 75–82.

Ito, L.M., de Araujo, L.A., Tess, V.L.C. *et al.* (2001) Self-exposure therapy for panic disorder. *Br J Psychiatry* **178**, 331–6.

Jacobson, E. (1938) *Progressive Relaxation*. University of Chicago Press, Chicago.

Jansson, L. & Ost, L.G. (1982) Behavioral treatments for agoraphobia: an evaluative review. *Clin Psychol Rev* **2**, 311–36.

Johnston, D.W., Lancashire, M., Mathews, A.M., Munby, M., Shaw, P.M. & Gelder, M.G. (1976) Imaginal flooding and exposure to real phobic situations: changes during treatment. *Br J Psychiatry* **129**, 372–7.

Jones, M.C. (1924) A laboratory study of fear: the case of Peter. *J Genet Psychol* **31**, 308–15.

Keane, T.M., Fairbank, J.A., Caddell, J.M. & Zimmering, R.T. (1989) Implosive (flooding) therapy reduces symptoms of PTSD in Vietnam combat veterans. *Behav Ther* **20**, 245–60.

Klosko, J.S., Barlow, D.H., Tassinari, R. & Cerny, J.A. (1990) A comparison between alprazolam and behavior therapy in the treatment of panic disorder. *J Consult Clin Psychol* **58**, 77–84.

Lang, P.J. & Lazovik, A.D. (1963) Experimental desensitization of a phobia. *J Abnorm Soc Psychol* **66**, 519–25.

Lang, P.J., Lozovik, A.D. & Reynolds, D.J. (1965) Desensitization, suggestibility and pseudotherapy. *J Abnorm Psychol* **70**, 395–402.

Lang, P.J., Melamed, B.G. & Hart, J. (1970) A psychophysiological analysis of fear modification using an automated desensitization procedure. *J Abnorm Psychol* **76**, 220–34.

Leary, M.R., Kowalski, R.M. & Campbell, C.D. (1988) Self-presentational concerns and social anxiety: the role of generalized impression expectancies. *J Res Personal* **22**, 308–21.

Leitenberg, H., Agras, W.S., Edwards, J.A., Thompson, L.E. & Wincze, J.P. (1970) Practice as a psychotherapeutic variable: an experimental analysis within single cases. *J Psychiatr Res* **7**, 215–25.

Levis, D.J. (1989) The case for a return to a two-factor theory of avoidance: the failure of non-fear interpretations. In: *Contemporary Learning Theories, Volume 1. Pavlovian Conditioning and the Status of Traditional Learning Theory* (S.B. Klein & R.R. Mowrer (eds, pp. 227–77) Lawrence Erlbuam Associates, Hillsdale, NJ.

Levis, D.J. (1991) A clinician's plea for a return to the development of nonhuman models of psychopathology: new clinical observations in need of laboratory study. In: *Fear Avoidance and Phobias: A Fundamental Analysis* (M.R. Denny (ed.), pp. 395–427). Lawrence Erlbaum Associates, Hillsdale, NJ.

Levis, D.J. & Boyd, T.L. (1979) Symptom maintenance: an infrahuman analysis and extension of the conservation of anxiety principle. *J Abnorm Psychol* **88**, 107–20.

Levis, D.J. & Stampfl, T.G. (1972) Effects of serial CS presentation on shuttlebox avoidance responding. *Learning and Motivation* **3**, 73–90.

Lindsay, M., Crino, R. & Andrews, G. (1997) Controlled trial of exposure and response prevention in obsessive-compulsive disorder. *Br J Psychiatry* **171**, 135–9.

Marchione, K.E., Michelson, L., Greenwald, M. & Dancu, C. (1987) Cognitive behavioral treatment of agoraphobia. *Behav Res Ther* **25**, 319–28.

Marks, I., Boulougouris, J. & Marset, P. (1971) Flooding versus desensitization in the treatment of phobic patients: A cross-over study. *Br J Psychiatry* **119**, 353–75.

Marks, I., Lovell, K., Noshirvani, H., Livanou, M. & Thrasher, S. (1998) Treatment of post-traumatic stress disorder by exposure and/or cognitive restructuring. *Arch Gen Psychiatry* **55**, 317–25.

Marks, I.M., Stern, R.S., Mawson, D., Cobb, J. & McDonald, R. (1980) Clomipramine and exposure for obsessive-compulsive rituals. *Br J Psychiatry* **136**, 1–25.

Masserman, J.H. (1943) *Behavior and Neurosis*. University of Chicago Press, Chicago.

Mathews, A.M. (1971) Psychophysiological approaches to the investigation of desensitization and related procedures. *Psychol Bull* **76**, 73–91.

Mathews, A.M., Johnston, D.W., Lancahsire, M., Mundy, M., Shaw, P.M. & Gelder, M.G. (1976) Imaginal flooding and exposure to real phobic situations: treatment outcome with agoraphobics. *Br J Psychiatry* **129**, 362–71.

Mattick, R. & Peters, L. (1988) Treatment of severe social phobia: effects of guided exposure with and without cognitive restructuring. *J Consult Clin Psychol* **56**, 251–60.

Mattick, R., Peters, L. & Clark, J. (1989) Exposure and cognitive restructuring for social phobia: a controlled study. *Behav Ther* **20**, 3–23.

Mavissakalian, M., Michelson, L., Greenwald, D., Kornblith, S. & Greenwald, M. (1983) Cognitive-behavioral treatment of agoraphobia: paradoxical intention versus self-statement training. *Behav Res Ther* **21**, 75–86.

McAllister, W.R., McAllister, D.E., Scoles, M.T. & Hampton, S.R. (1986). Persistence of fear-reducing behavior: relevance for the conditioning theory of neurosis. *J Abnorm Psychol* **95**, 365–72.

McGlynn, F.D. (1973) Graded imagination and relaxation as components of experimental desensitization. *J Nerv Ment Dis* **156**, 377–85.

McGlynn, F.D., Mealiea, W.L. & Landau, D.L. (1981) The current status of systematic desensitization. *Clin Psychol Rev* **1**, 149–79.

Meyer, V. (1966) Modification of expectations in cases with obsessional rituals. *Behav Res Ther* **4**, 273–80.

Meyer, V. & Levy, R. (1973) Modification of behavior in obsessive-compulsive disorders. In: *Issues and Trends in Behavior Therapy* (H.E. Adams & P. Urnikel (eds), pp. 77–136). Charles C. Thomas, Springfield, IL.

Meyer, V., Levy, R. & Schnurer, A. (1974) A behavioral treatment of obsessive-compulsive disorders. In: *Obsessional States* (H.R. Beech (ed.), pp. 233–58) Methuen, London.

Mowrer, O.H. (1947) On the dual nature of learning: a reinterpretation of "conditioning" and "problem-solving." *Harvard Educational Review* **17**, 102–48.

Orwin, A. (1973) "The running treatment": a preliminary communication on a new use for an old therapy (physical activity) in the agoraphobic syndrome. *Br J Psychiatry* **122**, 175–9.

Ost, L.G., Ferebee, I. & Furmark, T. (1997) One-session group therapy of spider phobia: direct versus indirect treatments. *Behav Res Ther* **8**, 721–32.

Paul, G.L. (1966) *Insight Versus Desensitization in Psychotherapy*. Stanford University Press, Stanford.

Paul, G.L. (1969) Outcome of systematic desensitization II: controlled investigations of individual treatment, technique variations, and current status. In: *Behavior Therapy: Appraisal and Status* (C.M. Franks (ed.), pp. 105–59). McGraw-Hill, New York.

Paunovic, N. & Ost, L.G. (2001) Cognitive-behavior therapy vs exposure in the treatment of PTSD in refugees. *Behav Res Ther* **39**, 1183–97.

Pitts, F.N. & McClure, J.N. (1967) Lactate metabolism and anxiety neurosis. *N Engl J Med* **277**, 1329–36.

Rabavilas, A.D., Boulougouris, J.C. & Stefanis, C. (1976) Duration of flooding sessions the treatment of obsessive-compulsive patients. *Behav Res Ther* **14**, 349–55.

Razran, G. (1961) The observable unconscious and the inferable conscious in current Soviet psychophysiology: interoceptive conditioning, semantic conditioning, and the orienting reflex. *Psychol Rev* **68**, 81–147.

Rothbaum, B.O., Hoges, L., Kooper, R., Opdyke, D., Williford, J.S. & North, M. (1995a) Effectiveness of computer-generated (virtual reality) graded exposure in the treatment of acrophobia. *Am J Psychiatry* **152**, 626–8.

Rothbaum, B.O., Hoges, L., Kooper, R., Opdyke, D., Williford, J.S. & North, M. (1995b) Virtual reality graded exposure in the treatment of acrophobia: a case report. *Behav Ther* **26**, 547–54.

Rothbaum, B.O., Hodges, L., Watson, B.A., Kessler, C.D. & Opdyke, D. (1996) Virtual reality exposure therapy in the treatment of fear of flying: a case report. *Behav Res Ther* **34**, 477–81.

Rothbaum, B.O., Hodges, L., Smith, S. & Lee, J.H. (2000) A controlled study of virtual reality exposure therapy for the fear of flying. *J Consult Clin Psychol* **68**, 1020–6.

Stampfl, T.G. (1987) Theoretical implications of the neurotic paradox as a problem in behavior theory: an experimental resolution. *Behav Anal* **10**, 161–73.

Stampfl, T.G. (1991) Analysis of aversive events in human psychopathology: fear and avoidance. In: *Fear Avoidance and Phobias: A Fundamental Analysis* (M.R. Denny (ed.), pp. 363–93). Lawrence Erlbaum Associates, Hillsdale, NJ.

Sherrington, C.S. (1961) [original publication 1906] *The Integrative Action of the Nervous System*. Yale University Press, New Haven, CT.

Stampfl, T.G. & Levis, D.J. (1967) Essentials of implosive therapy: a learning-theory-based psychodynamic behavioral therapy. *J Abnorm Psychol* **72**, 496–503.

Sue, D. (1975) The effect of duration of exposure on systematic desensitization and extinction. *Behav Res Ther* **13**, 55–60.

Tarrier, N., Pilgrim, H., Sommerfield, C. *et al.* (1999) A randomized trial of cognitive therapy and imaginal exposure in the treatment of chronic post-traumatic stress disorder. *J Consult Clin Psychol* **67**, 13–18.

Taylor, S. (1996) Meta-analysis of cognitive-behavioral treatments for social phobia. *J Behav Ther Exp Psychiatry* **27**, 1–9.

Telch, M.J., Lucas, J.A., Schmidt, N.B. *et al.* (1993) Group cognitive-behavioral treatment of panic disorder. *Behav Res Ther* **31**, 279–87.

Wallace, S.T. & Alden, L.E. (1991) A comparison of social standards and perceived ability in anxious and nonanxious men. *Cognit Ther Res* **15**, 237–54.

Watson, J.P. & Marks, I.M. (1971) Relevant and irrelevant fear in flooding—a crossover study of phobic patients. *Behav Ther* **2**, 275–93.

Watson, J.B. & Rayner, R. (1920) Conditioned emotional reactions. *J Exp Psychol* **3**, 1–14.

Wiederhold, B.K., Gevirtz, R. & Wiederhold, M.D. (1998) Fear of flying: a case report using virtual reality therapy with physiological monitoring. *Cyberpsychology and Behavior* **1**, 91–103.

Williams, S.L. (1990) Guided mastery treatment of agoraphobia: beyond stimulus exposure. *Prog Behav Mod* **26**, 89–121.

Williams, S.L., Dooseman, G. & Kleifield, E. (1984) Comparative effectiveness of guided mastery and exposure treatments for intractable phobias. *J Consult Clin Psychol* **52**, 505–18.

Williams, S.L. & Rappaport, A. (1983) Cognitive treatment in the natural environment for agoraphobics. *Behav Ther* **14**, 299–313.

Williams, S.L., Turner, S.M. & Peer, D.F. (1985) Guided mastery and performance desensitization treatments for severe acrophobia. *J Consult Clin Psychol* **53**, 237–47.

Williams, S.L. & Zane, G. (1989) Guided mastery and stimulus exposure treatments for severe performance anxiety in agoraphobics. *Behav Res Ther* **27**, 237–45.

Wolpe, J. (1958) *Psychotherapy by Reciprocal Inhibition.* Stanford University Press, Stanford, CA.

Woods, S.W., Charney, D.S., Goodman, W.K. & Henninger, G.R. (1987) Carbon dioxide-induced anxiety: behavioral, physiologic, and biochemical effects of 5% CO_2 in panic disorder patients and 5% and 7.5% CO_2 in healthy subjects. *Arch Gen Psychiatry* **44**, 365–75.

25 Anxiety Disorders: Alternative Drug Treatments

N. Laufer, S. Gur, R. Gross-Isseroff & A. Weizman

Panic disorder

Although standard agents, such as tricyclic antidepressants (TCAs), benzodiazepines, monoamine oxidases, and selective serotonin reuptake inhibitors, with or without cognitive behavioral therapy have demonstrated a high rate of response (70–90%), in panic disorder (PD) efficacy may be more limited in the presence of multiple symptom domains and comorbidities and/or when side-effects are present. The results for some alternative pharmacologic treatments for PD have been encouraging, although the number and range of controlled double-blind studies in this area are limited.

Noradrenergic agents

A relationship between noradrenergic activity and anxiety was first suggested by Redmond and Haung (1979); who noted that stimulation of the locus coeruleus (LC) in primates caused an anxiety reaction similar to a panic attack (PA). Challenge studies measuring physiological, anxiogenic and metabolite responses have indicated that abnormal β- and α_2-adrenergic function may be part of the underlying mechanism (Charney & Heninger 1986; Charney *et al.* 1987).

An early open trial of propranolol 20–80 mg daily in 10 patients with PAs (six with PD) demonstrated a suppression of symptoms in patients with a history of disease of 6 months or less (Heiser & Defrancisco 1976). A later double-blind placebo-controlled crossover study with propranolol showed a reduction of both somatic and psychic symptoms in 17 of 26 patients with chronic anxiety disorders, including of 19 with PD or agoraphobia with PAs (Kathol *et al.* 1980).

In 1985, Munjack *et al.* (1985) conducted a 6-week crossover comparative trial between imipramine and propranolol with a blind assessor in 38 patients. About half the patients with PD achieved complete remission with both drugs, and a further third were partially responsive although a large drop-out rate (40%) and absence of double-blind conditions should be noted. Although Ravaris *et al.* (1991) found propranolol and alprazolam to be equally effective, with an improvement rate of over 75%, a similar study by Noyes *et al.* (1984) ($N = 20$) with propranolol and diazepam showed that diazepam induced a moderate improvement in symptoms in most patients whereas propranolol was beneficial in only one-third. In one of the very sparse double-blind, placebo-controlled trials reported (Munjack *et al.* 1989), the propranolol and placebo groups had a similar response rate (43% and 40%, respectively).

These contrasting results might be partially explained by differences in the clinical characteristics of the studied population, the study design, the length of trial and the dose-titration. The patient sample in the study of Munjack *et al.* (1989) comprised primarily of nonagoraphobic patients with a shorter duration of illness compared to the study of Ravaris *et al.* (1991), where 65% of the patients had moderate to severe agoraphobia and a longer duration of illness. As agoraphobia and long-duration of PD have been shown to predict a positive preferential response to propranolol, this might explain positive results in the latter study. Further, Noyes *et al.* (1984) used a rapid dosage incrementation and noted significant side-effects, whereas Munjack *et al.* (1985) used gradual dose increases and noted no side-effects, which might also be relevant in view of the presence of side-effects predicting a poor response. Furthermore, in view of the known placebo response rate variability, the lack of placebo washout or placebo control in most of the studies limits the conclusions that can be drawn.

There are some data to suggest that the combination of β-blockers with other treatments may be useful. Two open-label studies combined propranolol with either diazepam (Hallstrom *et al.* 1984) or alprazolam (Shehi & Patterson 1984) and found that the combination was superior to propranolol alone and/or allowed the use of lower doses of each drug.

Pindolol is a β-blocker with additional antagonistic serotonergic properties (5-HT1A receptor blockade). It has been shown in some studies to augment the antidepressant response to treatment in patients with major depression. A double-blind placebo-controlled study ($N = 25$) suggests that it might also be efficacious in patients with PD who failed to respond to fluoxetine (20 mg for 8 weeks) and who were treated previously with at least two antidepressant medications (response to latter medications not described: Hirschmann *et al.* 2000).

Although recommendations regarding the use of β-blockers in PD cannot yet be made, propranolol has been considered the drug of choice for panic symptoms associated with mitral valve prolapse (Venkatesh *et al.* 1980). It may also be the rational choice in PD patients with medical comorbidities that require treatment with β-blockers, such as hypertension. However, clinicians should remember that β-blockers can be harmful, especially in patients with asthma and diabetes and may provoke or exacerbate depression.

Clonidine

Clonidine is an α_2-adrenergic receptor agonist that inhibits the spontaneous firing of norepinephrine (noradrenaline) neurones in the LC, a site known to be important in the mediation of anxiety (Svensson *et al.* 1975). Many studies have shown that intravenous administration of clonidine hydrochloride in single doses of 1.5–2.0 μg/kg acutely decreases anxiety in patients with PD (Charney & Heninger 1986; Nutt 1989; Uhde *et al.* 1989). However, Coplan *et al.* (1992) failed to confirm these findings.

Liebowitz *et al.* (1981) conducted an 8-week open trial in patients with PD or agoraphobia with PAs. They found that only four out of 11 subjects had a good response at doses of 0.2–0.5 mg/day, whereas the remainder had only transient responses despite dose increases (up to 1.0 mg/day) or intolerable side-effects. Hoehn-Saric *et al.* (1981), in a 4-week double-blind placebo crossover study reported only a moderate clinical effect with the same doses. There was a significant improvement in the 1st week in psychic symptoms of anxiety, but only a transient decrease in somatic symptoms. Moreover, in 3/14 patients symptoms worsened, and treatment had to be discontinued. It should be noted, though, that this patient population has been previously treated for PD with other medications (not described), so they might represent a treatment refractory sample.

The administration of oral clonidine to 18 patients in a 10-week double-blind flexible-dose, placebo-controlled trial yielded anxiolytic effects in some panic and anxiety measures in some patients, but not in the group as a whole (Uhde *et al.* 1989). By contrast, in a small 6-week crossover, placebo trial clonidine hydrochloride (4–5 μg/kg/day) was found to be more effective than imipramine hydrochloride (100 mg/day) in reducing anxiety stimulated by phobic exposure (Ko *et al.* 1983).

Most of the studies reported significant side-effects in the majority of subjects, such as sedation, fatigue and loss of motivation. The greater usefulness shown by short-term over long-term anxiolytic treatment might be explained by tolerance, which has also been reported for clonidine's sedative and analgesic properties (Drew *et al.* 1979). This is supported by the relatively consistent finding of transient responses in some patients across the studies. Tolerance to the anxiolytic effect of chronic clonidine treatment has been postulated to be due to desensitization of the LC α_2-autoreceptors.

Anticonvulsants

PD and epilepsy, particularly temporal lobe epilepsy share some common phenomenology (Gloor *et al.* 1982) and high reported rates of comorbidity have been described (McNamara & Fogel 1990). Both have been shown to involve abnormalities in distinct common brain regions, namely the temporal/limbic, by magnetic resonance imaging and positron emission tomography studies. Further electroencephalographic (EEG) abnormalities have been reported in 16–40% of patients with PD, suggesting that some "epileptiform" activity may play a role in the disorder (Stein & Uhde 1989).

Valproic acid (sodium valproate)

A small number of case reports have described anti-panic effects of valproic acid (Roy-Byrne 1988; McElroy *et al.* 1991). In three open trials of valproic acid with a total of 36 patients, 28 showed moderate to marked improvement in PAs and general anxiety, with varying but less improvement demonstrated in phobic symptoms (Primeau *et al.* 1990; Keck *et al.* 1993; Woodman & Noyes 1994). Generally, there was a rapid response in the 1st week, with further, gradual improvement for up to 6 weeks.

The only double-blind placebo-controlled, randomized crossover study in this area was conducted in patients with PD after withdrawal (7-day washout) from benzodiazepines (Lum *et al.* 1991). Treatment with valproic acid led to a significant improvement in scores in the length and intensity of the PAs, and in the psychic and somatic anxiety scores. The relevance of the findings to drug-naive or benzodiazepine non-responders remains to be determined.

Ontiveros and Fontaine (1992) reported a case series of four patients unresponsive to antidepressants and/or benzodiazepine, in whom valproate was added to ongoing clonazepam treatment, with a marked improvement in symptoms within 4 weeks. Although a decrease in the clonazepam dose resulted in a recurrence of the PAs, valproate was gradually decreased and stopped without relapse in two cases. The authors speculated that the beneficial effect of this drug combination was attributable to an increase in γ-aminobutyric acid (GABA) transmission via the different mechanisms of actions of the two agents.

In most studies valproic acid was reasonably well tolerated. Patients experienced few side-effects that limited treatment, although some reported gastro-intestinal dysfunction, dizziness and sleepiness (Lum *et al.* 1991).

Carbamazepine

Carbamazepine (CBZ) has been reported to be effective in ameliorating PAs in patients with EEG abnormalities (McNamara & Fogel 1990; Dantendorfer *et al.* 1995). In an open trial (Tondo *et al.* 1989) with 34 patients treated for a year with CBZ, a good response, measured by number of attacks, degree of avoidance behavior, and active functioning was noted in 58.8% of patients, with a significant correlation between response and the duration of treatment and drug dose. However, Klein *et al.* (1982) in a study of 10 patients treated with CBZ, reported a decrease in help-seeking behaviors and dysphoria, but no decrease of PAs.

In the only controlled study conducted to date, CBZ was not found to be significantly superior to placebo with regard to frequency of attacks, global severity index, phobic anxiety and depression subscales, although a statistically significant decrease in anxiety scores was noted on several measures (Uhde *et al.* 1988). Four of the original 18 subjects dropped out of the study, three because of significant side-effects and the fourth because of a dramatic response and a demand for treatment on an open basis. The presence of either EEG abnormalities or prominent psychosensory symptoms did not predict response to CBZ. The results of this study are tempered by the small sample size and the lack of exclusion of placebo responders. Furthermore, the length of treatment may have been inadequate, in view of the findings of the open study of Tondo *et al.* (1989), where a good response was correlated with the administration of CBZ for periods longer than an average of 7.2 months (a clinically questionable and very lengthy latency period).

Although CBZ has been shown to be efficacious in assisting alprazolam withdrawal (Klein *et al.* 1994), the 53% discontinuation rate ($N = 36$) contrasts with the successful discontinuation of a variety of benzodiazepines in the valproic acid study ($N = 12$: Lum *et al.* 1991). Furthermore, in the CBZ study, PD symptoms were not measured, and other factors, known to play a significant role in determining the success of withdrawal, such as current and past benzodiazepine treatment, dose detitration, and different pharmacokinetics of the specific benzodiazepines discontinued, may have contributed to the differences in efficacy.

Gabapentin

Gabapentin is a novel anticonvulsant agent. Its mechanism of action is unknown, although there is some evidence of an increase in GABA synthesis and release and alteration in monoamine neurotransmitter release (Taylor *et al.* 1998). Preclinical behavioral tests have shown a dose-dependent anxiolytic effect, comparable to that of the benzodiazepines (Singh *et al.* 1996).

In a randomized, double-blind, placebo-controlled, parallel-group study, 103 patients received treatment with gabapentin or placebo for 8 weeks (Pande *et al.* 2000). Although no overall between-group difference was observed in scores on the Panic and Agoraphobia Scale (PAS), posthoc analysis of the most severely ill patients showed a significant improvement in PAS score compared to placebo, but only in women. Side-effects were consistent with the known side-effect profile of gabapentin and included somnolence, headaches and dizziness.

The apparent differential efficacy of clonazepam and possible preliminary efficacy of valproic acid and gabapentin, compared with CBZ, at least as shown in open trials, might be explained by the differential effects on the activity of the GABA-benzodiazepine-chloride ionophore macromolecular complex at the central rather than the peripheral benzodiazepine receptors. The follow-up compound to gabapentin, pregabalin, is now in clinical trials for PD.

Baclofen

Since several studies have suggested that antianxiety and antidepressant drugs that produce antipanic effects also augment GABA transmission, Breslow *et al.* (1989) studied the effect of baclofen, a selective GABA$_B$ agonist, in PD. Nine medication-free patients with PD were treated with 30 mg/day of oral baclofen for 4 weeks in a double-blind, placebo-controlled, crossover trial. Baclofen was significantly more effective than placebo in reducing the number of PAs and anxiety but had no effect on depressive symptoms. A few side-effects were reported.

Lithium

Two case reports and one case series of five patients with PD showing a response to lithium augmentation of tetracyclic antidepressants (Cournoyer 1986; Feder 1988; Carmara 1990) support the role of lithium in the treatment of PD. Like in depression, the response occurred within 10 days. It is noteworthy that none of the patients had a history of mood disorder.

Neuropeptides

An anxiogenic role for cholecystokinin was suggested by deMontigny (1989), who observed that its intravenous injection in the tetrapeptide form (CCK-4) induced realistic panic-like attacks in healthy volunteers. Later studies showed that patients with PD have an increased sensitivity to CCK-4 (Bradwejn *et al.* 1991) and that CCK-4-induced PAs could be prevented by the administration, in a dose-related manner, of L-365,260, a compound with specific and high-affinity antagonist activity for the CCK-B receptor subtype, located primarily in the brain (Bradwejn *et al.* 1994). However, the CCK-B receptor antagonist CI-988 did not show these properties (Van Megen *et al.* 1996).

In a multicenter placebo-controlled double-blind trial of L-365,260 in the treatment of PD with or without agoraphobia, 40 patients received L-365,260 (120 mg/day) and 43 placebo following a 1-week single-blind placebo period (Kramer *et al.* 1995). At the dose tested, there were no clinically significant differences between the groups in global improvement, anxiety scores, PA frequency, intensity or disability measures. Thereafter, using a similar design, Pande *et al.* (1999a) found no difference on an interim analysis (when about half the 80 patients had been enrolled) in the weekly rate of PAs when CI-988 was added. In both these studies, the authors noted that the results did not rule out the role of cholecystokinin in PD for several reasons. First, the potential site of action of the medications are not known, and they may not have been distributed to the regions involved in the prevention of endogenous PAs. Second, although peak levels were constant at a value known to counteract the majority of CCK-4-induced PAs (Van Megen *et al.* 1997), trough levels may have been insufficient. Furthermore, pretreatment with 50 mg L365,260, which has been shown to prevent CCK-4-induced PAs in PD patients, did not block sodium-lactate-induced PAs (Van Megen *et al.* 1996) compared to clinically established antipanic agents (Coplan *et al.* 1992). This indicates that cholecystokinin may be involved in PD in a manner other than as a final common pathway.

Peptides related to the pituitary adrenocorticotrophic hormone (ACTH), including the ACTH(4–9) analog ORG 2766, had a similar effect to benzodiazepines in the social interaction animal model of anxiety (File 1981). However, a double-blind placebo-controlled study in 20 patients showed no reduction in PAs in either group, or significant differences in anxiety and depression score reduction (den Boer *et al.* 1989).

Dopaminergic agents

Although some challenge and metabolite studies have suggested a possible role for dopamine in PD, results have been mixed (Johnson *et al.* 1994). A survey of psychiatrists (El-Khayat & Baldwin 1998) and the recent 15-center World Health Organization Study (Ustun & Sartorius 1995) on psychological problems in general health care has shown significant, although variable, frequency of antipsychotic prescription for anxiety disorders. However, no studies have demonstrated unequivocal efficacy in PDs (Johnson *et al.* 1995).

Bupropion, a dopamine uptake inhibitor, was found in one study to be ineffective in treating PAs (Sheehan *et al.* 1983). However, monoamine oxidase inhibitors (MOIs), which possess a combined noradrenergic, serotonergic and dopaminergic activity, are established antipanic agents. Additional research is needed to determine whether dopamine is involved in the antipanic effect of these agents.

Calcium channel blockers

A small open study of calcium channel blockers (verapamil 240 mg/day or diltiazem 180 mg/day) demonstrated a favourable response in four of seven patients with pathological anxiety and PAs (Goldstein 1985), and a 16-week double-blind crossover study in 11 patients showed a statistically significant, though clinically modest, reduction in the number of PAs and anxiety rating scores, but not in agoraphobia (Klein & Uhde 1988). Four patients rated themselves as having markedly benefited from the drug, three had a marginal response, and four were complete nonresponders.

A different blocker, nifedipine, however, was ineffective in a single dose in the treatment of PD (N = 6: Klein *et al.* 1990).

It is of interest that in a study of basilar artery flow in nine PD patients, a significantly greater decrease in comparison to controls was demonstrated in response to hyperventilation. Two patients with the greatest decrease in blood flow in response to hyperventilation showed symptom reduction concomitant to normalization of blood flow response after 4 weeks nimodipine treatment (Gibbs 1992). This study suggests that the possible beneficial effect of calcium channel blockers in PD may be mediated by increased cerebral blood flow.

However other possible mechanisms of action might include inhibition of neurotransmitter (e.g. norpine-

phrine) release (Callanan & Kennan 1983), or relief of autonomic manifestations of anxiety, namely tachycardia, palpitations and increased blood pressure. However, limited trials, differences in study design, patient samples and medications, limit conclusions.

Second-messenger agents: inositol

Inositol is an isomer of glucose and a key metabolic precursor of the phosphatidylinositol cycle, itself a precursor of the intracellular second-messenger system for numerous neurotransmitters (Holub 1986). No disturbance of inositol levels has yet been reported in PD. However, it is considered a promising agent because of its proven effectiveness in the treatment of depression (Levine *et al.* 1995), and the effectiveness of antidepressants in the treatment of PD. Accordingly, Benjamin *et al.* (1995) studied patients with PD with and without agoraphobia given inositol 12 g or placebo in 4-week treatment phases. The inositol group showed a significant improvement over the placebo group in the number of PAs, panic scores and phobia scores, although no difference was found in anxiety and depression scores. Although the authors allowed the concomitant use of 1 mg of the benzodiazepine, lorazepam prn this was equally true for both phases, and lorazepam did not appear to interact with the beneficial effect of inositol.

Generalized anxiety disorder

Benzodiazepines represent the most classical and effective anxiolytic treatment for patients with generalized anxiety disorder (GAD), although problems of side-effects, dependence and misuse in the last 10 years has reduced their use. Buspirone, as well as TCAs, selective serotonin reuptake inhibitors (SSRIs), and newer antidepressants have also demonstrated efficacy in a number of trials. Most studies have been short-term and long-term studies would be important given the chronicity and course of the condition. It is also worth noting that patients with GAD often have comorbidity including mood disorders and substance, hypnotic or alcohol abuse/dependence.

β-blockers

Use of β-adrenergic blockers in the treatment of anxiety began when it was shown that propranolol might be beneficial in decreasing the autonomic symptoms of anxiety, especially cardiovascular manifestations (Granville-Grossman & Turner 1966).

Most studies of β-blockers were carried out in the 1970s and propranolol is the most studied β-blocker, although the results were conflicting. Although no benefit was shown in two placebo-controlled crossover trials (Ramsey *et al.* 1973; Kellner *et al.* 1974), some advantage was shown in other studies (Tanna *et al.* 1977) with a superior advantage for somatic symptoms (Kathol *et al.* 1980). In comparison to an active antianxiety drug (benzodiazepine) one study showed equal efficacy (Wheatley 1969), but two studies showed less efficacy although again somatic symptoms showed some benefit (Tyrer & Lader 1974a; Tyler & Lader 1974b). With respect to other β-blockers, positive results were reported for practolol versus placebo but only one rating scale was used to assess response and most patients were taking concurrent medications (Bonn *et al.* 1972). The study of sotalol versus placebo produced mixed results and although physicians' rating of improvement scales showed some advantage, patient ratings showed no difference (Tyrer & Lader 1973). In the remaining three studies (Burrows *et al.* 1977; Silverstone 1974; Johnson *et al.* 1976) the efficacy of oxprenolol versus placebo or an active antianxiety drug was evaluated. While the active antianxiety drug showed advantage over placebo, no significant difference between oxprenolol and placebo was found. Furthermore no advantage for somatic symptoms was shown in two of the studies (Burrows *et al.* 1977; Johnson *et al.* 1976). With respect to mechanism, a peripheral site of action was suggested, given the efficacy of D-propranolol (Bonn & Turner 1971) and efficacy of nonlipid soluble β-blockers, such as practolol. However a small double-blind placebo-controlled crossover 3-week trial (King *et al.* 1987: $N = 11$) of a selective β_2-adrenoreceptor antagonist (ICI 118551) (receptors present only peripherally) in chronic anxiety, as well as to determine whether β_1- or β_2-receptor blockade was important, showed equal improvement of symptoms when the selective antagonist was given in comparison to both propranolol and placebo. In this study, eight of the 11 patients were continued on benzodiazepines to which they were partially or wholly unresponsive. Thus under conditions of this study, no beneficial effects of either selective or nonselective β-blockade on chronic anxiety could be demonstrated.

Interestingly, another more recent 3-week double-blind study ($N = 196$) comparing propranolol, diclordiazepoxide and placebo showed advantage of the active groups at week 1; at week 2 advantage only for propranolol; and at the end, no differences due to improvement in all three groups. In this study, propranolol caused greater improvement in psychic than somatic symptoms of anxiety (Meibach *et al.* 1987).

The most recently published study of a β-blocker showed a dramatic improvement within 2 days in response to betaxolol, a centrally acting agent with a long half-life, in 29 out of 31 patients (including 27 GAD patients), although this was an open trial (Swartz 1998) and concurrent medication was continued. The authors postulated possible advantages of this agent to include no intrinsic sympathomimetic activity, and thus a greater effect against somatic manifestations of anxiety, such as tachycardias and coronary vasospasm, as well as no alteration of sleep architecture. However, efficacy will need to be substantiated with placebo-controlled studies.

Differences in results may be accounted for by heterogeneous samples including acute and chronic anxiety with varying severity and duration in many studies, lack of placebo washout in view of high placebo response, and the nonavoidance of concurrent medications. Inadequate duration of many studies with the majority under 3 weeks duration might be important in light of the improved response at 3 weeks in the longer studies, although the longer placebo response should also be noted (Meibach *et al.* 1987). Inadequate dosage, small sample sizes with the majority less than 20, might also be relevant limitations. Further, the influence of order of treatment in the crossover studies (which represent the majority) may be significant given the waxing and waning course and spontaneous improvements in this patient group. Another factor to consider might be β-blocker action to improve benzodiazepine withdrawal symptoms in the positive studies where this medication was stopped, generally 1 week before the study. Withdrawal symptoms seem to peak between 3 and 7 days and continue for 2–4 weeks (Petursson & Lader 1981) and, since propranolol has been shown to decrease these withdrawal symptoms that are predominantly somatic in type (Tyrer *et al.* 1981), this may partly explain the beneficial results in some of these trials. Although some authors have suggested the importance of non-specific factors accounting for treatment response, β-blockers might represent a third or fourth line treatment in nonresponders to other treatments, or when side-effects present a problem, particularly where somatic symptoms dominate.

Peptides

Based on the evidence that infusions of CCK-4 tetrapeptide in animals and humans (Bradwejn *et al.* 1991) has been shown to evoke anxiety and PAs, a 4-week double-blind, placebo-controlled study of the CCK-4 receptor antagonist CI-988 in patients ($N = 88$) with GAD was carried out (Bammert-Adams *et al.* 1995) following a 1–2 week placebo washout. CI-988 (300 mg/day) did not demonstrate anxiolytic effect superior to placebo. However, the observed treatment by center interaction and the variable placebo response rate observed among the three centers, where two centers had a very high placebo response as well as possibly inadequate dose, may limit interpretation of the results.

Treatment with ORG 2766 a MSH/ACTH analog in a double-blind placebo-controlled trial showed no significant reduction in anxiety in 12 GAD patients (den Boer *et al.* 1992). The parallel finding in PD and social phobia raises questions regarding the predictive value of the social interaction model in rodents for predicting anxiolytic activity although sample sizes were small.

Antipsychotic drugs

Antipsychotic drugs were known in the past as "major tranquilizers." Although a survey of psychiatrists and study in primary care suggested a significant rate of prescription, there are only a few studies to support their role in the treatment of nonpsychotic anxiety. Many early studies of a variety of antipsychotics suffered from several flaws, such as study population characterization, lack of exclusion of comorbidities, high drop-out rates, and inadequate washout with use of concomitant medications, and so conclusions were limited (for a review see El-Khayat & Baldwin 1998). In more recent, well-designed studies, a 6-week double-blind study including 106 patients, flusprilene in doses up to 1.5 mg/week was found to be effective in reducing both the somatic and psychic elements of generalized anxiety (Wurthmann *et al.* 1995). There was a positive dose–response relationship and in another study (of 205 patients) it was noted that there is a relationship between positive outcome and the lack of side-effects (Wurthmann *et al.* 1997). The paucity of side-effects of new atypical antipsychotic drugs may stimulate studies with these agents in the treatment of GAD.

Post-traumatic stress disorder

Post-traumatic stress disorder (PTSD) is quite resistant to antidepressants, and treatment is often complicated by side-effects related to the antidepressant drugs (Ballenger *et al.* 2000; Friedman 2000). Despite these facts, there have not been many large-scale double-blind controlled studies of nonantidepressant medications.

Anticonvulsant and mood stabilizers

As a group, the anticonvulsants are the most studied alternative treatment for PTSD (Ford 1996; Ballenger *et al.* 2000). The rationale for using anticonvulsants stems from the kindling model, which has been implicated in the etiology of PTSD (Hertzberg *et al.* 1999; Friedman 2000) and has been postulated as a mechanism for the efficacy in bipolar disorder.

In a double-blind comparison to placebo, 10 patients received lamotrigine at doses up to 50 mg/day. Lamotrigine was shown to be superior to placebo in improving both re-experiencing and avoidance/numbing symptoms (Hertzberg *et al.* 1999). In an open-label trial, 16 patients treated with divalproex had a significant decrease of intrusion and hyperarousal symptoms, but no change of avoidance/numbing symptoms (Clark *et al.* 1999). Other case reports also support the use of valproic acid in PTSD (Fesler 1991; Berigan & Holzgang 1995). CBZ is also reported to be useful in PTSD (Looff *et al.* 1995; Lipper *et al.* 1986).

Anticonvulsants such as gabapentin and vigabatrin (Macleod 1996; Brannon *et al.* 2000) were also used with some benefit, each in a single PTSD patient. Lithium was noted to decrease irritability in two PTSD patients (Forster *et al.* 1995).

Antipsychotics

Antipsychotic medications are also used for the treatment of PTSD and were occasionally reported as beneficial in some case reports (Bleich *et al.* 1986; Dillard *et al.* 1993). There are case reports that the novel atypical antipsychotic drug risperidone is also useful in controlling specific symptoms of PTSD such as flashbacks and nightmares (Leyba & Wampler 1998), irritable aggression (Monnelly & Ciraulo 1999), and intrusive thoughts and emotional reactivity (Krashin & Oates 1999).

Adrenergic agents

Various noradrenergic mechanisms have been suggested to play a role in the pathophysiology of PTSD and its typical disturbances of arousal and memory (Southwick *et al.* 1999; Coupland 2000; Raskind *et al.* 2000). Patients with PTSD have increased α_2 receptor sensitivity as shown by challenge tests (e.g., yohimbine challenge: Southwick *et al.* 1999).

Treatment with betaxolol, a long-acting β_1-adrenergic blocker, led to a decrease of anxiety in several PTSD patients (Swartz 1998). The α_1-adrenergic antagonist prazosin was shown to ameliorate nightmares in four PTSD patients, with a dose-dependent effect (5 mg/day being more effective than 2 mg/day) (Raskind *et al.* 2000). A similar response was noted with the use of the α_2-agonist guanfacine (Horrigan 1996; Horrigan & Barnhill 1996). Propranolol, a β-blocker, and clonidine, an α_2-agonist, both of which have a suppressive effect on noradrenergic activity, were shown to be effective in treating the re-experiencing and hyperarousal symptoms in open trials (Famularo *et al.* 1988; Kinzie & Leung 1989; Harmon & Riggs 1996; Southwick *et al.* 1999). All these trials were with a relatively small number of patients, the largest was 11 and in most trials the subjects were children.

Opiate antagonists

Opiate antagonists, including nalmefene and naltrexone, were also reported as beneficial in reducing flashbacks in a few cases of PTSD (Bills & Kreisler 1993; Glover 1993).

Inositol

Inositol, a signal transduction modulator, was used with some benefit in the treatment of PTSD in a small trial (Kaplan *et al.* 1996).

Obsessive-compulsive disorder

Obsessive compulsive (OC) symptoms in up to 40–60% of patients are unimproved with classical treatment (TCAs such as clomipramine [CMI] and SSRIs). Most studies of alternative treatments were tried on treatment-resistant patients. This has to be borne in mind as these patients may not represent all patients seeking treatment and may, in some cases, represent specific subtypes of the psychopathology in question. Many of the studies employ small samples and are open-labeled. Therefore replication on larger samples in a double-blind design are needed.

Antipsychotics

Although O'Regan (1970) reported two patients who had a beneficial response to haloperidol alone, another study could not replicate this finding (Hussain & Ahad 1970). However, based on case reports on the efficacy of combined neuroleptic/SSRI treatment in obsessive-compulsive disorder (OCD) patients with comorbid tic disorders, such as Tourette's syndrome (Riddle *et al.* 1988; Delgado *et al.* 1990), an open trial in 17 patients showed efficacy of classical neuroleptic addition in the treatment of OCD patients who did not response to an adequate trial of fluvoxamine with or without lithium (McDougle *et al.* 1990). A further double-blind, placebo-controlled study of haloperidol addition (up to 10 mg) to fluvoxamine nonresponders showed a significant improvement in OC symptoms in comparison to placebo (McDougle *et al.* 1994). In both studies comorbid tic disorder was associated with a positive response, with a total of 20 out of 21 patients with the comorbid condition achieving a response in contrast to nine out of 27 without this diagnosis. Although the classical neuroleptics were well-tolerated, anticholinergics were given to all subjects and propranolol where akathisia developed.

The most commonly reported adjunctive treatment of OCD consists of the atypical antipsychotic agents, as either monotherapy or augmentation of SSRIs.

Risperidone, a 5-HT2A/D2 antagonist, has been tried either alone (Dryden-Edwards & Reiss 1996) or in combination with a SSRI (McDougle *et al.* 1995; Stein *et al.* 1997; Agid & Lerer 1999; Fitzgerald *et al.* 1999); in a number of cases the results are contradictory. While in some patients a clinically significant improvement in OC symptoms was noted (McDougle *et al.* 1995; Stein *et al.* 1997; Agid & Lerer 1999; Fitzgerald *et al.* 1999), others reported exacerbation of these symptoms with risperidone (Dryden-Edwards

& Reiss 1996). All of these studies were open-label studies on a limited number (one to eight) patients. Recently, two relatively large-scale studies on risperidone augmentation in OCD were published. One was a double-blind placebo-controlled study of risperidone augmentation of SSRIs and reported a significant amelioration of OC symptoms in the treated group ($N = 18$) as compared to the placebo group (McDougle et al. 2000). The second study was an open-label risperidone augmentation study ($N = 20$) (Pfanner et al. 2000) and it also reported a significant decrease in OC symptoms. There is still a need for large-scale double-blind, placebo-controlled trials.

Olanzapine, a 5-HT2, D1, D2, D3 and D4 antagonist with α_1-adrenergic and muscarinic antagonist activity, has also been tried in some drug-resistant OCD patients in the treatment of OCD as either monotherapy (Degner et al. 2000; Ohaeru 2000) or in combination with SSRIs (Potenza et al. 1998; Weiss et al. 1999; Bogetto et al. 2000). It seems that this drug is well-tolerated and has a beneficial effect on OC symptoms. Again, we still lack the benefit of large-scale, double-blind, placebo-controlled studies, as the reported trials were carried out on four to 10 patients and were open-label studies.

Clozapine, which has a similar pharmacological profile to olanzapine except for a lower affinity to D2 receptors, was similarly tried for the alleviation of OC symptoms (Steinert et al. 1996; Strous et al. 1999; Tibbo & Gendemann 1999) with good results. However, as with other atypical neuroleptics, clozapine can also aggravate pre-existing OCD, or even precipitate obsessive symptoms in symptom-free patients who suffer from other disorders (De Haan et al. 1999). It is important to note again, that trials with clozapine were open-label case histories and, to the best of our knowledge, there are no placebo-controlled double-blind studies of this medication.

It is important to note that, in this context, in most studies the atypical antipsychotic agents were tried in OCD patients refractory to serotonin reuptake inhibitor (SRI) treatment, or those with comorbid diagnoses such as personality disorder, tic disorder and schizophrenia. These groups may turn out to be specific subtypes of OCD. It is noteworthy that olanzapine has been demonstrated to possess antiobsessive activity in some schizophrenic patients with OC symptoms (Poyurovsky et al. 2000).

Adrenergic agents

Pindolol, a β-adrenergic/5-HT1A blocker was tried in a few studies in augmentation of SRIs. In a case series of eight patients showing limited response to SSRI, the addition of pindolol in doses between 7.5 and 10 mg caused remission in one patient only when given for between 2 and 10 weeks (Koran et al. 1996). A placebo-controlled double-blind study to determine the efficacy of pindolol addition to fluvoxamine at the beginning of the treatment in 15 patients showed no difference in response and no shortening of response latency (Mundo et al. 1998). However, a more recent double-blind study in 14 treatment-resistant OCD patients showed a significant improvement in OC symptoms at 4 weeks when added to paroxetine at a dose of 7.5 mg (given t.i.d.) (Dannon et al. 2000). These studies were performed after it had been found that pindolol augmentation in major depressive disorder was successful. A possible reason for the discrepant findings with the Koran et al. (1996) study might be related to inadequate dosage frequency in the latter study (which was given b.i.d. to improve compliance). This may have produced inadequate plasma levels in view of the short half-life of pindolol of 3–4 h. These conflicting studies need large-scale replication, as well as basic studies to elucidate the mechanism of interaction between pindolol and SSRIs. It is possible that the antagonistic activity of pindolol at the somatodendritic 5-HT1A receptor enables serotonergic neurotransmission (Blier et al. 1998; Haddjeri et al. 1999).

Clonidine, an α_2-adrenergic agonist has been used in OCD as both a pharmacological challenge (Brambilla et al. 1997a,b) and as a therapeutic agent (Hewlett et al. 1992; Dolfus 1993; Jenike 1993). OCD patients have a blunted growth hormone response to clonidine (Brambilla et al. 1997a). This suggests a subsensitivity of α_2-adrenergic receptors. Since these receptors are thus implicated in the pathophysiology of OCD it seems reasonable to try treatments that interfere with them. Clonidine was therefore tried as a treatment of OCD with contradictory results. A double-blind placebo-controlled crossover study has found no beneficial effects of clonidine in OCD (Hewlett et al. 1992). On the other hand, clonidine was found to be beneficial in Tourette-related OCD (Dolfus 1993) and as augmentation in treatment-resistant OCD (Jenike 1993).

Opioid agents

Two open-label trials with the opioid agent tramadol were reported (Shapira *et al.* 1997; Goldsmith *et al.* 1999). Tramadol is a mixed SRI and μ-antagonist. Both studies reported amelioration in OCD symptoms. An earlier trial on two patients administered naloxone, a nonselective opioid antagonist, to OCD patients and found exacerbation of OC symptoms (Insel & Pickar 1983). Though the mechanism of action is unclear, it is tempting to speculate that these effects are due to interactions between the opioid system and the serotonergic system. It is of interest in this context, that plasma beta-endorphin levels were found to be decreased in untreated OCD patients (Weizman *et al.* 1990).

Antiandrogens and adrenal steroids

Based on case series and case reports that have described a reduction in OC symptoms during treatments that antagonized gonadal steroids (Casas *et al.* 1986; Leonard 1989; Weiss *et al.* 1995; Chouinard *et al.* 1996; Eriksson 2000: total $N = 10$) and on the hypothesis that gonadal hormones play a role in the pathogenesis of OCD, the antiandrogen treatment flutamide, was given to determine the role of androgen receptor activation in OCD exacerbation by gonadal steroids. This open study with eight patients found no reduction in OC symptoms and anxiety, although reduction in aggressive feelings was observed (Altemus *et al.* 1999). These results seem to suggest a limited role of androgen receptor activation although double-blind placebo-controlled studies would be important to rule out efficacy. The lack of response to an androgen receptor antagonist only, might suggest that exacerbation of OCD symptoms may be mediated through estrogen receptors or receptor-independent mechanisms. Estrogen receptors might be important due to the interaction demonstrated between gonadal hormones and the serotonergic system (Toren *et al.* 1996). Furthermore, in the positive case reports and series cited, the agents used also reduced synthesis of circulatory estrogens: cypoterone acetate due to suppression of luteinizing hormone release (Casas *et al.* 1986; Weiss *et al.* 1995); testolactone due to aromatase inhibition (Leonard 1989); aminoglutethimide due to global steroid biosynthesis inhibition (Chouinard *et al.* 1996); and triptorelin, a long-acting gonadotrophin-releasing hormone analog due to reduction in circulating androgens and estrogens (Eriksson 2000).

Peptides

Oxytocin may play a role in the pathogenesis of some forms of OCD. This assumption is based on elicited OC-like behaviors in rats on oxytocin administration, as well as reports of exacerbations of OC symptoms in pregnancy or puerperium. OC symptoms might represent pathological correlates of exaggerated maternal behavior as a result of CSF oxytocin changes or raised CSF oxytocin levels as was reported in OCD patients in comparison to controls (Leckman *et al.* 1994). However, although a case report detailed symptomatic improvement in one man treated with intramuscular oxytocin for 4 weeks, other case reports ($N = 3$ and $N = 2$) showed no improvement although these were in single doses (Charles *et al.* 1989; Salzberg & Swedo 1992). A randomized double-blind placebo-controlled trial in 12 patients for 6 weeks also showed no benefit (den Boer & Westenberg *et al.* 1992), and a further randomized double-blind, placebo-controlled cross-over trial in 7 patients using higher doses showed no benefit (Epperson *et al.* 1996). However, the study length of 1 week was suggested as a possible limitation and reason for failure to respond.

Hallucinogenic agents

Lately it has been noted in a series of cases that hallucinogenic agents, such as lysergic acid diethylamide (LSD), a 5-HT2 partial antagonist, can alleviate OC symptoms for a period of time exceeding their use (Moreno & Delgado 1997). Most probably these agents act directly on the serotonergic system, though the mechanism of action on OC symptoms remains to be elucidated. Controlled trials of these agents are presently underway (Delgado, pers. comm.).

Mood stabilizers

Two double-blind trials of lithium as an augmentation to serotonergic drugs did not produce conclusive evidence of the effectiveness of such a regimen. In a placebo-controlled trial of lithium augmentation to fluvoxamine there was a small reduction in OCD symptoms after 2 weeks (20 patients) but not after 4 weeks (10 patients: McDougle *et al.* 1991). A similar augmentation to clomipramine treatment was ineffective in 16 patients (Piggot et al. 1991).

However another mood stabilizer and anticonvulsant, gabapentin, was reported to be of beneficial effect in case reports (Cora-Locatelli et al. 1998a). In other case reports, valproate (Cora-Locatelli et al. 1998b) and CBZ (Koopowitz & Berk 1997) were found to be effective in reducing OC symptoms, specifically in patients with comorbid epilepsy.

Inositol

Inositol, a molecule involved in cellular signal transduction, has been tried as both monotherapy (N = 13: Fux et al. 1996) and in combination with SRIs (N = 10) (Seedat & Stein 1999), with relatively good results. Even though these studies were double-blind, a replication in a larger sample is needed.

Autoimmune aspects

A subgroup of paediatric OCD patients belong to the category of pediatric autoimmune neuropsychiatric disorders associated with streptococcal infections (PANDAS). A pilot study of penicillin prophylaxis for children suffering such OCD (N = 37) failed to produce positive results (Garvey et al. 1999). On the other hand, plasma exchange (N = 10) was found to significantly reduce OC symptoms as compared to an appropriate placebo group (Perlmutter et al. 1999).

Social phobia

Social phobia (SP) is a common disabling condition often associated with other psychiatric comorbidities. It may be categorized into the more common and more severe generalized type and the performance type. In the last 10 years monoamine inhibitors, benzodiazepines and, most recently, SSRIs have shown promise as treatment agents, although the efficacy and side-effects vary. Studies in the now classical treatments are just beginning to be replicated, so studies in alternative medication are limited.

Noradrenergic agents

There is some evidence suggesting an autonomic nervous system dysfunction in SP. Behavioral challenge studies have reported higher heart rate responses in patients with performance phobia compared to patients with generalized phobia (Heimberg et al. 1990; Levin et al. 1993). Stein et al. (1992) found that orthostatic challenge in patients with SP led to higher plasma norepinephrine levels, but this was not replicated in another study by the same group (Stein et al. 1994). Potts et al. (1996) demonstrated an increase in social anxiety in response to yohimbine in a placebo-controlled crossover study in six patients.

Of the analog studies—all in nonpatient samples that examined the effect of β-blockers on anxiety during observed performance, which shares many features with performance phobia—eight studies found β-blockers to be superior to placebo in reducing some aspects of performance anxiety, whereas three did not (Liebowitz et al. 1985). Ten of the 11 studies involved nonselective β-blockers, but one used atenolol, a cardioselective β-blocker that penetrates the central nevous system less well than propranolol. This study found atenolol efficacious, indicating a peripheral mode of action in performance anxiety.

A small placebo-controlled trial of the β-blocker propranolol in the treatment of SP revealed no differences with placebo. However, all the patients were concomitantly receiving social skills training (Falloon et al. 1981). Gorman et al. (1985), in an open clinical trial reported a good response in patients with SP to atenolol, but this was not supported in subsequent double-blind studies (Liebowitz et al. 1991, 1992). In the latter, the sample was comprised predominantly of patients with generalized SP, and the number of patients with performance-type phobia was too small for a separate analysis.

In a case report, clonidine demonstrated a good response in a patient unresponsive to other pharmacological treatments and psychotherapy where a possible mechanism involving thermoregulation was postulated (Goldstein 1987).

Anticonvulsants

The only anticonvulsant study to date in the treatment of SP is gabapentin. In a randomized, double-blind, placebo-controlled trial (Pande et al. 1999b), 69 patients were randomized to receive gabapentin (900–3600 mg daily) or placebo for 14 weeks. Changes in symptoms of SP were evaluated by clinician and patient rating scales. The results showed a progressive decline in scores on the Leibowitz Social Anxiety Scale (LSAS) until week 10, with plateauing at the same time the maximum dose was reached. The drug/placebo difference was greater for men and older patients. Side-effects included dizziness and dry mouth; and somnolence, nausea, flatulence, and decreased libido occurred more frequently in the study group, although the difference from controls was not statistically significant. Both arms had significant attrition, due mostly, in the gabapentin group, to adverse events. The conclusions of the study were limited by the strict inclusion criteria (low rate of comorbidity and LSAS score of 50+), which might explain why a significant number of patients continued to have high scores on the LSAS, yielding lower response rates than for clonazepam or phenelzine in other studies. Clinical trials are currently taking place for the follow-up compound to gabapentin, pregabalin in social anxiety disorder.

Dopaminergic agents

Involvement of the dopaminergic system in SP is suggested by several findings:

1 High rates of SP have been noted in Parkinson's disease, a condition known to be associated with abnormal brain dopaminergic function (Stein *et al.* 1990). Furthermore, some patients with social phobic symptoms have been treated successfully with dopamine agonists (Mikkelsen *et al.* 1981).

2 Patients with PD and SP have lower levels of cerebrospinal fluid homovanillic acid than patients with PD alone (Johnson *et al.* 1994). Accordingly increased homovanillic acid levels have been associated with measures of extraversion in depressed patients (Moller *et al.* 1996).

3 MOIs have been found to be effective in the treatment of SP, whereas TCAs have not (Liebowitz *et al.* 1987; Heimberg *et al.* 1998). MOIs differ from tetracyclic antidepressants in their more potent effects on the dopaminergic system.

4 A single photon emission computed tomography (SPECT) study using a specific ligand for the dopamine transporter noted reduced dopamine binding to the basal ganglia in patients with SP (Tiihonen *et al.* 1997). Another SPECT study using a D2 receptor radio-tracer showed reduced binding in the striatum in comparison to controls (Schneier *et al.* 2000). Further a positron emission tomography (PET) study revealed that dopamine D2 receptor binding to the putamen was associated with the presence of detachment, a personality trait that may be relevant to SP (Farde *et al.* 1997).

5 In animal models, social status has been shown to be reflected in differences in dopamine D2 striatal density (Grant *et al.* 1998). Only one case series of a pure dopaminergic agent has so far been published (Villarreal *et al.* 2000). Four subjects with generalized SP were given pergolide, a potent D1 and D2 dopamine agonist, for 12 weeks. Two dropped out after 4 weeks, one because of drug side-effects and lack of efficacy, and the other was lost to follow-up. No change was found in SP symptoms in any of the subjects.

Neuropeptides

In a small double-blind, placebo-controlled study, treatment with ORG 2766 (ACTH [4–9] analog) in 12 patients resulted in only a small decrease in scores on the avoidance and anxiety subscale of the SP scale, with no significant difference compared to placebo (den Boer *et al.* 1994).

Acknowledgements

The authors thank Ms. Gloria Ginzach and Ms. Marian Propp for their editorial and secretarial assistance.

References

Agid, O. & Lerer, B. (1999) Risperidone augmentation of paroxetine in a case of severe, treatment-refractory obsessive-compulsive disorder without comorbid psychopathology. *J Clin Psychiatry* **60**, 55–6.

Altemus, M., Greenberg, B.D., Keuler, D., Jacobson, K.R. & Murphy, D.L. (1999) Open trial flutamide for treatment of obsessive-compulsive disorder. *J Clin Psychiatry* **60**, 442–5.

Ballenger, J.C., Davidson, J.R.T., Lecurbier, Y. & Nutt, D.M. (2000) Consensus statement on post-traumatic stress disorder from the International Consensus Group of Depression and Anxiety. *J Clin Psychiatry* **61** (Suppl. 5), 60–6.

Bammert-Adams, J., Pyke, R.E., Costa, J. *et al.* (1995) A double-blind, placebo-controlled study of CCK-B receptor antagonist, CI-988 in patients with generalized anxiety disorder. *J Clin Psychopharmacol* **15**, 428–34.

Benjamin, J., Levine, J., Fux, M., Aviv, A., Levy, D. & Belmaker, R.H. (1995) Double-blind, placebo controlled, crossover trial of inositol treatment for panic disorder. *Am J Psychiatry* **152**, 1004–6.

Berigan, T.R. & Holzgang, A. (1995) Valproate as an alternative in post-traumatic stress disorder: a case report. *Mil Med* **160**, 318.

Bills, L.J. & Kreisler, K. (1993) Treatment of flashbacks with naltrexone. *Am J Psychiatry* **150**, 1430.

Bleich, A., Siegel, B. & Garb, R. (1986) Post-traumatic stress disorder following combat exposure: clinical features and psychopharmacological treatment. *Br J Psychiatry* **149**, 365–9.

Blier, P., Pineyro, G., El Mansari, M., Bergeron, R. & de Montigny, C. (1998) Role of somatodendritic 5-HT auto-receptors in modulating 5-HT neurotransmission. *Annals of the New York Academy of Science* **861**, 204–16.

den Boer, J.A., van Vliet, I.M. & Westenberg, H.G.M. (1994) Recent advances in the psychopharmacology of social phobia. *Prog Neuropsychopharmacol Biol Psychiatry* **18**, 625–45.

den Boer, J.A., Westenberg, H.G.M. & de Vries, H. (1992) The MSH/ACTH analog ORG 2766 in anxiety disorders. *Peptides* **13**, 109–12.

den Boer, J.A. & Westernberg, H.G.M. (1992) Oxytocin in obsessive-compulsive disorder. *Peptides* **13**, 1083–5.

den Boer, J.A., Westernberg, H.G.M., Mastenbrock, B. & van Ree, J.M. (1989) The ACTH (4–9) analog ORG 2766 in panic disorder: a preliminary study. *Psychopharmacol Bull* **2**, 204–8.

Bogetto, F., Bellino, S., Vaschetto, P. & Ziero, S. (2000) Olanzapine augmentation of fluvoxamine-refractory obsessive-compulsive disorder (OCD): a 12-week open trial. *Psychiatry Res* **92**, 91–8.

Bonn, J.A. & Turner, P. (1971) D-propranolol and anxiety. *Lancet* **I**, 1355–6.

Bonn, J.A., Turner, P. & Hicks, D.C. (1972) β-adrenergic-receptor blockade with practolol in treatment of anxiety. *Lancet* **I**, 814–5.

Bradwejn, J., Koszycki, D., Couetoux-du Tertre, A., van Megen, H., den Boer, J. & Westenberg, H. (1994) The panicogenic effects of cholecystokinin-tetrapeptide are antagonized by L-365,260, a central cholecystokinin receptor antagonist, in patients with panic disorder. *Arch Gen Psychiatry* **51**, 486–93.

Bradwejn, J., Koszycki, D. & Shriqui, C. (1991) Enhanced sensitivity to cholecystokinin tetrapeptide in panic disorder. *Arch Gen Psychiatry* **48**, 603–10.

Brambilla, F., Bellodi, L., Perna, G. *et al.* (1997b) Noradrenergic receptor sensitivity in obsessive-compulsive disorder. II. Cortisol response to acute clonidine administration. *Psychiatry Res* **69**, 163–8.

Brambilla, F., Perna, G., Bellodi, L. *et al.* (1997a) Noradrenergic receptor sensitivity in obsessive-compulsive disorders. I. Growth hormone response to clonidine stimulation. *Psychiatry Res* **69**, 155–62.

Brannon, N., Labbate, L. & Huber, M. (2000) Gabapentin treatment for post-traumatic stress disorder. *Can J Psychiatry* **45**, 84.

Breslow, M.F., Fankhauser, M.P., Potter, R.L., Meredith, U.E., Misinszeh, J. & Hope, D.G. (1989) Role of GABA in antipanic drug efficacy. *Am J Psychiatry* **146**, 353–6.

Burrows, G.D., Davies, B., Fail, L., Poynton, C. & Stevenson, H. (1976) A placebo controlled trial of diazepam and oxprenolol for anxiety. *Psychopharmacology* **50**, 177–9.

Callanan, K.M. & Kennan, A.K. (1983) Differential effects of D600, nifedipine and dantrolene sodium on excitation-secretion coupling and presynaptic β-adrenergic responses in rat atria. *Br J Pharmacol* **83**, 841–7.

Carmara, E.G. (1990) Lithium potentiation of antidepressant treatment in panic disorder. *J Clin Psychopharmacol* **19**, 225–6.

Casas, M., Alvarez, E., Duro, P. *et al.* (1986) Antiandrogenic treatment of obsessive-compulsive neurosis. *Acta Psychiatr Scand* **73**, 221–2.

Charles, G., Guillaume, R., Schittecatte, M., Pholien, P., Van Wettere, P. & Wilmotte, J. (1989) Oxytocin in the treatment of obsessive-compulsive disorder: a report on two cases. *Psychiatry and Psychobiology* **4**, 111–15.

Charney, D.S. & Heninger, G.R. (1986) Abnormal regulation of noradrenergic function in panic disorder: effects of clonidine in healthy subjects and patients with agoraphobia and panic disorder. *Arch Gen Psychiatry* **43**, 1042–55.

Charney, D., Woods, S., Goodman, W. & Heninger, G.R. (1987) Neurobiological mechanisms of panic anxiety: biochemical and behavioral correlates of yohimbine-induced panic attacks. *Am J Psychiatry* **144**, 1030–36.

Chouinard, G., Belanger, M.C., Beauclair, L., Sultan, S. & Murphy, B.E. (1996) Potentiation of fluoxetine by aminoglutethimide, an adrenal steroid suppressant, in obsessive-compulsive disorder resistant to SSRIs: a case report. *Prog Neuropsychopharmacol Biol Psychiatry* **20**, 1067–79.

Clark, R.D., Canive, J.M., Calais, L.A., Qualls, C. & Tuason, V.B. (1999) Divalproex in post-traumatic stress disorder: an open-label clinical trial. *J Trauma Stress* **12**, 395–401.

Coplan, J.D., Liebowitz, M.R., Gorman, J.M. *et al.* (1992) Noradrenergic function in panic disorder: effects of intravenous clonidine pretreatment on lactate-induced panic. *Biol Psychiatry* **31**, 135–46.

Cora-Locatelli, G., Greenberg, B.D., Martin, J. & Murphy, D.L. (1998a) Gabapentin augmentation for fluoxetine-treated patients with obsessive-compulsive disorder. *J Clin Psychiatry* **59**, 480–1.

Cora-Locatelli, G., Greenberg, B.D., Martin, J. & Murphy, D.L. (1998b) Valproate monotherapy in an SRI-intolerant OCD patient. *J Clin Psychiatry* **59**, 82.

Coupland, N.J. (2000) Brain mechanisms and neurotransmitters. In: *Post-traumatic Stress Disorder—Diagnosis, Management and Treatment* (D.M. Nutt, J.R.T. Davidson & J. Zohar (eds), pp. 69–100). Martin Duniz, London.

Cournoyer, J. (1986) Rapid response of a disorder to the addition of lithium carbonate: panic resistant to tricyclic antidepressants. *Can J Psychiatry* **31**, 335–8.

Dannon, P.N., Sasson, Y., Hirschmann, S., Iancu, I., Grunhaus, L.J. & Zohar, J.K. (2000) Pindolol augmentation in treatment-resistant obsessive-compulsive disorder: a double-blind placebo-controlled trial. *Eur Neuropsychopharmacol* **10**, 165–9.

Dantendorfer, K., Amering, M., Baischer, W. *et al.* (1995) Is there a pathophysiological and therapeutic link between panic disorder and epilepsy? *Acta Psychiatr Scand* **91**, 430–2.

De Haan, L., Linszen, D.H. & Gorsira, R. (1999) Clozapine and obsessions in patients with recent-onset schizophrenia and other psychotic disorders. *J Clin Psychiatry* **60**, 364–5.

Degner, D., Bleich, S., Kornhuber, J. & Ruther, E. (2000) Olanzapine treatment of obsessive-compulsive disorder. *Can J Psychiatry* **45**, 393.

Delgado, P.L., Goodman, W.K., Price, L.H., Heninger, G.R. & Charney, D.S. (1990) Fluvoxamine/pimozide treatment of concurrent Tourette's and obsessive-compulsive disorder. *Br J Psychiatry* **157**, 762–5.

Dillard, M.L., Bendfeldt, F. & Jernigan, P. (1993) Use of thioridazine in post-traumatic stress disorder. *South Med J* **86**, 1276–8.

Dolfus, S. (1993) Indications for clonidine in child psychiatry. *Encephale* **19**, 83–7.

Drew, G.M., Gower, A.J. & Marriott, A.S. (1979) α_2-adrenoreceptors mediate clonidine-induced sedation in the rat. *Br J Pharmacol* **67**, 133–41.

Dryden-Edwards, R.C. & Reiss, A.L. (1996) Differential response of psychotic and obsessive symptoms to risperidone in an adolescent. *J Child Adolesc Psychopharmacol* **6**, 139–45.

El-Khayat, R. & Baldwin, D.S. (1998) Antipsychotic drugs for nonpsychotic patients: assessment of the benefit/risk ratio in generalized anxiety disorder. *J Psychopharmacol* **12**, 323–9.

Epperson, C.N., McDougle, C.J. & Price, L.H. (1996) Intranasal oxytocin in obsessive-compulsive disorder. *Biol Psychiatry* **40**, 547–9.

Eriksson, T. (2000) Antiandrogenic treatment for obsessive-compulsive disorder. *Am J Psychiatry* **157**, 483.

Falloon, I.R., Lloyd, G.G. & Harpin, R. (1981) The treatment of social phobia. *J Nerv Ment Dis* **169**, 180–4.

Famularo, R., Kunscherff, R. & Fenton, T. (1988) Propranolol treatment for childhood post-traumatic stress disorder, acute type. *American Journal of Diseases of Childhood* **142**, 1244–7.

Farde, L., Gustavsson, J.P. & Jönsson, E. (1997) D2 dopamine receptors and personality traits. *Nature* **385**, 590.

Feder, R. (1988) Lithium augmentation of clomipramine. *J Clin Psychiatry* **49**, 458.

Fesler, R.A. (1991) Valproate in combat-related post-traumatic stress disorder. *J Clin Psychiatry* **52**, 361–4.

File, S.E. (1981) Contrasting effects of ORG 2766 and alpha-MSH on social and exploratory behavior in the rat. *Peptides* **2**, 255–60.

Fitzgerald, K.D., Stewart, C.M., Tawile, V. & Rosenberg, D.R. (1999) Risperidone augmentation of serotonin reuptake inhibitor treatment of pediatric obsessive-compulsive disorder. *J Child Adolesc Psychopharmacol* **9**, 115–23.

Ford, N. (1996) The use of anticonvulsants in post-traumatic stress disorder: case study and overview. *J Trauma Stress* **9**, 857–63.

Forster, P.L., Shoenfeld, F.B., Marmar, C.R. & Lang, A.J. (1995) Lithium for irritability in post-traumatic stress disorder. *J Trauma Stress* **8**, 143–9.

Friedman, M.J. (2000) What might the psychobiology of post-traumatic stress disorder teach us about future approaches to pharmacotherapy? *J Clin Psychiatry* **61** (Suppl. 7), 44–51.

Fux, M., Levine, J., Aviv, A. & Belmaker, R.H. (1996) Inositol treatment of obsessive-compulsive disorder. *Am J Psychiatry* **153**, 1219–21.

Garvey, M.A., Perlmutter, S.J., Allen, A.J. *et al.* (1999) A pilot study of penicillin prophylaxis for neuropsychiatric exacerbations triggered by streptococcal infections. *Biol Psychiatry* **45**, 1564–71.

Gibbs, D.M. (1992) Hyperventilation-induced cerebral ischemia in panic disorder and effect of nimodipine. *Am J Psychiatry* **149**, 1589–91.

Gloor, P., Olivier, A., Quesney, L.F., Andermann, F. & Horowitz, S. (1982) The role of the limbic system in experimental phenomena of temporal lobe epilepsy. *Ann Neurol* **12**, 129–44.

Glover, H. (1993) A preliminary trial of nalmefene for the treatment of emotional numbing in combat veterans with post-traumatic stress disorder. *Isr J Psychiatry Relat Sci* **30**, 255–63.

Goldsmith, T.B., Shapira, N.A. & Keck, P.E. Jr (1999) Rapid remission of OCD with tramadol hydrochloride. *Am J Psychiatry* **156**, 660–1.

Goldstein, J.A. (1985) Calcium channel blockers in the treatment of panic disorder. *J Clin Psychiatry* **46**, 546.

Goldstein, S. (1987) Treatment of social phobia with clonidine. *Biol Psychiatry* **2**, 369–72.

Gorman, J.M., Liebowitz, M.R., Fyer, A.J., Campeas, R. & Klein, D. (1985) Treatment of social phobia with atenolol. *J Clin Psychopharmacol* **5**, 669–77.

Grant, K.A., Shively, C.A., Nader, M.A. *et al.* (1998) Effect of social status on striatal dopamine D2 receptor binding characteristics in cynomolgus monkeys assessed with positron emission tomography. *Synapse* **29**, 80–3.

Granville-Grossman, K.L. & Turner, P. (1966) The effect of propranolol on anxiety. *Lancet* **I**, 788–90.

Haddjeri, N., de Montigny, C. & Blier, P. (1999) Modulation of the firing activity of rat serotonin and noradrenaline neurons by (+/–) pindolol. *Biol Psychiatry* **45**, 1163–9.

Hallstrom, C., Treasaden, I., Edwards, J.G. & Lader, M. (1984) Diazepam, propranolol and their combination in the management of chronic anxiety. *Br J Psychiatry* **139**, 417–21.

Harmon, R.J. & Riggs, P.D. (1996) Clonidine for post-traumatic stress disorder in preschool children. *J Am Acad Child Adolesc Psychiatry* **35**, 1247–9.

Heimberg, R.G., Hope, D.A., Dodge, C.S. *et al.* (1990) DSM-III-R subtypes of social phobia: comparison of generalized social phobics and public speaking phobics. *J Nerv Ment Dis* **173**, 172–9.

Heimberg, R.G., Liebowitz, M.R., Hope, D.A. *et al.* (1998) Cognitive behavioral group therapy versus phenelzine therapy for social phobia: 12 week outcome. *Arch Gen Psychiatry* **55**, 1133–41.

Heiser, J.F. & Defrancisco, D. (1976) The treatment of pathological panic states with propranolol. *Am J Psychiatry* **133**, 1389–94.

Hertzberg, M.A., Butterfield, M.I., Feldman, M.E. *et al.* (1999) A preliminary study of lamotrigine for the treatment of post-traumatic stress disorder. *Biol Psychiatry* **45**, 1226–9.

Hewlett, W.A., Vinogradov, S. & Agras, W.S. (1992) Clomipramine, clonazepam, and clonidine treatment of obsessive-compulsive disorder. *J Clin Psychopharmacol* **12**, 420–30.

Hirschmann, S., Dannon, P.N., Iancu, I., Dolberg, O.T., Zohar, J. & Grunhaus, L. (2000) Pindolol augmentation in patients with treatment-resistant panic disorder: a double-blind placebo-controlled trial. *J Clin Psychopharmacol* **20**, 556–9.

Hoehn-Saric, R., Merchant, A.F., Keyser, M.L. & Smith, V.K. (1981) Effects of clonidine on anxiety disorders. *Arch Gen Psychiatry* **38**, 1273–8.

Holub, B.J. (1986) Metabolism and function of myoinositol and inositol phospholipid. *American Review of Nutrition* **6**, 653–97.

Horrigan, J.P. (1996) Guanfacine for PTSD nightmares. *J Am Acad Child Adolesc Psychiatry* **35**, 975–6.

Horrigan, J.P. & Barnhill, L.J. (1996) The suppression of nightmares with guanfacine. *J Clin Psychiatry* **57**, 371.

Hussain, M.Z. & Ahad, A. (1970) Treatment of obsessive-compulsive neurosis. *CMAJ* **103**, 648–56.

Insel, T.R. & Pickar, D. (1983) Naloxone administration in obsessive-compulsive disorder: report of two cases. *Am J Psychiatry* **140**, 1219–20.

Jenike, M.A. (1993) Augmentation strategies for treatment-resistant obsessive-compulsive disorder. *Harv Rev Psychiatry* **1**, 17–26.

Johnson, M.R., Lydiard, B. & Ballenger, J.C. (1995) Panic disorder: pathophysiology and drug treatment. *Drugs* **69**, 328–44.

Johnson, M.R., Lydiard, R.B., Zealberg, J., Fossey, M.D. & Ballenger, J.C. (1994) Plasma and CSF HVA levels in panic patients with comorbid social phobia. *Biol Psychiatry* **36**, 425–7.

Johnson, G., Singh, B. & Leeman, M. (1976) Controlled evaluation of the β-adrenoreceptor blocking drug oxprenolol in anxiety. *Med J Aust* **1**, 909–12.

Kaplan, Z., Amir, M., Swarz, M. & Levine, J. (1996) Inositol treatment of post-traumatic stress disorder. *Anxiety* **2**, 51–2.

Kathol, R., Noyes, R. Jr, Slymen, D.J., Crowe, R.R., Clancy, J. & Kerber, R.E. (1980) Propranolol in chronic anxiety disorders: a controlled study. *Arch Gen Psychiatry* **37**, 1361–5.

Keck, P.E., Taylor, V.E., Tugrul, K.C., McElroy, S.L. & Bennett, J.A. (1993) Valproate treatment of panic disorder and lactate-induced panic attacks. *Biol Psychiatry* **33**, 542–6.

Kellner, R., Collins, A.C., Shulman, R.S. & Pathak, D. (1974) Short-term antianxiety effects of propranolol HCl. *J Clin Pharmacol* **14**, 301–4.

King, D.J., Devaney, N.M. & Gilbert, J.K. (1987) A double-blind placebo-controlled trial of a selective β_2-adrenoceptor antagonist (ICI 118551) in chronic anxiety. *Int Clin Psychopharmacol* **2**, 191–200.

Kinzie, J.D. & Leung, P. (1989) Clonidine in Cambodian patients with post-traumatic stress disorder. *J Nerv Ment Dis* **177**, 546–50.

Klein, E., Colin, V., Stolk, J. & Lenox, R.H. (1994) Alprazolam withdrawal in patients with panic disorder and generalized anxiety disorder. Vulnerability and effect of carbamazepine. *Am J Psychiatry* **151**, 1760–6.

Klein, E., Geraci, M. & Uhde, T.W. (1990) Inefficacy of single-dose nifedipine in the treatment of phobic anxiety. *Isr J Psychiatry Relat Sci* **27**, 1589–91.

Klein, E. & Uhde, T. (1988) Controlled study of verapamil for treatment of panic disorder. *Am J Psychiatry* **145**, 431–44.

Klein, E., Uhde, T.W., Post, R.M. (1982) Reply to a letter—carbamazepine, alprazolam withdrawal and panic disorder. *Am J Psychiatry* **144**, 266.

Ko, G.N., Elsworth, J.D., Roth, R.H., Rifkin, B.G., Leigh, H. & Redmond, E. (1983) Panic-induced elevation of plasma MHPG levels in phobic-anxious patients: effects of clonidine and imipramine. *Arch Gen Psychiatry* **40**, 425–30.

Koopowitz, L.F. & Berk, M. (1997) Response of obsessive-compulsive disorder to carbamazepine in two patients with comorbid epilepsy. *Ann Clin Psychiatry* **9**, 171–3.

Koran, L.M., Mueller, K. & Maloney, A. (1996) Will pindolol augment the response to a serotonin reuptake inhibitor in obsessive-compulsive disorder? *J Clin Psychopharmacol* **16**, 253–4.

Kramer, M.S., Cutler, N.R., Ballenger, J.C. *et al.* (1995) A placebo controlled trial of L-365,260, a CCK_B antagonist in panic disorder. *Biol Psychiatry* **37**, 462–6.

Krashin, D. & Oates, E.W. (1999) Risperidone as an adjunct therapy for post-traumatic stress disorder. *Military Medicine* **164**, 605–6.

Leckman, J.F., Goodman, W.R., North, W.C. *et al.* (1994) Elevated cerebrospinal fluid levels of oxytocin in obsessive-compulsive disorder: Comparison with Tourette's syndrome and healthy controls. *Arch Gen Psychiatry* **51**, 782–92.

Leonard, H.L. (1989) Drug treatment of obsessive-compulsive disorder. In: *Obsessive-Compulsive Disorder in Children and Adolescents* (J.L. Rapoport (ed.), pp. 217–36). American Psychiatric Press, Washington, D.C.

Levin, A.P., Saoud, J.B., Gorman, J.M., Fyer, A.J., Crawford, R. & Liebowitz, M.R. (1993) Responses of generalized and discrete social phobias during public speaking challenge. *J Anxiety Disord* 7, 207–21.

Levine, J., Barak, Y., Gonsalves, M. *et al.* (1995) Double-blind controlled trial of inosital treatment of depression. *Am J Psychiatry* 152, 792–4.

Leyba, C.M. & Wampler, T.P. (1998) Risperidone in PTSD. *Psychiatr Serv* 49, 245–6.

Liebowitz, M.R., Campeas, R. & Hollander, E. (1987) MAOIs: impact on social behavior. *Psychiatry Res* 22, 89–90.

Liebowitz, M.R., Fyer, A.J., McGrath, P. & Klein, D.F. (1981) Clonidine treatment of panic disorder. *Psychopharmacol Bull* 17, 122–3.

Liebowitz, M.R., Gorman, J.H., Fyer, A.J. & Klein, D.F. (1985) Social phobia. *Arch Gen Psychiatry* 42, 729–36.

Liebowitz, M.R., Schneier, F., Campeas, R. *et al.* (1992) Phenelzine versus atenolol in social phobia. *Arch Gen Psychiatry* 49, 290–300.

Liebowitz, M.R., Schneier, F.R., Hollander, E. *et al.* (1991) Treatment of social phobia with drugs other than benzodiazepines. *J Clin Psychiatry* 52 (Suppl. 11), 10–15.

Lipper, S., Davidson, J.R.T. & Grady, T.A. (1986) Preliminary study of carbamazepine in post-traumatic stress disorder. *Psychosomatics* 27, 849–54.

Looff, D., Grimley, P., Kuller, R., Martin, A. & Shonfield, L. (1995) Carbamazepine for PTSD. *J Am Acad Child Adolesc Psychiatry* 34, 703–4.

Lum, M., Fontaine, R., Elie, R. & Ortiveros, A. (1991) Probable interaction of sodium divalproate with benzodiazepines. *Prog Neuropsychopharmacol Biol Psychiatry* 15, 269–73.

Macleod, A.D. (1996) Vigabatrin and post-traumatic stress disorder. *J Clin Psychopharmacol* 16, 190–1.

McDougle, C.J., Epperson, C.N., Pelton, G.H., Wasylink, S. & Price, L.H. (2000) A double-blind, placebo-controlled study of risperidone addition in serotonin uptake inhibitor-refractory obsessive-compulsive disorder. *Arch Gen Psychiatry* 57, 794–801.

McDougle, C.J., Fleischmann, R.L., Epperson, C.N., Wasylink, S., Leckman, J.F. & Price, L.H. (1995) Risperidone addition in fluvoxamine-refractory obsessive-compulsive disorder: three cases. *J Clin Psychiatry* 56, 526–8.

McDougle, C.J., Goodman, W.K., Leckman, J.F., Lee, N.C., Heninger, G.R. & Price, L.H. (1994) Haloperidol addition in fluvoxamine-refractory obsessive-compulsive disorder. *Arch Gen Psychiatry* 51, 302–8.

McDougle, C.J., Goodman, W.K., Price, L.H. *et al.* (1990) Neuroleptic addition in fluvoxamine-refractory obsessive-compulsive disorder. *Am J Psychiatry* 147, 652–4.

McDougle, C.J., Price, L.H., Goodman, W.K., Charney, D.S. & Heninger, G.R. (1991) A controlled trial of lithium augmentation in fluvoxamine-refractory obsessive-compulsive disorder: lack of efficacy. *J Clin Psychopharmacol* 11, 175–84.

McElroy, S.L., Keck, P.E. & Lawrence, J.L. (1991) Treatment of panic disorder and benzodiazepine withdrawal with valproate. *J Neuropsychiatry Clin Neurosci* 2, 232–3.

McNamara, M.E. & Fogel, B.S. (1990) Anticonvulsant-responsive panic attacks with temporal lobe EEG abnormalities. *J Neuropsychiatry Clin Neurosci* 2, 193–6.

Meibach, R.C., Dunner, D., Wilson, L.G., Ishiki, D. & Dager, S.R. (1987) Comparative efficacy of propranolol, chlordicazepoxide and placebo in the treatment of anxiety: a double blind trial. *J Clin Psychiatry* 48, 355–8.

Mikkelsen, E.T., Deltor, J. & Cohen, D.J. (1981) School avoidance and social phobia triggered by haloperidol in patients with Tourette's disorder. *Am J Psychiatry* 138, 1572–6.

Moller, S.E., Mortensen, E.L., Breum, L. *et al.* (1996) Aggression and personality: association with amino acids and moneamin metabolites. *Psychol Med* 26, 323–31.

Monnelly, E.P. & Ciraulo, D.A. (1999) Risperidone effects on irritable aggression in post-traumatic stress disorder. *J Clin Psychopharmacol* 19, 377–8.

deMontigny, C. (1989) Cholecystokinin tetrapeptide induces panic-like attacks in healthy volunteers. *Arch Gen Psychiatry* 46, 511–17.

Moreno, F.A. & Delgado, P.L. (1997) Hallucinogen-induced relief of obsessions and compulsions. *Am J Psychiatry* 154, 1037–8.

Mundo, E., Guglielmo, E. & Bellido, L. (1998) Effect of adjuvant pindolol on the antiobsessional response to fluvoxamine: a double-blind, placebo-controlled study. *International Clinics of Psychopharmacology* 13, 219–24.

Munjack, D.J., Crocker, B., Cabe, D. *et al.* (1989) Alprazolam, Propranolol, and placebo in the treatment of panic disorder and agoraphobia with panic attacks. *J Clin Psychopharmacol* 9, 22–7.

Munjack, D.J., Rebal, R., Shaner, R., Staples, F., Brown, R. & Leonard, M. (1985) Imipramine versus propranolol for the treatment of panic attacks: a pilot study. *Compr Psychiatry* 26, 80–9.

Noyes, R.J., Anderson, D.J., Clancy, J. *et al.* (1984) Diazepam and propranolol in panic disorder and agoraphobia. *Arch Gen Psychiatry* 41, 287–92.

Nutt, D. (1989) Altered central α_2-adrenoreceptor sensitivity in panic disorder. *Arch Gen Psychiatry* 46, 165–9.

O'Regan, J.B. (1970) Treatment of obsessive-compulsive neurosis with haloperidol. *CMAJ* 103, 167–8.

Ohaeru, J.U. (2000) Naturalistic study of olanzapine in treatment-resistant schizophrenia and acute mania, depression and obsessional disorder. *East Afr Med J* 77, 86–92.

Ontiveros, A. & Fontaine, R. (1992) Sodium valproate and clonazepam for treatment resistant panic disorder. *J Psychiatry Neurosci* **17**, 78–80.

Pande, A.C., Davidson, J.R.T., Jefferson, J.W. *et al.* (1999b) Treatment of social phobia with gabapentin: a placebo controlled study. *J Clin Psychopharmacol* **19**, 341–438.

Pande, A.C., Greiner, M., Adams, J.B., Lydiard, R.B. & Pierce, M.W. (1999a) Placebo-controlled trial of the CCK-B antagonist CI-988 in panic disorder. *Biol Psychiatry* **46**, 860–2.

Pande, A.C., Pollack, M.K., Corchatt, J. *et al.* (2000) Placebo-controlled study of gabapentin treatment of panic disorder. *J Clin Psychopharmacol* **20**, 467–71.

Perlmutter, S.J., Leitman, S.F., Garvey, M.A. *et al.* (1999) Therapeutic plasma exchange and intravenous immunoglobulin for obsessive-compulsive disorder and tic disorders in childhood. *Lancet* **354**, 1153–8.

Petursson, H. & Lader, M.H. (1981) Withdrawal from long-term benzodiazepine treatment. *BMJ* **283**, 643–5.

Pfanner, C., Marazziti, D., Dell'Osso, L. *et al.* (2000) Risperidone augmentation in refractory obsessive-compulsive disorder: an open-label study. *International Clinics of Psychopharmacology* **15**, 297–301.

Piggot, T.A., Pato, M.T., L'Heureux, F. *et al.* (1991) A controlled comparison of adjuvant lithium carbonate of thyroid hormone in clomipramine-treated patients with obsessive-compulsive disorder. *J Clin Psychopharmacol* **11**, 242–8.

Potenza, M.N., Wasylink, S., Longhurst, J.G., Epperson, C.N. & McDougle, C.J. (1998) Olanzapine augmentation of fluoxetine in the treatment of refractory obsessive-compulsive disorder. *J Clin Psychopharmacol* **18**, 423–4.

Potts, N.L., Book, S. & Davidson, J.R. (1996) The neurobiology of social phobia. *Int Clin Psychopharmacol* **11** (Suppl. 3), 43–8.

Poyurovsky, M., Dorfman-Etrog, P., Hermesh, H., Tollefson, G.D. & Weizman, A. (2000) Beneficial effect of olanzapine in schizophrenic patients with obsessive-compulsive symptoms. *Int Clin Psychopharmacol* **15**, 169–73.

Primeau, F., Fontaine, R. & Beauclair, L. (1990) Valproic acid and panic disorder. *Can J Psychiatry* **35**, 248–50.

Ramsey, I., Greer, S. & Bagley, C. (1973) Propranolol in neurotic and thyrotoxic anxiety. *Br J Psychiatry* **122**, 555–60.

Raskind, M.A., Dobie, D.J., Kanter, E.D., Petrie, E.C., Thompson, C.E. & Peskind, E.R. (2000) The α-adrenergic antagonist prazosin ameliorates combat trauma nightmares in veterans with post-traumatic stress disorder: a report of four cases. *J Clin Psychiatry* **61**, 129–33.

Ravaris, C.I., Friedman, M.J., Hauri, P.J. & McHugo, G.J. (1991) A controlled study of alprazolam and propranolol in panic-disordered and agoraphobic outpatients. *J Clin Psychopharmacol* **11**, 344–50.

Redmond, D. & Huang, Y. (1979) Current concepts. II. New evidence for a locus coeruleus-norepinephrine connection with anxiety. *Life Sci* **25**, 2149–62.

Riddle, M.A., Leckman, J.F., Hardin, M.T., Anderson, G.M. & Cohen, D.J. (1988) Fluoxetine treatment of obsessions and compulsions in patients with Tourette's syndrome. *Am J Psychiatry* **145**, 1173–4.

Roy-Byrne, P.P. (1988) Anticonvulsants in anxiety and withdrawal syndromes: Hypotheses for future research. In: *Use of Anticonvulsants in Psychiatry: Recent Advances* (S.L. McElroy & H.G. Pope (eds), pp. 155–68). Oxford Health Care, Clifton, NJ.

Salzberg, A.D. & Swedo, S.E. (1992) Oxytocin and vasopressin in obsessive-compulsive disorder. *Am J Psychiatry* **149**, 713–14.

Schneier, F.R., Liebowitz, M.R., Abi-Dargham, A., Zea-Ponce, Y., Lin, S.H. & Laruelle, M. (2000) Low dopamine D2 receptor binding potential in social phobia. *Am J Psychiatry* **157**, 457–9.

Seedat, S. & Stein, D.J. (1999) Inositol augmentation of serotonin reuptake inhibitors in treatment-refractory obsessive-compulsive disorder: an open trial. *International Clinics of Psychopharmacology* **14**, 353–6.

Shapira, N.A., Keck, P.E. Jr, Goldsmith, T.D., McConville, B.J., Eis, M. & McElroy, S.L. (1997) Open-label pilot study of tramadol hydrochloride in treatment-refractory obsessive-compulsive disorder. *Depress Anxiety* **6**, 170–3.

Sheehan, D., Davidson, J. & Manshreck, T. (1983) Lack of efficacy of a new antidepressant (bupropion) in the treatment of panic disorder with phobias. *J Clin Psychopharmacol* **3**, 28–31.

Shehi, M. & Patterson, W.M. (1984) Treatment of panic attacks with alprazolam and propranolol. *Am J Psychiatry* **141**, 900–1.

Silverstone, J.T. (1974) Some new approaches to the treatment of anxiety. *Psychopharmacol Bull* **10**, 10–11.

Singh, L., Field, M.J., Ferris, P. *et al.* (1996) The antiepileptic agent gabapentin (Neurontin) possesses anxiolytic-like and antinociceptive actions that are reversed by D-serine. *Psychopharmacology (Berlin)* **127**, 1–9.

Southwick, S.M., Bremner, J.D., Rasmusson, A., Morgan, C.A., Arnsten, A. & Charney, D.S. (1999) Role of norepinephrine in the pathophysiology and treatment of post-traumatic stress disorder. *Biol Psychiatry* **46**, 1192–204.

Stein, M.B., Asmundson, G.J.G. & Chartier, M. (1994) Autonomic responsivity in generalized social phobia. *J Affect Disord* **31**, 211–21.

Stein, D.J., Bouwer, C., Hawkridge, S. & Emsley, R.A. (1997) Risperidone augmentation of serotonin reuptake inhibitors in obsessive-compulsive and related disorders. *J Clin Psychiatry* **58**, 119–22.

Stein, M.B., Heuser, I.J., Juncos, J.L. & Uhde, T.W. (1990) Anxiety disorders in patients with Parkinson's disease. *Am J Psychiatry* **147**, 217–20.

Stein, M.B., Tancer, M.E. & Uhde, T.W. (1992) Physiologic and plasma norepinephrine responses to orthostasis in patients with panic disorder and social phobia. *Arch Gen Psychiatry* **49**, 311–17.

Stein, M.B. & Uhde, T.W. (1989) Infrequent occurrence of EEG abnormalities in panic disorder. *Am J Psychiatry* **146**, 517–20.

Steinert, T., Schmidt-Michel, P.O. & Kaschka, W.P. (1996) Considerable improvement in a case of obsessive-compulsive disorder in an emotionally unstable personality disorder, borderline type under treatment with clozapine. *Pharmacopsychiatry* **29**, 111–14.

Strous, R.D., Patel, J.K., Zimmet, S. & Green, A.I. (1999) Clozapine and paroxetine in the treatment of schizophrenia and obsessive-compulsive features. *Am J Psychiatry* **156**, 973–4.

Svensson, T.J., Bunney, B.S. & Aghajanian, G.K. (1975) Inhibition of both noradrenergic and serotonergic neurons in brain by the α-adrenergic agonist clonidine. *Brain Res* **92**, 291–306.

Swartz, C.M. (1998) Betaxolol in anxiety disorders. *Ann Clin Psychiatry* **10**, 9–14.

Tanna, V.T., Penningroth, R.P. & Woolson, R.F. (1977) Propranolol in the treatment of anxiety neurosis. *Compr Psychiatry* **18**, 319–26.

Taylor, C.P., Gee, N.S., Su, T.Z. *et al.* (1998) A summary of mechanistic hypotheses of gabapentin pharmacology. *Epilepsy Res* **29**, 233–49.

Tibbo, P. & Gendemann, K. (1999) Improvement of obsessions and compulsions with clozapine in an individual with schizophrenia. *Can J Psychiatry* **44**, 1049–50.

Tiihonen, J., Kuikka, J., Bergstrom, K., Lepola, U., Koponen, H. & Leinonen, E. (1997) Dopamine reuptake site densities in patients with social phobia. *Am J Psychiatry* **154**, 239–42.

Tondo, L., Burrai, C., Scamonatti, L. *et al.* (1989) Carbamazepine in panic disorder. *Am J Psychiatry* **146**, 558–9.

Toren, P., Dor, J., Rehavi, M. & Weizman, A. (1996) Hypothalamic–pituitary–ovarian axis and mood. *Biol Psychiatry* **40**, 1051–5.

Tyrer, P.J. & Lader, M.H. (1973) Effects of β-adrenergic blockade with sotalol in chronic anxiety. *Clinical Pharmacology and Therapeutics* **14**, 418–26.

Tyrer, P.J. & Lader, M.H. (1974a) Response to propranolol and diazepam in somatic and psychic anxiety. *BMJ* **2**, 14–16.

Tyrer, P.J. & Lader, M.H. (1974b) Physiological responses to propranolol and diazepam in chronic anxiety. *British J Clin Pharmacol* **1**, 387–90.

Tyrer, P.J., Rutherford, D. & Huggett, T. (1981) Benzodiazepine withdrawal symptoms and propranolol. *Lancet* **1**, 520–2.

Uhde, T.W., Stein, M.B. & Post, R.M. (1988) Lack of efficacy of carbamazepine in the treatment of panic disorder. *Am J Psychiatry* **145**, 1104–9.

Uhde, T.W., Stein, M.B., Vittone, B.J. *et al.* (1989) Behavioral and physiological effects of short-term and long-term administration of clonidine in panic disorder. *Arch Gen Psychiatry* **46**, 170–7.

Ustun, T.B. & Sartorius, N. (eds) (1995) *Mental Illnesses In General Health Care. An International Study*. John Wiley, Chichester.

Van Megen, J.J., Westenberg, J.G. & den Boer, J.A. (1996) Effect of the cholecystokinin B receptor antagonist L-365,260 on lactate-induced panic attacks in panic disorder patients. *Biol Psychiatry* **40**, 804–6.

Van Megen, K.J.G.M., Westenberg, K.G.M., den Boer, J.A., Slacy, B., van Es-Radhakishun, F. & Parde, A.C. (1997) The cholecystokinin-β receptor antagonist CI-988 failed to affect CCK-4 induced symptoms in panic disorder patients. *Psychopharmacology* **129**, 243–8.

Venkatesh, A., Pauls, D.J., Crowe, R.R. *et al.* (1980) Mitral valve prolapse in neurosis (panic disorder). *Am Heart J* **100**, 302–5.

Villarreal, G., Johnson, M.R., Rubey, R., Lydiard, R.B. & Ballanger, J.C. (2000) Treatment of social phobia with the dopamine agonist pergolide. *Depress Anxiety* **11**, 45–7.

Weiss, M., Baerg, E., Wisebord, S. *et al.* (1995) The influence of gonadol hormones on periodicity of obsessive-compulsive disorder. *Can J Psychiatry* **40**, 205–7.

Weiss, E.L., Potenza, M.N., McDougle, C.J. & Epperson, C.N. (1999) Olanzapine addition in obsessive-compulsive disorder refractory to selective serotonin reuptake inhibitors: an open-label case series. *J Clin Psychiatry* **60**, 524–7.

Weizman, R., Gil-Ad, I., Hermesh, H., Munitz, H. & Laron, Z. (1990) Immunoreactive beta-endorphin, cortisol, and growth hormone plasma levels in obsessive-compulsive disorder. *Clin Neuropharmacol* **13**, 297–302.

Wheatley, D. (1969) Comparative effects of propranolol and chlordiazepoxide in anxiety states. *Br J Psychiatry* **115**, 1411–12.

Woodman, C.L. & Noyes, R. (1994) Panic disorder: treatment with valproate. *J Clin Psychiatry* **55**, 134–6.

Wurthmann, C., Klieser, E. & Lehmann, E. (1997) Side effects of low-dose neuroleptics and their impact on clinical outcome in generalized anxiety disorder. *Prog Neuropsychopharmacol Biol Psychiatry* **21**, 601–9.

Wurthmann, C., Klieser, E., Lehmann, E. & Pester, U. (1995) Test therapy in the treatment of generalized anxiety disorders with low-dose fluspirilene. *Prog Neuropsychopharmacol Biol Psychiatry* **19**, 1049–60.

26 Physical Treatments

T.E. Schlaepfer & B.D. Greenberg

Introduction

It should be clear that pharmacologic somatic treatments and special forms of psychotherapy have an important role to play in patients suffering from anxiety disorders. This chapter on physical treatments will focus on different methods of brain stimulation, which have mostly been only very recently introduced in the research on anxiety disorders and are at the moment far from a widespread introduction into the treatment armamentarium. Although they currently are most valuable as research tools in the elucidation of the underlying neurobiology of these disorders, these techniques may very well mature into treatment options for patients that are resistant to conventional interventions.

The methods discussed here are electroconvulsive therapy, repetitive transcranial magnetic stimulation, functional neurosurgery and vagus nerve stimulation. In terms of diagnostic categories we will focus mainly on obsessive-compulsive disorder because of the relative lack of efficacy of conventional treatments for a substantial proportion of patients suffering from severe forms of this disorder. Obsessive-compulsive disorder has a lifetime population prevalence of about 2% in a number of countries. An estimated five to six million people are affected in the US alone. Patients typically experience symptoms for prolonged periods, which can substantially impair social and occupational functioning (Rasmussen & Eisen 1992; Eisen *et al.* 1999; Malizia 1999).

Hypothesized brain circuit abnormalities in anxiety disorders

Association between basal ganglia disease and obsessive-compulsive symptoms, plus evolving knowledge of ganglia function, led to proposals that this was a likely locus of dysfunction in obsessive-compulsive disorder (OCD: Pitman *et al.* 1987; Rapoport & Wise 1988). Neuroimaging studies using different structural and functional imaging techniques have found: (i) abnormal basal ganglia volume in patients (e.g., Luxenberg *et al.* 1988; Robinson *et al.* 1995; Rosenberg *et al.* 1997), although not always consistently (Aylward *et al.* 1996); (ii) Other studies noted that, even with normal striatal volume, other abnormalities, such as low N-acetyl-aspartate concentrations on magnetic resonance spectroscopy were found, presumably representing reduced basal ganglia neuronal integrity (Ebert *et al.* 1997; Bartha *et al.* 1998).

Since OCD may in theory arise from dysfunction in several brain regions, perhaps most likely at different points in corticobasal circuits, structural measures may find abnormalities in any given region inconsistently. For example, prefrontal cortex dysfunction is also likely to play a role in OCD (Flor-Henry *et al.* 1979; Ward 1988; Otto 1992). However, initial studies of prefrontal volume found no differences between OCD patients and volunteers (Insel *et al.* 1983; Behar *et al.* 1984; Jenike *et al.* 1996). One early study, using a different magnetic resonance imaging (MRI) technique, found prolonged MRI T1 relaxation times in right prefrontal white matter in OCD patients, and an abnormally greater right–left T1 difference in patients. The degree of asymmetry was correlated with symptom severity in that study (Garber *et al.* 1989). In general, since volumetric differences between patients and healthy individuals may be relatively modest, they may be difficult to find in the relatively small samples typically studied. Complicating matters further, the etiology of OCD is likely heterogeneous.

The results of functional neuroimaging studies have been more consistent. Photon emission tomography (PET) and single photon emission computerized tomography (SPECT) studies have found abnormalities at various points within the corticobasal loops described by Alexander *et al.* (1986). For example, several fluorodeoxyglucose positron emission tomography (FDG-PET) studies of OCD patients at rest (when no effort was made to provoke symptoms) found increased metabolism, most commonly in the caudate nuclei, orbitofrontal cortex, and cingulate gyrus (Baxter *et al.* 1987, 1988; Nordahl *et al.* 1989; Swedo *et al.* 1989). One of these studies also found increased lateral prefrontal metabolism (Swedo *et al.* 1989). HMPAO-SPECT studies found enhanced medial and dorsolateral prefrontal perfu-sion in untreated OCD patients compared to controls (Hoehn-Saric *et al.* 1991; Harris *et al.* 1994). On PET during experimental OCD symptom provocation, activation of orbitofrontal cortex, caudate nucleus, and the cingulate gyrus was observed, and changes in thalamic activity approached significance (Rauch *et al.* 1994). Furthermore, effective medication or behavioral treatment was associated with activity reductions in the same structures, including caudate (Baxter 1994), orbitofrontal cortex (Swedo *et al.* 1992), and in a putative network including orbitofrontal cortex, caudate, and anterior cingulate (Schwartz *et al.* 1996). Interestingly, the response to treatment has been most often associated with reduced metabolism in the right cerebral hemisphere.

These findings are generally consistent with the earlier views of possible neuroanatomic substrates of OCD (Rapoport & Wise 1988). They have also influenced more detailed models of how a failure of normal inhibitory modulation within the parallel corticobasal loops might be involved in the illness (Modell *et al.* 1989; Baxter *et al.* 1990; Rauch & Baxter 1998). One working hypothesis is that obsessive-compulsive symptoms arise when the processing of cortical input to the basal ganglia is defective. The resulting dysregulated thalamocortical excitatory drive would likely further exacerbate abnormal basal ganglia function. Excessive and abnormally modulated activity throughout these circuits could result. As noted, studies using functional and structural neuroimaging support this view. Data from a recent study using the paired-pulse transcranial magnetic stimulation (pTMS) technique are also congruent with this hypothesis (Greenberg *et al.* 2000).

Reports of neurosurgical operations used in a small number of treatment-refractory OCD patients also are consistent with the current anatomical models of pathophysiology. Despite important methodological difficulties with these studies, neurosurgical procedures, including stereotactic anterior cingulotomy and capsulotomy, have been reported to have the common effect of reducing anxiety and core OCD symptom severity in at least some severely affected patients. All of the procedures described in the literature would be expected to have either direct or indirect effects on cortical–striatal–thalamic–pallidal circuits. Different procedures may have different effects, and reduced symptoms could occur as a direct consequence of the lesions made, or of secondary degeneration and consequent functional plasticity in other parts of the brain. While this possibility has yet to be systematically investigated, a preliminary investigation found that OCD symptoms and prefrontal metabolism appeared to be reduced in tandem after stereotactic anterior capsulotomy (Mindus *et al.* 1986).

Electroconvulsive therapy

Electroconvulsive therapy (ECT) is the somatic treatment with the longest history of continuous use in psychiatry. Cerletti and Bini had already introduced it as a clinical treatment in 1937 (Fink 1984). Significant improvements in the technique of ECT have been made since then, including the use of synthetic muscle relaxants, like succinylcholine, the anaesthesia of patients with short-acting agents, preoxygenation of the patient, the use of electroencephalogram (EEG) recording and significantly improved stimulators, all measures which lead to greatly reducing the morbidity associated with the treatment. Despite these advances, the popularity of ECT decreased in the 1960s and 1970s, due to the use of more effective neuroleptics and as a result of a strong antiECT movement. However, ECT has gained popularity again in the last 15 years due to its efficacy, and it is the only somatic therapy from the 1930s that remains in widespread use today. Between 100 000 and 150 000 patients are subjected to ECT every year in the US, under strictly defined medical conditions. The efficacy of ECT has been well-established in major depression and, to a lesser degree, in mania and schizophrenia (Fink 1985).

OCD was considered particularly resistant to ECT treatment, but more recent data have called this dogma into question (Khanna *et al.* 1988; Goodman *et al.* 1993; Husain *et al.* 1993; Maletzky *et al.* 1994). This is especially true for patients suffering from concomitant affective symptoms.

Clinically, it is reasonable to consider ECT in patients with concomitant depression and OCD or other anxiety disorders, but its efficacy in pure, refractory OCD remains an open question, which would merit careful study in larger treatment trials. ECT is likely already used fairly often in intractably ill OCD patients, most of whom have comorbid mood disorders. And, as is the case for other neuropsychiatric disorders, case studies or experimental trials of ECT in patients with severe OCD who did not respond would probably not be reported.

In any case, like with all chronic psychiatric disorders, adequate planning should be made with regards to the treatment strategy following ECT if the patient's condition responds, like new medication regimens or maintenance ECT.

Repetitive transcranial magnetic stimulation

Repetitive transcranial magnetic stimulation (rTMS) has been used in neurology as a method of investigation for almost two decades. Its application as a putative treatment in neuropsychiatric disorders, particularly affective and anxiety disorders, is much more recent. There is now abundant evidence for the involvement of the prefrontal cortex in affective processes. rTMS allows for an extremely focal and relatively noninvasive stimulation of cortical tissue and therefore interference of those brain circuits, and looks like an excellent tool for investigation of the neurobiology of anxiety disorders, foremost OCD, in which a large amount of data on local brain abnormalities has been obtained from neuroimaging studies. rTMS appears to have focal and selective excitatory or inhibitory (depending on stimulation frequency) cortical effects, as a function of stimulation parameters, thereby offering the capacity to probe both the anatomic localization and the neurophysiological

alterations that result in psychiatric manifestations or symptomatic improvement. Research with this new tool has contributed to our understanding of a variety of clinical and basic research issues.

Methodology of transcranial magnetic stimulation

Transcranial magnetic stimulation (TMS) uses the physical principle of inductance to transmit energy transcranially across scalp and skull without the painful side-effects of direct transcranial electrical stimulation. TMS involves placing a small coil of wire on the scalp and passing a very powerful current through it (Barker *et al.* 1985; Roth *et al.* 1991). This produces a magnetic field that passes largely unimpeded through the tissues of the head (in contrast to electric fields, which are diffused by head tissue). Oscillations in the magnetic field induce an electrical current in the brain. The strength of the induced current is largely a function of the rate of change of the magnetic field, which varies with the current in the coil. Other factors are the strength of the current and the coil geometry and the number of windings in the coil (Cohen *et al.* 1990; Rothwell *et al.* 1991). In order to induce enough current to depolarize neurones in the brain, the current passed through the stimulating coil must start and stop or reverse its direction within about 300 ms.

rTMS in OCD

As noted, brain circuit models of OCD have in common certain functionally linked brain areas, principally prefrontal cortex (orbitofrontal cortex and dorsolateral prefrontal cortex), "paralimbic" structures (anterior cingulate, anterior temporal, parahippocampal, and insular cortex), basal ganglia (caudate nucleus, putamen, globus pallidus), and thalamus (Modell *et al.* 1989; Leckman *et al.* 1997). Prefrontal cortex is consistently implicated in the symptomatic state in OCD by functional neuroimaging (Hoehn-Saric & Greenberg 1997). The region is further implicated because it plays an important role in functions, e.g., response inhibition, verifying operations, and mood regulation. These processes are very likely to be important in the elaboration of OCD symptoms. rTMS of the prefrontal cortex may provide further evidence of the importance of this region in OCD symptoms.

We performed a preliminary controlled study of rTMS as a probe of prefrontal cortex involvement in

OCD (Greenberg *et al.* 1997). Most of the 12 patients with OCD were moderately ill (the mean entry Yale–Brown Obsessive Compulsive Scale score was 20); two more severely ill individuals were included. Single sessions of high frequency (20 Hz) stimulation were administered, in a randomized design, to left and right dorsolateral prefrontal cortex, and to a parieto-occipital control site. The prefrontal locations were 5 cm anterior and 2 cm inferior to the hand area of primary motor cortex on each side; the parieto-occipital control site, which also received active stimulation, was 10 cm posterior to primary motor cortex in the midline. Each site was stimulated, 2 days apart, with 20 Hz trains of 2 s each, once per minute for 20 min (800 pulses total per session) with a figure eight-shaped focal coil attached to a Cadwell High Speed Magnetic Stimulator (Cadwell Laboratory, Kennewick, WA). rTMS intensity was 80% of abductor pollicis brevis twitch threshold.

The data indicated a selective reduction in compulsive urges only after right prefrontal rTMS. The symptom reduction lasted at least 8 h. These OCD patients, who were not clinically depressed as a group, also reported significant mood elevation 30 min after right prefrontal stimulation, but this was more transient than the reduction in compulsive urges.

The laterally specific effect was unexpected but interesting in light of several lines of evidence (Greenberg *et al.* 1997; Lippitz *et al.* 1999). These include studies finding that provocation of OCD symptoms (primarily compulsive urges) was associated with increased perfusion in the right caudate (Rauch *et al.* 1994) and in the right orbitofrontal cortex (McGuire *et al.* 1994) on PET. In contrast, another study found orbitofrontal perfusion increased bilaterally after provocation (Rauch *et al.* 1994).

Even more intriguing is that effects of treatment are preferentially associated with changes in right hemisphere activity. Improvement after pharmacological or behavioral treatment has been associated with reduction in right medial prefrontal or right orbitofrontal metabolism (Baxter *et al.* 1992; Swedo *et al.* 1992) or perfusion (Hoehn-Saric *et al.* 1991; Harris *et al.* 1994) with reduction in metabolic rates in the right caudate nucleus (Baxter *et al.* 1992), with normalized metabolic rates in the right prefrontal cortex (Benkelfat *et al.* 1990), and with reduction in an abnormally high pretreatment correlation between metabolic rates in the right prefrontal cortex and the right caudate nucleus (Baxter *et al.* 1992; Schwartz *et al.* 1996).

More tentative evidence of hemispheric selectivity in OCD comes from an open neurosurgical study in which the position of right- but not left-sided anterior capsulotomy lesions appeared to influence efficacy in intractable OCD (Lippitz *et al.* 1999). The findings above lend some support to the view that laterality of activity in corticobasal circuits may be important in OCD. It is also possible that findings implicating right-sided abnormalities in OCD are important although not specific to the illness. The data preferentially supporting right hemisphere activity in OCD may, for example, relate to a large literature implicating right hemisphere activity in the experience of negative emotion (Davidson *et al.* 1999), and in emotional processing more generally.

Our initial study of rTMS in OCD suggested that a single stimulation session might have reduced compulsions by affecting prefrontal function for longer than the immediate stimulation period (Greenberg *et al.* 1997). Further testing in studies combining rTMS with functional neuroimaging, and with cognitive probes of regional brain activity in OCD, are needed to establish this relationship more definitively.

The effects of prefrontal rTMS on OCD symptoms, which developed rapidly after stimulation, contrast with the much more gradual symptom improvement after neurosurgery discussed above, and with the effects of conventional medication treatment and behavior therapy. A likely reason for this difference in time course is that the therapeutic effects of neurosurgery, and conventional treatment depend on ongoing neural plasticity in brain circuits affected, perhaps primarily within cortico–striato–thalamo–cortical loops. The contrasting acute effects of prefrontal rTMS in OCD suggest a more immediate, and transient, disruption of activity necessary for the elaboration of compulsive urges. In theory, this could occur via a direct rTMS-induced disruption of prefrontal activity necessary for symptoms, or indirectly, via enhancement of activity in brain pathways that modulate OCD symptoms.

rTMS in anxiety disorders other than OCD

Treatment studies in other anxiety disorders have been largely impressionistic. McCann *et al.* (1998) reported that two patients with post-traumatic stress disorder showed improvement during open treatment with 1 Hz rTMS over the right frontal cortex. Grisaru *et al.* (1998) stimulated 10 patients suffering from post-traumatic stress disorder over the motor cortex and reported decreased anxiety. It is very likely that rTMS will be most useful in the study of neuronal circuits involved in anxiety disorders of it is coupled with other measures of cerebral function.

Vagus nerve stimulation

Another, less invasive means of directly affecting central function is to stimulate the cranial nerves that are direct extensions of the brain with chronically implanted electrical stimulators in the chest wall and stimulating leads placed over the left vagus. This can be used instead of neurosurgery to achieve functional alteration of networks for therapeutic benefit in central pain syndromes and movement disorders. For years, scientists have been interested in whether and how autonomic functions modulate activity in the limbic system and higher cortex. Numerous studies have identified extensive projections of the vagus nerve via its sensory afferent connections in the nucleus tractus solitarius (NTS) to many brain areas (Bailey & Bremer 1938; MacLean 1990). Vagus nerve stimulation (VNS) is currently used in the treatment of complex partial seizures (Ben-Menachem *et al.* 1995; Handforth *et al.* 1998). These studies in a total of 313 treatment-resistant patients demonstrated a mean decline of overall seizure frequency of about 25–30% compared to baseline. Some evidence in this patient group pointed toward the possible benefit of VNS as an antidepressant or mood-stabilizing treatment. These included clinical observations of mood improvement in epilepsy patients (Elger *et al.* 2000), anatomic afferent connections of the left vagus nerve to the central nervous system (CNS) and to structures relevant to mood regulation, the anticonvulsant activity of VNS taken in the context of the role of anticonvulsant medications or ECT in treating mood disorders, neurochemical studies indicating VNS effects on key neurotransmitters involved in mood regulation, and evidence that VNS changes the metabolic activity of key limbic system structures (George *et al.* 2000). This evidence led to an initial open trial of left-sided VNS in a group of treatment resistant patients described in the companion article in this journal (Rush *et al.* 2000). This clinical open trial demonstrated that VNS might be a new method for treating patients with severe treatment-resistant depression. It showed that 40% of

the 30 treated patients displayed at least a 50% or greater improvement in their condition as assessed with the Hamilton Rating Scale for Depression. Half the patients also had at least a 50% improvement on the Montgomery Asberg Depression Rating Scale.

In December 2000, the US Food and Drug Administration (FDA) granted Cyberonics Inc. an unconditional investigational device exemption (IDE) for a pilot study of VNS with the NCP® system in treating patients with OCD, panic disorder and adult onset post-traumatic stress disorder. Up to 30 patients at four study sites will be implanted with the NCP® system and stimulated with left cervical (neck area) vagus nerve stimulation. Additional study sites will be initiated through 2002.

Functional neurosurgery

Functional neurosurgery in psychiatry is used to alter the physiology of specific neural systems to treat specific disorders (Diering & Bell 1991). Previously referred to as psychosurgery, functional neurosurgery is currently conducted on a small number of patients with treatment-resistant mood, anxiety, and other psychiatric disorders (Yudofsky & Ovsiew 1990). Although originally used extensively in schizophrenia, functional neurosurgery has generally been found to be more effective in major depression and OCD.

Early studies by Papez (1937) identified limbic circuits as key to emotion regulation, and it is these limbic structures that have been the targets of most neurosurgical approaches in psychiatry. Attempts to refine early surgical approaches led to the use of less extensive lesions (Fulton 1949) and stereotactic procedures with enhanced anatomical specificity. More targeted procedures included the thalamotomy (Spiegel *et al.* 1950), cingulotomy (Cassidy *et al.* 1965), subcaudate tractotomy (Knight 1965), and limbic leukotomy (combination of cingulotomy and subcaudate tractotomy: Kelly *et al.* 1973).

Current stereotactic neurosurgical procedures for psychiatric disorders

Modern stereotactic approaches have reduced morbidity and produce only transient effects on attention, without reported long-term effects on neurological status, higher brain functions, or personality (Maxwell

1993). Nonetheless, a significant percentage of patients may have a new onset seizure disorder following these surgical interventions. Two of the more common procedures (cingulotomy, anterior capsulotomy) are described below (Mindus & Jenike 1992). Other procedures include amygdalotomy (for aggression), hypothalamotomy, thalamotomy, and surgery for various combinations of limbic structures. While modern stereotactic technique and standardized psychiatric diagnosis have improved the generalizability of these studies, most remain uncontrolled and retrospective.

Anterior cingulotomy

Anterior cingulotomy refers to the bilateral severing of the anterior supracallosal fibers of the anterior cingulate, altering connections within the limbic system. This procedure has been reported to be efficacious not only in the treatment of mood disorders and intractable pain but also in anxiety disorders (Ballantine *et al.* 1977). Therapeutic results are generally better in the treatment of major depression (about 60%) than in OCD and, importantly, appear only after some considerable postsurgery delay. Ballantine *et al.* (1977) reported that 75% of 154 patients with mood disorder improved after bilateral cingulotomy. A retrospective review by Jenike *et al.* (1991) found that 25–30% of OCD patients benefited substantially from cingulotomy. This therapeutic effect in OCD is thought to be due to interruption of abnormal fronto–striatal–thalamic activity, as suggested by PET imaging studies (Martuza *et al.* 1990). The claim that destruction of the anterior cingulate is associated with antidepressant effects is compatible with some findings from imaging studies of sleep deprivation (Wu *et al.* 1992) and pharmacological treatment (Bench *et al.* 1995), indicating reduced functional activity in this region to be correlated with antidepressant response.

Anterior capsulotomy

Anterior capsulotomy entails the destruction of the anterior limb of the internal capsule, which severs thalamo–orbitofrontal fibers (Hay *et al.* 1993). This may be accomplished via radiofrequency heat lesions or gamma irradiation using the gamma knife, a stereotactic gamma irradiation unit (Sabatini *et al.* 1994).

This procedure has been reported to have efficacy in OCD with about a 70% success rate (Martuza *et al.* 1990).

Conclusions

The literature on using surgical ablation techniques in the treatment of psychiatric disorders is quite small, and since all procedures other than gamma irradiation involve opening the skull, there has been little opportunity for sham-controlled investigation. Both the retrospective nature of the studies and the seriousness of the intervention, limit the certainty about claims of therapeutic efficacy. At the same time, it should be recognized that patients who receive these procedures almost invariably have chronic and severe mood disorders or OCD, and often other comorbid illnesses. They have virtually exhausted their options for other forms of treatment. Modern criteria for use of functional neurosurgery are especially rigorous in selecting for highly treatment-resistant patients. Therefore, reports of significant improvement in a substantial percentage of patients deserve attention.

In general, the literature on functional neurosurgery in anxiety disorders supports the role of limbic structures in these syndromes. While the specific anatomical targets for the various neurosurgical approaches have varied, all the procedures affect limbic networks, directly or indirectly. This may result in alterations in the relative activity of various structures in this network. In addition, the injury to fronto–limbic connections may alter serotonergic and dopaminergic transmission at sites remote from the lesion (Corkin *et al.* 1979). The association between the time course of mood changes and the appearance of thalamic atrophy following frontal leukotomy supports the importance of these remote effects.

Acknowledgements

This chapter is supported in part by grants from the Swiss National Science Foundation (3200–047130, 4038–044046 and 3231–044523, Dr. Schlaepfer), and an Independent Investigator Award from the National Alliance for Research on Schizophrenia and Depression (Dr. Greenberg).

References

Alexander, G.E., DeLong, M.R. & Strick, P.L. (1986) Parallel organization of functionally segregated circuits linking basal ganglia and cortex. *Annu Rev Neurosci* **9**, 357–81.

Aylward, E.H., Reiss, A.L., Reader, M.J. *et al.* (1996) Basal ganglia volumes in children with attention-deficit hyperactivity disorder. *J Child Neurol* **11**(2), 112–15.

Bailey, P. & Bremer, F. (1938) A sensory cortical representation of the vagus nerve. *J Neurophysiol* 405–12.

Ballantine, H., Levy, B., Dagi, T. & Giriunas, I. (1977) Cingulotomy for psychiatric illness: report of 13 years' experience. In: *Neurosurgical Treatment in Psychiatry, Pain, and Epilepsy* (W. Sweet, S. Obrador & J. Martin-Rodriguez (eds)), pp. 333–54). University Park Press.

Barker, A.T., Jalinous, R. & Fresston, I.L. (1985) Non-invasive magnetic stimulation of human motor cortex. *Lancet* **1**(2), 1106–7.

Bartha, R., Stein, M.B., Williamson, P.C. *et al.* (1998) A short echo 1H spectroscopy and volume tric MRI study of the corpus striatum in patients with obsessive-compulsive disorder and comparison subjects. *Am J Psychiatry* **155**, 1584–91.

Baxter, L.R.J. (1994) Positron emission tomography studies of cerebral glucose metabolism in obsessive-compulsive disorder. *J Clin Psychiatry* **55**(10) (Suppl.), 54–9.

Baxter, L.R., Jr. Phelps, M.E., Mazziotta, J.C., Guze, B.H., Schwartz, J.M. & Selin, C.E. (1987) Local cerebral glucose metabolic rates in obsessive-compulsive disorder. A comparison with rates in unipolar depression and in normal controls. *Arch Gen Psychiatry* **44**, 211–18.

Baxter, L.R., Jr. Schwartz, J.M., Guze, B.H., Bergman, K. & Szuba, M.P. (1988) Cerebral glucose metabolic rates in nondepressed patients with obsessive-compulsive disorder. *Am J Psychiatry* **145**, 1560–3.

Baxter, L.R., Jr. Schwartz, J.M., Mazziotta, J.C. *et al.* (1990) PET imaging in obsessive-compulsive disorder with and without depression. *J Clin Psychiatry* **51** (Suppl.), 61–9; discussion 70.

Baxter, L.R., Jr. Schwartz, J.M. & Bergman, K.S. (1992) Caudate glucose metabolic rate changes with drug and behavior therapy for obsessive-compulsive disorder. *Arch Gen Psychiatry* **49**, 681–9.

Behar, D., Rapoport, J.L., Berg, C.J. *et al.* (1984) Computerized tomography and neuropsychological test measures in adolescents with obsessive-compulsive disorder. *Am J Psychiatry* **141**(3), 363–9.

Bench, C., Frackowiak, R. & Dolan, R. (1995) Changes in regional cerebral blood flow on recovery from depression. *Psychol Med* **25**, 247–61.

Benkelfat, C., Nordahl, T.E. & Semple, W.E. (1990) Local cerebral glucose metabolic rates in obsessive-compulsive disorder: patients treated with clomipramine. *Arch Gen Psychiatry* **47**, 840–8.

Ben-Menachem, E., Hamberger, A., Hedner, T., Hammond, E., & Uthman, B. (1995) Effects of vagus nerve stimulation on amino acids and other metabolites in the CSF of patients with partial seizures. *Epilepsy Res* **20**, 221–7.

Cassidy, W., Ballantine, H. & Flanagan, N. (1965) Frontal cingulotomy for affective disorders. *Biol Psychiatry* **8**, 269.

Cohen, L.G., Roth, B.J., Nilsson, J. *et al.* (1990) Effects of coil design on delivery of focal magnetic stimulation. Technical considerations. *Electroencephalogr Clin Neurophysiol* **73**, 350–7.

Corkin, S., Twitchell, T. & Sullivan, E. (1979) Safety and efficacy of cingulotomy for pain and psychiatric disorders. In: *Modern Concepts in Psychiatric Surgery* (E. Hitchcock & H. Ballantine (eds)). Elsevier/North-Holland Biomedical Press, New York.

Davidson, R.J., Abercrombie, H., Nitschke, J.B. & Putnam, K. (1999) Regional brain function, emotion and disorders of emotion. *Curr Opin Neurobiol* **9**(2), 228–34.

Diering, S. & Bell, W. (1991) Functional neurosurgery for psychiatric disorders: a historical perspective. *Stereotact Funct Neurosurg* **57**, 175–94.

Ebert, D., Speck, O., Konig, A., Berger, M., Hennig, J. & Hohagen, F. (1997) 1H-magnetic resonance spectroscopy in obsessive-compulsive disorder: evidence for neuronal loss in the cingulate gyrus and the right striatum. *Psychiatry Res* **74**(3), 173–6.

Eisen, J.L., Goodman, W.K., Keller, M.B. *et al.* (1999) Patterns of remission and relapse in obsessive-compulsive disorder: a 2-year prospective study. *J Clin Psychiatry* **60**(5), 346–51; quiz 352.

Elger, G., Hoppe, C., Falkai, P., Rush, A. & Elger, C. (2000) Vagus nerve stimulation is associated with mood improvements in epilepsy patients. *Epilepsy Res* **42**(2–3), 203–10.

Fink, M. (1984) Meduna and the origins of convulsive therapy. *Am J Psychiatry* **141**, 1034–41.

Fink, M. (1985) *Convulsive Therapy*. Raven Press, New York.

Flor-Henry, P., Yeudall, L.T., Koles, Z.J. & Howarth, B.G. (1979) Neuropsychological and power spectral EEG investigations of the obsessive-compulsive syndrome. *Biol Psychiatry* **14**(1), 119–30.

Fulton, J. (1949) *Functional Localization in Relation to Frontal Lobotomy*. Oxford University Press, Oxford.

Garber, H., Ananth, J., Chiu, L., Griswald, V. & Oldendorf, W. (1989) Nuclear magnetic resonance study of obsessive-compulsive disorder. *Am J Psychiatry* **146**, 1001–5.

George, M., Sackeim, H., Rush, A. *et al.* (2000) Vagus nerve stimulation: a new tool for brain research and therapy. *Biol Psychiatry* **47**(4), 287–95.

Goodman, W., McDougle, C., Barr, L., Aronson, S. & Prices, L. (1993) Biological approaches to treatment-resistant obsessive-compulsive disorder. *J Clin Psychiatry* 54 (Suppl.), 16–26.

Greenberg, B.D., George, M.S., Martin, J.D. *et al.* (1997) Effect of prefrontal repetitive transcranial magnetic stimulation in obsessive-compulsive disorder: a preliminary study. *Am J Psychiatry* 154(6), 867–9.

Greenberg, B.D., Ziemann, U., Cora-Locatelli, G. *et al.* (2000) Altered cortical excitability in obsessive-compulsive disorder. *Neurology* 54, 142–7.

Grisaru, N., Amir, M., Cohen, H. & Kaplan, Z. (1998) Effect of transcranial magnetic stimulation in post-traumatic stress disorder: a preliminary study. *Biol Psychiatry* 44(1), 52–5.

Handforth, A., DeGiorgio, C., Schachter, S., Uthman, B., Naritoku, D. & Tecoma, E. (1998) Vagus nerve stimulation therapy for partial-onset seizures: a randomized active control trial. *Neurology* 51, 48–55.

Harris, G.J., Hoehn-Saric, R., Lewis, R., Pearlson, G.D. & Steeter, C. (1994) Mapping of SPECT regional cerebral perfusion abnormalities in obsessive-compulsive disorder. *Human Brain Mapping* 237–48.

Hay, P., Sachdev, P., Cumming, S. *et al.* (1993) Treatment of obsessive-compulsive disorder by psychosurgery. *Acta Psychiatr Scand* 87, 197–207.

Hoehn-Saric, R. & Greenberg, B.D. (1997) Psychobiology of obsessive-compulsive disorder: anatomical and physiological considerations. *Int Rev Psychiatry* 9, 15–30.

Hoehn-Saric, R., Pearlson, G.D., Harris, G.J., Machlin, S.R. & Camargo, E.E. (1991) Effects of fluoxetine on regional cerebral blood flow in obsessive-compulsive patients. *Am J Psychiatry* 148, 1243–5.

Husain, M., Lewis, S. & Thronton, W. (1993) Maintenance ECT for refractory obsessive-compulsive disorder. *Am J Psychiatry* 150(12), 1899–900.

Insel, T.R., Murphy, D.L., Cohen, R.M., Alterman, I., Kilts, C. & Linnoila, M. (1983) Obsessive-compulsive disorder: a double-blind trial of clomipramine and clorgyline. *Arch Gen Psychiatry* 40, 605–12.

Jenike, M.A., Baer, L., Ballantine, T. *et al.* (1991) Cingulotomy for refractory obsessive-compulsive disorder. A long-term follow-up of 33 patients [see comments]. *Arch Gen Psychiatry* 48(6), 548–55.

Jenike, M.A., Breiter, H.C., Baer, L. *et al.* (1996) Cerebral structural abnormalities in obsessive-compulsive disorder. A quantitative morphometric magnetic resonance imaging study [see comments]. *Arch Gen Psychiatry* 53(7), 625–32.

Kelly, D., Richardson, A. & Mitchell-Heggs, N. (1973) Stereotactic limbic leucotomy: neurophysiological aspects and operative techniques. *Br J Psychiatry* 123, 133.

Khanna, S., Gangadhar, B., Sinha, V., Rajendra, P. & Channabasavanna, S. (1988) Electroconvulsive therapy in obsessive-compulsive disorder. *Convulsive Ther* 4, 314–20.

Knight, G. (1965) Stereotactic tractotomy in the surgical treatment of mental illness. *J Neurol Neurosurg Psychiatry* 28, 304.

Leckman, J.F., Grice, D.E., Boardman, J. *et al.* (1997) Symptoms of obsessive-compulsive disorder. *Am J Psychiatry* 154(7), 911–17.

Lippitz, B.E., Mindus, P., Meyerson, B.A., Kihlstrom, L. & Lindquist, C. (1999) Lesion topography and outcome after thermocapsulotomy or gamma knife capsulotomy for obsessive-compulsive disorder: relevance of the right hemisphere [In process citation]. *Neurosurgery* 44(3), 452–8; discussion 458–60.

Luxenberg, J.S., Swedo, S.E., Flament, M.F., Friedland, R.P., Rapoport, J. & Rapoport, S.I. (1988) Neuroanatomical abnormalities in obsessive-compulsive disorder detected with quantitative X-ray computed tomography. *Am J Psychiatry* 145(9), 1089–93.

MacLean, P. (1990) *The Triune Brain in Evolution: Role in Paleocerebral Functions*. Plenum Press, New York.

Maletzky, B., McFarland, B. & Burt, A. (1994) Refractory obsessive-compulsive disorder and ECT. *Convulsive Ther* 10(1), 34–42.

Malizia, A. (1999) What do brain imaging studies tell us about anxiety disorders? *J Psychopharmacol* 13, 372–8.

Martuza, R.L., Chiocca, E.A., Jenike, M.A., Giriunas, I.E. & Ballantine, H.T. (1990) Stereotactic radio-frequency thermal cingulotomy for obsessive-compulsive disorder [see comments]. *J Neuropsychiatry Clin Neurosci* 2(3), 331–6.

Maxwell, R. (1993) *Behavioral Modification. Brain Surgery: Complication Avoidance and Management*. Churchill Livingstone, New York.

McCann, U.D., Kimbrell, T.A., Morgan, C.M. *et al.* (1998) Repetitive transcranial magnetic stimulation for post-traumatic stress disorder. *Arch Gen Psychiatry* 55(3), 276–9.

McGuire, P.K., Bench, C.J., Frith, C.D., Marks, I.M., Frackowiak, R.S. & Dolan, R.J. (1994) Functional anatomy of obsessive-compulsive phenomena. *Br J Psychiatry* 164, 459–68.

Mindus, P., Bergstrom, K., Thuomas, K.A. & Hindmarsh, T. (1986) Magnetic resonance imaging of stereotactic radiosurgical lesions in the internal capsule. *Acta Radiol suppl* 369, 614–17.

Mindus, P. & Jenike, M. (1992) Neurosurgical treatment of malignant obsessive-compulsive disorder. *Psychiatr Clin North Am* 15, 921–38.

Modell, J.G., Mountz, J.M., Curtis, G.C. & Greden, J.F. (1989) Neurophysiologic dysfunction in basal ganglia/limbic striatal and thalamocortical circuits as a pathogenetic mechanism of obsessive-compulsive disorder. *J Neuropsychiatry Clin Neurosci* 1, 27–36.

Nordahl, T.E., Benkelfat, C. & Semple, W.E. (1989) Cerebral glucose metabolic rates in obsessive-compulsive disorder. *Neuropsychopharmacology* 2, 23–8.

Otto, M.W. (1992) Normal and abnormal information processing. A neuropsychological perspective on obsessive-compulsive disorder. *Psychiatr Clin North Am* **15**(4), 825–48.

Papez, J.W. (1937) A proposed mechanism of emotion. *Arch Neurol Psychiat* **38**, 725–43.

Pitman, R.K., Green, R.C., Jenike, M.A. & Mesulam, M.M. (1987) Clinical comparison of Tourette's disorder and obsessive-compulsive disorder. *Am J Psychiatry* **144**(9), 1166–71.

Rapoport, J.L. & Wise, S.P. (1988) Obsessive-compulsive disorder: evidence for basal ganglia dysfunction. *Psychopharmacol Bull* **24**(3), 380–4.

Rasmussen, S.A. & Eisen, J.L. (1992) The epidemiology and clinical features of obsessive-compulsive disorder. *Psychiatr Clin North Am* **15**(4), 743–58.

Rauch, S.L. & Baxter, L.R. (1998) Neuroimaging of OCD and related disorders. In: *Obsessive-Compulsive Disorders: Practical Management* (M.A. Jenike, L. Baer & W.E. Minichiello (eds), pp. 289–317). Mosby, Boston.

Rauch, S.L., Jenike, M.A., Alpert, N.M. *et al.* (1994) Regional cerebral blood flow measured during symptom provocation in obsessive-compulsive disorder using oxygen 15-labeled carbon dioxide and positron emission tomo-graphy [see comments]. *Arch Gen Psychiatry* **51**(1), 62–70.

Robinson, D., Wu, H., Munne, R.A. *et al.* (1995) Reduced caudate nucleus volume in obsessive-compulsive disorder. *Arch Gen Psychiatry* **52**(5), 393–8.

Rosenberg, D.R., Keshavan, M.S., Dick, E.L., Bagwell, W.W., MacMaster, F.P. & Birmaher, B. (1997) Corpus callosal morphology in treatment-naive pediatric obsessive-compulsive disorder. *Prog Neuropsychopharmacol Biol Psychiatry* **21**(8), 1269–83.

Roth, B., Cohen, L. & Hallett, M. (1991) The electric field induced during magnetic stimulation. In: *Magnetic Motor Stimulation: Basic Principles and Clinical Experience (EEG Suppl. 43)* (W. Lecy, R. Cracco, A. Barker & J.

Rothwell (eds), pp. 268–78). Elsevier Science Publishers, Amsterdam.

Rothwell, J.C., Thompson, P.D., Day, B.L., Boyd, S. & Marsden, C.D. (1991) Stimulation of the human motor cortex through the scalp. *Exp Physiol* **76**, 159–200.

Rush, A., George, M., Sackeim, H., Marangell, L., Husain, M. & Giller, C. (2000) Vagus nerve stimulation (VNS) for treatment-resistant depressions: a multicenter study. *Biol Psychiatry* **47**, 276–86.

Sabatini, U., Toni, D., Pantano, P. *et al.* (1994) Motor recovery after early brain damage. A case of brain plasticity. *Stroke* **25**(2), 514–17.

Schwartz, J.M., Stoessel, P.W., Baxter, L.R. Jr, Martin, K.M. & Phelps, M.E. (1996) Systematic changes in cerebral glucose metabolic rate after successful behavior modification treatment of obsessive-compulsive disorder. *Arch Gen Psychiatry* **53**(2), 109–13.

Spiegel, E., Wycis, H. & Freed, H. (1950) Thalamotomy in mental disorders. *Archives of Neurology and Psychiatry* **64**, 595–8.

Swedo, S.E., Leonard, H.L., Kruesi, M.J.P. *et al.* (1992) Cerebrospinal fluid neurochemistry in children and adolescents with obsessive-compulsive disorder. *Arch Gen Psychiatry* **49**, 29–36.

Swedo, S.E., Rapoport, J.L., Cheslow, D.L. *et al.* (1989) High prevalence of obsessive-compulsive symptoms in patients with Sydenham's chorea. *Am J Psychiatry* **146**(2), 246–9.

Ward, C.D. (1988) Transient feelings of compulsion caused by hemispheric lesions: three cases. *J Neurol Neurosurg Psychiatry* **51**(2), 266–8.

Wu, J.C., Gillin, J.C., Buchsbaum, M.S., Hershey, T., Johnson, J.C. & Bunney, W.E. (1992) Effect of sleep deprivation on brain metabolism of depressed patients. *Am J Psychiatry* **149**, 538–43.

Yudofsky, S. & Ovsiew, F. (1990) Neurosurgical and related interventions for the treatment of patients with psychiatric disorders. *J Neuropsychiatry Clin Neurosci* **2**, 253–5.

27 Herbal Therapy and Anxiety

M. Bourin

Introduction

Generalized anxiety disorder (GAD) is one of the most common of the anxiety disorders. Its prevalence in the general population varies between 5% and 15% depending on the criteria used to define it. GAD corresponds to severe anxiety, characterized according to the Diagnostic Statistical Manual, third edition revised (DSM-III-R: American Psychiatric Association 1987) chronic cognitive disorders (Angst & Vollrath 1991). Several investigators have questioned the validity of the diagnosis (Breier *et al.* 1985; Barlow *et al.* 1986). The pattern of illness in patients with DSM-IV defined GAD with 6-month duration criterion tends to be fairly chronic, although with fluctuating symptom severity. A large percentage of patients present with short-term anxiety disorders that are related to stressors. In the DSM-III-R this kind of anxiety disorder is classified as adjustment disorder with anxious mood (ADAM) as opposed to GAD. According to the DSM-III-R, the essential feature of this disorder is a maladaptive reaction to an identifiable psycho-social stressor. It is one of the most frequent psychiatric diagnoses made in seriously physically ill patients (Schatzberg 1990) and in older patients (Tueth 1993).

Many questions are currently raised by the treatment of ADAM, particularly the question of choice of drug treatment. Benzodiazepines have been widely used in the treatment of ADAM. Certain rules should be observed when they are prescribed: prescribe for short periods (4–6 weeks) using the minimum effective dose (often difficult to determine in advance); be careful when prescribing for drug addicts; avoid issuing repeat prescriptions; during long-term treatment re-evaluate

whether it is still necessary to prescribe benzodiazepines; decrease the dose very gradually when treatment is withdrawn (Ashton 1989; Tyrer 1989). Routine observance of these rules is essential in practice in the outpatient management of anxious patients. There has been a search for therapeutic alternatives in the treatment of anxiety, notably in the chronic or recurrent forms, where the risks of dependence related to benzodiazepines are markedly increased (Curran 1991).

One alternative is to use psychological therapies. These can be effective when given by skilled therapists but, on the other hand, constraints on resource and even time may render psychological interventions impracticable. It is estimated that alternative or complementary treatment is used by 20% to 30% of the North American population (Eisenberg *et al.* 1993). The goal of the present chapter is to evaluate the efficacy of different medicines used in treating anxiety defined as GAD or ADAM, as there have been few if any trials in other forms of anxiety. Focus will be on the kava plant (*Piper methysticum*) and the passion flower (*Passiflora incarnata*).

Kava plant

Preparations made from the rhizome of the kava plant have been used extensively by the people of the South Pacific (Singh & Blumenthal 1997). Traditionally kava was used to treat anxiety but was known to have anticonvulsant sedative and muscle relaxant properties (Bone 1993/1994), as well as to treat of a variety of ailments such as gonorrhea (Lebot *et al.* 1992).

Among a number of agents extracted from kava, kavain which is an α-pyrone seems to be one of the most pharmacologically active agents. There is some evidence regarding the affinity of kavalactones on γ-aminobutyric acid (GABA) or benzodiazepine-binding sites (Davies *et al.* 1992; Jussogie *et al.* 1994). On the other hand, kava extract has been reported to produce changes on the electroencephalogram similar to those induced by diazepam (Gebner & Cnota 1994).

The conflicting evidence of pharmacological activity of kava extracts led researchers to design clinical trials with kava extracts containing mainly 100–200 mg of kavalactones for daily utilization. A recent systematic review and meta-analysis for treating anxiety by kava extract clearly proved its efficacy (Pittler & Ernst 2000). Systematic literature searches were performed to identify all randomized controlled trials of kava for the treatment of anxiety. All publications were blinded before assessment by someone not involved in the study. Data were extracted in a standardized, pre-defined fashion independently by two reviewers. The methodological quality of all trials was assessed and the superiority of kava extracts over placebo was suggested by all seven trials. The meta-analysis of three trials suggests a significant difference in the reduction of the total score on the Hamilton Rating Scale for Anxiety (HAM-A: Hamilton 1959) in favor of kava extract.

The main problem with the meta-analysis is that there are few indications in terms of anxiety diagnosis; it was performed using trials that were homogenous in terms of drug quality. The authors of this meta-analysis used a quality score from 0 to 5 based on randomization, double-blind design, description of withdrawals and drop-outs. All studies were performed in Germany except one in the US. For all studies there was no control group, it was a comparison between kava and placebo.

Three of the clinical trials had a quality score of 5, two of them were from gynecology practices, one from a university outpatient clinic (Kinzler *et al.* 1991). The publication of five out of seven of the studies were in German and so it is not very easy to compare the kind of patients included. In three of the seven studies all the patients were female. The conclusions of the authors of the meta-analysis (Pittler & Ernst 2000) suggest that kava extract is relatively safe and more efficacious than placebo in the symptomatic treatment of anxiety. In the author's opinion the lack of information on the true diagnosis of patients is an important limitation to the meta-analysis.

In different studies the adverse effects reported most frequently were gastrointestinal complaints, allergic skin reactions, headaches and photosensitivity (for review see Warnecke *et al.* 1990). Table 27.1 shows the only two trials with the highest quality score of 5 using HAM-A.

The clinical trial (Volz & Kleser 1997) in general practice seems more realistic, even if it had a quality score of 3 in the meta-analysis of Pittler and Ernst (2000) because of the lack of description of the method generating the sequence of randomization as well as the method of double-blind. The scale of the placebo effect is in relation with the one found in these kind of trials on anxiety (Bourin 2000) contrasting with the poor placebo effect of the two trials described in Table 27.1. The most important data are found in two postmarketing surveillance studies (Siegers *et al.* 1992; Hofmann & Winter 1996): 2.3% and 1.5% of

Table 27.1 Double-blind randomized placebo-controlled trials of kava for anxiety.

Author	Study patients kava extract/placebo [Mean age/years]	Adverse effect
Kinzler *et al.* (1991)	Outpatients with anxiety syndrome Of nonpsychotic origin HAM-A ≥ 19 N = 58 [44/42]	None
Warnecke (1991)	Female patients with anxiety syndrome HAM-A ≥ 19 N = 40 [45–60]	Restlessness, stomach complaints, drowsiness, tremor (four patients)

patients given a daily dose of 120–240 mg kava extract and 105 mg kavapyrone, respectively, complained of the adverse effects mentioned previously.

Passion flower

The *Passiflora incarnata* component contains flavonoids, maltol, hydroxycoumarins and alkaloids belonging to the beta-carboline family. These compounds, including harmane, harmine, harmol, and harmalol (Bennati 1967; Bennati & Fedeli 1968), are present in the plant at levels up to 0.032% and are known to act on central benzodiazepines receptors.

No clinical studies of *Passiflora incarnata* alone were reported and so Bourin *et al.* (1997) performed a randomized, controlled trial that used a commercial preparation EUPHYTOSE® (EUP) containing *Passiflora incarnata* in addition to *Valeriana officinalis*, *Crataegus oxyacantha*, *Ballota foetida*, *Paullinia cupana*, and *Cola nitida*.

Valeriana officinalis is traditionally used as a neuro-sedative. Its components contain various iridoid triesters belonging to the valepotriate family (Foerster *et al.* 1984), which are generally considered as responsible for the sedative activity attributed to valerian preparations (Von Eicksted & Rahman 1969); *Ballota foetida* and hawthorn are also used traditionally as anxiolytics.

Cola nitida has long been used as a mild stimulant, the nut extract containing a water-soluble complex including caffeine and kolatine. *Paullinia cupana* is also known as a stimulant, mainly in South America where it is consumed as a traditional drink. As with *Cola nitida*, *Paullinia cupana* extracts contains a high level of caffeine (around 4%). This latter compound, as well as kolatine, may counteract the sedative effects of the other components (Herman 1982). Previous studies conducted in mice have shown that EUP was able to increase significantly the number of punished passages (from 33% to 42% depending on the dose) in the four-plates test, which is normally considered to be a predictive test for anxiolytics (Aron *et al.* 1971).

Moreover, binding studies with various types of cerebral receptor have shown that EUP was able to displace the binding of the tritiated ligand to central benzodiazepine receptors in a dose-dependent manner with an IC50 of 37,1 µg/mL. Another action that has been discovered is that of agonist at muscarinic receptors (M1), which are known to have a role in memory-related phenomena. The IC_{50} for these M1 receptors was 30 µg/mL (Valli *et al.* 1991). In addition, a study of psychometric effects in healthy volunteers (images test, number-symbol pair test, flicker-fusion test, reaction-choice test) showed that there was no difference from placebo on day (D) 3, D7 or D14 (Bourin 1994); EUP presented neither sedative nor stimulant properties. Unfortunately there is little pharmacokinetic data about this drug because of its complex composition.

All these preliminary results justified the carrying out of a controlled clinical study in patients presenting with ADAM, comparing EUP with a placebo. The study was a multicenter-controlled general practice study against placebo, with randomization into two parallel groups of patients followed-up as outpatients with ADAM criteria (limiting the duration of the anxiety to at least 6 weeks). Thirty-one general practitioners participated in this study which was coordinated by psychiatrists in four regions in France. All investigators of a regional group participated in sponsor-initiated, prestudy, multicenter meetings led by the regional co-ordinator in order to ensure uniformity in the selection, supervision and evaluation of study patients. They were trained by expert coordinators to employ a diagnostic algorithm for including patients presenting with ADAM and excluding patients with other psychiatric illnesses. The period of actual treatment was preceded by a pre-inclusion period of 7 days during which patients were treated single-blind with placebo. In order to be definitely included, patients had to continue to fulfil the selection criteria at the end of the placebo period and have a HAM-A Scale score of more than 20, with less than 10% difference between the HAM-A score on D-7 and the HAM-A score at D0. When included, all patients received two tablets three times a day (placebo or EUP) over 28 days.

Evaluation criteria were therefore HAM-A Scale on D0, D7, D14 and D28, Covi Scale scores on D0, D14 and D28 (Covi *et al.* 1979), and Sheehan Self-Evaluation Scale scores on D0, D14 and D28 (Sheehan *et al.* 1996). Compliance was assessed by counting the tablets on each day of evaluation and at the end of the study.

Homogenity of the two treatment groups was studied with regard to patient characteristics (i.e., sex, age, previous treatment with anxiolytic drugs). Patients analysed were those who conformed to the protocol with the exception of two patients who did not fulfil the inclusion criteria. The HAM-A Rating Scale was

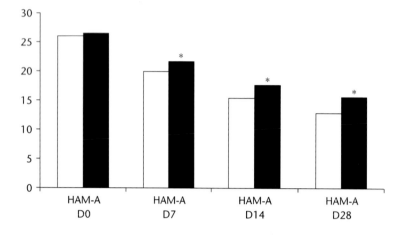

Fig. 27.1 Quantitative analysis of principal judgement criterion Hamilton Rating Scale for Anxiety (HAM-A). □ Plant extracts ($n = 91$); ■ Placebo ($n = 91$). *Analysis of contrasts, significant difference on day (D) 7, D14 and D28 ($P = 0.05$).

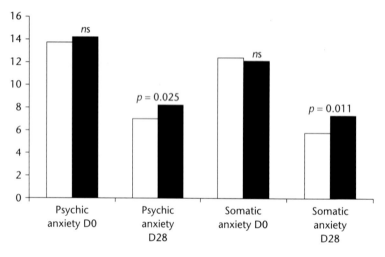

Fig. 27.2 Comparison of scores for psychic and somatic anxiety on the Hamilton Rating Scale for Anxiety (HAM-A). □ Plant extracts ($n = 91$); ■ Placebo ($n = 91$).

used in a quantitative and qualitative manner. For qualitative analysis, patients were ascribed as "responders" or "nonresponders," analyses were performed using the chi-2 test. Quantitative analysis was performed using the Student's t-test, comparing the groups mean HAM-A rating scores at D28 of the trial. Covi scores were also evaluated with the Student's t-test. The Sheehan Self-evaluation Scale was used to assess each item—work, family life, social life—compared with D0 of the trial. Intergroup comparisons on D14 and D28 were performed using Mann–Whitney's statistical test for nonparametric data because there were less patients in each group and because of ordinal values.

A total of 182 patients who fulfilled the criteria for ADAM were included (18 preselected patients were excluded from the study at the time of definite inclu-

sion), 91 were allocated at random to the placebo group and 91 to the EUP group. There were no significant differences in terms of age and sex between the groups at the time of inclusion. Compliance was good in the two groups, medication was taken completely even by patients with side-effects. There were no patient dropouts in the study, probably because of the careful selection of patients (see earlier) and the low incidence of side-effects (Figs. 27.1, 27.2; Table 27.2–27.5).

Although no evaluation of its efficacy has been performed previously, EUP is an old, marketed, widely used drug in France. The present study demonstrated the better efficacy of EUP over placebo in adult outpatients with ADAM. The principal criterion of HAM-A score on D28, analysed either qualitatively (responder/nonresponder of success/failure) or quantitatively

Table 27.2 Qualitative analysis of the principal judgement criterion (patients counted as improved or cured).

D28	Plant extracts	Placebo
HAM-A < 14	52 (57.1%)	35 (38.5%)
HAM-A = 14	39 (42.9%)	56 (61.5%)
Total	91	91
	χ^2: P = 0.011	
HAM-A < 10	39 (42.9%)	23 (25.3%)
HAM-A = 10	52 (57.1%)	68 (74.7%)
Total	91	91
	χ^2: P = 0.012	

D, day.

Table 27.3 Change in scores on the Covi Scale.

	Plant extracts (N = 91)	Placebo (N = 91)
Covi D0	6.11 ± 1.9	5.85 ± 1.8
Covi D14	3.24 ± 1.7	3.54 ± 1.9
Covi D28	2.25 ± 1.9	2.88 ± 2.4*

D, day.
*Analysis of contrasts, significant difference on D14 and D28 (P = 0.05).

showed a statistically significant difference in favor of EUP.

However, these results were obtained in a population in which the severity of the anxiety was relatively minor: 52% of patients included had a HAM-A score on D0 of between 20 and 25, and only 25% of patients

Table 27.5 Adverse events probably related to treatment.

Event	Plant extracts (N = 91)	Placebo (N = 91)
Dry mouth	1	1
Headache	1	0
Constipation	1	2
Stomach pain	0	3
Drowsiness	1	2

had been treated in the previous 3 months with an anxiolytic, generally a benzodiazepine.

This population included a high proportion of "nervous subjects" often seen for the first time, perhaps the inclusion criteria for the study limited the start of symptoms 6 weeks prior to the study. The most important result of this study was that it showed there were more patients counted as "cured" (HAM-A score <10) in treated patients than in placebo group (42.9% vs. 25.3%).

An analysis, which took account of the effect for each center, did not reveal any region/treatment interaction, proving that the superiority of EUP was the same wherever patients were from.

The Covi Scale scores which also evaluated the severity of the anxiety gave similar results to those obtained with the HAM-A score. However, there was no significant difference on D14 in change over time, but only on D28. This result may be explained by a greater sensitivity of the HAM-A scale compared with the Covi Scale.

The scale for self-evaluation by the patient (work, family and social life) measured on D0, D14 and D28

Table 27.4 Change in scores on the Sheehan Self-evaluation Scale.

Work	Plant extracts (N = 67)	Placebo (N = 65)	Mann–Whitney
D0–D14	1.58 ± 1.7	1.58 ± 1.9	NS
D0–D28	2.34 ± 2.2	2.13 ± 2.3	NS
Family	Plant extracts (N = 85)	Placebo (N = 84)	Mann–Whitney
D0–D14	1.87 ± 1.9	1.54 ± 2.1	NS
D0–D28	3.00 ± 2.4	2.41 ± 2.4	P = 0.065
Social life	Plant extracts (N = 85)	Placebo (N = 84)	Mann–Whitney
D0–D14	1.60 ± 1.9	1.13 ± 2.1	P = 0.019
D0–D28	2.62 ± 2.2	2.01 ± 2.6	P = 0.034

D, day; NS, not significant.

revealed a greater improvement in the item "social life" from D14, indicating early resumption of social and leisure activities in the EUP-treated group. Results for the item "family life" were at the threshold of significance on D28. There was no significant difference in the item "work" on D14 or D28. There was no evidence of sedation as found with valerian extracts (Gerhard et al. 1996), probably because there is a good equilibrium between the mild sedative compounds and the mild stimulant compounds. In addition, there was no greater effect on the sleep items than on anxiety items.

The global evaluation of efficacy by investigators also demonstrated the superiority of EUP over placebo (results not shown in previous tables). The study also confirmed that EUP is very well tolerated. There was no difference in the number of adverse events between the two treatment groups. No event required treatment to be withdrawn, and no events were judged to be serious. This confirms what had been demonstrated in healthy volunteers where the psychometric performance of volunteers treated with EUP did not differ from the performance of volunteers treated with placebo (Bourin 1994).

Further clinical studies to explore the effects of EUP versus a benzodiazepine and a placebo over a longer period (3–6 months) in the treatment of chronic GAD, with a follow-up of several weeks after withdrawal of treatment, should make it possible to investigate rebound and withdrawal phenomena (Murphy et al. 1989). This type of study would be part of the current trend in pharmacological treatment of anxiety, which is trying to reduce the side-effects of treatment (especially cognitive side effects) and dependence (Bourin et al. 1993). The advantages of such studies would be the long-term evaluation of the effects of treatment on the prevention of relapse and attenuation of the chronic nature of chronic anxiety (Lader 1994).

It would also be interesting to use a checklist of somatic symptoms (Guelfi et al. 1983) to further understand which symptoms EUP improves. This scale could be used to differentiate the anxiety symptoms and the side-effects of drugs (Bourin & Malinge 1995).

The main difficulty with plant extract combinations is to know which extracts are truly active on anxiety disorders. The European Community registers only four-extract combinations and so, in the case of EUP, it is difficult to know which four extracts to keep among the six.

Further research is needed to if *Passiflora incarnata* is the most active among the six extracts used in EUP? We already know that in *Passiflora incarnata* as well as in *Passiflora caerula* (Wolfman et al. 1994) there are flavonoid derivatives like chrysine that displaces [3H] flunitrazepam binding to the central benzodiazepine receptors in mice. In elevated plus maze in mice, chrysine (1 mg/kg) induces increase in the number of entries into the open arms and in the time spent on the open arms consistent with an anxiolytic action (Bourin 1997). The effects of chrysine on the elevated plus maze mice were abolished by pretreatment with the specific benzodiazepine antagonist flumazenil (3 mg/kg).

Conclusion

Systematic literature searches were performed in the computerized databases MEDLINE and EMBASE, but there was only few randomized double-blind studies using herbal therapy in the field of anxiety disorders. The studies using kava extract are reviewed in a paper by Pittler and Ernst (2000) and there is another paper by Bourin et al. (1997) that uses plant extracts, including passion flower and valerian (along with other extracts). The results are not all positive, and the main problem is the lack of a control drug like a benzodiazepine.

To use kava or passion flower extracts in common practice for treating GAD we need a titration in kavain and chrysine respectively. It seems that the active compounds work by binding with benzodiazepine receptors but with lower effect than benzodiazepines. So, instead of using herbal therapy, we must reconsider the use of low doses of benzodiazepine (Bourin et al. 1995, 1998).

It is possible that the combination of some plant extracts are useful, but we need to have well-designed clinical trials to be sure of the efficacy. It would be interesting to add valerian to kava or passion flower because it has mild sedative effects in healthy volunteers (Kuhlmann et al. 1999). In the author's experience (Bourin 1994), EUP did not modify the psychometric performance of healthy volunteers.

To date there are large national differences in the regulatory status of herbal remedies. In various countries, such as the US and the UK, herbal remedies can circumvent the regulatory premarket drug evaluation by posing as dietary supplements (De Smet 1993). Yet the European guideline for regulatory evaluation of anxiolytics requires a pharmacokinetic exploration as part of the application for marketing authorization.

A final consideration (De Smet & Brouwers 1997) is that the pharmacokinetic evaluation for a herbal preparation will only provide clinical information when there is sufficient evidence that the studied components are responsible for therapeutic effects.

References

Angst, J. & Vollrath, M. (1991) The natural history of anxiety disorders. *Acta Psychiatr Scand* **84**, 446–52.

American Psychiatric Association (1987) *Diagnostic Statistical Manual of Mental Disorders*, 3rd edn revised. American Psychiatric Association, Washington, D.C.

Aron, C., Simon, P., Larousse, C. & Boissier, J.R. (1971) Evaluation of a rapid technique detecting minor tranquilizers. *Neuropharmacology* **10**, 459–69.

Ashton, M. (1989) Risk of dependence on benzodiazepine drugs: a major problem of long-term treatment. *BMJ* **298**, 103–4.

Barlow, D.H., Blanchard, E.B., DiNardo, P.A., Vermileya, J.A. & Vermileya, B.B. (1986) Generalized anxiety and generalized anxiety disorder. Description and reconceptualization. *Am J Psychiatry* **143**, 40–4.

Bennati, E. (1967) Identification by thin layer chromatography of liquid extract of *Passiflora incarnata*. *Boll Chim Farm* **106**, 756–60.

Bennati, E. & Fedeli, E. (1968) Gas chromatography of fluid extract of *Passiflora incarnata*. *Boll Chim Farm* **107**, 716–20.

Bone, K. (1993/1994) Kava: a safe herbal treatment for anxiety. *Br J Physother* **3**, 147–53.

Bourin, M. (1994) Etude des effets de l'euphytose sur les performances psychométriques du volontaire sain. *Psychol Med* **26**, 1471–8.

Bourin, M. (1997) Animal models of anxiety: are they suitable for predicting drug action in humans? *Pol J Pharmacol* **49**, 79–84.

Bourin, M. (2000) Clinical methodology for testing anxiolytic drugs. *Therapie* **55**, 147–53.

Bourin, M., Bougerol, T., Guitton, B. & Broutin, E. (1997) A combination of plant extracts in the treatment of outpatients with adjustment disorder with anxious mood: controlled study versus placebo. *Fundam Clin Pharmacol* **11**, 127–32.

Bourin, M., Colombel, M.C. & Guitton, B. (1998) Alprazolam 0.125 mg twice a day improves aspects of psychometric performance in healthy volunteers. *J Clin Psychopharmacol* **18**, 364–72.

Bourin, M., Colombel, M.C. & Malinge, M. (1995) Lorazepam 0.25 mg twice a day improves aspects of psychometric performance in healthy volunteers. *J Psychopharmacol* **9**, 251–7.

Bourin, M., Couëtoux du Tertre, A. & Payeur, R. (1993) Evaluation of safety and side effects in the process of antianxiety drug development. *Eur Psychiatry* **8**, 285–91.

Bourin, M. & Malinge, M. (1995) Controlled comparison of the effects and abrupt discontinuation of buspirone and lorazepam. *Prog Neuropsychopharmacol Biol Psychiatry* **19**, 567–75.

Breier, A., Charnen, D.S. & Heninger, G.R. (1985) The diagnostic validity of anxiety disorders and their relationship to depressive illness. *Am J Psychiatry* **142**, 787–96.

Covi, L., Lipman, M.C., Nair, D.M. & Crezlinsky, T. (1979) Symptomatic volunteers in multicenter drug trials. *Prog Neuropsychopharmacol Biol Psychiatry* **3**, 521–8.

Curran, H.V. (1991) Benzodiazepines memory and mood: a review. *Psychopharmacology* **105**, 1–8.

Davies, L., Drew, C., Duffield, P., Johnston, G.A. & Jamieson, D.D. (1992) Kava pyrones and resin studies on GABA (A), GABA (B) and benzodiazepine binding sites in the rodent brain. *Pharmacol Toxicol* **71**, 120–6.

De Smet, P.A.G.M. (1993) Legislatory outlook on the safety of herbal remedies. In: *Adverse Effects of Herbal Drugs*, Vol. 2 (P.A.G.M. De Smet, K. Hänsel, K. Keller *et al.* (eds), pp. 1–90). Springer-Verlag, Heidelberg.

De Smet, P.A.G.M. & Brouwers, J.R.B.J. (1997) Pharmacokinetic evaluation of herbal remedies: basic introduction, applicability, current status and regulatory need. *Clin Pharmacokinet* **32**, 427–36.

Eisenberg, D.M., Kessler, R.C., Foster, C., Norlock, F.E., Calkins, D.R. & Delbanco, T.L. (1993) Unconventional medicine in the United States: prevalence, costs and patterns of use. *N Engl J Med* **328**, 246–52.

Foerster, W., Becker, H. & Rodriguez, E. (1984) HPLC analysis and valepotriates in the North American *Genera plectritis* and *Valeriana*. *Planta Med* **1**, 7–9.

Gebner, B. & Cnota, P. (1994) Extract of kava-kava rhizome in comparison with diazepam and placebo. *Zeitscrift für Phytother* **15**, 30–7.

Gerhard, U., Linnenbrink, N., Georghiadon, C. & Hobi, V. (1996) Vigilance-reducing effects of two herbal hypnotics. *Schweiz Rundsch Med Prax* **85**, 473–81.

Guelfi, J.D., Pull, C.B., Guelfi, C., Ruschel, S. & Dreyfus, J.F. (1983) La CHESS. Utilisation dans la pathologie anxieuse et dépressive. Structure factorielle. *Ann Med Psychol* **141**, 257–77.

Hamilton, M. (1959) The assessment of anxiety states by rating. *Br J Med Psychol* **32**, 50–5.

Herman, A.R. (1982) Pharmacological properties of *Paullinia cupana*. *J Ethnopharmacol* **6**, 311–38.

Hofmann, R. & Winter, U. (1996) Therapeutische möglich-keiten mit kava-kava bei angsterkrankungen. *Psycho* **22**, 51–3.

Jussogie, A., Schinz, A. & Hiencke, C. (1994) Kavapyrone extract enriched from *Piper methysticum* as modulator of the GABA binding site in different regions of the rat brain. *Psychopharmacology* **116**, 469–74.

Kinzler, E., Kröner, J. & Lehmann, E. (1991) Wirksamkeit eines kava-spezial-extraktes bei patieinten mit magst, spannungs und erregunszuständem nicht-psychrtischen genese. *Arzneimittelforschung* **41**, 584–8.

Kuhlmann, J., Berger, W., Podzweit, H. & Schmidt, U. (1999) The influence of valerian treatment in "reaction time, alertness and concentration" in volunteers. *Pharmacopsychiatry* **32**, 235–41.

Lader, M. (1994) Diagnosis and treatment of generalized anxiety disorder in current therapeutic approaches to panic and other anxiety disorders. In: *International Academy for Biomedical and Drug Research*, Vol. 8 (G. Darcourt, G. Mendlewicz, G. Racagni & N. Brunello (eds), pp. 113–20). Karger, Basel.

Lebot, V., Merlin, M. & Lindstrom, L. (1992) *Kava, the Specific Drug*. Yale University Press, New Haven, CT.

Murphy, S.M., Owen, R. & Tyrer, P. (1989) Comparative assessment of efficacy and withdrawal symptoms after 6 and 12 weeks' treatment with diazepam or buspirone. *Br J Psychiatry* **154**, 528–34.

Pittler, M.H. & Ernst, E. (2000) Efficacy of kava extract for treating anxiety: systematic review and meta-analysis. *J Clin Psychopharmacol* **20**, 84–9.

Schatzberg, A.F. (1990) Anxiety and adjustment disorder. A treatment approach. *J Clin Psychiatry* **51** (Suppl. 11), 20–4.

Sheehan, D.V., Harnett-Sheehan, K. & Raj, B.A. (1996) The measurement of disability. *Int Clin Psychopharmacol* **11** (Suppl. 3), 89–95.

Siegers, C.P., Honold, E., Krall, B., Meng, G. & Habs, M. (1992) Ergebnisse einer anwendungsbeobachtung L1090 mit Laitan® kapseln. *Arztl Forsch* **39**, 7–11.

Singh, Y. & Blumenthal, M. (1997) Kava: an overview. *Herbalgram* **39**, 34–54.

Tueth, M.J. (1993) Anxiety in the older patient: differential diagnosis and treatment. *Geriatrics* **48**, 51–4.

Tyrer, P. (1989) Risk of dependence on benzodiazepine drugs. The importance of patient selection. *BMJ* **298**, 104–5.

Valli, M., Paubert-Braquet, M., Pilot, S., Fabre, R., Lefrançois, G. & Rod, D. (1991) Euphytose, an association of plant extracts with anxiolytic activity: investigation of its mechanism of action by an *in vitro* binding study. *Phytother Res* **5**, 241–4.

Volz, H.P. & Kleser, M. (1997) Kava-kava extract WS 1400 versus placebo in anxiety disorders: a randomized placebo-controlled 25 week outpatient trial. *Pharmacopsychiatry* **30**, 1–5.

Von Eicksted, K.W. & Rahman, S. (1969) Psychopharmacologic effects of valepotriates. *Arzneimittel Forschung* **19**, 316–19.

Warnecke, G. (1991) Psychosomatische dysfunktionen im weiblichen klimakterium. *Fortschr Med* **109**, 119–22.

Warnecke, G., Pfaender, H., Gerster, G. & Graeza, E. (1990) Wirksamkeit von kava-kava-extract beim klimakterischen syndrom. *Z Phytoher* **11**, 81–6.

Wolfman, C., Viola, H., Peladini, A., Dajhas, F. & Medina, J.H. (1994) Possible anxiolytic effects of chrysine, a central benzodiazepine receptor ligand isolated from *Passiflora coerulea*. *Pharmacological Biochemistry and Behavior* **47**, 1–4.

PART FIVE

CONCLUSION

28 Anxiety Disorders: Current Needs and Future Prospects

D. Nutt & J. Ballenger

Some key unanswered questions

What we will try to do in this chapter is build on the great body of clinical and research data presented in the previous chapters by highlighting where we feel the key unresolved issues are. These issues seem to us to be critical in the understanding of anxiety and in the action of treatments of these disorders and may help direct the research agenda in anxiety. Clearly there are many more research questions relating for anxiety disorders than we can discuss here so the ones we focus on reflect our own expertise and interests to some extent.

How long to treat?

There is good evidence in depression that long-term treatment with antidepressants leads to a better outcome. Indeed some patients who have had three or more episodes may require lifelong treatment to prevent relapse. The situation in the anxiety disorders is much less well understood. There have been few long-term studies of drug treatment and perhaps a few more on long-term effects of psychological treatments (see the respective chapters on treatments). There are various reasons for this lack of knowledge which include the fact that the anxiety disorders have only become the subject of intervention studies quite recently, perhaps reflecting a perceived bias in medical circles that they are not "real" illnesses.

In this regard the new European registration guidelines that recommend at least one maintenance-of-efficacy study of at least 6 months duration should provide some welcome data over the next few years.

There is already evidence for the prolonged efficacy of paroxetine in panic disorder (PD), social anxiety disorder, obsessive-compulsive disorder (OCD), and generalized anxiety disorder (GAD). Sertraline has long-term data in OCD and PD, and venlafaxine has at least 6-month data in GAD. In some disorders, especially OCD and social anxiety disorder, improvement appears to continue beyond 6 months and even at 1 year the drug response may not have reached a plateau.

Perhaps one of the most intriguing and potentially important observations are the new findings in GAD that extending treatment up to 1 year continues to lead to progressive improvements in symptom resolution and life quality. The recent studies with paroxetine and venlafaxine have showed that although there were significant and clinically meaningful improvements with both drugs at 3 weeks, patients continued to improve for the remainder of the period of study. Indeed in the paroxetine studies the improvement in response in the second 6 months was similar in magnitude to that in the first 6 months. Such research findings are mirrored by clinical experience in the treatment of other anxiety disorders, especially social anxiety disorder, and argue that the minimum duration of treatment might be a year, possibly longer. Of course these results also raise the issue of how long we should treat before deciding that a treatment is not working. It may be as well to warn patients that they should be prepared to stay in therapy for several months before they may experience significant benefit from antidepressant therapy and, if some benefit is seen, that they should continue with the treatment for at least 6 months to maximize the gains in symptom relief and quality of life.

However sustained efficacy does not give direct information about the risks of relapse on stopping; only discontinuation studies can do this. There is evidence that relapse rates are about three times as high on stopping selective serotonin reuptake inhibitors (SSRIs) than continuing on them in OCD and PD, and we would expect that over the next decade similar evidence will accrue for the other anxiety disorders.

Withdrawal reactions from antidepressants are well-recognized and it will be of interest to determine whether patients with anxiety disorders are more or less susceptible to them than depressed patients. Certainly some of the symptoms of withdrawal from both tricyclic antidepressants (TCAs) and SSRIs can mimic anxiety so disentangling this issue will not be easy.

The optimal dose of antidepressant

One intriguing issue in the drug treatment of anxiety is that of optimal dose. It appears that this may vary from drug to drug and from disorder to disorder. However several general themes are beginning to emerge, especially for the newer antidepressants where we have more complete data sets across the different disorders. For example, there is a fair body of data that the efficacious dose of SSRI in PD is somewhat greater than that required in depression. For example, with paroxetine in flexible-dose studies the mean dose for PD ended up at just over 30 mg/day, whereas in depression it is just over 20 mg/day, and in the fixed-dose trial only the 40 mg dose, and not the 20 mg one, separated from placebo. Similar findings in PD exist for fluvoxamine and citalopram (see Chapter 18).

In OCD the picture is similar and the limited data in GAD are in the same direction. The only exception may be for sertraline where there is less good trial evidence, although in clinical practice few patients are maintained on the lowest licensed dose of 50 mg/day.

The data for the TCAs is more equivocal (see Chapter 19). The TCA most studied in anxiety is probably clomipramine, which has a strong data set in OCD and PD. In OCD higher doses do seem to have better efficacy whereas in PD the position is less clear. Early data suggested that high doses might be needed but others have suggested lower ones are equally effective (Lotufo-Neto *et al.* 2001). With imipramine there is a general feeling from US studies that higher doses show more efficacy (Mavissakalian & Perel 1988) and that

therapeutic gains on factors such as quality of life can be obtained at doses over and above those needed to stop panic attacks.

What do these data tell us about the mode of action of antidepressants in anxiety disorders? We believe they help to dispel the notion that the anxiety disorders are but a variant of depression. In addition the fact that the anxiety disorders themselves show differential dose and time responses to the various antidepressants argues against their being different expressions of the same disorder. Further evidence in support of neurochemical differences comes from the differential dose–response to benzodiazepines. Patients with PD generally need higher doses than those with GAD or social anxiety disorder whereas PTSD and OCD may respond hardly at all.

One or two neurotransmitters? A growing role for mixed action agents?

It is becoming accepted that in the treatment of severe in-patient depression antidepressants that act on both the 5-hydroxtryptamine (5-HT) and norepinephrine (noradrenaline) systems may have greater efficacy than those that are selective to one only. There is no evidence for such an assertion in any of the anxiety disorders and indeed the limited evidence from early OCD and PD studies rather argues against this idea. For example, in OCD drugs with fairly balanced norepinephrine and 5-HT uptake blocking affinity, e.g., imipramine seem less efficacious than those that are relatively 5-HT selective, e.g., clomipramine. Selective norepinephrine uptake blockers such as desipramine are without effect or of limited efficacy (Leonard *et al.* 1991).

In PD there is good evidence that imipramine is highly efficacious but as well as having mixed uptake-blocking properties it is metabolized to desipramine. A study that examined the relationship between the plasma concentrations of imipramine and desipramine in successfully treated PD patients found that the plasma concentration of imipramine was the better predictor of good outcome (Mavissakalian & Perel 1988), which suggests that 5-HT is more important in the therapeutic response. Whether a similar picture holds for mixed agents of nonTCA structure needs to be properly evaluated as there are two drugs that fall into this class of uptake blocker (venlafaxine and milnacipram) as well as other dual acting agents that work in other ways, e.g., mirtazapine. Already there is a body of evidence that venlafaxine is effective in GAD as well as in depression and long-term studies in GAD have shown that it might achieve a remission rate that compares favorably with that produced by the SSRIs (see Chapter 22). There are now several open studies of venlafaxine in other anxiety disorders including social anxiety disorder and PD which show efficacy. (Nutt & Johnson 1998). What is currently lacking are well-powered comparator studies of venlafaxine versus the SSRIs of the sort that were so helpful in highlighting the greater efficacy of this mixed agent in depression (Anderson 2001).

Similarly there are no proper reports on the efficacy of the other mixed agents mirtazapine and milnacipram in anxiety disorders. Mirtazapine might be expected to have some direct anxiolytic actions because it is also a potent antihistamine (H1 blocker) and a good 5-HT2 antagonist—two pharmacological features that are associated with anxiety reduction (see Nutt 1998a and Chapter 21). Milnacipram is a balanced 5-HT+ norepinephrine reuptake blocker with a slight preference for the norepinephrine site. It has a treatment profile in depression that suggests similar efficacy to venlafaxine though with a somewhat different side-effect profile (less nausea). Given the lack of strong theoretical basis for predicting that norepinephrine enhancing antidepressants would be anxiolytic, it may be that the required clinical trials are not carried out by the companies and so we may have to rely on clinical experience to carry this issue forward. However some progress has been made in disentangling the exact contribution that norepinephrine makes to the action of antidepressants which might readily be transferred to studies on anxiety and this is discussed below.

How do treatments work?

This presents one of the most interesting issues in the biology of the anxiety disorders at present because of the recent evidence that has allowed the unravelling of this issue in depression. This work centers around the use of depletion techniques to interfere with the production of the key amine transmitters, especially 5-HT and norepinephrine. The impact of reducing the synaptic availability of these transmitters on the therapeutic effect of the drug treatments gives a great insight into their mode of action. For instance, in depression the issue of whether antidepressants work by increasing synaptic concentrations of amines or by down-regulating postsynaptic receptor function has been a matter of debate for several decades. The now classic studies of Yale group (Delgado *et al.* 1990, 1999; see Bell *et al.* 2001) using tryptophan depletion have clearly established that removing the availability of 5-HT by limiting precursor access leads to relapse of depression. This effect was found with antidepressant drugs that act on the 5-HT system (the SSRIs and monoamine oxidase inhibitors [MAOIs]) but not with those that act on norepinephrine system such as desipramine and mazindol. Conversely the norepinephrine synthesis inhibitor α-methyl-*p*-tyrosine (αMPT) reversed the therapeutic actions of norepinephrine acting drugs such as desipramine but had no effect in patients who were well treated on 5-HT acting ones.

Taken together these data strongly support the view that the critical mode of action of antidepressants is to make more amine available in the synapse rather than to change postsynaptic receptor function. A critical question is whether the same holds true for the anxiety disorders?

So far there have been only a few studies that have attempted to address this issue. The first was in OCD where tryptophan depletion was found not to result in relapse (Barr *et al.* 1994; Smeraldi *et al.* 1996). More recently we have conducted a study of tryptophan depletion in PD patients who were well and recovered but still taking paroxetine (Forshall *et al.* 2000; Bell *et al.* 2002). We used the panic challenge agent flumazenil to evoke susceptibility to panic attacks in those patients both on the control and on the tryptophan depletion day. The findings were quite clear. Treatment with paroxetine almost completely blocked the panicogenic actions of flumazenil as indicated by the lack of response on the control day. However, on the depleted day the flumazenil challenge resulted in a significant number of patients having increases in anxiety and panic attacks. This finding suggests that paroxetine (and presumably other SSRIs) act to increase synaptic 5-HT function and this then restrains panic. Such an explanation fits well with the panic mechanism theory of Deakin and Graeff (1991) who postulated that an increase in 5-HT in the region of the periaqueductal gray region of the brain stem would inhibit panic. We presume on the basis of this study of inpatients that paroxetine acts to increase 5-HT in this region and so inhibits panic and that tryptophan depletion releases this brake.

Several questions remain to be resolved. Perhaps the most critical is whether the antianxiety effects of antidepressants in other anxiety disorders is similarly susceptible to tryptophan depletion. Very new data suggest that trytophan depletion will cause relapse in social anxiety disorder patients reported on SSRIs. Indeed, it would be interesting to know if other antianxiety treatments such as the benzodiazepines could have their therapeutic actions undone by tryptophan depletion as there is some evidence that they also act on the 5-HT system (Nutt & Cowen 1987). In the specific instance of PD it would be fascinating to establish if tryptophan depletion would also reverse the effects of the SSRIs to block the panicogenic actions of other challenges such as carbon dioxide, CCK-4, sodium lactate, etc. It has already been shown that antidepressant treatments that are effective in PD will block the actions of a number of these panicogens but if this is a 5-HT mediated effect is not yet known (see Bradwejn & Koszycki 1994 and Chapter 15).

A related issue is to what extent is the failure of tryptophan depletion to reverse the antiOCD actions of SSRIs confounded by the experimental design? In our study (Bell *et al.* 2002) anxiety did not change significantly until the patients were challenged with flumazenil, although mood did drop prior to this. Perhaps the OCD study should be repeated using an anxiety provocation after tryptophan depletion. This is a feasible option given the fact that many patients can have their symptoms provoked by exposure *in-vivo*.

Norepinephrine depletion?

As yet there appear not to have been any studies of norepinephrine depletion in the anxiety disorders either before or after treatment. This is of some importance for several reasons. The new data on the treatment efficacy of venlafaxine in GAD suggests some extra therapeutic benefit at a dose of 125 mg/day or above as compared with lower doses. It is now clear that venlafaxine exhibits a dose–effect relationship on brain neurotransmitters with blockade of 5-HT reuptake being seen at the lowest therapeutic dose of 37.5 mg. Significant norepinephrine blockade doesn't appear until a dose equivalent to of 125 mg in a 70 kg person is reached (Melichar *et al.* 2001).

The role of norepinephrine in the symptoms of GAD is only beginning to be understood but there is some evidence that it may play a part (see review by Nutt 2001 and Chapter 11). It would therefore be of some interest to determine if blockade of norepinephrine synthesis by αMPT would undo some or all of the effect of venlafaxine and what symptoms might preferentially be induced. αMPT is an inhibitor of tyrosine hydroxylase which limits its conversion to L-dopa and so reduces norepinephrine synthesis. It has been shown to undo the therapeutic actions of antidepressants such as desipramine that act predominantly on the norepinephrine system (Miller *et al.* 1996). If venlafaxine becomes established as a treatment for other anxiety disorders the same questions will be relevant to those.

How does buspirone work?

We now have some idea about the mode of action of the two major treatment modalities for anxiety, the benzodiazepines and the antidepressants, but the mode of action of buspirone is still somewhat of a mystery. This is not just a theoretical issue because an understanding of this could lead to a new class of treatment. Moreover a number of similar drugs have been made and tested with little success so it may be that there is a lesson here in terms of specific pharmacology (see Levine & Potter 2000 and Chapter 20).

The conventional teaching is that buspirone is a selective 5-HT1A partial agonist that acutely inhibits 5-HT neuronal firing. Under the 5-HT excess theory of anxiety this would then be directly anxiolytic in conditions such as GAD but would worsen other disorders such as PD (Deakin & Graeff 1991). Although buspirone itself does not seem to worsen PD, more recent analogs such as flesinoxan, which are full agonists of this receptor, do increase anxiety in PD (van Vleit *et al.* 1996). However the raphe inhibiting actions of buspirone are immediate whereas as with the antidepressants the therapeutic effects take some time to emerge, which suggests that other factors are important. Perhaps the most obvious target is the postsynaptic 5-HT1A receptor, which is found in high densities in forebrain areas implicated in such as the hippocampus, septum and temporal cortex (Pike *et al.* 1996). Stimulation of these receptors is thought to lift depression and it may be that anxiety responds similarly. There is provisional evidence that in PD these receptors are down-regulated in a similar manner to that found in depression (Sargent *et al.* 2000: Fig. 28.1) and so per-

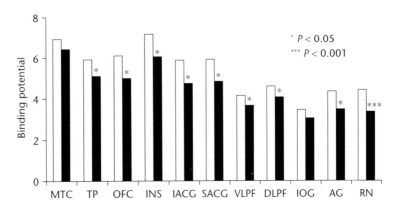

Fig. 28.1 Density of 5-HT1A receptors in various brain regions in patients with panic disorder: a 11C-WAY 100635 positron emission tomography (PET) study. MTC, medial temporal cortex; OFC, orbitofrontal cortex; RN, raphe nucleus; ROI, region of interest; TP, temporal cortex. □ volunteers; ■ panic disorders.

haps stimulation by an agonist increases their function and is anxiolytic. It would also be of some interest to see if the anxiolytic actions of buspirone were vulnerable to tryptophan depletion.

Chemistry or cognitions?

Perhaps the most acrimonious debate in psychiatric research in resent years has been about the relative contribution of cognitions and neurochemistry to the nature and treatment of the anxiety disorders. At one extreme is the cognitive view that as all anxiety is a cognitive experience then abnormal cognitions must cause anxiety. This then treats all the biological elements to anxiety as being simply mediators of cognitions. In its purest sense this view is illustrated in Fig. 28.2 for PD. Panicogenic challenges are seen as causing symptoms that patients perceive as unpleasant and frightening. This then leads to a pathognomonic cognitive experience (the so-called catastrophic cognition) of the patient who experiences thoughts such as "I'm dying" or "I'm going to faint" and then panics.

The growth of this cognitive theory, which now has been applied to all the anxiety disorders, has been accompanied by a much bigger movement in applied psychology—cognitive therapy. This is undoubtedly an effective and powerful series of procedures (see Chapter 23) but may not work exactly according to the theory that underpins it, and some have suggested that cognitive therapy works more through exposure than through a direct effect on cognitions (e.g., Marks 2002).

Our own view is that cognitive factors clearly have a role to play in any human anxiety paradigm, and may be critical in some. For example the panicogenic actions of the β-adrenoceptor agonist isoproterenol (isoprenaline), which does not cross the blood–brain barrier, are likely to be indirectly mediated perhaps by cognitive responses to peripheral sensations. However, most anxiogenic agents do enter the brain and we suspect that some of these may provoke anxiety directly whereas other may act through changing cognitions (Fig. 28.3).

What of the clinical situation? There is good evidence that in some anxiety disorders patients display specific biases to certain classes of cognitions. In PD these are thoughts or ideas of harm and illness. In GAD

Challenge (drug, lactate, ↑pCO_2 etc)

↓

Symptom

↓

Catastrophic misinterpretation of threat

↓

Panic attack

Fig. 28.2 Cognitive mediation of anxiety.

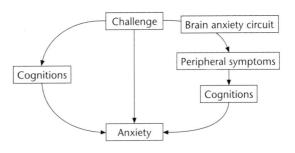

Fig. 28.3 Routes to anxiety.

505

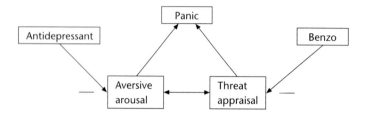

Fig. 28.4 Possible mechanisms of drug effects in panic disorder. (Middleton *et al.* 1991.) —, reduces.

they tend to be nonspecific worries about uncontrollable future mishaps whereas in social anxiety disorder they relate to experiences of shame and humiliation (see Chapter 7). These biases can be elicited by presentation of provoking ideas, for example in the form of sentences or statements that can be displayed on a computer screen. Patients with PD show greater responses (as revealed by interference with ongoing performance measures) when having to process a harm-related sentence than with a one describing public humiliation. The converse is true for patients with social anxiety disorder who demonstrate greater interference from the social threat statements than from the physical harm ones. Such cognitive biases are the substrate on which cognitive therapy works, and as patients improve these biases disappear. But what do drugs do to them?

One theory is that of Middleton (1991) (Fig. 28.4). He postulated that the two main antipanic agents, the antidepressants and the benzodiazepines, work in quite different ways. He suggested that the antidepressants act to reduce the aversive physiological sensations or "cognitive" response to a panic threat (e.g., that experienced when entering a supermarket that had previously been avoided) whereas the benzodiazepines attenuate the ability of the person to detect

that the threat is present. This theory is potentially testable which, to some extent, we have done. Using threat statements in the from of sentences displayed on a computer screen in the guise of a performance task we were able to show that threat statements indeed disrupted the performance of patients with PD (Weinstein & Nutt 1995) so revealing the predicted cognitive bias. More important was the observation that after successful treatment with an SSRI in the absence of any cognitive or, indeed, any formal psychological intervention this bias was normalized. This is consistent with the observations that medication effective in social anxiety disorder also reduces abnormal social cognitions (Davidson *et al.* 1994). These data suggest that the cognitions of PD are state markers and rather call into question the primacy of their role in the pathogenesis of the condition. It would be of great interest to see if similar changes in cognitions could be induced by effective drug treatment across the other anxiety disorders.

Future therapies

There has been major progress in the treatment of anxiety disorders in the past decade (see Table 28.1),

Table 28.1 A comparison of key treatment aspects of the different anxiety disorders.

Disorder	Dose	Response rate	Onset worsening	Mixed 5-HT/NAD-299 drugs work?	Relapse after tryptophan depletion
Panic	High	Good	Yes	?	Yes
GAD	Normal	Moderate	Rare	Yes	?
SAD	Normal	Moderate	Rare	? Probably	?Probably
PTSD	Normal	Poor	Yes	?	?
OCD	High	Poor	No	?No	No

GAD, generalized anxiety disorder; OCD, obsessive-compulsive disorder; PTSD, post-traumatic stress disorder; SAD, social anxiety disorder.

Table 28.2 Potential future treatments for anxiety disorders.

Type of approach	Examples	Comments
Modify current treatments	Modify SSRIs, e.g., adding 5-HT1A/5-HT2 blocking	?No better efficacy but better tolerability
5-HT1 receptor antagonists	5-HT1A/1B blockers, e.g. NAD-299*	In depression trials
5-HT2 receptor antagonists	Deramciclane = 2C	In phase 2 for depression ?Also in anxiety
Agomelatine	5-HT 2C antagonist + melatonin agonist	In clinical trials
Subtype selective GABA$_A$ receptor agonists/partial agonists	Pagoclone α_2 and α_3 subtype agonists	Some +ve data in PD Less S/Es than traditional benzodiazepines
Novel GABA modulators	Pregabalin May work on Ca channels	Some clinical data
Antistress agents	CRF antagonist	Animal tests +ve Under trials for depression
Substance P antagonists (NK1 receptor antagonists)	MK 869	Reduce anxiety in depression trials
Glutamate antagonists	NMDA antagonists	Stop conditioned anxiety, e.g., PTSD in animals
Reduce glutamate release	MGLUr1 agonists	Work in animal models Broad range of therapeutic indications

Ca, calcium; PTSD, post-traumatic stress disorder; SSRIs, selective serotonin reuptake inhibitors.
* Johansson *et al.* 1997.

which is fitting since some had called the 1990s the decade of anxiety. However there is still a long way to go. For many of the anxiety disorders the prognosis is still poor and even with optimal therapy many patients remain only partly recovered. In many studies the percentage of patients recovered varies from between 35% and 60% (Ballenger 1999). Moreover all currently used medications have side-effects which are limiting in a proportion of patients. So where and what are the future therapies for anxiety?

Our view of the future of this field is given in Table 28.2. This should give cause for hope as there are many new compounds in development and some are targeted at receptor systems that have only recently become implicated in anxiety.

Perhaps the most obviously exciting are the γ-aminobutirric acid-A (GABA$_A$) receptor subtype agonists as these have very focal actions in the brain and in animal tests at least show excellent separation of anxiolytic and sedative actions (McKernan *et al.* 2000; Nutt & Malizia 2001). What is not yet clear is which subtype, the α_2 or the α_3 GABA$_A$ receptor, mediates anxiety and it may be that there are subtleties that could soon emerge. For instance, both α_2 and α_3 subtype agonists are anxiolytic but it may be that one acts more on conditioned and one on unconditioned forms of anxiety. An extra degree of potential sophistication is offered by the prospect of partial agonists at one or both of these receptors.

Support for the potential utility of GABA$_A$ receptor partial agonists comes from the early studies with pagoclone. This is a partial agonist at some subtypes of the GABA$_A$ receptor, as has recently been demonstrated by physiological studies (Wilson *et al.* 1997) and by PET (Lingford-Hughes *et al.* 2000). Pagoclone has also been shown to have some efficacy in PD where it reduced panic attacks (Sandford *et al.* 2001).

Much of the drive in the development of peptide therapeutics has come from the desire to attack depression at its presumed source—the central and peripheral stress axis. For nearly a decade now we have known that blocking central corticotropin releasing factor (CRF) receptors will reduce stress in animals although these experiments initially relied on directly injecting a peptide analog of CRF (a-helical CRF) into the brain. More recently stable small molecule antagonists have been discovered and studies with these have confirmed that central CRF mediates many of the behavioral responses to stress in animals (Gutman *et al.* 2001). One antagonist, R121919, has been put into pilot trials of human depression with some promising results (Zobel *et al.* 2001) but these had to be stopped for reasons of drug safety. New compounds are in the pipelines of many drug companies so this finding may soon be replicated. It appears that depression rather than anxiety disorders has been targeted because of the evidence of cortisol dysregulation in depression but it might well be the case that anxiety disorders might also respond, especially conditions with established cortisol abnormalities such as PTSD.

Other peptide antagonists especially the substance P (NK1 receptor) blockers have caused a lot of excitement in recent years with the finding that MK869 was effective in depression (Kramer *et al.* 1998; Nutt 1998b; Argyropoulos & Nutt 2000). Many companies have made high affinity agonists with high selectivity for the NK1 receptor. Some of these new antagonists have been tested in anxiety disorders, such as social anxiety disorder, as well as in depression but as yet there are no data in the public domain.

Finally the potential of glutamate as a target should not be overlooked. This is the key excitatory transmitter in the human brain and so is critically involved in all learning and memory as well as performance. The role of glutamate in anxiety has been discussed in a number of recent publications where a particular involvement in PTSD seems likely (O'Brien & Nutt 1998; Nutt 2000). In essence the glutamate theory of anxiety suggests that the learning of anxiety is a consequence of glutamate-mediated learning. It is possible to block glutamate transmission by postsynaptic antagonists such as dizocilpine (MK801) but these tend to produce problematic alterations in consciousness and so could only really be contemplated as a short-term and immediate intervention. Intriguingly it is also possible to reduce glutamate function by decreasing release by inhibiting presynaptic cell activity.

One way of doing this is with a specific presynaptic glutamate agonist that acts on the glutamate auto receptor. One such compound has been made by Lilly and shown to have activity in a number of animal models in which anxiety is prominent including drug and alcohol withdrawal and conflict tests. As there are many other potential indications for this sort of compound, including schizophrenia, the field is one that is likely to grow and it may soon be possible for clinical trials in anxiety to start.

In conclusion, there appears to be a growing list of potential new pharmacological approaches to the treatment of the anxiety disorders. Some are improvements on established therapies and others have novel—even radical—modes of action. We are confident that some of these new approaches will translate into clinical benefit in the next decade or two. Similarly the novel treatments of repetitive transcutaneous magnetic stimulation (rTMS) and vagal nerve stimulation hold considerable promise (see Chapter 26).

A number of empirically demonstrated effective psychotherapies, either cognitive or behavioral based, are now available but not yet well studied in some conditions, especially GAD, PTSD and, to a lesser extent, social anxiety disorder. Also significantly, more work is required to understand potential additive or even synergistic effects of combining these treatments with drug therapies.

References

Anderson, I. (2001) Meta-analytical studies on new antidepressants. *Br Med Bull*, **57**, 161–78.

Argyropoulos, S.V. & Nutt, D.J. (2000) Substance P antagonists: novel agents in the treatment of depression. *Expert Opin Investig Drugs* **9**(8), 1871–5.

Ballenger, J.C. (1999) Current treatments of the anxiety disorders in adults. *Biol Psychiatry* **46**(11), 1579–94.

Barr, L.C., Goodman, W.K., McDougle, C.J. *et al.* (1994) Tryptophan depletion in patients with obsessive-compulsive disorder who respond to serotonin reuptake inhibitors. *Arch Gen Psychiatry* **51**, 309–17.

Bell, C., Abrams, J. & Nutt, D.J. (2001) Tryptophan depletion and its implications for psychiatry. *Br J Psychiatry* **178**, 399–405.

Bell, C., Forshall, S., Adrover, M. *et al.* (2002) Does 5-HT restrain panic? A tryptophan depletion study in panic disorder patients recovered on paroxetine. *J Psychopharmacol* **16**(1), 5–14.

Bradwejn, J. & Koszycki, D. (1994) Imipramine antagonism of the panicogenic effects of cholecystokinin tetrapeptide in panic disorder patients. *Am J Psychiatry* **151**, 261–3.

Davidson, J.R., Tupler, L.A. & Potts, N.L. (1994) Treatment of social phobia with benzodiazepines. *J Clin Psychiatry* **55** (Suppl.), 28–32.

Deakin, J.F.W. & Graeff, F.G. (1991) 5-HT and mechanisms of defence. *J Psychopharmacol* **5**(4), 305–15.

Delgado, P.L., Charney, D.S., Price, L.H., Aghajanian, G.K., Landis, H. & Heninger, G.R. (1990) Serotonin function and the mechanism of antidepressant action: reversal of antidepressant induced remission by rapid depletion of plasma tryptophan. *Arch Gen Psychiatry* **47**, 411–18.

Delgado, P.L., Miller, H.L., Salomon, R.M. *et al.* (1999) Tryptophan-depletion challenge in depressed patients treated with desipramine or fluoxetine. Implications for the role of serotonin in the mechanism of antidepressant action. *Biol Psychiatry* **46**, 212–20.

Forshall, S., Bell, C. & Nutt, D.J. (2000) Relapse of panic symptoms after rapid depletion of tryptophan. *J Psychopharmacol* **14**(3) (Suppl.), A30–33.

Gutman, D.A., Owens, M.J. & Nemeroff, C.B. (2001) CRF receptor antagonists: a new approach to the treatment of depression. *Pharmaceutical News* **8**, 18–25.

Johansson, L., Sohn, D., Thorberg, S. *et al.* (1997) The pharmacological characterization of a novel selective 5-hydroxytryptamine 1A receptor antagonist. *NAD-299 The J Pharmacol Exp Ther* **283**(1), 216–25.

Kramer, M.S., Cutler, N., Feighner, J. *et al.* (1998) Distinct mechanism for antidepressant activity by blockade of central substance P receptors. *Science* **281** (5383), 1640–5.

Leonard, H.L., Swedo, S.E., Lenane, M.C. *et al.* (1991) A double-blind desipramine substitution during long-term clomipramine treatment in children and adolescents with obsessive-compulsive disorder. *Arch Gen Psychiatry* **48**(10), 922–27.

Levine, L.R. & Potter, W.Z. (2000) The 5-HT1A receptor: an unkept promise? In: *Anxiolytics* (M. Briley & D.J. Nutt (eds), pp. 95–104). Birkhauser Verlag, Switzerland.

Lingford-Hughes AR, Uh1 N, Feeney AJ, Wilson SJ, Grasby PG, D'Orlando K, Gammans R, Nutt DJ. (2000). Is pagoclone a partial agonist at the central GABA-benzodiazepine receptor: A [11C]-flumazenil positron emission tomography study? *Int J Neuropsychopharm* **3**, S288.

Lotufo-Neto, F., Bernik, M., Ramos, R.T. *et al.* (2001) A dose-finding and discontinuation study of clomipramine in panic disorder. *J Psychopharmacol* **15**, 13–17.

Marks, I.M. (2002) The maturing of therapy: Some brief psychotherapies help anxiety/depressive disorders but mechanisms of action are unclear. *Br J Psychiatry* **180**, 200–4.

Mavissakalian, M. & Perel, I.M. (1988) Imipramine dose–response relationship in panic disorder with agoraphobia. *Arch Gen Psychiatry* **46**, 127–31.

McKernan, R.M., Rosahl, T.W., Reynolds, D.S. *et al.* (2000) Sedative but not anxiolytic properties of benzodiazepines are mediated by the GABA$_A$ receptor α_1 subtype. *Nat Neurosci* **3**, 587–92.

Melichar, J.K., Haida, A., Rhodes, C., Reynolds, A.H., Nutt, D.J. & Malizia, A.L. (2001) Venlafaxine occupation at the noradrenaline reuptake site: *in vivo* determination in healthy volunteers. *J Psychopharmacol* **15**(1), 9–12.

Middleton, H.C. (1991) 5-HT and mechanisms of defence. *J Psychopharmacol* **5**(4), 281–5.

Miller, H.L., Delgado, P.L., Salomon, R.M. *et al.* (1996) Clinical and biochemical effects of catecholamine depletion on antidepressant-induced remission of depression. *Arch Gen Psychiatry* **53**(2), 117–28.

Nutt, D.J. (1998a) Efficacy of mirtazapine in clinically relevant subgroups of depressed patients. *Depress Anxiety* **7**(1), 7–10.

Nutt, D.J. (1998b) Substance-P antagonists: a new treatment for depression? *Lancet* **352**, 1644–6.

Nutt, D.J. (2000) The psychobiology of post-traumatic stress disorder. *J Clin Psychiatry* **61**(5), 24–32.

Nutt, D.J. (2001) Neurobiological mechanisms in generalized anxiety disorder. *J Clin Psychiatry* **62**(11), 22–7.

Nutt, D.J. & Cowen, P.J. (1987) Diazepam alters brain 5-HT function in man. Implications for the acute and chronic effects of benzodiazepines. *Psychol Med* **17**, 601–7.

Nutt, D.J. & Johnson, F.N. (1998) Potential applications of venlafaxine. *Reviews in Contemporary Pharmacotherapy* **9**(5), 321–31.

Nutt, D.J. & Malizia, A.L. (2001) New insights into the role of the GABA$_A$ benzodiazepine receptor. *Br J Psychiatry* **179**, 390–6.

O'Brien, M. & Nutt, D.J. (1998) Loss of consciousness and PTSD a clue to aetiology and treatment? *Br J Psychiatry* **173**, 102–4.

Pike, V.W., McCarron, J.A., Lammertsma, A.A. *et al.* (1996) Exquisite delineation of 5-HT1A receptors in human brain with PET and [carbonyl-11 C]WAY-100635. *Eur J Pharmacol* **301**, 1–3.

Sandford, J.J., Forshall, S., Bell, C., Argyropoulos, S., D'Orlando, K.J., Gammans, R.E. & Nutt, D.J. (2001) Cross-over trial of partial agonist pagoclone and placebo in patients with DSM-IV panic disorder. *J Psychopharm* **15**(3), 205–8.

Sargent, P.A., Nash, J., Hood, S. *et al.* (2000) 5-HT1A receptor binding in panic disorder; comparison with depressive disorder and healthy volunteers using PET and [11C]WAY-100635. *Neuroimage*, **11**(5), 189.

Smeraldi, E., Diaferia, G., Erzegovesi, S., Lucca, A., Bellodi, L. & Moja, E.A. (1996) Tryptophan depletion in obsessive-compulsive patients. *Biol Psychiatry* **40**, 398–402.

van Vliet, I.M., Westenberg, H.G. & den Boer, J.A. (1996) Effects of the 5-HT1A receptor agonist flesinoxan in panic disorder. *Psychopharmacology (Berl)* **127**(2), 174–80.

Weinstein, A.M. & Nutt, D.J. (1995) A cognitive dysfunction in anxiety and its amelioration by effective treatment with SSRIs. *J Psychopharm* **9**(2), 83–9.

Wilson, S.J., Birnie, A., Sheridan, B. & Nutt, D.J. (1997) Sleep effects of pagoclone, a new benzodiazepine partial agonist. British Sleep Society meeting.

Zobel, A.W. *et al.* (2001) Effects of the high affinity corticotropin-releasing hormone receptor 1 antagonist R121919 in major depression: the first 20 patients treated. *J Psychiatr Res* **34**, 171–81.

Index

United States (US)
  generalized anxiety disorder 51
    studies 53
  herbal remedies 496
  obsessive-compulsive disorder studies 86–7
    costs 91
  panic disorder studies 346, 347
  social anxiety disorder studies 101
United States Air Force Academy, panic attack studies 143
University Hospital of Ghent (Belgium) 399–400
urticaria 399, 401
  hydroxyzine treatment 402, 406
US (unconditioned stimulus) 448–50

V

vagal tone 305–6
vagus nerve stimulation (VNS) 485, 508
valepotriates 493
Valeriana officinalis (valerian) 493, 496
valproate 46, 274, 327, 473
valproic acid 323, 469
  and benzodiazepines compared 465
  panic disorder treatment 465
Valsalva's maneuver 103, 189, 304
variable number of tandem repeats (VNTR) 241
vasoconstriction 276, 305
vasopressin 86
VBR (ventricle-to-brain ratio) 206
venlafaxine 348, 349, 501, 502–3, 504
  activity 418
  anxiety disorder treatment 418–22
  clinical use 419–22
  drug interactions 419
  extended release 418
  and fluoxetine compared 422
  immediate release 418
  overdose 419
  pharmacokinetics 418–19
  safety issues 419
  side-effects 419
  toxicity 419
  withdrawal 419
venlafaxine hydrochloride 419
ventral medulla 260
ventricle-to-brain ratio (VBR) 206
verapamil 324, 385, 467
Verdun Target Symptom Rating Scale (VTSRS) 404
vertigo 12, 325
  comorbidity 43
veterans (war) *see* war veterans
vicarious learning 106
victimization, and post-traumatic stress disorder 74, 426
Vietnam veterans 217
  dopamine studies 193
  fluoxetine studies 350
  sertraline studies 351
  venlafaxine studies 421
vigabatrin 469
violence, and post-traumatic stress disorder 73
virtual reality, and exposure therapy 457

Vistaril *see* hydroxyzine
VNS (vagus nerve stimulation) 485, 508
VNTR (variable number of tandem repeats) 241
VTSRS (Verdun Target Symptom Rating Scale) 404

W

waitlist conditions 438, 447, 451, 453, 455–6
war neuroses
  etiology 15
  treatment 15
war veterans
  dopamine studies 193
  exposure therapy 452
  flashbacks 272
  post-traumatic stress disorder 14–15, 77, 172–3, 216, 350–1, 375–6
  rapid eye movement studies 128
  sex differences 77
  see also Vietnam veterans
washing, and obsessive-compulsive disorder 83–4, 452
water, fear of 29
Watson, John Broadus (1878–1958) 9, 445–6
WAY 100635 213, 238, *505*
Wechsler Verbal Memory 215
Westphal, Carl (1833–90) 14
white matter 202, 203, 206, 219
WHO *see* World Health Organization (WHO)
Williams syndrome 102
witches, execution 7
Wittenborn Psychiatric Rating Scale (WPRS) 404
Wolpe, Joseph (1915–97) 446, 447, 448
World Health Organization (WHO) 3, 10
  anxiety disorder studies 44, 53, 467
  primary care study 33
  psychiatric disorder studies 115
World War I (1914–18), shell shock 14–15
World War II (1939–45) 9
  resistance fighters 350
worry 51–2
  definition 54
  excessive 17
  and generalized anxiety disorder 54
worry exposure 429
WPRS (Wittenborn Psychiatric Rating Scale) 404

X

xenon, in brain imaging 204, 210

Y

Yale (US) 217–18, 503
Yale–Brown Obsessive Compulsive Scale (Y-BOCS) 168, 171, 340, 341, 342
  obsessive-compulsive disorder studies 371, 372, 373, 390, 484
Y-BOCS *see* Yale–Brown Obsessive Compulsive Scale (Y-BOCS)
yohimbine 58, **187**, 189, 211, 218
  anxiety induction 188
  panicogenicity 279–80